Cutaneous Malignancy of the Head and Neck

A Multidisciplinary Approach

Cutaneous Malignancy of the Head and Neck

A Multidisciplinary Approach

Randal S. Weber, MD, FACS
Brian A. Moore, MD, FACS

Plural Publishing Inc.
San Diego
Oxford
Brisbane

PLURAL PUBLISHING INC.

5521 Ruffin Road
San Diego, CA 92123

e-mail: info@pluralpublishing.com
Web site: http://www.pluralpublishing.com

49 Bath Street
Abingdon, Oxfordshire OX14 1EA
United Kingdom

Typeset in 10½/13 Palatino by Flanagan's Publishing Services, Inc.
Printed in Malaysia

Library of Congress Cataloging-in-Publication Data:

Cutaneous malignancy of the head and neck : a multidisciplinary approach / [edited by] Randal S. Weber & Brian A. Moore.
p. ; cm.
Includes bibliographical references and index.
ISBN-13: 978-1-59756-338-3 (alk. paper)
ISBN-10: 1-59756-338-2 (alk. paper)
1. Head—Cancer. 2. Neck—Cancer. 3. Skin—Cancer. I. Weber, Randal S. II. Moore, Brian A. (Brian Andrew), 1972-
[DNLM: 1. Head and Neck Neoplasms—diagnosis. 2. Head and Neck Neoplasms—surgery. 3. Reconstructive Surgical Procedures—methods. 4. Skin Neoplasms—diagnosis. 5. Skin Neoplasms—surgery. WE 707]
RC280.H4C88 2010
616.99'491—dc22
2010045804

CONTENTS

Foreword by Helmuth Goepfert *ix*
Acknowledgments *xi*
Contributors *xiii*

1 **Skin Anatomy** **1**
Richard O. Wein and Randal S. Weber

2 **Clinical Evaluation** **11**
Christina J. Yang, Brian A. Moore, and Randal S. Weber

3 **Psychosocial Impact of Skin Cancer Treatment** **29**
Michelle C. Fingeret

4 **Screening, Surveillance, and Prevention** **41**
Sharon R. Hymes and Carol R. Drucker

5 **Ultraviolet Carcinogenesis and Immune Suppression** **57**
Stephen E. Ullrich

6 **Histopathology of Nonmelanoma Skin Cancer** **79**
Jonathan L. Curry, Carlos A. Torres-Cabala, and Victor G. Prieto

7 **Epidemiology, Staging, and Prognosis of Nonmelanoma Skin Cancer** **101**
Carsten E. Palme, Mark C. Smith, and Michael J. Veness

8 **Aggressive Nonmelanoma Skin Cancer** **119**
Christian P. Hasney, Nandita Guha-Thakurta, Brian A. Moore, and Randal S. Weber

9 **Surgical Management of Locoregional Disease** **143**
Stephen Y. Lai and Randal S. Weber

10 **Special Considerations: Periauricular Lesions** **155**
Paul W. Gidley

11 **Special Considerations: Periorbital and Ocular Adnexal Cutaneous Lesions** **173**
Bita Esmaeli and Aaron Savar

12 **Special Considerations: Neurosurgical Management** 183
Franco DeMonte

13 **Radiotherapy for Cutaneous Squamous and Basal Cell Carcinoma** 191
William M. Mendenhall, Robert J. Amdur, and Nancy P. Mendenhall

14 **Photodynamic Therapy for Nonmelanoma Skin Cancer** 205
Joseph P. Housel and Nathalie C. Zeitouni

15 **Therapeutic Horizons for Cutaneous Malignancies** 215
Michael E. Kupferman, Randal S. Weber, and Eben L. Rosenthal

16 **Adnexal Tumors** 223
Amy C. Hessel

17 **Merkel Cell Carcinoma** 233
Cecelia E. Schmalbach

18 **Dermatofibrosarcoma Protuberans** 247
Thomas D. Shellenberger and Erich M. Sturgis

19 **Angiosarcoma** 257
Amy C. Hessel, Brian A. Moore, and Erich M. Sturgis

20 **Melanoma: Epidemiology, Staging, and Prognosis** 269
Audrey B. Erman and Carol R. Bradford

21 **Molecular Biology and Genetics of Melanoma/Mechanisms of Spread** 281
Helmut Schaider, Susan E. Zabierowski, and Meenhard Herlyn

22 **Immunobiology and Immunotherapy of Melanoma** 297
Lauren L. Levy, Johnny Kao, and Andrew G. Sikora

23 **Histology of Melanoma and Precursor Lesions** 317
A. Hafeez Diwan, Doina Ivan, and Victor G. Prieto

24 **Local Management of Melanoma** 333
Benjamin L. Judson and Dennis H. Kraus

25 **Regional Management of Melanoma in the Clinically Node-Negative Neck** 343
Jeffrey E. Gershenwald, Matthew T. Ballo, and Jeffrey N. Myers

26 **Regional Management of Melanoma in the Clinically Node-Positive Neck** 373
Jesus E. Medina

27 **Role of Chemotherapy, Biochemotherapy, and Targeted Systemic Therapies in the Treatment of Metastatic Melanoma** 387
Sapna P. Patel, Richard W. Joseph, and Kevin B. Kim

28 **Ocular Melanoma** 409
Dan S. Gombos

29 **Mucosal Melanoma** 413
Snehal G. Patel and Jatin P. Shah

30 **Microscopically Oriented Histographic Surgery (MOHS): Indications, Principles, and Technique** 425
Michael R. Migden

31 **Mohs Surgery: Adjunctive Treatment of Skin Cancer** 441
Valencia D. Thomas and Kimberly Thomas

32 **Principles of Head and Neck Cutaneous Reconstruction** 455
Roxanna Baratelli, Brian A. Moore, and Matthew M. Hanasono

33 **Nasal Reconstruction** 471
Matthew M. Hanasono, Robert L. Walton, and Elisabeth K. Beahm

34 **Lip Reconstruction** 487
Howard N. Langstein and Hani Sbitany

35 **Periorbital Reconstruction** 505
Stephen R. Klapper, Charles N.S. Soparkar, and James R. Patrinely

36 **Auricular Reconstruction** 531
Lok Huei Yap, Sean G. Boutros, and Charles E. Butler

37 **Scalp Reconstruction** 557
Melissa A. Crosby

38 **Reconstruction of the Cheek** 575
Anuja K. Antony and Babak J. Mehrara

39 **Prosthetic Rehabilitation** 587
Theresa M. Hofstede, Patricia C. Montgomery, Rhonda F. Jacob, Peggy J. Wesley, Jack W. Martin, and Mark S. Chambers

Index *601*

FOREWORD

Cutaneous malignancy is a broad subject, encompassing a range of histologies that extends far beyond the more frequently encountered entities: basal cell carcinoma, squamous cell carcinoma, and melanoma. Similarly, a wide range of health care providers diagnose and treat skin cancer on a regular basis. From rural primary care clinics to urban dermatologic surgery practices to international cancer centers, a subset of these malignancies prove to be diagnostic and treatment challenges, potentially leading to morbidity and even mortality. Cutaneous malignancy represents a growing worldwide public health problem, with a rapidly rising incidence, decreasing age at presentation, and significant health care costs to society.

As the largest organ of the body, the skin weighs approximately 3 kilograms and covers 7,600 square centimeters of our anatomy. Rugged, waterproof, and continuously regenerating, it defends against foreign substances, helps to regulate body temperature, and protects against the effects of UV light through the diverse tissues of its harmonious architecture. These diverse histologic tissues can fall subject to malignant transformation from exposure to the very entities from which they serve to protect us, giving rise to neoplasms with diverse biologic behavior. The vast majority of cutaneous malignancies, namely, basal cell carcinoma and squamous cell carcinoma, can effectively be treated through a variety of means when diagnosed early; certain nonmelanoma skin cancers and melanoma merit more aggressive evaluation and treatment by a multidisciplinary team of experts in cutaneous oncology.

No single publication discusses the unique oncologic, functional, and aesthetic demands presented by cutaneous malignancy of the head and neck. This timely textbook fills that void with practical information and detailed, color images that are invaluable for the practioner who is called upon by his or her patient to manage these malignancies in a comprehensive fashion providing the best opportunity for cure and cosmetic and functional restoration. The central tenet of the text is that patients with aggressive and potentially life-threatening cutaneous malignancies of the head and neck, melanoma and certain nonmelanoma cancers, are best treated in a multidisciplinary setting.

The senior editor, Randal Weber, has proven expertise as a clinician and investigator and leads a multidisciplinary team of physicians who manage patients with the spectrum of cutaneous malignancies. Dr. Weber previously edited a multiauthored textbook, *Basal and Squamous Cell Skin Cancer of the Head and Neck*. By partnering for this more comprehensive text with Brian Moore, an oncologic and reconstructive surgeon, the broader scope of the current text includes not only malignant melanoma and adenexal tumors but also an entire section devoted to reconstruction and rehabilitation adhering to a defect-based approach.

Dr. Weber and Dr. Moore have assembled a cadre of contributors from numerous disciplines that are leaders in the care of patients with head and neck malignancy. Dr. Carsten Palme from Australia is known for his contributions to our understanding of the prognostic impact of lymph node metastasis and immunosuppresion in patients with cutaneous squamous cell carcinoma. Similarly, Drs. Paul Gidley and Franco DeMonte discuss their vast experience with temporal bone and skull base involvement from these aggressive lesions. Leading dermatologic surgeons such as Drs. Deborah MacFarlane, Nathalie Zeitouni, and Michael Migden graciously provide detailed information about some of the techniques employed in managing advanced skin malignancy. Prominent figures in the melanoma literature, including Drs. Carol Bradford and Jeffrey Gershenwald, deliver practical, cutting-edge information, with staging updates and a contemporary assessment of sentinel lymph node biopsy, a technique that is integral to the appropriate management of head and neck cutaneous melanoma.

A defect-based approach to head and neck cutaneous reconstruction is detailed through the efforts of highly respected plastic surgeons, oculoplastic surgeons, and facial plastic surgeons, including Drs. Robert Walton, Elisabeth Beahm, Howard Langstein, and Charles Butler. For patients with advanced malignancy requiring radiation or systemic therapy, the insights of figures such as Drs. William Mendenhall and Kevin Kim nicely complement the other chapters with helpful background information appreciated by the non-oncologist or radiotherapist, as well as innovative approaches to complex situations.

This unique book covers all aspects of multidisciplinary management from low-impact disease, such as small basal cell carcinoma, to the potentially life-threatening entities such as angiosarcoma and advanced melanoma, helping the reader to identify risk factors for aggressive disease. The reader will find a rich table of contents, with content ranging from screening and prevention through clinical evaluation and management; important topics in cancer biology and immunology are included to explain the underlying mechanisms of carcinogenesis, invasion, and metastasis. Despite its broad scope the chapter content is focused and concise, with excellent images and readily accessible tables and figures to illustrate key learning points.

Over the years the management of skin malignancies has evolved, and the dynamic nature of advanced cutaneous malignancy is reflected in the blend of established, senior contributors, and emerging leaders in the field. The experience of interdisciplinary cooperation among experts with differing specialty backgrounds has evolved. Whereas in the past, competition existed among treating disciplines, a complementary and collaborative approach is now the standard. The selection of treatment has been refined with the goals being cure and preservation or restoration of form and function. Evolving research has produced exciting new approaches such as targeted molecular therapy that hold promise for patients with aggressive disease.

Truly believing that no one discipline can provide comprehensive care for advanced cutaneous malignancy, the editors have assembled contributors who bring special expertise from multiple disciplines including dermatology, dermatologic surgery, head and neck surgery, surgical oncology, radiation and medical oncology, ophthalmology, neurosurgery, reconstructive surgery, prosthodontry, pathology, radiology, epidemiology, psychology, and basic science. The editors have collated what clinicians in the field need to know to in a textbook intended to serve us all—a management guide that is well assembled and very timely.

Priorities for health care delivery today mandate demonstration of value in the care rendered; treatment needs to be evidenced-based with an emphasis on quality, safety, and cost-effectiveness. Multidisciplinary teams will evolve into integrated care units where the patient's treatment is planned prospectively and coordinated among providers thus facilitating efficiency and cost-effectiveness. *Cutaneous Malignancy of the Head and Neck: A Multidisciplinary Approach* incorporates these principles and guides us in this direction.

Helmuth Goepfert, MD, FACS

ACKNOWLEDGMENTS

No words can truly express our gratitude to Mariann Crapanzano, JD, ELS, the coordinator of publications for the Department of Head and Neck Surgery at the University of Texas MD Anderson Cancer Center. Mariann was instrumental in the completion of this text, as she marshalled contributors (and the editors) toward deadlines and provided key editorial insight throughout the process. Simply put, this textbook would not have happened without her support and efforts.

We are deeply indebted to our section editors, Jeffrey N. Myers, MD, PhD, Deborah MacFarlane, MD, and Matt Hanasono, MD, for their unparalleled efforts in designing the content, identifying experienced contributors from a multitude of clinical disciplines, and ensuring timely delivery of quality chapters.

We also thank Judy Meyer, Sandy Doyle, Kelsey Marrujo, and the entire editorial and production staff at Plural Publishing for their vision in supporting this text, and for their patience in completing it.

CONTRIBUTORS

SECTION EDITORS

Matthew M. Hanasono, MD
Associate Professor
Department of Plastic Surgery
The University of Texas MD Anderson Cancer Center
Houston, Texas
Chapters 32–39

Deborah MacFarlane, MD
Professor
Department of Dermatology
Director, Fellowship in Procedural Dermatology and Mohs Surgery
MD Anderson Cancer Center
Chapters 30–31

Jeffrey N. Myers, MD, PhD, FACS
Hubert L. and Olive Stringer Distinguished Professorship in Cancer Research
Director of Research and Deputy
Chair for Academic Programs
Department of Head and Neck Surgery
The University of Texas MD Anderson Cancer Center
Houston, Texas
Chapters 20–29

AUTHORS

Robert J. Amdur, MD
Professor
Department of Radiation Oncology
Shands Hospital at the University of Florida
Gainesville, Florida
Chapter 13

Anuja Kandanatt Antony, MD, MPH
Assistant Professor and Director of Microsurgery
Division of Plastic, Reconstructive and Cosmetic Surgery
University of Illinois at Chicago
Chicago, Illinois
Chapter 38

Matthew T. Ballo, MD
Associate Professor
Department of Radiation Oncology
The University of Texas MD Anderson Cancer Center
Houston, Texas
Chapter 25

Roxanna Baratelli, MD
Department of Otolaryngology
Tulane University
New Orleans, Louisiana
Chapter 32

Elisabeth K. Beahm, MD, FACS
Professor
Department of Plastic Surgery
The University of Texas MD Anderson Cancer Center
Houston, Texas
Chapter 33

Sean G. Boutros, MD, FACS
Houston Plastic and Craniofacial Surgery
Houston, Texas
Chapter 36

Carol R. Bradford, MD, FACS
Professor and Chair
Department of Otolaryngology-Head and Neck Surgery
University of Michigan
Ann Arbor, Michigan
Chapter 20

Charles E. Butler, MD, FACS
Professor
Department of Plastic Surgery
The University of Texas MD Anderson Cancer Center
Houston, Texas
Chapter 36

Mark S. Chambers, DMD, MS
Professor and Chief, Section of Oncologic Dentistry and Prosthodontics
Director, Clinical Research Program (HNS)
Department of Head and Neck Surgery
The University of Texas MD Anderson Cancer Center
Houston, Texas
Chapter 39

Melissa A. Crosby, MD, FACS
Assistant Professor
Department of Plastic Surgery
The University of Texas MD Anderson Cancer Center
Houston, Texas
Chapter 37

Jonathan L. Curry, MD
Assistant Professor, Mary Beth Pawelek Chair in Neurosurgery
Department of Pathology & Dermatology
The University of Texas MD Anderson Cancer Center
Houston, Texas
Chapter 6

Franco DeMonte, MD, FRCSC, FACS
Professor of Neurosurgery and Head and Neck Surgery
The University of Texas MD Anderson Cancer Center
Houston, Texas
Chapter 12

Abdul Hafeez Diwan, MD, PhD
Associate Professor and Chief of Dermatopathology
Baylor College of Medicine
Departments of Pathology & Immunology and Dermatology
Houston, Texas
Chapter 23

Carol R. Drucker, MD
Associate Professor
Associate Medical Director
Cancer Prevention Clinic
The University of Texas MD Anderson Cancer Center
Houston, Texas
Chapter 4

Audrey B. Erman, MD
Department of Otolaryngology-Head and Neck Surgery
University of Michigan
Ann Arbor, Michigan
Chapter 20

Bita Esmaeli, MD, FACS
Professor of Ophthalmology
Director, Ophthalmic Plastic and Reconstructive Surgery Fellowship Program
Section of Ophthalmology

Department of Head and Neck Surgery
The University of Texas MD Anderson Cancer Center
Houston, Texas
Chapter 11

Michelle C. Fingeret, PhD
Assistant Professor
Department of Behavioral Science
The University of Texas MD Anderson Cancer Center
Houston, Texas
Chapter 3

Jeffrey E. Gershenwald, MD, FACS
Professor
Department of Surgical Oncology
Medical Director, Melanoma and Skin Center
The University of Texas MD Anderson Cancer Center
Houston, Texas
Chapter 25

Paul W. Gidley, MD, FACS
Associate Professor
Otology-Neurotology
Department of Head and Neck Surgery
The University of Texas MD Anderson Cancer Center
Houston, Texas
Chapter 10

Dan S. Gombos, MD, FACS
Associate Professor of Ophthalmology
Department of Head and Neck Surgery
Section of Ophthalmology
The University of Texas M. D. Anderson Cancer Center
Houston, Texas
Chapter 28

Nandita Guha-Thakurta, MD
Assistant Professor
Section Neuroradiology
Department of Diagnostic Imaging
The University of Texas MD Anderson Cancer Center
Houston, Texas
Chapter 8

Matthew M. Hanasono, MD
Associate Professor
Department of Plastic Surgery
The University of Texas MD Anderson Cancer Center
Houston, Texas
Chapters 32 and 33

Christian P. Hasney, MD
Resident
Tulane University School of Medicine
Department of Otolaryngology-Head and Neck Surgery
New Orleans, Louisiana
Chapter 8

Meenhard Herlyn, DVM, DSc
Professor and Leader
Program of Molecular and Cellular Oncogenesis
The Wistar Institute
Philadelphia, Pennsylvania
Chapter 21

Amy C. Hessel, MD
Associate Professor and Surgeon
The University of Texas MD Anderson Cancer Center
Houston, Texas
Chapters 16 and 19

Theresa M. Hofstede, DDS, BSc
Assistant Professor of Dental Oncology
Prosthodontist (Maxillofacial)
Department of Head and Neck Surgery
The University of Texas MD Anderson Cancer Center
Houston, Texas
Chapter 39

Joseph P. Housel, MD
Dermatology Resident
Roswell Park Cancer Institute and University at Buffalo
Buffalo, New York
Chapter 14

Sharon R. Hymes, MD
Professor
Associate Medical Director- Melanoma & Skin Clinic
The University of Texas MD Anderson Cancer Center
Houston, Texas
Chapter 4

Doina Ivan, MD
Assistant Professor of Pathology and Dermatology
Dermatopathology Section
The University of Texas MD Anderson Cancer Center
Houston, Texas
Chapter 23

Rhonda F. Jacob, DDS, MS, FACP
Professor of Dental Oncology-Maxillofacial Prosthodontist
Diplomate and Examiner, Board of Prosthodontics
Director, Implants and Imaging Program
The University of Texas MD Anderson Cancer Center
Houston, Texas
Chapter 39

Richard W. Joseph, MD
Fellow, Hematology/Oncology
The University of Texas MD Anderson Cancer Center
Houston, Texas
Chapter 27

Benjamin L. Judson, MD, MPA
Assistant Professor
Department of Surgery, Section of Otolaryngology
Yale University School of Medicine
New Haven, Connecticut
Chapter 24

Johnny Kao, MD
Assistant Professor
Department of Radiation Oncology
New York, New York
Chapter 22

Stephen R. Klapper, MD, FACS
Klapper Eyelid & Facial Plastic Surgery
Carmel, Indiana
Chapter 35

Kevin B. Kim, MD
The University of Texas MD Anderson Cancer Center
Houston, Texas
Chapter 27

Dennis H. Kraus, MD
Attending Surgeon, Head and Neck Service
Department of Surgery and Director of Speech, Hearing and Rehabilitation Center Memorial Sloan-Kettering Cancer Center
Professor, Department of Otorhinolaryngology-Head and Neck Surgery
Cornell University Medical Center
New York, New York
Chapter 24

Michael E. Kupferman, MD
Assistant Professor
Department of Head and Neck Surgery
The University of Texas MD Anderson Cancer Center
Houston, Texas
Chapter 15

Stephen Y. Lai, MD, PhD, FACS
Assistant Professor
Department of Head and Neck Surgery
Department of Molecular and Cellular Oncology

The University of Texas MD Anderson Cancer Center
Houston, Texas
Chapter 9

Howard N. Langstein, MD, FACS
Chief, Division of Plastic and Reconstructive Surgery
University of Rochester
Rochester, New York
Chapter 34

Lauren L. Levy
Mount Sinai School of Medicine
New York, New York
Chapter 22

Jack W. Martin, DDS, MS
Professor, Section of Oncologic Dentistry and Prosthodontics
Director, Maxillofacial Prosthetics and Oncologic Dentistry Fellowship Program
Department of Head and Neck Surgery
The University of Texas MD Anderson Cancer Center
Houston, Texas
Chapter 39

Jesus E. Medina, MD
Paul & Ruth Jonas Professor
The University of Oklahoma Health Sciences Center
Oklahoma City, Oklahoma
Chapter 26

Babak Joseph Mehrara, MD, FACS
Department of Surgery
Memorial Sloan-Kettering Cancer Center
Associate Professor of Surgery (Plastic)
Weill-Cornell Medical Center
New York, New York
Chapter 38

Nancy P. Mendenhall, MD
Professor, Department of Radiation Oncology
Shands Hospital at the University of Florida
Gainesville, Florida
Medical Director
University of Florida Proton Therapy Institute
Jacksonville, Florida
Chapter 13

William M. Mendenhall, MD
Department of Radiation Oncology
University of Florida College of Medicine
Gainesville, Florida
Chapter 13

Michael R. Migden, MD
Assistant Professor
Department of Dermatology and Plastic Surgery
The University of Texas MD Anderson Cancer Center
Houston, Texas
Chapter 30

Patricia C. Montgomery
Anaplastologist, Section of Oncologic Dentistry and Prosthodontics
The University of Texas MD Anderson Cancer Center
Houston, Texas
Chapter 39

Brian A. Moore, MD, FACS
Director, Head and Neck Surgical Oncology
Vice Chairman of Otolaryngology
Ochsner Medical Center
New Orleans, Louisiana
Chapters 2, 8, 19, and 32

Jeffrey N. Myers, MD, PhD, FACS
Hubert L. and Olive Stringer Distinguished Professorship in Cancer Research
Director of Research and Deputy
Chair for Academic Programs
Department of Head and Neck Surgery
The University of Texas MD Anderson Cancer Center
Houston, Texas
Chapter 25

Carsten E. Palme, MB, BS, FRACS
Staff Surgeon and Clinical Senior Lecturer
Otolaryngology Head and Neck Surgery
Westmead Hospital
University of Sydney
Sydney, Australia
Chapter 7

Sapna P. Patel, MD
Assistant Professor, Melanoma Medical Oncology
The University of Texas MD Anderson Cancer Center
Houston, Texas
Chapter 27

Snehal G. Patel, MD, FRCS
Attending Surgeon, Head and Neck Service
Memorial Sloan-Kettering Cancer Center
Associate Professor, Weill-Cornell Medical School
New York, New York
Chapter 29

James R. Patrinely, MD, FACS
Clinical Associate Professor of Plastic Surgery
Clinical Associate Professor of Ophthalmology
Baylor College of Medicine
Houston, Texas
Chapter 35

Victor G. Prieto, MD, PhD
Professor of Pathology and Dermatology and Section Chief of Dermatopathology
Director of Dermatopathology Fellowship
Houston, Texas
Chapters 6 and 23

Eben L. Rosenthal, MD
Julius Hicks Professor of Surgery
Division of Otolaryngology
University of Alabama at Birmingham
Birmingham, Alabama
Chapter 15

Aaron Savar, MD
Fellow in Ophthalmic and Plastic Reconstructive Surgery
Section of Ophthalmology
Department of Head and Neck Surgery
The University of Texas MD Anderson Cancer Center
Houston, Texas
Chapter 11

Hani Sbitany, MD
Chief Resident
Division of Plastic and Reconstructive Surgery
University of Rochester
Rochester, New York
Chapter 34

Helmut Schaider, MD
Assistant Professor
Department of Dermatology
Medical University of Graz
Graz, Austria
Chapter 21

Cecelia E. Schmalbach, MD, FACS
Lt. Colonel, USAF-MC
Chief, Head and Neck Microvascular Surgery
Department of Otolaryngology
Wilford Hall Medical Center
Lackland Air Force Base, Texas
Chapter 17

Jatin P. Shah, MD, PhD (Hon), FACS, FRCS (Hon), FRACS (Hon), FDSRCS (Hon)
Elliot W. Strong Chair in Head and Neck Oncology
Chief, Head and Neck Service
Memorial Sloan-Kettering Cancer Center
Professor of Surgery
Weill Cornell Medical College
New York, New York
Chapter 29

Thomas D. Shellenberger, DMD, MD
Head and Neck Surgical Oncologist
MD Anderson Cancer Center
Orlando, Florida
Adjunct Assistant Professor
Department of Head and Neck Surgery
The University of Texas MD Anderson Cancer Center
Houston, Texas
Chapter 18

Andrew Gregory Sikora, MD, PhD
Assistant Professor and Director of Head and Neck Translational Research
Department of Otolaryngology-Head and Neck Surgery
Immunobiology, Oncological Sciences, Dermatology
Mount Sinai School of Medicine
New York, New York
Chapter 22

Mark C. Smith, MB, BS, BSc (Med) FRACS
Clinical Fellow
Otolaryngology-Head and Neck Surgery
Westmead
Sydney, Australia
Chapter 7

Charles N. S. Soparkar, MD, PhD, FACS
Clinical Assistant Professor Plastic Surgery & Ophthalmology
Baylor College of Medicine
Clinical Specialist, Department of Head and Neck Surgery
The University of Texas MD Anderson Cancer Center
Plastic Eye Surgery Associates
Houston, Texas
Chapter 35

Erich M. Sturgis, MD, MPH
Associate Professor
Department of Head and Neck Surgery and Department of Epidemiology
The University of Texas MD Anderson Cancer Center
Houston, Texas
Chapters 18 and 19

Kimberly Thomas, MS
MD Candidate
University of Texas Southwestern Medical School
Dallas, Texas
Chapter 31

Valencia D. Thomas, MD
Assistant Professor
MD Anderson Cancer Center
University of Texas at Houston School of Medicine
Houston, Texas
Chapter 31

Carlos A. Torres-Cabala, MD
Assistant Professor
Departments of Pathology and Dermatology
The University of Texas MD Anderson Cancer Center
Houston, Texas
Chapter 6

Stephen E. Ullrich, PhD
Professor of Immunology
Dallas/Fort Worth "Living Legends" Professor
The University of Texas MD Anderson Cancer Center
Houston, Texas
Chapter 5

Michael J. Veness, MB, BS, MD, MMed, FRANZCR
Clinical Associate Professor, University of Sydney
Department of Radiation Oncology
Westmead Hospital, Westmead
Sydney, Australia
Chapter 7

Robert L. Walton, MD, FACS
Professor of Surgery (Plastic)
Northwestern University Feinberg School of Medicine
Chicago, Illinois
Chapter 33

Randal S. Weber, MD, FACS
Professor and Chairman, Department of Head and Neck Surgery
John Brooks Williams and Elizabeth Williams
Distinguished University Chair in Cancer Medicine
The University of Texas MD Anderson Cancer Center
Houston, Texas
Chapters 1, 2, 8, 9, and 15

Richard O. Wein, MD, FACS
Associate Professor
Department of Otolaryngology-Head and Neck Surgery
Tufts Medical Center
Boston, Massachusetts
Chapter 1

Peggy J. Wesley, LVN
Anaplastologist, Section of Oncologic Dentistry and Prosthodontics
The University of Texas MD Anderson Cancer Center
Houston, Texas
Chapter 39

Christina J. Yang, MD
Department of Otolaryngology-Head and Neck Surgery
Tulane University School of Medicine
New Orleans, Louisiana
Chapter 2

Lok Huei Yap, MD, FRCS (Plast), FRCS(Ed), MB Bch BAO
Consultant Plastic, Reconstructive & Aesthetic Surgeon
University Hospitals Birmingham NHS Trust
Queen Elizabeth Hospital
Birmingham, West Midlands
United Kingdom
Chapter 36

Susan E. Zabierowski, PhD
Program of Molecular and Cellular Oncogenesis
The Wistar Institute
Philadelphia, Pennsylvania
Chapter 21

Nathalie C. Zeitouni, MDCM, FRCPC
Interim Chair, Department of Dermatology
Chief, Dermatologic Surgery
Associate Professor of Dermatology
Roswell Park Cancer Institute and
State University of New York at Buffalo
Chapter 14

Randal S. Weber, MD, FACS:
To our patients afflicted with cutaneous malignancies who have taught us so much;
To my wife, Jane, and children, Austin and Sophie, who provide love, support, and understanding;
To my teachers, mentors, and colleagues who have imparted their wisdom and guidance that have so greatly benefited me and my patients.

Brian A. Moore, MD, FACS:
To my children, who are proof that miracles happen;
To my wife, who has made it all possible;
To my parents, who provided the opportunities;
To my patients and mentors, who taught and trusted;
Thank you.

1

SKIN ANATOMY

RICHARD O. WEIN
RANDAL S. WEBER

Introduction

The purpose of this chapter is to aid the future discussions within this text concerning the diagnosis and management of skin cancer of the head and neck. To better understand the tendencies of specific tumors, an understanding of the anatomy of the skin of the face and the associated lymphatic pathways of the head and neck is critical. With this information, the clinician can stratify patients at greatest risk for developing a skin cancer, understand the areas of the face where local recurrence is most common, and appreciate the anatomic pathways that malignancies may take that can lead to treatment failure.

Anatomy and Physiology

The skin is the heaviest human organ in the body. It is dynamic, metabolic, and responsive to the local environment. The composition of the skin of the face is variable and dependent on age, sex, anatomic location, previous sun exposure, and traumatic injury. The skin has the ability to provide a protective barrier to fluid loss and mechanical injury, has the capacity for thermoregulation, has a role in immunologic surveillance, and provides sensory perception.

The skin is divided into three components: epidermis, basement membrane, and dermis, as depicted in Figure 1–1.[1]

Epidermis

The epidermis is composed of four layers in which immature keratinocytes migrate from deep to superficial levels, maturing as stratified squamous epithelial cells. As the cells migrate superficially, they lose their mitotic capacity and ability to synthesize cytokines. The thickness of this layer ranges from 0.075 to 0.15 mm, and the keratinocyte transit time can vary from 40 to 56 days.[2]

The layers of the epidermis (from deep to superficial) include the following: stratum germinatinum/basale, stratum spinosum, stratum granulosum, and stratum corneum.

Stratum Germinativum/Basale

This is the basal layer. It is mitotically active and the least differentiated. Cells in this layer are attached to each other by desmosomes and to the basement membrane by hemidesmosomes. This layer contains keratin intermediate filaments also called tonofilaments that form a cytoskeleton. Melanocytes are present in this level.

Stratum Spinosum

This also is known as the prickle cell or spinous layer. It is composed of polyhedral cells arranged parallel to the basal layer that is 5 to 10 cell layers thick. The tonofilaments associated with desmosomal attachments are prominently noted on hematoxylin and eosin (H&E) staining in the level.

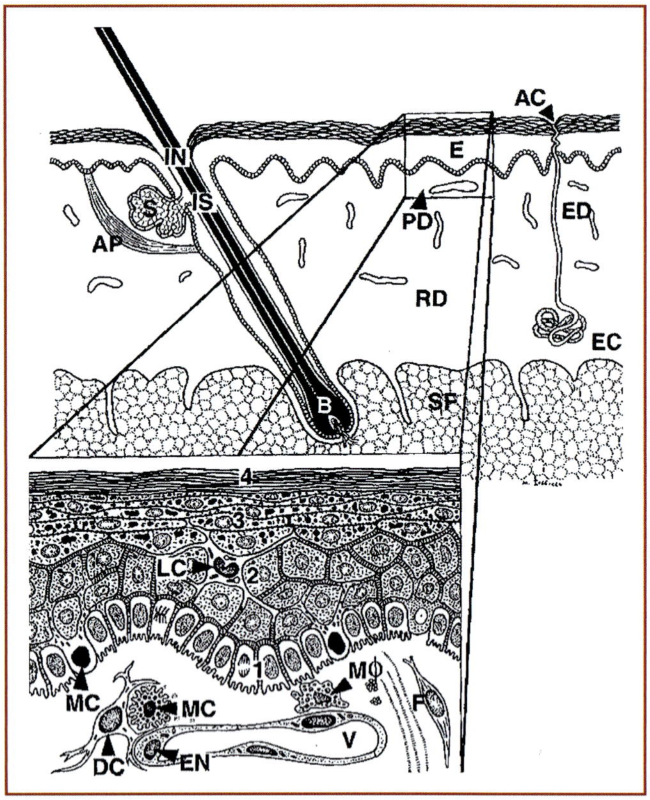

Figure 1–1. Schematic overview of the architecture and cytologic constituents of normal human skin. Projection demonstrates cellular components of epidermis and superficial dermis in greater detail, with epidermal strata denoted numerically (*1*, stratum basalis; *2*, stratum spinosum; *3*, stratum granulosum; *4*, stratum corneum); *E*, epidermis; *PD*, papillary dermis; *RD*, reticular dermis; *SF*, subcutaneous fat; *LC*, Langerhans cell; *M*, melanocyte; *IN*, follicular infundibulum; *IS*, follicular isthmus; *B*, follicular bulb; *AP*, arrector pili muscle; *S*, sebaceous gland; *AC*, eccrine acrosyringium; *ED*, dermal eccrine gland; *EC*, coil of eccrine gland; *V*, vessel; *EN*, endothelial cell; *MC*, mast cell; *Mø*, macrophage; *DC*, perivascular dendritic cell; *F*, fibroblast with adjacent extracellular matrix. (Courtesy of Michael Loffreda.) (Murphy GF. Histology of the skin. In: Elder D, Elenitsas R, Jaworsky C, Johnson Jr B, eds. *Lever's Histopathology of the Skin.* 8th ed. Philadelphia, PA: Lippincott-Raven; 1997:7. Reprinted with permission.)

Stratum Granulosum

This level, also known as the granular layer, is characterized by cells with a flattened appearance that contain deeply basophilic keratohyalin granules. The thickness of this layer is proportional to the thickness of the overlying stratum corneum. An inverse relationship exists with the thickness of this layer and the presence of parakeratosis.

Stratum Corneum

Also known as the horny layer, this level is devoid of nuclei and its cells appear flattened as they form plates of keratin. This is the primary protective barrier of the epidermis. This layer appears eosinophilic on H&E staining with cells demonstrating large intracellular spaces in an interlacing basket-weave pattern.

Other Cell Types

Numerous cell types, beyond the keratinocyte, are found in these layers and include melanocytes, Langerhans cells, and neuroendocrine cells.

Melanocytes are responsible for the production of melanin, an endogenous screen against ultraviolet light. Melanocytes are considered to arise from neural crest origin. In sun-exposed areas, they are found in a 1 to 4 ratio to keratinocytes. This ratio changes to 1 to 30 in nonexposed sites. When melanocytes produce melanin, it accumulates in organelles called melanosomes. Melanosomes are transported through the epidermis in the dendritic projections of the melanocyte to the stratum spinosum. The transfer and degradation of the melanosome to the keratinocytes determines the degree of skin pigmentation categorized clinically by Fitzpatrick and depicted in Table 1–1.[3]

Melanin production increases in response to sun exposure and various hormones (melanocyte stimulating hormone/MSH, adrenocorticotropic hormone/ACTH, estrogens, and progesterone). Variations in pigmentation relate to variations in melanosome size rather than number of melanocytes. The number of melanocytes present within the epidermis decreases with age.

Langerhans cells are dendritic histiocytic cells that process antigens. They are of bone marrow origin. Langerhans cells are responsible for contact hypersensitivity and express class II major histocompatibility (MHC) antigens. They are found in the stratum basale, spinosum, and granulosum layers.

Table 1–1. Fitzpatrick's Classification (1988) of Sun-Reactive Skin Types[3]

I:	White or freckled skin, always burns/never tans
II:	White skin, usually burn/tan less than average
III:	Olive skin, mild burn/tan average
IV:	Light brown skin, burns minimally/tans easily
V:	Dark brown skin, rarely burns/tans easily
VI:	Black skin, never burns/always tans

Fitzpatrick.[3]

Neuroendocrine cells, also known as Merkel cells, assemble in a neurocellular complex and function in pressure sensing for light touch. These cells are considered to be of neural crest origin.

The epidermis contains no dedicated blood vessels.

Basement Membrane Zone

Also known as the dermoepidermal junction, the basement membrane is the site of nutrient delivery and waste disposal from the dermis to the epidermis.[1] It is composed of two layers, the lamina lucida and the lamina densa. The lamina lucida is thinner and superficial, and it lies in contact with basal layer of epidermis. Conversely, the lamina densa is in contact with dermis.

The basement membrane is the target of immunologic attack with bullous diseases of the skin. Photoaging is associated with flattening with of this dermal-epidermal junction.

Dermis

The primary function of the dermis is to sustain and support the epidermis. It has numerous components that include collagen, elastic tissue, ground substance, cellular components (fibroblasts), and a dedicated nerve and vascular supply. The fibroblast is the major cell type of this layer and has the capacity to produce procollagen and elastic fibers.

Collagen makes up 70% of the weight of the dermis (85% type I, 15% type III), and elastic fibers contribute to less than 1% of the weight of the dermis. Despite this representing only a minority of this volume, elastic fibers play an important role in the deformational capacity of this layer. Cross-linked type I collagen fibers provide the tensile strength of the dermis and epidermis. The extracellular matrix of the dermis is composed of fibrous proteins and glycoproteins embedded in a hydrated ground substance of glycosaminoglycans and proteoglycans that is secreted by fibroblasts.[1]

The dermis is composed of two layers. The papillary dermis is the superficial layer that is made up of loose connective tissue with elastic fibers, reticular fibers, collagen, and interdigitating mesenchymal cones. The reticular dermis constitutes the deeper layer, which is thicker and composed of dense connective tissue with downward invaginations. The reticular dermis has larger vessels, nerve endings, lymphatics, and epidermal appendages. Interlaced elastic fibers and parallel arrangements of bundles of collagen fibers also are in this layer. This area contains mast cells that contribute to the synthesis of ground substance and produce histamine, potentially explaining the pruritis associated with scar formation.

Additional cellular elements found in the dermis include the pilosebaceous appendages, apocrine glands, and eccrine glands. Pilosebaceous units are intradermal epithelial structures lined with epithelial cells. Sebaceous glands open within the hair follicle and secrete sebum that lubricates the skin and provides a moisture barrier. Arrector pili muscles connect the deep portion of the follicle to the superficial dermis and are under sympathetic control. The pilosebaceous unit contains a reservoir of pluripotential stem cells that are critical in epidermal reproductivity after trauma or surgical care such as with the harvest of a split-thickness skin graft.

The apocrine glands are located in specialized regions such as the external auditory canal (as ceruminous glands) and the eyelid (as Moll's glands). Their secretions produce odor and are considered to have a vestigial function in pheromone production. Eccrine glands, also known sweat glands, are not found on the vermilion border of the lip or the external auditory canal. Their activity is under the control of sympathetic nerves from the thermoregulatory centers in the hypothalamus.

Blood Supply

Vascularity becomes more prominent in the dermis, as opposed to other layers of the skin, which has a significant impact as it relates to postsurgical reconstruction. Vertical vascular channels interconnect two horizontal dermal plexuses (one within papillary dermis; the other at the dermal-subcutaneous channel). The deep subcutaneous perforating vessels supply the dermal-subcutaneous plexus.

The angiosome concept, first described by Taylor and Palmer in 1987,[4] demonstrated that three-dimensional vascular territories are supported by source arteries and veins that communicate with other angiosomes via choke vessels and true anastamotic arteries. Performing a detailed anatomic study of the angiosome concept in the head and neck, Houseman et al[5] noted that individual angiosomes are connected at junctional zones within tissues (muscle, skin, or specialized organs/glands) rather than between tissues. Midline anastomoses were noted to be rich in the skin of scalp, forehead, and lips yet poor in oral cavity sites such as the tongue and palate. Thirteen angiosomes were identified in the head and neck that are supplied by the carotid (internal and external) and subclavian arteries. The predominant arterial supply to the face and scalp was noted to be from skin perforators of source vessels including the ophthalmic, superficial temporal, posterior auricular, occipital, and facial arteries. Only three territories, supplied by the vertebral, lingual, and ascending pharyngeal arteries, did not supply the skin and were isolated to supplying only to deeper tissue.[5]

Lymphatic Drainage

Our understanding of the lymphatic spread of skin cancers of the head and neck has benefited significantly over the last decade with the widespread use of lymphoscintigraphy and sentinel node biopsy for cutaneous melanoma. Lymph node spread for cutaneous malignancies follows relatively predictable patterns of spread. Pathak et al[6] demonstrated this clinically by predicting the location of lymph node spread of cutaneous malignant melanoma of the head and neck in 92% of 169 patients studied prospectively. The results of this study are outlined in Table 1–2.[6] The issue of assessing for lymphatic

Table 1–2. Clinical Predictions of the Locations for Lymphatic Metastases from Head and Neck Cutaneous Malignancy, with Noted Variations

Primary Location	Clinical Prediction (Actual Spread %)	Location of Variant Spread
Forehead	Parotid, levels I–III (94%)	Level IV
Upper face	Parotid, levels I–III (91%)	Level IV, Level V
Lower face	Parotid, levels I–III (100%)	None reported
Upper anterior neck	Levels I–IV (89%)	Level V
Coronal scalp	Parotid, levels I–V (85%)	Level IV, postauricular
Ear	Parotid, levels I–V (100%)	None reported
Periauricular	Parotid, levels I–V (100%)	None reported
Upper coronal neck	Levels I–V (100%)	None reported
Posterior scalp	Levels II–V, occipital (89%)	Level I, postauricular
Upper posterior neck	Levels II–V, occipital (100%)	None reported
Lower posterior neck	Levels II–V, occipital (84%)	External jugular

Source: Used with permission from Pathak et al, *Head Neck.* 2001.[6] Copyright John Wiley and Sons, 2001.

spread is equally important in nonmelanoma skin cancer, as rates of lymphatic spread of cutaneous squamous cell carcinoma have been reported to be as high as 20%.[7]

However, in discussing regional metastasis, one needs to reconcile that assessing a specific primary site for a cutaneous head and neck lesion can be difficult because of the lack of a uniform system that clearly defines regions. As such, any review of the literature on this topic requires some caution if formal anatomic boundaries defining regions such as the cheek versus temple are not utilized. In an attempt to promote such standardization, Vauterin[8] divided the cutaneous head and neck primary sites into the following anatomic regions depicted in Figure 1–2: anterior scalp, posterior scalp, forehead, temple, periorbital, pinna, postauricular, nose, cheek, chin, and neck.

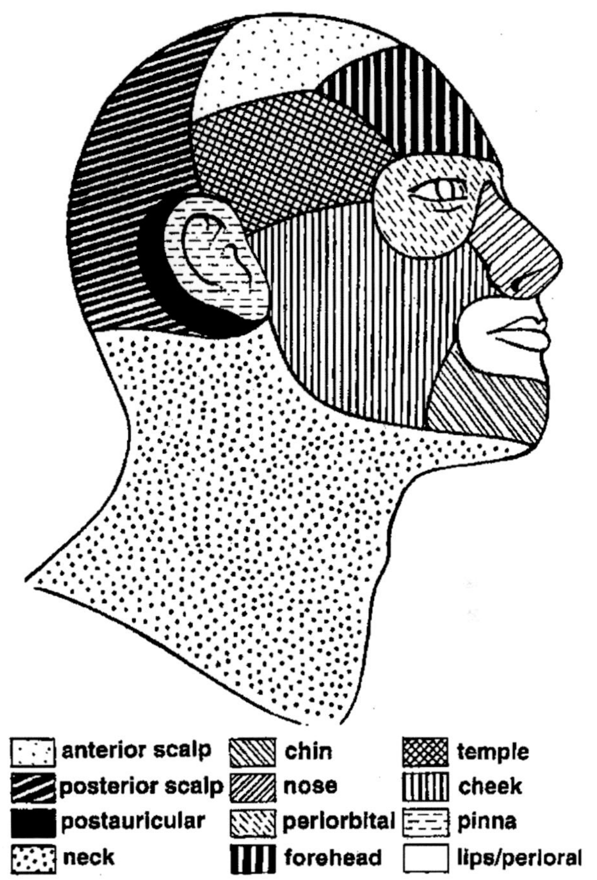

Figure 1–2. Anatomic zones of the head and neck. (Vauterin TJ, Veness NJ, Morgan GJ, et al. Patterns of lymph node spread of cutaneous squamous cell carcinoma of the head and neck. *Head Neck.* 2006;28:786. Reprinted with permission.)

Nodal Drainage Patterns

Lymphatic nodal basins of the head and neck that have been described relative to the spread of cutaneous malignancies include the following nodal groups, as illustrated in Figure 1–3.

Periauricular Lymphatics

This region is composed of three subsites. The preauricular lymph nodes follow the course of the superficial temporal artery and drain the anterior scalp, forehead, temple, pinna, periorbital region, cheek, and lateral nose. Parotid lymph nodes provide a drainage basin similar to preauricular group. Postauricular lymph nodes drain the posterior scalp and pinna.

Suboccipital Lymphatics

The posterior scalp and upper posterior neck drain to suboccipital lymph nodes. If a vertical line is drawn through external auditory canal, lesions posterior to the line may spread to this region.

External Jugular Lymphatics

There are a limited number of nodes superficial to sternocleidomastoid muscle and adjacent to greater auricular nerve. This area drains lateral cheek/chin, pinna, and upper neck. O'Brien[9] has emphasized the importance of this overlooked region that accounts for some of the periparotid nodal drainage.

Buccinator/Perifacial Lymphatics

These nodes follow the nasolabial path of the facial artery and preferentially drain the lateral nose, upper lip, medial cheek, and nasolabial fold. Bilateral drainage is possible in midline lesions.

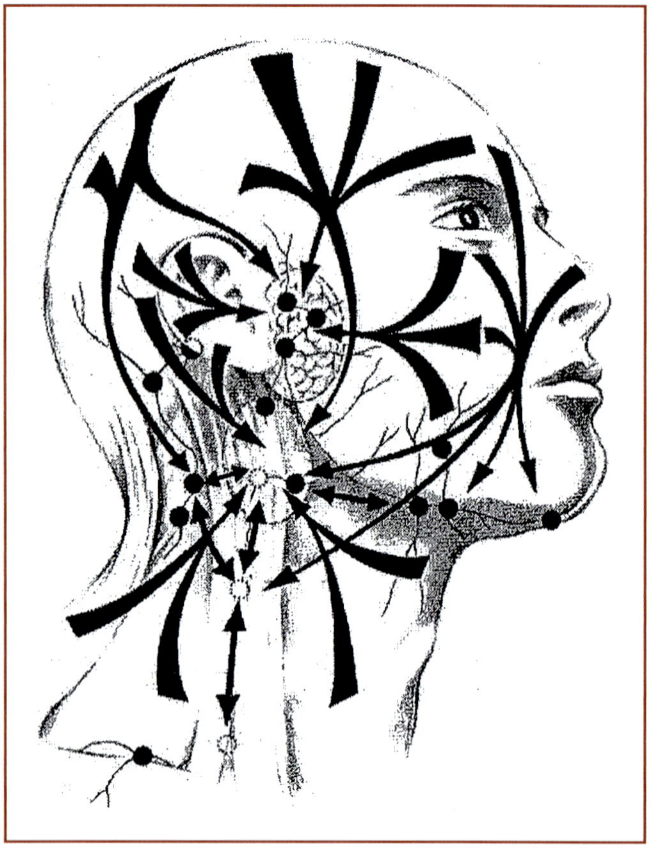

Figure 1–3. Patterns of lymph node spread of cutaneous squamous cell carcinoma of the head and neck. Vauterin TJ, Veness NJ, Morgan GJ, et al. Patterns of lymph node spread of cutaneous squamous cell carcinoma of the head and neck. *Head Neck.* 2006;28:786. Reprinted with permission.)

Cervical Lymphatic Basins

The skin of the head and neck also drains to the traditional cervical lymph node basins often involved by lesions of the upper aerodigestive tract. For this reason, a skin cancer primary (or history thereof) should be considered when evaluating a patient who presents with an isolated lymph node metastasis with an unclear primary site of origin.

Lymph nodes in the submental triangle (Level Ia) constitute the draining basin for the upper and lower lips, nasal vestibule, and skin of the chin. Submandibular (Level Ib) nodes provide lymphatic drainage for the cheek, chin, nose, and nasolabial region. The posterior triangle (Level V) carries lymphatic drainage for the neck, pinna, and posterior scalp. The jugular chain lymph nodes (Levels II, III, and IV) remain important in cutaneous malignancy because all sites of the head and neck may drain to this area. Finally, supraclavicular lymph nodes parallel the transverse cervical artery and drain the regions of the lower neck and upper chest.

A recurrent theme that has been reported by multiple authors on the spread of cutaneous malignancies of the lateral aspect of the face and head (cheek, pinna and temple) is the predilection for these tumors to metastasize to the periauricular/parotid lymph nodes and upper neck lymphatics (levels II/III).[6–11] The impact of this common pattern of presentation and spread, with certain subsites demonstrating a higher rate of regional metastases, has clinical significance when considering surgical management of these cancers and may warrant parotidectomy and neck dissection to optimize regional control (Table 1–3).

Nerve Supply

Perineural invasion (PNI) is an important means of spread for cutaneous malignancies of the head and neck that requires attention at initial evaluation and during operative management. Pain followed by anesthesia in the distribution of a nerve should alert the practitioner to the possibility of perineural invasion.[12] However, the majority of patients (60–70%) with PNI present without symptoms.[13] Identification of perineural invasion is associated with an increased risk for local recurrence and frequently constitutes an indication for adjuvant therapy.[14] Perineural invasion most commonly affects the trigeminal and facial nerves, potentially serving as a pathway for extension to the skull base and intracranial spread.[15]

Cutaneous tumors that exhibit neurotropism include squamous cell carcinoma, keratoacanthoma, basal cell carcinoma, malignant melanoma, primary cutaneous adenoid cystic carcinoma, microcystic adnexal carcinoma, and eccrine epithelioma.[13] The anterior scalp or temporoparietal region and the midface frequently have been described as a tumor

Table 1–3. Location of Probable Skin Lesion of Origin in Patients with Metastatic Cutaneous SCC

Index Lesion Location	Lymph Node (+) *N* = 40	Lymph Node (–) *N* = 153
Periauricular (%)	12 (30%)	47 (30.7%)
Forehead and temple	9 (22.5%)	30 (19.6%)
Cheek	5 (12.5%)	22 (14.4%)
Nose	5 (12.5%)	14 (9.2%)
Scalp	3 (7.5%)	13 (8.5%)
Neck	3 (7.5%)	9 (5.9%)
Lower (nonmucosal) lip	2 (5.0%)	7 (4.6%)
Periorbital	0	8 (5.2%)
Upper lip	1 (2.5%)	3 (2.0%)

Source: Modified with permission from Moore BA et al, *Laryngoscope* 2005.[7]

site that is prone to manifesting perineural invasion. For scalp lesions, the nerves at greatest risk for perineural invasion include the supraorbital and frontal branches of the facial nerve. For midface (cheek and periorbital) lesions, invasion of the supraorbital, supratrochlear, infraorbital, and distal branches of the facial nerve have been reported most frequently. Goepfert et al[14] demonstrated a 14% incidence of perineural invasion in a single institutional review of 520 patients. In his review, the trigeminal and facial nerves were the most commonly involved. Of note, greater than 40% of patients with perineural invasion in the series had involvement of the maxillary division of the trigeminal nerve.

Special Considerations

The H-zone, as described by Baker et al,[16] includes the midface structures of the upper lip, nose, and medial canthus. This region extends from the lower eyelids horizontally to the preauricular region. From the temple, the H-zone extends to the level of the angle of the mandible and includes the ear and postauricular sulcus. Skin cancers, in particular basal cell carcinomas, arising in this region demonstrate a higher reported risk for local recurrence (Fig 1–4). This region is a site of embryonic fusion planes that are perpendicular to the skin surface and allow for deeper extension of tumor.[16] Tumors, both basal cell and squamous cell carcinoma in particular, may invade more deeply in the region of the midfacial embryonic fusion planes prior to exhibiting greater superficial growth.[17]

Periorbital skin cancers require additional consideration for assessment relative to the orbital septum. Midfacial and medial canthal tumors should be evaluated for possible nasolacrimal duct extension or cribriform plate invasion with deeply invasive lesions.

Environmental Exposure and Risk Stratification

The majority of solar and tanning bed ultraviolet (UV) radiation is UVA (320–400 nm). UVB (290–320 nm) radiation is the primary source of sunburn injury and the primary focus of sunscreens. Exposure to UVB radiation results in the formation of thymidine dimers in the p53 tumor suppressor gene within keratinocyte DNA. This mutation can alter the cell's ability to undergo apoptosis and ultimately lead to uncontrolled growth and tumor formation.[18] Reduced DNA

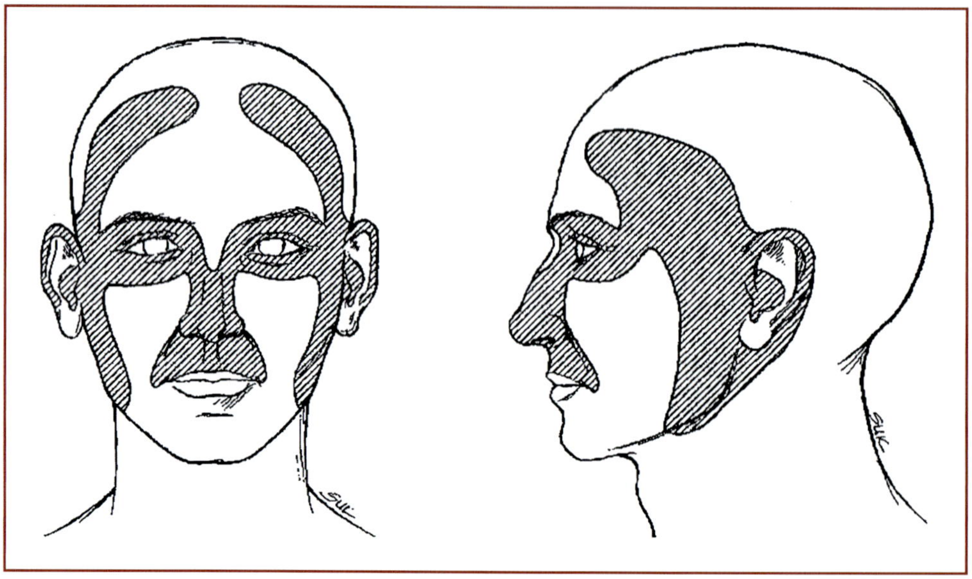

Figure 1–4. The H-zone includes the midface structure, upper lip, nose, and medial canthus. This region extends from the lower eyelid horizontally to the preauricular region. From the temple, the H-zone extends to the level of the mandible and includes the ear and postauricular sulcus. Skin cancers arising in this region are felt to have a higher risk for local recurrence. (Reprinted with permission from Baker SR, Swanson NA, Grekin RC. An interdisciplinary approach to the management of basal cell carcinoma of the head and neck. *J Dermatol Surg Oncol.* 1987; 13(10): 1096.)

repair capacity is an independent risk factor for nonmelanoma skin cancers, but reduced UVB mutagen sensitivity does not appear to play a role in the development of cutaneous malignant melanoma.[19,20]

Risk factors for skin cancer include exposure to ultraviolet radiation and skin pigmentation. Individuals with skin types characteristic of Fitzpatrick Type I and II skin are at higher risk for developing a skin cancer than those with skin types with greater pigmentation. The most prevalent locations where skin cancers present are the cheek and pinna, followed by temple and forehead. Areas on the lateral aspect of the head made up the majority of the primary lesions.[6–8]

Changes in the normal appearance of nevi of the skin should elicit concern for biopsy. The ABCD (asymmetry, border irregularity, color variegation, Diameter less than 6 mm) criterion was established to aid in screening for lesions that require additional evaluation. Addition of an "E" to the acronym (evolving with respect to size, shape, shades of color, surface features or symptoms) has also been advocated.[21]

The risk factors for developing cutaneous malignancy of the head and neck, as well as the evaluation and management of patients with such lesions, are discussed in greater detail in subsequent chapters.

Conclusions

Skin cancer of the head and neck is a growing worldwide epidemic. Knowledge of the anatomy and physiology of the skin is fundamental to the assessment and management of patients with cutaneous malignancy of the head and neck. In particular, an appreciation of the rich lymphatic drainage of the skin of the head and neck constitutes the foundation for the clinical assessment and potential diagnostic and therapeutic interventions for both aggressive nonmelanoma skin cancer and melanoma.

References

1. Murphy GF. Histology of the skin. In: Elder D, Elenitsas R, Jaworsky C, Johnson Jr B, eds. *Lever's Histopathology of the Skin*. 8th ed. Philadelphia, PA: Lippincott-Raven; 1997:5–50.
2. Nemes Z, Steinert PM. Bricks and mortar of the epidermal barrier. *Exp Mol Med*. 1999;31(1):5–19.
3. Fitzpatrick TB. The validity and practicality of sun-reactive skin types I through VI. *Arch Dermatol*. 1988;124(6):869–871.
4. Taylor GI, Pan WR. Angiosomes of the leg: anatomic study and clinical implications. *Plast Recon Surg*. 1998; 102(3):599–616.
5. Houseman ND, Taylor GI, Pan WR. The angiosomes of the head and neck: anatomic study and clinical applications. *Plast Reconstr Surg*. 2000;105(7):2287–2313.
6. Pathak I, O'Brien CJ, Peterson-Schaeffer K, et al. Do nodal metastases from cutaneous melanoma of the head and neck follow a clinically predictable pattern? *Head Neck*. 2001;23(9):785–790.
7. Moore BA, Weber RS, Prieto V, et al. Lymph node metastases from cutaneous squamous cell carcinoma of the head and neck. *Laryngoscope*. 2005;115:1561–1567.
8. Vauterin TJ, Veness NJ, Morgan GJ, et al. Patterns of lymph node spread of cutaneous squamous cell carcinoma of the head and neck. *Head Neck*. 2006;28:785–791.
9. O'Brien CJ, Shah P, Balm AJ. Neck dissection and parotidectomy for melanoma. In: Thompson JF, Morton DL, Kroon BB, eds. *Textbook of Melanoma*. London, UK: Martin Dunitz; 2004:296–306.
10. Jol JA, van Velthuysen ML, Hilgers FJ, et al. Treatment results of regional metastases from cutaneous head and neck squamous cell carcinoma. *Eur J Surg Oncol*. 2002;29: 81–86.
11. Jackson GL, Ballantyne AJ. Role of parotidectomy for skin cancer of the head and neck. *Am J Surg*. 1981;142: 464–469.
12. Padya TA, Cornelius RS, Athavale SM, et al. Perineural extension to the skull base from early cutaneous malignancies of the midface. *Otolaryngol Head Neck Surg*. 2007; 137:742–746.
13. Feasel AM, Brown TJ, Bogle MA, Tschen JA, Nelson BR. Perineural invasion of cutaneous malignancies. *Dermatol Surg*. 2001;27(6):531–542.
14. Goepfert H, Dicktel WJ, Medina JE, et al. Perineural invasion in squamous cell carcinoma of the head and neck. *Am J Surg*. 1984;148:542–547.
15. Ballantyne AJ, McCarten AB, Ibanez ML. The extension of cancer of head and neck through peripheral nerves. *Am J Surg*. 1963;106:651–667.
16. Baker SR, Swanson NA, Grekin RC. An interdisciplinary approach to the management of basal cell carcinoma of the head and neck. *J Dermatol Surg Oncol*. 1987;13(10): 1095–1106.
17. Panje WR, Ceilley RI. The influence of embryology of the mid-face on the spread of epithelial malignancies. *Laryngoscope*. 1979;89:1914–1920.
18. Alam M, Ratner D. Cutaneous squamous cell carcinoma. *New Engl J Med*. 2001;344(13):975–983.
19. Wang L, Li C, Strom SS, et al. Repair capacity for UV light-induced DNA damage associated with risk of non-melanoma skin cancer and tumor progression. *Clin Cancer Res*. 2007;13(21):6532–6539.
20. Wang LE, Xiong P, Strom SS, et al. In vitro sensitivity to ultraviolet B light and skin cancer risk: a case-control analysis. *J Natl Cancer Inst*. 2005;97(24):1822–1831.
21. Abbasi NR, Shaw HM, Rigel DS, et al. Early diagnosis of cutaneous melanoma: revisiting the ABCD criteria. *JAMA*. 2004;292:2771–2776.

2

CLINICAL EVALUATION

CHRISTINA J. YANG
BRIAN A. MOORE
RANDAL S. WEBER

Introduction and Epidemiology

Cutaneous malignancies are the most frequently encountered cancer in the United States, and basal cell carcinoma (BCC) and squamous cell carcinoma (SCC) constitute the most common types of skin cancer. Although the skin of the head and neck accounts for only 9% of the total body surface area, a large portion of cutaneous malignancies occur in this region due to its near constant exposure to ultraviolet radiation.[1–3] The annual incidence of nonmelanoma skin cancer in the United States is estimated at more than 1.3 million cases, with basal cell carcinoma diagnosed about four times more often than squamous cell carcinoma.[1–2] This incidence increases with age and has a male predominance.[3] The estimated lifetime risk of developing skin cancer in the United States is 1 in 2, and that for cutaneous malignant melanoma, 1 in 55.[1]

Malignant melanoma (MM) comprises 3% to 5% of all skin cancers but leads to 75% of skin cancer deaths and 4% of all cancer deaths in the United States.[1–2] After a rapid increase in the incidence of melanoma during the 1970s, the rate of increase stabilized at roughly 3% per year since 1990, but is still increasing faster than any other malignancy worldwide.[1,4] In 2009, 69,000 new cases of MM were diagnosed in the United States, affecting 39,000 men and 30,000 women.[2] About 15 to 30% of these cases arise in the head and neck, reflecting both a greater melanocyte density in and greater UV exposure to this anatomic region.[1,2,4–6]

Key Patient History Aspects

Ultraviolet Exposure

The single most important etiologic factor for the development of skin cancer is ultraviolet radiation (UVA and UVB) exposure. The cumulative amount of chronic sun exposure is more closely associated with SCC than with BCC, whereas episodic UV exposure carries an increased risk of developing melanoma later in one's lifetime.[4,7–9] Increases in outdoor leisure time, social desirability of a tan, trends toward wearing lesser amounts of clothing while outdoors, and widespread use of tanning booths contribute to an increased amount of UV exposure, often beginning at an early age. Such lifestyle choices may help explain the increasing incidence of skin cancer.[3,7,10–11] This is particularly true for individuals with sun sensitivity, identified by a history of sunburning easily, multiple or severe sunburns, and difficulty tanning, in addition to traits such as male sex, natural blonde or red hair color, blue eyes, and fair skin (Fitzpatrick grade I/II).[5,12–15]

More than five sunburns may double one's lifelong melanoma risk.[14,16] Therefore, it is imperative to enquire about the patient's sun exposure history, focusing on tanning behaviors, a history of sunburns, and even occupation, as outdoor workers are at greater risk for skin cancer.

Geography

Another important risk factor for development of skin cancer is geography: individuals living closer to the equator carry a higher risk.[9,11] There is a north-south gradient of skin cancer incidence in the United States, along with very high rates of skin cancer in Australia.[9,11,17,18] This geographical correlation is less apparent for melanoma than for SCC and BCC.[4,9] Finally, stratospheric ozone depletion may increase levels of UVB radiation at the earth's surface and may also contribute to increasing skin cancer incidence, particularly for malignant melanoma.[19–20]

Other Risk Factors

Exposure to ionizing radiation (whether therapeutic or occupational) also increases the risk of developing BCC and SCC.[4,21,22] Other risk factors for nonmelanoma skin cancer include a past medical history of any type of skin cancer, immunosuppression, genetic syndromes such as xeroderma pigmentosum (autosomal recessive) and nevoid basal cell nevus syndrome (autosomal dominant), trauma (burns, ulcers, and scars such as the Marjolin, or postburn, ulcer), chronic stasis ulcers and sinus tracts, and exposure to coal tar, pitch, creosote, arsenic compounds, radiation, or mustard gas.[2,23,24]

Large (over 20 cm) congenital nevi, dysplastic nevi, personal nevus count greater than 50, history of melanoma or nonmelanoma skin cancers, oculocutaneous albinism, and xeroderma pigmentosum are also significant risk factors for invasive cutaneous malignant melanoma.[7,24] A family history of melanoma also increases one's risk of developing melanoma, as a quarter of families with melanoma carry heritable germline mutations in the tumor suppressor gene CDKN2A/p16 on chromosome 9p21.[5,7] Genetic abnormalities involving cyclin-dependent kinase 4 (CDK4) and the melanocortin-1 receptor (MC1R) also have been linked to susceptibility to MM.

The risk factors for cutaneous malignancy are summarized in Table 2–1.

Clinical Implications

It is imperative to maintain a high index of suspicion for skin cancer in patients with these personal, family, occupational, and environmental risk factors. When evaluating a patient with a suspicious cutaneous lesion, particular attention must be devoted to potential recreational or occupational exposures, use (if any) of sun-protective behaviors, past history of skin lesions, a family history of skin cancer, particularly aggressive disease, and comorbid conditions, especially immunosuppression.

When a lesion is present, several questions are essential, and these are listed in Table 2–2: how long has the lesion been there; has it changed (and if so, how); what about is concerning to the patient; are there any others; is it painful; does it bleed; is there regional numbness or paresthesia; does it itch or feel as if bugs or ants are crawling on it (formication)? The presence of formication is worrisome for perineural invasion and warrants closer investigation with anatomic imaging.[25,26]

Patients presenting with a neck or parotid mass should be queried for any personal history of skin lesions or malignancy. Often, the patient may not know that a particular lesion was, in fact, cancer, so it is imperative to ask if there have been any skin lesions previously treated in the head and neck. Metastatic skin cancer may present in the parotid gland, and patients with parotid lesions should be asked if they have been treated for an ipsilateral skin lesion, especially in the temporal region. Interestingly, the most common parotid malignancy in Australia is metastatic skin cancer.[27,28]

Squamous Cell Carcinoma

Squamous cell skin cancers arise from a common progenitor, the keratinocyte. Common premalignant lesions are actinic keratosis (also known as

Table 2–1. Risk Factors in Tumorigenesis of BCC, SCC, and MM of the Head and Neck

Risk Factors	BCC	SCC	MM
Genetic factors	xeroderma pigmentosum, albinism, basal cell nevus syndrome (autosomal dominant)[24,33]	xeroderma pigmentosum, albinism, HPV, epidermodysplasia verruciformis[24,33]	xeroderma pigmentosum, oculocutaneous albinism[24,33] positive family history
Molecular factors	impaired DNA excision/repair	impaired DNA excision/repair	impaired DNA excision/repair
	UV carcinogenesis: tumor initiation, promotion, progression after radiation- or chemically induced DNA damage, impaired apoptosis	UV carcinogenesis: tumor initiation, promotion, progression after radiation- or chemically induced DNA damage, impaired apoptosis	increased cellular growth factor, melanin reactive oxygen species[17]
	p53, p21, c-Ha-ras, and K-ras mutations[22,24]	p53, p21, c-Ha-ras, and K-ras mutations; HPV[22,24]	heritable CDKN2A/p16 and CDK4 mutations[5,7,17]
		precursor lesions; tissue injury (radiation, burns, ulcers, and scars [Marjolin ulcer])	high melanocyte density in head and neck region[5]
Host/Environmental factors	chronic UV exposure (occupational and/or recreational), geography (low latitude)	chronic UV exposure (occupational and/or recreational), geography (low latitude)	intense UV radiation[5,17]
	immunosuppression, trauma, burns, chronic stasis ulcers and sinus tracts, chronic dermatoses, and exposure to coal tar, pitch, creosote, arsenic compounds, radiation, paraffin, or mustard gas[23]	immunosuppression, trauma, burns, chronic stasis ulcers and sinus tracts, chronic dermatoses, cigarette smoking, and exposure to coal tar, pitch, creosote, arsenic compounds, radiation, paraffin, or mustard gas[23]	immunosuppression, occupational exposures, redox-active metal exposure, and smoking[21]

Table 2–2. Key Historical Questions

How long has the lesion been present?
Has it changed (and if so, how)?
What about the lesion is concerning to the patient?
Are there any others?
Is it painful?
Does it bleed?
Is there regional numbness or tingling (paresthesias)?
Does it itch or feel as if bugs or ants are crawling on it (formication)?

solar keratosis) and Bowen's disease (squamous cell carcinoma in situ), with keratoacanthoma a frequent imitator.

Actinic keratoses present as multiple red-to-tan macules or scales on sun-exposed areas of the head and neck such as the forehead, scalp (in alopecic males), nose, malar eminences, and helix (Fig 2–1). These lesions are extremely common in fair-skinned, middle-aged men and mark an individual's cumulative lifetime UVB exposure.[1,4] Actinic keratoses have a risk of malignant degeneration to SCC of 0.075% to 0.096% per lesion per year (10–20% of actinic keratoses over 10–25 years), but there are no reliable predictors of which cases will progress.[29]

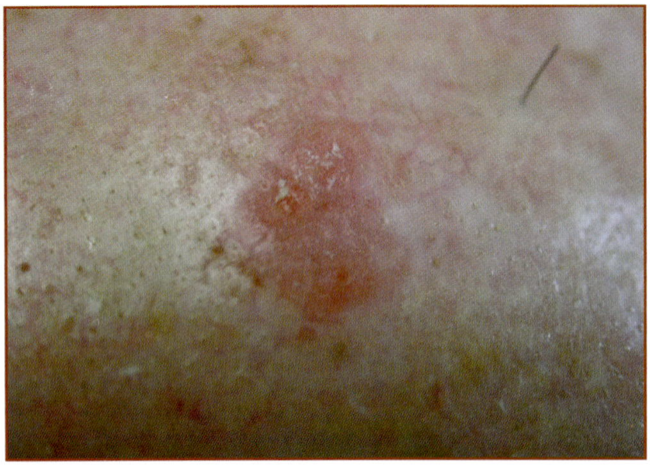

Figure 2–1. Actinic keratosis of the cheek in a 57-year-old man. Note the scaly, reddish macule and surrounding evidence of sun damage. Photo courtesy David J. MacGregor, MD.

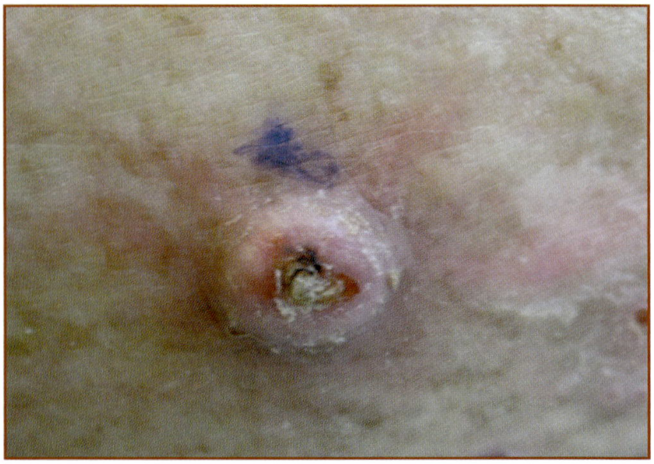

Figure 2–2. Keratoacanthoma of the head and neck. Note the well-circumscribed nodule with central keratin-filled crater. Photo courtesy David J. MacGregor, MD.

Bowen's disease usually appears as single or multiple erythematous plaques, patches, or papules, resembling psoriatic lesions, eczematous patches, viral warts, or superficial basal cell carcinoma. Some of these lesions (3%) precede development of invasive SCC by many years.[30]

By contrast, keratoacanthoma is a rapidly growing rounded nodule that develops a central keratin-filled crater over 2 to 6 months and may spontaneously involute (Fig 2–2). Keratoacanthoma may be histologically indistinguishable from well-differentiated SCC.

Invasive SCC may be described by the patient as an enlarging or nonhealing sore. It is usually first seen as a firm erythematous lesion with elevated borders and central ulceration which may exhibit indistinct margins (Fig 2–3). When preceded by actinic changes, these lesions tend to remain localized.[29] By comparison, lesions arising de novo or induced by ionizing irradiation, thermal injury, or chemical burns are more locally aggressive and may have a higher incidence of regional metastasis. In general, cutaneous SCC spreads by local, centrifugal expansion and infiltration, then shelving or skating along the path of least resistance, along planes of fascia, perichrondrium, or periosteum. However, aggressive squamous cell skin cancers (particularly of the spindle and adenosquamous variants) can invade deeply early in their course to involve subcutaneous tissue including nerve, cartilage, bone, or muscle and sometimes spread by distant metastasis.[25,27,31] Regional lymph node metastasis, most frequently within the parotid gland, occur in less than 5% of cases, more often in poorly differentiated tumors, those exhibiting perineural invasion, lymphovascular invasion, inflammation, or

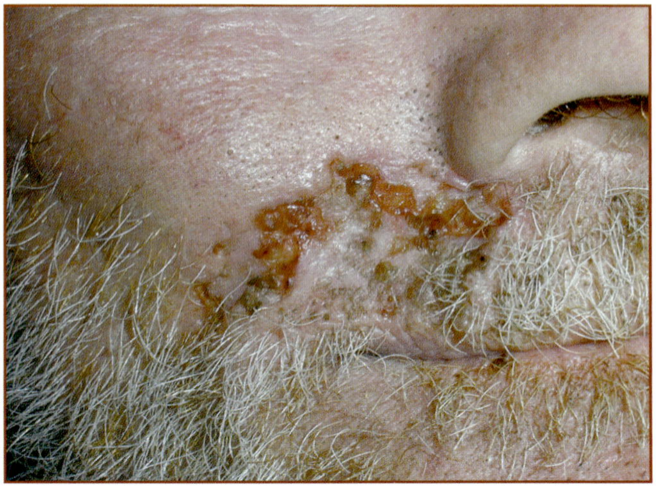

Figure 2–3. Squamous cell carcinoma of the cheek and upper lip in 49-year-old man. This infiltrating lesion had been neglected for some time prior to presentation.

invasion deeper than subcutaneous fat, large (>2 cm diameter) and deeply invasive (Clark level IV and V) lesions, and periauricular SCCs.[25–28,31,32]

Basal Cell Carcinoma

Basal cell skin cancers arise de novo from basal keratinocytes of the epidermis and adnexal structures; they have no precursor lesion. Histologically, these tumors grow in a circumscribed pattern of interanastomosing lobules with pushing margins, nuclear palisading at the periphery, and surrounding dermal retraction. The malignant cells closely resemble the basal cell layer of the skin and occasionally will display squamoid differentiation.

Clinically, basal cell carcinomas have four histomorphologic growth patterns: nodular or noduloulcerative (the most common type, 80% of BCCs), morpheaform (sclerosing or infiltrative), superficial multicentric, and metatypical (basosquamous). The nodular type appears as a pearly, pink, raised, well-circumscribed papule or nodule with rolled borders and overlying telangiectasias (Fig 2–4). They may bleed spontaneously or with minimal trauma (Fig 2–5). Longstanding or neglected nodular BCCs may exhibit central ulceration; these "rodent ulcers" appear similar clinically to SCCs.[33]

Infiltrative, or morpheaform, BCC, the least common and most invasive type, occurs in 10% of patients and appears as a yellow-to-white, fibrotic, firm plaque with indistinct margins that may resemble a scar (Fig 2–6).[33] These tumors tend to be deeply invasive and often extend peripherally beyond the apparent clinical margin. Noncon-tiguous projections of tumor extend outward and are surrounded by sclerotic bands of collagen, a pattern to be considered when planning treatment.

Superficial multicentric BCCs arise from the epidermis in multiple areas as tiny, red, scaling patches with threadlike irregular borders and clinically resemble chronic dermatitis; they generally do not invade deeply but may be associated with extensive areas of lateral involvement.[33]

Metatypical (basosquamous) BCC may present as rapidly growing ulcerative lesions. Rapid, aggressive local growth may be associated with perineural spread. As its name implies, this variant can behave similarly to SCC and is categorized under SCC in the current National Comprehensive Cancer Network (NCCN) guidelines.[34]

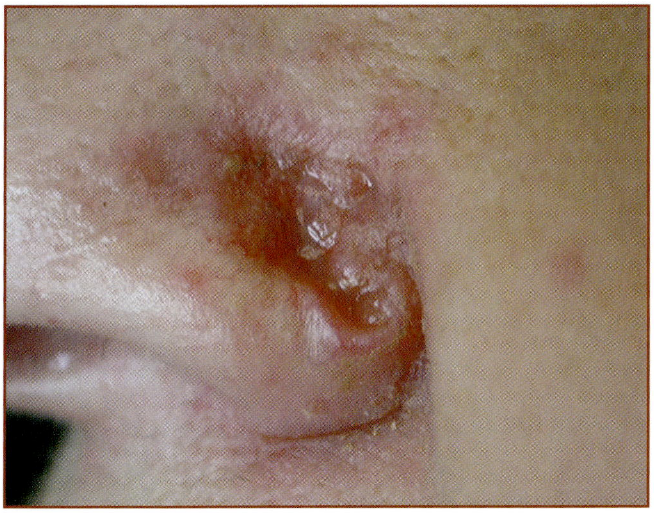

Figure 2–4. Basal cell carcinoma of the left nasal ala in a 53-year-old woman. Note the pearly appearance of this papule, as well as the central ulceration, imparting the appearance of a "rodent ulcer." Photo courtesy David J. MacGregor, MD.

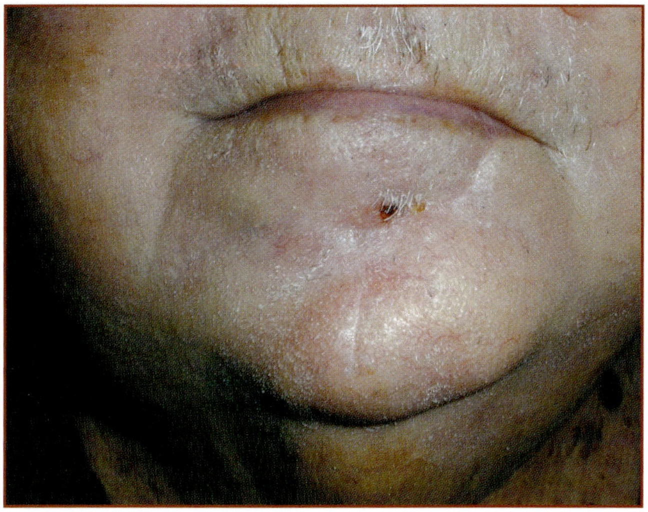

Figure 2–5. Recurrent basal cell carcinoma of the mentum in an 84-year-old man. Tumor clearance required resection of the mandibular periosteum and complex lip reconstruction.

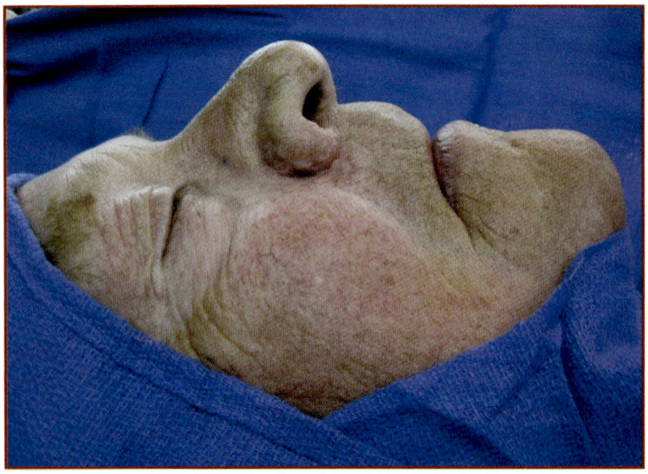

Figure 2–6. Infiltrative basal cell carcinoma of the right nasal ala and melolabial fold. Reconstruction was deferred until a second stage to guarantee negative margins on permanent section.

BCC tends to spread along the path of least resistance, along perichondrium, periosteum, or fascia, rather than invading cartilage, bone, or muscle. Embryonic fusion planes such as the nasolabial fold, retroauricular sulcus, preauricular area, and canthus offer little resistance to tumor spread; the resulting "iceberg phenomenon" of subclinical spread helps explain the high recurrence rates (30–40%) for BCC of the nose, ear, scalp, and periocular area.[27] Unlike squamous cell carcinoma, metastasis from basal cell carcinoma is extremely rare. Risk factors include perineural invasion, infiltrative type, and multiple local recurrences. Regional metastasis from these tumors is usually a precursor to distant spread (to the bone, lung, or liver), which may present 9 to 10 years after treatment of the regional disease.

Melanoma

Melanoma classically presents as a pigmented skin lesion that changes over weeks to months; the ABCDE paradigm (asymmetry, borders, color, diameter, evolution) was designed for early diagnosis of the most common type of melanoma, the superficial spreading type.[35] This subtype accounts for 65% to 75% of all melanomas. It exhibits asymmetry, as the borders of the raised lesion are irregular, with both smooth and ragged contours (Fig 2–7). Clark noted that superficial spreading melanoma lesion margins tend to be indented, flattened, or show peninsular protrusions (scalloped edges).[36] Melanoma may be heterogeneous in color, but typically is tan, brown, or black. Red, white, and blue coloration is a worrisome sign. Irregular color variation, including black, dark brown, tan, and blue-gray pigmentation, is commonly observed in the superficial spreading type.[5] Depigmentation within or around an irregular, disorganized pigmented lesion (as a halo) is pathognomonic for malignant melanoma.[36] Diameter greater than 6 mm is considered significant. These lesions may evolve over weeks to months with further changes in appearance, or they may be associated with common symptoms such as itching.[37]

Beyond the ABCDE paradigm, any lesion that appears different from surrounding nevi should also be considered suspicious for malignancy. Symptoms like bleeding, ulceration, paresthesias, and pain tend to present with advanced disease; the 2002 AJCC staging system upstaged all stage I to III disease exhibiting ulceration, and this persists in the 2010 staging system.[38] Staging is especially important considering the apparent lack of correlation between time to diagnosis of MM and tumor thickness.[37]

After superficial spreading melanoma, the other common subtypes are lentigo maligna (melanoma in situ), nodular, acral lentiginous, and desmoplastic melanoma. Lentigo maligna melanoma is considered to be the precursor to invasive lentigo malignant melanoma, which is commonly found in the head and neck region of older individuals. Unlike superficial spreading malignant melanoma, which has a border with some smooth, arc-shaped contour, the borders of lentigo maligna are entirely irregular. It appears flat on gross examination and exhibits slow radial growth along the dermo-epidermal junction (Fig 2–8). Lentigo maligna is most commonly brown in color and occurs commonly in the head and neck region.

Nodular melanoma is a relatively uniform, dark blue-to-black nodular lesion occurring on both sun-exposed and non-sun-exposed anatomic regions.[39] Differential diagnosis includes hemangioma, blue nevus, pyogenic granuloma, and pigmented BCC.

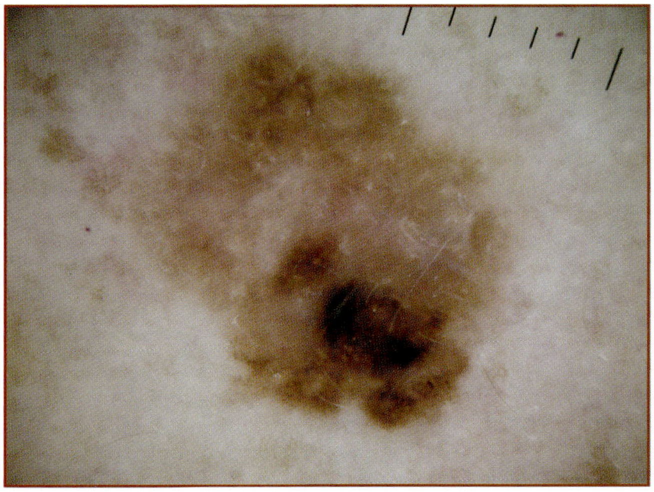

Figure 2–7. Dermoscopic view of a 7-mm in maximum dimension malignant melanoma of the forehead. Note the asymmetry and irregular borders, as well as the color heterogeneity. The lesion had grown larger and manifest pigmentation changes over the preceding 3 months, thereby meeting all of the "ABCDE" criteria. Photo courtesy of David J. MacGregor, MD.

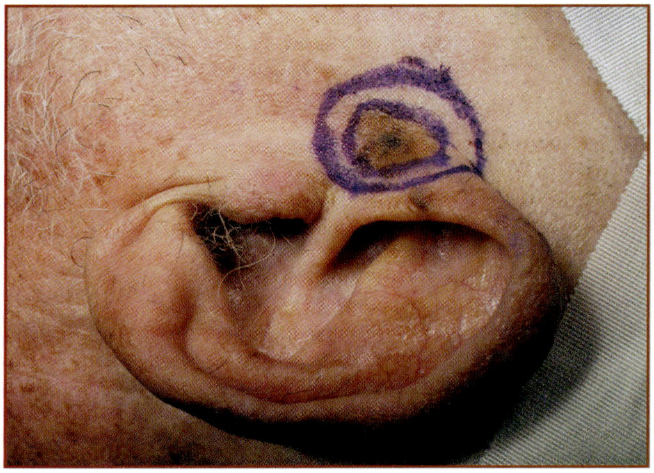

Figure 2–8. Lentigo maligna of the left preauricular region, with margins of resection mapped.

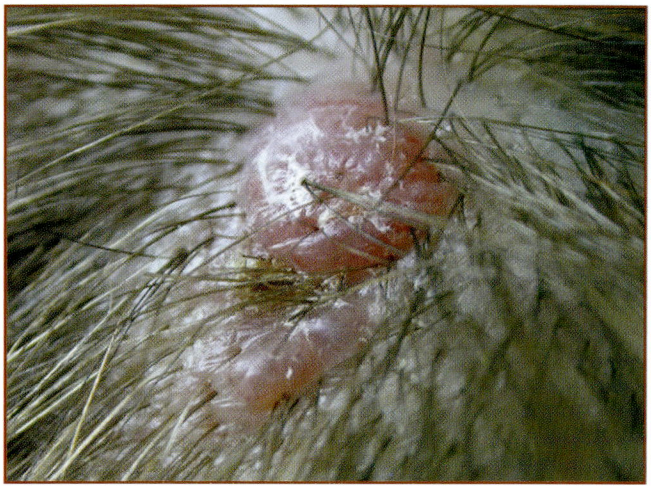

Figure 2–9. Amelanotic melanoma of the scalp in a 49-year-old patient. Photo courtesy David J. MacGregor, MD.

The majority of these lesions are advanced (Clark's level III, IV, and V) at the time of presentation and carry a poorer prognosis than other clinicopathologic subtypes.[5]

Desmoplastic melanoma is a rare melanoma subtype, but three-fourths of cases occur in the head and neck. This subtype is frequently amelanotic (Fig 2–9) and may resemble benign lesions on inspection, commonly presenting as a hard, fibrous, subcutaneous lesion within a lentigo maligna lesion.[5,17,37] A subset of desmoplastic melanoma demonstrates perineural spread and a high recurrence rate, meriting further categorization as desmoplastic-neurotropic melanoma.[5]

Acral lentiginous melanoma is the most common subtype in nonwhites and tends to occur on the palms of the hands, soles of the feet, and oral/anogenital mucosa. Primary mucosal melanoma is a separate disease entity with different risk factors and pathophysiology from the above malignant melanoma subtypes and is not addressed in this chapter.

Physical Examination

As with all conditions, the physical examination begins with thorough inspection and palpation of the skin of the head and neck, including the scalp, for any suspicious lesions and old scars. If a lesion is detected, care should be given to record the size with accurate lateral measurements, depth or fixation to underlying structures, margins (clearly defined or not), and the presence of bleeding or ulceration.

In conjunction with a basic naked-eye examination, dermoscopy has been shown to improve the sensitivity of early melanoma detection and secondary prevention, such as for early, thin nodular melanomas that may not meet clinical ABCD criteria.[39] Sequential digital dermoscopy, performed at a three-month follow-up interval, may be a useful and cost-effective tool for early melanoma detection, specifically in the surveillance of atypical lesions without suspicion of melanoma in high-risk groups (those with familial atypical mole and multiple melanoma syndrome, atypical mole syndrome, and multiple nevi with a history of melanoma).[40] Patients with common nevi and no other risk factors are not good candidates for this surveillance technique.

Cranial nerve exam is paramount to detect clinical evidence of perineural invasion, which is an ominous prognostic sign. Cranial nerves V and VII are most commonly affected.[25,26] Sensation must be checked in all branches of the trigeminal nerve, and subtle clues of facial weakness should be sought, such as loss of the forehead crease, lip weakness, and flattening of the nasolabial fold (Fig 2–10).[25,26] Additionally, diplopia or proptosis may suggest involvement of cranial nerves III, IV, or VI, if not direct orbital infiltration. Otoscopy and hearing assessment are important for auricular and periauricular lesions to gauge the extent of temporal bone involvement.

The neck and parotid regions should be evaluated for lymphadenopathy, with close attention paid to the "high-risk" basins for the lesion in question. The parotid gland constitutes the primary lymphatic drainage basin for the temporoparietal region and lateral face, and other areas drain in a logical fashion to external jugular, deep jugular chain, and occipital or posterior cervical nodes.[27] Central or midface lesions exhibit bilateral drainage to the facial and level I nodes. The specifics on lymphatic drainage patterns of the skin of the head and neck are discussed elsewhere in this text. It is imperative to search for a concurrent skin lesion (or evidence of prior excision) in a patient who presents with a neck malignancy, even if an upper aerodigestive tract primary is possible.

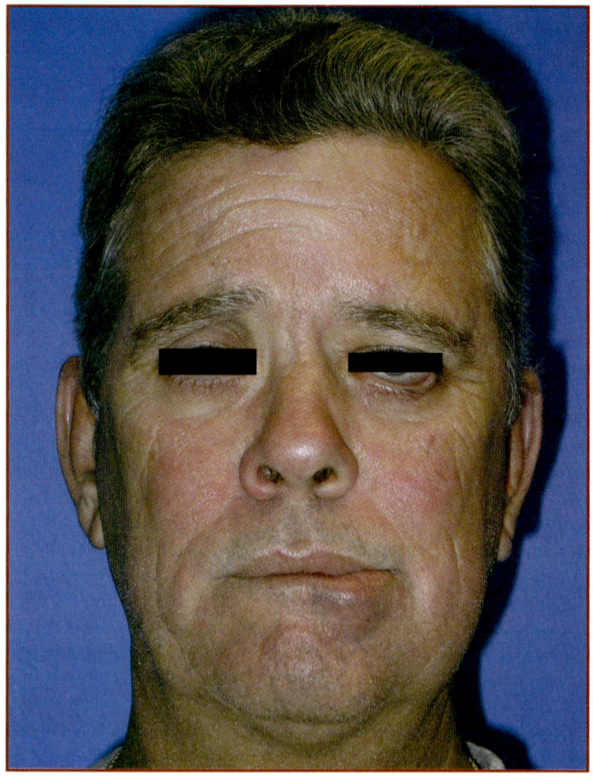

Figure 2–10. This 53-year-old man had undergone prior resection of a squamous cell carcinoma of the left lower (hair-bearing) lip. He developed lancinating left lower facial pain, then lower lip weakness, and finally complete facial nerve paresis, coincident with the onset of recurrent lower lip swelling. Note the loss of forehead wrinkles, ectropion, blunting of the left melolabial fold, and lower lip asymmetry. Extensive perineural invasion was identified in all branches of the facial nerve and in the mental/inferior alveolar nerve. The entire extratemporal facial nerve was resected en bloc with the lower lip recurrence.

Evaluation of Suspicious Lesions

Biopsy

Any suspicious skin lesion should be biopsied in order to establish pathologic diagnosis, assess tumor depth, and evaluate for ulceration, mitotic rate, and vascular or perineural invasion.[5,38] For smaller, well-defined BCC and SCC lesions, simple excisional biopsy with 3- to 5-mm margins is sufficient, whereas 1-cm margins should be planned for larger or poorly defined lesions. Mohs excision, including assessment of margins, and other treatment modalities, are discussed in later chapters.

Small lesions suspicious for melanoma may be assessed by full-thickness excisional biopsy with 1- to 2-mm margins of normal appearing skin. Larger lesions, which are not amenable to excisional biopsy without causing significant deformity, should undergo full-thickness incisional biopsy through the thickest part of the lesion for diagnosis.

Punch biopsy remains one of the more common techniques due to its rapidity, technical ease, and minimal morbidity. This may be subject to sampling error, so repeat biopsy is indicated if the original biopsy does not offer adequate diagnostic information. It cannot be overemphasized that shave biopsies, fine-needle aspiration, or any other partial thickness biopsy should specifically be avoided for skin lesions suspicious for malignancy, as these methods do not adequately assess tumor depth and margins of excision.[38] Biopsy results then guide further staging and treatment, which may include wide local excision and sentinel lymph node biopsy (SLNB).[37,42]

Imaging

Although most early basal and squamous cell skin cancers and malignant melanomas are successfully controlled with a single attempt at local therapy, a subset of biologically aggressive skin cancers displays rapid growth, invades muscle, cartilage, or bone, spreads along peripheral cutaneous nerves, and metastasizes to regional lymph nodes.[25–28,44] For this latter group, and for stage III and IV malignant melanomas, diagnostic imaging studies are important.

If there is evidence of regional disease, chest x-ray and serum lactate dehydrogenase (LDH) are recommended by the American Joint Committee on Cancer (AJCC) for staging purposes in melanoma.[38,41] Chest x-ray is rapid and easily obtained, but subject to false positives and exposure to ionizing radiation.

High-resolution computed tomography (CT) with bone windows should be obtained when bony invasion or perineural invasion is suspected, with irregularities in the cortex and widened neural foramina respectively suggesting these features (Fig 2–11).[26] A contrast-enhanced CT of the neck also is useful for evaluation of regional or disseminated disease, particularly for aggressive squamous cell carcinoma (which may metastasize to lung and bone) and advanced malignant melanoma (Fig 2–12).[34,41]

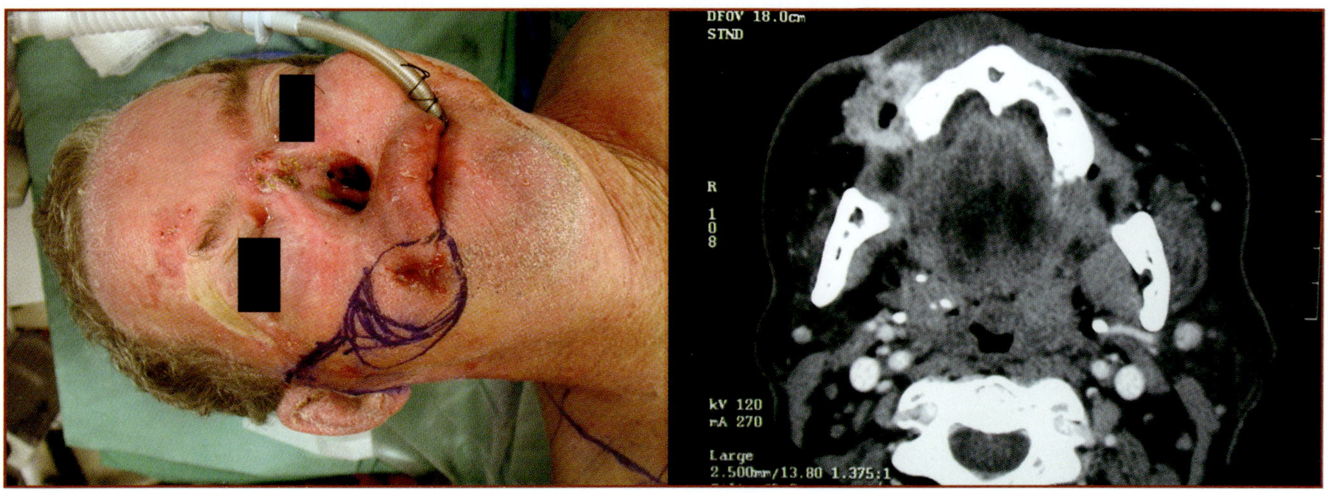

Figure 2–11. Recurrent SCC in an immunocompromised patient. Note the extensive evidence of prior surgery, including rhinectomy. A CT scan revealed invasion of this lesion to the maxilla. The lesion was resected en bloc with an infrastructure maxillectomy.

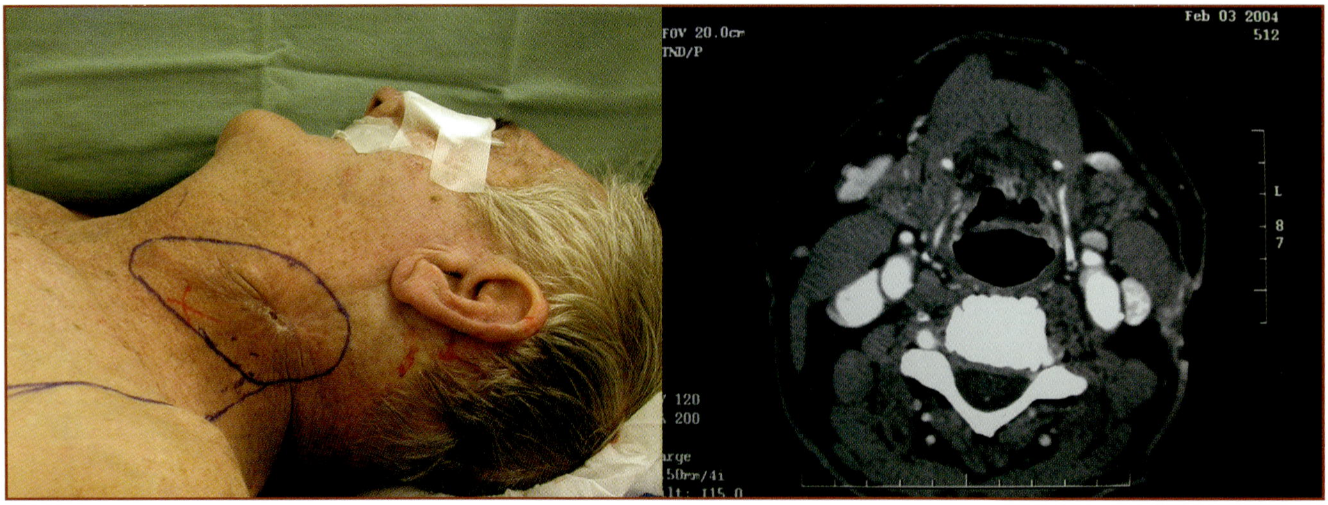

Figure 2–12. Deeply invasive recurrent SCC of the cervical skin, with infiltration of the sternocleidomastoid muscle evident on preoperative CT scan.

Lymph nodes 1.5 cm or larger in size with a hypodense center and peripheral enhancement on CT should be considered positive for malignancy. The disadvantages of CT include a low positive predictive value for smaller lesions without clinical signs of bony invasion, cost, additional radiation exposure, nephrotoxic effects of the iodinated contrast bolus, and a high false-positive rate.[28]

Magnetic resonance imaging (MRI) is the imaging modality of choice when intraorbital/intracranial extension or perineural invasion is suspected.[26] Although more costly and more challenging to perform than CT, it provides excellent, multiplanar soft tissue detail without exposing the patient to ionizing radiation. Gadolinium contrast is not associated with the same risks as iodinated contrast commonly used with CT but has been associated with systemic sclerosis.

High-resolution ultrasound examination of regional lymph nodes as a primary tool for nonmelanoma skin cancer (NMSC) or MM staging is not useful due to the modality's inherent limitations; most nodal foci that are not palpable clinically will be less than 4 mm in size and therefore not reliably detectable by ultrasound.[28] However, it is an excellent screening tool; and its low cost, widespread availability, and low-risk profile make it a reasonable choice in the evaluation of regional disease. High-resolution ultrasound-fine needle aspiration (FNA) is a highly specific modality for the preoperative evaluation of sentinel lymph nodes prior to sentinel lymph node biopsy for stage I/II cutaneous malignant melanoma. Limitations of ultrasound-FNA include operator dependence, the need for rapid cytopathologic analysis of FNA specimens (ideally within 24 hours to permit timely sentinel lymph node biopsy), and low sensitivity, the latter being the main argument against its use as a substitute for sentinel lymph node dissection (SLNB).[43,44]

Positron-emission tomography (PET), often fused with CT scan images, has been advocated recently in the diagnostic workup of stage III malignant melanoma, as it may influence management in 15% of cases.[38,43–45] It also may be useful in detecting locally aggressive tumor behavior for larger (>3 cm) nonmelanoma skin cancers, especially nodular BCC lesions. However, this modality is somewhat limited in the analysis of poorly vascularized or smaller (<1 cm) lesions, and study of suspicious cutaneous lesions of the head and neck may be limited by the normal high uptake in the brain.[45,46] Other disadvantages include cost and false positives due to infection and other regional hypermetabolic activity.

Staging and Treatment Considerations

Squamous Cell Carcinoma and Basal Cell Carcinoma

Current staging for cutaneous carcinomas, according to the 2010 AJCC Guidelines (including squamous cell and basal cell carcinoma), is summarized in Tables 2–3 and 2–4.

Squamous Cell Carcinoma

Following complete history and physical, full thickness biopsy, and imaging studies as indicated for suspicion of extensive disease, an SCC lesion is classified as local or involving regional lymph nodes (by clinical examination or imaging studies). The former category is further stratified into low- versus high-risk categories. Local, low-risk SCC lesions may be treated by curettage and electrodesiccation, excision with postoperative margin assessment (4- to 6-mm clinical margins), or radiation therapy (for nonsurgical candidates). Curettage and electrodesiccation is permitted for superficial lesions in non-hair-bearing sites; if subcutaneous fat is reached, then curettage is aborted and surgical excision performed instead. If positive margins are found following initial excision, then the lesion is further treated with Mohs excision, reexcision with complete circumferential peripheral and deep margin assessment (frozen or permanent section) or radiation therapy.[34]

Local, high-risk SCC skin lesions of the head and neck should initially undergo Mohs excision, resection with complete circumferential peripheral and deep margin assessment (frozen or permanent section), or radiation therapy (for nonsurgical candidates).[34,44] Lesions exhibiting positive margins, extensive perineural or large-nerve involvement should be further treated with adjuvant radiation therapy.

Suspicious regional lymph nodes, whether palpable on clinical examination or radiologically abnormal, that are associated with a SCC lesion should undergo FNA. If FNA is negative, consider clinical, radiographic, cytopathologic (whether by repeat FNA or open biopsy) reanalysis; if re-evaluation produces a second negative result, the algorithm proceeds as for limited local disease. There is an evolving role for sentinel lymph node mapping and biopsy in aggressive nonmelanoma skin cancer. For positive results, imaging is ordered (if not already accomplished) to further determine the size, number, and location of involved lymph nodes and ultimately evaluate for surgical candidacy versus radiation therapy or observation. Surgical treatment, including selective neck dissection for N1 disease, comprehensive neck dissection for N2 disease (bilateral for N2c), and superficial parotidectomy for involved parotid lymph nodes, with possible adjuvant radiation with or without chemotherapy, are discussed in later chapters.

Follow-up with complete history and physical should occur every 3 to 6 months for 2 years, then every 6 to 12 months for 3 years, then annually for life for local disease and more frequently—every 1 to 3 months for the first year, every 2 to 4 months for year 2, every 4 to 6 months for years 3 to 5, then every 6 to 12 months annually for life—for regional disease.[34]

N1S3 staging developed in Australia by Palme and Veness[18,28,47] focuses on the number and maximal size of involved lymph nodes and also incorporates the parotid gland as one of the regional cervical levels, at least for the purpose of predicting disease-related outcomes in head and neck cutaneous SCC.

Basal Cell Carcinoma

Following complete history and physical, full thickness biopsy, and imaging studies as indicated, a BCC lesion is then stratified as low or high risk (see Table 2–3): primary treatment options for low risk lesions include curettage and electrodesiccation (for a specific subset of lesions described below), excision with postoperative margin assessment, or radiation therapy (for nonsurgical candidates). Curettage and electrodesiccation of low-risk BCC skin lesions are permitted by NCCN guidelines under the following conditions: nonhair-bearing site, superficial lesion (if the subcutaneous layer is reached, then curettage is aborted and surgical excision performed instead),

Table 2–3. TNM Staging for Cutaneous Squamous Cell Carcinoma and Other Cutaneous Carcinomas (2010 AJCC staging criteria)[38]

T (primary tumor)	
Tx	Cannot be assessed
T0	No evidence of primary tumor
Tis	Carcinoma in situ
T1	≤2 cm greatest dimension with <2 high-risk features*
T2	>2 cm or any size with ≥2 high-risk features*
T3	With invasion of maxilla, mandible, orbit, or temporal bone
T4	With invasion of skeleton (axial or appendicular) or perineural invasion of skull base
N (regional lymph nodes)	
Nx	Cannot be assessed
N0	No regional lymph node metastases
N1	Single ipsilateral lymph node ≤3 cm
N2	
N2a	Single ipsilateral lymph node 3 to 6 cm
N2b	Multiple ipsilateral lymph nodes ≤6 cm
N2c	Bilateral or contralateral lymph nodes ≤6 cm
N3	Lymph node >6 cm
M (distant metastasis)	
M0	No distant metastases
M1	Distant metastases
T staging excludes cSCC of the eyelid.	
*High risk features for T staging	
Depth/ invasion	>2 mm thickness
	Clark level ≥4
	Perineural invasion
Anatomic location	Primary site ear or non-hair-bearing lip
Differentiation	Poorly differentiated or undifferentiated

and biopsy results are acquired if not previously performed.[34] Head and neck BCC lesions with positive margins on excision should undergo Mohs excision, resection with complete circumferential peripheral and deep margin assessment (frozen or permanent section), or radiation therapy.

Table 2–4. 2010 AJCC Staging for Cutaneous Squamous Cell Carcinoma and Other Cutaneous Carcinomas: TNM Staging and Histologic Grade[38]

Anatomic Stage/Prognostic Groups			
Stage 0	Tis	N0	M0
Stage I	T1	N0	M0
Stage II	T2	N0	M0
Stage III	T3	N0	M0
	T1	N1	M0
	T2	N1	M0
	T3	N1	M0
Stage IV	T1	N2	M0
	T2	N2	M0
	T3	N2	M0
	Any T	N3	M0
	T4	Any N	M0
	Any T	Any N	M1

Histologic Grade (G)	
Gx	Cannot be assessed
G1	Well differentiated
G2	Moderately differentiated
G3	Poorly differentiated
G4	Undifferentiated

Used with the permission of the American Joint Committee on Cancer (AJCC), Chicago, Illinois. The original source for this material is the AJCC Cancer Staging Manual, Seventh Edition (2010) published by Springer Science and Business Media LLC, www.springer.com.

For high-risk BCC of the head and neck, primary treatment consists of Mohs excision, resection with complete circumferential peripheral and deep margin assessment (frozen or permanent section), or radiation therapy (for nonsurgical candidates). For those lesions with positive margins or extensive perineural or large nerve involvement, adjuvant radiation therapy also is recommended.

Follow-up includes lifelong screening with complete skin exam every 6 to 12 months. Local recurrences follow the primary treatment algorithms; regional or distant metastases warrant a multidisciplinary approach including tumor board consultation and coordination of therapeutic plan.

Melanoma

The AJCC staging criteria apply to cutaneous melanoma but not to mucosal or ocular melanomas. Tables 2–5 and 2–6 summarize the 2010 AJCC melanoma staging classification.

When a suspicious pigmented skin lesion is biopsy-confirmed melanoma, pathology is reviewed for Breslow thickness, ulceration status, mitotic rate, deep and peripheral margin status, presence or absence of satellitosis, and Clark level (for lesions ≤1 mm) for clinical staging. As for SCC, workup includes a complete history and physical, with attention to locoregional area and draining lymph nodes as well as historical risk factors (described earlier in this chapter). Among the major changes with the 2009 AJCC staging system, tumor mitotic rate has replaced Clark's level in defining T1b disease.[36,38,48,49] Furthermore, all patients with microscopic nodal metastases (specifically including micrometastases detected on immunohistochemical staining), regardless of the extent of tumor burden, are classified as stage III.[38]

For stages IA, IB, and IIA disease, imaging (CT, PET, or MRI) is warranted only to evaluate specific signs or symptoms prior to wide excision with or without sentinel lymph node biopsy. Sentinel lymph node biopsy is recommended for stage IA lesions exhibiting adverse features: thickness ≥0.75 mm, positive deep margins, lymphovascular invasion, and younger age.

For stage IIB-IIC disease, chest x-ray is optional and routine imaging not recommended except as clinically indicated. Workup of stage III disease may include chest x-ray, CT (possible PET-CT), and/or MRI for staging, and FNA or open lymph node biopsy for clinically positive or in-transit nodal metastasis.[44] Pelvic CT may also be pursued if inguinofemoral nodes are positive. Stage IV (metastatic) disease workup should include FNA (preferred, if feasible) or open biopsy, serum lactate dehydrogenase (LDH) measurement, as well as imaging (CT of chest/abdomen/pelvis, MRI brain, and/or PET) as clinically indicated.[41]

Adjuvant treatment options include clinical trials, observation, interferon alfa, and/or radiation therapy to the nodal basin with multiple involved

Table 2–5. TNM Staging for Cutaneous Melanoma (2010 AJCC staging criteria)[38]

T Classification	**Thickness (mm)**	**Ulceration Status/Mitoses**
Tis	NA	NA
T1	≤1.00	a: Without ulceration and mitosis <1/mm^2 b: With ulceration or mitoses ≥1/mm^2
T2	1.01–2.00	a: Without ulceration b: With ulceration
T3	2.01–4.00	a: Without ulceration b: With ulceration
T4	>4.00	a: Without ulceration b: With ulceration
N	**No. of metastatic nodes**	**Nodal metastatic burden**
N0	0	NA
N1	1	a: Micrometastasis b: Macrometastasis
N2	2–3	a: Micrometastasis b: Macrometastasis c: In transit metastases/satellites without metastatic nodes
N3	4+ metastatic nodes, or matted nodes, or in transit metastases/satellites with metastatic nodes	
M	**Site**	**Serum LDH**
M0	No distant metastases	NA
M1a	Distant skin, subcutaneous, or nodal metastases	Normal
M1b	Lung metastases	Normal
M1c	All other visceral metastases Any distant metastases	Elevated

NA: not applicable, LDH: lactate dehydrogenase.

Micrometastases are diagnosed after sentinel lymph node biopsy.

Macrometastases are defined as clinically detectable nodal metastases confirmed pathologically.

Used with the permission of the American Joint Committee on Cancer (AJCC), Chicago, Illinois. The original source for this material is the AJCC Cancer Staging Manual, Seventh Edition (2010) published by Springer Science and Business Media LLC, www.springer.com.

nodes or extranodal extension. Nonsurgical primary treatment options include hyperthermic melphalan perfusion/infusion, intralesional BCG or interferion (IFN) injection, local ablation therapy, radiation therapy, systemic chemotherapy, or topical imiquimod.[41]

Table 2-6. Anatomic Stage Groupings for Cutaneous Melanoma[38]

Clinical Staging				Pathologic Staging			
	T	N	M		T	N	M
0	Tis	N0	M0	0	Tis	N0	M0
IA	T1a	N0	M0	IA	T1a	N0	M0
IB	T1b	N0	M0	IB	T1b	N0	M0
	T2a	N0	M0		T2a	N0	M0
IIA	T2b	N0	M0	IIA	T2b	N0	M0
	T3a	N0	M0		T3a	N0	M0
IIB	T3b	N0	M0	IIB	T3b	N0	M0
	T4a	N0	M0		T4a	N0	M0
IIC	T4b	N0	M0	IIC	T4b	N0	M0
III	Any T	N > N0	M0	IIIA	T1-4a	N1a	M0
					T1-4a	N2a	M0
				IIIB	T1-4b	N1a	M0
					T1-4b	N2a	M0
					T1-4a	N1b	M0
					T1-4a	N2b	M0
					T1-4a	N2c	M0
				IIIC	T1-4b	N1b	M0
					T1-4b	N2b	M0
					Any T	N2c	M0
					Any T	N3	M0
IV	Any T	Any N	M1	IV	Any T	Any N	M1

Clinical staging includes microstaging of the primary melanoma and clinical/ radiologic evaluation for metastases. By convention, it should be used after complete excision of the primary melanoma with clinical assessment for regional and distant metastases.

Pathologic staging includes microstaging of the primary melanoma and pathologic information about the regional lymph nodes after partial (ie, sentinel node biopsy) or complete lymphadenectomy. Pathologic stage 0 or stage IA patients are the exception; they do not require pathologic evaluation of their lymph nodes.

Conclusion

Early detection of cutaneous squamous cell carcinoma, basal cell carcinoma, and malignant melanoma of the head and neck requires a high index of suspicion for lesions exhibiting ulceration, large size, fixation to adjacent structures, or any of the ABCDE characteristics, particularly in fair-skinned patients with chronic or intense intermittent UV exposure, those with carcinogenic or radiation exposure, and those with high-risk genetic syndromes. Excisional or full-thickness incisional biopsy should be performed to confirm pathologic diagnosis and guide treatment. Imaging studies such as CT scan, MRI, ultrasound, and PET-CT also may be valuable in evaluation and staging of more advanced and aggressive lesions.

Patients with aggressive skin malignancies benefit from evaluation and treatment by a multidisciplinary team—this evaluation and workup will provide the necessary information for the team to make evidence-based recommendations for surgical and adjuvant therapy.

References

1. Skin Cancer Foundation. *Skin Cancer Facts 2009*. Retrieved Mar 18 2010 from http://www.skincancer.org/skin-cancer-facts .
2. American Cancer Society. *Cancer Facts & Figures 2009*. Atlanta, GA: American Cancer Society; 2009.
3. Christenson LJ, Borrowman TA, Vachon CM, et al. Incidence of basal cell and squamous cell carcinomas in a population younger than 40 years. *JAMA*. 2005;294(6):681–690.
4. Rigel DS. Cutaneous ultraviolet exposure and its relationship to the development of skin cancer. *J Am Acad Dermatol*. 2008;58(5 suppl 2):S129–S132.
5. Schmalbach CE, Johnson TM, Bradford CR. The management of head and neck melanoma. *Curr Prob Surg*. 2006;43(11):781–835.
6. Stadelmann WK, McMasters K, Digenis AG, Reintgen DS. Cutaneous melanoma of the head and neck: advances in evaluation and treatment. *Plast Reconstr Surg*. 2000;105(6):2105–2126.
7. Bataille V, de Vries E. Melanoma—Part 1: epidemiology, risk factors, and prevention. *Br Med J* (Clinical research ed). 2008;337:a2249.
8. Mocellin S, Nitti D. Vitamin D receptor polymorphisms and the risk of cutaneous melanoma: a systematic review and meta-analysis. *Cancer*. 2008;113(9):2398–2407.
9. Qureshi AA, Laden F, Colditz GA, Hunter DJ. Geographic variation and risk of skin cancer in US women. Differences between melanoma, squamous cell carcinoma, and basal cell carcinoma. *Arch Int Med*. 2008;168(5):501–507.
10. Coups EJ, Manne SL, Heckman CJ. Multiple skin cancer risk behaviors in the U.S. population. *Am J Prev Med*. 2008;34(2):87–93.
11. Harrison SL, Buettner PG, MacLennan R. Body-site distribution of melanocytic nevi in young Australian children. *Arch Dermatol*. 1999;135(1):47–52.
12. Hall HI, Saraiya M, Thompson T, Hartman A, Glanz K, Rimer B. Correlates of sunburn experiences among U.S. adults: results of the 2000 National Health Interview Survey. *Pub Health Rep*. 2003;118(6):540–549.
13. Qiu D, Tanaka S. International comparisons of cumulative risk of skin cancer, from Cancer Incidence in Five Continents Vol. VIII. *Jap J Clin Oncol*. 2006;36(8):533–534.
14. Solomon CC, White E, Kristal AR, Vaughan T. Melanoma and lifetime UV radiation. *Cancer Causes Control*. 2004;15(9):893–902.
15. Zanetti R, Rosso S, Martinez C, et al. The multicentre south European study "Helios." I: skin characteristics and sunburns in basal cell and squamous cell carcinomas of the skin. *Br J Cancer*. 1996;73(11):1440–1446.
16. Pfahlberg A, Kolmel KF, Gefeller O. Timing of excessive ultraviolet radiation and melanoma: epidemiology does not support the existence of a critical period of high susceptibility to solar ultraviolet radiation- induced melanoma. *Br J Dermatol*. 2001;144(3):471–475.
17. Thompson JF, Scolyer RA, Kefford RF. Cutaneous melanoma. *Lancet*. 2005;365(9460):687–701.
18. Forest VI, Clark JJ, Veness MJ, Milross C. N1S3: a revised staging system for head and neck cutaneous squamous cell carcinoma with lymph node metastases: results of 2 Australian Cancer Centers. *Cancer*. 2010;116(5):1298–1304.
19. Lloyd SA. Stratospheric ozone depletion. *Lancet*. 1993;342(8880):1156–1158.
20. Mettlin CJ. Skin cancer and ozone depletion: the case for global action. *J Surg Oncol*. 2001;77(2):76–78.
21. Mabruk MJ, Toh LK, Murphy M, Leader M, Kay E, Murphy GM. Investigation of the effect of UV irradiation on DNA damage: comparison between skin cancer patients and normal volunteers. *J Cut Pathol*. 2009;36(7):760–765.
22. Murphy M, Mabruk MJ, Lenane P, et al. The expression of p53, p21, Bax and induction of apoptosis in normal volunteers in response to different doses of ultraviolet radiation. *Br J Dermatol*. 2002;147(1):110–117.
23. Emadi SN, Mortazavi M, Mortazavi H. Late cutaneous manifestations 14 to 20 years after wartime exposure to sulfur mustard gas: a long-term investigation. *Arch Dermatol*. 2008;144(8):1059–1061.
24. Somoano B, Niendorf KB, Tsao H. Hereditary cancer syndromes of the skin. *Clin Dermatol*. 2005;23(1):85–106.
25. Goepfert H, Dichtel WJ, Medina JE, et al. Perineural invasion in squamous cell skin carcinoma of the head and neck. *Am J Surg*. 1984;148(4):542–547.
26. Mendenhall WM, Amdur RJ, Hinerman RW, et al. Skin cancer of the head and neck with perineural invasion. *Am J Clin Oncol*. 2007;30(1):93–96.
27. Moore BA, Weber RS, Prieto V, et al. Lymph node metastases from cutaneous squamous cell carcinoma of the head and neck. *Laryngoscope*. 2005;115(9):1561–1567.
28. Veness MJ, Porceddu S, Palme CE, Morgan GJ. Cutaneous head and neck squamous cell carcinoma metastatic to parotid and cervical lymph nodes. *Head Neck*. 2007;29(7):621–631.
29. Fu W, Cockerell CJ. The actinic (solar) keratosis: a 21st-century perspective. *Arch Dermatol*. 2003;139:66–70.

30. Cox NH, Eedy DJ, Morton CA. Guidelines for management of Bowen's disease: 2006 update. *Br J Dermatol.* 2007;156:11–21.
31. Veness MJ, Palme CE, Morgan GJ. High-risk cutaneous squamous cell carcinoma of the head and neck: results from 266 treated patients with metastatic lymph node disease. *Cancer.* 2006;106(11):2389–2396.
32. Smeets NW, Krekels GA, Ostertag JU, et al. Surgical excision vs Mohs' micrographic surgery for basal-cell carcinoma of the face: randomised controlled trial. *Lancet.* 2004;364(9447):1766–1772.
33. Madan V, Lear JT, Szeimies R-M. Nonmelanoma skin cancer. *Lancet.* 2010;375:673–685.
34. National Comprehensive Cancer Network. NCCN Clinical Practice Guidelines in Oncology. Basal cell and squamous cell cancers, v.1.2010. Retrieved Mar 20 2010 from http://www.nccn.org .
35. Rigel DS, Friedman RJ, Kopf AW, Polsky D. ABCDE—an evolving concept in the early detection of melanoma. *Arch Dermatol.* 2005;141(8):1032–1034.
36. Clark WH, Jr., From L, Bernardino EA, Mihm MC. The histogenesis and biologic behavior of primary human malignant melanomas of the skin. *Cancer Res.* 1969;29(3): 705–727.
37. Demierre MF, Sabel MS, Margolin KA, Daud AI, Sondak VK. State of the science 60th anniversary review: 60 years of advances in cutaneous melanoma epidemiology, diagnosis, and treatment, as reported in the journal Cancer. *Cancer.* 2008;113(7 suppl):1728–1743.
38. Balch CM, Gershenwald JE, Soong S-j, et al. Final version of 2009 AJCC melanoma staging and classification. *J Clin Oncol.* 2009;27(36):6199–6206.
39. Kalkhoran S, Milne O, Zalaudek I, et al. Historical, clinical, and dermoscopic characteristics of thin nodular melanoma. *Arch Dermatol.* 2010;146(3):311–318.
40. Haenssle H, Korpas B, Hansen-Hagge C, et al. Selection of patients for long-term surveillance with digital dermoscopy by assessment of melanoma risk factors. *Arch Dermatol.* 2010;146(3):257–264.
41. National Comprehensive Cancer Network. NCCN Clinical Practice Guidelines in Oncology. Melanoma, v.2.2010. Retrieved 20 Mar 2010 from http://www.nccn.org .
42. Chen SL, Iddings DM, Scheri RP, Bilchik AJ. Lymphatic mapping and sentinel node analysis: current concepts and applications. *CA: A Cancer J for Clinicians.* 2006;56(5): 292–309; quiz 16–17.
43. Sanki A, Uren RF, Moncrieff M, et al. Targeted high-resolution ultrasound is not an effective substitute for sentinel lymph node biopsy in patients with primary cutaneous melanoma. *J Clin Oncol.* 2009;27(33):5614–5619.
44. Voit C, van Akkooi AC, Schafer-Hesterberg G, et al. Rotterdam criteria for sentinel node (SN) tumor burden and the accuracy of ultrasound (US) -guided fine-needle aspiration cytology (FNAC): can US-guided FNAC replace SN staging in patients with melanoma? *J Clin Oncol.* 2009;27:4994–5000.
45. Tyler DS, Onaitis M, Kherani A, et al. Positron emission tomography scanning in malignant melanoma. *Cancer.* 2000;89(5):1019–1025.
46. Fosko SW, Hu W, Cook TF, Lowe VJ. Positron emission tomography for basal cell carcinoma of the head and neck. *Arch Dermatol.* 2003;139(9):1141–1146.
47. Palme CE, O'Brien CJ, Veness MJ, et al. Extent of parotid disease influences outcome in patients with metastatic cutaneous squamous cell carcinoma. *Arch Otolaryngol Head Neck Surg.* 2003;129:750–753.
48. Breslow A. Thickness, cross-sectional areas and depth of invasion in the prognosis of cutaneous melanoma. *Ann Surg.* 1970;172(5):902–908.
49. Azzola MF, Shaw HM, Thompson JF, et al. Tumor mitotic rate is a more powerful prognostic indicator than ulceration in patients with primary cutaneous melanoma: an analysis of 3661 patients from a single center. *Cancer.* 2003;97(6):1488–1498.

3

PSYCHOSOCIAL IMPACT OF SKIN CANCER TREATMENT

MICHELLE C. FINGERET

Introduction

For reasons that are unclear, there has been extremely limited attention in the scientific literature to examining the specific psychosocial needs of patients with cutaneous malignancies. Although there has been at least some focus on psychosocial issues for patients with malignant melanoma, psychological adjustment in patients with nonmelanoma skin cancer (NMSC) essentially has been neglected.[1–4] Greater interest may be generated for psychosocial outcomes in melanoma due to the aggressive nature of this tumor that frequently metastasizes to distant sites and comprises major cause of mortality among skin malignancies.[5] Consideration of psychosocial issues is also highly relevant for individuals with less lethal cutaneous cancers, as there are still long-term implications for quality of life.

Patients with cutaneous malignancies of the head and neck encounter particularly salient challenges because these tumors affect a highly visible and socially significant part of the body. Admittedly, there will be a wide range of psychosocial outcomes in this patient population, it is important to consider that some patients with cutaneous malignancies experience devastating consequences involving facial disfigurement and functional impairment when portions of or entire facial structures must be removed. Body image and appearance-related concerns may also dominate the clinical picture—even for patients experiencing less obvious forms of disfigurement. This chapter describes what is known about the broad, as well as disease-specific, psychosocial issues encountered by patients with cutaneous malignancies of the head and neck. Additionally, a model for the effective delivery of psychosocial health services are described that can be incorporated into clinical practice.

Psychosocial Issues and Cancer

Numerous psychosocial concerns are central to the cancer experience. Considerable attention has been given to the psychological distress which the National Comprehensive Cancer Network (NCCN) defines as "a multifactorial, unpleasant emotional experience of a psychological (cognitive, behavioral, emotional), social, and/or spiritual nature that may interfere with the ability to cope effectively with cancer, its physical symptoms, and its treatment."[6] The prevalence of psychological distress has been found to vary by type of cancer, time since diagnosis, degree of physical and role impairment, amount of pain, prognosis, and other variables. A commonly cited study by Zabora[7] reports rates of significant psychological distress ranging between 29% and 43% across a large pool of cancer patients. These data are consistent with other studies reporting elevated rates of psychological symptoms and significant mental health problems such as depression, anxiety, and posttraumatic stress disorders for cancer patients relative to the general population.[8–11] Within this context, suicide/suicidality amongst cancer patients merits special consideration. According to a recent study conducted with data from the Surveillance, Epidemiology, and Ends Results (SEER) program of the National Cancer Institute, patients with cancer in the United States were found to have nearly twice the incidence of suicide than the general population. Suicide rates vary significantly among patients with cancers of different anatomical sites, with the highest relative increase in suicide risk in the first 5 years after diagnosis. Patients with cancer in the head and neck region were found to be among the groups with the highest overall suicide rate.[12]

The 2007 Institute of Medicine (IOM) report, *Cancer Care for the Whole Patient: Meeting Psychosocial Health Needs,* identified a number of other emotional and mental health concerns not necessarily tied to psychiatric syndromes. This report mentions the importance of recognizing generalized worry, feelings of loss of control, sadness, anger, confusion and fear, isolation, heightened sense of vulnerability, changes in sexual function and reproductive ability, and spiritual and existential issues in cancer patients. Family members of cancer patients are also affected, with fear of losing the loved one, concern about suffering, and grief. Moreover, psychosocial problems extend beyond mental health, promoting physical stressors such as health impairment and disability, fatigue, and pain. Additional social and financial stressors identified related to low income, high cost of health care, lack of health insurance, reduced employment, and lack of transportation to healthcare appointments.[13]

Psychosocial Issues for Patients with Skin Cancer of the Head and Neck

Despite the wide variation in clinical presentation, functional sequelae, and treatment-specific issues based on disease type and stage, one of the most important features shared by patients with skin cancer of the head and neck is that they all experience some degree of physical change to a highly visible and socially significant part of their body. The facial region is recognized as being intimately tied with one's sense of self and has a profound influence on impressions formed by others.[14,15] Change, whether through disease or therapy, fosters adverse psychosocial responses because of the social significance of the face and its association with identity, communication abilities, and interpersonal functioning.

Facial Disfigurement

Research with a broad range of patient groups has consistently demonstrated that the predominant difficulties of individuals experiencing facial disfigurement lie in social interaction.[16–19] Though many psychosocial difficulties identified by patients with facial disfigurement are not dissimilar to those already described above for cancer patients, it is important to recognize that the source of depression, anxiety, social avoidance/isolation, and impaired sexuality is directly linked to appearance-related and bodily changes. Understanding this link is critical for developing targeted psychotherapeutic interventions that alleviate distress associated with skin cancer.

Complicating this evaluation is the wide variability in psychological adjustment to acquired disfigurement. It has been consistently shown that individual response to disfigurement cannot be adequately explained by disease characteristics or severity of disfigurement alone.[17,20–22] Macgregor,[15] who conducted over 30 years of work on the social effects of disfigurement, has observed, counterintuitively, that adjustment can sometimes be easier for individuals with a more severe form of disfigurement compared to those with less obvious forms of disfigurement. She reasoned that those with more obvious forms of disfigurement tend to experience reliable and predictable negative social responses to their facial appearance which allow them to effectively anticipate and psychologically prepare for certain types of situations. However, the social response to less obvious forms of disfigurement is not nearly as predictable, promoting a constant sense of uncertainty and heightened levels of anxiety in social situations. Clearly, patients with skin cancer in the head and neck region experience a wide range of clinical outcomes involving perceived "noticeability" of their facial changes. That patients with even small and unnoticeable facial changes can experience significant distress, whereas those with extensive facial defects can adjust poorly or well to their bodily changes, suggests that the patient's psychological reaction demands attention from the treatment team regardless of disease characteristics or readily observable changes.

Body Image

Central to the discussion of psychosocial issues for patients with skin cancer in the head and neck region is the construct of body image. Body image reflects much more than one's view of his or her physical appearance; it is a multifaceted concept involving perceptions, thoughts, and feelings about the entire body and its functioning.[19] When one conceptualizes body image in this comprehensive manner, it is clear that the range of bodily changes skin cancer patients can undergo during the process of or following treatment in terms of scarring, swelling, skin discoloration, hair loss, tooth loss, sensory changes (eg, numbness, tingling, burning), and functional loss/alterations (eg, changes in speech, swallowing, articulation, hearing, eyesight), are encompassed here. A fundamental element of body image experiences are that they are inherently subjective and as such do not reflect objective reality of the body.[23] The degree to which an individual is invested in his or her appearance and holds specific body image ideals is important to consider, as are the methods individuals use to manage or cope with body image changes. The complex nature of body image functioning is further reflected by the notion that individuals may not only have their own personal concerns about bodily changes but also concerns about how others in their social network respond and react to these changes.

Within the oncology setting, it is useful to consider a continuum of body image concerns (Fig 3–1). This model is consistent with previous work describing a broader array of medical patients, and assumes that the majority of medically ill patients experience body image discomfort related to their disease and treatment.[23] At one extreme of this continuum are patients who experience a great deal of distress around their body image, significantly disrupting their daily life. In addition to body image-focused concerns, these patients are very likely to exhibit broader psychosocial difficulties and high levels of depression and/or anxiety. At the other extreme are patients with no apparent body image concerns. Within this group of patients are individuals who may experience minimal to no observable changes in their body image as a result of treatment as well as those who experience considerable changes but generally are not concerned about or invested in their appearance. It is possible that some patients experience positive adaptation to bodily changes (eg, consider cancer to be a "blessing in disguise"). However, it also is important to consider that a portion of these patients may be minimizing their concerns about body image. These patients may be reluctant to share these concerns with their medical team for a variety of reasons, chief among these may be embarrassment and shame. In the middle of this continuum are those who acknowledge what are considered to be a normative or average amount of body image concerns. Although these individuals may not be overwhelmed by their concerns, body image issues can have a moderately negative impact on quality of life regardless of their intensity and are important to address within the context of the medical provider-patient relationship.

Due to the centrality of body image issues for skin cancer patients, further attention is being given to discussing the variety of factors that shape and sustain body image experiences and reactions for this population. A widely recognized model of body image development delineated by Thomas Cash identifies a number of historical and development influences, as well as proximal events and processes, that contribute to body image concerns.[24] Early in life, a number of historical factors predispose one's thoughts, feelings, and behaviors related to body image. This includes cultural socialization concerning values and standards of appearance, experiences tied to social interactions, and one's

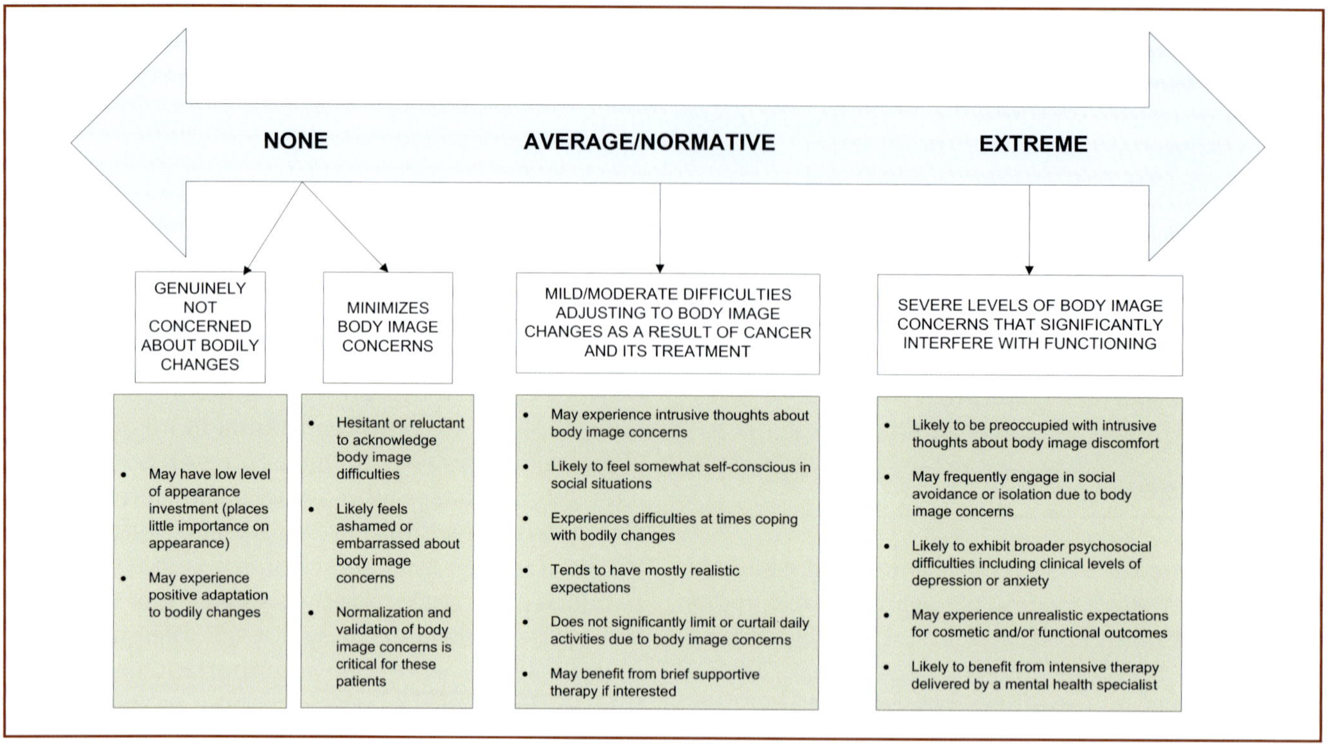

Figure 3–1. Continuum of body image (BI) concerns in the oncology setting. (Fingeret MC. Body image and disfigurement. In: Duffy J, Valentine A, eds. *MD Anderson Manual of Psychosocial Oncology*. Figure 21–1. McGraw-Hill. Reprinted with permission.)

actual physical characteristics. Proximal processes entail current events that trigger and maintain body image experiences. A diagnosis of skin cancer and subsequent treatment represent proximal events that trigger self-evaluations of one's physical appearance and bodily functioning. This can be especially problematic for individuals who place a high degree of importance on physical attributes (ie, those with a high degree of appearance investment) as they are more likely to direct attention, encode, and interpret stimuli related to bodily experiences in a negative fashion. White[25] explains that cancer patients with perceived or actual appearance changes that threaten their personal body image ideals will experience negative appearance-related assumptions, thoughts, emotions, and behaviors if the discrepancy between their perceived and body image ideals relates to a physical attribute in which they have significant personal investment. In other words, patients who value the way their face looks will have trouble adjusting to any alterations (whether perceived or actual) that deviate from their ideal self-image. A negative evaluation of one's body image can result from and lead to a variety of problematic thoughts, behaviors, and emotions. Maladaptive thought processes involve distortions and assumptions about appearance that can lead to intense feelings of shame, anxiety, and depression. Among the problematic behavioral strategies that can be used to cope with body image changes are social isolation and avoidance, concealment/camouflaging of body parts, and excessive reassurance seeking from others.

Other Disease-Specific Psychosocial Issues

Additional psychosocial concerns specific to patients with skin cancer of the head and neck involve the nature and clinical course of the disease. Patients with skin cancer have a lifelong risk of developing second primary tumors that can require repeated surgical resections and reconstructive procedures.[26] Moreover, many skin tumors are prone to both recurrence and metastasis.[27] Fears of recurrence, spread, and development of additional cancers thus are highly salient and pronounced for this population, perhaps even more so than with other cancer groups. Emotional difficulties tied to the clinical course of facial skin cancer have been recognized as a critical element of quality of life in this patient group. Recurrence anxiety has been recognized as a dominant force for melanoma patients once they have completed initial cancer therapy, and particular concerns have been raised about whether this fear can result in patient noncompliance with or avoidance of continued surveillance.[2] Specific concerns about the disease process also have been found to be a fundamental issue for patients with NMSC, and are included in the only known, validated, disease-specific quality of life measure in this patient group. The Skin Cancer Index (SCI) is a 15-item measure designed to address relevant psychosocial issues for NMSC patients not adequately captured by other instruments.[28,29] This measure has a distinct Emotional Subscale that focuses on worry about recurrence, spread, and future cancers as well as more generalized feelings of anxiety and frustration.

Meeting Psychosocial Needs of Patients With Skin Cancer

The 2007 IOM report, mentioned earlier in this chapter, reviewed evidence supporting the effectiveness of a range of services that can help patients and their families manage the psychological/behavioral and social aspects of cancer.[13] Ultimately, this report concluded: "Attending to psychosocial needs should be an integral part of quality cancer care" (p. 8). Despite the availability of effective resources, it appears that psychosocial health-care needs often are not well addressed in the oncology setting. In addition to being dissatisfied with information they receive about their diagnosis and available treatment, many patients report that their care providers do not understand their psychosocial needs and are unaware of psychosocial health resources.[30] Additional research indicates that physicians tend to underestimate oncology patients' psychological distress and that oncologists themselves acknowledge frequent failure to attend to the psychosocial needs of their patients.[13,31,32] Various barriers to providing appropriate psychosocial care have been identified, including inadequate education/training on strategies for addressing psychosocial health issues, perceived lack of time to address psychosocial concerns, shortages and suboptimal distribution of health personnel, poor coordination of care across providers, lack of awareness of appropriate allied health professionals for referral and quality information resources, and difficulties stemming from the payment and policy environment.[13,33] Schoefield et al[33] identified a number of strategies that can be used to overcome barriers to providing psychosocial care. Chief among these strategies is to correct misperceptions among health-care providers that addressing psychosocial issues is excessively time-consuming. Research demonstrates that an additional 40 seconds of clinical time spent in acknowledging the psychosocial difficulties associated with cancer can reduce anxiety.[34]

Considerable attention is given in the 2007 IOM report to the adverse consequences of unmet psychosocial needs. Emotional distress, limited financial resources, and inadequate social support have been associated with increased morbidity, mortality, and decreased functional status.[13] Research on the manner in which psychosocial problems influence health continues to emerge, with a great deal of focus on the links between stress and disease. Stress is known to have harmful effects on the immune, cardiovascular, and neuroendocrine system, and chronic stress has been found to influence the progression and recurrence of cancer.[35]

To address the psychosocial health issues of cancer patients, the IOM has put forth a unifying model that involves the following components: (1) identifying patients with psychosocial health needs that are likely to affect their health or health care, (2) linking patients and their families to appropriate health services, (3) supporting patients in managing their illness, (4) coordinating psychosocial and biomedical health care, and (5) following up on care delivered to monitor the effectiveness of services and make modifications as needed.[13] This model cannot be implemented without the core element of effective patient-provider communication. A substantial body of literature exists to support the benefits of interventions aimed at improving provider communication and patient involvement in care that is beyond the scope of this chapter. Interested readers should review the National Cancer Institute report, *Patient-Centered Communication in Cancer Care*, for more information on the basic principles of effective communication in cancer care.[36] The key processes and outcomes of a patient-centered approach to communication involve: (a) eliciting, understanding, and validating the patient's perspective, (b) reaching a shared understanding of the patient's problem and its treatment, and (c) helping the patient become meaningfully involved in choices related to his or her health.

Identification of Psychosocial Needs

As discussed in the 2007 IOM report, relying on patients to volunteer information about their psychosocial needs is woefully inadequate.[13] Healthcare providers are urged to directly inquire about whether patients are experiencing psychosocial concerns, and to routinely incorporate this process into their clinical practice. It is argued here that the best method for identifying psychosocial needs is to utilize a brief validated screening instrument and to follow up with the patient during the clinic visit on any items that have been endorsed. This approach not only conveys to the patients that their psychosocial needs are important and relevant, but also provides a structured way to systematically evaluate various emotional and social difficulties.

To be conducive to the clinic setting, effective screening tools must be brief and easily administered. Several tools that have either been specifically developed for cancer patients or have been widely used with this population are available. The Distress Thermometer (DT) is a well-known screening tool recommended for routine use in the NCCN "Practice Guidelines in Oncology for Distress Management."[6] This measure should be administered to patients in the waiting room prior to each clinic visit. The DT consists of a primary item asking patients to rate their level of distress on a scale from 1 (no distress) to 10 (extreme distress) using a visual analogue scale with a picture of a thermometer. This approach mirrors one that has been widely adopted to measure pain in many clinic and hospital settings. On the same page as the thermometer is a 35-item Problem List, which encourages patients to identify specific difficulties they are having in relation to practical, family, emotional, spiritual/religious, and physical domains. This tool can be helpful in identifying a broad range of psychosocial difficulties and can prompt direct referrals to community resources and/or different types of health care professionals (eg, social worker, spiritual counselor, psychologist) depending on which items are endorsed. On the DT, a clinical cutoff of 4 has been empirically established to denote patients requiring further evaluation for moderate or severe levels of distress.

In contrast to the DT, which focuses on identifying psychosocial concerns that are not necessarily tied to mental health disorders, other screening tools that have been used in the oncology setting focus more specifically on detecting problems such as anxiety, depression, adjustment disorders, and posttraumatic stress disorder. Four of the more commonly used screening tools to evaluate mental health issues in cancer patients are discussed below.

The Brief Symptom Inventory 18 (BSI 18) evaluates depression, anxiety, somatic complaints, and overall psychological distress in medical and community populations.[37] It can be completed in approximately 4 minutes. Because of its extensive psychometric testing with cancer patients, oncology norms are available. The Hospital Anxiety and Depression Scale (HADS) also has been widely used with cancer patients and has the advantage of being specifically designed for use in a medical setting.[38] Unlike other measures of depression and anxiety developed for the general population, the 14-item HADS excludes questions about somatic complaints such as fatigue or pain so that physical symptoms directly related to cancer will not contribute to depression scores. The Beck Depression Inventory-II (BDI-II) is composed of 21 items and is recognized as one of the most widely used self-report screening measures of depression.[39] Considerable data have been gathered on its validity and reliability across diverse patient groups. However, standard cut-points probably are not relevant for cancer patients as somatic complaints contribute to the overall score. The Patient Health Questionnaire-9 (PHQ-9) is similar to the BDI-II in that it was developed to identify the presence of depressive symptoms consistent with diagnostic criteria for depression used by mental health professionals.[40] The PHQ-9 has been validated for use in primary care, and can easily be used repeatedly to monitor depression over time. Each item of the PHQ-9 directly corresponds to the 9 DSM-IV criteria for a depressive episode.[41]

Strategies for Addressing Psychosocial Health Issues

Within the context of routine care, the primary oncology team can effectively manage mild distress and certain psychosocial concerns. Physicians and other health-care professionals must take the time to discuss normative fears, worries, uncertainty about the future, concerns about illness, and treatment side effects. NCCN clinical practice guidelines specifically recommend providing enough time for the patient to ask questions, to ensure that patients are placed at ease, and specifically to acknowledge that this is a difficult experience for the patient and that distress is normal and to be expected.[6] When moderate to severe levels of distress are identified (for example, with a DT score ≥4) or psychosocial concerns are identfied that cannot be appropriately addressed by the health-care team, it is critical to be able to offer resources or provide referrals to directly address these difficulties.

A core element of the IOM's health-care model discussed above involves appropriate care planning.[13] It is critical for providers to be familiar with community resources and establish relationships with providers specializing in psychosocial health care. Table 3–1 provides a list of a variety of organizations and/or programs providing psychosocial services that are relevant to patients with cutaneous malignancies of the head and neck.

Particular consideration is given to services available for individuals with appearance-related concerns stemming from facial disfigurement. The Changing Faces program and the American Cancer Society (ACS) Look Good . . . Feel Better program both offer support to these patients. Changing Faces is a national organization based in the United Kingdom that has a variety of educational handouts available for purchase that can be provided to patients on critical psychosocial topics such as how to handle other people's reaction to facial disfigurement and how to talk with health-care professionals about disfigurement. The ACS Look Good . . . Feel Better program provides hands-on sessions as well as interactive videos on their Web site to help patients with cancer feel more comfortable with their appearance and improve their self-esteem.

Finally, oncologists are urged to establish close collegial relationships with mental health providers and other allied health professionals that deliver psychosocial services. Clinical integration of psychosocial services with on-site professionals is described as an ideal health-care model in the 2007 IOM report because this is believed to facilitate patient follow-through on referrals and improves treatment outcomes.[13] Moreover, this approach promotes optimal collaborative care and management of patients and allows treating physicians to obtain rapid feedback on psychosocial concerns and behavioral health issues of referred patients. Regardless of whether psychosocial services are integrated into the medical care setting or referred to providers off-site, follow-up with patients after a referral is a critical element of quality care that must not be overlooked. This can involve a routinely scheduled phone call, standard questioning as part of a scheduled outpatient visit, or even possibly the use of Internet or Web-based technology. Regardless of the method used, incorporation of follow-up activities must be planned and routinely carried out to assist with monitoring psychosocial difficulties, to determine whether services provided are benefiting the patient, or to develop a new care plan to ensure that patient's psychosocial needs are being met.

Table 3–1. List of Community Resources

Organization/Program	Services Provided	Way to Contact
American Cancer Society (ACS)	ACS provides different support groups for cancer survivors and their families at centers around the country. They also offer access to a breadth of cancer information and educational materials	http://www.cancer.org 1-800-227-2345
ACS: Look Good . . . Feel Better program	A free, national public service administered by ACS designed to assist individuals having difficulty coping with appearance-related changes. Small group programs, one-on-one salon consultations, and self-help materials are available for women and men.	http://www.lookgoodfeelbetter.org 1-800-395-5665
American Psychosocial Oncology Society (APOS)	APOS is a professional society that aims to advance the science and practice of psychosocial care for people with cancer. This organization provides a national toll-free hotline as a resource to help people with cancer and their caregivers find counseling services in their own community	http://www.apos-society.org Toll-Free Hotline: 1-866-276-7443
Cancer*Care*	Cancer*Care* is a national nonprofit organization that provides free, professional services to anyone affected by cancer. This includes online, telephone, and face-to-face counseling, education, financial assistance, and practical help. Cancer*Care* also has Telephone Educational Workshops and booklets that provide the latest cancer information straight from the experts.	http://www.cancercare.org 1-800-813-HOPE (4673)
Gilda's Club	Gilda's Club is an organization that offers support and networking groups, seminars, workshops, specialized children's programs, and social events in a nonresidential homelike setting. Affiliate clubhouses are located in numerous cities around the US.	http://www.gildasclub.org 1-888-GILDA-4-U
Lance Armstrong Foundation (LAF)	LAF is a nonprofit organization that provides practical information and tools people with cancer need to live their life on their own terms. Specific information on coping with physical and emotional effects on cancer and practical tips on adapting to body image changes are available	http://www.livestrong.org 1-866-673-7205
LAF SurvivorCare Program	A Lance Armstrong Foundation program available to help individuals deal with their cancer experience that provides counseling and referrals to local resources, help addressing information on financial and insurance concerns, and information on clinical trials matching to new treatments in development	1-866-467-7205
National Cancer Institute (NCI), Cancer Information Service	This service provides education about cancer prevention, risk factors, early detection, symptoms, diagnosis, and treatment. It includes information specialists that can answer questions by telephone, TTY, instant messaging and e-mail. They can also provide printed and electronic NCI publications.	http://www.cancer.gov 1-800-4-CANCER

Table 3–1. *continued*

Organization/Program	Services Provided	Way to Contact
National Coalition for Cancer Survivorship (NCCS)	NCCS is the oldest survivor-led cancer advocacy organization in the county, advocating for quality cancer care for all Americans and empowering cancer survivors. NCCS has a free-audio program named the Cancer Survivor Toolbox that teaches skills to help people with cancer meet the challenges of their illness	http://www.canceradvocacy.org 1-877-622-7937
People Living with Cancer	A patient information Web site of the American Society of Clinical Oncology (ASCO) that provides timely oncologist-approved information to help patients and families make informed healthcare decisions. Specific information on coping with emotional and physical matters is available	http://www.plwc.org 1-866-651-3038
The Wellness Community	The Wellness Community has centers around the country that offer special groups and wellness classes for cancer survivors and family members, and now is also offering some online support groups. Their Web site offers a virtual kitchen and nutrition center that provides resources and information on general nutrition. Additional resources related to relaxation/visualization, stress management, exercise and healing are also available.	http://www.the wellnesscommunity.org 1-888-793-WELL
Changing Faces	A national charity organization based in the UK that supports and represents people who have disfigurements of the face or body from any cause. This organization provides support for children, young people, adults and families by providing advice, information (booklets, videos, self-help guides), and counseling	http://www.changingfaces.org.uk
Let's Face It (University of Michigan)	A Web site designed to advance knowledge about, by, and for people with facial differences and to promote their full and equal participation in society. This site provides links to relevant resources and related organizations, as well as educational information on a variety of conditions causing facial disfigurement	http://www.dent.umich.edu/faceit
About Face USA	An organization designed to provide information and emotional support to individuals with facial differences and their families and increase public understanding through awareness programs and education on behalf of those they serve	http://www.aboutfaceusa.org 1-800-665-FACE (3223)

Conclusions

Patients with cutaneous malignancy of the head and neck are at risk for a variety of adverse psychosocial outcomes. These patients encounter specific challenges due to the centrality of body image issues in their disease and subsequent treatment. Although this chapter summarizes what is known about the psychosocial difficulties of skin cancer patients, we are limited by the scant available research. It is incumbent on all those who treat patients with cutaneous malignancies of the head and neck to further examine psychosocial issues and to elucidate the factors that contribute to significant distress and psychosocial impairment in these patients. A model for the effective delivery of psychosocial care, outlined here, can readily be incorporated into the clinic setting. In the comprehensive care of these patients, available assessment tools can be used to identify the psychosocial needs of patients. Once recognized, patients and providers alike will benefit from the treatment resources in the community, examples of which are listed in Table 3–1.

References

1. Trask PC, Paterson AG, Hayasaka S, Dunn RL, Riba M, Johnson T. Psychosocial characteristics of individuals with non-stage IV melanoma. *J Clin Oncol.* 2001;19(11):2844–2850.
2. Boyle DA. Psychological adjustment to the melanoma experience. *Semin Oncol Nurs.* 2003;19(1):70–77.
3. Brandberg Y, Mansson-Brahme E, Ringborg U, Sjoden PO. Psychological reactions in patients with malignant melanoma. *Eur J Cancer.* 1995;31A(2):157–162.
4. Cassileth BR, Lusk EJ, Tenaglia AN. Patients' perceptions of the cosmetic impact of melanoma resection. *Plast Reconstr Surg.* 1983;71(1):73–75.
5. Fisher DF, Kwong LN, Chin L. Melanoma. In: DeVita VT, Lawrence TS, Rosenberg SA, eds. *Cancer: Principles and Practices of Oncology.* Philadelphia, PA: Lippincott Williams & Wilkins; 2008:1889–1897.
6. The NCCN Clinical Practice Guidelines in Oncology™ Distress management (Version 2.2009). © 2009 National Comprehensive Cancer Network, Inc. Available at: http://www.NCCN.org. Retrieved June 26, 2009. To view the most recent completed version of the NCCN Guidelines, go online to http://www.NCCN.org .
7. Zabora J, BrintzenhofeSzoc K, Curbow B, Hooker C, Piantadosi S. The prevalence of psychological distress by cancer site. *Psychooncology.* 2001;10(1):19–28.
8. Spiegel D, Giese-Davis J. Depression and cancer: mechanisms and disease progression. *Biol Psychiatry.* 2003;54(3):269–282.
9. Kangas M, Henry JL, Bryant RA. Posttraumatic stress disorder following cancer. A conceptual and empirical review. *Clin Psychol Rev.* 2002;22(4):499–524.
10. Sellick SM, Crooks DL. Depression and cancer: an appraisal of the literature for prevalence, detection, and practice guideline development for psychological interventions. *Psychooncology.* 1999;8(4):315–333.
11. Derogatis LR, Morrow GR, Fetting J, et al. The prevalence of psychiatric disorders among cancer patients. *JAMA.* 1983;249(6):751–757.
12. Misono S, Weiss NS, Fann JR, Redman M, Yueh B. Incidence of suicide in persons with cancer. *J Clin Oncol.* 2008;26(29):4731–4738.
13. Institute of Medicine. *Cancer Care for the Whole Patient: Meeting Psychosocial Health Needs.* Washington DC: National Academic Press; 2008.
14. MacGregor FC. Some psycho-social problems associated with facial deformities. *Am Sociolog Rev.* 1951;16:629–638.
15. Macgregor FC. Facial disfigurement: problems and management of social interaction and implications for mental health. *Aesthetic Plast Surg.* 1990;14(4):249–257.
16. Clarke A. Psychosocial aspects of facial disfigurement: problems, management and the role of a lay-led organization. *Psychol, Health Med.* 1999;4(2):127–142.
17. Rumsey N, Harcourt D. Body image and disfigurement: issues and interventions. *Body Image.* 2004;1(1):83–97.
18. Newell R. *Body Image and Disfigurement Care.* New York, NY: Taylor & Francis Group; 2000.
19. Pruzinsky T. Social and psychological effects of facial disfigurement: quality of life, body image and surgical reconstruction. In: Weber RW, Goepfert H, Miller MJ, eds. *Basal and Squamous Cell Carcinomas Skin Cancers of the Head and Neck.* Philadelphia, PA: Williams & Wilkins; 1996:357–362.
20. Clarke A, Rumsey N, Collin JR, Wyn-Williams M. Psychosocial distress associated with disfiguring eye conditions. *Eye.* 2003;17(1):35–40.
21. Thompson A, Kent G. Adjusting to disfigurement: processes involved in dealing with being visibly different. *Clin Psychol Rev.* 2001;21(5):663–682.
22. Rumsey N, Clarke A, White P, Wyn-Williams M, Garlick W. Altered body image: appearance-related concerns of people with visible disfigurement. *J Adv Nurs.* 2004;48(5):443–453.
23. Pruzinsky T. Enhancing quality of life in medical populations: a vision for body image assessment and rehabilitation as standards of care. *Body Image: Int J Res.* 2004;1(1):71–81.
24. Cash TF, Strachan MD. Cognitive-behavioral approaches to changing body image. In: Cash TF, Pruzinsky T, eds. *Body Image: A Handbook of Theory, Research and Clinical Practice.* New York, NY: Guilford Press; 2002:478–486.
25. White CA. Body image dimensions and cancer: a heuristic cognitive behavioural model. *Psychooncology.* 2000;9(3):183–192.
26. Clayman GL, Lee JJ, Holsinger FC, et al. Mortality risk from squamous cell skin cancer. *J Clin Oncol.* 2005;23(4):759–765.
27. Rudolph R, Zelac DE. Squamous cell carcinoma of the skin. *Plast Reconstr Surg.* 2004;114(6):82e–94e.
28. Rhee JS, Matthews BA, Neuburg M, Burzynski M, Nattinger AB. Creation of a quality of life instrument for nonmelanoma skin cancer patients. *Laryngoscope.* 2005;115(7):1178–1185.

29. Rhee JS, Matthews BA, Neuburg M, Logan BR, Burzynski M, Nattinger AB. Validation of a quality of life instrument for nonmelanoma skin cancer patients. *Arch Facial Plast Surg*. 2006(8):314–318.
30. President's Cancer Panel. *Living Beyond Cancer: Finding a New Balance* (President's Cancer Panel 2003–2004 annual report). Bethesda, MD: National Cancer Institute, National Institutes of Health, Department of Health and Human Services; 2004.
31. Fallowfield L, Ratcliffe D, Jenkins V, Saul J. Psychiatric morbidity and its recognition by doctors in patients with cancer. *Br J Cancer*. 2001;84(8):1011–1015.
32. Keller M, Sommerfeldt S, Fischer C, et al. Recognition of distress and psychiatric morbidity in cancer patients: a multi-method approach. *Ann Oncol*. 2004;15(8):1243–1249.
33. Schofield P, Carey M, Bonevski B, Sanson-Fisher R. Barriers to the provision of evidence-based psychosocial care in oncology. *Psychooncology*. 2006;15(10):863–872.
34. Fogarty LA, Curbow BA, Wingard JR, McDonnell K, Somerfield MR. Can 40 seconds of compassion reduce patient anxiety? *J Clin Oncol*. 1999;17(1):371–379.
35. Thaker PH, Lutgendorf SK, Sood AK. The neuroendocrine impact of chronic stress on cancer. *Cell Cycle*. 2007; 6(4):430–433.
36. Epstein RM, Street RL. Patient Centered Communication in Cancer Care: Promoting Healing and Reducing Suffering (NIH Publication No 07-6225; 2007). Bethesda, MD: National Cancer Institute.
37. Zabora J, BrintzenhofeSzoc K, Jacobsen P, et al. A new psychosocial screening instrument for use with cancer patients. *Psychosomatics*. 2001;42(3):241–246.
38. Zigmond AS, Snaith RP. The hospital anxiety and depression scale. *Acta Psychiatr Scand*. 1983;67(6):361–370.
39. Beck AT, Steer RA, Brown GK. *Manual for the Beck Depression Inventory-II*. San Antonio, TX: Psychological Corporation; 1996.
40. Kroenke K, Spitzer RL, Williams JB. The PHQ-9: validity of a brief depression severity measure. *J Gen Intern Med*. 2001;16(9):606–613.
41. Spitzer RL, Kroenke K, Williams JB. Validation and utility of a self-report version of PRIME-MD: the PHQ primary care study. Primary Care Evaluation of Mental Disorders. Patient Health Questionnaire. *JAMA*. 1999;282(18): 1737–1744.

4

SCREENING, SURVEILLANCE, AND PREVENTION

SHARON R. HYMES
CAROL R. DRUCKER

Introduction

Skin cancer is the most common form of cancer in the United States, with more than one million cases diagnosed annually.[1] Approximately 1 in 5 Americans will develop skin cancer in their lifetime.[2] The two most common types, basal cell carcinoma (BCC) and squamous cell carcinoma (SCC), are highly curable and uncommonly metastasize or lead to death when diagnosed early. Conversely, malignant melanoma (MM) accounts for approximately 3% of skin cancer cases but causes more than 75% of skin cancer-related deaths.[3–5] One in 55 people will be diagnosed with melanoma during their lifetime, and this rate is expected to increase.[3,6] Although the incidence of many cancers is falling, the incidence of nonmelanoma skin cancer (NMSC) and melanoma continues to rise.[3,5]

These concerning statistics have prompted investigators to evaluate how and when to screen for skin cancer. Skin cancer screening and surveillance are easy to perform, even during routine medical examinations. Surveillance, or continued serial examination, may be warranted in select populations who are at high risk for developing new or recurrent skin malignancies. This chapter reviews the subject of skin screening and surveillance, and discusses approaches aimed at the prevention of both melanoma and nonmelanoma skin cancer.

Screening

Unlike screening for the four other major early detectable cancers (breast, colon, prostate, and cervical), skin cancer screening requires no invasive imaging, technological studies, or blood work. The target organ can be seen and evaluated with the trained eye. Enhanced imaging tools in various stages of development may be utilized to increase the true positive findings and decrease false negatives. Through meticulous physical examination and judicious use of newer technologies, skin cancer screening will become more accurate and cost effective, with fewer unnecessary biopsies. Nevertheless, the most critical tool in the examination is and will remain the skill of the screener.

The characteristics of a good cancer screening program are summarized in Table 4–1.[7] Because of, the prevalence of the disease, the ease of screening, and the impact of early detection on outcome, that skin cancer screening meets these criteria. Furthermore, screening for NMSC can be done simultaneously with melanoma screening at no additional cost.

Despite the relative ease of skin cancer screening, the U.S. Preventive Services Task Force (USPSTF), Department of Health and Human Services (DHHS) has not recommended routine physician skin cancer screening, rating it "I" for insufficient evidence. The

Table 4–1. Characteristics of a Good Cancer Screening Program

✓ Screening should be highly sensitive and specific
✓ The prevalence of the disease should be high enough to warrant screening
✓ The health implications should be high enough to warrant screening
✓ The disease should not be immediately life-threatening
✓ The screening procedure should be simple, inexpensive, and acceptable to the population
✓ The disease should be one for which early diagnosis results in improved prognosis
✓ Screening should lead to more effective treatment at an earlier stage

USPSTF concludes that "the current evidence is insufficient to assess the balance of benefits and harm of screening for skin cancer by primary care clinicians or patient skin self-examination (SSE). The evidence is insufficient (lack of studies) to determine whether early detection of skin cancer reduces mortality or morbidity"[8] In its previous review in 2001, USPSTF also rated skin screening as "I." At that time they found that, although total-body skin examination can increase the detection of thin melanoma, controlled studies were needed to see if this would have an important effect on mortality. Additional investigation was advocated to address the impact of early detection on those at risk for thin melanoma.[9,10]

These statements require careful and accurate interpretation. This recommendation does not find that skin screening is ineffectual, but rather recognizes problems in the design and implementation of prior studies. Skin screening studies have lacked adequately powered, population-based, prospective, randomized controlled trials, as well as direct evidence linking skin cancer screening to improved health outcomes.[11] In addition, many studies have failed to consider the training of the screener or have failed to identify high-risk patients with a prescreening history of premalignant or malignant skin lesions.[12] An evaluation of the American Academy of Dermatology's Skin Cancer Screening Program from 1992 to 1994 found that, when dermatologist screening took place, a higher percentage of melanoma was found in earlier stages than in cases documented in the Surveillance, Epidemiology and End Results (SEER) registry. The authors concluded that access to dermatologists, particularly for older patients, may represent one approach to improving melanoma-related health outcomes.[13,14]

Mathematical models have demonstrated that a one-time melanoma screening of people over 50 years and screening siblings of melanoma patients every 2 years is cost effective.[15] Perhaps the most important message is that full skin examination, even when patients are seen for other medical problems, may lead to early detection of skin cancer. Most melanomas found in a general practice dermatology clinic were found as a result of dermatologist-initiated full body skin examination, even when patients were seen for other problems. These incidentally detected malignancies were more likely to be thin, with associated decreased mortality.[16,17]

Although there is no consensus about melanoma screening, the American Cancer Society has recommended total skin screening as part of a cancer-related checkup for people age 20 or older since 1993.[18,19] As results from adequate trials may not be imminent, many leaders advocate for skin cancer screening, assuming that future well-designed studies will support this decision.[12] The American Academy of Dermatology not only supports skin screening, but initiated a free, yearly screening program in 1985, which continues to this day.[20] This national program is staffed by dermatologists who perform complete skin screening in most major American cities, focusing on those with suboptimal access to dermatologic care.

Screening Techniques

Self-Screening Examination (SSE)

Based on the premise that SSE may aid in early detection, there are ongoing efforts designed to educate the community about known risk factors of MM and NMSC, and to encourage this practice.[21] The lay public plays an important role in identifying skin cancer, with estimates that 72% of all melanomas are detected by nonphysicians such as patients, families, or friends.[20,22] In a large Australian study, almost half of melanomas were detected by the patients themselves, and one fifth were detected by their partners. Physicians, however, were more likely to identify thinner lesions and second primary melanomas.[23]

The practice of SSE blossomed in 1985 with the development of the ABCD acronym, alerting patients that asymmetry, border irregularity, color variation, and diameter (greater than 6 mm) of pigmented lesions may be risk factors for melanomas.[24] The "E" was added in 2005 and represents "evolving," meaning a change in size, shape, surface, color, or symptoms.[25] The E is considered by many dermatologists to be the most significant sign, especially in the pediatric population, because the most common presentation of childhood melanoma may be a rapidly growing pink or amelanotic papule. Figure 4–1 demonstrates a melanoma exhibiting the classic ABCDE criteria.

Taken together, these criteria have proved to be reasonably sensitive and specific, although glaring exceptions exist, such as dysplastic nevi, amelanotic melanomas, or melanomas less than 6 mm in diameter.[26,27] Also, some common benign lesions like seborrheic keratoses frequently exhibit all of the ABCDE characteristics.

Studies have shown that even people at increased risk for skin malignancy do not always perform SSE, and efforts have been implemented to improve both compliance and accuracy.[28] Furthermore, even when performed, there seems to be a gender difference in how people recognize skin changes. Women tend to recognize color variation, whereas men identified irregular borders, suggesting a partnership may be helpful.[26,29] High-risk patients who were taught SSE along with their partners were more prone to perform the examinations.[30] In support of this, other studies have shown that key predictors of the performance of SSE were the presence of a partner, the use of a wall mirror, mole mapping diagrams, and body photographs.[31–33] Active teaching programs illustrating the ABCDE criteria, along with SSE utilizing a lighted hand magnifying glass and a millimeter ruler, may be more efficient in eliciting a behavioral change than distributing color brochures alone.[34] Using sample photographs, an instructional video, hand mirror, shower card, and American Cancer Society brochure, the "check it out" trial found increased performance of SSE.[35] Other factors affecting compliance were attitude, history of skin biopsies, risk perception, and knowledge of the disease.[36] Importantly, SSE also establishes teamwork between the patient and the physician, to aid in early melanoma detection.[37]

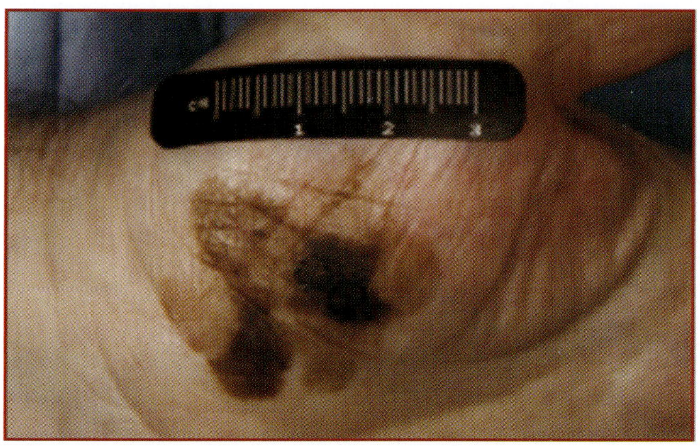

Figure 4–1. ABCDE criteria demonstrated in a slowly growing melanoma.

Physician Screening

Physicians and other health professionals may benefit from continuing education programs that stress how, why, and on whom to perform full body examinations. Some medical schools now include skin evaluation as a permanent part of their curricula, but it remains to be seen whether behaviors actually change after graduation.[38] Specialist training also may be important, as dermatologists demonstrate better diagnostic accuracy than primary care physicians (PCPs). Therefore, more innovative strategies are needed to better train PCPs and enhance skin cancer screening skills.[39,40]

Thoroughness is the cornerstone of physician screening. Less visible areas such as the scalp, back, fingers, toes, nails, oral cavity, buttock folds, and perineum should be checked. Melanomas are found more often in patients who were completely undressed for their skin exam versus those who were not, and makeup and nail polish should be removed.

How difficult is it to screen for melanoma and nonmelanoma skin cancer? In the average patient with banal or small numbers of nevi, screening is not difficult. However, examination of patients with multiple, atypical appearing nevi (Fig 4–2) is daunting. In these challenging cases, it usually is possible to find a mole phenotype that is distinctive to the individual. Multiple nevi that manifest similar morphology in one individual are called signature nevi.[41] Although individually each may seem atypical, the recurring pattern is reassuring (Fig 4–3). These lesions may exhibit a variety of patterns and colors such as pink, two-tone, eclipse, targetoid, small and uniformly dark, or even resembling a "fried egg" with a central dark papule surrounded by macular hyperpigmentation.[37] In patients with many nevi, finding a nevus that does not exhibit the signature pattern may narrow down the number of lesions that need closer evaluation.[42] This phenotypically different nevus, or "ugly duckling" mole, merits further scrutiny or biopsy as it may represent an early melanoma (Fig 4–4).[43,44]

Figure 4–2. Many atypical moles in a patient with multiple melanomas.

Screening Tools

Screening tools are increasingly available to health professionals, although their impact on the early diagnosis of melanoma and NMSC remains undetermined. The use of the handheld dermatoscope has become commonplace in screening examinations performed by dermatologists. This is a noninvasive tool that magnifies, illuminates, and allows visualization of structures within the epidermis, dermal epidermal junction, and superficial dermis. Der-

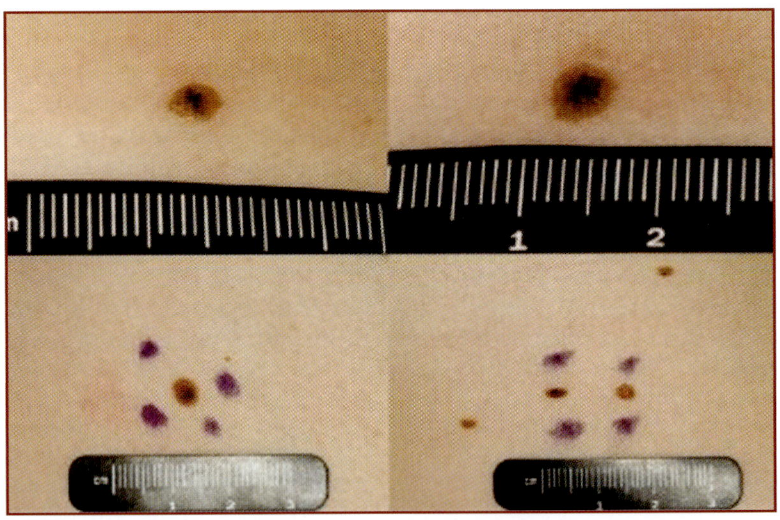

Figure 4–3. Signature nevi. Although each lesion appears atypical with a dark, hyperpigmented center, this "fried egg" phenotype was found in all of this patient's benign nevi.

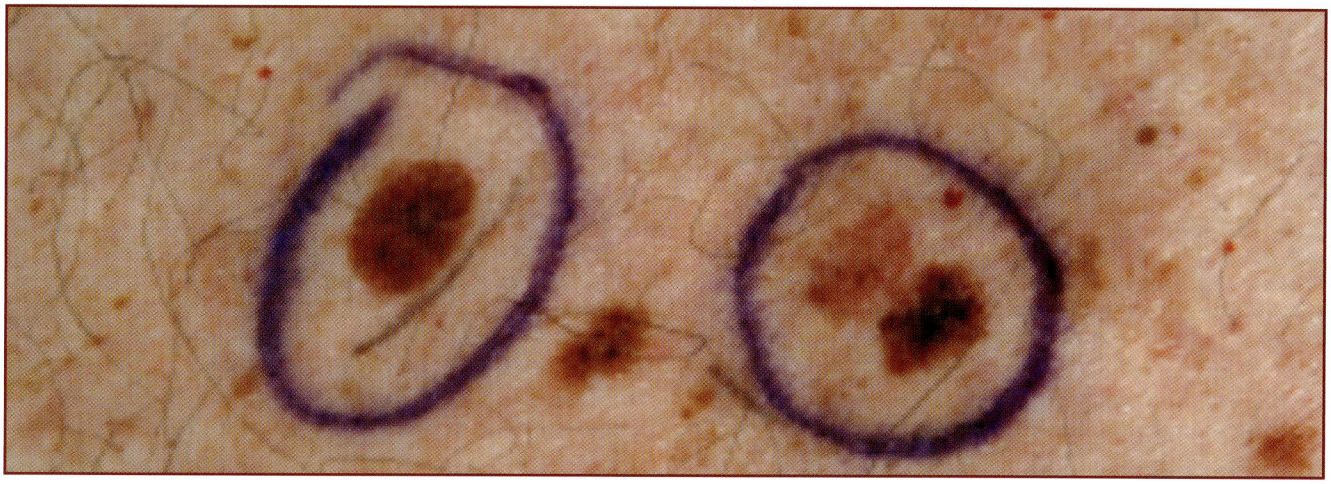

Figure 4–4. Ugly duckling mole. This patient's signature mole also has a dark center surrounded by macular hyperpigmentation. The red macule in the right circle is phenotypically different and proven to be melanoma after biopsy.

moscopy, also called dermatoscopy, skin surface microscopy, or epiluminescence microscopy, originally was performed holding the instrument on a fluid interface like oil, water, or alcohol, which stayed on the skin. In the United States, a small handheld unit utilizing polarized light has become increasing popular, as it eliminates the need for contact on the skin, a potential source of nosocomial infections.[45]

Educational courses about dermoscopy are readily available for health professionals interested in skin screening. This noninvasive tool also helps to identify subtle pigmentation patterns, vascular features, and even areas of regression within a suspect lesion, allowing for more accurate identification. The technique helps distinguish between melanocytic and nonmelanocytic tumors, and it may increase accuracy in diagnosing melanomas.[46,47] In large lesions, it is used to identify the most suspicious area to be sampled, if the whole lesion is not to be excised. Its accuracy depends, not surprisingly, on the experience of the user.[48,49] With practice, complete skin examination using the dermatoscope increased the median examination time by only 72 seconds.[50] Teledermoscopy, or sharing images on the Internet, allows multiple clinicians to consult on a problematic case. Similarly, digital dermoscopy employs an attached digital camera to produce sequential images that can be followed or used for consultation.

Whole body photography with mapping pictures of suspect lesions also has also proved helpful for screening and surveillance. The use of baseline photography with or without dermatoscopy is associated with lower biopsy rates and earlier melanoma detection.[51–54] Photographic equipment may vary from instant Polaroid or 35-mm film to sophisticated digital images, but the quality and ease of storage and retrieval is very important.[55] Various computer storage systems are available, which vary in their ease of use. Although sophisticated computer software that captures both digital and dermatoscopic images is available, software does not improve the diagnostic accuracy for melanoma detection above that of a dermatologist.[55–57] Therefore, no matter how sophisticated, this software remains a tool of the screener, and should not be used alone. Multispectral digital dermoscopy may provide information about lesions not evident to the naked eye by combining images taken at different wavelengths and a range of depths that subsequently are analyzed by a computer.[37,55]

Reflectance confocal scanning laser microscopy (CSLM) is a sophisticated imaging system that allows visualization of the epidermis and papillary dermis at high resolution by focusing a low-power laser beam and detecting the light reflected through a pinhole-sized spatial filter. This beam is scanned over a 2-dimensional grid to obtain an instant, noninvasive horizontal microscopic section at variable depths.[55,58] Unfortunately, high costs currently limit the routine use of CSLM for screening purposes.

Surveillance

Once a lesion is identified as suspicious for either NMSC or MM, it should be biopsied or excised. In cases in which surgical removal is inadvisable or declined, periodic surveillance may be planned, usually with sequential examination utilizing mapping images or photography.

Some individuals or groups can be identified as high risk for developing melanoma and NMSC, and they may be well served by a surveillance program.[59] Although certain features are shared by both MM and NMSC, these features are summarized in the following section.

Surveillance Candidates for Malignant Melanoma

A melanoma risk tool is available at http://www.cancer.gov/melanomarisktool/, but needs to be validated in different populations.[60]

Phenotype

Patients at risk include those with light skin color, poor tanning ability, light eyes, and blond or red hair.[61,62]

Exposure to Ultraviolet Radiation (UVR)

UVR is a known carcinogen.[63] Questions about the exact relationship of melanoma to UVR remain, but there is sufficient evidence for carcinogenicity.[64,65] Increased risk also appears to be related to intermittent sunburns, both in childhood and adulthood.[66] Comparisons of skin cancer data from Norway and Australia/New Zealand indicate that squamous cell carcinoma and basal cell carcinoma are related mainly to annual solar UVB fluences, whereas UVA fluences play a larger role for MM.[67] Exposure to UVR via tanning or sun-beds also may increase the risk of melanoma development, especially when the first exposure occurs before 35 years of age.[68–70] This is not surprising because UVR plays a significant modifying role in nevus development, despite a potential genetic predisposition.[71]

Family History and Genetic Factors

A positive family history of MM in a first-degree relative affords patients an approximately twofold increase in risk of melanoma.[61] Germline mutations in 3 different genes have been shown to influence the risk of melanoma: cyclin-dependent kinase inhibitor 2A (CDKN2A), cyclin-dependent kinase 4 (CDK4), and melanocortin-1 receptor (MC1R).[72,73] Certain allelic variants of MC1R, namely, R151C, R160W, and D294H, are strongly associated with red hair phenotype and increased melanoma susceptibility. Natural expression of 2 of these variants may sensitize melanocytes to the cytotoxic effect of UV, thereby increasing the burden of DNA damage and oxidative stress.[74,75]

Other hereditary conditions associated with an increased melanoma risk include retinoblastoma (from prior treatment), oculocutaneous albinism, and xeroderma pigmentosum (XP), one of a group of autosomal recessive disorders characterized by defects in DNA repair.[76] The incidence of NMSC and MM are markedly increased in XP, particularly if these individuals are not protected from the sun from birth.[77]

Nevi, or Pigmented Lesions

An increased number of nevi, even if they are common and not dysplastic, is a notable risk factor for MM.[78] The prototypic dysplastic nevus is often larger than 5 mm, has a prominent flat component, an irregular or asymmetric outline, indistinct borders, and variable pigmentation.[79] Histologic features include a disordered growth pattern with lymphocytic host response and random cytologic atypia in melanocytes.[80] With common, nondysplastic nevi, there is a relative risk for progression to melanoma of 1.6 ($p = 0.43$) for 11 to 25 nevi, 4.4 ($p = 0.01$) for 26 to 50 nevi, 5.4 ($p = 0.008$) for 51 to 100 nevi, and 9.8 ($p = 0.001$) for more than 100 lesions.[62] The presence of atypical or dysplastic nevi further increases the melanoma risk, with relative risks of 3.8 ($p = 0.001$) for 1 to 5 dysplastic nevi and 6.3 ($p = 0.003$) for 6 or more of these lesions.[62,78] Evolving or new melanocytic lesions in patients over 50 years of age carry an increase risk of malignancy, even when not dysplastic.[54]

Ionizing Radiation

People exposed to ionizing radiation may be at increased risk of developing melanoma, although alternative explanations are possible. Accordingly, future epidemiological studies on the long-term effects of ionizing radiation should include melanoma as an outcome of interest.[81]

Immunosuppression

The incidence pattern and risk factor profile for melanoma after transplantation strongly suggest that the intensity, and possibly the duration, of iatrogenic immunosuppression increases melanoma risk that is perhaps compounded by personal sun exposure and sensitivity. These findings suggest the marked influence of immunologic control over melanoma incidence.[82] The incidence of MM in transplant recipients may be up to 0 to 8 times higher than seen in the general populations.[83,84]

Congenital Nevi

The risk of malignant melanoma depends on the size of the lesion and is highest in those nevi traditionally designated as garment nevi, as seen in Figure 4–5.[85]

Personal History of Melanoma

Patients with a history of a single melanoma have a lifelong 5% to 8% risk of developing a second melanoma.[86,87]

Miscellaneous/Behavioral

Tobacco smoking in older populations is an independent risk factor for cutaneous melanoma in the elderly.[88]

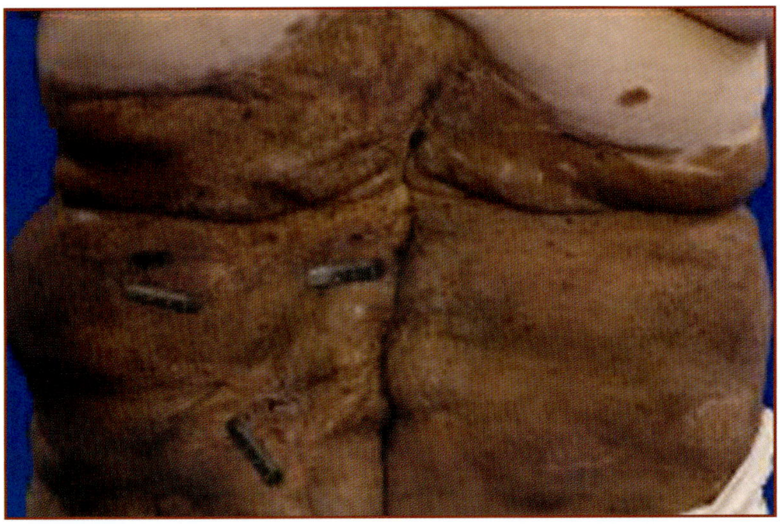

Figure 4–5. Congenital bathing trunk nevus that developed multiple sites of atypical melanocytic hyperplasia and melanoma.

Surveillance Candidates for Nonmelanoma Skin Cancer

Phenotype

Similar to that of melanoma, light-haired and light-skinned individuals who burn easily are at risk. A history of cutaneous melanoma significantly increases the risk of basal cell and squamous cell skin cancer.[89]

Exposure to Ultraviolet Radiation

There is a strong correlation with the average annual UVR exposure and incidence of skin cancer, as well as a direct relationship between the incidence of NMSC and latitude. For SCC, chronic long-term exposure carries more risk; however, BCC may be slightly different with intermittent intense burns being more important.[90] Women have a greater frequency of BCC on the lower extremity, whereas men have more ear lesions, possibly related to fashion and hairstyle.[90] Furthermore, tanning bed use not only increases the risk of melanoma as already discussed, but also of nonmelanoma skin cancer.[70]

Ionizing Radiation

Exposure to ionizing radiation produces a threefold increased risk of NMSC.[91] In genetic diseases characterized by reduced cellular DNA repair capability such as XP, ionizing radiation is contraindicated, as it may result in the development of malignant skin tumors.[92]

Precursor Lesions

Actinic keratoses (AK) are a potential precursor and marker for developing invasive NMSC.[93] Actinic keratoses, sometimes called solar keratoses, are considered premalignant because of their characteristic atypical keratinocytes and their relationship with SCC. An individual AK may evolve into SCC at a rate of .075% to .096% per lesion per year, and affected individuals tend to have many actinic keratoses.[90]

A nevus sebaceous is a congenital lesion that may undergo malignant transformation, usually to BCC, in childhood or adolescence. Hence, they often are excised, with the timing of the procedure determined by weighing the small risk of malignant transformation against the morbidity associated with excision and anesthesia.[94]

Occupational, Environmental, and Behavioral Concerns

There is an increased incidence of BCC and SCC in outdoor workers compared to indoor workers, modified by their skin type, simply because of UVR exposure.[95] Interestingly, airline pilots are at risk for both BCC and SCC because of exposure to cosmic radiation.[96] Chemical exposure involving pesticides, asphalt, tar, and polycyclic aromatic hydrocarbons is associated with the development of cutaneous SCC.[97] Systemic arsenic has been shown to act as a tumor promoter for both BCC and SCC with a latency period from exposure of 20 to 40 years.[98,99] Similar to melanoma, smoking is associated with a twofold increase in developing cutaneous SCC.[100] Diets high in fat, thermal burns, and chronic, nonhealing wounds also predispose patients to the development of NMSC.[90]

Genetic Syndromes

Xeroderma pigmentosum and oculocutaneous albinism demand strict UV avoidance for life.[90] Patients with epidermodysplasia verruciformis, a recessive inherited disorder with widespread colonization of the skin by multiple subtypes of human papillomavirus (HPV), are at higher risk to develop SCC, usually in sun-exposed areas.[90] Dystrophic epidermolysis bullosa, a blistering genetic disorder present from birth, can result from dominant and recessive mutations. Cutaneous SCC is more common in the recessive form, and aggressive tumors are the most common cause of death.[90,101] Nevoid basal cell carcinoma syndrome, or Gorlin syndrome, is an autosomal dominant disorder due to a mutation in the human PTCH gene.[102] Patients often present with BCC in childhood, as well as other phenotypic abnormalities. Ultraviolet radiation exposure needs to be minimized, and ionizing or therapeutic radiation is contraindicated.[92] Rarer dermatologic syndromes such as Bazex or Rombo syndrome also carry an increased risk of BCC.[90]

Immunosuppression

Immunosuppressed individuals demonstrate a marked risk for the development of cutaneous neoplasms that is up to 65 times higher than the general population, with associated morbidity and mortality. Prevention, prompt recognition, and effective treatment of skin cancer in this population are vital.[103,104] Organ transplant recipients have high rates of NMSC, primarily SCC but also BCC, and this is compounded by skin type, sun exposure, age at transplantation, and length of immunosuppression.[90] The relative risk of SCC in organ transplant recipients is approximately 100-fold higher than in the immunocompetent population. Not only can they develop multiple lesions, but also they are more prone to recurrence and metastases. Likewise, the incidence of BCC is increased "only" by a factor of 10.[105] Although 10% of actinic keratoses become SCC during a 5- to 10-year time frame in the immunocompetent, the rate of progression in organ transplant patients is increased, and the time to progression is decreased.[106,107]

Patients with HIV, despite highly active antiretroviral therapy (HAART), also may be at increased risk for cutaneous SCC.[108] Oral glucocorticoids increase the risk of BCC, even in nontransplant recipients, raising the possibility that these medications may allow skin cancer to emerge from immunosurveillance—this risk does not extend to inhaled steroids.[109,110] The presence of HPV, especially oncogenic strains in immunosuppressed individuals, increases the risk of NMSC. Bowenoid papulosis, a type of SCC in situ, usually is found in wartlike genital lesions and may occur in conjunction with oncogenic HPV.[108]

Miscellaneous

Patients undergoing treatment for other malignancies with multikinase inhibitors that suppress the actions of Raf kinase and vascular endothelial growth factor, such as sorafenib and tipifarnib, recently have shown a concerning predisposition for developing multiple cutaneous SCC.[112]

Surveillance Methods

How should these "high-risk" patients be followed? The risks and morbidity of intervention must be carefully weighed against the risks and morbidity, if not mortality, of inaction. Removing all nevi will not prevent melanoma, as malignant lesions arise de novo and from preexisting nevi.[51,113] Close follow-up is imperative, as short-term monitoring studies show that some melanomas exhibit observable dermatoscopic changes over 3 to 6 months.[114–116] Symptoms such as ulceration, bleeding or itching may also indicate the need for biopsy, as does a patient's concern about the appearance of a new mole.

Although practitioners should strongly consider removing any lesion the patient thinks has changed, we should bear in mind that nevi are not static. Pigmented lesions may appear spontaneously with advancing age, and benign nevi may even regress in younger patients.[117,118] Eruptive nevi have occurred in association with the onset of blistering diseases, as well as following organ transplantion and HIV infection.[119-121] Generally, the likelihood that new lesions represent melanoma increases over age 50.[54]

Patients at high risk may be better followed by dermatologists than generalists, as they may be able to detect these cancers earlier and when thinner.[23,122] Even though patients detected 45% of the initial primary melanomas (98/218), dermatologists discovered 80% of the second primary tumors.[122] Periodic skin examination in high-risk patients with photomapping can help monitor high risk lesions.[123,124]

Patients at risk for melanoma, especially if they have many nevi, are difficult to screen and follow. These patients may benefit from participation in a specialized pigmented lesion clinic staffed by personnel with experience in serial photographic mapping, dermoscopy, and surgical excisions. This format may outperform less specialized care with a lower false negative biopsy rate and increased sensitivity for malignant lesions.[125–127]

Prevention

The purpose of screening and surveillance is to identify skin cancer early and recognize populations at risk. Prevention aims to anticipate the problem and create ways to avoid it, within genetic and environmental parameters. Prevention may involve environmental or behavioral modifications, with education as the cornerstone. Although counseling should be a priority for high-risk patients, dermatologists are more likely to instruct patients on skin cancer prevention strategies than family physicians or providers in other specialties.[128] Primary care providers and other health care professionals should play a key role not only in screening for skin cancer, but also in providing patient education and access to skin specialists when necessary.[129–131]

Photoprotection complements education in efforts to prevent skin cancer, and it includes wearing UV protective clothing, avoiding the sun at peak hours, seeking shade, and wearing sunscreens. Such sun-protective behavior can start at an early age and be reinforced in school by building shade structures, encouraging kids to wear wide-brimmed hats, and limiting student sun exposure, especially in susceptible individuals.[132] Such early steps are imperative in melanoma, as UV-induced formation of melanocytic nevi takes place in early childhood, and the increased number of UV-induced nevi may boost the relative risk for development of MM by nearly a factor of 7.[133,134] Educational programs geared to the public such as SunWise (sun protection education for young children) and SunSmart (population-based prevention programs incorporating substantial television advertising) have been created, and the early results seem promising from an economic and health point of view.[135,136]

Adolescents may merit a special approach. Despite Australia's rigorous sun protection message, the majority of Australian adolescents prefer to get a tan and resist wearing sun-protective clothing or sunscreens or even seeking out shade.[137] New educational sites on the Internet and YouTube have been created to reach this age group.[138] For those who crave a tan, "sunless tanning" by the application of dihydroxyacetone (DHA) temporarily darkens the skin. However, DHA is not UV protective, and other photoprotection should be used. Increased advocacy by celebrities or authority figures, positive peer pressure, innovations, or incorporation of protective fabrics into contemporary clothing by the fashion industry, and improved, more appealing, sun protection products gradually may trigger more compliance with sun-protective behaviors among adolescents.[139]

Education alone cannot stop tanning behavior in some high-risk individuals who seek out indoor tanning. There is accumulating evidence that UVR exposure in tanning parlors can be addictive, and the use of indoor tanning is growing despite public health warnings.[140] Additionally, there is an overall lack of regulation on pediatric tanning bed use.[141] Physicians must capitalize on their position as the most trusted source of information for young persons and actively counsel patients against tanning beds and excessive exposure.[142]

Genetic counseling should be considered for high-risk populations, such as melanoma-prone families. Patients who were identified as carriers of high-risk genes, such as CDKN2A mutations, reported significantly reduced anxiety and reduced depression scores after receipt of the results compared to those who declined testing. Carriers also reported a significantly greater frequency of clinical skin examination at 12-month follow-up compared with decliners.[143]

For patients at high risk for NMSC after prolonged immunosuppression, ionizing radiation, or organ transplantation, skin screening and educational programs that emphasize avoidance of high-risk behaviors like sunbathing should become an integral part of their care, along with regular surveillance. Premalignant lesions such as AK also should be addressed aggressively. When a small number of well-defined keratoses are present, localized destruction with cryosurgery is useful, but this is impractical with large numbers of ill-defined lesions. In this circumstance, therapy needs to be directed at a larger field, perhaps the whole face or extremities. Depending on the patient's underlying condition, topical modalities like 5-fluorouracil cream, imiquimod, or photodynamic therapy may be offered. Skin malignancies should be identified early and definitively treated, followed by continued intense surveillance for recurrence or new malignancies. In organ transplant patients, the vast majority of skin cancer recurrences and metastases occur within 3 years after the incident high-risk tumor—these patients may be candidates for ongoing research protocols on novel agents.

Despite close surveillance, patients with certain genodermatoses, as well as transplant or immunosuppressed patients, may develop numerous and extensive NMSC. When chronic immunosuppressive drugs cannot be stopped, the use of topical and systemic retinoids may be considered. In 1988, Kraemer et al[144] prospectively studied oral isotretinoin in 5 patients with XP and found that it effectively prevented additional skin cancers, and isotretinoin may also be helpful in some cases of basal cell nevus syndrome.[144,145] Organ transplant recipients on retinoids may have fewer SCC and keratotic lesions, with the effect most pronounced in those who have had previous skin cancers. Studies suggest that patients with the highest propensity to develop skin cancer or those with more antecedent lesions have the most significant response.[105] The beneficial prophylactic effects are quickly lost when the medication is discontinued, followed by a rapid increase of new NMSC.[130] Retinoids exhibit some significant side effects, such as xerosis, fatigue, poor wound healing, elevated triglycerides, and possible retinoid-related depression, that require discontinuation with potential loss of benefit.[146] Potentially, topical retinoids may decrease actinic keratoses in high-risk patients, without the systemic side effects.[147,148]

Summary

As the incidence of MM and NMSC continues to increase, education of both the public and the medical community about screening, surveillance, and prevention becomes increasingly important. Good tools are available to teach patients techniques of self-screening examination, and practitioners have access to excellent continuing education programs. Complete skin evaluations readily can be performed when patients are evaluated for other nonskin-related problems. This becomes even more important when the patient is immunosuppressed, especially in the presence of preexisting actinic damage. Patients at high risk for skin cancer may benefit from a team approach that features counseling, screening, and surveillance by dedicated professionals.

References

1. American Cancer Society. *Cancer Facts & Figures 2009.* Atlanta, GA: American Cancer Society; 2009.
2. Robinson JK. Sun exposure, sun protection, and vitamin D. *JAMA.* 2005;294:1541–1543.
3. The Skin Cancer Foundation. Skin Cancer Facts. 2009; Available from: http://www.skincancer.org/skin-cancer-facts.
4. American Cancer Society. How Many People Get Melanoma Skin Cancer? 13 May 2008.
5. National Center for Chronic Disease Prevention and Health Promotion. The Burden of Skin Cancer. 13 May 2008.
6. The National Cancer Institute. Melanoma of the Skin. Available from: http://seer.cancer.gov/statistics/.
7. McDonald CJ. Status of screening for skin cancer. *Cancer.* 1993;72(3 suppl):1066–1070.
8. U.S. Preventive Services Task Force. Screening for skin cancer: U.S. Preventive Services Task Force recommendation statement. *Ann Intern Med.* 2009;150(3)188–193.
9. U.S. Preventive Services Task Force. Screening for skin cancer: recommendations and rationale. *Am J Prev Med.* 200;20(3 suppl):44–46.
10. Helfand M, Mahon SM, Eden KB, Frame PS, Orleans CT. Screening for skin cancer. *Am J Prev Med.* 2001;20 (3 suppl):47–58.
11. Wolff T, Tai E, Miller T. Screening for skin cancer: an update of the evidence for the U.S. Preventive Services Task Force. *Ann Intern Med.* 2009;150(3):194–198.
12. Federman DG, Concato J, Kirsner RS. Screening for skin cancer: absence of evidence. *Arch Dermatol.* 2009;145(8): 926–927.
13. Geller AC, Zhang Z, Sober AJ, et al. The first 15 years of the American Academy of Dermatology skin cancer screening programs: 1985–1999. *J Am Acad Dermatol.* 2003;48(1):34–41.
14. Pennie ML, Soon SL, Risser JB, Veledar E, Culler SD, Chen SC. Melanoma outcomes for Medicare patients: association of stage and survival with detection by a dermatologist vs a nondermatologist. *Arch Dermatol.* 2007;143(4):488–494.
15. Losina E, Walensky RP, Geller A, et al. Visual screening for malignant melanoma: a cost-effectiveness analysis. *Arch Dermatol.* 2007;143(1):21–28.
16. Kantor J, Kantor DE. Routine dermatologist-performed full-body skin examination and early melanoma detection. *Arch Dermatol.* 2009;145(8):873–876.

17. Schneider JS, Moore DH, II, Mendelsohn ML. Screening program reduced melanoma mortality at the Lawrence Livermore National Laboratory, 1984 to 1996. *J Am Acad Dermatol.* 2008;58(5):741–749.
18. Koh HK. Melanoma screening: focusing the public health journey. *Arch Dermatol.* 2007;143(1):101–103.
19. Smith RA, Cokkinides V, Eyre HJ. American Cancer Society guidelines for the early detection of cancer, 2006. *CA Cancer J Clin.* 2006;56(1):11–25.
20. Terushkin V, Halpern AC. Melanoma early detection. *Hematol Oncol Clin North Am.* 2009;23(3):481–500, viii.
21. Carli P, De Giorgi V, Palli D, et al. Dermatologist detection and skin self-examination are associated with thinner melanomas: results from a survey of the Italian Multidisciplinary Group on Melanoma. *Arch Dermatol.* 2003;139(5):607–612.
22. Brady MS, Oliveria SA, Christos PJ, et al. Patterns of detection in patients with cutaneous melanoma. *Cancer.* 2000;89(2):342–347.
23. McPherson M, Elwood M, English DR, Baade PD, Youl PH, Aitken JF. Presentation and detection of invasive melanoma in a high-risk population. *J Am Acad Dermatol.* 2006; 54(5):783–792.
24. Friedman RJ, Rigel DS, Kopf AW. Early detection of malignant melanoma: the role of physician examination and self-examination of the skin. *CA Cancer J Clin.* 1985;35(3):130–151.
25. Abbasi NR, Shaw HM, Rigel DS, et al. Early diagnosis of cutaneous melanoma: revisiting the ABCD criteria. *JAMA.* 2004;292(22):2771–2776.
26. Heymann WR. Screening for melanoma. *J Am Acad Dermatol.* 2007;56(1):144–145.
27. Branstrom R, Hedblad MA, Krakau I, Ullen H. Laypersons' perceptual discrimination of pigmented skin lesions. *J Am Acad Dermatol.* 2002;46(5):667–673.
28. Carli P, De Giorgi V, Palli D, et al. Self-detected cutaneous melanomas in Italian patients. *Clin Exp Dermatol.* 2004;29(6):593–596.
29. Robinson JK, Turrisi R. Skills training to learn discrimination of ABCDE criteria by those at risk of developing melanoma. *Arch Dermatol.* 2006;142(4):447–452.
30. Robinson JK, Turrisi R, Stapleton J. Efficacy of a partner assistance intervention designed to increase skin self-examination performance. *Arch Dermatol.* 2007;143(1):37–41.
31. Weinstock MA, Risica PM, Martin RA, et al. Reliability of assessment and circumstances of performance of thorough skin self-examination for the early detection of melanoma in the Check-It-Out Project. *Prev Med.* 2004;38(6):761–765.
32. Chiu V, Won E, Malik M, Weinstock MA. The use of mole-mapping diagrams to increase skin self-examination accuracy. *J Am Acad Dermatol.* 2006;55(2):245–250.
33. Oliveria SA, Chau D, Christos PJ, Charles CA, Mushlin AI, Halpern AC. Diagnostic accuracy of patients in performing skin self-examination and the impact of photography. *Arch Dermatol.* 2004;140(1):57–62.
34. Robinson JK, Ortiz S. Use of photographs illustrating ABCDE criteria in skin self-examination. *Arch Dermatol.* 2009;145(3):332–333.
35. Lee KB, Weinstock MA, Risica PM. Components of a successful intervention for monthly skin self-examination for early detection of melanoma: the "Check It Out" trial. *J Am Acad Dermatol.* 2008;58(6):1006–1012.
36. Robinson JK, Fisher SG, Turrisi RJ. Predictors of skin self-examination performance. *Cancer.* 2002;95(1):135–146.
37. Goodson AG, Grossman D. Strategies for early melanoma detection: approaches to the patient with nevi. *J Am Acad Dermatol.* 2009;60(5):719–735; quiz 736–718.
38. Doshi DN, Firth K, Mintz M, Ehrlich A. Pilot study of a skin cancer education curriculum for medical students. *J Am Acad Dermatol.* 2007;56(1):167–169.
39. Epstein DS, Lange JR, Gruber SB, Mofid M, Koch SE. Is physician detection associated with thinner melanomas? *JAMA.* 1999;281(7):640–643.
40. Chen SC, Pennie ML, Kolm P, et al. Diagnosing and managing cutaneous pigmented lesions: primary care physicians versus dermatologists. *J Gen Intern Med.* 2006;21(7):678–682.
41. Schaffer JV, Glusac EJ, Bolognia JL. The eclipse naevus: tan centre with stellate brown rim. *Br J Dermatol.* 2001;145(6):1023–1026.
42. Bolognia JL. Too many moles. *Arch Dermatol.* 2006;142(4):508.
43. Grob JJ, Bonerandi JJ. The 'ugly duckling' sign: identification of the common characteristics of nevi in an individual as a basis for melanoma screening. *Arch Dermatol.* 1998;134(1):103–104.
44. Scope A, Dusza SW, Halpern AC, et al. The "ugly duckling" sign: agreement between observers. *Arch Dermatol.* 2008;144(1):58–64.
45. Stauffer F, Kittler H, Forstinger C, Binder M. The dermatoscope: a potential source of nosocomial infection? *Melanoma Res.* 2001;11(2):153–156.
46. Bafounta ML, Beauchet A, Aegerter P, Saiag P. Is dermoscopy (epiluminescence microscopy) useful for the diagnosis of melanoma? Results of a meta-analysis using techniques adapted to the evaluation of diagnostic tests. *Arch Dermatol.* 2001;137(10): 1343–1350.
47. Binder M, Puespoeck-Schwarz M, Steiner A, et al. Epiluminescence microscopy of small pigmented skin lesions: short-term formal training improves the diagnostic performance of dermatologists. *J Am Acad Dermatol.* 1997;36(2 pt 1):197–202.
48. Binder M, Schwarz M, Winkler A, et al. Epiluminescence microscopy. A useful tool for the diagnosis of pigmented skin lesions for formally trained dermatologists. *Arch Dermatol.* 1995;13(3):286–291.
49. Kittler H, Pehamberger H, Wolff K, Binder M. Diagnostic accuracy of dermoscopy. *Lancet Oncol.* 2002;3(3):159–165.
50. Zalaudek I, Kittler H, Marghoob AA, et al. Time required for a complete skin examination with and without der-

moscopy: a prospective, randomized multicenter study. *Arch Dermatol.* 2008;144(4):509–513.
51. Kelly JW, Yeatman JM, Regalia C, Mason G, Henham AP. A high incidence of melanoma found in patients with multiple dysplastic naevi by photographic surveillance. *Med J Aust.* 1997;167(4):191–194.
52. Feit NE, Dusza SW, Marghoob AA. Melanomas detected with the aid of total cutaneous photography. *Br J Dermatol.* 2004;150(4):706–714.
53. Wang SQ, Kopf AW, Koenig K, Polsky D, Nudel K, Bart RS. Detection of melanomas in patients followed up with total cutaneous examinations, total cutaneous photography, and dermoscopy. *J Am Acad Dermatol.* 2004;50(1):15–20.
54. Banky JP, Kelly JW, English DR, Yeatman JM, Dowling JP. Incidence of new and changed nevi and melanomas detected using baseline images and dermoscopy in patients at high risk for melanoma. *Arch Dermatol.* 2005;141(8):998–1006.
55. Marghoob AA, Swindle LD, Moricz CZ, et al. Instruments and new technologies for the in vivo diagnosis of melanoma. *J Am Acad Dermatol.* 2003;49(5):777–797; quiz 798–799.
56. Binder M, Kittler H, Dreiseitl S, Ganster H, Wolff K, Pehamberger H. Computer-aided epiluminescence microscopy of pigmented skin lesions: the value of clinical data for the classification process. *Melanoma Res.* 2000;10(6):556–561.
57. Rosado B, Menzies S, Harbauer A, et al. Accuracy of computer diagnosis of melanoma: a quantitative meta-analysis. *Arch Dermatol.* 2003;139(3):361–367; discussion 366.
58. Rajadhyaksha M, Grossman M, Esterowitz D, Webb RH, Anderson RR. In vivo confocal scanning laser microscopy of human skin: melanin provides strong contrast. *J Invest Dermatol.* 1995;104(6):946–952.
59. Fears TR, Guerry DT, Pfeiffer RM, et al. Identifying individuals at high risk of melanoma: a practical predictor of absolute risk. *J Clin Oncol.* 2006;24(22):3590–3596.
60. Tucker MA. Melanoma epidemiology. *Hematol Oncol Clin North Am.* 2009;23(3):383–395, vii.
61. Gandini S, Sera F, Cattaruzza MS, et al. Meta-analysis of risk factors for cutaneous melanoma: III. Family history, actinic damage and phenotypic factors. *Eur J Cancer.* 2005;41(14):2040–2059.
62. Holly EA, Kelly JW, Shpall SN, Chiu SH. Number of melanocytic nevi as a major risk factor for malignant melanoma. *J Am Acad Dermatol.* 1987;17(3):459–468.
63. US Department of Health and Human Services. National Toxicology Program. Report on Carcinogens. December 10, 2007.
64. World Health Organization. IARC monographs on the evaluation of carcinogenic risks to humans. Solar and ultraviolet radiation. *IARC Monogr Eval Carcinog Risks Hum.* 1992;55:1–316.
65. Gandini S, Sera F, Cattaruzza MS, et al. Meta-analysis of risk factors for cutaneous melanoma: II. Sun exposure. *Eur J Cancer.* 2005;41(1):45–60.
66. Dennis LK, Vanbeek MJ, Beane Freeman LE, Smith BJ, Dawson DV, Coughlin JA. Sunburns and risk of cutaneous melanoma: does age matter? A comprehensive meta-analysis. *Ann Epidemiol.* 2008;18(8):614–627.
67. Moan J, Porojnicu AC, Dahlback A. Ultraviolet radiation and malignant melanoma. *Adv Exp Med Biol.* 2008;624:104–116.
68. Gallagher RP, Spinelli JJ, Lee TK. Tanning beds, sunlamps, and risk of cutaneous malignant melanoma. *Cancer Epidemiol Biomarkers Prev.* 2005;14(3):562–566.
69. IARC Working Group. The association of use of sunbeds with cutaneous malignant melanoma and other skin cancers: a systematic review. *Int J Cancer.* 2007;120(5):1116–1122.
70. The association of use of sunbeds with cutaneous malignant melanoma and other skin cancers: A systematic review. *Int J Cancer.* 2007;120(5):1116–1122.
71. Wachsmuth RC, Turner F, Barrett JH, et al. The effect of sun exposure in determining nevus density in UK adolescent twins. *J Invest Dermatol.* 2005;124(1):56–62.
72. Hussussian CJ, Struewing JP, Goldstein AM, et al. Germline p16 mutations in familial melanoma. *Nat Genet.* 1994;8(1):15–21.
73. Zuo L, Weger J, Yang Q, et al. Germline mutations in the p16INK4a binding domain of CDK4 in familial melanoma. *Nat Genet.* 1996;12(1):97–99.
74. Abdel-Malek ZA, Knittel J, Kadekaro AL, Swope VB, Starner R. The melanocortin 1 receptor and the UV response of human melanocytes—a shift in paradigm. *Photochem Photobiol.* 2008;84(2):501–508.
75. Greinert R. Skin cancer: new markers for better prevention. *Pathobiology.* 2009;76(2):64–81.
76. Kleinerman RA, Tucker MA, Tarone RE, et al. Risk of new cancers after radiotherapy in long-term survivors of retinoblastoma: an extended follow-up. *J Clin Oncol.* 2005;23(10):2272–2279.
77. Somoano B, Niendorf KB, Tsao H. Hereditary cancer syndromes of the skin. *Clin Dermatol.* 2005;23(1):85–106.
78. Bataille V, Bishop JA, Sasieni P, et al. Risk of cutaneous melanoma in relation to the numbers, types and sites of naevi: a case-control study. *Br J Cancer.* 1996;73(12):1605–1611.
79. Tucker MA, Goldstein AM. Melanoma etiology: where are we? *Oncogene.* 2003;22(20):3042–3052.
80. Elder DE, Clark WH, Jr., Elenitsas R, Guerry Dt, Halpern AC. The early and intermediate precursor lesions of tumor progression in the melanocytic system: common acquired nevi and atypical (dysplastic) nevi. *Semin Diagn Pathol.* 1993;10(1):18–35.
81. Fink CA, Bates MN. Melanoma and ionizing radiation: is there a causal relationship? *Radiat Res.* 2005;164(5):701–710.
82. Vajdic CM, van Leeuwen MT, Webster AC, et al. Cutaneous melanoma is related to immune suppression in kidney transplant recipients. *Cancer Epidemiol Biomarkers Prev.* 2009;18(8):2297–2303.

83. Lindelof B, Sigurgeirsson B, Gabel H, Stern RS. Incidence of skin cancer in 5356 patients following organ transplantation. *Br J Dermatol.* 2000;143(3):513–519.
84. Le Mire L, Hollowood K, Gray D, Bordea C, Wojnarowska F. Melanomas in renal transplant recipients. *Br J Dermatol.* 2006;154(3):472–477.
85. Krengel S, Hauschild A, Schafer T. Melanoma risk in congenital melanocytic naevi: a systematic review. *Br J Dermatol.* 2006;155(1):1–8.
86. Goggins WB, Tsao H. A population-based analysis of risk factors for a second primary cutaneous melanoma among melanoma survivors. *Cancer.* 2003;97(3):639–643.
87. Dummer R, Panizzon R, Bloch PH, Burg G. Updated Swiss guidelines for the treatment and follow-up of cutaneous melanoma. *Dermatology.* 2005;210(1):39–44.
88. Nagore E, Hueso L, Botella-Estrada R, et al. Smoking, sun exposure, number of nevi and previous neoplasias are risk factors for melanoma in older patients (60 years and over). *J Eur Acad Dermatol Venereol.* 2010;24(1):50–57.
89. Kroumpouzos G, Konstadoulakis MM, Cabral H, Karakousis CP. Risk of basal cell and squamous cell carcinoma in persons with prior cutaneous melanoma. *Dermatol Surg.* 2000;26(6):547–550.
90. Rigel DS CC, Carucci J, Wharton J, eds. *Actinic Keratosis, Basal Cell Carcinoma and Squamous Cell Carcinoma,* 2nd ed. Barcelona, Spain: Mosby Elsevier; 2008.
91. Lichter MD, Karagas MR, Mott LA, Spencer SK, Stukel TA, Greenberg ER. Therapeutic ionizing radiation and the incidence of basal cell carcinoma and squamous cell carcinoma. The New Hampshire Skin Cancer Study Group. *Arch Dermatol.* 2000;136(8):1007–1011.
92. Hymes SR, Strom EA, Fife C. Radiation dermatitis: clinical presentation, pathophysiology, and treatment 2006. *J Am Acad Dermatol.* 2006;54(1):28–46.
93. Chen GJ, Feldman SR, Williford PM, et al. Clinical diagnosis of actinic keratosis identifies an elderly population at high risk of developing skin cancer. *Dermatol Surg.* 2005;31(1):43–47.
94. Rosen H, Schmidt B, Lam HP, Meara JG, Labow BI. Management of nevus sebaceous and the risk of basal cell carcinoma: an 18-year review. *Pediatr Dermatol.* 2009;26(6):678–681.
95. Radespiel-Troger M, Meyer M, Pfahlberg A, Lausen B, Uter W, Gefeller O. Outdoor work and skin cancer incidence: a registry-based study in Bavaria. *Int Arch Occup Environ Health.* 2009;82(3):357–363.
96. Ott C, Huber S. [The clinical significance of cosmic radiation in aviation]. *Praxis (Bern 1994).* 2006;95(4):99–106.
97. Lei U, Masmas TN, Frentz G. Occupational non-melanoma skin cancer. *Acta Derm Venereol.* 2001;81(6):415–417.
98. Simeonova PP, Luster MI. Mechanisms of arsenic carci - nogenicity: genetic or epigenetic mechanisms? *J Environ Pathol Toxicol Oncol.* 2000;19(3):281–286.
99. Wong SS, Tan KC, Goh CL. Cutaneous manifestations of chronic arsenicism: review of seventeen cases. *J Am Acad Dermatol.* 1998;38(2 pt 1):179–185.
100. Grodstein F, Speizer FE, Hunter DJ. A prospective study of incident squamous cell carcinoma of the skin in the nurses' health study. *J Natl Cancer Inst.* 1995; 87(14):1061–1066.
101. Fine JD, Johnson LB, Weiner M, Li KP, Suchindran C. Epidermolysis bullosa and the risk of life-threatening cancers: the National EB Registry experience, 1986–2006. *J Am Acad Dermatol.* 2009;60(2):203–211.
102. Kimonis VE, Goldstein AM, Pastakia B, et al. Clinical manifestations in 105 persons with nevoid basal cell carcinoma syndrome. *Am J Med Genet.* 1997;69(3): 299–308.
103. Kovach BT, Stasko T. Skin cancer after transplantation. *Transplant Rev (Orlando).* 2009;23(3):178–189.
104. Guenova E, Lichte V, Hoetzenecker W, et al. Nodular malignant melanoma and multiple cutaneous neoplasms under immunosuppression with azathioprine. *Melanoma Res.* 2009;19(4):271–273.
105. Berg D, Otley CC. Skin cancer in organ transplant recipients: Epidemiology, pathogenesis, and management. *J Am Acad Dermatol.* 2002;47(1):1–17; quiz 18–20.
106. Ulrich C, Degen A, Patel MJ, Stockfleth E. Sunscreens in organ transplant patients. *Nephrol Dial Transplant.* 2008;23(6):1805–1808.
107. Johnson TM, Rowe DE, Nelson BR, Swanson NA. Squamous cell carcinoma of the skin (excluding lip and oral mucosa). *J Am Acad Dermatol.* 1992;26(3 Pt 2):467–484.
108. Clifford GM, Polesel J, Rickenbach M, et al. Cancer risk in the Swiss HIV Cohort Study: associations with immunodeficiency, smoking, and highly active antiretroviral therapy. *J Natl Cancer Inst.* 2005;97(6): 425–432.
109. Karagas MR, Cushing GL, Jr., Greenberg ER, Mott LA, Spencer SK, Nierenberg DW. Non-melanoma skin cancers and glucocorticoid therapy. *Br J Cancer.* 2001;85(5): 683–686.
110. Jensen AO, Thomsen HF, Engebjerg MC, et al. Use of oral glucocorticoids and risk of skin cancer and non-Hodgkin's lymphoma: a population-based case-control study. *Br J Cancer.* 2009;100(1):200–205.
111. Freiman A, Bird G, Metelitsa AI, Barankin B, Lauzon GJ. Cutaneous effects of smoking. *J Cutan Med Surg.* 2004;8(6):415–423.
112. Hong DS, Reddy SB, Prieto VG, et al. Multiple squamous cell carcinomas of the skin after therapy with sorafenib combined with tipifarnib. *Arch Dermatol.* 2008;144(6):779–782.
113. Bevona C, Goggins W, Quinn T, Fullerton J, Tsao H. Cutaneous melanomas associated with nevi. *Arch Dermatol.* 2003;139(12):1620–1624; discussion 1624.
114. Menzies SW, Gutenev A, Avramidis M, Batrac A, McCarthy WH. Short-term digital surface microscopic monitoring of atypical or changing melanocytic lesions. *Arch Dermatol.* 2001;137(12):1583–1589.
115. Kittler H, Guitera P, Riedl E, et al. Identification of clinically featureless incipient melanoma using sequential

dermoscopy imaging. *Arch Dermatol.* 2006;142(9):1113–1119.
116. Altamura D, Avramidis M, Menzies SW. Assessment of the optimal interval for and sensitivity of short-term sequential digital dermoscopy monitoring for the diagnosis of melanoma. *Arch Dermatol.* 2008;144(4):502–506.
117. MacKie RM, English J, Aitchison TC, Fitzsimons CP, Wilson P. The number and distribution of benign pigmented moles (melanocytic naevi) in a healthy British population. *Br J Dermatol.* 1985;113(2):167–174.
118. Siskind V, Darlington S, Green L, Green A. Evolution of melanocytic nevi on the faces and necks of adolescents: a 4 y longitudinal study. *J Invest Dermatol.* 2002;118(3):500–504.
119. Soltani K, Bernstein JE, Lorincz AL. Eruptive nevocytic nevi following erythema multiforme. *J Am Acad Dermatol.*1979;1(6):503–505.
120. Szepietowski J, Wasik F, Szepietowski T, Wlodarczyk M, Sobczak-Radwan K, Czyz W. Excess benign melanocytic naevi in renal transplant recipients. *Dermatology.* 1997;194(1):17–19.
121. Duvic M, Lowe L, Rapini RP, Rodriguez S, Levy ML. Eruptive dysplastic nevi associated with human immunodeficiency virus infection. *Arch Dermatol.* 1989;125(3):397–401.
122. Fisher NM, Schaffer JV, Berwick M, Bolognia JL. Breslow depth of cutaneous melanoma: impact of factors related to surveillance of the skin, including prior skin biopsies and family history of melanoma. *J Am Acad Dermatol.* 2005;53(3):393–406.
123. Halpern AC. The use of whole body photography in a pigmented lesion clinic. *Dermatol Surg.* 2000;26(12):1175–1180.
124. Nehal KS, Oliveria SA, Marghoob AA, et al. Use of and beliefs about baseline photography in the management of patients with pigmented lesions: a survey of dermatology residency programmes in the United States. *Melanoma Res.* 2002;12(2):161–167.
125. Carli P, Nardini P, Crocetti E, De Giorgi V, Giannotti B. Frequency and characteristics of melanomas missed at a pigmented lesion clinic: a registry-based study. *Melanoma Res.* 2004;14(5):403–407.
126. Osborne JE, Chave TA, Hutchinson PE. Comparison of diagnostic accuracy for cutaneous malignant melanoma between general dermatology, plastic surgery and pigmented lesion clinics. *Br J Dermatol.* 2003;148(2):252–258.
127. Johnson TM, Chang A, Redman B, et al. Management of melanoma with a multidisciplinary melanoma clinic model. *J Am Acad Dermatol.* 2000;42(5 Pt 1):820–826.
128. Feldman SR, Fleischer AB, Jr. Skin examinations and skin cancer prevention counseling by US physicians: a long way to go. *J Am Acad Dermatol.* 2000;43(2 pt 1):234–237.
129. Halpern AC, Mandal SK. Role of dermatologists in treating melanoma. *J Natl Compr Canc Netw.* 2006;4(7):695–702.
130. Edman RL, Wolfe JT. Prevention and early detection of malignant melanoma. *Am Fam Physician.* 2000;62(10):2277–2285.
131. Eide MJ, Weinstock MA, Clark MA. The association of physician-specialty density and melanoma prognosis in the United States, 1988 to 1993. *J Am Acad Dermatol.* 2009;60(1):51–58.
132. Hunter S, Wells KJ, Jacobsen PB, et al. Assessment of elementary school students' sun protection behaviors. *Pediatr Dermatol.* 2010;27(2):182–188.
133. Dulon M, Weichenthal M, Blettner M, et al. Sun exposure and number of nevi in 5- to 6-year-old European children. *J Clin Epidemiol.* 2002;55(11):1075–1081.
134. Gandini S, Sera F, Cattaruzza MS, et al. Meta-analysis of risk factors for cutaneous melanoma: I. Common and atypical naevi. *Eur J Cancer.* 2005;41(1):28–44.
135. Kyle JW, Hammitt JK, Lim HW, et al. Economic evaluation of the US Environmental Protection Agency's SunWise program: sun protection education for young children. *Pediatrics.* 2008;121(5):e1074–e1084.
136. Dobbinson SJ, Wakefield MA, Jamsen KM, et al. Weekend sun protection and sunburn in Australia trends (1987–2002) and association with SunSmart television advertising. *Am J Prev Med.* 2008;34(2):94–101.
137. Dobbinson S, Wakefield M, Hill D, et al. Prevalence and determinants of Australian adolescents' and adults' weekend sun protection and sunburn, summer 2003–2004. *J Am Acad Dermatol.* 2008;59(4):602–614.
138. Hossler EW, Conroy MP. YouTube as a source of information on tanning bed use. *Arch Dermatol.* 2008;144(10):1395–1396.
139. Paul C, Tzelepis F, Parfitt N, Girgis A. How to improve adolescents' sun protection behavior? Age and gender issues. *Am J Health Behav.* 2008;32(4):387–398.
140. Weinstock MA. The struggle for primary prevention of skin cancer. *Am J Prev Med.* 2008;34(2):171–172.
141. Westerdahl J, Ingvar C, Masback A, Jonsson N, Olsson H. Risk of cutaneous malignant melanoma in relation to use of sunbeds: further evidence for UV-A carcinogenicity. *Br J Cancer.* 2000;82(9):1593–1599.
142. Robinson JK, Kim J, Rosenbaum S, Ortiz S. Indoor tanning knowledge, attitudes, and behavior among young adults from 1988–2007. *Arch Dermatol.* 2008;144(4):484–488.
143. Kasparian NA, Meiser B, Butow PN, Simpson JM, Mann GJ. Genetic testing for melanoma risk: a prospective cohort study of uptake and outcomes among Australian families. *Genet Med.* 2009;11(4):265–278.
144. Kraemer KH, DiGiovanna JJ, Moshell AN, Tarone RE, Peck GL. Prevention of skin cancer in xeroderma pigmentosum with the use of oral isotretinoin. *N Engl J Med.* 1988;318(25):1633–1637.
145. Goldberg LH, Hsu SH, Alcalay J. Effectiveness of isotretinoin in preventing the appearance of basal cell

carcinomas in basal cell nevus syndrome. *J Am Acad Dermatol.* 1989;21(1):144–145.
146. Martinez JC, Otley CC, Euvrard S, Arpey CJ, Stasko T. Complications of systemic retinoid therapy in organ transplant recipients with squamous cell carcinoma. *Dermatol Surg.* 2004;30(4 Pt 2):662–666.
147. Thorne EG. Long-term clinical experience with a topical retinoid. *Br J Dermatol.* 1992;127(Suppl 41): 31–36.
148. Euvrard S, Verschoore M, Touraine JL, et al. Topical retinoids for warts and keratoses in transplant recipients. *Lancet.* 1992;340(8810):48–49.

5

ULTRAVIOLET CARCINOGENESIS AND IMMUNE SUPPRESSION

STEPHEN E. ULLRICH

Introduction

Skin cancer is the most prevalent cancer diagnosed in the industrialized world. Estimates suggest approximately 1.5 million new cases of skin cancer will be diagnosed in the United States this year. Approximately 1 of 5 Americans will be diagnosed with a skin cancer during their lifetime. Melanoma now is the most common cancer reported in young adults 25 to 29 years old. Estimates suggest that 100,000 to 150,000 new cases of melanoma will be diagnosed in 2010, and approximately 11,000 Americans a year die from skin cancer (see The American Academy of Dermatology Web site http://www.aad.org/media/background.factsheets/fact_skincancer.html) for latest skin cancer statistics).[1] Skin cancer ranks among the top 5 most costly cancers to treat in America, presenting a major public health problem.[2,3]

Early during the 20th century, it was recognized that sunlight plays a role in skin cancer induction, and by the middle of the century, it was recognized that the ultraviolet (UV) radiation in sunlight was responsible for inducing nonmelanoma skin cancer.[4] UV-induced mutations in important tumor suppressor genes, such as *p53* and *ptch1*, play critical roles in the induction of squamous and basal cell carcinoma.[5,6] Epidemiologic data strongly suggest that intermediate sunlight exposure, especially early in life, is associated with melanoma induction.[7–10] In addition to its direct carcinogenic effect, UV exposure contributes to skin cancer induction by suppressing the immune response. This was first recognized by Margaret Kripke and colleagues in the early 1970s.[11] Since these early studies were published, the phenomenon of UV-induced immune suppression has been reproduced in a variety of experimental animal systems by a variety of laboratories around the world. UV exposure also has been found to suppress certain aspects of the immune response in humans, at doses similar to those that induce immune suppression in mice.[12] This chapter reviews the association between UV-induced immunosuppression and carcinogenesis, concentrating on the mechanisms involved.

The Role of Sunlight in Skin Cancer Induction

During the latter part of the 19th and the early part of the 20th centuries, dermatologists recognized the skin cancer-promoting properties of sunlight.[13,14] Subsequent animal experiments confirmed the carcinogenic properties of UV radiation,[15] and by the last third of the 20th century, it was well accepted that the UV radiation in sunlight causes skin cancer.[4,16]

Skin Cancer Action Spectrum

An important contribution to our understanding of the role that UVB radiation plays in skin cancer induction was provided by the skin cancer action spectrum. An action spectrum is the rate of a physiologic activity plotted against wavelength of light causing the effect. It shows which wavelengths of light are the most effective at inducing the biologic effect in question. Investigators from the Photobiology Unit at the Skin Cancer Hospital in Philadelphia and the Dermatology Department at the University of Utrecht generated an action spectrum to investigate the most effective wavelengths at inducing skin cancer in SKH:HR1 hairless mice. The so-called SCUP (Skin Cancer Utrecht-Philadelphia) action spectrum demonstrated maximal effectiveness at skin cancer induction in the UVB region of the solar spectrum (maximal activity at 293 nm).[17]

Signature Mutations

The second critical piece of data implicating UVB radiation in photocarcinogenesis was the existence of UVB "signature mutations" in tumor suppressor genes. Carcinogens induce characteristic mutations in cancer-related genes. UVB radiation induces two types of photolesions in irradiated DNA: cyclobutane pyrimidine dimers and pyrimidine (6-4) pyrimidone photoproducts (ie, 6-4 photoproducts). These photolesions result in covalent links between adjacent pyrimidines, and the miscoding that results during DNA replication induces either a single C to T or a double CC to TT transition. Because no other carcinogen induces these mutations, they are known as UVB signature mutations. Approximately 90% of human squamous cell carcinomas and 50% of basal cell carcinomas have UV signature mutations in the *p53* tumor suppressor gene.[18–20] Similarly, UVB signature mutations are found in a high proportion in UV-induced murine skin cancers.[21,22]

UVB signature mutations in the *ptch1* tumor suppressor gene have also been found in a high proportion of human basal cell carcinomas.[23] This "molecular epidemiology profile" provides powerful support for the role of UVB radiation in nonmelanoma skin cancer induction. The role of *p53* and *ptch1* in the signaling pathways that control tumor growth and the alterations of their function by solar UV radiation are not reviewed here. For excellent reviews, please see papers by Epstein, Ananthaswamy, and de Gruijl.[6,24,25]

The molecular alterations caused by UVB radiation that lead to melanoma induction are not as clear. It has been recognized for years that intermediate sun exposure and a history of sunburns is a leading risk factor for melanoma development.[9] However, UV signature mutations in genes that play a critical role in melanogenesis, such as *BRAF* and *NRAS* are not prominent. Hocker and Tsao[26] performed a "molecular meta-analysis" on the published literature to shed some light on this problem. They note that mutations in the *BRAF* oncogene, first reported by Davis and colleagues,[27] accounted for almost half of the melanoma mutations reported in the literature. The primary *BRAF* mutation reported (c1799 T to A transversion pVal600Glu) is not a UV signature mutation, nor were UV signature mutations prominent in mutated *NRAS*. Indeed, their analysis found that four highly recurrent, non-UVB mutations accounted for most of the mutations in *BRAF* and *NRAS*. UV signature mutations accounted for a significantly higher proportion of mutations in tumor suppressor genes (*CDKN2A*, *p53*). The authors conclude that their mutational analysis provided supportive evidence for UVB participation in mutating the tumor suppressor genes *CDKN2A* and *p53*, but less so for mutations in the oncogenes, *BRAF* and *NRAS*.[26]

A recent paper from Kraemer's group[28] supports the idea that UVB mutations in tumor suppressor genes play a role in melanoma. They analyzed mutations in the tumor suppressor gene *PTEN* (phosphatase and tensin homologue), one of the most frequently mutated human cancer genes. Laser microdissection was used to capture melanoma cells from cutaneous melanomas isolated from DNA repair-deficient xeroderma pigmentosum patients. A high proportion of the tumors (56%) had mutations in the *PTEN* gene, and 91% of those mutations were "UV signature" mutations occurring at dipyrimidine sites. The frequency of UV signature mutations in *PTEN* was significantly higher than that predicted by chance. Moreover, the observed mutations, primarily the mis-sense mutations found in exons 5 and 8, inactivate *PTEN* tumor suppressor function. These findings provide the first direct molecular evidence that UV-induced alterations in the tumor suppressor gene *PTEN* play an important role in human melanoma induction.[28]

Indirect DNA Damage

Indirect DNA damage may also be involved.[29] Both UVB and UVA activate reactive oxygen species and the subsequent induction of DNA damaging products such as 8-oxo-7, 8-dihydro-2'-deoxygaunosine (8-oxo-dG). 8-oxo-dG adducts can produce the transversions that ultimately result in the *BRAF v600* mutation so prominent in human melanoma. This idea is supported to a degree by animal data showing that UVA radiation can induce melanoma in zebra fish, and may explain melanoma production in UVA-irradiated opossums.[30–32] On the other hand, data generated using a mouse model suggests that UVB, and not UVA is the relevant wavelength for inducing melanoma.[33] Unlike nonmelanoma skin cancer, where a role for UVB signature mutations in the tumor suppressor genes *p53* and *ptch1* is clear, the UV wavelengths involved in melanoma induction, and the molecular lesions involved, remain elusive.

UV-Induced Immune Suppression

The phenomena and mechanisms that underlie UV-induced immune suppression have been studied intensely over the past 4 decades because UV-induced immune suppression represents a major risk factor for sunlight induced skin cancer. Three major pieces of information support the role of photoimmune suppression in photocarcinogenesis. First was the work by Kripke[11] that demonstrated that subcarcinogenic exposure to UV radiation allowed for the progressive growth of the highly antigenic UV-induced skin cancers.[11] In her initial experiments, Kripke attempted to transplant UV-induced skin cancers into age- and sex-matched syngeneic recipient animals. None of the tumor transplants took, and she was only able to successfully transplant the UV-induced skin cancers when the recipient mice were immunocompromised. This indicated that the UV-induced skin cancers were highly antigenic, and they were rejected by the immune system of the recipient mice. However, Kripke also found that she could successfully transplant UV-induced skin cancers into recipient mice that were exposed to a subcarcinogenic regimen of UV radiation.[11] This suggested that a short course of UV exposure suppressed the immune response. In subsequent studies, Kripke and colleagues demonstrated not only that UV radiation suppresses certain aspects of the immune response, but also that immune regulatory T cells are induced by UV exposure and they play a critical role in the induction of skin cancer in the primary UV-irradiated host.[34–38]

The second indication came from the increased prevalence of skin cancers on sun-exposed sites of immunosuppressed organ transplant patients. This observation, initially made in kidney transplant recipients, has now been confirmed with a variety of organ transplant recipients, and the data indicate a progressive increase in cancer frequency that is associated with the duration of immunosuppression.[39–42] Finally, Streilein and colleagues[43] reported that close to 100% of biopsy-proven skin cancer patients were susceptible to the immune suppressive effects of UV radiation, compared to 40% to 50% of the general population. This suggests that those more susceptible to immune suppression are more likely to develop skin cancers.

Contact Hypersensitivity and Delayed Type Hypersensitivity Studies

Much of what we know about the mechanisms underlying UV-induced immune suppression comes from experiments using mice. Although the initial tumor immunology experiments involved chronic long-term UV irradiation, two simpler in vivo assay systems have been employed to dissect the mechanisms involved: contact hypersensitivity (CHS) and classic delayed type hypersensitivity (DTH). These assays are shorter in duration, employ environmentally relevant doses of UV radiation that can be delivered in one exposure, and use defined antigens. For example, Elmets and colleagues[44] showed that it was possible to suppress CHS after a single low dose of UV radiation and he could transfer immune suppression to a nonirradiated mouse by transferring T cells. Similar results were obtained when DTH was used as the immunologic endpoint.[45,46] The action spectrum for UV-induced suppression, using CHS as the endpoint, indicated that the critical wavelengths were found in the UVB region of the solar spectrum.[47] UV exposure, at least when DTH was used as the endpoint, could suppress both the induction and the elicitation of immunity (ie, could suppress when given before immunization or before challenge), and could suppress secondary immune reactions.[48,49] We now know that the inability of UV to suppress the elicitation reaction when CHS is the endpoint is related to the inability of the T regulatory cells to traffic to the site of antigenic challenge (the ear).[50] Although it is clear that wavelengths in the UVB region of the solar spectrum are primarily responsible for suppressing primary immune reactions, UVA plays a critical role in suppressing secondary immune reactions and suppressing the memory response.[47,49,51]

Role of T Helper Cells

Three T helper cell subsets, T helper 1 (Th1), T helper 2 (Th2), and Interleukin (IL)-17 secreting T cells (Th17) have been identified based on their cytokine secretion pattern, transcriptional regulators, and the types of immune reactions they control. Th1 cells secrete interferon-gamma (IFN-γ) but not IL-4, and help in the production of complement fixing antibodies and the immune response to intracellular pathogens. The lineage specific transcription factors T-bet and HLX play a role in their development. Th2 cells secrete IL-4 but not IFN-γ, help with the production of non-complement-fixing antibodies and are generally involved in helping the immune response to parasites. The lineage specific transcription factors GATA-3 and MAF play a role in their development. Th17 cells, the newest described subset of T helper cells, secrete IL-17, help the immune response to extracellular bacteria and play a critical role in the induction of autoimmunity. The lineage specific transcription factors RORγτ and RORα are involved in the development of Th17 cells, which was recently reviewed by Dong.[52]

UV radiation suppresses Th1-driven immune reactions. UV exposure promotes the production of Th-2 cytokines, such as IL-4 and IL-10, and neutralizing their function blocks UV-induced immune suppression.[53–55] Injecting the Th1 promoting cytokine, IL-12, into mice reverses UV-induced immune suppression, reverses the activation of T regulatory cells and reverses tolerance induction.[56–59] Also, UV exposure suppresses the induction of complement fixing antibodies, suppresses the immune response to intracellular pathogens, such as tuberculosis, but does not effectively suppress an anti-parasite immune response.[60–62] The effect of UV radiation on Th17-mediated immune reactions remains to be seen.

Epidermal UV Photoreceptors

To induce a biologic effect, the electromagnetic energy of UV radiation must be absorbed by an epidermal photoreceptor and converted into a biologically recognizable signal. Experimental evidence suggests that 3 distinct UV photoreceptors are found in the skin: DNA, *trans*-urocanic acid (UCA), and membrane lipids (Fig 5–1).

DNA

Experimental data supporting DNA as the photoreceptor for immune suppression comes primarily from data generated by Kripke and colleagues. Kripke used two different approaches. In the first she employed *Monodelphis domestica*, the South American opossum, as her experimental model. These animals are unique, and very much different from mice and humans in that they possess an endogenous DNA repair enzyme that binds to pyrimidine dimers in UV-damaged DNA. When activated by visible photoreactivating light, the repair enzyme splits the dimer and returns the DNA to its original conformation. These marsupials are susceptible to the immune suppressive effects of UV radiation, as evidenced by the fact that their CHS response was suppressed by UVB radiation in a dose-dependant fashion. When the endogenous repair enzyme system was activated with visible light following UV exposure, the immune suppression was abrogated.

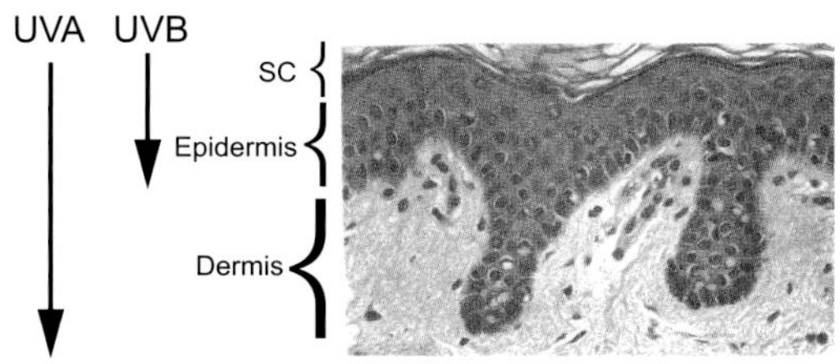

Chromophore	Origin	Mode of Action	Potential Targets	Ref #
cis-UCA	SC	Cytokine release APC function	DC or Mast Cells	73,81,83
DNA damage	Epidermis	Cytokine release APC function	DC or KC	65,66,68
bioactive lipids	Epidermis	Cytokine release	KC or Mast cells	84,93,119,120
tryptophan	Epidermis	metabolites bind AhR receptor and induce cytokine release	APC or Mast cells	92

Figure 5–1. UV-photoreceptors. To induce a biological effect, the electromagnetic energy contained within UV radiation must be absorbed by a photoreceptor and converted into a recognizable signal. UVB does not penetrate past the dermal-epidermal junction, yet system-wide immune suppression occurs. The receptors for UVB radiation, their location in the skin, mode of action and potential targets are depicted here. AhR, arylhydrocarbon receptor; APC, antigen presenting cell; cis-UCA, cis-urocanic acid; DC, dendritic cell; KC, keratinocytes; SC, stratum corneum.

When the sequence of events was reversed (visible light before UV radiation) no reversal of immune suppression was observed.[63]

The second approach used mice and liposomes to deliver an exogenous DNA repair enzyme, bacteriophage DNA repair enzyme T4 endonuclease 5 (T4N5), to the skin of UV-irradiated animals. Electron microscopy demonstrated that liposome encapsulated gold-labeled T4N5 could transverse keratinocyte membranes, and migrate into the nucleus of the target cells.[64] When liposomes containing the T4N5 were applied to the skin of UV-irradiated mice, the number of cyclobutane pyrimidine dimers in the irradiated skin was reduced, the suppression of CHS was reversed, and the induction of suppressor cells was abrogated.[65] Furthermore, applying the liposomes to UV-irradiated keratinocyte cultures reversed UV-induced IL-10 secretion.[66]

One consequence of UV exposure on epidermal Langerhans cells is an inhibition of their ability to present antigen to T cells.[67] Kripke wanted to know if UV-induced pyrimidine dimer formation was involved in this well-known UV-induced defect. Fluorescein isothiocyanate (FITC) positive draining lymph node cells from UV-irradiated FITC painted mice (presumably migrating epidermal Langerhans cells) were isolated. These cells then were treated with liposomes containing photolyase, a pyrimidine dimer specific repair enzyme purified from *Anacystis nidulans*. The mode of action of photolyase is similar to that of the *M. domestica* photorepair enzyme. The enzyme binds to pyrimidine dimers, and on subsequent exposure to photoreactivating light, the dimer splits, and the DNA returns to its original confirmation. Treating the FITC-positive draining lymph node cells with photolyase and photoreactivating light restored their antigen-presenting cell function, in that when the cells were injected into normal recipient mice, a vigorous CHS reaction to FITC was induced. Reversing the treatment, photoreactivating light before photolyase, had no restorative effect.[68]

Subsequently, these findings were confirmed using human volunteers. Wolf and colleagues[69,70] report that UV irradiation of human skin upregulates the production of epidermal IL-10 and Tumor Necrosis Factor-alpha (TNF-α) mRNA and protein, and applying T4N5–containing liposomes to the skin immediately after UV exposure reverses cytokine production. Stege and colleagues[71] applied the photolyase from *A. nidulans* to the skin of UV-irradiated human volunteers. Applying photoreactivating light after the photolyase (but not before) diminished the numbers of pyrimidine dimers in the skin of the UV-irradiated individuals and reversed the UV-induced suppression of the elicitation of CHS to nickel. Kuchel and colleagues[72] report similar findings in regard to solar simulated-induced suppression to recall reactions in humans. These studies provide compelling evidence supporting the hypothesis that DNA is a major epidermal photoreceptor for UV-induced immune suppression.

Trans-UCA

Based on similar action spectrums for UV-induced immune suppression of CHS and the absorption of UVB radiation by *trans*-urocanic acid, De Fabo and Noonan[73] proposed that *trans*-UCA serves as an epidermal photoreceptor for UV-induced immune suppression. Further they suggested that the photoisomerized product, *cis*-UCA could serve as an immunosuppressive mediator. These provocative insights prompted many photobiologists to examine the immunosuppressive properties of *cis*-UCA. A series of early papers showed that applying *cis*-UCA to mice by a variety of routes (IV, topical, or intradermal) resulted in immune suppression.[74–76] An action spectrum for isomerization of UCA in the skin was generated showing maximal isomerization by UVB wavelengths.[77]

Cis-UCA was found in the serum of UV-irradiated mice and antibodies to *cis*-UCA could reverse UV-induced suppression of DTH, whereas the suppression of CHS was less sensitive to reversal by monoclonal anti-*cis*-UCA.[78–80] Perhaps more importantly, antibodies to *cis*-UCA can delay skin cancer formation in UV-irradiated mice.[81] These findings confirm the important role *cis*-UCA plays in the generation of immune suppression.[82,83]

Although much is known about *cis*-UCA-induced immune suppression, little is known about the molecular events that lead to immune suppression. A particular vexing problem is identifying the receptor to which *cis*-UCA binds to initiate immune suppression. Previous studies indicated that a cytokine cascade was involved in the pathway of events leading to immune suppression, and one of the first steps in the cascade was the UV-induced secretion of the lipid mediator of inflammation, platelet-activating factor (PAF), by irradiated keratinocytes.[55,84]

It is theorized that PAF receptor binding plays a role in *cis*-UCA induced immune suppression. We employed a series of selective PAF receptor antagonists to block binding. We also injected *cis*-UCA treated mice with ketanserin, a serotonin (5-HT) receptor antagonist that was included as a negative control. To our surprise, ketanserin blocked *cis*-UCA and UV-induced immune suppression. This prompted an in-depth examination of serotonin receptor binding in *cis*-UCA and UV-induced immune suppression. First, we noted that the structure of serotonin and *cis*-UCA in aqueous solution were similar. Second, we found that serotonin specific antibody immuno-precipitated *cis*-UCA, and *cis*-UCA specific antibody immuno-precipitated serotonin. Furthermore, antibodies to serotonin blocked *cis*-UCA-induced immune suppression, and antibodies to *cis*-UCA blocked serotonin-induced immune suppression. Third, *cis*-UCA bound to the human 5-HT_{2A} receptor with relatively high affinity (K_d = 4.6 nM) and *cis*-UCA activated calcium flux when added to 5-HT_{2A} positive cells lines. Calcium flux was inhibited when the cells were pretreated with ketanserin. Finally, we noted that *cis*-UCA induced immune suppression was preferentially inhibited by 5-HT_{2A}, and not 5-HT_1, or 5-HT_{2C} receptor antagonists. These findings support the hypothesis that *cis*-UCA mediates immune suppression by binding to the serotonin receptor.[85] Studies by Slominski and colleagues[86] have indicated that serotonin is secreted by epidermal cells following UV irradiation. Our findings suggest that UV-induced epidermal serotonin may play a role in cutaneous immune regulation.

Lipids

UV-irradiation of keratinocytes activates a variety of transcription factors, which induces cytokine secretion.[66,87] Evidence exists suggesting that a DNA-independent pathway can play a role in activating transcription. Devary and colleagues UV-irradiated enucleated HeLa cells and found that both AP-1 and NF-Îb, two transcription activators that activate cytokine production, were activated.[88,89] These findings were confirmed by others, using a keratinocyte-like cell line and UVB rather than UVC radiation.[90,91]

Osmotic shock, which causes membrane damage independent of DNA, also activates NF-kb and AP-1.[89] Rosette and Karin[89] suggested that membrane growth factor receptor activation was the signal that initiated non-nuclear UVB activation of cells. Fritsche and colleagues[92] have recently discovered that the receptor involved is the arylhydrocarbon receptor. Their data indicates that tryptophan acts as a UV chromophore, and following UV irradiation, a tryptophan derivative, 6-formylindolo[3,2-b] carazole is formed. This intracellular photoproduct then activates the arylhydrocarbon receptor, which in turn activates prostaglandin synthase-2 (also know as cyclooxygenase-2: COX-2). No activation of 6-formylindolo[3,2-b]carazole was found in tryptophan-starved cells, nor was COX-2 expression up regulated in UV-irradiated arylhydrocarbon receptor knockout mice. Further support for the role of lipids as a photoreceptor comes from the observations that treating keratinocytes with UV-irradiating phosphatidylcholine activates IL-10 production and that injecting the irradiated phospholipid into mice induces apoptosis and immune suppression.[84,93]

Cellular Targets in the Skin

The ability of UV radiation to penetrate into the skin is limited. Almost all of the UVB is absorbed in the epidermis and the UVA, which can penetrate deeper, is mostly absorbed in the upper layers of the dermis (Fig 5–2). Regardless, UV exposure has systemic

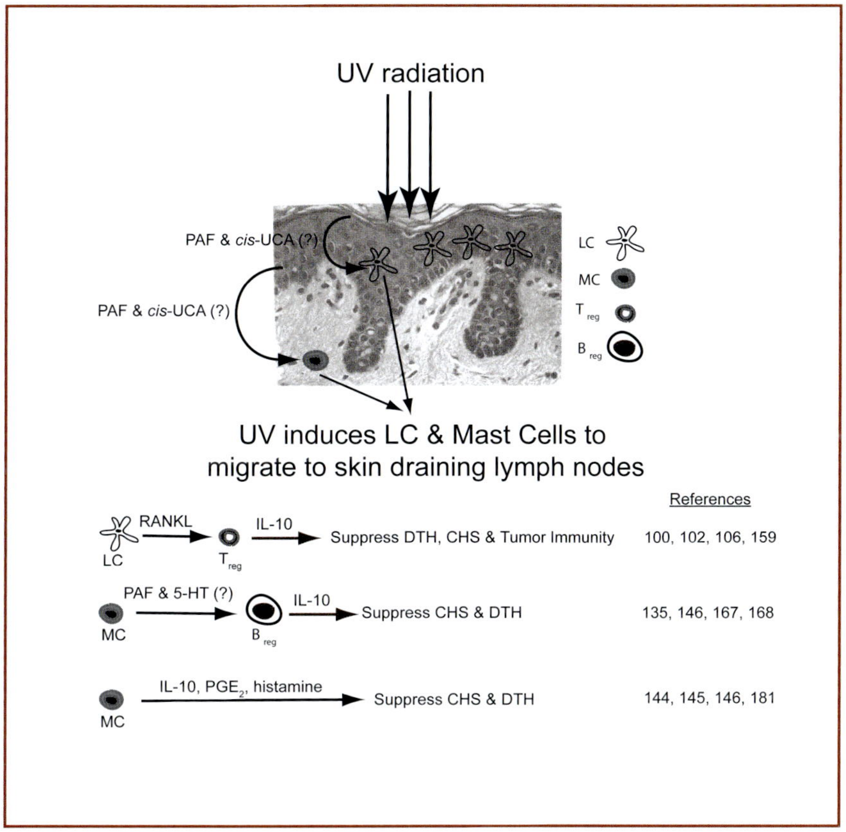

Figure 5–2. UV-induced migration of immune regulatory Langerhans cells (LC) and mast cells (MC) provides one mechanism to transmit the immune suppressive signal from the skin to the immune system. For example, UV-induced cis-UCA, PAF and RANK ligand (RANKL) are probably involved in inducing LC and MC migration. Once in the lymph nodes LC and MC may activate other regulatory elements (T regulatory cells-T_{regs}; B regulatory Cells-B_{regs}) to induce immune suppression. Alternatively, the products released by UV-activated MC and LC (IL-10, histamine, PGE_2,) may directly interact with effector cells to suppress their function.

effects. This is best illustrated by the fact that UV-irradiation at one body site suppresses the immune response to haptens or antigens introduced at distant un-irradiated sites.[45,94] Cellular migration in vivo explains how the immune suppressive signal is transmitted from the skin to distant immune organs.

Langerhans Cells

The traditional textbook definition of Langerhans cells suggests that they are the primary antigen-presenting cells found in the skin. They reside as immature cells in the epidermis, and on encountering antigen, they migrate from the skin to the draining lymph nodes, become mature, and present antigen to T cells. However, newer studies on Langerhans cell function have led immunologists to question and redefine the role of Langerhans cells.[95] This re-evaluation of Langerhans cell function resulted primarily from data published in 3 independent studies in 2005.[96–98] In these experiments, the investigators expressed a diphtheria toxin receptor driven by the langerin (CD207) promoter, thereby making a transgenic mouse that selectively expressed the diphtheria toxin receptor in Langerhans cells. Mice normally do not express the diphtheria toxin receptor, so mice are impervious to the toxic effects of diphtheria. Injecting diphtheria toxin into the langerin-diphtheria-toxin receptor positive mice resulted in a Langerhans cell-deficient animal. The Langerhans cell-l- mice were then sensitized with a contact allergen, and the immune response was measured. Contrary to expected results, contact sensitization of Langerhans-depleted mice resulted in an CHS response. This indicated that Langerhans cells were not essential for inducing cutaneous immunity to contact allergens and another cell must be involved. Dermal dendritic cells may in fact represent the critical dermal antigen presenting cells.[98,99] The exact role of epidermal Langerhans cell is not clear, but they could serve primarily as immune regulatory cells.[97]

Immune regulation by Langerhans cells is a recognized function. UV exposure destroys the dendritic Langerhans cells network in the skin, and immunization through UV-irradiated skin results in the induction of immune tolerance.[44,100] Furthermore, FITC positive, Ia+ cells isolated from the lymph nodes of UV-irradiated mice fail to induce CHS when injected into recipient mice.[67,68] When Ia+ Langerhans cells isolated from the skin were exposed to UV radiation in vitro, and then conjugated with hapten, they failed to induce immunity when injected into normal recipient mice.[101,102] UV-irradiated Langerhans cells preferentially activate Th2 cells and induce clonal anergy in Th1 cells.[103–105]

A molecular mechanism links UV-induced alterations in Langerhans cell function to immune modulation in distant lymph organs.[106] UV-irradiation of keratinocytes upregulates a wide variety of gene products such as growth factors, cytokines and inflammatory mediators. The transcription factor NF-κb is activated following UV exposure as is the *R*eceptor *A*ctivator of *N*F-κb (RANK) and its ligand, RANKL. Based on these observations, and the finding that RANKL is over expressed in psoriatic skin, Loser and colleagues[106] generated transgenic mice expressing RANKL in the skin under the control of the keratin-14 promoter. CHS in these transgenic animals was significantly depressed, and the numbers of T regulatory cells in the lymph nodes of the transgenic mice was significantly increased. Co-culturing Langerhans cells (which normally express RANKL) isolated from the RANKL-transgenic mice with wild-type CD4+ CD25+ T cells activated the proliferation of the T regulatory cells. Furthermore, when these RANKL-transgenic mice were treated with monetason fourate, a chemical that depletes epidermal Langerhans cells, a significant depletion of lymph node T regulatory cells was observed.

To link RANKL expression on the Langerhans cells with UV-induced immune suppression, 2 experiments were performed. In the first, UV irradiated mice were injected with RANK-Fc, which blocks RANK binding to its receptor. Treating the mice with RANK-Fc totally blocked UV-induced immune suppression. In addition, skin was obtained from RANKL deficient mice, or wild-type controls, and the skin was grafted onto the backs of age- and sex-matched wild-type recipients. Hapten sensitization through UV-irradiated RANKL+/+ skin (normal skin) resulted in immune suppression. However, when the mice that received RANKL−/− skin were exposed to UV and sensitized with hapten, no immune suppression was found. These data indicate that RANKL plays a role in the induction of immune suppression. Furthermore, they support the hypothesis that

UV-irradiated Langerhans cells transmit the suppressive signal from the skin to the lymph nodes, where they activate T regulatory cells.[106]

Keratinocytes

The release of a variety of immune regulatory factors by UV-irradiated keratinocytes represents another mechanism by which an immunosuppressive signal is transmitted from the skin to the immune system. Keratinocyte-derived PAF, prostaglandin E_2, 5-HT, histamine, calcitonin gene related peptide (CGRP), a-melanocyte stimulating hormone, IL-10, and IL-4, are examples of immune regulatory factors released following UV exposure that play a role in UV-induced immune suppression. [53,54,84,85,107–110] The exact mechanism through which each of these factors contributes to immune suppression is not exactly clear.[55] Data generated in my lab indicate that one of the first steps in the pathway leading to immune suppression is the secretion of the lipid mediator of inflammation, PAF.[84] As its name implies, PAF activates a wide variety of cells including platelets, monocytes, mast cells, and polymorphonuclear leukocytes. It is a transcriptional activator that turns on the transcription of genes involved in UV-induced immune suppression (ie, PGE_2 and IL-10).[111] PAF is secreted in response to keratinocyte damage, such as occurs following UV irradiation, oxidative stress, or chemical toxicity.[112–114]

PAF plays a role in the induction of apoptosis and cytokine secretion following UV irradiation of the skin and in UV-induced sensitivity to pain.[115–117] Because PAF upregulates the production of PGE_2 a factor that is critical for the induction of immune suppression, we tested the hypothesis that PAF activates cytokine production and drives UV-induced immune suppression.[107,118] PAF activates COX-2 production and activates the transcription of IL-10. We found that treating mice with selective PAF-receptor antagonists blocked UV-induced immune suppression.[84] Moreover, when PAF receptor deficient mice were exposed to UV, no immune suppression was observed.[119] Similarly, when UV-irradiated oxidized phosphatidylcholine was injected into mice, immune suppression was activated, it was blocked when the mice were pretreated with a selective PAF receptor antagonist.[84] Subsequent studies have confirmed the immune suppressive function of PAF, and that PAF and PAF-like oxidized phospholipids contribute to UV-induced cutaneous damage.[93,120,121]

The production of PAF is under tight regulation, and PAF-acetylhydrolase serves as an anti-inflammatory molecule by rapidly degrading PAF.[122] Keratinocytes accumulate the osmolyte taurine and upregulate the expression of its transporter, TAUT, in response to osmotic stress and UV radiation.[123,124] TAUT−/− mice are highly susceptible to the immunosuppressive effects of UV radiation, and injecting these mice with PAF receptor antagonists blocks UV-induced immune suppression. UV may damage cellular membranes, releasing PAF, which results in immune suppression. Taurine may serve as a endogenous factor that protects cytoplasmic membranes from stress, and in doing so, modulates PAF production and interferes with immune suppression.[125] Not only do these data further confirm the immune suppressive function of PAF, but they also further indicate the important role that UV-induced modulation of membrane lipid function plays in the induction of immune suppression.

It is not entirely clear what the cellular targets of the immunomodulatory cytokines and factors released by UV-irradiated keratinocytes are. Langerhans cells are an obvious target, and UV-induced factors such as IL-10 suppress Langerhans cells antigen presenting cell function.[126] Histamine and PGE_2 suppress the differentiation of Th1 cells, while promoting the differentiation of Th2 cells (a consequence of total body UV exposure), in part by modulating dendritic cell function.[128–130] Similarly CGRP, which is released by nerve endings in UV-irradiated skin, inhibits Langerhans cell antigen presenting function; alpha-melanocyte stimulating hormone, through its ability to stimulate IL-10 production, does the same.[110,131,132]

Mast Cells

Mast cells were initially described as "Mastzellen" (well-fed cells) based on their granular appearance and metachromatic staining. Mast cells are derived from bone marrow CD34+ hematopoietic stem cells. Mast cell precursors circulate in the blood, and undergo final maturation/differentiation after they migrate into the peripheral tissue in which they ultimately reside.[133] The conventional wisdom regarding mast cell function is that they serve primarily as effector cells in IgE-mediated allergic inflammation, in part through the release of preformed mediators on degranulation. It now is clear that this view of mast cell function is very limited, and we know that mast cells regulate adaptive immune reactions, in part through the regulated release of immune regulatory cytokines and factors.[134]

Some of the very first data to suggest that mast cells can regulate adaptive immunity were generated by photoimmunologists. Streilein and colleagues[109] observed that UV-induced CGRP suppressed the induction of CHS. They further noted that CGRP mediated its effect by activating mast cells to release TNF-α, and suggested that "calcitonin gene related peptide *or UV radiation* impairs CHS via an effect on mast cells." Hart and colleagues[135] later observed that mast cell deficient mice were immune competent, in that they were capable of generating a vigorous CHS reaction when hapten was applied to the skin. But when these mice were exposed to UV radiation prior to contact sensitization, no immune suppression was noted. Furthermore, when wild-type bone marrow derived mast cells were injected into the dermis of the mast cell deficient mice, and the reconstituted animals were exposed to UV radiation, immune suppression was restored. Failure to see immune suppression in the mast cell deficient mice, and reconstituting the effect in the "mast cell knock-in" mice, provided compelling evidence that mast cells are critical for UV-induced immune suppression.[135–137] Mast cell derived IL-10 has recently been shown to regulate skin pathology and the chronic inflammation associated with UV exposure.[138]

Mast cells also play a role in UVA-induced immune suppression. In most of the studies described so far, the investigators have exposed immunologically naïve mice to UVB radiation, and then immunized them with antigen (either a contact allergen or a classic DTH-inducing antigen) and measured the effect UV exposure had on the induction of an immune response. As mentioned above, UVA is the major component of UV radiation in sunlight and can have deleterious effect on human health. Studies in mice and humans have shown that UVA suppresses secondary and memory immune reactions.[49,51,139–141] Mast cells are involved in UVA-induced immune suppression in that no immune suppression was found in UVA-irradiated mast cell deficient mice.[142]

Because mast cells are located in the dermis, direct irradiation by UVB wavelengths is not possible, suggesting an indirect mechanism must be involved in activation. There is evidence that *cis*-UCA is involved by inducing mast cell degranulation, but this remains controversial.[143,144] Some have suggested that UV irradiation of the skin activates sensory nerves to secrete neuropeptides such as CGRP, substance P, alpha-melanocyte stimulating hormone, which then modulate mast cell function.[131] The absence of immune suppression in UV-irradiated mice pretreated with capsaicin, a chemical that depletes neuropeptides from sensory nerves in vivo, supports this hypothesis.[145]

Regardless of the mechanism by which mast cells are activated following UV exposure, ultimately, the immunosuppressive signal must be transmitted from the skin to the draining lymph node. Recent data indicate that unconventional mast cell migration provides yet another mechanism linking the UV-irradiated skin to the immune system. Inflammatory signals recruit mast cell precursors from the circulation to the periphery, where they mature and become effector cells. Within 6 hours of UV irradiation, dermal mast cells numbers increase as part of the inflammatory response. Surprisingly, within 24 hours of UV exposure, the mast cell number in the skin returns to baseline while the number in lymph nodes doubles—indicating mast cell migration from the skin to the lymph nodes.

To prove this, skin from green fluorescent protein (GFP) positive mice was grafted onto the backs of mast cell deficient animals, and the grafted mice were exposed to UV radiation. GFP+ mast cells were found in the draining lymph nodes of the UV-irradiated mast cell deficient recipient mice. Mast cell migration was required for immune suppression. Mast cells express CXCR4 on their surface and total body UV-irradiation up-regulates lymph node expression of CXCL12, the ligand for CXCR4. When UV-irradiated wild-type mice were injected with AMD3100, an antileukemia drug that is a CXCR4 antagonist, both mast cell migration and UV-induced immune suppression was abrogated. These findings indicate that UV-induced mast cell migration from the skin to the lymph nodes serves as one mechanism to transmit the immune suppressive signal from the skin to the immune system.[146]

Mast cells have been implicated in skin cancer susceptibility. Increased mast cell number is a bad prognostic indicator for melanoma, Merkel cell carcinoma, and nonmelanoma skin cancer.[147–150] It is assumed that the immunosuppressive ability of dermal mast cells influences tumor cell growth and progression, but this remains to be proven.

UV-Induced Immune Regulatory Cells

One of the hallmarks of UV-induced immune suppression is the ability to transfer immune suppression from the irradiated host to an unirradiated recipient. Early studies indicated that immune suppression was transferred by suppressor T cells, which are now known as T regulatory cells.[34,151,152]

T Regulatory Cells

T cells transfer immune suppression. Treating spleen cells isolated from UV-irradiated mice with anti-thymocyte serum and complement abrogates the suppression of tumor immunity by a Lyt1+2– T cell.[34,153,154] The cell responsible for UV-induced suppression of CHS was also shown to be a Lyt1+2– T cell.[44] Subsequent studies with newer reagents indicated that the UV-induced suppressor T cell was a CD4+, CD8– T cell.[155] Unfortunately, suppressor T cell research became stagnant, due in part to the inability to clone T suppressor cells, the failure to clone I-J, the putative suppressor T cell restriction factor, the failure to find any suppressor cell specific cell surface receptor, and the failure to identify any of the putative suppressor factors that were evoked to play a role in turning off immunity.

The breakthrough that revitalized the field was Sakaguchi's work demonstrating that removing the thymus of 3-day-old mice activates autoimmune disease when the mice grow to maturity. This suggested that self-reactive T cells were removed by thymectomy, and these cells controlled the induction of autoimmunity. To identify the cell responsible, different populations of T cells were injected into nude mice and the development of autoimmunity was monitored in the recipient mice. Injecting CD4+/CD25+ cells, but not CD4+/CD25– cells into mice suppressed the induction of autoimmunity.[152] Subsequent studies demonstrated that the newly described T regulatory cells were activated through a bona fide alpha beta (α/β) T cell receptor (TcR), and once activated, these cells secreted cytokines (IL-10 and TGF-β) associated with immune regulation.[156] UV-induced suppressor T cells were shown to be bona fide T cells. The CD4+, CD8– cells expressed the (α/β) TcR, were major histocompatibility complex restricted, and secreted IL-10. These cells blocked antigen-presenting cell function in vitro and transferred immune suppression, in an antigen-specific fashion, when injected into naïve recipient mice.[157]

IL-10 secreting T cells which expressed the negative co-stimulatory molecule CTLA-4, and exhibited negative regulatory function were isolated from the lymph nodes of UV-irradiated mice.[158] Neutralizing anti-IL-10 antibody blocked the suppressive function of these cells; subsequent studies demonstrated that the suppressor cells express the classic T regulatory cell phenotype (ie, CD4+/CD25+) and could not be induced in IL-10 knockout mice.[158,159] Similarly, Ghoreishi and Dutz[160] found that epicutaneous application of antigen through UV-irradiated skin, activates CD4+/CD25+ IL-10 secreting T regulatory cells. Of equal importance was the observation that the UV-induced T regulatory cells express FOXP3, the master controller of T regulatory cell development and activity.[161,162]

Natural Killer T (NKT) Cells

Moodycliffe et al[163] found that NKT cells could also transfer UV-induced immune suppression. These lymphocytes were originally called NKT cells because they expressed cell surface markers that are found on both T cells (CD4, α/β T cell receptor) and NK cells (NK1.1 in mice or CD161 in humans). NKT cells are unique in that they are restricted by CD1, a nonpolymorphic major histocompatibility complex-like molecule, and express a limited diversity of the

T cell antigen receptor on their surface. Also NKT cells secrete cytokines within hours of activation, which is believed to contribute to their ability to regulate, either positively or negatively, adaptive immune reactions.[164] NKT cells are further marked by the expression of T cell (CD4) and NK cell (Ly49b/DX5) markers on the surface, plus CD1 restriction and the secretion of a large amount of IL-4 and IL-10 within hours of activation.[163] These cells also play a role in UVA-induced immune suppression.[51] More recent findings indicate that the cells bind CD1-tertramers, suggesting that they are invariant NKT cells[165] Whether they directly suppress tumor rejection in vivo, or activate other cells to become T regulatory cells, by virtue of IL-10 secretion, remains to be seen.

B Cells

A third cell type that can transfer immune suppression from a UV-irradiated host to a nonirradiated recipient is the B cell. Although the immune regulatory role of B cells is not as widely appreciated as that of T regulatory cells, a growing number of papers in the literature document immune regulation by B cells.[166,167] As expected, lymph node cellularity was increased in UV-irradiated mice, with increased numbers of B cells and dendritic cells. Both cell subsets were isolated and conjugated with hapten. The cells were then injected into age- and sex-matched recipients, and the effect this treatment had on CHS was measured. Transferring the CD11c dendritic cells from the lymph node of normal or UV-irradiated mice generated a vigorous immune reaction. When the B cells from the UV-irradiated mice were mixed with normal dendritic cells, and the mixture was injected into a normal recipient, CHS was suppressed. No suppression was seen when hapten-conjugated B cells isolated from normal mice were mixed with CD11c dendritic cells isolated from either normal or UV-irradiated recipients. Byrne and Halliday[168] also noted that the B cells secreted IL-10, which suppresses dendritic cell function.

Both PAF and 5-HT are involved in the generation of the suppressor B cells. No transfer of immune suppression is found when the B cells were isolated from mice injected with PAF and 5-HT receptor antagonists.[168] The critical role that IL-10 plays in UV-induced immune suppression was confirmed by demonstrating no immune suppression when B cells were transferred from UV-irradiated IL-10–/– mice.[168]

Human Photoimmunology

When toxicologists consider regulatory limits on immunotoxicant exposure levels, they often suggest a tenfold increase above the amount that causes immune suppression in animals primarily because of the uncertainty involved.[169] When it comes to UV radiation, the immunotoxin that all humans are exposed to on a daily level, there is little uncertainty about the dose of UV that modulates immune function in humans. That is because the effect of UV on the human immune system is well known. As in mice, UV exposure suppresses DTH and CHS in irradiated human volunteers.[139,170–174]

The photoreceptors in humans are similar to those described in mice. The action spectrum for UV-induced suppression of antigen-presenting cell function and erythema in humans shows similar wavelengths are involved.[175,176] Also, as mentioned above, applying liposomes containing DNA repair enzymes to human skin overcomes UV-induced immune suppression, supporting a role for DNA as a UV photoreceptor.[69–72] Similarly, *cis*-UCA is found in human skin following UV exposure, and there is ample evidence that *cis*-UCA suppresses human immune function.[12,177,178] UV-irradiation of human skin results in the production of many of the immune regulatory cytokines that play a role in UV-induced immune suppression in animal studies, including IL-10, PGE_2, TNF-α, although the exact cell that secretes IL-10 in humans following UV exposure needs clarification.[179–185] Experimental data demonstrate that the dose of UV needed to induce immune suppression in animals and humans is comparable.[94,186]

Sunscreen Photobiology

In the area of sunscreen photobiology, studies with human volunteers led to valuable insights into the wavelengths and immune reactions involved rather than just confirming data first generated using experimental animal systems. Because no UVC radiation reaches the earth's surface, the chemical filters used in sunscreens are designed to block UVB and more recently UVA but not UVC. Unfortunately, many early sunscreen studies using mice irradiated with UVC-containing FS-40 sunlamps came to the erroneous conclusion that sunscreens do not block UV-induced immune suppression.[188]

Another important consideration involved the type of immune response used as the endpoint. For practical, ethical, and financial reasons, it is more appropriate to measure the effect UV exposure has on recall reactions in humans, rather than studying the effect UV has on the induction of the immune response. When Moyal and colleagues[139] and Damian and co-workers[173] measured the effect of sunscreens on the UV-induced suppression of the recall reaction, they found that narrow spectrum UVB-blocking sunscreens had little effect, whereas broad-spectrum UVA-absorbing sunscreens provided maximal protection. These findings led to an intense examination of the wavelengths that suppress secondary immune reactions, and confirmed that UVA suppresses secondary and memory reactions in humans.[140,141,174,189,190] UVA radiation is immune suppressive, an observation that was generally overlooked by mouse photoimmunologists who were looking primarily at the effects of UVB on the induction of the immune response.

On the other hand, other studies suggest that UVA exposure is immune protective. Exposure to a large nonimmunosuppressive dose of UVA followed by an immunosuppressive dose of UVB resulted in no immune suppression.[191] This immune protection may be due to the modulation of cytokine and heme oxygenase production in the skin of mice first exposed to UVA radiation and then exposed to UVB.[192–194] Similar findings have been reported in humans first exposed to UVA and then UVB radiation.[172]

The question that arises is: is this a laboratory artifact or does UVA protection occur in nature, due to the fact that most of solar UV radiation is UVA? Although the answer is not clear, two things must be kept in mind. First, the shape of the dose response curve for UVA immune suppression is not linear, but rather a bell-shaped one, and no immune suppression is found at the high UVA doses.[195] Second, until very recently, most sunscreens provide maximal UVB protection and minimal protection in the UVA region of the solar spectrum. Using such a sunscreen to prevent sunburn may provide the high UVA exposure that conceivably could protect against immune suppression on subsequent exposure to UVB radiation.

Prevention and Early Interventional Strategies

Sun Avoidance and Sunscreen Use

This chapter reviewed the literature concerning the mechanisms underlying UV-induced immunosuppression and carcinogenesis. Understanding the mechanisms involved is important in order to generate new therapies to fight skin cancer. Clearly, sun avoidance is the best way to go, and the success of the Australia campaign of promoting sun avoidance and sunscreen use is having a positive effect.[196,197] Sunscreen usage prevents skin cancer induction in mice, and humans, in part by preventing immune suppression, and the formation of UV signature mutations in the *p53* gene in murine and/or human skin.[5,49,139,196–199] Sunscreen usage also blocks the formation of sunlight induced benign melanocyte nevi, a strong surrogate marker for melanoma risk.[200,201] The major problems with sunscreen use are that insufficient amounts are applied to the skin, most users fail to reapply the sunscreen during prolonged sun exposure, not all sunscreens provide broad-spectrum (both UVB and UVA) protection, and they work only when applied before sun exposure.

Interventional Horizons

If prevention is not achieved, it is possible to repair the damage after exposure. Liposomes containing DNA repair enzymes could be applied to UV-irradiated skin.[202] Applying T4N5-containing liposomes to xeroderma pigmentosum patients significantly reduced the annualized rate of new actinic keratoses compared to that found in patients treated with a placebo, suggesting that repairing pyrimidine dimer formation after UV exposure may contribute to preventing skin cancer in humans.[203]

There are a number of "downstream mediators" that play a prominent role in UV-induced immune suppression and photocarcinogenesis. Targeting many of them could result in skin cancer prevention. Treating UV-irradiated mice with selective PAF receptor antagonists has blocked skin cancer induction and progression. Similarly, administering selective serotonin receptor antagonists to UV-irradiated mice can block photocarcinogenesis, and the PAF and 5-HT receptor antagonists work synergistically to prevent skin cancer induction.[204] One of the downstream effects of UV-induced PAF is the upregulation of COX-2 activity. Treating UV-irradiated mice with selective COX-2 inhibitors blocks skin cancer induction and progression.[181,205] Another important UV-induced immune modulatory factor is IL-10. UV-induced carcinogenesis is severely impaired in IL-10-deficient mice.[159] Moreover, UV-induced T regulatory cells express the negative costimulatory factor CTLA-4 on their surface, and injecting UV-irradiated mice with antibodies to CTLA-4 significantly suppresses tumor induction.[206]

Nutritional supplements also modulate UV-induced immune suppression and carcinogenesis.[207] One that has been extensively studied is epigallocatechin-3-gallate, a polyphenol found in green tea. It prevents UV-induced photocarcinogenesis and UV-induced immune suppression.[208,209] The mechanism, interestingly enough, involves a novel function of the immune stimulatory cytokine, IL-12. IL-12 reverses UV-induced immune suppression, the activation of T regulatory cells, and UV-induced tolerance induction.[56,58,59,210] In addition to driving the activation of Th1 cells, IL-12 also accelerates DNA repair. Schwarz and colleagues noted that IL-12 treatment reduced UV-induced apoptosis in vitro and sunburn cells formation in vivo, reduced the formation of pyrimidine dimers following UV exposure and upregulated the expression of nucleotide excision repair genes. Furthermore, they observed that IL-12 was not able to reverse UV-induced immune suppression when injected into UV-irradiated DNA repair deficient mice.[211,212] Subsequent studies indicated that green tea polyphenols induce the secretion of IL-12 by keratinocytes, which suppresses apoptosis, immune suppression, and carcinogenesis by activating DNA repair.[213,214] These are just a few examples of how a better understanding of the basic mechanisms underlying photocarcinogenesis and photoimmune suppression can provide tangible benefits.

References

1. Bickers DR, Lim HW, Margolis D, et al. The burden of skin diseases: 2004 a joint project of the American Academy of Dermatology Association and the Society for Investigative Dermatology. *J Am Acad Dermatol.* 2006; 55(3):490–500.
2. Chen JG, Fleischer AB, Smith ED, et al. Cost of non-melanoma skin cancer treatment in the United States. *Dermatol Surg.* 2001;27(12):1035–1038.
3. Housman TS, Feldman SR, Williford PM, et al. Skin cancer is among the most costly of all cancers to treat for the Medicare population. *J Am Acad Dermatol.* 2003; 48(3):425–429.
4. Urbach F. Evidence and epidemiology of UV-induced carcinogenesis in man. *Natl Cancer Inst Monogr.* 1978; 50:5–10.
5. Benjamin CL, Ullrich SE, Kripke ML, Ananthaswamy HN. p53 tumor suppressor gene: a critical molecular target for UV induction and prevention of skin cancer. *Photochem Photobiol.* 2008;84(1):55–62.
6. Epstein EH. Basal cell carcinomas: attack of the hedgehog. *Nat Rev Cancer.* 2008;8(10):743–754.
7. Kricker A, Armstrong BK, Goumas C, et al. Ambient UV, personal sun exposure and risk of multiple primary melanomas. *Cancer Causes Control.* 2007;18(3):295–304.
8. Lea CS, Scotto JA, Buffler PA, Fine J, Barnhill RL, Berwick M. Ambient UVB and melanoma risk in the United States: a case-control analysis. *Ann Epidemiol.* 2007;17(6): 447–453.
9. Elwood JM, Jopson J. Melanoma and sun exposure: an overview of published studies. *Int J Cancer.* 1997;73(2): 198–203.
10. Gilchrest BA, Eller MS, Geller AC, Yaar M. The pathogenesis of melanoma induced by ultraviolet radiation. *N Engl J Med.* 1999;340(17):1341–1348.
11. Kripke ML. Antigenicity of murine skin tumors induced by ultraviolet light. *J Natl Cancer Inst.* 1974; 53(5):1333–1336.
12. Norval M, McLoone P, Lesiak A, Narbutt J. The effect of chronic ultraviolet radiation on the human immune system. *Photochem Photobiol.* 2008;84(1):19–28.
13. Unna PG. *Die Histopathologie der Hautkrankheiten.* Berlin, Germany: A. Hirschwald; 1894.
14. Hyde JN. On the influence of light in the production of cancer of the skin. *Am J Med Sci.* 1906;131(1):1–10.

15. Findley GM. Ultraviolet light and skin cancer. *Lancet.* 1928;2:1070–1073.
16. Urbach F. Ultraviolet radiation and skin cancer of humans. *J Photochem Photobiol.* 1997;40(1):3–7.
17. de Gruijl FR, Sterenborg HJCM, Forbes PD, et al. Wavelength dependence of skin cancer induction by ultraviolet irradiation of albino hairless mice. *Cancer Res.* 1993; 53(1):53–60.
18. Brash DE, Rudolf JA, Simon JA, et al. A role for sunlight in skin cancer: UV-induced p53 mutations in squamous cell carcinoma. *Proc Natl Acad Sci U S A.* 1991;88: 10124–10128.
19. Ziegler A, Jonason AS, Leffell DJ, et al. Sunburn and p53 in the onset of skin cancer. *Nature.* 1994;372(6508): 773–776.
20. Rady P, Scinicariello F, Wagner RF, Jr., Tyring SK: p53 mutations in basal cell carcinomas. *Cancer Res.* 1992;52(13):3804–3806.
21. Kanjilal S, Pierceall WE, Cummings KK, Kripke ML, Ananthaswamy HN. High frequency of p53 mutations in ultraviolet radiation-induced murine skin tumors: evidence for strand bias and tumor heterogeneity. *Cancer Res.* 1993;53(13):2961–2964.
22. Ananthaswamy HN, Fourtanier A, Evans RL, et al. p53 Mutations in hairless SKH-hr1 mouse skin tumors induced by a solar simulator. *Photochem Photobiol.* 1998; 67(2):227–232.
23. Bodak N, Queille S, Avril MF, et al. High levels of patched gene mutations in basal-cell carcinomas from patients with xeroderma pigmentosum. *Proc Natl Acad Sci U S A.* 1999;96(9):5117–5122.
24. Matsumura Y, Ananthaswamy HN. Toxic effects of ultraviolet radiation on the skin. *Toxicol Appl Pharmacol.* 2004; 195(3):298–308.
25. de Gruijl FR, Rebel H. Early events in UV carcinogenesis —DNA damage, target cells and mutant p53 foci. *Photochem Photobiol.* 2008;84(2):382–387.
26. Hocker T, Tsao H. Ultraviolet radiation and melanoma: a systematic review and analysis of reported sequence variants. *Hum Mutat.* 2007;28(6):578–588.
27. Davies H, Bignell GR, Cox C, et al. Mutations of the BRAF gene in human cancer. *Nature.* 2002;417(6892): 949–954.
28. Wang Y, Digiovanna JJ, Stern JB, et al. Evidence of ultraviolet type mutations in xeroderma pigmentosum melanomas. *Proc Natl Acad Sci U S A.* 2009;106(15): 6279–6284.
29. Besaratinia A, Pfeifer GP. Sunlight ultraviolet irradiation and BRAF V600 mutagenesis in human melanoma. *Hum Mutat.* 2008;29(8):983–991.
30. Setlow RB, Grist E, Thompson K, Woodhead AD. Wavelengths effective in induction of malignant melanoma. *Proc Natl Acad Sci U S A.* 1993;90:6666–6670.
31. Wood SR, Berwick M, Ley RD, Walter RB, Setlow RB, Timmins GS. UV causation of melanoma in Xiphophorus is dominated by melanin photosensitized oxidant production. *Proc Natl Acad Sci U S A.* 2006;103(11): 4111–4115.
32. Ley RD. Ultraviolet radiation A-induced precursors of cutaneous melanoma in Monodelphis domestica. *Cancer Res.* 1997;57(17):3682–3684.
33. De Fabo EC, Noonan FP, Fears T, Merlino G. Ultraviolet B but not ultraviolet A radiation initiates melanoma. *Cancer Res.* 2004;64(18):6372–6376.
34. Fisher MS, Kripke ML. Systemic alteration induced in mice by ultraviolet light irradiation and its relationship to ultraviolet carcinogenesis. *Proc Natl Acad Sci U S A.* 1977;74(4):1688–1692.
35. Kripke ML, Lofgreen JS, Beard J, Jessup JM, Fisher MS. In vivo immune responses of mice during carcinogenesis by ultraviolet irradiation. *J Natl Cancer Inst.* 1977; 59(4):1227–1230.
36. Jessup JM, Hanna N, Palaszynski E, Kripke ML. Mechanisms of depressed reactivity to dinitrochlorobenzene and ultraviolet-induced tumors during ultraviolet carcinogenesis in BALB/c mice. *Cell Immunol.* 1978;38(1): 105–115.
37. Fisher MS, Kripke ML. Further studies on the tumor-specific suppressor cells induced by ultraviolet radiation. *J Immunol.* 1978;121(3):1139–1144.
38. Fisher MS, Kripke ML. Suppressor T lymphocytes control the development of primary skin cancers in ultraviolet-irradiated mice. *Science.* 1982;216(4550):1133–1134.
39. Penn I. Cancers following cyclosporine therapy. *Transplantation.* 1987;43:32–35.
40. Caforio AL, Fortina AB, Piaserico S, et al. Skin cancer in heart transplant recipients: risk factor analysis and relevance of immunosuppressive therapy. *Circulation.* 2000; 102(19 Suppl 3):222–227.
41. Fortina AB, Caforio AL, Piaserico S, et al. Skin cancer in heart transplant recipients: frequency and risk factor analysis. *J Heart Lung Transplant.* 2000;19(3):249–255.
42. Tremblay F, Fernandes M, Habbab F, Edwardes MD, Loertscher R, Meterissian S. Malignancy after renal transplantation: incidence and role of type of immunosuppression. *Ann Surg Oncol.* 2002;9(8):785–788.
43. Yoshikawa T, Rae V, Bruins-Slot W, Van den Berg JW, Taylor JR, Streilein JW. Susceptibility to effects of UVB radiation on induction of contact hypersensitivity as a risk factor for skin cancer in humans. *J Invest Dermatol.* 1990;95(5):530–536.
44. Elmets CA, Bergstresser PR, Tigelaar RE, Wood PJ, Streilein JW. Analysis of the mechanism of unresponsiveness produced by haptens painted on skin to low dose UV radiation. *J Exp Med.* 1983;158:781–794.
45. Ullrich SE. Suppression of the immune response to allogeneic histocompatibility antigens by a single exposure to ultraviolet radiation. *Transplantation.* 1986;42(3):287–291.
46. Ullrich SE, Azizi E, Kripke ML. Suppression of the induction of delayed-type hypersensitivity reactions in mice by a single exposure to ultraviolet radiation. *Photochem Photobiol.* 1986;43(6):633–638.

47. Elmets CA, LeVine MJ, Bickers DR. Action spectrum studies for induction of immunologic unresponsiveness to dinitrofluorobenzene following in vivo low dose ultraviolet radiation. *Photochem Photobiol.* 1985;42(4): 391–397.
48. Magee MJ, Kripke ML, Ullrich SE. Suppression of the elicitation of the immune response to alloantigen by ultraviolet radiation. *Transplantation.* 1989;47(6):1008–1013.
49. Nghiem DX, Kazimi N, Clydesdale G, Ananthaswamy HN, Kripke ML, Ullrich SE. Ultraviolet a radiation suppresses an established immune response: implications for sunscreen design. *J Invest Dermatol.* 2001;117(5): 1193–1199.
50. Schwarz A, Maeda A, Schwarz T. Alteration of the migratory behavior of UV-induced regulatory T cells by tissue-specific dendritic cells. *J Immunol.* 2007;178(2): 877–886.
51. Nghiem DX, Kazimi N, Mitchell DL, et al. Mechanisms underlying the suppression of established immune responses by ultraviolet radiation. *J Invest Dermatol.* 2002;119(3):600–608.
52. Dong C. TH17 cells in development: an updated view of their molecular identity and genetic programming. *Natl Rev Immunol.* 2008;8(5):337–348.
53. Rivas JM, Ullrich SE. Systemic suppression of delayed-type hypersensitivity by supernatants from UV-irradiated keratinocytes. An essential role for keratinocyte-derived IL-10. *J Immunol.* 1992;149(12):3865–3871.
54. El-Ghorr AA, Norval M. The role of interleukin-4 in ultraviolet B light-induced immunosuppression. *Immunology.* 1997;92(1):26–32.
55. Shreedhar V, Giese T, Sung VW, Ullrich SE. A cytokine cascade including prostaglandin E2, IL-4, and IL-10 is responsible for UV-induced systemic immune suppression. *J Immunol.* 1998;160(8):3783–3789.
56. Schmitt DA, Owen-Schaub L, Ullrich SE. Effect of IL-12 on immune suppression and suppressor cell induction by ultraviolet radiation. *J Immunol.* 1995;154(10): 5114–5120.
57. Schmitt DA, Walterscheid JP, Ullrich SE. Reversal of ultraviolet radiation-induced immune suppression by recombinant interleukin-12: suppression of cytokine production. *Immunology.* 2000;101(1):90–96.
58. Schwarz A, Grabbe S, Aragane Y, et al. Interleukin-12 prevents ultraviolet B-induced local immunosuppression and overcomes UVB-induced tolerance. *J Invest Dermatol.* 1996;106:1187–1191.
59. Müller G, Salonga J, Germann T, Schuler G, Knopp J, Enk AH. IL-12 as mediator and adjuvant for the induction of contact sensitivity in vivo. *J Immunol.* 1995;155: 4661–4668.
60. Brown EL, Rivas JM, Ullrich SE, Young CR, Norris SJ, Kripke ML. Modulation of immunity to Borrelia burgdorferi by ultraviolet irradiation: differential effect on Th1 and Th2 immune responses. *Eur J Immunol.* 1995;25(11):3017–3022.
61. Jeevan A, Gilliam K, Heard H, Kripke ML. Effects of ultraviolet radiation on the pathogenesis of Mycobacterium lepraemurium infection in mice. *Exp Dermatol.* 1992;1(3):152–160.
62. Jeevan A, Evans R, Brown EL, Kripke ML. Effect of local ultraviolet irradiation on infections of mice with Candida albicans, Mycobacterium bovis BCG, and Schistosoma mansoni. *J Invest Dermatol.* 1992;99(1):59–64.
63. Applegate LA, Ley RD, Alcalay J, Kripke ML. Identification of the molecular target for the suppression of contact hypersensitivity by ultraviolet radiation. *J Exp Med.* 1989;170(4):1117–1131.
64. Yarosh D, Bucana C, Cox P, Alas L, Kibitel J, Kripke M. Localization of liposomes containing a DNA repair enzyme in murine skin. *J Invest Dermatol.* 1994;103(4): 461–468.
65. Kripke ML, Cox PA, Alas LG, Yarosh DB. Pyrimidine dimers in DNA initiate systemic immunosuppression in UV-irradiated mice. *Proc Natl Acad Sci U S A.* 1992; 89(16):7516–7520.
66. Nishigori C, Yarosh DB, Ullrich SE, et al. Evidence that DNA damage triggers interleukin 10 cytokine production in UV-irradiated murine keratinocytes. *Proc Natl Acad Sci U S A.* 1996;93(19):10354–10359.
67. Okamoto H, Kripke ML. Effector and suppressor circuits of the immune response are activated in vivo by different mechanisms. *Proc Natl Acad Sci U S A.* 1987; 84(11):3841–3845.
68. Vink AA, Moodycliffe AM, Shreedhar V, et al. The inhibition of antigen-presenting activity of dendritic cells resulting from UV irradiation of murine skin is restored by in vitro photorepair of cyclobutane pyrimidine dimers. *Proc Natl Acad Sci U S A.* 1997;94(10):5255–5260.
69. Wolf P, Cox P, Yarosh DB, Kripke ML. Sunscreens and T4N5 liposomes differ in their ability to protect against ultraviolet-induced sunburn cell formation, alterations of dendritic epidermal cells, and local suppression of contact hypersensitivity. *J Invest Dermatol.* 1995;104(2): 287–292.
70. Wolf P, Maier H, Mullegger RR, et al. Topical treatment with liposomes containing T4 endonuclease V protects human skin in vivo from ultraviolet-induced upregulation of interleukin-10 and tumor necrosis factor-alpha. *J Invest Dermatol* 2000;114(1):149–156.
71. Stege H, Roza L, Vink AA, et al. Enzyme plus light therapy to repair DNA damage in ultraviolet-B-irradiated human skin. *Proc Natl Acad Sci U S A.* 2000;97:1790–1795.
72. Kuchel JM, Barnetson RS, Halliday GM. Cyclobutane pyrimidine dimer formation is a molecular trigger for solar-simulated ultraviolet radiation-induced suppression of memory immunity in humans. *Photochem Photobiol Sci.* 2005;4(8):577–582.
73. De Fabo EC, Noonan FP. Mechanism of immune suppression by ultraviolet irradiation in vivo. I. Evidence for the existence of a unique photoreceptor in skin and its role in photoimmunology. *J Exp Med.* 1983;157:84–98.

74. Ross JA, Howie SEM, Norval M, Maingay J. Systemic administration of urocanic acid generates suppression of the delayed type hypersensitivity response to herpes simplex virus in a murine model of infection. *Photodermatology.* 1988;5:9–14.
75. Ross JA, Howie SEM, Norval M, Maingay J, Simpson TJ. Ultraviolet-irradiated urocanic acid suppresses delayed type hypersensitivity to herpes simplex virus in mice. *J Invest Dermatol.* 1986;87:630–633.
76. Kondo S, Sauder DN, McKenzie RC, et al. The role of cis-urocanic acid in UVB-induced suppression of contact hypersensitivity. *Immunol Lett.* 1995;48(3):181–186.
77. Gibbs NK, Norval M, Traynor NA, Wolf M, Johnson BE, Crosby J. Action spectra for the trans to cis photoisomerisation of urocanic acid in vitro and in mouse skin. *Photochem Photobiol.* 1993;57(3):584–590.
78. Moodycliffe AM, Norval M, Kimber I, Simpson TJ. Characterization of a monoclonal antibody to cis-urocanic acid: detection of cis-urocanic acid in the serum of irradiated mice by immunoassay. *Immunology.* 1993;79:667–672.
79. El-Ghorr AA, Norval M. A monoclonal antibody to *cis*-urocanic acid prevents the UV-induced changes in Langerhans cells and DTH responses in mice, although not preventing dendritic cell accumulation in lymph nodes draining the site of irradiation and contact hypersensitivity responses. *J Invest Dermatol.* 1995;105:264–268.
80. Moodycliffe AM, Bucana CD, Kripke ML, Norval M, Ullrich SE. Differential effects of a monoclonal antibody to cis-urocanic acid on the suppression of delayed and contact hypersensitivity following ultraviolet irradiation. *J Immunol.* 1996;157(7):2891–2899.
81. Beissert S, Ruhlemann D, Mohammad T, et al. IL-12 prevents the inhibitory effects of cis-urocanic acid on tumor antigen presentation by Langerhans cells: implications for photocarcinogenesis. *J Immunol.* 2001;167(11):6232–6238.
82. Norval M, Gibbs NK, Gilmour J. The role of urocanic acid in UV-induced immunosuppression: Recent advances (1992–1994). *Photochem Photobiol.* 1995;62:209–217.
83. Norval M, El-Ghorr AA. Studies to determine the immunomodulating effects of cis-urocanic acid. *Methods.* 2002;28(1):63–70.
84. Walterscheid JP, Ullrich SE, Nghiem DX. Platelet-activating factor, a molecular sensor for cellular damage, activates systemic immune suppression. *J Exp Med.* 2002;195(2):171–179.
85. Walterscheid JP, Nghiem DX, Kazimi N, et al. Cis-urocanic acid, a sunlight-induced immunosuppressive factor, activates immune suppression via the 5-HT_{2A} receptor. *Proc Natl Acad Sci U S A.* 2006;103(46):17420–17425.
86. Nordlind K, Azmitia EC, Slominski A. The skin as a mirror of the soul: exploring the possible roles of serotonin. *Exp Dermatol.* 2008;17(4):301–311.
87. O'Connor A, Nishigori C, Yarosh D, et al. DNA double strand breaks in epidermal cells cause immune suppression in vivo and cytokine production in vitro. *J Immunol.* 1996;157(1):271–278.
88. Devary Y, Rosette C, DiDonato JA, Karin M. NF-kB activation by ultraviolet light is not dependent on a nuclear signal. *Science.* 1993;261:1442–1445.
89. Rosette C, Karin M. Ultraviolet light and osmotic stress: activation of the JNK cascade through multiple growth factor and cytokine receptors. *Science.* 1996;274(5290):1194–1197.
90. Simon MM, Aragane Y, Schwarz A, Luger TA, Schwarz T. UVB light induces a nuclear factor κB (NFκB) activity independently from chromosomal DNA damage in cell-free cytosolic extracts. *J Invest Dermatol.* 1994;102(4):422–427.
91. Kulms D, Pöppelmann B, Yarosh D, Luger TA, Krutmann J, Schwarz T. Nuclear and cell membrane effects contribute independently to the induction of apoptosis in human cells exposed to UVB radiation. *Proc Natl Acad Sci U S A.* 1999;96(14):7974–7979.
92. Fritsche E, Schafer C, Calles C, et al. Lightening up the UV response by identification of the arylhydrocarbon receptor as a cytoplasmatic target for ultraviolet B radiation. *Proc Natl Acad Sci U S A.* 2007;104(21):8851–8856.
93. Marathe GK, Johnson C, Billings SD, et al. Ultraviolet B radiation generates platelet-activating factor-like phospholipids underlying cutaneous damage. *J Biol Chem.* 2005;280(42):35448–354457.
94. Damian DL, Halliday GM. Measurement of ultraviolet radiation-induced suppression of recall contact and delayed-type hypersensitivity in humans. *Methods.* 2002;28(1):34–45.
95. Asahina A, Tamaki K. Role of Langerhans cells in cutaneous protective immunity: is the reappraisal necessary? *J Dermatol Sci.* 2006;44(1):1–9.
96. Bennett CL, van Rijn E, Jung S, et al. Inducible ablation of mouse Langerhans cells diminishes but fails to abrogate contact hypersensitivity. *J Cell Biol.* 2005;169(4):569–576.
97. Kaplan DH, Jenison MC, Saeland S, Shlomchik WD, Shlomchik MJ. Epidermal Langerhans cell-deficient mice develop enhanced contact hypersensitivity. *Immunity.* 2005;23(6):611–620.
98. Kissenpfennig A, Henri S, Dubois B, et al. Dynamics and function of Langerhans cells in vivo: dermal dendritic cells colonize lymph node areas distinct from slower migrating Langerhans cells. *Immunity.* 2005;22(5):643–654.
99. Fukunaga A, Khaskhely NM, Sreevidya CS, Byrne SN, Ullrich SE. Dermal dendritic cells, and not Langerhans cells, play an essential role in inducing an immune response. *J Immunol.* 2008;180(5):3057–3064.
100. Toews GB, Bergstresser PR, Streilein JW. Epidermal Langerhans cell density determines whether contact hypersensitivity or unresponsiveness follows skin painting with DNFB. *J Immunol.* 1980;124:445–449.

101. Cruz PD, Nixon-Fulton J, Tigelaar RE, Bergstresser PR. Disparate effects of in vitro UVB irradiation in intravenous immunization with purified epidermal cell subpopulations for the induction of CHS. *J Invest Dermatol.* 1989;92:160–165.
102. Cruz PD, Tigelaar RE, Bergstresser PR. Langerhans cells that migrate to skin after intravenous infusion regulate the induction of contact hypersensitivity. *J Immunol.* 1990;144:2486–2492.
103. Akdis CA, Simons FE. Histamine receptors are hot in immunopharmacology. *Eur J Pharmacol.* 2006;533(1–3): 69–76.
104. Simon JC, Cruz PC, Bergstresser PR, Tigelaar RE. Low dose ultraviolet B-irradiated Langerhans cells preferentially activate CD4+ cells of the T helper 2 subset. *J Immunol.* 1990;145:2087–2091.
105. Simon JC, Tigelaar RE, Bergstresser PR, Edelbaum D, Cruz PD. Ultraviolet B radiation converts Langerhans Cells from immunogenic to tolerogenic antigen-presenting cells: induction of specific clonal anergy in CD4+ T helper 1 cells. *J Immunol.* 1991;146:485–491.
106. Loser K, Mehling A, Loeser S, et al. Epidermal RANKL controls regulatory T-cell numbers via activation of dendritic cells. *Nat Med.* 2007;12(12):1372–1379.
107. Chung H-T, Burnham DK, Robertson B, Roberts LK, Daynes RA. Involvement of prostaglandins in the immune alterations caused by the exposure of mice to ultraviolet radiation. *J Immunol.* 1986;137:2478–2484.
108. Hart PH, Jaksic A, Swift G, Norval M, El-Ghorr AA, Finlay-Jones JJ. Histamine involvement in UVB-and cis-urocanic acid-induced systemic suppression of contact hypersensitivity responses. *Immunology.* 1997;91(4): 601–608.
109. Niizeki H, Alard P, Streilein JW. Cutting edge: calcitonin gene-related peptide is necessary for ultraviolet B-impaired induction of contact hypersensitivity. *J Immunol.* 1997;159(11):5183–5186.
110. Grabbe S, Bhardwaj RS, Mahnke K, Simon MM, Schwarz T, Luger TA. α-melanocyte-stimulating hormone induces hapten-specific tolerance in mice. *J Immunol.* 1996; 156(2):473–478.
111. Zimmerman GA, McIntyre TM, Prescott SM, Stafforini DM. The platelet-activating factor signaling system and its regulators in syndromes of inflammation and thrombosis. *Crit Care Med.* 2002;30(5 Suppl):S294–S301.
112. Sheng Y, Birkle DL. Release of platelet activating factor (PAF) and eicosanoids in UVC-irradiated corneal stromal cells. *Curr Eye Res.* 1995;14(5):341–347.
113. Alappatt C, Johnson CA, Clay KL, Travers JB. Acute keratinocyte damage stimulates platelet-activating factor production. *Arch Dermatol Res.* 2000;292(5):256–259.
114. Ramos G, Kazimi N, Nghiem DX, Walterscheid JP, Ullrich SE. Platelet activating factor receptor binding plays a critical role in jet fuel-induced immune suppression. *Toxicol Appl Pharmacol.* 2004;195(3):331–338.
115. Barber LA, Spandau DF, Rathman SC, et al. Expression of the platelet-activating factor receptor results in enhanced ultraviolet B radiation-induced apoptosis in a human epidermal cell line. *J Biol Chem.* 1998;273(30): 18891–18897.
116. Dy LC, Pei Y, Travers JB. Augmentation of ultraviolet B radiation-induced tumor necrosis factor production by the epidermal platelet-activating factor receptor. *J Biol Chem.* 1999;274(38):26917–26921.
117. Zhang Q, Sitzman LA, Al-Hassani M, et al. Involvement of platelet-activating factor in ultraviolet B-induced hyperalgesia. *J Invest Dermatol.* 2009;129(1):167–174.
118. Pei Y, Barber LA, Murphy RC, et al. Activation of the epidermal platelet-activating factor receptor results in cytokine and cyclooxygenase-2 biosynthesis. *J Immunol.* 1998;161(4):1954–1961.
119. Wolf P, Nghiem DX, Walterscheid JP, et al. Platelet-activating factor is crucial in psoralen and ultraviolet A-induced immune suppression, inflammation, and apoptosis. *Am J Pathol.* 2006;169(3):795–805.
120. Zhang Q, Mousdicas N, Yi Q, et al.. Staphylococcal lipoteichoic acid inhibits delayed-type hypersensitivity reactions via the platelet-activating factor receptor. *J Clin Invest.* 2005;115(10):2855–2861.
121. Yao Y, Wolverton JE, Zhang Q, et al. Ultraviolet B radiation generated platelet-activating factor receptor agonist formation involves EGF-R-mediated reactive oxygen species. *J Immunol.* 2009;182(5):2842–2848.
122. Biancone L, Cantaluppi V, Del Sorbo L, Russo S, Tjoelker LW, Camussi G. Platelet-activating factor inactivation by local expression of platelet-activating factor acetyl-hydrolase modifies tumor vascularization and growth. *Clin Cancer Res.* 2003;9(11):4214–4220.
123. Marques M, Pei Y, Southall MD, et al. Identification of platelet-activating factor acetylhydrolase II in human skin. *J Invest Dermatol.* 2002;119(4):913–919.
124. Warskulat U, Reinen A, Grether-Beck S, Krutmann J, Haussinger D. The osmolyte strategy of normal human keratinocytes in maintaining cell homeostasis. *J Invest Dermatol.* 2004;123(3):516–521.
125. Rockel N, Esser C, Grether-Beck S, Warskulat U, et al. The osmolyte taurine protects against ultraviolet B radiation-induced immunosuppression. *J Immunol.* 2007;179(6):3604–3612.
126. Beissert S, Hosoi J, Grabbe S, Asahina A, Granstein RD. IL-10 inhibits tumor antigen presentation by epidermal antigen-presenting cells. *J Immunol.* 1995;154(3): 1280–1286.
127. Lagier B, Lebel B, Bousquet J, Pene J. Different modulation by histamine of IL-4 and interferon-gamma (IFN-gamma) release according to the phenotype of human Th0, Th1 and Th2 clones. *Clin Exp Immunol.* 1997;108(3): 545–551.
128. Morelli AE, Thomson AW. Dendritic cells under the spell of prostaglandins. *Trends Immunol.* 2003;24(3):108–111.

129. Ullrich SE. Does exposure to UV radiation induce a shift to a Th-2-like immune reaction? *Photochem Photobiol.* 1996;64(2):254–258.
130. Kalinski P, Vieira PL, Schuitemaker JH, de Jong EC, Kapsenberg ML. Prostaglandin E_2 is a selective inducer of interleukin-12 p40 (IL-12p40) production and an inhibitor of bioactive IL-12p70 heterodimer. *Blood.* 2001;97(11):3466–3469.
131. Seiffert K, Granstein RD. Neuropeptides and neuroendocrine hormones in ultraviolet radiation-induced immunosuppression. *Methods.* 2002;28(1):97–103.
132. Hosoi J, Murphy GF, Egan CL, et al. Regulation of Langerhans cell function by nerves containing calcitonin gene-related peptide. *Nature.* 1993;363:159–163.
133. Galli SJ, Nakae S, Tsai M. Mast cells in the development of adaptive immune responses. *Nat Immunol.* 2005;6(2): 135–142.
134. Kalesnikoff J, Galli SJ. New developments in mast cell biology. *Nat Immunol.* 2008;9(11):1215–1223.
135. Hart PH, Grimbaldeston MA, Swift GJ, Jaksic A, Noonan FP, Finlay-Jones JJ. Dermal mast cells determine susceptibility to Ultraviolet B-induced systemic suppression of contact hypersensitivity responses in mice. *J Exp Med.* 1998;187(12):2045–2053.
136. Alard P, Kurimoto I, Niizeki H, Doherty JM, Streilein JW. Hapten-specific tolerance induced by acute, low-dose ultraviolet B radiation of skin requires mast cell degranulation. *Eur J Immunol.* 2001;31(6):1736–1746.
137. Alard P, Niizeki H, Hanninen L, Streilein JW. Local ultraviolet B irradiation impairs contact hypersensitivity induction by triggering release of tumor necrosis factor-alpha from mast cells. *Br J Invest Dermatol.* 1999; 113:983–990.
138. Grimbaldeston MA, Nakae S, Kalesnikoff J, Tsai M, Galli SJ. Mast cell-derived interleukin 10 limits skin pathology in contact dermatitis and chronic irradiation with ultraviolet. *Nat Immunol.* 2007;8(10):1095–1104.
139. Moyal D, Courbière C, Le Corre Y, de Lacharrière O, Hourseau C: Immunosuppression induced by chronic solar-simulated irradiation in humans and its prevention by sunscreens. *Eur J Dermatol.* 1997;7(3):223–225.
140. Moyal DD, Fourtanier AM. Broad-Spectrum sunscreens provide better protection from the suppression of the elicitation phase of delayed-type hypersensitivity response in humans. *J Invest Dermatol.* 2001;117: 1186–1192.
141. Fourtanier A, Gueniche A, Compan D, Walker SL, Young AR. Improved protection against solar-simulated radiation-induced immunosuppression by a sunscreen with enhanced ultraviolet A protection. *J Invest Dermatol.* 2000;114:620–627.
142. Ullrich SE, Nghiem DX, Khaskina P. Suppression of an established immune response by UVA—a critical role for mast cells. *Photochem Photobiol.* 2007;83(5): 1095–1100.
143. Wille JJ, Kydonieus AF, Murphy GF. cis-urocanic acid induces mast cell degranulation and release of preformed TNF-alpha: A possible mechanism linking UVB and cis-urocanic acid to immunosuppression of contact hypersensitivity. *Skin Pharmacol Appl Skin Physiol.* 1999; 12(1–2):18–27.
144. Hart PH, Townley SL, Grimbaldeston MA, Khalil Z, Finlay-Jones JJ. Mast cells, neuropeptides, histamine, and prostaglandins in UV-induced systemic immunosuppression. *Method.s* 2002;28(1):79–89.
145. Khalil Z, Townley SL, Grimbaldeston MA, Finlay-Jones JJ, Hart PH. cis-Urocanic acid stimulates neuropeptide release from peripheral sensory nerves. *J Invest Dermatol.* 2001;117(4):886–891.
146. Byrne SN, Limon-Flores AY, Ullrich SE. Mast cell migration from the skin to the draining lymph nodes upon ultraviolet irradiation represents a key step in the induction of immune suppression. *J Immunol.* 2008; 180(7):4648–4655.
147. Grimbaldeston MA, Pearce AL, Robertson BO, et al. Association between melanoma and dermal mast cell prevalence in sun-unexposed skin. *Br J Dermatol.* 2004; 150(5):895–903.
148. Grimbaldeston MA, Green A, Darlington S, et al. Susceptibility to basal cell carcinoma is associated with high dermal mast cell prevalence in non-sun-exposed skin for an Australian population. *Photochem Photobiol.* 2003;78(6):633–639.
149. Grimbaldeston MA, Skov L, Baadsgaard O, et al. Communications: high dermal mast cell prevalence is a predisposing factor for basal cell carcinoma in humans. *J Invest Dermatol.* 2000;115(2):317–320.
150. Beer TW, Ng LB, Murray K. Mast cells have prognostic value in Merkel cell carcinoma. *Am J Dermatopathol.* 2008;30(1):27–30.
151. Daynes RA, Spellman CW. Evidence for the generation of suppressor cells by UV radiation. *Cell Immunol.* 1977;31:182–187.
152. Sakaguchi S, Sakaguchi N, Asano M, Itoh M, Toda M. Immunologic self-tolerance maintained by activated T cells expressing IL-2 receptor alpha-chains (CD25). Breakdown of a single mechanism of self-tolerance causes various autoimmune diseases. *J Immunol.* 1995; 155(3):1151–1164.
153. Spellman CW, Daynes RA. Modification of immunological potential by ultraviolet radiation. II. Generation of suppressor cells in short-term UV-irradiated mice. *Transplantation.* 1977;24:120–126.
154. Ullrich SE, Kripke ML. Mechanisms in the suppression of tumor rejection produced in mice by repeated UV irradiation. *J Immunol.* 1984;133(5):2786–2790.
155. Ullrich SE, Magee MJ. Specific suppression of allograft rejection after treatment of recipient mice with UV radiation and allogeneic spleen cells. *Transplantation.* 1988; 46:115–119.

156. Sakaguchi S, Wing K, Miyara M: Regulatory T cells—a brief history and perspective. *Eur J Immunol.* 2007;37 (Suppl 1):S116–S123.
157. Shreedhar VK, Pride MW, Sun Y, Kripke ML, Strickland FM. Origin and characteristics of ultraviolet-B radiation-induced suppressor T lymphocytes. *J Immunol.* 1998; 161(3):1327–1335.
158. Schwarz A, Beissert S, Grosse-Heitmeyer K, et al. Evidence for functional relevance of CTLA-4 in ultraviolet-radiation-induced tolerance. *J Immunol.* 2000;165: 1824–1831.
159. Loser K, Apelt J, Voskort M, et al. IL-10 controls ultraviolet-induced carcinogenesis in mice. *J Immunol.* 2007;179(1):365–371.
160. Ghoreishi M, Dutz JP. Tolerance induction by transcutaneous immunization through ultraviolet-irradiated skin is transferable through CD4+CD25+ T regulatory cells and is dependent on host-derived IL-10. *J Immunol.* 2006;176(4):2635–2644.
161. Gorman S, Kuritzky LA, Judge MA, et al. Topically applied 1,25-dihydroxyvitamin D3 enhances the suppressive activity of CD4+CD25+ cells in the draining lymph nodes. *J Immunol.* 2007;179(9):6273–6283.
162. Hori S, Nomura T, Sakaguchi S. Control of regulatory T cell development by the transcription factor Foxp3. *Science.* 2003;299(5609):1057–1061.
163. Moodycliffe AM, Nghiem D, Clydesdale G, Ullrich SE. Immune suppression and skin cancer development: regulation by NKT cells. *Nat Immunol.* 2000;1(6):521–525.
164. Kronenberg M, Gapin L. The unconventional lifestyle of NKT cells. *Nat Rev Immunol.* 2002;2(8):557–568.
165. Fukunaga A, Khaskhley NM, Ma Y, Sreevidya CS, Taguchi K, Nishigori C, Ullrich SE. Langerhans cells serve as immunoregulatory cells by activating NKT cells. J. Immunol. 2010; 185(8):4633–4640.
166. Mizoguchi A, Bhan AK. A case for regulatory C cells. *J Immunol.* 2006;176(2):705–710.
167. Byrne SN, Halliday GM. B cells activated in lymph nodes in response to ultraviolet irradiation or by interleukin-10 inhibit dendritic cell induction of immunity. *J Invest Dermatol.* 2005;124(3):570–578.
168. Matsumura Y, Byrne SN, Nghiem DX, Miyahara Y, Ullrich SE. A role for inflammatory mediators in the induction of immunoregulatory B cells. *J Immunol.* 2006; 177(7):4810–4817.
169. Selgrade MK. Use of immunotoxicity data in health risk assessments: uncertainties and research to improve the process. *Toxicology.* 1999;133(1):59–72.
170. Cestari TF, Kripke ML, Baptista PL, Bakos L, Bucana CD. Ultraviolet radiation decreases the granulomatous response to lepromin in humans. *J Invest Dermatol.* 1995; 105(1):8–13.
171. Damian DL, Halliday GM, Taylor CA, Barnetson RS. Ultraviolet radiation induced suppression of Mantoux reactions in humans. *J Invest Dermatol.* 1998;110(5): 824–827.
172. Skov L, Hansen H, Barker JNWN, Simon JC, Baadsgaard O. Contrasting effects of ultraviolet-A and ultraviolet-B exposure on induction of contact sensitivity in human skin. *Clin Exp Immunol.* 1997;107(3):585–588.
173. Damian DL, Halliday GM, Barnetson RSC. Broad-spectrum sunscreens provide greater protection against ultraviolet-radiation-induced suppression of contact hypersensitivity to a recall antigen in humans. *J Invest Dermatol.* 1997;109(2):146–151.
174. Kelly DA, Seed PT, Young AR, Walker SL. A commercial sunscreen's protection against ultraviolet radiation-induced immunosuppression is more than 50% lower than protection against sunburn in humans. *J Invest Dermatol.* 2003;120(1):65–71.
175. Hurks HM, Out-Luiting C, Vermeer BJ, Claas FH, Mommaas AM: In situ action spectra suggest that DNA damage is involved in ultraviolet radiation-induced immunosuppression in humans. *Photochem Photobiol.* 1997;66(1):76–81.
176. Young AR, Chadwick CA, Harrison GI, Nikaido O, Ramsden J, Potten CS. The similarity of action spectra for thymine dimers in human epidermis and erythema suggests that DNA is the chromophore for erythema. *J Invest Dermatol.* 1998;111(6):982–988.
177. Kammeyer A, Pavel S, Asghar SS, Bos JD, Teunissen MB. Prolonged increase of cis-urocanic acid levels in human skin and urine after single total-body ultraviolet exposures. *Photochem Photobiol.* 1997;65(3):593–598.
178. Sleijffers A, Kammeyer A, de Gruijl FR, et al. Epidermal cis-urocanic acid levels correlate with lower specific cellular immune responses after hepatitis B vaccination of ultraviolet B-exposed humans. *Photochem Photobiol.* 2003;77(3):271–275.
179. Enk CD, Sredni D, Blauvelt A, Katz SI. Induction of IL-10 gene expression in human keratinocytes by UVB exposure in vivo and in vitro. *J Immunol.* 1995;154: 4851–4856.
180. Grewe M, Gyufko K, Krutmann J. Interleukin-10 production by cultured human keratinocytes: regulation by UVB and UVA1 radiation. *J Invest Dermatol.* 1995; 104:3–6.
181. Buckman SY, Gresham A, Hale P, et al. COX-2 expression is induced by UVB exposure in human skin: implications for the development of skin cancer. *Carcinogenesis.* 1998;19(5):723–729.
182. Brink N, Szamel M, Young AR, Wittern KP, Bergemann J. Comparative quantification of IL-1beta, IL-10, IL-10r, TNF-alpha and IL-7 mRNA levels in UV-irradiated human skin in vivo. *Inflamm Res.* 2000;49(6):290–296.
183. Grewe M, Duvic M, Aragane Y, Schwarz T, Ullrich SE, Krutmann J. Lack of induction of IL-10 expression in human keratinocytes—reply. *J Invest Dermatol.* 1996; 106(6):1330–1331.
184. Teunissen MB, Koomen CW, Jansen J, et al. In contrast to their murine counterparts, normal human keratinocytes and human epidermoid cell lines A431 and

HaCaT fail to express IL-10 mRNA and protein. *Clin Exp Immunol.* 1997;107(1):213–223.
185. Kang K, Gilliam AC, Chen G, Tootell E, Cooper KD. In human skin, UVB initiates early induction of IL-10 over IL-12 preferentially in the expanding dermal monocytic/macrophagic population. *J Invest Dermatol.* 1998; 110(1):31–38.
186. Stoebner PE, Rahmoun M, Ferrand C, Meunier L, Yssel H, Pene J. A single sub-erythematous exposure of solar-simulated radiation on the elicitation phase of contact hypersensitivity induces IL-10-producing T-regulatory cells in human skin. *Exp Dermatol.* 2006;15(8):615–624.
187. Kim TH, Ananthaswamy HN, Kripke ML, Ullrich SE. Advantages of using hairless mice versus haired mice to test sunscreen efficacy against photoimmune suppressions. *Photochem Photobiol.* 2003;78(1):37–42.
188. Ullrich SE, Kim TH, Ananthaswamy HN, Kripke ML. Sunscreen effects on UV-induced immune suppression. *J Invest Dermatol Symp Proc.* 1999;4(1):65–69.
189. Poon TS, Barnetson RS, Halliday GM. Prevention of immunosuppression by sunscreens in humans is unrelated to protection from erythema and dependent on protection from ultraviolet A in the face of constant ultraviolet B protection. *J Invest Dermatol.* 2003;121(1): 184–190.
190. Baron ED, Fourtanier A, Compan D, Medaisko C, Cooper KD, Stevens SR. High ultraviolet A protection affords greater immune protection confirming that ultraviolet A contributes to photoimmunosuppression in humans. *J Invest Dermatol.* 2003;121(4):869–875.
191. Reeve VE, Bosnic M, Boehm-Wilcox C, Nishimura N, Ley RD. Ultraviolet A radiation (320–400 nm) protects hairless mice from immunosuppression induced by ultraviolet B radiation (280–320 nm) or cis-urocanic acid. *Int Arch Allergy Immunol.* 1998;115(4):316–322.
192. Reeve VE, Tyrrell RM. Heme oxygenase induction mediates the photoimmunoprotective activity of UVA radiation in the mouse. *Proc Natl Acad Sci U S A.* 1999; 96(16):9317–9321.
193. Reeve VE, Bosnic M, Nishimura N. Interferon-gamma is involved in photoimmunoprotection by UVA (320–400 nm) radiation in mice. *J Invest Dermatol.* 1999;112(6): 945–950.
194. Shen J, Bao S, Reeve VE. Modulation of IL-10, IL-12, and IFN-gamma in the epidermis of hairless mice by UVA (320–400 nm) and UVB (280–320 nm) radiation. *J Invest Dermatol.* 1999;113:1059–1064.
195. Byrne SN, Spinks N, Halliday GM. Ultraviolet A irradiation of C57BL/6 mice suppresses systemic contact hypersensitivity or enhances secondary immunity depending on dose. *J Invest Dermatol.* 2002;119(4):858–864.
196. Green A, Williams G, Neale R, et al. Daily sunscreen application and betacarotene supplementation in prevention of basal-cell and squamous-cell carcinomas of the skin: a randomised controlled trial. *Lancet.* 1999; 354(9180):723–729.
197. van der Pols JC, Williams GM, Pandeya N, Logan V, Green AC. Prolonged prevention of squamous cell carcinoma of the skin by regular sunscreen use. *Cancer Epidemiol Biomarkers Prev.* 2006;15(12):2546–2548.
198. Ananthaswamy HN, Ullrich SE, Mascotto RE, et al. Inhibition of solar simulator-induced p53 mutations and protection against skin cancer development in mice by sunscreens. *J Invest Dermatol.* 1999;112(5):763–768.
199. Ananthaswamy HN, Loughlin SM, Cox P, Evans RL, Ullrich SE, Kripke ML. Sunlight and skin cancer: inhibition of p53 mutations in UV-irradiated mouse skin by sunscreens. *Nat Med.* 1997;3(5):510–514.
200. Gallagher RP, Rivers JK, Lee TK, Bajdik CD, McLean DI, Coldman AJ. Broad-spectrum sunscreen use and the development of new nevi in white children: A randomized controlled trial. *JAMA.* 2000;283(22):2955–2960.
201. Chang YM, Newton-Bishop JA, Bishop DT, et al. A pooled analysis of melanocytic nevus phenotype and the risk of cutaneous melanoma at different latitudes. *Int J Cancer.* 2009;124(2):420–428.
202. Yarosh D, Alas LG, Yee V, et al. Pyrimidine dimer removal enhanced by DNA repair liposomes reduces the incidence of UV skin cancer in mice. *Cancer Res.* 1992;52(15):4224–4231.
203. Yarosh D, Klein J, O'Connor A, Hawk J, Rafal E, Wolf P. Effect of topically applied T4 endonuclease V in liposomes on skin cancer in xeroderma pigmentosum: a randomised study. Xeroderma Pigmentosum Study Group. *Lancet.* 2001;357(9260):926–929.
204. Sreevidya CS, Khaskhely NM, Fukunaga A, Khaskina P, Ullrich SE. Inhibition of photocarcinogenesis by platelet-activating factor or serotonin receptor antagonists. *Cancer Res.* 2008;68(10):3978–3984.
205. Fischer SM, Lo HH, Gordon GB, et al. Chemopreventive activity of celecoxib, a specific cycloogenase-2 inhibitor, and indomethacin against ultraviolet-light induced skin carcinogenesis. *Mol Carcinogenesis.* 1999;25:231–240.
206. Loser K, Scherer A, Krummen MB, et al. An important role of CD80/CD86-CTLA-4 signaling during photocarcinogenesis in mice. *J Immunol.* 2005;174(9):5298–5305.
207. Katiyar SK. UV-induced immune suppression and photocarcinogenesis: chemoprevention by dietary botanical agents. *Cancer Lett.* 2007;255(1):1–11.
208. Wang ZY, Agarwal R, Bickers DR, Mukhtar H. Protection against ultraviolet B radiation-induced photocarcinogenesis in hairless mice by green tea polyphenols. *Carcinogenesis.* 1991;12(8):1527–1530.
209. Katiyar SK, Challa A, McCormick TS, Cooper KD, Mukhtar H. Prevention of UVB-induced immunosuppression in mice by the green tea polyphenol (–)-epigallocatechin-3-gallate may be associated with alterations in IL-10 and IL-12 production. *Carcinogenesis.* 1999;20:2117.
210. Schmitt DA, Ullrich SE. Exposure to ultraviolet radiation causes dendritic cells/macrophages to secrete immune suppressive IL-12p40 homodimers. *J Immunol.* 2000;165:3162–3167.

211. Schwarz A, Maeda A, Kernebeck K, van Steeg H, Beissert S, Schwarz T. Prevention of UV radiation-induced immunosuppression by IL-12 is dependent on DNA repair. *J Exp Med.* 2005;201(2): 173–179.
212. Schwarz A, Stander S, Berneburg M, et al. Interleukin-12 suppresses ultraviolet radiation-induced apoptosis by inducing DNA repair. *Nat Cell Biol.* 2002;4(1):26–31.
213. Schwarz A, Maeda A, Gan D, Mammone T, Matsui MS, Schwarz T. Green tea phenol extracts reduce UVB-induced DNA damage in human cells via interleukin-12. *Photochem Photobiol.* 2008;84(2):350–355.
214. Meeran SM, Akhtar S, Katiyar SK. Inhibition of UVB-induced skin tumor development by drinking green tea polyphenols is mediated through DNA repair and subsequent inhibition of inflammation. *J Invest Dermatol.* 2009;129(5):1258–1270.

6

HISTOPATHOLOGY OF NONMELANOMA SKIN CANCER

JONATHAN L. CURRY
CARLOS TORRES-CABALA
VICTOR G. PRIETO

Introduction

The histopathology of nonmelanoma skin tumors encompasses a heterogeneous group of neoplasms and conditions. Although the two most common types of nonmelanoma skin cancer are widely recognized to be basal cell carcinoma (BCC) and squamous cell carcinoma (SCC), even these basic histologies include numerous variants and permutations. In general, cutaneous pathology may be broken down by the cell or embryologic tissue of origin: epithelium, mesenchyme, adnexal structures, neuroendocrine cells, and even lymphoid tissue. Due to the variability and sheer volume of cutaneous pathologies, the dermatopathologist is an integral member of the multidisciplinary cutaneous oncology team. This chapter provides an overview of the more frequently encountered nonmelanocytic neoplasms of cutaneous origin.

Epithelial Proliferations of the Skin

Actinic Keratosis

Actinic keratosis (AK) is an intraepidermal proliferation of basal keratinocytes that occurs on sun-damaged ("actinic") skin of the face and neck with scale or keratin formation ("keratosis"). There is much debate whether AKs are premalignant or fully malignant lesions.[1] Investigations have demonstrated that the ability of AKs to develop into SCC requires accumulation of additional mutations in initiated clones of atypical basal keratinocytes, therefore supporting their interpretation as premalignant.[2,3]

The histologic findings include hyperkeratosis and parakeratosis with an underlying proliferation of atypical basal keratinocytes between segments of follicular and eccrine ostia. Atypical keratinocytes demonstrate enlarged, hyperchromatic nuclei with pleomorphism. The cells are arranged in small epithelial buds that project into the papillary dermis. The border between the clusters of atypical keratinocytes and normal-appearing follicular keratinocytes is often well demarcated. Atypical keratinocytes are confined to the basal and suprabasal layers of the epidermis and may involve skin adnexa, but do not involve all layers of the epidermis, as seen in SCC in situ (SCIS). Dermal solar elastosis from chronic sun exposure is microscopically composed of aggregates of basophilic ("elastotic") material, which chemically resembles elastic tissue and that is newly synthesized from altered dermal fibroblasts (Fig 6–1A).[4]

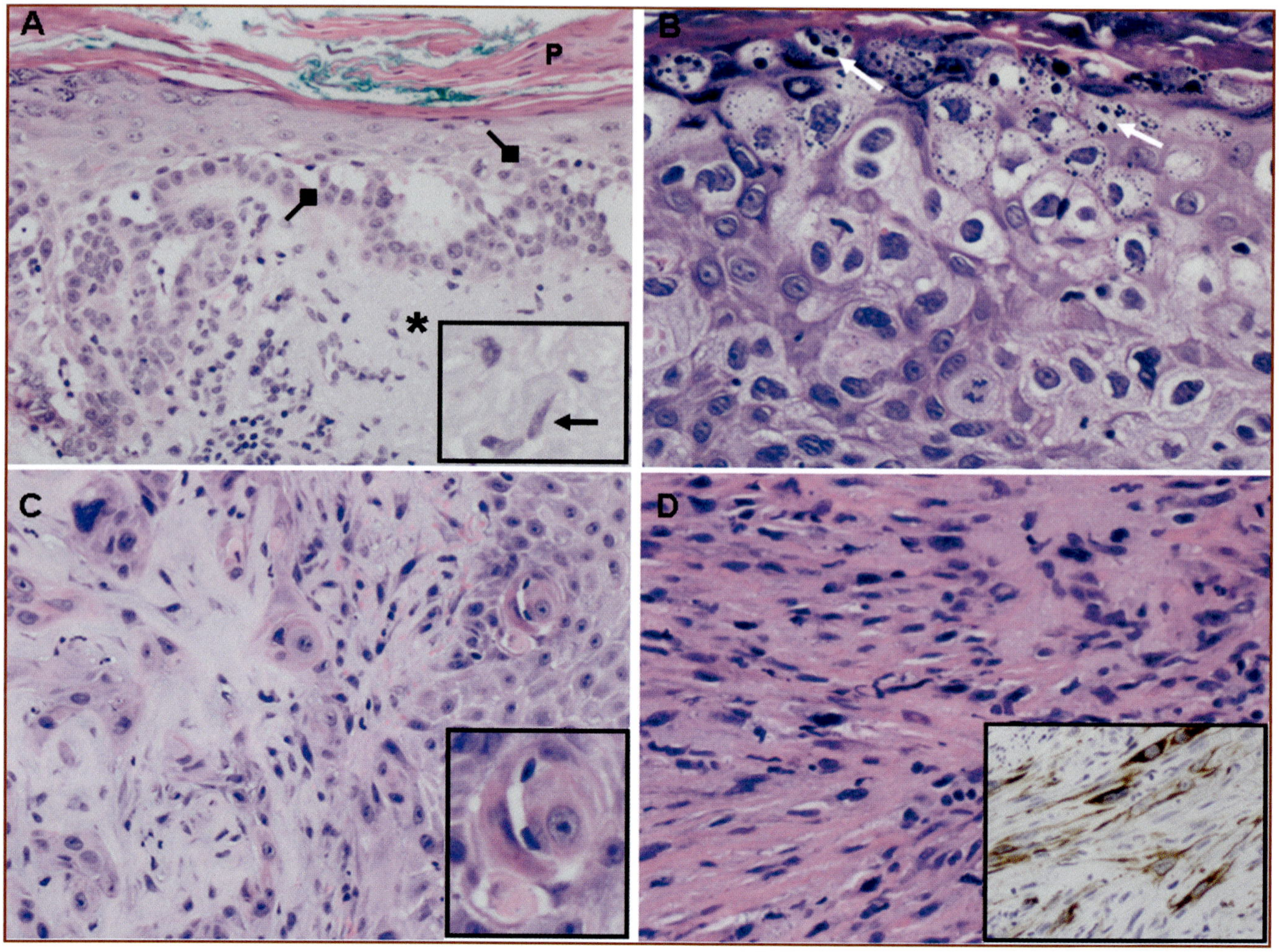

Figure 6–1. A. Actinic keratosis with acantholytic pattern. Sun-damaged skin with hyperkeratosis, parakeratosis (P), and proliferation of atypical basaloid keratinocytes projecting into the papillary dermis. Some of the atypical keratinocytes are acantholytic or separated from each other (*diamond arrows*). Dermis with basophilic elastotic material (*) synthesized by altered fibroblast (*inset, single arrow*). B. Squamous cell carcinoma (SCC) in situ. Full thickness involvement of the epidermis by atypical keratinocytes with clear, pale cytoplasm. Some of the atypical keratinocytes contain coarse keratohyaline granules in the cytoplasm (*arrows*). C. Invasive SCC with keratinization and formation of concentric layers of abnormal keratinocytes or keratin pearls (*inset*). D. Invasive sarcomatoid SCC. Atypical spindle shaped cells are poorly differentiated with absence of keratinization. Tumor cells are reactive with anti-pankeratin cocktail (cytokeratin AE1/AE3, MNF116, Zym5.2, and Cam5.2) by immunohistochemistry (IHC) (*inset*).

Histologic Variants of Actinic Keratosis

There are several histologic variants of actinic keratosis, that may lead to a differential diagnosis of other neoplastic or inflammatory skin disorders.

Hyperplastic actinic keratosis (HAK) is characterized by prominent epidermal hyperplasia or acanthosis.

Pigmented actinic keratosis may histologically resemble lentigo maligna as it has atypical pigmented keratinocytes and increased melanocytes in a background of chronic sun damage. Evaluation with immunohistochemical studies such as Mart-1, HMB-45, and Mitf-1 in these problematic cases is useful to better delineate the melanocytes along the dermal-epidermal junction.[5]

Acantholytic actinic keratosis shows individual, atypical keratinocytes separated from each other due to loss of intercellular cohesion. The differential diagnosis includes focal acantholytic dyskeratosis or Darier disease; however, the presence of cytologic atypia allows distinction from these entities.

Lichenoid actinic keratosis contains epidermal changes of actinic keratosis (eg, hyperkeratosis, parakeratosis, and cytologic atypia of basal keratinocytes) in addition to a bandlike or "lichenoid" infiltrate of lymphocytes and macrophages in the papillary dermis that obscures the dermal-epidermal junction. Lichen planus or benign lichenoid keratosis (lichen planuslike keratosis) would be considered in the differential diagnosis.[6]

Actinic chelitis shows solar damage to the lip with histologic features of hyperkeratosis, parakeratosis, hypergranulosis, and atypia of basal keratinocytes in the squamous mucosa.

Squamous Cell Carcinoma (SCC)

Cutaneous SCC of the head and neck commonly arises from the epidermis on sun-exposed skin. SCC in situ (SCIS; called Bowen disease when occurring on non-sun-exposed skin) is characterized by atypia of keratinocytes involving all layers of an acanthotic epidermis that otherwise lacks keratinocyte maturation (ie, with hypogranulosis and parakeratosis). Mitotic figures, nuclear pleomorphism with vesicular or hyperchromatic nuclei, prominent nucleoli, and randomly dispersed dyskeratotic cells are common histopathologic features.[7] Atypical keratinocytes are confined to the epidermis with an intact basement membrane zone. Some cases of SCIS will demonstrate intraepidermal collections of atypical keratinocytes (Borst-Jadassohn pattern) or contain atypical, pagetoid-appearing cells with abundant pale, clear cytoplasm.[8] A histologic clue for a keratinocytic process is the presence of coarse keratohyline granules in the atypical pagetoid-appearing cells (Fig 6–1B).

Invasive squamous cell carcinoma (SCC) consists of a proliferation of atypical keratinocytes which have destructively grown into the dermis. The basement membrane zone around the infiltrating nests or cords of tumor cells may be retained; thus it cannot be the sole histologic criteria for invasion.[9] Histologic grading of SCCs is based on the degree of keratinization and maturation of infiltrating tumor cells: well-, moderately, and poorly differentiated.[7]

Well-differentiated SCC is composed of polygonal shaped cells with intercellular bridges and abundant glassy, eosinophilic cytoplasm. Features of keratinization with parakeratotic material or keratin pearls are evident in the center of concentric layers of abnormal keratinocytes (Fig 6–1C). Moderately differentiated SCC demonstrates less eosinophilic cytoplasm and keratin-pearl formation. Poorly differentiated SCC shows a minimal degree of keratinization, lacks keratin pearls, and exhibits greater nuclear pleomorphism and a higher risk of perineural invasion. As in other cutaneous malignancies, there typically is an infiltrate of lymphocytes, plasma cells and eosinophils.[10] The depth of invasion (measured from the top of the granular cell layer to the deepest portion of the tumor) and perineural invasion reportedly influence biologic potential of tumors.[11]

Cutaneous SCC cells are positive for high-molecular-weight cytokeratins: cytokeratin 5 and 6 (CK5/6) and p63. Well- and moderately differentiated SCCs will display features of keratinization by light microscopy; therefore, routine use of immunohistochemical studies typically is not necessary for diagnosis. Immunohistochemical studies are utilized for poorly differentiated tumors with minimal features of keratinization.

Histologic Variants of Squamous Cell Carcinoma

Certain histologic variants of invasive SCC are associated with either a propensity for recurrence and greater risk for metastasis or a more indolent clinical course.

Adenoid or acantholytic SCC typically occurs on the head and neck of older age males. The tumor is composed of invasive lobules of squamous cells with acantholysis arranged in a tubular or alveolar-like pattern reminiscent of glandular structures. Continuity with the epidermis and absence of labeling with carcinoembryonic antigen (CEA) in these pseudoglandular structures by immunohistochemistry help differentiate these lesions from other malignancies (eg, epithelioid angiosarcoma or metastatic adenocarcinoma). Acantholytic SCC tends to have a slightly higher rate of metastatic potential of 2.0% compared with the standard invasive SCC which is less than 0.5%.[7]

Spindle cell or sarcomatoid SCC occurs in the setting of chronic sun-damaged skin or at sites of prior radiation exposure. These tumors have a propensity to occur on the head and neck of older Caucasian males and are often deeply infiltrative at time of presentation. Spindle cell SCC related to radiation therapy has a more aggressive clinical course and greater metastatic potential. Histologically, the tumor is composed of invasive bundles of poorly differentiated, atypical, spindle-shaped cells with hyperchromatic, pleomorphic nuclei admixed with scattered, bizarre-shaped, giant cells. There may be extension into the subcutis and fascia and perineural invasion (Fig 6–1D). In the absence of an epidermal connection, keratinization, and dyskeratosis, the differential diagnosis would include melanoma, atypical fibroxanthoma (AFX), and other malignant spindle cell tumors of the skin. Reactivity for CK5/6, with MNF116 (which detects cytokeratin 5, 6, 8, 17, and 19) and anti-p63 confirms the diagnosis of SCC.[12–14]

Verrucous carcinoma (VC) is a low grade, well-differentiated squamous proliferation that commonly occurs in the oral cavity, genitocrual region (designated as giant condyloma acuminatum or Buschke-Lowenstein tumor), and the plantar surfaces of the foot (referred to as epithelioma cuniculatum). On rare occasions, verrucous carcinoma can occur in other cutaneous sites, including the scalp.[15] Microscopically the tumors are composed of well-differentiated squamous cells arranged in broad, bulbous, blunt, cellular tongues with a pushing border at the frontal edge. The epidermis shows marked papillomatosis, hyperkeratosis, and acanthosis. Perineural invasion is infrequent, and the risk for metastasis is low. VC are associated with different types of human papillomavirus (HPV): HPV types 6 and 11, 16, and 18, and 16 are associated with lesions on the oral cavity, genitocrual areas, and foot, respectively. HPV 33 have been described in VC of the scalp, and HPV 11, 18, and 1 in VC on other cutaneous sites.[16] Differential diagnosis includes verruca vulgaris and pseudoepitheliomatous hyperplasia. In uncertain cases, evaluation of the entire lesion will help differentiate VC from these entities.

Keratoacanthoma (KA) has been described as either a low-grade squamous neoplasm or SCC with borderline or low malignant potential. Keratoacanthomas commonly occur on the face and extremities. Multiple KAs or KA-like epithelial proliferations have been described in association with Muir-Torre syndrome, immunosuppression, and patients treated with multikinase inhibitors.[17,18] Keratoacanthomas are characterized by a nodular, circumscribed, keratin filled, crateriform proliferation of well-differentiated squamous cells with abundant glassy, eosinophilic cytoplasm. The border of the lesion is smooth, lacking the infiltrative border of SCC. There are neutrophilic and eosinophilic microabscesses, plus a mixed infiltrate along the base of the lesion. Fibrosis and a giant cell reaction indicate areas of regression (Fig 6–2). The differential diagnosis includes well-differentiated invasive SCC with central keratinization. In general, KA usually presents as a very rapidly growing lesion that may spontaneously regress. In the absence of a full-thickness biopsy to evaluate the base of the lesion, a SCC cannot be excluded; additional biopsy or excision usually is recommended.

Basal Cell Carcinoma (BCC)

Basal cell carcinoma is an epithelial proliferation that arises from the basal layer of the epidermis or the infudibular portion of the hair follicles. Basal cell

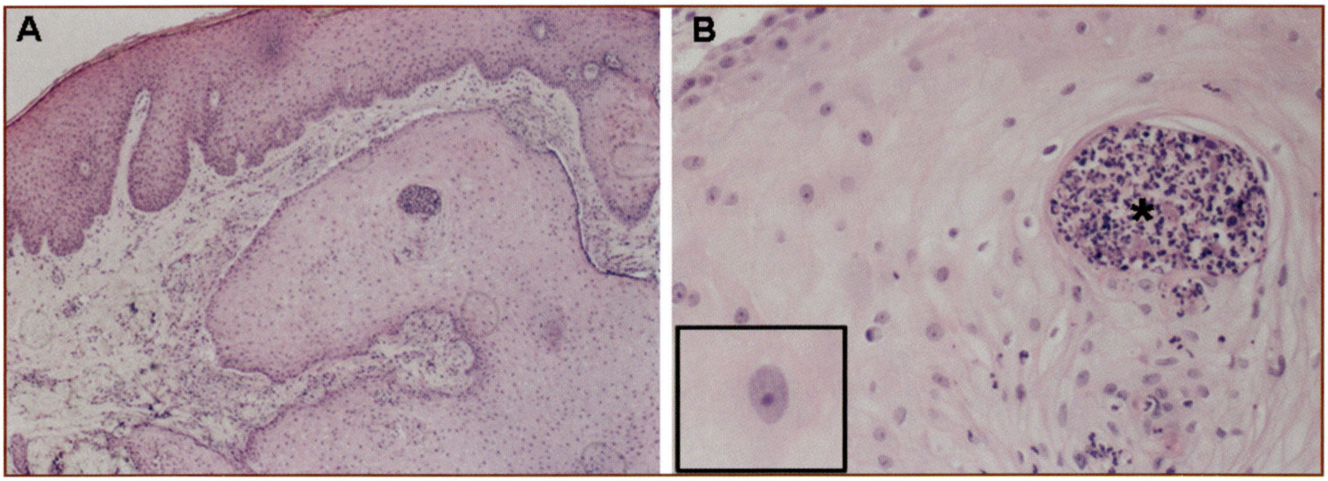

Figure 6–2. A. Keratoacanthomas with nodular, circumscribed, keratin filled, crateriform proliferation of well-differentiated squamous cells. **B.** Tumor cells contain abundant glassy, eosinophilic cytoplasm (*inset*) and intraepithelial mircoabscesses (*) are commonly present.

carcinomas are a common cutaneous malignancy encountered in the sun-exposed skin of the head and neck. Tumors typically occur in individuals beyond the fourth decade and classically present as a flesh-colored, translucent papule with telangiectasia. Corresponding to the various histologic patterns, other clinical presentations include erythematous or scarlike plaques.[19] Basal cell carcinomas tend to be locally infiltrative, and, if lesions are allowed to persist, they may become ulcerated, "rodent ulcers." Metastasis is infrequent and may correlate with size of tumor, depth of invasion, prior radiation therapy, and pattern of actin expression.[20] Basal cell carcinoma can occur in the pediatric population, which may reflect a genodermatosis (eg, xeroderma pigmentosa) or basal cell nevus syndrome (Gorlin-Goltz syndrome). Mutations in the human homologue of *Drosophila* patched gene (PTCH) or defects in the hedgehog signaling pathway are responsible for both sporadic and inherited forms of basal cell carcinoma.[21]

Histologically, BCC are composed of small tumor cells with basophilic nuclei and scant cytoplasm arranged in cords, nests, or nodules with continuous rows of tumor cells at the periphery in a palisaded arrangement. Surrounding the cells there is mucinous material as well as retraction spaces due to shrinkage from tissue processing. Mitotic figures and apoptotic bodies are common features. The immature tumor stroma is more cellular and less fibrous compared to typical dermal collagen; in addition, it has a mucinous appearance due to increased hyaluronic acid. These qualities give a characteristic bluish tinctorial appearance to the tumor stroma on hematoxylin and eosin (H&E) stained sections (Fig 6–3, A–C). Tumor cells in the center may break down and disappear through apoptosis and formation of cyst-like structures (so called nodulocystic BCC). At times empty halos are histologic clues for tumor nest drop out of the tissue sample.[22] It is not uncommon to detect amorphous eosinophilic keratin-type amyloid in the stroma. Basal cell carcinomas stain positive for low-molecular-weight cytokeratins 8, 17, 19 and with berEP4.[23,24]

Histologic Variants of Basal Cell Carcinoma

Several histologic variants of basal cell carcinoma are recognized, and some of them are associated with a more aggressive clinical course. Other BCC variants may simulate histologically other cutaneous neoplasms encountered in the head and neck (Table 6–1).

Histologic variants of BCC that impact biologic behavior are superficial, micronodular, and infiltrative or morpheaform, as well as tumors with squamous differentiation. Superficial pattern BCC contains nests

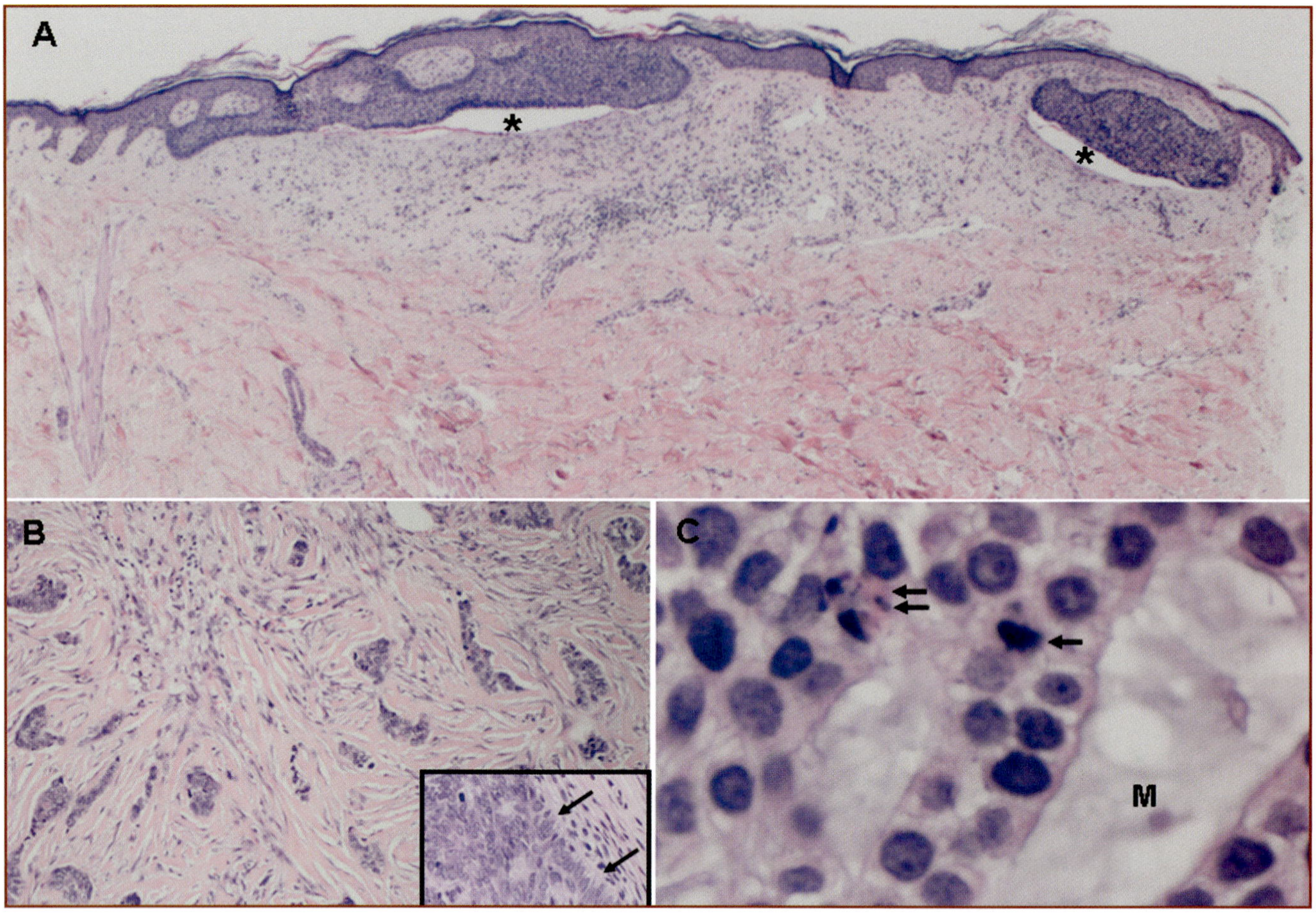

Figure 6–3. A. Basal cell carcinoma (BCC) with superficial pattern. Buds of basaloid tumor cells connected to the epidermis with clear retraction spaces (*) between the tumor cells and stroma. **B.** BCC with infiltrative/morpheaform pattern. Cords and nests of basaloid tumor cells in a sclerotic, eosinophilic stroma. Palisade arrangement of tumor cells nuclei in rows at the periphery of the tumor nodule (*inset, arrows*). **C.** Mitoses (*single arrow*), apoptoses (*double arrows*) and mucinous stroma (M) are all characteristic histologic features of BCC.

of basaloid cells with peripheral palisading, and they are attached to the basal layer of the epidermis in multiple places. Tumor cells seldom extend beyond the papillary dermis, and retraction spaces, mitoses, and apoptosis separated by areas of regression and fibrosis are routine features. The multifocality of this variant accounts for higher clinical rate of recurrence.[22]

Histologically, the micronodular BCC is composed of small tumor nests of basaloid cells in a myxoid stroma. Tumor nodules often may extend into the deep dermis and subcutaneous tissue, and these lesions reportedly have a higher rate of recurrence.[25]

Basal cell carcinoma with squamous features (also called metatypical BCC) demonstrates classic histologic features of BCC combined with areas which show prominent squamous differentiation of tumor cells (cytoplasmic keratinization or keratin pearls). These tumors tend to be locally aggressive and, on rare instances, may metastasize with the squamous component more frequently seen at the site of metastasis.[20]

Infiltrative and morpheaform BCC are aggressive tumors that demonstrate a downward, irregular extension of small cords or clusters of tumor cells at the advancing border of growth. Thin strands of

Table 6–1. Histologic Variants of Basal Cell Carcinoma (BCC)

Type	Microscopic Features	Recurrence	Metastasis
Superficial	Multifocal connection of basaloid tumor cells to the epidermis.	F	I
Nodular	Large nests of basaloid tumor cells in the dermis.	I	I
Micronodular	Small basaloid tumor nests involving deep dermis and subcutis.	F	I
Infiltrative/morpheaform	Irregular, cords and cluster of basaloid tumor cells in a dense connective tissue stroma.	F	I
Squamous differentiation	BCC with areas that show keratinization or keratin pearls.	F	I
Hamartomatous	BCC with abortive hair follicle like structures or papillary mesenchymal bodies and a cellular stroma.	I	I
Adenoid	Basaloid tumor cells with cribriform pattern of growth.	I	I

F = frequent, I = infrequent.

tumor cells embedded in a dense connective tissue stroma may extend into the reticular dermis and subcutis. Peripheral nuclear palisading is not readily apparent, and stromal retraction is inconspicuous.

Histologic variants of BCC with no significant impact on prognosis, but which may mimic other cutaneous neoplasms encountered in the head and neck, are the hamartomatous type, which includes keratotic, infundibulocystic, follicular, and other specific cell lineages of differentiation, and adenoid type.

Basal cell carcinoma with hamartomatous features may show abortive hair folliclelike structures, pilar-type keratinization, or cornification with parakeratosis. Differentiation from trichoepithelioma may be difficult. BCC usually has at least focal mucinous stroma and peripheral clefting.[26] The absence of labeling of the tumor stroma with CD34 may be helpful in identifying BCC. At any rate, in cases that extend to the deep tissue edge, it is usually recommended to re-excise and evaluate the entire lesion.[27]

Adenoid BCC is composed of cells arranged in rows around small mucin-filled spaces, with a cribriform and glandlike pattern of growth. Histologic features that distinguish this tumor from true glandular tumors (eg, adenoid cystic carcinoma) include a connection to the epidermis, peripheral palisading of nuclei, and retraction artifact.

Extramammary Paget Disease

Extramammary Paget disease (EMPD) is a neoplasm that normally affects apocrine gland-bearing skin of the axillary and anogenital regions. However, on rare occasions, EMPD can occur on facial skin.[28] Lesions may clinically appear as an eczemalike rash, SCC, or superficial basal cell carcinoma.

Histologically, EMPD is composed of atypical, large, round cells with prominent nucleoli and abundant pale cytoplasm at all levels of the epidermis and follicular epithelium. Tumor cells often are separated by a basal layer of keratinocytes along the dermal-epidermal junction (known as the "eye-liner sign"). The differential diagnosis includes SCIS and melanoma in-situ. Tumor cells of EMPD are positive for cytokeratin 7 and CEA and may demonstrate intracytoplasmic mucin which can be detected with mucicarmine stain (Fig 6–4, A–B).

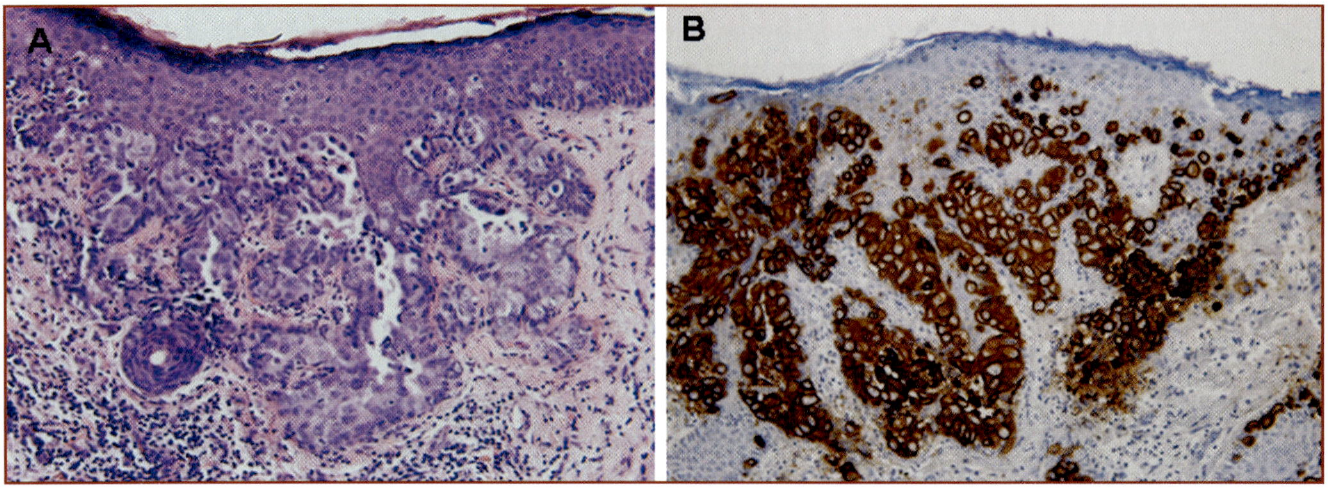

Figure 6–4. A. Extrammamary Paget disease. Atypical, large, round tumor cells with prominent nucleoli and abundant pale cytoplasm at all levels of the epidermis and follicular epithelium. **B.** Tumor cells positive for cytokeratin 7.

Mesenchymal Neoplasms

Fibrohistiocytic Proliferations

Fibrohistiocytic tumors of the skin can be categorized as benign, intermediate, or malignant and are characterized by aggressive local growth, propensity to recur if incompletely excised, and a low risk of metastatic potential in most cases.[29] The diagnosis relies on a constellation of histologic and cytologic features with immunophenotyping of the tumor cells for confirmation. Immunohistochemical markers utilized to diagnose soft tissue tumors of the skin include factor XIIIA, CD34, CD68, and CD10, in addition to absence of epithelial and melanocytic markers.[30,31]

Benign Fibrous Histiocytoma (Dermatofibroma) and Indeterminate Fibrohistiocytic Lesion

Dermatofibromas are common, benign, soft tissue neoplasms of the skin that typically occur on the extremities. Lesions that present on the head and neck are frequently referred to as benign fibrous histiocytoma (BFH).

Histologically, BFH is a well-circumscribed, dermal-based neoplasm composed of short spindle-shaped cells arranged in storiform fascicles that infiltrate thick, sclerotic bundles of collagen. The overlying epidermis is acanthotic with increased pigment of basal keratinocytes, and, at the periphery of the lesion, the spindle-shaped cells surround or entrap bundles of collagen. There is a mixture of cell types, including fibroblasts, histiocytes, and Touton or floret-type of multinucleated giant cells, xanthoma cells, and siderophages. Mitotic figures are commonly seen, but there is no significant cytologic atypia. On occasion, scattered large atypical or "monster" cells may be encountered, but they should only account for a minor population of cells.

Lesions with increased cellularity (cellular fibrous histiocytomas) often extend into the deep reticular dermis and superficial portions of the subcutaneous tissue. Benign cellular fibrous histiocytomas are more likely to recur if incompletely excised and may even metastasize. Immunohistochemically, fibrous histiocytoma are positive for factor XIIIA and negative for CD34.

At times, fibrohistiocytic tumors may express immunophenotypic features of a fibrous histiocytoma and dermatofibrosarcoma protuberans (DFSP). These indeterminate fibrous histiocytic lesions histologically appear similar to cellular fibrous histiocytomas and are composed of cellular fascicles with a storiform pattern that frequently extends into superficial portions of the subcutaneous tissue. Indeterminate fibrous histiocytic lesions are composed of a dual population of factor XIIIa and CD34-positive tumor cells and have a propensity to recur (Fig 6–5, A–B).[32]

Dermatofibrosarcoma Protuberans (DFSP)

Dermatofibrosarcoma protuberans of the head and neck are associated with a higher rate of recurrence than tumors at other cutaneous sites, and they typically occur on the forehead and scalp.[33] DFSP occur in adults; the variant giant cell fibroblastoma (GCF) is more commonly encountered in children.

DFSP is a deep dermal and subcutaneous neoplasm composed of a cellular proliferation of a uniform population of spindle-shaped cells in a storiform arrangement that infiltrates into the subcutaneous adipose tissue in a "honeycomb" or "string of pearls" pattern. There are minimal cellular pleomorphism and infrequent mitoses. Siderophages and xanthoma cells are not a characteristic cellular component. Tumor cells are positive for CD34 and negative for factor XIIIa (Fig 6–6, A–C).

Giant cell fibroblastoma (GCF) histologically demonstrates a proliferation of stellate-shaped spindle cells with areas of angiectoid, interconnecting pseudovascular spaces often lined by floret-type multinucleated giant cells. Tumor cells are also CD34 positive. Both DFSP and GCF contain COL1A1/PDGFβ transcripts. Therefore, some authors have recommended the use of anti-PDGF medications, such as Gleevec, for tumors not amenable to surgery.[34]

Atypical Fibroxanthoma (AFX)

Atypical fibroxanthoma is a low-grade soft tissue neoplasm which typically occurs on the sun-exposed skin of the head and neck in elderly men. Adequate surgical excision is often curative and the risk for recurrence or metastasis is low.

AFX is a dermal neoplasm composed of large, pleomorphic, spindle, and stellate-shaped tumor cells with hyperchromatic, irregular, vesicular nuclei and prominent nucleoli. Bizarre-shaped multinucleated tumor cells and abnormal mitotic figures are common features (Fig 6–7, A–B). A narrow grenz zone of normal dermal collagen separates the tumor from the overlying epidermis. Rarely, there is infiltration into the subcutaneous adipose tissue. Tumor cells are positive for CD68 and CD10 and negative for epithelial and melanocytic markers.[31]

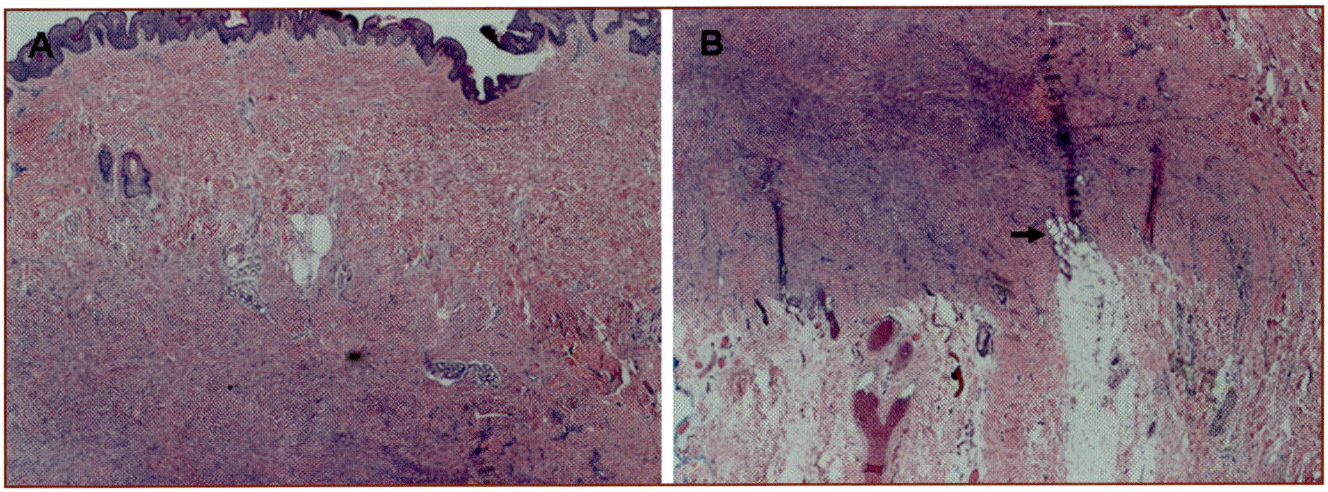

Figure 6–5. A. Indeterminate fibrous histiocytic lesion. Cellular fascicles of spindle cells in the dermis. **B.** Involvement of the superficial aspect of subcutis (*arrow*) is a common feature.

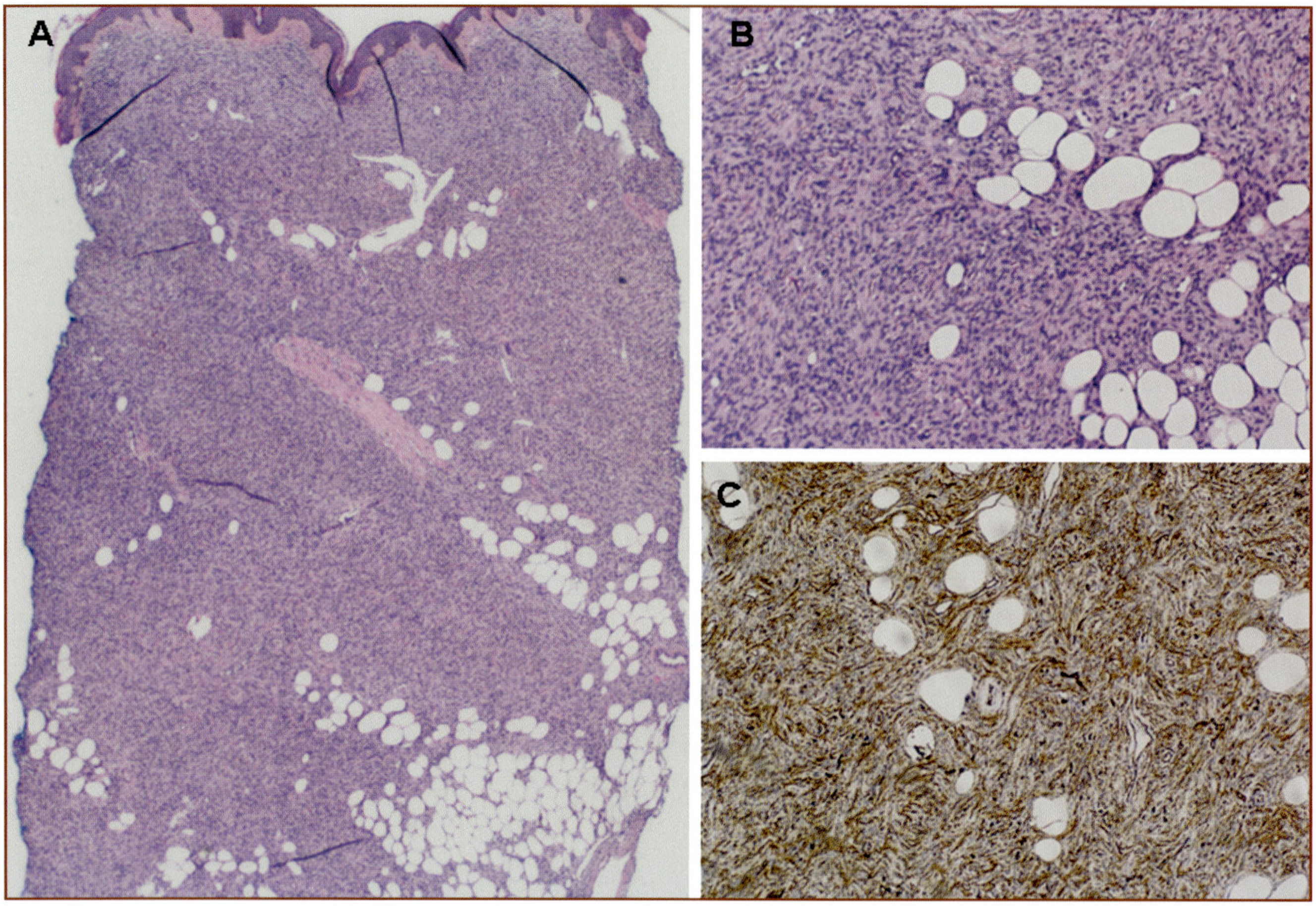

Figure 6–6. **A.** Dermatofibrosarcoma protuberans (DFSP). Cellular proliferation of short, fusiform-shaped spindle cells in the dermis and subcutis. **B.** Tumor cells infiltrate adipose tissue in a "honeycomb" pattern. **C.** Tumor cells are positive for CD34.

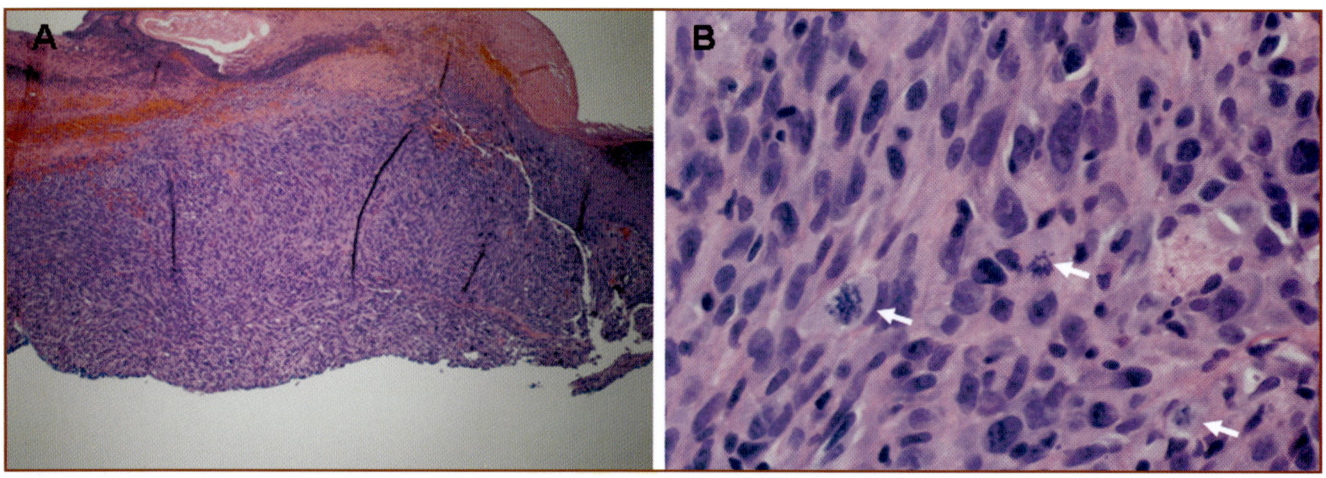

Figure 6–7. **A.** Atypical fibroxanthoma (AFX). Ulcerated, cellular tumor nodule in the dermis. **B.** Cytologically malignant epithelioid and spindle-shaped cells with abnormal mitotic figures (*arrows*).

Malignant Fibrous Histiocytoma (MFH)

Malignant fibrous histiocytoma is a deep soft tissue neoplasm in adults, which shares histologic and immunohistochemical features with AFX. The location in the skin (AFX is confined to dermis while MFH involves subcutaneous tissue) and tumor size (AFX average size 2.0 cm versus MFH average size 4.0 cm) help to differentiate these entities. Upward extension of the tumor cells into the dermis can be seen in the superficial type of MFH.[35] Despite the similar histologic and immunohistochemical features, the biologic behavior of these tumors drastically differs. AFX commonly is cured by complete excision, whereas MFH typically recurs and even metastasizes.

Vascular Tumors

Kaposi Sarcoma

Kaposi sarcoma (KS) is a spindle cell neoplasm associated with human herpes virus (HHV)-8 and represents one of the most common skin tumors in transplanted, Mediterranean, and HIV-positive subjects.[36] HHV-8 is necessary, but not sufficient, to cause KS.[37]

The histopathologic findings of usual lesions are associated with disease progression: patch, plaque, and nodular stage.[38] The earliest lesions, corresponding to the patch stage, are the most difficult to diagnose. Newly formed slitlike or irregular vascular spaces are seen at high power magnification; these neoplastic channels may surround pre-existing capillaries, resulting in the so-called promontory sign. Plaque and nodular stages exhibit more cellular infiltrates composed of spindle cells arranged in fascicles. Extravasated red blood cells are present. There usually are intracytoplasmic bodies (also referred as "autolumination" or Dorfman bodies) that correspond to fragments of phagocytized erythrocytes. Immunohistochemical studies for HHV-8, LNA-1, D2-40, CD31, and CD34 may be useful for diagnosis. Rare variants include anaplastic, lymphangioma-like, micronodular, and intravascular.[39–42] Partially regressed lesions following antiretroviral therapy reveal a significant reduction in the number of spindle cells in the intervening stroma and a few residual spindle cells around native vessels.[38]

Angiosarcoma

About 50% of cutaneous angiosarcoma (AS) cases occur on the head and neck, especially on the scalp of elderly men.[43] Rarely, it involves intra-oral, pharyngeal, or maxillary locations.[44]

The early stages are characterized by a proliferation of small, thin-walled vessels that dissect collagen bundles in the reticular dermis. As the lesion progresses, the newly formed blood vessels appear to branch and anastomose with conspicuous, protuberant endothelial cells showing atypical nuclei. Plaques can develop into nodules composed of closely attached tumor cells, making the vascular nature of the neoplasm less obvious (Fig 6–8). Histological grading goes from well-differentiated neoplasms to very poorly differentiated ones, in which the distinction from spindle cell squamous cell carcinoma, melanoma, and KS may be difficult. In such cases, immunohistochemical studies that may help in the diagnosis are CD31, CD34, D2-40, factor VIII-related antigen, Ulex europaeus lectin, and laminin.[45] Traditionally, the degree of differentiation of this neoplasm has not been considered important for prognosis, as correlation with outcome could not be demonstrated.[46] A recent report, however, has postulated that epithelioid morphology and necrosis, combined with clinical features such as age, may define a subgroup of higher risk angiosarcomas.[46]

Smooth Muscle and Neural Tumors

Leiomyosarcoma

Cutaneous leiomyosarcoma is a malignant neoplasm composed of cells that show diffuse or focal expression of smooth muscle differentiation markers. Cutaneous leiomyosarcoma usually presents as a solitary lesion, classically described as situated mostly on the extremities.[47] It recently has been reported, however, that more cutaneous leiomyosarcomas present on the head and neck than any other location of the body.[48] The tumor rarely metastasizes, although it may recur in about 40% of the cases.[49]

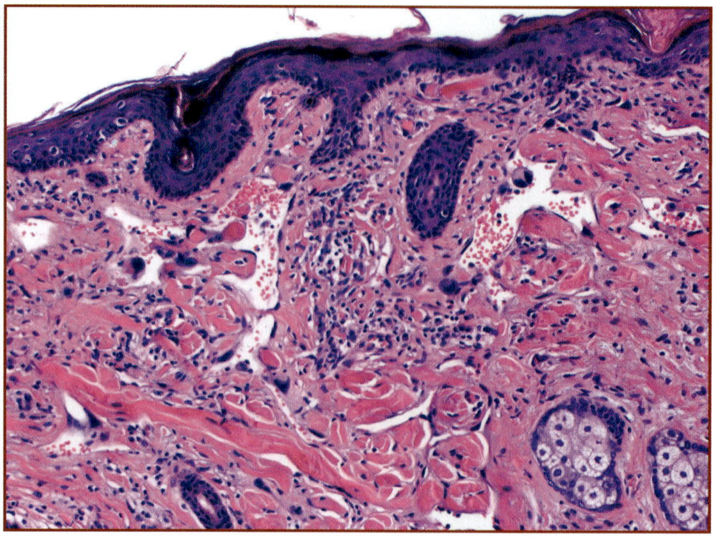

Figure 6–8. Angiosarcoma. Abnormal anastomosing dermal blood vessels lined by atypical endothelial cells. The neoplastic vessels dissect collagen bundles.

Histologically, cutaneous leiomyosarcomas are located in the dermis and may extend into the superficial subcutis. The neoplastic cells form interlacing fascicles; the cells show spindle shape, eosinophilic cytoplasm, elongated nuclei with blunt ends, and small to prominent nucleoli.[50] Bizarre cells and mitotic figures may be present. Cytologic atypia and at least one mitotic figure per 10 HPF are enough for a diagnosis of malignancy. Two types of growth patterns have been described: nodular and diffuse.[47] Other histologic variants also have been reported in the literature, including a desmoplastic one.[51] Most of the cases are positive, at least focally, for desmin, smooth muscle actin, and vimentin. Occasionally, they may show focal expression of S-100 protein, leading to possible confusion with spindle cell melanoma.[50]

Malignant Peripheral Nerve Sheath Tumor

Malignant peripheral nerve sheath tumor (MPNST, neurofibrosarcoma) is a malignant tumor originating from or differentiating toward cells of the peripheral nerve sheath. MPNSTs are mostly located on the trunk and extremities; head and neck sites are involved in 8 to 20% of cases.[52] The tumors located on the head and neck frequently involve the fifth cranial nerve and arise in association with neurofibromas, with or without von Recklinghausen disease.[53,54]

The tumors are highly cellular, spindle cell neoplasms. The tumor cells show wavy, comma-shaped nuclei and frequent mitotic figures. A fascicular pattern of growth is characteristic, as well as an alternation of areas of high and low cellular density; the latter ones often showing myxoid stroma. The myxoid areas frequently demonstrate a perivascular arrangement of tumor cells. If extensive necrosis is present, it tends to spare the perivascular tumor cells, giving the tumor a "peritheliomatous" appearance. As with other neural tumors, MPNST has vessels with prominent endothelial cells. Patchy (not diffuse) immunohistochemical positivity for S-100 protein is characteristic.

Among the many variants of MPNST that have been described, those tumors composed of round cells (epithelioid) and also tumors displaying mesenchymal components (rhabdomyoblastoma, chondrosarcoma, osteosarcoma, angiosarcoma), as they mimic other tumors, may pose considerable diagnostic difficulty. Plexiform schwannoma (a tumor showing a predilection for the head and neck region), especially the cellular subtype, may be difficult to distinguish from MPNST. However, cellular schwannomas show diffuse positivity for S-100 protein in contrast with the patchy pattern seen in MPNST.[55]

Granular Cell Tumor

Granular cell tumor (GCT, also known as Abrikossoff tumor) is a benign lesion of neural origin. The head and neck region is affected in up to 65% of the cases, and, of these, 70% are intraoral.[56] The malignant counterpart of GCT remains rare and accounts for less than 2% of the cases.[57]

GCTs are solitary or multiple, small, poorly circumscribed nodules located in the dermis, subcutis or submucosa. The overlying squamous epithelium can show acanthosis (skin) or pseudoepitheliomatous hyperplasia (oral mucosa) mimicking a squamous cell carcinoma. The tumor cells tend to cluster in nests, ribbons, or in a plexiform pattern and are rounded to spindle with an eosinophilic cytoplasm containing granules that are PAS-positive, diastase-resistant.[58] These granules are phagolysosomes containing myelin and mitochondria. The nuclei vary from small and dark to large with vesicular chromatin. A mild to moderate amount of nuclear atypia is normal within these tumors. In older lesions, collagen may represent the larger volume of the tumor, and only a few scattered nests of granular cells can be observed.

The tumor cells show an immunohistochemical panel that confirms their neural origin: S-100, neuron-specific enolase, and laminin are often positive. The lysosomal granules are also positive for CD68, whereas neurofilament and glial fibrillary acidic protein (GFAP) are negative.[59–62] The differential diagnosis of GCT includes rhabdomyoma, hibernoma, fibroxanthoma and reactive changes associated with surgical trauma. As mentioned above, the areas of epidermal hyperplasia above the lesion should not be confused with squamous cell carcinoma.

Malignant GCT are histologically similar to their benign counterpart but show three or more of the following features: greater than two mitoses per 10 HPF, pleomorphism, necrosis, prominent nucleoli, diffuse spindling, and high nucleus/cytoplasm ratio. Tumors with intermediate features are termed "atypical granular cell tumor." Recurrence of the tumor occurs usually within 1 year. Metastases take several years to appear and mainly involve the lymph nodes, lung and liver.[57] Other tumors that can show focal granular changes are leiomyosarcoma, malignant fibrous histiocytoma, and angiosarcoma.

Malignant Adnexal Neoplasms

Malignant adnexal neoplasms are epithelial tumors that show differentiation toward the pilosebaceous unit, the sebaceous glands, or the eccrine/sebaceous glands.

Follicular Neoplasms

Trichilemmal Carcinoma

Trichilemmal carcinoma (TC) is a neoplasm that differentiates toward the external root sheath of the hair follicle.[63] TC arises in hair-bearing, sun-exposed areas, especially the face, scalp and ears. It is still unknown whether they originate de novo or from a preexistent trichilemmoma.[64] In general, TC exhibits indolent clinical behavior, although local recurrences have been described.[65]

Microscopically, TC shows a lobular growth pattern with invasion of the reticular dermis. There are focal cells with clear, glycogen-rich cytoplasm and abrupt keratinization without a granular layer ("trichilemmal-type" keratinization). There may be mitotic figures, atypia, and individual cell necrosis. Peripheral palisading of nuclei with basal vacuolization is sometimes present. The tumor is connected to the epidermis and the follicular epithelium. The differential diagnosis includes trichilemmoma, malignant pilar tumor, clear cell squamous cell carcinoma, clear cell basal cell carcinoma, metastatic clear cell renal carcinoma, and cutaneous adnexal carcinomas with divergent differentiation.

Malignant Pilar Tumor

Pilar tumors (proliferating trichilemmal tumor) are tumors that differentiate toward the isthmus region of the external root sheath of the hair follicle. The scalp represents the most common location for these tumors. Classification into benign, low-grade malignant, and high-grade malignant has been proposed based on the degree of nuclear atypia, mitoses, invasion and necrosis present in the lesion.[66]

Malignant pilar tumors (MPT) may occur within a preexisting benign pilar tumor or a trichilemmal cyst. Histologically, MPT show nuclear pleomorphism, high mitotic activity, and an invasive growth pattern. Low-grade MPT show irregularly shaped nests of cells that infiltrate the deep dermis. High-grade MPT show individual cell cords and stromal desmoplasia. Occasionally there are abrupt keratinization, compact eosinophilic keratin (typical of trichilemmal cysts), and focal matrical differentiation (represented by shadow/"ghost" cells).[67]

Eccrine Neoplasms

This section includes neoplasms with a predominant differentiation toward the eccrine ducts or glands. Usually, eccrine carcinomas occur de novo, although they occasionally can arise from a pre-existing benign tumor.

Porocarcinoma

Porocarcinoma is the malignant counterpart of poroma, a neoplasm that differentiates toward the eccrine duct. Most cases of porocarcinoma occur in the lower extremities; 18% of cases occur in the head and neck.[68] Porocarcinoma has the potential to develop regional and distant metastases, and it may be fatal.[69]

Microscopically, porocarcinoma consists of cords and nests of keratinocytes that, although connected to the epidermis, demonstrate a sharp demarcation from it. These cords and nests infiltrate the dermis, producing a desmoplastic stromal reaction. The lesions contain ducts that are reactive to CEA and EMA. Severe atypia and a high mitotic rate are frequently identified. Epidermotropism is not rare, and the appearance can simulate extramammary Paget's disease.[70] Occasionally, there are squamous and clear cell differentiation, as well as melanin pigmentation. The tumor is positive for pancytokeratin by immunohistochemistry.[71]

Hidradenocarcinoma

Hidradenocarcinoma usually is a dermal or subcutaneous nodule that can emerge in any area of the body. This carcinoma can metastasize extensively and be lethal.

Microscopically, hidradenocarcinoma consists of one or several nodules with massive necrosis and focal ductal structures. The nodules are composed of clear, squamous or mucinous cells with focal atypia, pleomorphic nuclei, and mitoses. The cells are positive for CAM 5.2 and cytokeratin 19. The ductular structures are CEA and EMA positive.[72]

Microcystic Adnexal Carcinoma

Microcystic adnexal carcinoma (MAC, also known as sclerosing sweat duct carcinoma) is a low-grade adenocarcinoma that forms ducts. Microcystic adnexal carcinoma is frequently located on the face and lip; it is locally infiltrative but does not metastasize.[73,74]

Histologically, the solid to cystic structures are located in the most superficial areas of the neoplasm; while in the deepest areas, the cells tend to form single-cell, elongated clusters ("Indian filing"). Sclerosis is common, and perineural invasion may be seen. The tumor cells are well differentiated and lack pleomorphism or mitotic figures—this feature is important for its distinction from squamous cell carcinoma or standard adenocarcinoma. MAC cells are positive to AE1/AE3, CK7, and Bcl-2; a low proliferation index is revealed by Ki-67.[75]

Malignant Mixed Tumor

Malignant mixed tumor (MMT, malignant chondroid syringoma) is the malignant counterpart of benign mixed tumors. It is a very rare neoplasm that shows a predilection for the trunk and extremities. Unlike benign mixed tumor, it is infrequent in the head and neck.[76]

Microscopically, MMT is a poorly circumscribed tumor with both epithelial and mesenchymal chondromyxoid components. The epithelial component forms cords, nests, and some tubules of one or two layers of cells. Atypia can be mild to severe, mitoses are numerous, and necrosis is common. Plasmacytoid differentiation of the epithelial cells is considered an indication of myoepithelial differentiation and may be important for the diagnosis of MMT. The cells of MMT can co-express S-100 and cytokeratin.[77,78]

Mucinous Carcinoma (MC)

Mucinous carcinoma is frequent on the scalp and the eyelids. The course of MC usually is indolent, and it tends to recur locally. However, it has the potential to metastasize, especially to regional lymph nodes.

Microscopically, MC is a dermal tumor with large pools of a basophilic mucin divided by fibrous septa that give it a honeycomb appearance. Within the mucin, nests of epithelial cells are frequent. Nuclei show little atypia and mitotic figures are rare. Immunohistochemically, the cells are positive for low molecular weight cytokeratins, and negative for CK20.[79] CEA, EMA, GCDFP-15, alpha-lactalbumin, salivary amylase, and beta-2-microglobulin are positive as well.[80] In the noninvasive areas, anti-p63 labels a rim of benign myoepithelial cells.[81]

The differential diagnosis includes metastatic mucinous carcinoma, usually from the breast or gastrointestinal tract. The lesions are histologically identical to primary mucinous carcinomas of the eyelid, although occasionally they are bilateral and anti-p63 fails to detect a rim of myoepithelial cells.

Sebaceous Neoplasms

Sebaceous Adenoma

Although a benign tumor, sebaceous adenoma (SA) is important to recognize as it frequently is located on the head and neck.[82] SA may be associated with Muir-Torre syndrome, a condition characterized by predisposition to malignancies of the colon, endometrium, urogenital, and upper gastrointestinal tracts.[83]

Microscopically, SA is a circumscribed and multilobulated tumor that shows a peripheral rim of basaloid cells and a predominance of mature sebaceous cells. Demonstration of microsatellite instability through immunohistochemical studies for DNA mismatch repair gene-encoded proteins (such as MLH-1, MSH-2, MSH-6, and PMS-2) is useful for the diagnosis of Muir-Torre syndrome.[84]

Sebaceous Epithelioma

Sebaceous epithelioma (sebaceoma) also occurs on the face and scalp and may also be found in association with Muir-Torre syndrome. The classic histologic description of sebaceous epithelioma is that of a well circumscribed nodule in which more than half of the cells are basaloid but still show mature sebaceous and transitional cells.[85]

Sebaceous Carcinoma

Sebaceous carcinoma (SC) is a neoplasm of sebaceous differentiation frequent in the head and neck. Based on its location, SC can be classified into ocular and extraocular categories.[86] SC recurs locally, can metastasize, and is lethal in 10 to 20% of cases.[87] SC also can be associated with the Muir-Torre syndrome, particularly when lesions are located outside the head and neck.[88,89]

Microscopically, the cells of SC are polygonal and show a multivacuolated clear cytoplasm. They are arranged in lobules, with a fibrovascular stroma. Characteristically, desmoplasia is not evident. Comedonecrosis may be seen. Pleomorphism and mitotic figures may be present and vary in severity and number (Fig 6–9, A–C). Grading of SC is based on growth patterns: from well-demarcated lobules (grade I) to sheets of cells with an invasive growth (grade III). Carcinoma in situ and extrammamary Paget disease of the sebaceous type can be associated with SC. SC is positive for pankeratin, EMA, CD15, and adipophilin.[90] Detection of p53 and proliferating cell nuclear antigen (PCNA) might be useful for prognosis.[91]

Merkel Cell Carcinoma

Merkel cell carcinoma (MCC) is a malignant neoplasm with epithelial and neuroendocrine differentiation. It has a high incidence of local recurrence, regional spread, and distant metastases. About 50% of MCC occur on the sun-exposed skin of the head and neck.[92] A new polyomavirus (so-called Merkel cell polyomavirus) has been associated recently with MCC; a causal relationship still needs to be proved.[93]

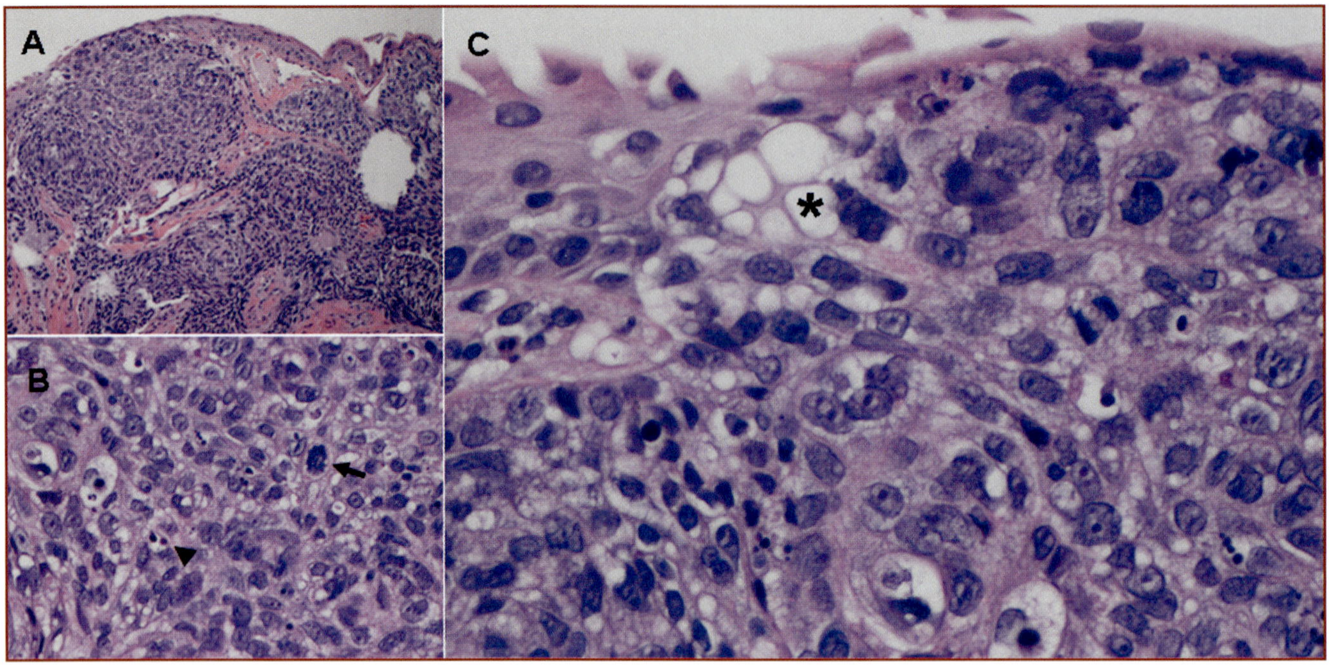

Figure 6–9. **A.** Sebaceous carcinoma. Infiltrating tumor lobules connected to the epidermis composed of basaloid cells. **B.** High grade tumor with prominent apoptosis (*arrowhead*) and mitoses (*arrow*). **C.** Tumor cells with sebaceous differentiation characterized by multivacuolated clear cytoplasm (*).

Histologically, MCC is composed of small uniform cells with round nuclei and scant cytoplasm ("blue cells") arranged in a solid pattern in the dermis and subcutaneous fat (Fig 6–10, A–B). Mitoses are frequent, and necrosis can be seen in large lesions. Intraepidermal pagetoid spread can also be present.[94] Occasionally, there may be areas of standard adenocarcinoma or squamous cell carcinoma, either in situ or invasive.[95]

The differential diagnosis includes basal cell carcinoma, lymphoma, poorly differentiated squamous cell carcinoma, eccrine carcinoma, peripheral primitive neuroectodermal tumor, metastatic neuroendocrine carcinoma, metastatic neuroblastoma and melanoma. In particular, the presence of the intraepidermal component may mimic the characteristic pagetoid upward migration of melanoma.

By immunohistochemistry, MCC shows paranuclear ("dotlike") or diffuse cytoplasmic staining for low molecular weight cytokeratins and cytokeratin 20. MCC also expresses markers of neuroendocrine differentiation such as chromogranin, synaptophysin, and neuron-specific enolase. MCC can be positive for CD99 and CD117 (c-KIT).[96,97]

Lymphoid Neoplasms and Selected Reactive Conditions

Lymphoid Hyperplasia (reactive)

Cutaneous Lymphoid Hyperplasia

Cutaneous lymphoid hyperplasia (CLH), also known as cutaneous "pseudolymphoma" or "lymphocytoma" cutis, is a reactive lymphoproliferative process induced by microbial, physical, or chemical irritants.[98] In the head and neck, the ear lobe is a frequent location of Borrelia-induced CLH (lymphadenosis benigna cutis). Other lesions may be

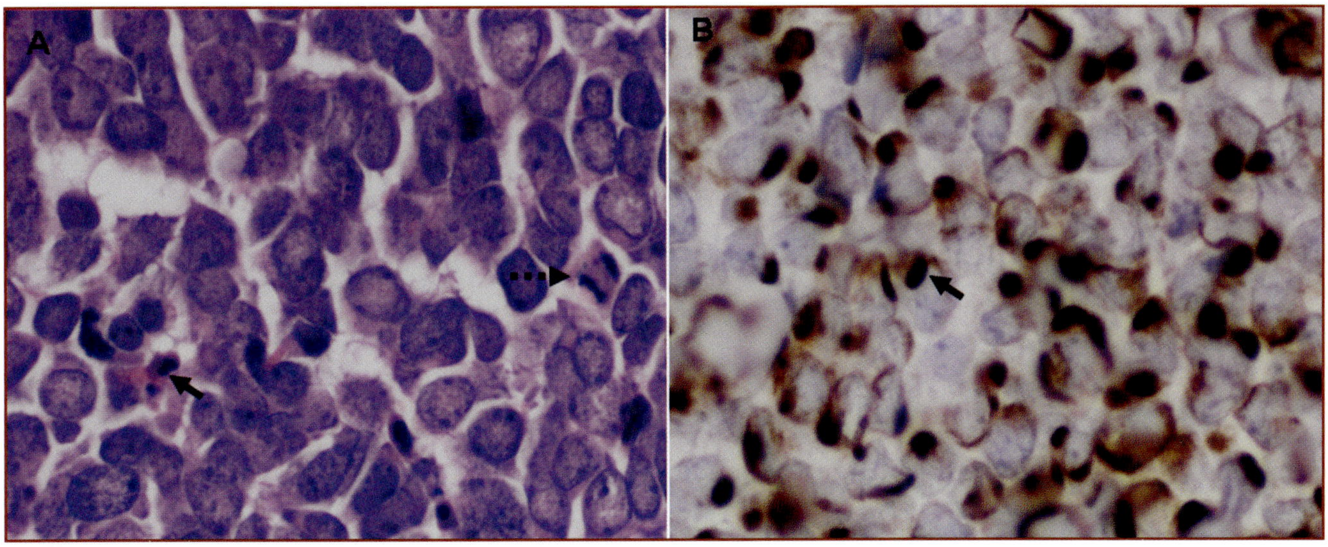

Figure 6–10. **A.** Merkel cell carcinoma composed of small uniform cells with round nuclei and scant cytoplasm in the dermis and subcutaneous tissue. Nuclei are granular with "salt and pepper" appearance and mitoses (*arrow*) and apoptosis (*dashed arrow*) are frequent. **B.** Tumor cells are positive with cytokeratin 20 with dot like perinuclear accentuation (*arrow*).

associated with arthropod bite reactions or herpes virus infection.[99,100]

Histologically, a mixed lymphocytic infiltrate surrounds the vessels of the upper and mid dermis in a nodular pattern. Eosinophils and macrophages may be seen. Commonly, there are reactive follicles that contain "tingible body macrophages" (macrophages with ingested nuclear debris), creating a "starry sky" appearance. The nodular infiltrate shows a concave, poorly demarcated border. The immunochemistry of CLH reveals a reactive pattern characterized by a polyclonal infiltration of B-cells that are positive for CD20 and CD79a, mature T-cells positive for CD3 and no restriction of light chain immunoglobulins, as confirmed by studies for kappa and lambda.

Angiolymphoid Hyperplasia with Eosinophilia

Angiolymphoid hyperplasia with eosinophilia (ALHE), also called epithelioid hemangioma (Rosai), is a benign tumor that occurs frequently on the skin of the head and neck, especially on the forehead, scalp, and around the ear. It probably is a reactive rather than neoplastic process.[101,102] These lesions are prone to recurrence.

Microscopically, ALHE is a lobulated dermal or subcutaneous proliferation of immature blood vessels and chronic inflammation with abundant eosinophils. A large vessel surrounded by small arborizing vessels is sometimes observed. The endothelial cells have a characteristic abundant eosinophilic cytoplasm that protrudes in the lumen. They are positive for CD31, CD34, and VWF, and mitoses are occasional. A mixture of B-cells, T-cells, and eosinophils is located between the vessels. There may be lymphoid follicles with reactive germinal centers.

Cutaneous Lymphomas

The skin can be involved by B- and T-cell lymphomas that are either primary or secondary.

Primary Cutaneous B-Cell Lymphomas

Primary cutaneous B-cell lymphomas include the following: cutaneous marginal zone B-cell lymphoma

(MALT-type), cutaneous follicle center lymphoma, and cutaneous diffuse large B-cell lymphoma. Secondary lesions include involvement by intravascular large B-cell lymphoma, lymphomatoid granulomatosis, chronic lymphocytic leukemia, mantle cell lymphoma, and Burkitt lymphoma. In general, primary cutaneous B-cell lymphomas tend to present with a nodular, triangular architecture with the base in the deep dermis or subcutis ("bottom heavy"). Perivascular cuffing is present and the epidermis is spared ("Grenz zone"). The neoplastic lymphocytes express CD19, CD20, and CD79a.

Primary cutaneous marginal zone B-cell lymphomas (MZL) show residual reactive lymphoid follicles and an interfollicular infiltrate composed of monocytoid cells.[103] The most important studies for confirmation of the diagnosis of MZL are those for the immunoglobulin kappa and lambda light chains, ki-67, and Bcl-6.[104]

Primary cutaneous follicle center lymphomas (FCL) display a spectrum of histologic patterns from follicular to diffuse. The tumor is composed of a mixture of centrocytes and centroblasts. FCL, follicular type, frequently occurs on the head and neck area. The neoplastic cells are positive for Bcl-6, CD10, and usually do not express Bcl-2.[105] Although it is said that the finding of Bcl-2 expression in a FCL in the skin should raise the strong suspicion of a secondary involvement by a systemic lymphoma, a number of cases of primary cutaneous FCL also express Bcl-2.[104]

Primary cutaneous diffuse large B cell lymphoma (DLBCL), leg-type, is the most common variant of DLBCL occurring in the skin. Although most of the cases present with multiple tumors on the legs, the head and neck region can be involved. The tumor shows a dense, monomorphous infiltrate composed of large cells (immunoblasts and centroblasts)[104] The tumor cells show strong positivity for Bcl-2, MUM-1, and Bcl-6[106]

Primary Cutaneous T-Cell Lymphomas

Primary T-cell lymphomas of the skin include: mycosis fungoides, Sezary syndrome, CD30-positive T-cell lymphoproliferative disorders of the skin, subcutaneous panniculitislike T-cell lymphoma, primary cutaneous peripheral T-cell lymphoma (PTL), extranodal NK/T-cell lymphoma (nasal type), adult T-cell leukemia/lymphoma, and angioimmunoblastic T-cell lymphoma.

Mycosis fungoides (MF) is the most common cutaneous lymphoma. The lesions usually occur on sun-protected areas; however, variants such as folliculotropic MF (associated with follicular mucinosis) may involve the head and neck region.[107] The diagnosis of early (patch) lesions is mainly based on subtle histopathologic findings such as the presence of a superficial patchy-lichenoid lymphocytic infiltrate, fibrotic papillary dermis, and epidermotropic haloed lymphocytes showing cytologic atypia. The infiltrating cells commonly show a CD3-, CD4-positive phenotype. Loss of expression of CD7 and molecular analyses demonstrating a clonal T-cell population may help in the diagnosis. Sezary syndrome may be indistinguishable from MF on histologic examination, although it tends to display less epidermotropism.[104]

Primary cutaneous CD30-positive T-cell lymphoproliferative disorders include a spectrum of lesions ranging from lymphomatoid papulosis (LYP) to primary cutaneous anaplastic large cell lymphoma (ALCL).[108] Whereas LYP typically shows a wedge-shaped infiltrate with variable numbers of large atypical CD30-positive cells arranged in small clusters, ALCL usually presents with sheets of CD30-positive tumor cells. Borderline lesions are frequent.

Subcutaneous panniculitis-like T–cell lymphoma involves the subcutis. The lesion shows marked necrosis and karyorrhexis. The tumor cells are usually CD8-positive and express cytotoxic markers, such as perforin, granzyme B, and TIA-1.[109]

Extranodal NK/T-cell lymphoma, nasal type, shows a characteristic angiocentric distribution and positivity for EBV.[110] The cells express CD2 and CD56. The hydroa vacciniformelike variant, more common in Asia and South America, presents with facial edema and crusted lesions on sun-exposed areas; the lymphoma cells are usually positive for CD3, CD8, and cytotoxic markers.[111]

Cutaneous adult T-cell leukemia/lymphoma is a CD4-positive lymphoma caused by HTLV-I virus, histologically very similar to MF. Skin involvement by angioimmunoblastic T-cell lymphoma is characterized by perivascular lymphocytic infiltrates admixed with eosinophils and plasma cells.

Conclusions

Nonmelanoma skin tumors represent an eclectic group of neoplasms, although basal cell carcinoma and squamous cell carcinoma are the most common lesions encountered clinically. Cutaneous lesions may arise from the epithelium, mesenchymal elements, neuroendocrine cells, adnexal structures, and even lymphoid aggregates with the skin. An appreciation of the variability and nuance in skin neoplasms is required by the clinician, and excisional or incisional/punch biopsy often provides confirmatory information to complete the clinical picture. Consultation with an experienced dermatopathologist is integral to the multidisciplinary management of patients with aggressive cutaneous malignancy.

References

1. Bhawan J. Squamous cell carcinoma in situ in skin: what does it mean? *J Cutan Pathol.* 2007;34(12):953–955.
2. Person JR. An actinic keratosis is neither malignant nor premalignant: it is an initiated tumor. *J Am Acad Dermatol.* 2003;48(4):637–638.
3. Knudson AG, Jr. Mutation and cancer: statistical study of retinoblastoma. *Proc Natl Acad Sci U S A.* 1971;68(4): 820–823.
4. Uitto J. The role of elastin and collagen in cutaneous aging: intrinsic aging versus photoexposure. *J Drugs Dermatol.* 2008;7(2 suppl):s12–16.
5. Prieto VG, Shea CR. Use of immunohistochemistry in melanocytic lesions. *J Cutan Pathol.* 2008;35 (suppl 2): 1–10.
6. Prieto VG, Casal M, McNutt NS. Lichen planus-like keratosis. A clinical and histological reexamination. *Am J Surg Pathol.* 1993;17(3):259–263.
7. Cassarino DS, Derienzo DP, Barr RJ. Cutaneous squamous cell carcinoma: a comprehensive clinicopathologic classification. Part one. *J Cutan Pathol.* 2006;33(3): 191–206.
8. Steffen C, Ackerman AB. Intraepidermal epithelioma of Borst-Jadassohn. *Am J Dermatopathol.* 1985;7(1):5–24.
9. Gusterson BA, Warburton MJ, Mitchell D, Kraft N, Hancock WW. Invading squamous cell carcinoma can retain a basal lamina. An immunohistochemical study using a monoclonal antibody to type IV collagen. *Lab Invest.* 1984;51(1):82–87.
10. Wolf IH, Kodama K, Cerroni L, Kerl H. Nature of inflammatory infiltrate in superficial cutaneous malignancies during topical imiquimod treatment. *Am J Dermatopathol.* 2007;29(3):237–241.
11. Clayman GL, Lee JJ, Holsinger FC, et al. Mortality risk from squamous cell skin cancer. *J Clin Oncol.* 2005; 23(4):759–765.
12. Prieto VG, Lugo J, McNutt NS. Intermediate- and low-molecular-weight keratin detection with the monoclonal antibody MNF116. An immunohistochemical study on 232 paraffin-embedded cutaneous lesions. *J Cutan Pathol.* 1996;23(3):234–241.
13. Sigel JE, Skacel M, Bergfeld WF, House NS, Rabkin MS, Goldblum JR. The utility of cytokeratin 5/6 in the recognition of cutaneous spindle cell squamous cell carcinoma. *J Cutan Pathol.* 2001;28(10):520–524.
14. Gleason BC, Calder KB, Cibull TL, et al. Utility of p63 in the differential diagnosis of atypical fibroxanthoma and spindle cell squamous cell carcinoma. *J Cutan Pathol.* 2009;36(5):543–547.
15. Pattee SF, Bordeaux J, Mahalingam M, Nitzan YB, Maloney ME. Verrucous carcinoma of the scalp. *J Am Acad Dermatol.* 2007;56(3):506–507.
16. Murao K, Kubo Y, Fukumoto D, Matsumoto K, Arase S. Verrucous carcinoma of the scalp associated with human papillomavirus type 33. *Dermatol Surg.* 2005;31(10): 1363–1365.
17. Hong DS, Reddy SB, Prieto VG, et al. Multiple squamous cell carcinomas of the skin after therapy with sorafenib combined with tipifarnib. *Arch Dermatol.* 2008;144(6): 779–782.
18. Ponti G, Ponz de Leon M. Muir-Torre syndrome. *Lancet Oncol.* 2005;6(12):980–987.
19. Lear W, Dahlke E, Murray CA. Basal cell carcinoma: review of epidemiology, pathogenesis, and associated risk factors. *J Cutan Med Surg.* 2007;11(1):19–30.
20. Uzquiano MC, Prieto VG, Nash JW, et al. Metastatic basal cell carcinoma exhibits reduced actin expression. *Mod Pathol.* 2008;21(5):540–543.
21. Manfredi M, Vescovi P, Bonanini M, Porter S. Nevoid basal cell carcinoma syndrome: a review of the literature. *Int J Oral Maxillofac Surg.* 2004;33(2):117–124.
22. Crowson AN. Basal cell carcinoma: biology, morphology and clinical implications. *Mod Pathol.* 2006;19 (suppl 2): S127–S147.
23. Yoshikawa K, Katagata Y, Kondo S. Biochemical and immunohistochemical analyses of keratin expression in basal cell carcinoma. *J Dermatol Sci.* 1998;17(1):15–23.
24. Yu L, Galan A, McNiff JM. Caveats in BerEP4 staining to differentiate basal and squamous cell carcinoma. *J Cutan Pathol.* 2009;36(10):1074–1076.
25. Hendrix JD, Jr., Parlette HL. Micronodular basal cell carcinoma. A deceptive histologic subtype with frequent clinically undetected tumor extension. *Arch Dermatol.* 1996;132(3):295–298.
26. Bettencourt MS, Prieto VG, Shea CR. Trichoepithelioma: a 19-year clinicopathologic re-evaluation. *J Cutan Pathol.* 1999;26(8):398–404.

27. Kirchmann TT, Prieto VG, Smoller BR. CD34 staining pattern distinguishes basal cell carcinoma from trichoepithelioma. *Arch Dermatol.* 1994;130(5):589–592.
28. Chilukuri S, Page R, Reed JA, Friedman J, Orengo I. Ectopic extramammary Paget's disease arising on the cheek. *Dermatol Surg.* 2002;28(5):430–433.
29. Colome-Grimmer MI, Evans HL. Metastasizing cellular dermatofibroma. A report of two cases. *Am J Surg Pathol.* 1996;20(11):1361–1367.
30. Prieto VG, Reed JA, Shea CR. Immunohistochemistry of dermatofibromas and benign fibrous histiocytomas. *J Cutan Pathol.* 1995;22(4):336–341.
31. Weedon D, Williamson R, Mirza B. CD10, a useful marker for atypical fibroxanthomas. *Am J Dermatopathol.* 2005;27(2):181.
32. Horenstein MG, Prieto VG, Nuckols JD, Burchette JL, Shea CR. Indeterminate fibrohistiocytic lesions of the skin: is there a spectrum between dermatofibroma and dermatofibrosarcoma protuberans? *Am J Surg Pathol.* 2000;24(7):996–1003.
33. Barnes L, Coleman JA, Jr., Johnson JT. Dermatofibrosarcoma protuberans of the head and neck. *Arch Otolaryngol.* 1984;110(6):398–404.
34. Kashima A, Yamashita A, Moriguchi S, et al. Detection of COL1A1-PDGFB fusion transcripts and platelet-derived growth factor alpha and beta receptors in giant cell fibroblastoma of the postsacrococcygeal region. *Br J Dermatol.* 2006;154(5):983–987.
35. Ly H, Selva D, James CL, Huilgol SC. Superficial malignant fibrous histiocytoma presenting as recurrent atypical fibroxanthoma. *Australas J Dermatol.* 2004;45(2): 106–109.
36. Buonaguro FM, Tomesello ML, Buonaguro L, et al. Kaposi's sarcoma: aetiopathogenesis, histology and clinical features. *J Eur Acad Dermatol Venereol.* 2003;17(2): 138–154.
37. Wilkins K, Turner R, Dolev JC, LeBoit PE, Berger TG, Maurer TA. Cutaneous malignancy and human immunodeficiency virus disease. *J Am Acad Dermatol.* 2006;54(2): 189–206; quiz 207–110.
38. Grayson W, Pantanowitz L. Histological variants of cutaneous Kaposi sarcoma. *Diagn Pathol.* 2008;3:31.
39. Craddock KJ, Labonte S, Ghazarian D. Anaplastic Kaposi sarcoma resembling epithelioid angiosarcoma in an HIV-positive man. *Eur J Dermatol.* 2008;18(3):358–359.
40. Ramirez JA, Laskin WB, Guitart J. Lymphangioma-like Kaposi sarcoma. *J Cutan Pathol.* 2005;32(4):286–292.
41. Kempf W, Cathomas G, Burg G, Trueb RM. Micronodular Kaposi's sarcoma—a new variant of classic-sporadic Kaposi's sarcoma. *Dermatology.* 2004;208(3):255–258.
42. Luzar B, Antony F, Ramdial PK, Calonje E. Intravascular Kaposi's sarcoma—a hitherto unrecognized phenomenon. *J Cutan Pathol.* 2007;34(11):861–864.
43. Morgan MB, Swann M, Somach S, Eng W, Smoller B. Cutaneous angiosarcoma: a case series with prognostic correlation. *J Am Acad Dermatol.* 2004;50(6):867–874.
44. Favia G, Lo Muzio L, Serpico R, Maiorano E. Angiosarcoma of the head and neck with intra-oral presentation. A clinico-pathological study of four cases. *Oral Oncol.* 2002;38(8):757–762.
45. Glickstein J, Sebelik ME, Lu Q. Cutaneous angiosarcoma of the head and neck: a case presentation and review of the literature. *Ear Nose Throat J.* 2006;85(10): 672–674.
46. Deyrup AT, McKenney JK, Tighiouart M, Folpe AL, Weiss SW. Sporadic cutaneous angiosarcomas: a proposal for risk stratification based on 69 cases. *Am J Surg Pathol.* 2008;32(1):72–77.
47. Kaddu S, Beham A, Cerroni L, et al. Cutaneous leiomyosarcoma. *Am J Surg Pathol.* 1997;21(9):979–987.
48. Annest NM, Grekin SJ, Stone MS, Messingham MJ. Cutaneous leiomyosarcoma: a tumor of the head and neck. *Dermatol Surg.* 2007;33(5):628–633.
49. Snowden RT, Osborn FD, Wong FS, Sebelik ME. Superficial leiomyosarcoma of the head and neck: case report and review of the literature. *Ear Nose Throat J.* 2001; 80(7):449–453.
50. Holst VA, Junkins-Hopkins JM, Elenitsas R. Cutaneous smooth muscle neoplasms: clinical features, histologic findings, and treatment options. *J Am Acad Dermatol.* 2002;46(4):477–490; quiz, 491–474.
51. Berzal-Cantalejo F, Sabater-Marco V, Perez-Valles A, Martorell-Cebollada M. Desmoplastic cutaneous leiomyosarcoma: case report and review of the literature. *J Cutan Pathol.* 2006;33(suppl 2):29–31.
52. Ducatman BS, Scheithauer BW, Piepgras DG, Reiman HM, Ilstrup DM. Malignant peripheral nerve sheath tumors. A clinicopathologic study of 120 cases. *Cancer.* 1986;57(10):2006–2021.
53. Hoffmann DF, Everts EC, Smith JD, Kyriakopoulos DD, Kessler S. Malignant nerve sheath tumors of the head and neck. *Otolaryngol Head Neck Surg.* 1988;99(3): 309–314.
54. Demir Y, Tokyol C. Superficial malignant schwannoma of the scalp. *Dermatol Surg.* 2003;29(8):879–881.
55. Berg JC, Scheithauer BW, Spinner RJ, Allen CM, Koutlas IG. Plexiform schwannoma: a clinicopathologic overview with emphasis on the head and neck region. *Hum Pathol.* 2008;39(5):633–640.
56. Becelli R, Perugini M, Gasparini G, Cassoni A, Fabiani F. Abrikossoff's tumor. *J Craniofac Surg.* 2001;12(1):78–81.
57. Fanburg-Smith JC, Meis-Kindblom JM, Fante R, Kindblom LG. Malignant granular cell tumor of soft tissue: diagnostic criteria and clinicopathologic correlation. *Am J Surg Pathol.* 1998;22(7):779–794.
58. Lee J, Bhawan J, Wax F, Farber J. Plexiform granular cell tumor. A report of two cases. *Am J Dermatopathol.* 1994; 16(5):537–541.
59. Nikkels AF, Arrese Estrada J, Pierard-Franchimont C, Pierard GE. CD68 and factor XIIIa expressions in granular-cell tumor of the skin. *Dermatology.* 1993; 186(2):106–108.

60. Mazur MT, Shultz JJ, Myers JL. Granular cell tumor. Immunohistochemical analysis of 21 benign tumors and one malignant tumor. *Arch Pathol Lab Med.* 1990; 114(7):692–696.
61. Billeret-Lebranchu V, Martin de la Salle E, Vandenhaute B, Lecomte-Houcke M. [Granular cell tumor and congenital epulis. Histochemical and immunohistochemical of 58 cases]. *Arch Anat Cytol Pathol.* 1999;47(1):31–37.
62. Hoshi N, Tsu-ura Y, Watanabe K, Suzuki T, Kasukawa R. Expression of immunoreactivities to 75 kDa nerve growth factor receptor, trk gene product and phosphotyrosine in granular cell tumors. *Pathol Int.* 1995;45(10): 748–756.
63. Headington JT, French AJ. Primary neoplasms of the hair follicle. Histogenesis and classification. *Arch Dermatol.* 1962;86:430–441.
64. Misago N, Tanaka T, Kohda H. Trichilemmal carcinoma occurring in a lesion of solar keratosis. *J Dermatol.* 1993; 20(6):358–364.
65. Allee JE, Cotsarelis G, Solky B, Cook JL. Multiply recurrent trichilemmal carcinoma with perineural invasion and cytokeratin 17 positivity. *Dermatol Surg.* 2003;29(8): 886–889.
66. Ye J, Nappi O, Swanson PE, Patterson JW, Wick MR. Proliferating pilar tumors: a clinicopathologic study of 76 cases with a proposal for definition of benign and malignant variants. *Am J Clin Pathol.* 2004;122(4): 566–574.
67. Noto G, Pravata G, Arico M. "Shadow" cells in proliferating trichilemmal tumors. *Am J Dermatopathol.* 1990; 12(3):319–320.
68. Huet P, Dandurand M, Pignodel C, Guillot B. Metastasizing eccrine porocarcinoma: report of a case and review of the literature. *J Am Acad Dermatol.* 1996;35 (5 pt 2):860–864.
69. Robson A, Greene J, Ansari N, et al. Eccrine porocarcinoma (malignant eccrine poroma): a clinicopathologic study of 69 cases. *Am J Surg Pathol.* 2001;25(6):710–720.
70. Gschnait F, Horn F, Lindlbauer R, Sponer D. Eccrine porocarcinoma. *J Cutan Pathol.* 1980;7(6):349–353.
71. Claudy AL, Garcier F, Kanitakis J. Eccrine porocarcinoma. Ultrastructural and immunological study. *J Dermatol.* 1984;11(3):282–286.
72. Ko CJ, Cochran AJ, Eng W, Binder SW. Hidradenocarcinoma: a histological and immunohistochemical study. *J Cutan Pathol.* 2006;33(11):726–730.
73. Goldstein DJ, Barr RJ, Santa Cruz DJ. Microcystic adnexal carcinoma: a distinct clinicopathologic entity. *Cancer.* 1982;50(3):566–572.
74. Yu JB, Blitzblau RC, Patel SC, Decker RH, Wilson LD. Surveillance, epidemiology, and end results (SEER) database analysis of microcystic adnexal carcinoma (sclerosing sweat duct carcinoma) of the skin. *Am J Clin Oncol.* 2010;33(2):196–197.
75. Smith KJ, Williams J, Corbett D, Skelton H. Microcystic adnexal carcinoma: an immunohistochemical study including markers of proliferation and apoptosis. *Am J Surg Pathol.* 2001;25(4):464–471.
76. Harrist TJ, Aretz TH, Mihm MC, Jr., Evans GW, Rodriquez FL. Cutaneous malignant mixed tumor. *Arch Dermatol.* 1981;117(11):719–724.
77. Bates AW, Baithun SI. Atypical mixed tumor of the skin: histologic, immunohistochemical, and ultrastructural features in three cases and a review of the criteria for malignancy. *Am J Dermatopathol.* 1998;20(1):35–40.
78. Webb JN, Stott WG. Malignant chondroid syringoma of the thigh. Report of a case with electron microscopy of the tumour. *J Pathol.* 1975;116(1):43–46.
79. Eckert F, Schmid U, Hardmeier T, Altmannsberger M. Cytokeratin expression in mucinous sweat gland carcinomas: an immunohistochemical analysis of four cases. *Histopathology.* 1992;21(2):161–165.
80. Carson HJ, Gattuso P, Raslan WF, Reddy V. Mucinous carcinoma of the eyelid. An immunohistochemical study. *Am J Dermatopathol.* 1995;17(5):494–498.
81. Ivan D, Hafeez Diwan A, Prieto VG. Expression of p63 in primary cutaneous adnexal neoplasms and adenocarcinoma metastatic to the skin. *Mod Pathol.* 2005;18(1): 137–142.
82. Massa MC, Medenica M. Cutaneous adnexal tumors and cysts: a review. Part I. Tumors with hair follicular and sebaceous glandular differentiation and cysts related to different parts of the hair follicle. *Pathol Annu.* 1985; 20(pt 2):189–233.
83. Ponti G, Ponz de Leon M, Losi L, et al. Different phenotypes in Muir-Torre syndrome: clinical and biomolecular characterization in two Italian families. *Br J Dermatol.* 2005;152(6):1335–1338.
84. Orta L, Klimstra DS, Qin J, et al. Towards identification of hereditary DNA mismatch repair deficiency: sebaceous neoplasm warrants routine immunohistochemical screening regardless of patient's age or other clinical characteristics. *Am J Surg Pathol.* 2009;33(6):934–944.
85. Troy JL, Ackerman AB. Sebaceoma. A distinctive benign neoplasm of adnexal epithelium differentiating toward sebaceous cells. *Am J Dermatopathol.* 1984;6(1):7–13.
86. Margo CE, Mulla ZD. Malignant tumors of the eyelid: a population-based study of non-basal cell and non-squamous cell malignant neoplasms. *Arch Ophthalmol.* 1998;116(2):195–198.
87. Crowson AN, Magro CM, Mihm MC. Malignant adnexal neoplasms. *Mod Pathol.* 2006;19 (suppl 2):S93–S126.
88. Machin P, Catasus L, Pons C, et al. Microsatellite instability and immunostaining for MSH-2 and MLH-1 in cutaneous and internal tumors from patients with the Muir-Torre syndrome. *J Cutan Pathol.* 2002;29(7):415–420.
89. Lazar AJ, Lyle S, Calonje E. Sebaceous neoplasia and Torre-Muir syndrome. *Curr Diagn Pathol.* 2007;13(4): 301–319.
90. Muthusamy K, Halbert G, Roberts F. Immunohistochemical staining for adipophilin, perilipin and TIP47. *J Clin Pathol.* 2006;59(11):1166–1170.

91. Hasebe T, Mukai K, Yamaguchi N, et al. Prognostic value of immunohistochemical staining for proliferating cell nuclear antigen, p53, and c-erbB-2 in sebaceous gland carcinoma and sweat gland carcinoma: comparison with histopathological parameter. *Mod Pathol.* 1994; 7(1):37–43.
92. Goessling W, McKee PH, Mayer RJ. Merkel cell carcinoma. *J Clin Oncol.* 2002;20(2):588–598.
93. Feng H, Shuda M, Chang Y, Moore PS. Clonal integration of a polyomavirus in human Merkel cell carcinoma. *Science.* 2008;319(5866):1096–1100.
94. LeBoit PE, Crutcher WA, Shapiro PE. Pagetoid intraepidermal spread in Merkel cell (primary neuroendocrine) carcinoma of the skin. *Am J Surg Pathol.* 1992;16(6): 584–592.
95. Walsh NM. Primary neuroendocrine (Merkel cell) carcinoma of the skin: morphologic diversity and implications thereof. *Hum Pathol.* 2001;32(7):680–689.
96. Su LD, Fullen DR, Lowe L, Uherova P, Schnitzer B, Valdez R. CD117 (KIT receptor) expression in Merkel cell carcinoma. *Am J Dermatopathol.* 2002;24(4):289–293.
97. Nicholson SA, McDermott MB, Swanson PE, Wick MR. CD99 and cytokeratin-20 in small-cell and basaloid tumors of the skin. *Appl Immunohistochem Mol Morphol.* 2000;8(1):37–41.
98. Caro WA, Helwig HB. Cutaneous lymphoid hyperplasia. *Cancer.* 1969;24(3):487–502.
99. Hwong H, Jones D, Prieto VG, Schulz C, Duvic M. Persistent atypical lymphocytic hyperplasia following tick bite in a child: report of a case and review of the literature. *Pediatr Dermatol.* 2001;18(6):481–484.
100. Burg G, Schmid MH, Kung E, Dommann S, Dummer R. Semimalignant ("pseudolymphomatous") cutaneous B-cell lymphomas. *Dermatol Clin.* 1994;12(2):399–407.
101. Henry PG, Burnett JW. Angiolymphoid hyperplasia with eosinophilia. *Arch Dermatol.* 1978;114(8):1168–1172.
102. Arnold M, Geilen CC, Coupland SE, et al. Unilateral angiolymphoid hyperplasia with eosinophilia involving the left arm and hand. *J Cutan Pathol.* 1999;26(9): 436–440.
103. Tomaszewski MM, Abbondanzo SL, Lupton GP. Extranodal marginal zone B-cell lymphoma of the skin: a morphologic and immunophenotypic study of 11 cases. *Am J Dermatopathol.* 2000;22(3):205–211.
104. Cerroni L. Lymphoproliferative lesions of the skin. *J Clin Pathol.* 2006;59(8):813–826.
105. Bergman R, Kurtin PJ, Gibson LE, Hull PR, Kimlinger TK, Schroeter AL. Clinicopathologic, immunophenotypic, and molecular characterization of primary cutaneous follicular B-cell lymphoma. *Arch Dermatol.* 2001;137(4):432–439.
106. Paulli M, Viglio A, Vivenza D, et al. Primary cutaneous large B-cell lymphoma of the leg: histogenetic analysis of a controversial clinicopathologic entity. *Hum Pathol.* 2002;33(9):937–943.
107. Fraser-Andrews E, Ashton R, Russell-Jones R. Pilotropic mycosis fungoides presenting with multiple cysts, comedones and alopecia. *Br J Dermatol.* 1999;140(1):141–144.
108. Paulli M, Berti E, Rosso R, et al. CD30/Ki-1-positive lymphoproliferative disorders of the skin—clinicopathologic correlation and statistical analysis of 86 cases: a multicentric study from the European Organization for Research and Treatment of Cancer Cutaneous Lymphoma Project Group. *J Clin Oncol.* 1995;13(6): 1343–1354.
109. Salhany KE, Macon WR, Choi JK, et al. Subcutaneous panniculitis-like T-cell lymphoma: clinicopathologic, immunophenotypic, and genotypic analysis of alpha/beta and gamma/delta subtypes. *Am J Surg Pathol.* 1998;22(7):881–893.
110. Mraz-Gernhard S, Natkunam Y, Hoppe RT, LeBoit P, Kohler S, Kim YH. Natural killer/natural killer-like T-cell lymphoma, CD56+, presenting in the skin: an increasingly recognized entity with an aggressive course. *J Clin Oncol.* 2001;19(8):2179–2188.
111. Barrionuevo C, Anderson VM, Zevallos-Giampietri E, et al. Hydroa-like cutaneous T-cell lymphoma: a clinicopathologic and molecular genetic study of 16 pediatric cases from Peru. *Appl Immunohistochem Mol Morphol.* 2002;10(1):7–14.

7

EPIDEMIOLOGY, STAGING, AND PROGNOSIS OF NONMELANOMA SKIN CANCER

CARSTEN E. PALME
MARK C. SMITH
MICHAEL J. VENESS

Introduction

Nonmelanoma skin cancer (NMSC) is the most common malignancy worldwide and is managed by a diverse group of clinicians including primary care physicians, dermatologists, otolaryngologist-head and neck surgeons, surgical oncologists, plastic and reconstructive surgeons, and radiation oncologists. Therefore, it is important that all treating clinicians have a clear understanding of the epidemiology, staging, and prognosis of this disease. NMSC is a heterogeneous group of malignancies encompassing more than 80 different histologic subtypes that each require different management and demonstrate widely varying prognosis.[1] These malignancies range from very common lesions such as basal cell carcinoma (BCC) and squamous cell carcinoma (SCC) to relatively uncommon lesions including Merkel cell carcinoma (MCC). Other rarer lesions include adnexal carcinomas and mesenchymal tumors including cutaneous angiosarcoma and Kaposi sarcoma (KS).

The most common NMSC is overwhelmingly BCC, which comprises 70 to 75% of all cases, followed by SCC (20–25%) and MCC with less than 5%. The other histologic subtypes make up the remainder.[2,3] Exposure to ultraviolet (UV) radiation is the main etiologic factor for the development of BCC, SCC, and MCC; consequently, they have a high propensity for developing on the sun-exposed areas of the head and neck and extremeties.[2]

Overall, NMSC has a good prognosis with a low recurrence rate and greater than 90% 5-year disease-specific survival. Despite this, NMSC, particularly a subset of patients with aggressive SCC, still can present a significant challenge for both patient and treating clinician due to the development of locally recurrent disease in around 10% and the propensity for metastatic nodal disease in 3 to 5% of patients.[4–7]

Epidemiology

NMSC is at epidemic rates in regions such as Australia, which has the highest incidence of skin cancer in the world.[8] Worldwide, there are widely differing rates of NMSC in various populations, and in most regions the incidence is increasing.[8–10]

In Australia, the incidence of NMSC increased significantly between 1985 and 2002, with the annual incidence of BCC increasing from 657 per 100,000 to 884 per 100,000 and SCC more than doubling from 166 per 100,000 to 387 per 100,000.[8] This increase also has been noted in other countries and strongly emphasizes the current and future major public health concern that this disease represents.[10,11] In 2002, the incidence of NMSC in Australia was more than 5 times that of all other cancers combined with an annual rate of 1170 per 100,000.[8] In the United States, over 1 million new cases of NMSC are diagnosed annually.[12]

Typically, NMSC develops in older (>60 years old) Caucasian males with a history of chronic sun exposure over their lifetime (Fig 7–1). The majority are either BCC or SCC and arise on the sun-exposed regions of the head and neck.[2] When considering the population at risk of developing NMSC, a number of factors are important. These include patient factors such as increasing age, male gender, caucasian background, chronic sun exposure, outdoor occupation, immunosuppression, and certain systemic diseases including epidermolysis bullosa, oculocutaneous albinism, and xeroderma pigmentosum.[1,13–15] Environmental exposure to UV radiation is the major etiologic factor that leads to the development of NMSC. Additional factors such as proximity to the equator, ozone layer depletion and both occupational and recreational exposure significantly increase this risk.[14] Both SCC and MCC can be considered immunogenic malignancies, in contrast to BCC. Patients diagnosed with either a SCC or MCC are at risk of developing metastatic disease and subsequently dying of their disease. Death resulting from a diagnosis of BCC is extremely rare.

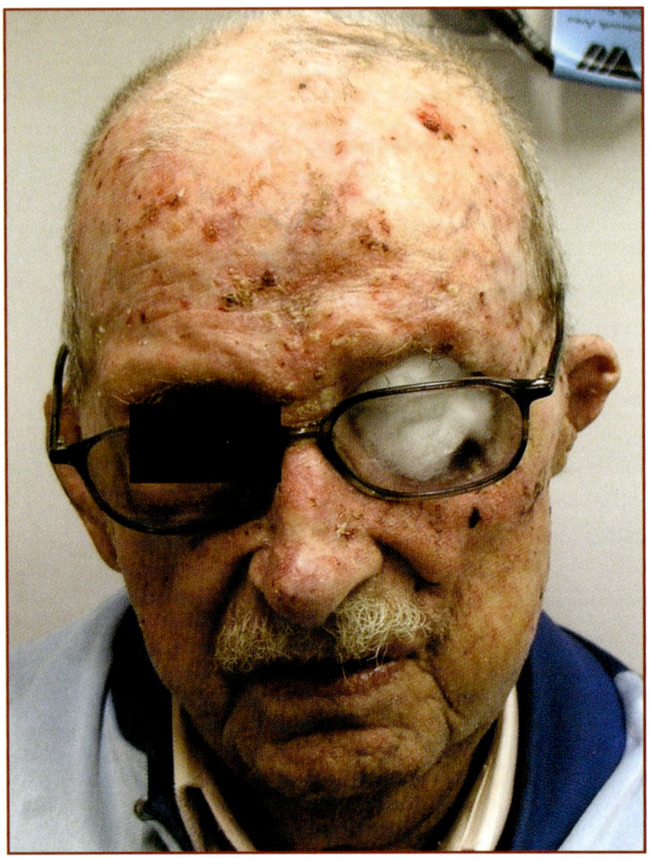

Figure 7–1. 80-year-old white male with widespread actinic changes secondary to chronic occupational sun exposure. Note loss of his left eye secondary to orbital invasion from SCC and also previous surgery to his right ear.

Basal Cell Carcinoma

In Caucasians, BCC is the most common malignancy.[16] In the United States, the annual incidence is estimated at 407 per 100,000 for men and 212 per 100,000 for women.[17] UV radiation is the main risk factor and, compared to other forms of NMSC, different patterns of UV radiation exposure appear to be important in the development of this tumor. Although chronic cumulative exposure to UV radiation is associated with an increased risk for SCC, for BCC intense intermittent exposure appears to be more closely associated with an increased incidence rather than the equivalent exposure over a longer period. A relationship between childhood and adolescent sunburn and the development of BCC also has been identified.[18]

Other important risk factors include male gender and increasing age. The presence of immunosuppression only marginally increases the risk of developing BCC and not to the same extent as is well documented in patients with SCC or MCC. Increased incidence of BCC also has been noted to occur after exposure to arsenic and coal tar. A number of genetic diseases predispose to BCC at a younger age including albinism, xeroderma pigmentosum, and Gorlin's syndrome.[17,18]

Squamous Cell Carcinoma

Australia leads the world in SCC with an annual incidence of 300 per 100,000. Townsville, a regional city in Northern Australia, has the highest rate of SCC in the world at 1300 per 100,000.[2,8] There is a significant variability in the incidence of SCC worldwide due to both population and environmental factors. In the United States, the incidence varies depending on location and ranges between 35 to 150 per 100,000.[15,19] SCC has an incidence of 16 per 100,000 in central Europe whereas Northern European countries are comparatively spared with a low incidence of 10 per 100,000.[19] When considering non-Caucasian populations, the rates are considerably lower. In Singapore, the rate for the population as a whole is 2.2 per 100,000; however, it was noted that there were differences between ethnic groups with the Chinese population having about twice the rate of Malays and Indians.[20] When considering differences between Caucasians and other ethnic groups with darker skin types, NMSC is 70 times more likely in fair skinned populations than in populations with darker skin. In populations with darker skin, SCC replaces BCC as the most common NMSC.[21]

Although there is significant variation in the incidence of SCC between countries, it has also been noted that, in many populations, there has been a steady increase in the incidence over the last 40 years. In Australia, North America, and Europe the incidence has increased by 3 to 8% per year since the 1960s.[3] de Vries et al[9] predicted that the incidence of NMSC in the Netherlands will increase over the next 10 years by nearly 80%. Various factors have been suggested as potential reasons for this increase over time. First, there has been an increase in the number of people at risk, with both an aging population and increasing numbers of immunosuppressed patients. Second, it has been proposed that there has been an increased exposure to more intense UV radiation due both to ozone layer depletion and increased exposure to sunlight through increased leisure time, fashion, and social trends. Finally, the increased incidence may be due in part to improved data collection and submission of specimens for thorough histopathologic evaluation due to increased awareness of SCC, on the part of both patients and clinicians alike.[6]

Risk Factors for SCC

Precursor Lesions. Precursor lesions are important in the development of SCC. These foremost include actinic keratosis (AK), which are dysplastic keratinocytic lesions arising within the epidermal layer of the skin induced by UV radiation.[13,22] Up to 50% of people in Australia over 40 yrs of age have one or more AK.[13] Although a substantial proportion (25–75%) of AK regress over time, a number eventually progress to invasive SCC. Estimates of the rate of progression of an individual AK to SCC have been reported at up to 20%. Despite this, two longitudinal studies recently reported a considerably lower annual rate of transformation. Marks et al[13] reported a rate of 0.096% per year whereas Criscione et al[22] reported an annual rate of 0.6% and 2.57% at 4 years. These studies reported that between 60% and 65% of SCC arose from pre-existing AK. Although the rate of an individual AK transforming into invasive SCC is low at risk, individuals usually have multiple AK, with one study documenting an average of 46.[22] This in part may explain the higher rate of transformation to SCC in some studies, given that the risk of developing SCC from one AK may be additive in those patients with multiple lesions. Similarly, patients who have a history of previous SCC are at significantly greater risk of developing further metachronous lesions, and this has been estimated at 10 times that of the general population.[23]

Environmental Exposure. Exposure to mutagenic UV radiation is the most significant causative factor for the majority of NMSC. Proximity to the equator is associated with a doubling in the incidence of SCC with every 8- to 10-degree latitude closer to the equator.[9] It has been proposed that thinning of the ozone layer has resulted in an increased incidence of diseases caused by UV radiation including NMSC. World Health Organization modeling estimates that for a 10% thinning in the ozone layer, there will be 300,000 more cases of NMSC worldwide per year.[24] Reductions in the density of the ozone layer have been measured of over 50% in southern Chile. These reductions in ozone layer density result in even greater increases in measured amount of UVB radiation.[25] A significant increase (approximately 38 times) in exposure to mutagenic radiation, (around 300 nm) has been reported based on the depletion of ozone. Exposure of the skin to UV radiation results in clearly defined mutagenic effects. The p53 tumor suppressor gene is believed to be an early target in the development of NMSC.[26]

Immunosuppression. Immunosuppression is one of the most important risk factors for the development of SCC and has a significant impact on both management and prognosis. Loss of immunocompetence can be either treatment or disease related and takes a number of different forms. Depending on its etiology, there are differing effects on the incidence of NMSC. Common causes of immunosuppression include solid organ transplantation, hematological malignancies such as non-Hodgkin's lymphoma (NHL) and chronic lymphocytic leukemia (CLL), and human immunodeficiency virus (HIV) infection.

Treatment-related immunosuppression, which classically occurs in solid organ transplant recipients, results in an increased rate of both SCC and, to a lesser extent, BCC. There is, however, a significantly greater increase in the rate of SCC resulting in an inversion in the proportion of BCC to SCC in Caucasians and, to a lesser extent, in populations that do not have a high background rate of SCC. In solid organ transplant recipients, there is between 65 to 250 times increased risk of developing SCC than in the general population and, furthermore, a greater risk of developing metastatic disease involving both regional and distant sites.[27–29] In the Australian transplant population, at least 45% of patients will develop a SCC within 10 years of transplantation; whereas patients from Europe have an incidence of 10 to 15% at 10 years after transplant.[30] Ramsay et al reported[31] that, in the renal transplant population in Queensland, the incidence of NMSC at 20 years was 81%, with 75% having invasive SCC.

Patients with CLL/NHL are at increased risk of NMSC secondary to disease-related impaired immunity. As with solid organ transplant recipients, the rate of SCC is markedly increased, resulting in a reversal in the ratio of BCC to SCC. In addition, SCC in this setting often behaves more aggressively, with increased rates of both local recurrence and metastatic disease compared to the general population. The rates for developing nodal metastases were increased to between 10 to 18%.[32,33]

Immunosuppression secondary to HIV has a different effect on NMSC. Wilkins et al reported[34] an approximately 5-fold increased risk of developing SCC in the HIV population compared with non-HIV controls.[34] Associated with this greater incidence is a propensity for aggressive SCC and an increased rate of spread to regional lymph nodes. Unlike other forms of immunosuppression, there does not appear to be an alteration in the ratio of BCC to SCC. Currently, it is unclear if CD4 count or HIV viral load affect the development of NMSC in HIV patients.[35]

Other Factors. There are current data to support a role for human papilloma virus (HPV) and the development of SCC. This association has been demonstrated in the immunocompromised population where up to 90% of tumors contain HPV DNA.[36] Interestingly, different HPV subtypes have been shown to have different mechanisms in the proposed pathway to tumor development. In a North American study, seropositivity to beta-HPV strains was associated with an increased risk for the development of SCC but not for BCC. Unlike cervical carcinoma or mucosal SCC in the head and neck, specific strains of HPV that have a particularly high risk for the development of cutaneous SCC have not been identified nor has causation been demonstrated.[37]

Cigarette smoking has been widely implicated in the development of many malignancies, although its role in the development of NMSC is controversial. A Dutch study showed a doubling of the risk of development of cutaneous SCC in smokers with an associated dose response.[38] Other studies have supported the association quoting increased rates of between 1.5 to 4 times whereas other studies have found no association. In contrast to the Dutch study, Odenbro et al,[39] in a large prospective study involving over 300,000 construction workers in Sweden, did not find any association between smoking and the development of SCC. Other less commonly reported risk factors for SCC include exposure to polycyclic aromatic hydrocarbons, arsenic, and exposure to other chemical carcinogens.[15]

Risk Factors for Metastatic Disease

The risk of developing metastatic spread in patients with BCC is almost negligible compared to SCC. In the latter, there exist well-defined and documented patient, tumor and treatment factors that predict the development of metastatic disease. The morbidity and mortality of patients with metastatic SCC are well known and the presence of regional disease has a significant impact on both management and prognosis (Fig 7–2). Studies suggest that the risk of developing nodal metastatic disease in patients with low risk SCC is 3 to 5%.[5–7,40] The incidence is significantly higher at approximately 10 to 15% among patients who present to tertiary head and neck cancer centers, many with high risk primary lesions.[4] The parotid gland is the most frequent site for developing metastatic SCC in patients with head and neck primaries with other regional basins such as the axilla or groin rarely involved. Most patients will have parotid and/or neck nodes involved with only a minority (20–30%) having only neck nodes. Although the majority of SCC does not metastasize, given the large number of patients with this disease worldwide, the absolute numbers of those who develop metastatic disease is highly significant and, therefore, make this a major current and future public health issue.

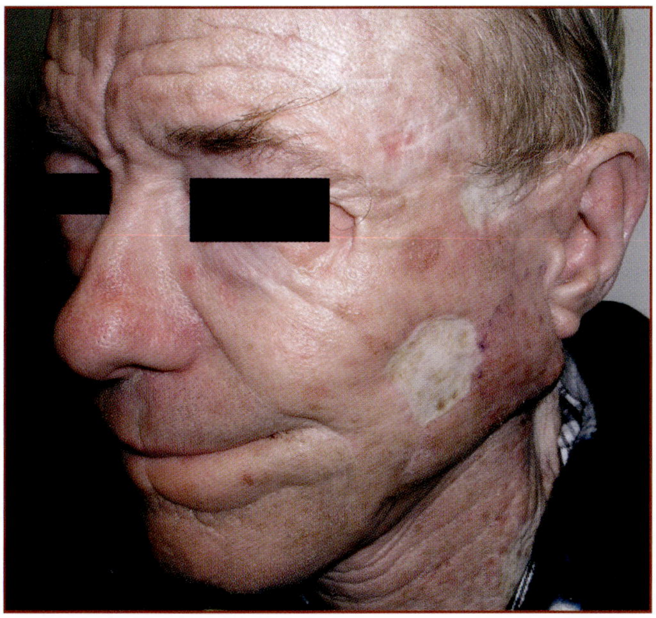

Figure 7–2. 60-year-old male with metastatic squamous cell carcinoma to his left parotid 12 months after excision of a SCC from his left cheek. He proceeded to nerve sparing parotidectomy and upper neck dissection followed by adjuvant radiotherapy (60 Gy in 30 fractions).

Patient factors that have shown to predict the development of metastatic disease include male gender, immunosuppression, and delayed presentation.[5,41] Tumor factors include tumor size, depth/thickness, invasion of adjacent tissue, location, the presence of perineural/lymphovascular invasion, tumor grade, and growth rate. Treatment factors that are important include inadequate primary treatment including incomplete resection and failure to consider re-excision or adjuvant external beam radiotherapy with subsequent persistent disease or development of local recurrence. Patients developing local recurrence are at a much higher risk of developing nodal meatastases.[4,6,42] Over 70% of metastatic nodal disease presents within 1 year of treatment of the primary lesion whereas few patients present with nodal metastatic disease after 5 years.[6]

Merkel Cell Carcinoma

MCC is a rare but aggressive primary cutaneous neuroendocrine (small cell) cancer. In the United States, the annual incidence for males and females is 0.34 per 100,000 and 0.17 per 100,000 respectively.[43] Similar to SCC, the incidence of MCC is rising, although this increase may be due in part to increased awareness and diagnosis. It is estimated that at least 1,500 new cases are diagnosed in the United States each year.[44] The majority of patients are elderly (70–80 yrs old) and almost always Caucasian, with the rate in the black population in the United States only 0.01 per 100,000 (Fig 7–3).[43] Chronic sun exposure is a major contributor to the development of MCC. An infectious etiology recently was proposed with Merkel cell polyomavirus identified in

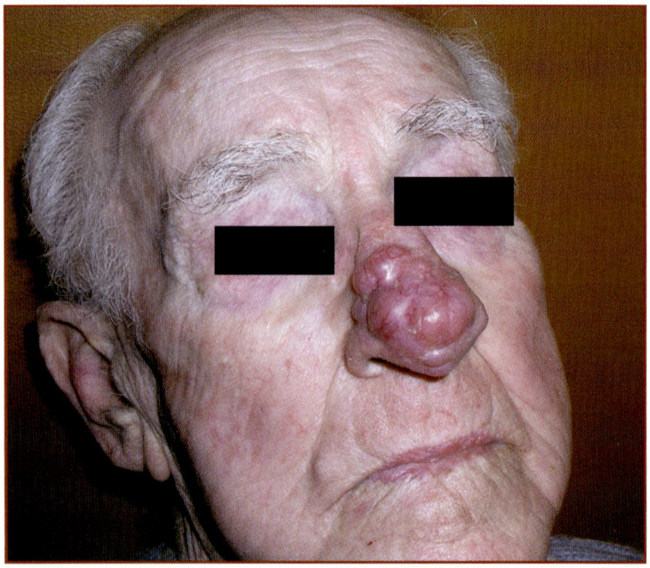

Figure 7–3. 83-year-old white male with a rapidly progressing nasal Merkel cell carcinoma. Note the nodular subcutaneous nature of the lesion and the typical red/purplish discoloration. The patient developed parotid nodal metastases shortly after radiotherapy to his nose.

the majority of lesions.[45] Ageli et al[43] noted that just under half of all lesions occurred in the head and neck. At the time of diagnosis 50% have localized disease with 25% of patients having metastatic nodal disease. Using sentinel node biopsy nearly 30 to 40% of clinically negative lymph nodes will harbor micrometastatic disease.[46]

Immunosuppressed patients have both an increased incidence and a more aggressive clinical course with an overall poorer prognosis.[46–48] The evidence suggests that many patients benefit from the addition of wide field adjuvant radiotherapy. Despite the high rate of distant metastases, the benefits and indications for chemotherapy remain unclear.

Staging

The importance of an accurate, clinically relevant, and universally applied staging system is that it allows patients to be appropriately classified according to the extent of disease and thus allow proper assessment, communication, management, and prognostication. Staging is a very important tool in the assessment of outcome, both within and across institutions, and it facilitates research and the development of targeted treatment regimens. The American Joint Committee on Cancer, Cancer Staging Manual (AJCC) tumor, node, metastasis (TNM) system is widely utilized in staging of patients with SCC.[1,49] MCC has been staged according to a system developed by Memorial Sloan Kettering Cancer Center (MSKCC), although the most recent edition of the AJCC staging manual introduces a new TNM system specifically for this rare tumor.[1,50]

Previous editions of the AJCC TNM classification did not differentiate on account of subtype of NMSC. Only horizontal size of the primary lesion was considered important when differentiating T stage (ie, T1–T3). Nodal disease was simply classified as either N0 or N1 to indicate regional involvement.[49] This flawed staging system did not usefully separate patients into prognostic groups. As such, a number of institutions and research groups proposed major improvements to the classification system, many of which have been adopted in the revised 7th edition of the AJCC manual.[1] The current edition also incorporates high-risk features when determining the stage of a lesion, which is a significant improvement compared with a purely anatomically based staging system (Table 7–1).

Table 7–1. High-Risk Features for Primary Tumor (T) Staging

Depth/Invasion	>2 mm thickness Clark level ≥IV Perineural invasion
Anatomic Location	Primary site ear Primary site non-hair-bearing lip
Differentiation	Poorly differentiated or undifferentiated

Source: Used with permission of the American Joint Committee on Cancer (AJCC), Chicago, Illinois. The original source for this material is the AJCC Cancer Staging Manual, Seventh Edition (2010) published by Springer Science and Business Media LLC, www.springer.com.

Squamous Cell Carcinoma

The current T classification differentiates early lesions (T1 or T2) based on size, and advanced lesions (T3, T4) based on the degree of invasion into surrounding tissues (Table 7–2). The new concept of including nonanatomic tumor characteristics to create prognostic groups also has allowed a number of additional factors to be incorporated into the staging system, including lesion site and differentiation. Despite improvements, there remain a number of concerns. First, a clear history of an obvious index lesion is absent in a minority of patients (20–30%) who present with clinically metastatic SCC of the head and neck.[42] Second, other high-risk features such as a history of recurrent or persistent disease are not considered in the current staging system for SCC.[4]

Horizontal tumor size is acknowledged as a risk factor for developing metastatic nodal disease, although it is probably a weak independent predictor. Cherpelis et al[51] reported a significant difference in the rate of lymph node metastasis using a 2-cm threshold (13 vs. 68%).[51] Similar reports in the literature confirmed a greater metastatic rate in lesions >2 cm in size (30%) when compared to smaller primary tumors (9%).[4] Despite this, recent studies have highlighted the limitation of simply applying two-dimensional tumor size as a sole prognostic factor. Veness et al[42] reported a series of 266 patients with metastatic nodal disease where 70% of lesions were <2 cm in size. In this study, tumor thickness was >4 mm in the majority of patients with T1 lesions, all of whom had nodal disease. There was a significant correlation between increasing tumor thickness and lesion size, suggesting these tumors had a propensity for both vertical and horizontal growth. The authors noted that not all large SCCs will metastasize, and it is possible that lesions that are horizontally large (2–3 cm), but not thick (ie, 2–3 mm), may lack the propensity to metastasize.

Brantsch and colleagues,[6] in a landmark study of 615 patients, considered prognostic factors in patients with SCC. The authors noted that, in addition to the factors which had been considered in the previous TNM classification, tumor thickness, anatomic sites, and histologic subtypes (desmoplasia) also were of prognostic importance. It was reported that tumor thickness >6 mm was a highly significant independent predictor for the development of metastases. Fourteen of 90 patients with tumors thicker than 6 mm developed nodal metastases, whereas no patients with lesions thinner than 2 mm developed regional disease. These findings prompted the authors to suggest a modification to the T classification and consider thickness of the primary tumor rather than the horizontal size with classifications of T1 <2 mm, T2 2–6 mm, and T3 >6 mm thick. Site of the primary lesion, immunosuppression and the horizontal size of the lesion were also found to be significant, but to a lesser extent.

Tumor thickness (4–5 mm) also has been associated with increased risk for the development of metastatic disease by others. Kraus et al[41] demonstrated that, while only one third of patients with SCC have lesions >4 mm thick, these accounted for >80% of lesions that develop metastatic nodal disease. Breuninger et al,[52] in a study involving more than 500 patients, reported no patients with a thickness of <2 mm developing disease whereas around 20% of patients with a lesion thicker than 5 mm developed regional nodal metastases. In keeping with tumor thickness, Clark levels also have been investigated and reported to be predictive. Rowe et al[4] reported that lesions measuring <4 mm thick or Clark level I through III had a metastatic rate of 6.7% whereas the rate for lesions >4 mm thick or Clark level IV or V was 45.7%.

Recurrent lesions are associated with a marked increase in the risk of developing metastases. Patients with inadequately excised lesions are at risk of both local recurrence and the development of nodal disease. Grover et al[53] noted that the risk of nodal metastasis was 15% in patients with recurrent lip SCC compared with 2% in those with de novo lesions.[4] In a review of the literature, the incidence of lymph node metastasis was 32% and 45% in the setting of recurrent lip and ear SCC, respectively.[41]

Poorly differentiated SCC is more likely to be associated with the development of regional metastases. Breuninger and colleagues[54] reported a significant difference in the rate of nodal metastasis between high- and low-grade SCC (17% vs 4%)· Other studies have supported a difference in tumor behavior

Table 7–2. Staging for Cutaneous SCC

Tumor		Nodes		Metastasis	
Tx	Primary tumor cannot be assessed.	**Nx**	Regional lymph nodes cannot be assessed.	**M0**	No distant metastasis.
T0	No evidence of primary tumor.	**N0**	No regional lymph node metastasis.	**M1**	Distant metastases.
Tis	Carcinoma in situ.	**N1**	Metastases in a single ipsilateral lymph node, 3 cm or less in greatest dimension.		
T1	Tumor thickness < 2 cm in greatest dimension with less than 2 high risk features.	**N2a**	Metastases in a single ipsilateral lymph node, more than 3 cm but not more than 6cm in greatest dimension.		
T2	Tumor thickness >2 cm in greatest dimension or any tumor with 2 or more high risk features.	**N2b**	Metastases in multiple ipsilateral lymph nodes, none more than 6 cm in greatest dimension.		
T3	Tumor with invasion of maxilla, mandible, orbit or temporal bone.	**N2c**	Metastases in bilateral or contralateral lymph nodes, none more than 6 cm in greatest dimension.		
T4	Tumor with invasion of skeleton (axial or appendicular) or perineural invasion of skull base.	**N3**	Metastases in a lymph node more than 6 cm in greatest dimension.		

Stage	T	N	M
Stage 0	Tis	N0	M0
Stage I	T1	N0	M0
Stage II	T2	N0	M0
Stage III	T3	N0	M0
	T1	N1	M0
	T2	N1	M0
	T3	N1	M0
Stage IV	T1	N2	M0
	T2	N2	M0
	T3	N2	M0
	T Any	N3	M0
	T4	N Any	M0
	T Any	N Any	M1

Source: Used with permission of the American Joint Committee on Cancer (AJCC), Chicago, Illinois. The original source for this material is the AJCC Cancer Staging Manual, Seventh Edition (2010) published by Springer Science and Business Media LLC, www.springer.com.

based on histologic grade, with the rate of poorly differentiated SCC increased in patients developing metastasis (44% vs 5%).[50] An Australian study also supported this finding with 46% of patients with nodal metastatic disease having moderately or poorly differentiated tumors, compared with 12% having a well-differentiated grade.[42]

Although the presence of perineural invasion in SCC is relatively uncommon, it leads to an increased risk of both local recurrence and metastatic disease. In one review, the rate of perineural invasion was reported to occur in approximately 5% of cases.[4] Geist et al[55] reported rates of perineural invasion in SCC of up to 14% in some series.[54] Goepfert[56] reported a 47% local recurrence rate and a metastatic rate of 34.8% in patients with perineural invasion treated surgically.[4] Lymphovascular invasion, at least in one study, also has been reported to increase the risk of developing nodal metastatic disease. Moore and colleagues[57] documented lymphovascular invasion as an independent risk factor with 40% of patients with nodal metastasis having lymphovascular invasion compared with only 8% of node negative subjects.

Specific anatomic subsites have been identified as having an increased risk. Patients with lesions draining to the parotid (eg, lateral scalp, temple, forehead, ear, or cheek) should be considered as high risk. Rowe et al[4] reported an increase rate of nodal disease in patients with primary lesions involving the external ear or the lip. Clark and Soutar[58] recently reviewed the literature with regard to nodal metastases from auricular primaries and reported a rate of 11.8%, which is more than double the rate for other subsites. An Australian study reviewed 130 patients treated for SCC of the lip and reported that recurrence at the primary site occurred in 13% of patients and nodal disease in 20%.[59] In a multi-institutional study considering patterns of lymph node spread, it was noted that, in patients who had metastatic nodal disease, the majority had primary lesions that were on the lateral sun-exposed side of the head.[60] Ebrahimi et al[61] considered the pattern of metastatic spread in the neck from primary SCC and found that nearly 40% were from the anterior part of the face, 15% were from the external ear, and 22% were from the posterior region of the head and neck, with around 25% of primary sites not identified.

Molecular markers such as epidermal growth factor receptor (EGFR) are emerging as potential biomarkers for aggressive SCC. Ch'ng et al[62] reported overexpression of EGFR present in 79% of primary lesions that subsequently developed nodal metastasis. However, Ch'ng noted that only 47% of metastatic deposits expressed EGFR. An Australian study reported that EGFR was expressed in only a minority of tumors and that it was not always activated.[63] These findings, along with a Phase II trial of an EGFR inhibitor that did not find an objective response, suggest that, although EGFR may be a marker of aggressive disease, further prospective research is required to establish its full significance in predicting the development of regional spread in patients with SCC.[64]

SCC Nodal Staging

Prior to the latest edition of the AJCC staging system, the classification for nodal disease consisted of only 3 categories: Nx, N0, and N1. All patients with regional cervical metastatic disease were staged as N1 irrespective of the extent of disease. For example, the N1 category would have included a patient with a single 2-cm lymph node in the parotid gland or large metastatic deposit causing facial nerve palsy or multiple nodes in the neck or skull base involvement. This system clearly did not adequately separate patients presenting with varying degrees of disease extent, and as such, was of limited clinical and prognostic usefulness.

O'Brien et al[65] recognized the significant limitation of the TNM system when proposing a novel staging system based on extent of metastatic regional disease involving the parotid and/or cervical nodes. Eight-seven patients who had been treated with curative intent for metastatic SCC of the head and neck were restaged according to this new system which separated nodal disease (size, number, and site) in the parotid (P) and neck (N) (Table 7–3). Multivariate analysis demonstrated that, although increasing P stage, positive margins and failure to have multimodality therapy were associated with increased risk of recurrence in the parotid, neither increased P stage nor type of therapy was significant for survival. However, both increasing N stage and

Table 7–3. O'Brien et al System for Clinical Staging of Metastatic Cutaneous SCC Involving the Parotid Gland +/– Neck

Parotid		Neck	
P1	Metastatic node up to 3 cm diameter.	N0	No clinical neck disease.
P2	Metastatic node more than 3 cm up to 6 cm in diameter or multiple parotid nodes.	N1	Single ipsilateral neck node up to 3 cm diameter.
P3	Metastatic node more than 6 cm in diameter or disease involving VII or contralateral nodes.	N2	Single node more than 3 cm diameter or multiple neck nodes or contralateral nodes.

Source: O'Brien CJ, McNeil EB, McMahon JD, Pathak I, Lauer CS, Jackson MA. Significance of clinical stage, extent of surgery and pathological findings in metastatic cutaneous squamous cell carcinoma of the parotid gland. *Head Neck.* 2002;24:417–422.

positive margins were found to be predictive of worse disease-specific survival.

Palme et al[66] subsequently tested this new P and N staging system on a separate group of patients from the Head and Neck Service, Westmead Hospital, Sydney. One hundred twenty-six patients with SCC metastatic to the parotid and/or neck were retrospectively restaged, and the results demonstrated that increasing P stage was associated with a reduction in local control and increased treatment failure within the parotid bed. Immunosuppression, single modality therapy and increasing P stage were all found on multivariate analysis to be significantly associated with decreased survival. However, unlike O'Brien's original paper, increasing N stage was not found to be significant.

Veness et al[67] reported the results of patients with metastatic cutaneous SCC involving only standard cervical lymph nodes groups (Level 1–5). Seventy-four patients were treated with curative intent. The majority, 52 of 74, were treated with both surgery and adjuvant radiotherapy, while 22 patients received single modality therapy only. The recurrence rate was 34%. This study demonstrated that increasing nodal size (≥3 cm), multiple nodal involvement, and extracapsular spread had a significant impact on outcome with a reduction in disease-specific survival.

Audet et al[68] reviewed the experience of treating metastatic SCC of the head and neck at a large Canadian head and neck unit. Fifty-six patients with a median age of 76 were eligible for inclusion in this study. All patients were retrospectively restaged according to O'Brien's P and N stage. The majority were treated with surgery and adjuvant radiotherapy (79%). The recurrence rate was 29% and the overall survival was 53%. Nodal size greater than 6 cm or facial nerve involvement (ie, P3) were significant predictors for a poor disease specific outcome.

The results from these studies prompted a multi-institutional international trial testing O'Brien's staging system on a cohort of patients from 6 institutions—3 from Australia and 3 from North America. In this study, data from 322 patients treated with curative intent were analyzed.[69] All patients had disease involving either the parotid and/or cervical lymph nodes and minimum of 2-year follow-up. The majority, 67%, had disease involving only the parotid gland, with 62 (19%) patients presenting with only cervical lymph nodes. Forty-three patients (13%) had disease in both parotid and cervical lymph node groups. The vast majority were treated with surgical resection (90%), with 236 receiving adjuvant external beam radiotherapy. The remainder was treated with radiotherapy only. Disease recurred in 105 cases (33%) with 42 occurring within the parotid bed, 33 within neck nodes, and 30 at distant sites. P stage did not affect local control. There was a trend toward worse survival in those patients with increasing P stage. However, when P2 and P3 (advanced disease), were grouped together and compared against P1 (early disease), there was a statistically significant difference with the former being associated with a worse survival. When considering nodal disease in the neck, there was no change in survival; however, when the patients were divided into clinically present or absent neck disease, a statistically significant survival difference was found favoring patients staged N0.[51]

Based on the results from the previous studies and those on the multi-institutional trial, O'Brien's staging system was subsequently used in preference to the 6th edition of the TNM classification by a number of authors. Although not yet ideal, it was a significant improvement on the existing staging system.

Forest et al[70] recently published a modification of the O'Brien staging, which includes the parotid with the rest of the neck nodes. The aim of this study was to include well accepted nodal factors such as size, location, and number in order to improve prognostication and simplify staging of patients with metastatic SCC of the head and neck. This proposed system was tested against a cohort of patients from the authors' institution and externally validated against a separate group from Westmead Hospital. In both instances, the stratifications were found to have prognostic significance. The nodal classification in the N1S3 system is similar to that of the current 7th edition of the AJCC, which was modified based on the results from O'Brien, Palme, Audet, and Andruchow.[65,66,68,69] The new system separates N positive disease into N1: single <3-cm node; N2: single node 3 to 6 cm or multiple ≤6 cm; and N3: >6 cm, and has acknowledged the universal concern that classifying all node-positive patients with metastatic SCC of the head and neck as N1 is inadequate for state of the art contemporary management, prognostication and research. The current 7th edition of the AJCC appears to be a much improved way of classifying patients with metastatic SCC in the head and neck.

Merkel Cell Carcinoma Staging

There are multiple staging systems for MCC, of which the most commonly used is that developed by the group at MSKCC. Yiengpruksawan[50] proposed a system in 2001 with 3 stages, with stage I subdivided into stage Ia and Ib. This staging system subsequently was modified with stage Ib becoming stage II and stage II and III becoming stage III and IV respectively (Table 7–4).

Clark et al[71] proposed a staging system modeled on the TNM system based on a patient cohort from 3 institutions, 2 Australian and 1 Canadian (Table 7–5). This system was found to be more predictive of the

Table 7–4. MSKCC Staging System for Merkel Cell Carcinoma

Stage I	Local disease <2 cm.
Stage II	Local disease >2 cm.
Stage III	Regional nodal disease.
Stage IV	Distant metastatic disease.

Source: Yiengpruksawan A, Coit DG, Thaler HT, et al. Merkel Cell Carcinoma Prognosis and Management. *Arch Surg.* 1991;126:1514–1519.

Table 7–5. Clark et al Merkel Cell Carcinoma Staging

Tumor		Nodes		Metastatis	
T1	Primary tumor <1 cm.	N0	Negative regional lymph nodes.	M0	No distant metastasis present.
T2	Primary tumor >1 cm.	N1	<2 cm positive regional lymph nodes.	M1	Distant metastasis.
		N2	>2 cm positive regional lymph nodes.		

Stage	T	N	M
Stage I	T1	N0	M0
Stage IIa	T1	N1	M0
Stage IIb	T2	N0	M0
Stage III	T Any	N2	M0
Stage IV	T Any	N Any	M1

Source: Clark JR, Veness MJ, Gilbert R, O'Brien C J, Gullane PJ. Merkel cell carcinoma of the head and neck: Is adjuvant radiotherapy necessary? *Head Neck.* 2007;29(3):249–257. Used with permission.

disease-specific survival, especially for patients who had stage I disease using the new system, whose 5-yr survival was noted to be 95%.

The 7th edition of the AJCC introduced a staging system specifically for MCC acknowledging differences from other cutaneous carcinomas in an attempt to have an accepted standardized staging system. The staging system developed by the AJCC was based on unpublished data from over 4,700 patients and a review of the available literature (Table 7–6). Considering the patient cohort on which the new staging system was developed, it was noted that there were survival differences when patients were stratified according to nodal status: nodes negative microscopically, nodes negative clinically, unknown nodal status, microscopic nodal disease, and macroscopic nodal disease. The importance of the pathologic assessment of the draining lymph nodes is emphasized in the AJCC staging system, which separates patients who have had clinical assessment only from those who have had both clinical and pathologic assessment.

Prognosis

Basal Cell Carcinoma

BCC is rarely life threatening. Disease-specific 5-year survival rates in excess of 95% are reported. The development of metastatic disease in either the nodal basin or distant disease is exceedingly rare, with reported rates ranging from 0.0028% to 0.55%.[17] Significant morbidity from BCC arises primarily from the potential for recurrence of incompletely excised disease. Wilson et al[72] showed that between 20 to 30% of incompletely excised BCC will develop local recurrence. Most patients will be successfully salvaged, although deeply recurrent midface lesions may require extensive surgery. The development of significant morbidity and mortality from BCC is due mainly to uncontrolled local invasion and destruction of critical areas, especially with lesions located around the anatomically complex and func-

Table 7–6. AJCC 7th Edition Merkel Cell Carcinoma Staging System

Tumor		Nodes		Metastasis	
TX	Primary tumor cannot be assessed	**NX**	Regional lymph nodes cannot be assessed	**M0**	No distant metastasis
T0	No evidence of primary tumor (eg, nodal/metastatic presentation without associated primary)	**N0**	No regional lymph nodes metastasis	**M1**	Metastasis beyond regional lymph nodes
Tis	In situ primary tumor	**cN0**	Nodes negative by clinical exam (no pathologic node exam performed)	**M1a**	Metastasis to skin, subcutaneous tissues or distant lymph nodes
T1	≤2 cm maximum tumor dimension	**pN0**	Nodes negative by pathologic exam	**M1b**	Metastasis to lung
T2	>2 cm but ≤5 cm maximum tumor dimension	**N1**	Metastasis in regional lymph node(s)	**M1c**	Metastasis to all other visceral sites
T3	>5 cm maximum tumor dimension	**N1a**	Micrometastasis		
T4	Primary tumor invades bone, muscle, fascia, or cartilage	**N1b**	Macrometastasis		
		N2	In transit metastasis		

Used with permission of the American Joint Committee on Cancer (AJCC), Chicago, Illinois. The original source for this material is the AJCC Cancer Staging Manual, Seventh Edition (2010) published by Springer Science and Business Media LLC, www.springer.com.

tionally important regions of the orbit, midface and skull base.

Squamous Cell Carcinoma

The majority of patients with primary SCC are cured following appropriate single modality treatment. Approximately 10% will develop local recurrence and 5% of patients will develop nodal metastases. Although the majority of immunocompetent patients with small, nonrecurrent superficial lesions can be considered to be at low risk for developing regional disease, there is a subset of patients who have unfavorable factors. In summary, these include tumor size, thickness, recurrence, grade, perineural and lymphovascular invasion, subsite, immunosuppression, and incomplete excision.[73]

Current state of the art therapy in patients who develop nodal metastases includes combined modality treatment involving surgical resection when possible and adjuvant external beam radiotherapy. Surgery or radiotherapy alone is associated with a significantly lower chance of achieving local control and disease-specific survival. Based on the current literature, the recurrence rates with single versus multimodality therapy are 20% versus 50%, respectively.[67] Despite contemporary best practice, 20 to 25% of patients subsequently succumb to their disease. Currently, there is a randomized, controlled trial being undertaken in Australia and New Zealand considering the benefit of adding platin-based chemotherapy as an adjuvant therapy in high-risk patients (posttrial). The usual first site of recurrence is locoregional (80%) rather than distant metastatic disease.[68,74] The majority of patients who fail therapy will have a combination of adverse features such as multiple involved nodes, increasing size of nodal disease (>3 cm), extracapsular spread, close/positive margins, or perineural invasion and therefore benefit from combined treatment.

Howle et al[75] reported on the aggressive nature of SCC arising from the scalp with nodal metastases, with nearly half of all patients recurring and 43% dead of disease within 5 years. The ear also has been noted to be a site associated with worse prognosis. Turner et al[76] reviewed the experience of the Westmead Hospital Group identifying 43 patients with metastatic SCC of the external ear. Although the majority of patients received combined modality treatment (74%), there was still significant morbidity with over one third of patients relapsing and 20% dying from their disease. It also was noted in this study that the median survival after relapse was 5.5 months.

Immunosuppression is a particularly poor prognostic factor in metastatic SCC of the head and neck. The Westmead Hospital Group, including the paper by Palme et al[66] considering the O'Brien staging system, were among the first to report this in the surgical literature. This landmark study found that the presence of immunosuppression was the most significant predictor of survival on multivariate analysis. Southwell et al[77] subsequently reported on a group of 49 patients with metastatic SCC with 9 cases having significant immunosuppression. Recurrence rates were significantly increased in this group at 56%. None of the 9 were alive at 2 years after curative treatment when compared with a disease-specific survival of 87% in immunocompetent patients.

The Westmead Hospital Group has recently published a 4-factor prognostic scoring system, the ITEM score, which considers *i*mmunosuppression, *t*reatment, *e*xtracapsular spread, and *m*argins.[78] In this study, a cohort of 250 patients was examined to identify relevant patient, tumor, and treatment factors that are prognostic in patients with metastatic SCC of the head and neck. Twenty-eight percent of patients developed recurrence. Those treated with combined modality had a lower recurrence rate than those treated with either surgery or radiotherapy alone (17% vs 48%, respectively). Regional recurrence was the first site of recurrence in 73% of patients, whereas distant metastatic disease as the first presentation of recurrence was uncommon and occurred in only 9 (13%) cases. Patients failing treatment did so with a median time of 8 months and 73% died of their disease demonstrating the importance of achieving nodal control.[78] Multivariate regression analysis reconfirmed that the presence of immunosuppression, extent of treatment—single modality versus multimodality, extracapsular spread, and margin status were the most important prognostic factors in patients with metastatic cutaneous SCC of the head and neck.

The importance of extranodal spread and positive surgical margin have been previously well documented as associated with a worse prognosis.[48,79,80] Using the coefficients of the ITEM variables as weights, risk scores were able to be calculated for each patient. The relative weights are: Immunosuppression Yes/No: 1.8/0; Treatment combined versus single modality: –1.8/0; Extracapsular spread Yes/No: 4.8/0; and Margin involved versus clear: 1.0/0. This allowed the development of risk groups based on cutoff scores. Patients with a score ≤2.6, >2.6 to ≤3, or >3 were classed respectively as low, medium, or high risk for dying of disease (Fig 7–4). These demonstrated that the chance of dying of disease according to this novel prognostic classification at 5 years was 6%, 24%, and 56%, respectively. This is a simple and easy system that can be used clinically to prognosticate, and it also may allow the precise identification of patients at significant risk of a poor outcome and, therefore, may prove useful when allocating and testing new and more targeted therapeutic regimes.

Merkel Cell Carcinoma

Prognosis in MCC is dependent on the stage of disease at presentation, with the presence of nodal metastases being the most powerful independent predictor of survival. Although early stage disease has a 60 to 90% 5-year survival, for stage IV disease this is 0%. On presentation, the majority of patients with MCC have localized disease (50–60%), with 20% to 30% presenting with regional nodal involvement. When first described, MCC was thought to have a good prognosis with only 3 deaths in the first 24 reported cases, but it subsequently has proved to be an aggressive disease, with cancer-specific death occurring in 25 to 50% of patients in some series.

Due to the high incidence of subclinical nodal disease, patients found to have pathologically negative lymph nodes have a better prognosis than patients who do not have pathologic evaluation of lymph node status.[81] Immunosuppression from chronic hematologic malignancy, organ transplantation, or HIV is associated with a much worse prognosis.[82,83]

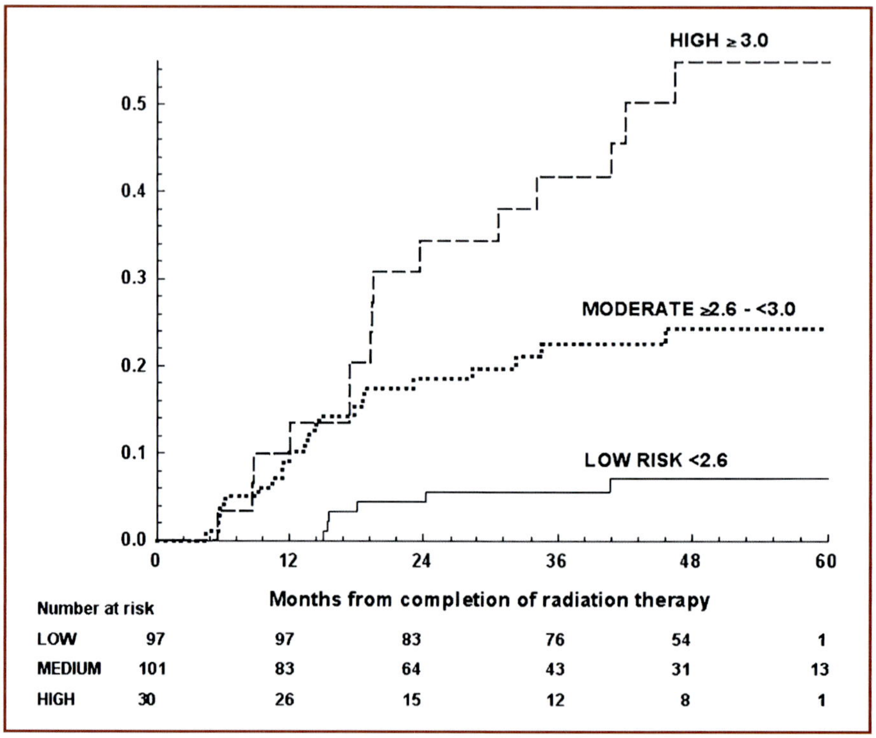

Figure 7–4. Survival based on risk: low, moderate, or high as per ITEM scoring.

MCC has high rates of locoregional recurrence (between 20–80%) and distant failure (25–30%). Up to 30% of patients who develop isolated regional recurrence are potentially curable. Patients who develop systemic recurrence are incurable with a median survival of between 3 and 6 months. Eng et al[84] reported on 46 patients with recurrent MCC with an overall survival of 37%; however, within this cohort, almost half had only local recurrence with regional and distant failure being 13% and 40%, respectively. Clark et al[71] reported 5-year survival based on their proposed staging system with stage I having 95% 5-year survival; stage IIa 68%; stage IIb 54%; stage III 35%; and stage IV 0%.[69]

Conclusion

Patients with BCC can expect to be cured of their disease. However, patients who develop either SCC or MCC are at a risk of morbidity and, in some cases, mortality. Although exposure to UV radiation is the most important risk factor for the development of NMSC, other factors including immunosuppression portend a poor outcome. A simple, accurate, and universally applied staging system is vital when managing these patients. Previous shortcomings in the AJCC TNM staging for NMSC largely have been addressed in the 7th edition. Ongoing research is needed to develop therapeutic strate-gies such as chemotherapy and targeted molecular therapy for patients with high-risk disease. Contemporary best practice management of primary and metastatic SCC of the head and neck includes a combination of surgery and/or external beam radiotherapy.

References

1. American Joint Committee on Cancer. Edge SB, Byrd DR, Compton CC et al, eds. *AJCC Cancer Staging Manual.* 7th ed. New York, NY: Springer; 2010.
2. Buettner PG, Raasch BA. Incidence of skin cancer in Townsville, Australia. *Int J Cancer.* 1998;78:587–593.
3. Diepgen TL, Mahler V. The epidemiology of skin cancer. *Br J Dermatol.* 2002;146(suppl 61):1–6.
4. Rowe DE, Carroll RJ, Day CL. Prognostic factors for local recurrence, metastasis and survival rates in squamous cell carcinoma of the skin ear and lip—implications for treatment modality selection. *J Am Acad Dermatol.* 1992; 26:976–90.
5. Joseph MG, Zulueta WP, Kennedy PJ. Squamous cell carcinoma of the skin of the trunk and limbs—the incidence of metastases and their outcome. *ANZ J Surg.* 1992;62: 697–701.
6. Brantsch KD, Meisner C, Schonfisch B, Trilling B, Wehner-Caroli J, Rocken M, Breuninger H. Analysis of risk factors determining prognosis of cutaneous squamous cell carcinoma: a prospective study. *Lancet Oncol.* 2008;9:713–720.
7. Czarnecki D, Staples M, Mar A, Giles G, Meehan C. Metastases from squamous cell carcinoma of the skin in southern Australia. *Dermatology.* 1994;189:52–54.
8. Staples MP, Elwood M, Burton RC, Williams JL. Nonmelanoma skin cancer in Australia: the 2002 national survey and trends since 1985. *Med J Aust.* 184:6–10.
9. de Vries E, van de Poll-Franse LV, Louwman WJ, de Gruijl FR, Coebergh JWW. Predictions of skin cancer incidence in the Netherlands up to 2015. *Br J Dermatol.* 2005;152:481–488.
10. Demers AA, Nugent Z, Michalcioiu C, Viseman MC, Kliewer EV. Trends of nonmelanoma skin cancer from 1960 through 2000 in a Canadian population. *J Am Acad Dermatol.* 2005;53:320–328.
11. Talmi YP. Problems in the Current TNM Staging of nonmelanoma skin cancer of the head and neck. *Head Neck.* 2007;29:525–527.
12. Holme SA, et al. Changing trends in non-melanoma skin cancer in South Wales 1988–1998. *Br J Dermatol.* 2000; 143(6):1224–1229.
13. Marks R, Rennie G. Malignant Transformation of solar keratoses to squamous cell carcinoma. *Lancet.* 1988;1: 795–797.
14. Ramirez CC Federman DG, Kirsner RS. Skin Cancer as an occupational disease: the effect of ultraviolet and other forms of radiation. *Int J Dermatol.* 2005;44:95–100.
15. Alam M, Ratner D. Cutaneous squamous cell carcinoma. *New Engl J Med.* 2001;344:975–983.
16. Diepgen TL, Mahler V. The epidemiology of skin cancer. *Br J Dermatol.* 2002;146:1–6.
17. Rubin AI, Chen EH, Ratner D. Basal cell carcinoma. *New Engl J Med.* 2005;353:2262–2269.
18. Zak-Prelich M, Narbutt J, Sysa-Jedrzejowska A. Environmental risk factors predisposing to the development of basal cell carcinoma. *Dermatol Surg.* 2004;30:248–252.
19. Stern RS. The mysteries of geographic variability in nonmelanoma skin cancer incidence. *Arch Dermatol.* 1999; 135:843–844.
20. Koh D, Wang H, Lee J, Chia KS, Lee HP, Goh CL. Basal cell carcinoma, squamous cell carcinoma and melanoma of the skin—analysis of the Singapore Cancer Registry data 1968–97. *Br J Dermatol.* 2003;148:1161–1166.

21. Gloster HM, Neal K. Skin cancer in skin of color. *J Am Acad Dermatol.* 2006;55;741–760.
22. Criscione VD, Weinstock MA, Naylor MF, et al. Actinic keratoses: natural history and risk of malignant transformation in the Veterans Affairs Topical Tretinoin Chemoprevention Trial. *Cancer.* 2009;115:2523–2530.
23. Marcil I, Stern RS. Risk of developing a subsequent nonmelanoma skin cancer in patients with a history of nonmelanoma skin cancer: a critical review of the literature and meta-analysis. *Arch Dermatol.* 2000;136:1524–1530.
24. World Health Organisation. WHO ultraviolet radiation and the INTERSUN programme. http://www.who.int/uv/uv_and_health/en/index.html. Retrieved 09/02/10.
25. Abarca JF, Casiccia CC. Skin cancer and ultraviolet-B radiation under the Antarctic ozone hole: southern Chile, 1987–2000. *Photodermatol Photoimmunol Photomed.* 2002; 18:294–302.
26. Rigel DS. Cutaneous ultraviolet exposure and its relationship to the development of skin cancer. *J Am Acad Dermatol.* 2008;58:S129–S132.
27. Hartevelt MM, Bavinck JN, Kootte AMM, Vermeer BJ, Vandenbroucke JP. Incidence of skin cancer after renal transplantation in the Netherlands. *Transplantation.* 1990; 49:506–509.
28. Lindelof B, Sigurgeirsson B, GabelH, Stern RS. Incidence of skin cancer in 5356 patients following organ transplantation. *Br J Dermatol.* 2000;143:513–519.
29. Cooper JZ, Brown MD. Special Concern about squamous cell carcinoma of the scalp in organ transplant recipients. *Arch Dermatol.* 2006;142:755–758.
30. Berg D, Otley C. Skin caner in organ transplant recipients: epidemiology pathogenesis and management. *J Am Acad Dermatol.* 2002;47:1–17.
31. Ramsay HM, Fryer AA, Hawley CM, et al. Nonmelanoma skin cancer risk in the Queensland renal transplant population. *Br J Dermatol.* 2002:147(5):950–956.
32. Mehrany K Weenig RH, Lee KK, Pittelkow MR, Otley CC. Increased metastasis and mortality from cutaneous squamous cell carcinoma in patients with chronic lympho - cytic leukemia. *J Am Acad Dermatol.* 2005;53:1067–1071.
33. Otley CC. Non-Hodgkin lymphoma and skin cancer: a dangerous combination. *Australas J Dermatol.* 2006;47: 231–236.
34. Wilkins K, Turner R, Dolev JC, LeBoit PE, Berger TG, Maurer TA. Cutaneous malignancy and human immu - nodeficiency virus disease. *J Am Acad Dermatol.* 2006;54: 189–206.
35. Crum Cianflone N, Huppler Hullsiek K, et al. Cutaneous malignancies among HIV infected persons. *Arch Intern Med,* 2009;169(12):1130–1138.
36. Majewski, S Jablonska S. Current views on the role of human papillomaviruses in cutaneous oncogenesis. *Int J Dermatol.* 2006;45:192–196.
37. Karagas MR, Nelson HN, Sehr P, et al. Human papillomavirus infection and incidence of squamous cell and basal cell carcinomas of the skin. *J Natl Cancer Inst.* 2006; 98(6):389–395.
38. De Hertog SAE, Wensveen CAH, Bastiaens MT, et al. Relation between smoking and skin cancer. *J Clin Oncol.* 2001;19:231–238.
39. Odenbro A, Bellocco R, Boffetta P, Lindelo B, Adami J. Tobacco smoking, snuff dipping and the risk of cutaneous squamous cell carcinoma: a nationwide cohort study in Sweden. *Br J Cancer.* 2005;92:1326–1328.
40. Nixon RL, Dorevitch AP, Marks R. Squamous cell carcinoma of the skin, accuracy of clinical diagnosis and outcome of follow-up in Australia. *Med J Australia.* 1986;144: 235–239.
41. Kraus DH, Carew JF, Harrison LB. Regional lymph node metastasis from cutaneous squamous cell carcinoma. *Arch Otolaryngol Head Neck Surg.* 1998;124:582–587.
42. Veness MJ, Palme CE, Morgan GJ. High risk cutaneous squamous cell carcinoma of the head and neck: results from 266 treated patients with metastatic lymph node disease. *Cancer.* 2006;106:2389–2396.
43. Ageli M, Clegg LX. Epidemiology of primary Merkel cell carcinoma in the United States. *J Am Acad Dermatol.* 2003;49:832–841.
44. Lemos B, Nghiem P. Merkel cell carcinoma: more deaths but still no pathway to blame. *J Invest Dermatol.* 2007; 127(9):2100–2103.
45. Feng H, Shuda M, Chang Y, Moore PS. Clonal integration of a polyomavirus in human merkel cell carcinoma. *Science.* 2008;319:1096–1100.
46. Veness MJ, Palme CE, Morgan GJ. Merkel cell carcinoma: a review of management. *Curr Opin Otolaryngol Head Neck Surg.* 2008;16:170–174.
47. Heath ML, Jaimes N, Lemos B, et al. Clinical characteristics of Merkel cell carcinoma at diagnosis in 195 patients: the AEIOU features. *J Am Acad Dermatol.* 2008;58(3): 375–381.
48. Nghiem P, et al. Merkel cell carcinoma, (chapter 30) In: Edge SB et al, eds. *AJCC Cancer Staging Manual,* 7th ed. New York, NY: Springer; 2010.
49. *AJCC Cancer Staging Manual,* 5th ed. New York, NY: Springer; 1996.
50. Yiengpruksawan A, Coit DG, Thaler HT et al. Merkel cell carcinoma prognosis and management. *Arch Surg.* 1991; 126:1514–1519.
51. Cherpelis BS, Marcusen C, Lang PG. Prognostic factors for metastasis in squamous cell carcinoma of the skin. *Dermatol Surg.* 2002:28:268–273.
52. Brueninger H, Black B Rassner G. Brief scientific statement: microstaging of squamous cell carcinomas. *Am J Clin Pathol.* 1990;94:624–627.
53. Grover R, Douglas RG, Shaw JH. Carcinoma of the lip in Auckland, New Zealand, 1969–1987. *Head Neck.* 1989; 11(3):264–268.
54. Breuninger H, Schaumberg-Lever G, Holzchuh J, Horny HP. Desmoplastic squamous cell carcinoma of the skin and vermilion surface a highly malignant subtype of skin cancer. *Cancer* 1997;79:915–919.
55. Geist DE, Garcia-Moliner M, Fitzek MM, Cho H, Rogers GS. Perineural invasion of cutaneous squamous cell

carcinoma and basal cell carcinoma: raising awareness and optimizing management. *Dermatol Surg.* 2008;34(12): 1642–1651.
56. Goepfert H, Dichtel WJ, Medina JE, Lindberg RD, Luna MD. Perineural invasion in squamous cell skin carcinoma of the head and neck. *Am J Surg.* 1984;148(4): 542–547.
57. Moore BA, Weber RS, Prieto V et al. Lymph node metastases from cutaneous squamous cell carcinoma of the head and neck. *Laryngoscope.* 2005;115:1561–1567.
58. Clark RR, Soutar DS, Lymph node metastases from auricular squamous cell carcinoma. A systematic review and meta-analysis. *J Plast Reconstr Aesthet Surg.* 2008;61: 1140–1147.
59. Babington S, Veness MJ Cakir B, Gebski VJ Morgan GJ. Squamous cell carcinoma of the lip: is there a role for adjuvant radiotherapy in improving local control following incomplete or inadequate excision. *ANZ J Surg.* 2003;73;621–625.
60. Vauterin TJ, Veness MJ, Morgan GJ, Poulsen MG, O'Brien CJ. Patterns of lymph node spread of cutaneous squamous cell carcinoma of the head and neck. *Head Neck.* 2006;28(9):785–791.
61. Ebrahimi A, Moncrieff MD, Clark JR, et al. Predicting the pattern of regional metastases from cutaneous squamous cell carcinoma of the head and neck based on location of the primary. *Head Neck.* 2010;32(10):1288–1294.
62. Ch'ng S, Low I, Ng D, Brasch H, Sullivan M, Davis P, Tan ST. Epidermal growth factor receptor: a novel biomarker for aggressive head and neck cutaneous squamous cell carcinoma. *Human Pathol.* 2008;39:344–349.
63. Fogarty GB, Conus NM, Chu J, McArthur G. Characterisation of the expression and activation of the epidermal growth factor receptor in squamous cell carcinoma of the skin. *Br J Dermatol.* 2007;156:92–98.
64. Glisson B, Kim E, Kiess M, et al. Phase II study of gefitinib in patients with metastatic/recurrent squamous cell carcinoma of the skin. *J Clin Oncol.* 2006;24(Abstract 5531).
65. O'Brien CJ McNeil EB, McMahon JD, Pathak I, Lauer CS, Jackson MA. Significance of clinical stage, extent of surgery and pathological findings in metastatic cutaneous squamous cell carcinoma of the parotid gland. *Head Neck.* 2002;24:417–422
66. Palme CE O'Brien CJ, Veness MJ, Mcneil EB, Bron LP, Morgan GJ. Extent of parotid disease influences outcome in patients with metastatic cutaneous squamous cell carcinoma. *Arch Otolaryngol Head Neck Surg.* 2003;113: 1070–1075.
67. Veness MJ, Palme CE, Smith M, et al. Cutaneous head and neck squamous cell carcinoma metastatic to cervical lymph nodes (non parotid): a better outcome with surgery and adjuvant radiotherapy. *Laryngoscope.* 2003;113: 827–833
68. Audet N, Palme CE, Gullane PJ, et al. Cutaneous metastatic squamous cell carcinoma to the parotid gland: analysis and outcome. *Head Neck.* 2004;26:727–732.
69. Andruchow JL, Veness MJ, Morgan GJ, et al. Implications for clinical staging of metastatic cutaneous squamous carcinoma of the head and neck based on a multicentre study of treatment outcomes. *Cancer.* 2006;106:1078–1083.
70. Forest VI, Clark JJ, Veness MJ, Milross C. N1S3: a revised staging system for head and neck cutaneous squamous cell carcinoma with lymph node metastases results of 2 Australian cancer centres. *Cancer.* 2010;116(5):1298–1304.
71. Clark JR, Veness MJ, Gilbert R, O'Brien C J, Gullane PJ. Merkel cell carcinoma of the head and neck: is adjuvant radiotherapy necessary? *Head Neck.* 2007;29(3):249–257.
72. Wilson AW, Howsam G, Santhanam V, Macpherson D, Grant J, Pratt CA, Townend JV. Surgical management of incompletely excised basal cell carcinomas of the head and neck. *Br J Oral Maxillofac Surg.* 2004;42(4):311–314.
73. Veness MJ, Porceddu S, Palme CE, Morgan GJ. Cutaneous head and neck squamous cell carcinoma metastatic to parotid and cervical lymph nodes. *Head Neck.* 2007;29: 621–631.
74. Veness MJ, Morgan GJ, Palme C, Gebski V. Cutaneous head and neck squamous cell carcinoma metastatic to cervical lymph nodes: surgery and adjuvant radiotherapy should be considered best practice. *Laryngoscope.* 2005;44:870–875.
75. Howle JR, Morgan GJ, Kalnins I, Palme CE, Veness MJ. Metastatic cutaneous squamous cell carcinoma of the scalp. *ANZ J Surg.* 2008;78:449–453.
76. Turner SJ, Morgan GJ, Palme CE, Veness MJ. Metastatic cutaneous squamous cell carcinoma of the external ear: a high risk cutaneous subsite. *J Laryngol Otol.* 2010;124: 36–31.
77. Southwell CE, Chaplin JM, Eisenberg RL, McIvor NP, Morton RP. Effect of immunocompromise on metastatic squamous cell carcinoma in the parotid and neck. *Head Neck.* 2006;28:244–248.
78. Oddone N, Morgan GJ, Palme CE, Perera L, Shannon J, Wong E, Gebski V, Veness MJ. Metastatic cutaneous carcinoma of the head and neck: the Immunosuppression, Treatment, Extranodal Spread and Margin status (ITEM) prognostic score to predict outcome and the need to improve survival. *Cancer.* 2009;115:1883–1891.
79. Ch'ng S, Maitra A, Allison RS, et al. Parotid and cervical nodal status predict prognosis for patients with head and neck metastatic cutaneous squamous cell carcinoma. *J Surg Oncol.* 2008;98:101–105.
80. Ch'ng S, Maitra A, Lea R, Brasch H, Tan ST. Parotid metastasis—an independent prognostic factor for head and neck cutaneous squamous cell carcinoma. *J Plast Reconstr Aesthet Surg.* 2006;59:1288–1293.
81. Gupta SG, Wang LC, Penas PF, Gellenthin M, Lee SJ, Nghiem P. Sentinel lymph node biopsy for evaluation and treatment of patients with Merkel cell carcinoma: the Dana-Farber experience and meta-analysis of the literature. *Arch Dermatol.* 2006;142(6):685–690.
82. Penn I, First MR. Merkel's cell carcinoma in organ recipients: report of 41 cases. *Transplantation.* 1999;68(11): 1717–1721.

83. Buell JF, Trofe J, Hanaway MJ, et al. Immunosuppression and Merkel cell cancer. *Transplant Proc.* 2002;34(5): 1780–1781.

84. Eng TY, Naguib M, Fuller CD, et al Treatment of recurrent Merkel cell carcinoma: an analysis of 46 cases. *Am J Clin Oncol.* 2004;24:576–583.

8

AGGRESSIVE NONMELANOMA SKIN CANCER

CHRISTIAN P. HASNEY
NANDITA GUHA-THAKURTA
BRIAN A. MOORE
RANDAL S. WEBER

Epidemiology

Skin cancer, including melanoma and nonmelanoma subtypes, represents the most common malignancy in the United States. In spite of widespread public health initiatives aimed at preventing cutaneous malignancies, the incidence of skin cancer continues to rise. Like other head and neck cancers, the management of cutaneous malignancy, especially those that are deemed aggressive, requires a multidisciplinary approach with appropriate use of surgery, radiation, chemotherapy, and, in select cases, targeted molecular therapy.

Although melanoma traditionally is considered the most lethal of skin malignancies, aggressive nonmelanoma skin cancers frequently fail standard surgical and nonsurgical dermatologic therapies. This chapter focuses on the biologic behavior and appropriate management of aggressive nonmelanoma skin cancer (NMSC). The histopathologic and clinical features of nonmelanoma skin malignancies are highlighted, as is their role in selecting the appropriate treatment modalities for these lesions. The surgical techniques that maximize local control while maintaining or restoring function and cosmesis are emphasized, along with the current strategies for addressing the cervical lymphatics. Finally, indications for systemic therapies and preventive strategies are described.

Nonmelanoma Skin Cancer

NMSC affects more than 1.3 million Americans each year with an estimated annual health care cost of greater than $426 million. The incidence of these lesions has increased steadily over the last 30 years.[1–3] Because the relationship between NMSC and ultraviolet radiation exposure is well described, these lesions tend to appear in sun-exposed areas of the body, with 75% appearing in the head and neck. Patients over 50 years of age, particularly men, are traditionally considered to be at greatest risk for NMSC. However, recent evidence has shown that the incidence of NMSC, and aggressive variants thereof, is on the rise in both women and younger patients.[4,5] Basal cell carcinoma (BCC) accounts for approximately 80% of NMSC, with squamous cell carcinoma (SCC) comprising the remaining 20%.

Ninety-five percent of these lesions are definitively addressed with a variety of ablative and nonablative therapies. However, there are aggressive variants of NMSC that are resistant to these traditional therapeutic measures. These lesions have a propensity for recurrence and metastasis, leading to approximately 2,500 deaths per year.[2]

Etiology of Nonmelanoma Skin Cancer

Ultraviolet light exposure has been identified as the most significant factor contributing to the development of cutaneous malignancies. Early, intense intermittent, and excessive sun exposure plays a vital role in carcinogenesis. The rising incidence of skin cancer may be partially attributed to the increased incidence of sunbathing and the use of artificial tanning beds, as a tanned complexion has taken a place of prominence within the Western ideal of beauty. Depletion of the ozone layer with increased ultraviolet exposure and public health programs that result in the detection of more malignant lesions also may play a role in the increasing incidence of skin cancer.[4]

Molecular Biology of Nonmelanoma Skin Cancer

Ultraviolet light, both UVB (290–320 nm) and UVA (320–400 nm), has long been established as a key factor in the pathogenesis of nonmelanoma skin cancer. UVA and UVB interact synergistically to cause mutations in keratinocyte DNA, most commonly through the formation of thymidine dimers in the p53 tumor suppressor gene and through the loss of Fas-Fas ligand interaction.[6] In the normal subject, these mutations are easily repaired. However, when DNA repair mechanisms fail, clonal expansion of mutated keratinocytes occurs, laying the foundation for the development of epithelioid cutaneous malignancy.[2]

Chronic ultraviolet light exposure causes the above events to occur on a larger scale and allows for accumulation of mutated and dysregulated cells until frank squamous cell carcinoma arises. Complicit in the oncogenesis of cutaneous squamous cell carcinoma is the activation of protooncogenes such as ras and the inactivation of tumor suppressor genes such as PTCH and INK4a/ARF. Aberrations in the PTCH tumor suppressor gene, along with derangements in the pathway of the protein sonic hedgehog, and abnormalities in the nuclear factor kappa B (NF-κB) signaling pathway have been linked to the development of basal cell carcinoma.[7]

Skin Cancer Syndromes

A number of genetic syndromes manifest with the development of NMSC in young patients. The most common syndromes are xeroderma pigmentosum, congenital basal cell nevus syndrome, and albinism.

Xeroderma Pigmentosum

Xeroderma pigmentosum (XP), an autosomal recessive DNA repair defect, is characterized by intense photosensitivity and often results in the development of NMSC or melanoma by 10 years of age. The initial symptoms of XP include photosensitivity and photodistributed lentigines that generally appear around 1 to 2 years of age. Actinic keratoses, BCC, SCC, and cutaneous melanoma appear within the first decade of life, with NMSC in sun-exposed areas being approximately 5% more frequent than melanoma.[8]

At the core of this disorder is the inability to repair pyrimidine dimers created by ultraviolet radiation exposure. Genetic lesions of this type, if unrepaired, may be propagated and result in carcinogenesis. Broadly speaking, the formation of tumors in XP results from the inactivation of tumor suppressor genes and the activation of oncogenes. Several recent studies implicate p53 and ras in the oncogenesis of XP, but many unidentified genes are targeted for mutations and complicit in tumor formation in XP.[9–12]

Patients with XP exhibit a 2000-fold increased risk of developing cutaneous BCC, SCC, and cutaneous melanoma when compared with normal patients of the same age. Survival of XP patients is greatly compromised by these lesions that are prone to recurrence and metastasis, with nearly 70% of those with XP perishing by age 40.[8]

Gorlin Syndrome

Congenital basal cell nevus (Gorlin) syndrome is an autosomal-dominant disease characterized by basal cell nevi and BCC early in life. Eighty to 90% of affected Caucasians will develop BCC by a median age of 20 years. Clinically, the characteristic BCC may appear as small brown papules resembling skin tags, benign nevi, and hemangiomas. Gorlin syndrome also is associated with a number of extracutaneous lesions, including odontogenic keratocysts of the mandible. Other extracutaneous neoplasms associated with this syndrome include ameloblastoma, medulloblastoma, meningioma, ovarian fibroma, fibrosarcoma, cardiac fibroma, and ovarian desmoid tumors.[8]

Through extensive genetic study, several investigators have mapped the gene for Gorlin syndrome to 9q22-31.[13–17] This locus is occupied by the patched (*PTCH*) gene which has been demonstrated to be abnormal in 15 to 39% of probands of Gorlin's families.[18–21] patched encodes the PTC protein, an important component in the inhibition of the smoothened (SMO) transmembrane protein.[22] This inhibitory action is critical for tumor suppression. Disruptions of this process lead to carcinogenesis and have been identified in Gorlin syndrome, sporadic medulloblastomas, breast carcinomas, meningiomas, and one colon cancer cell line.[23–26]

Albinism

Albinism, a collective term for a spectrum of genetic syndromes resulting from abnormalities in the production and processing of melanin, is another genetic abnormality that predisposes the affected individual to skin cancer. The most commonly occurring types of albinism, oculocutaneous albinism types 1 and 2, display an autosomal-recessive pattern of inheritance. Clinical findings in oculocutaneous albinism types 1 and 2 include a lack of pigmentation of the skin, hair, and eyes, decreased visual acuity, and spontaneous nystagmus. SCC is the most common cutaneous malignancy in albinos, occurring approximately twice as frequently in this cohort than in the normal population.[27]

The genetic basis of albinism is quite complex and variable across the spectrum of the disease. Oculocutaneous albinism type 1 results from mutations of the gene encoding the enzyme tyrosinase on the long arm of chromosome 11. More than 70 mutations resulting in defective production of tyrosinase have been identified. With the array of genetic abnormalities that may result in oculocutaneus albinism type 1, many of the afflicted display compound heterozygosity at this locus with two different recessive alleles resulting in the albino phenotype.[28–30]

Muir-Torre Syndrome

Muir-Torre syndrome (MTS) is an autosomal-dominant disorder characterized by sebaceous tumors and visceral malignancy. Sebaceous tumors tend to present in the fifth to sixth decade of life with sebaceous adenoma representing the most common tumor and sebaceous carcinoma as the second most common. The face is the most common site of sebaceous tumors in MTS. Interestingly, nearly 20% of those with MTS are found to have one or more keratoacanthomas, although the presence of a keratoacanthoma and a visceral malignancy in the absence of a sebaceous lesions does not establish a diagnosis of MTS.[8,31]

Colorectal carcinoma represents the majority of visceral malignancies in those with MTS. Unlike other syndromes associated with colorectal cancer, MTS does not manifest with diffuse colonic polyposis but with hereditary carcinoma in the context of limited benign colon polyps. The age of diagnosis of colon cancer in those with MTS is approximately 10 years younger than the general population.[31]

The genetics of MTS bear a striking similarity to those of hereditary nonpolyposis colon cancer (HNPCC). Linkage analysis revealed common mutations between these syndromes localized to the short arm of chromosome 2.[32–34] These genes, *hMSH2* and *hMLH1*, play a role in DNA mismatch repair and are commonly disrupted in both of these syndromes.[35,36] As a hallmark of a dysfunctional DNA repair system, stretches of repetitive DNA sequences serve as the genetic signature of HNPCC tumors. These repetitive sequences of HNPCC also have been identified in keratoacanthomas and sebaceous tumors of those with MTS.[37–40]

Precursor Lesions

The astute clinician should be mindful that both existing and precursor lesions play a pivotal role in the development of NMSC. Squamous cell carcinoma of the skin commonly arises from actinic keratoses (AK), scaly lesions that may appear pink, brown, or skin-colored. An individual AK has a 0.025% to 20% risk per year of malignant transformation. The mere presence of AKs imparts a 6 to 10% cumulative lifetime risk of developing cutaneous squamous cell carcinoma.[2] Other lesions identified as precursors of cutaneous squamous cell carcinoma include Bowen's disease, Bowenoid papulosis, and epidermodysplasia verruciformis.

Previous Skin Malignancy

As with malignancies of the upper aerodigestive tract, a history of cutaneous cancer of the head and neck increases the individual risk of developing future cutaneous malignancy. In cases of both squamous and basal cell carcinoma, there exists, respectively, an 18% and 40% risk of developing second primary skin malignancies within three years of initial treatment. These risks are 10 times greater than for those of the general population.[41]

Human Papillomavirus (HPV)

The initial link between HPV and carcinoma of the skin was made in patients with a rare genetic disease called epidermodysplasia verruciformis (EV) in the 1920s.[42] EV is characterized by the presence of multiple flat warts and macular skin lesions that frequently progress to SCC.[43,44] Also, EV confers a diminution of cell-mediated immunity, leaving these patients susceptible to HPV infection.[45]

HPV has two predominant genotypes, with those virus particles carrying the alpha genotype infecting mucosal surfaces and those with the beta genotype infecting skin.[46] Among the Beta-HPV strains, HPV-5 and HPV-8 are the two most strongly associated with SCC.[47] Beta-HPV DNA has been detected in up to 50% of SCC from immunocompetent patients and in up to 90% of lesions in the immunocompromised.[48,49]

As is clear from studies of EV patients, HPV appears to play a role in the pathogenesis of cutaneous SCC in the immunocompromised.[43] The variable detection rate of HPV in cutaneous SCC may be technique dependent, and early work did not account for potential confounding variables in the development of cutaneous SCC such as sun exposure history, chemical exposure, or personal history of skin malignancy. A recent case-control study took these confounders into account and found that, although there is a high prevalence of HPV DNA in the skin of the general population, Beta-HPV is differentially expressed in cutaneous SCC. These findings suggest a possible causative role of HPV in the pathogenesis of cutaneous SCC in immunocompetent patients.[50]

Other Risk Factors

Aside from ultraviolet light exposure, a number of genetic, environmental, and pre-existing conditions may predispose one to develop aggressive NMSC.[2,7] Exposure to ionizing radiation imparts a significant risk of developing NMSC. An analysis of patients who had undergone radiotherapy for childhood malignancies revealed a 6.3-fold increased risk of developing NMSC, particularly basal cell carcinoma. Most NMSC occurred within the radiation field, and survivors were also more likely to develop NMSC at a younger age than the general population. NMSC has been identified as the most common second malignancy to affect this cohort of patients.[51]

Immunosuppressed patients, especially those who have undergone organ transplantation and those with hematologic malignancies, are at a significantly increased risk for developing NMSC. Squamous cell carcinoma with aggressive features, such as local recurrence and nodal metastases, has been described in individuals receiving intensive immunosuppressive therapy following cardiac transplantation.[52] The significance of immunosuppression on the development, presentation, and treatment of aggressive NMSC is discussed later in this chapter.

Histopathology

Basal Cell Carcinoma

There are several distinct histologic subtypes of BCC: superficial, nodular, infiltrative, and micronodular. Superficial BCC tend to occur on the trunk and appear as well-defined plaquelike lesions. Nodular BCC present as the characteristic "rodent ulcer," with raised, rolled edges and central ulceration, and they display an affinity for the skin of the head and neck. Histologically, these types of BCC are characterized by peripheral palisading. Superficial and nodular BCC are considered generally indolent neoplasms which respond to traditional therapies such as local excision and even topical medications.[7,53] Infiltrative and micronodular BCC are considered aggressive variants and are discussed later in this chapter.

Squamous Cell Carcinoma

The classic SCC lesion of the skin is a pale pink, firm, textured lesion with or without accompanying scaling or hyperkeratosis. These lesions frequently arise from a pre-existing AK. Differential diagnosis of SCC includes AK, BCC, and keratoacanthoma (KAC). KAC is a rapidly growing ulceronodular lesion that resembles SCC histologically but is distinguished by its natural history of rapid growth and spontaneous involution. Histologic variants of SCC include the slow-growing, exophytic verrucous carcinoma, spindle cell SCC, desmoplastic SCC, and basosquamous SCC.[2]

Aggressive Nonmelanoma Skin Cancer

It is imperative to remember that not all nonmelanoma skin cancer exhibits indolent behavior. Aggressive variants of BCC and SCC exist. These lesions display an increased rate of local recurrence, as well as regional and distant metastases, that belie their common name. These aggressive neoplasms typically fail to respond to traditional ablative and nonablative dermatologic interventions and, consequently, become the domain of the head and neck surgeon. The clinical and pathologic features of aggressive nonmelanoma skin cancer are enumerated in Table 8–1.[54,55] The remainder of this chapter focuses on the pathophysiology, diagnosis and management, and prognostic implications of aggressive NMSC.

Table 8–1. Features of Aggressive Nonmelanoma Skin Cancer and Risk Factors for Regional Metastases

Clinical Features	Pathologic Features	Risk Factors
Recurrent lesions	Poor differentiation	Recurrent lesion
Regional metastases	Histology	Size >2.0 cm
Size >2 cm	Desmoplastic SCC	Invasion into subcutaneous tissues
Rapid growth	Spindle cell SCC	Poor differentiation
Location	Basosquamous carcinoma	Pre-existing scar
Central H-zone of the face	Infiltrative BCC	Ear or lip location
		Perineural invasion
		Lymphovascular invasion
		Inflammation

Aggressive Squamous Cell Carcinoma

Although well-differentiated squamous cell carcinoma may exhibit aggressive features, several histologic subtypes of SCC exist that are defined as aggressive lesions. These subtypes include: spindle cell carcinoma, desmoplastic SCC, and basosquamous carcinoma. Due to their propensity for recurrence and metastasis, adjuvant therapy often is indicated in the management of these malignancies.

Spindle Cell Squamous Carcinoma

Cutaneous spindle cell carcinoma is an aggressive variant that is prone to perineural invasion, local recurrence, and regional metastases. Histologically, this lesion is characterized by spindle cells surrounded by a collagenous stroma. The diagnosis may be clinched with electron microscopy and immunohistochemical staining for cytokeratins.[56]

Desmoplastic Squamous Cell Carcinoma

Desmoplastic SCC bears the characteristic histologic pattern of fine branches of tumor cells in the periphery and desmoplasia in the surrounding stroma. These lesions most commonly are found on the skin of the ear and have been noted to be thicker and more advanced at presentation than nondesmoplastic SCC, with poorly differentiated features on microscopic exam. Prospective studies have demonstrated a 6 times greater risk of metastasis and 10 times greater risk of local recurrence when compared with nondesmoplastic lesions.[57]

Basosquamous Carcinoma

Basosquamous carcinoma is an aggressive variant of SCC characterized by features of both BCC and SCC. Histologically, these lesions demonstrate malignant basal cells with peripheral palisading nuclei and aggregates of squamous cells with eosinophilic cytoplasm. There is a notable lack of transition between BCC and SCC components. These lesions notoriously display lymphatic and perineural invasion with frequent local recurrence and metastases.[58]

Aggressive Basal Cell Carcinoma

Infiltrative, formerly known as morpheaform, and micronodular BCC represent the aggressive subtypes of BCC. These lesions are relatively infrequent with infiltrative BCC comprising 2% to 5% of all BCC and micronodular BCC representing 15% of the larger nodular histologic subtype. These neoplasms display a marked tendency for local recurrence. Infiltrative lesions, in particular, demonstrate a significant incidence of subclinical spread due to the presence of tumor islands and ill-defined projections. Micronodular lesions are so-called due to their appearance as small tumor nodules with the characteristic peripheral palisading.[7,53]

Aggressive BCC is defined as lesions with an initial diameter of greater than 1 cm, those that have recurred twice despite treatment with apparently adequate therapies, and extension into deeper, noncutaneous tissues.[59] Distantly metastatic BCC is a rare entity occurring in less than 1% of cases. BCC, however, is notorious for locally aggressive behavior and may cause significant morbidity if left unchecked. BCC lesions occasionally display more than one histologic pattern. In these cases, therapy is targeted toward the more aggressive pattern.

Features of Aggressive NMSC

Lesion Size

Size of the primary lesion over 2 cm is considered an independent predictor for the development of nodal metastases. Rowe et al[60] set forth that the risk of nodal metastasis in patients with SCC lesions larger than 2 cm in size was 30% compared to 9% in those with lesions less than 2 cm in greatest dimension. More recent work has suggested that lesions as small as 1.5 cm may carry an increased risk of nodal metastases.[61,62] These results suggest that factors beyond lesion size contribute to the development of metastatic disease. A prospective study by Clayman et al[63] suggested that larger lesions (>4 cm) carry an increased risk of mortality, specifically a decrease in 3-year disease-free survival from 93 to 67% when compared with smaller lesions.

Tumor Thickness

If one considers the gross dimensions of the primary lesion to be of prognostic significance, it is a logical assumption that the microscopic depth of disease would also bear clinical import. Depth of invasion over 4 to 5 mm is considered a predictor of metastases in aggressive NMSC. A large prospective study of nearly 600 cutaneous SCC patients revealed an overall 4% rate of nodal metastases. Only 2.9% of patients with lesions less than 5 mm thick developed nodal metastases, compared to 17.5% of those with tumors more than 5 mm thick. This study boasted an extended follow-up period with a mean follow-up of 4 years.[57]

Recurrence

Nearly half of all cutaneous SCC patients with a positive margin on initial excision will develop a local recurrence.[64] Those with recurrent disease are particularly prone to develop nodal metastases. Grover et al[65] examined the risk of nodal metastasis in patients experiencing recurrent SCC of the lip. Their results indicated that 15% of those with recurrent lesions developed nodal disease, compared to 2% of those who were recurrence-free. A study of cutaneous SCC metastatic to cervical nodes identified 51% of patients developing nodal disease as individuals with recurrent local disease.[66]

Perineural Invasion (PNI)

PNI occurs in approximately 5% of patients with cutaneous SCC of the head and neck. The mechanism by which PNI occurs is direct invasion of tumor into the potential space surrounding individual nerve fibers (Fig 8–1). Although PNI generally is an incidental histopathologic finding, clinical symptoms may be present and include formication, pain, dysesthesia or anesthesia, diplopia, or facial paralysis. Goepfert et al[67] identified V_2 as the cranial nerve most commonly affected by PNI.

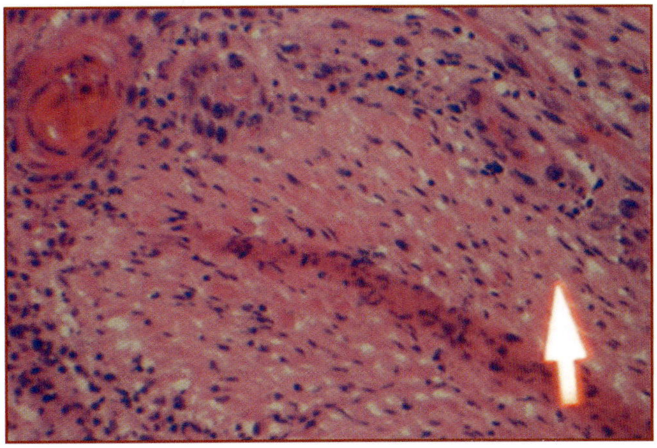

Figure 8–1. Photomicrograph of perineural invasion by cutaneous SCC.

PNI carries a significant association with nodal and distant metastases, overall, disease-specific, and relapse-free survival. A large study from MD Anderson Cancer Center showed statistically significant increases in both regional and distant metastases in patients with PNI when compared to those without.[68] Comparing patients with PNI over a 12-month period, Moore et al[69] identified an worsened overall survival (60% vs 80%), disease-specific survival (65% vs 95%) and relapse-free survival (65% vs 85%) in those with PNI compared to those without PNI.

Location

The site of the primary lesion, especially with respect to the central H-zone of the face and the periparotid skin, seems to influence the aggressiveness of cutaneous malignancies. The central H-zone of the face represents a site of particularly aggressive lesions. It is notable that aggressive BCC is of particular concern in this region. Skin cancers found at this site often present with nodal metastases and are prone to local recurrence.[70]

The anatomy of the central H-zone may offer some explanations for these findings. First, the central H-zone contains an abundance of nerves closely apposed to the skin that may be particularly vulnerable to early PNI. Second, there is a close apposition of deep structures to the skin surface, which may allow for early deep spread. Finally, the embryologic fusion planes of the midface are hypothesized to form distinct barriers to the superficial spread of cutaneous malignancies. Lesions within this region tend to spread to the deep tissues early, with invasion restricted to or between respective fusion planes. It is not until the lesion has established roots within the deep planes that superficial spread becomes apparent.[55]

Lesions located on the temporal and preauricular skin, which primarily drains to the parotid nodes, are associated with an increased risk of regional metastases. The potential for parotid metastases and catastrophic PNI of the facial nerve with progression to the skull base is obvious with lesions of this region. The significance of disease metastatic to the parotid was highlighted by O'Brien et al[71] in a 2002 prospective study. This study set forth the concept that the existing TNM staging system for cutaneous SCC was inadequate and should include a separate P stage representing the status of the parotid. P1 lesions are lesions metastatic to the parotid up to 3 cm, P2 are lesions between 3 and 6 cm, and P3 lesions are lesions larger than 6 cm or with facial nerve or skull base involvement. Patients with parotid metastases are more likely to develop a regional recurrence than those without intraparotid disease, and those with advanced (P2-P3) disease exhibit a diminished survival when compared to those with early (P1) disease.[71,72]

The impact of regional metastases in NMSC on prognosis was addressed in the 2010 American Joint Committee on Cancer (AJCC) staging update. This updated staging schema and the appropriate management of the parotid gland and its associated nodes are discussed later in this chapter.

Immunosuppression

Immunosuppression, particularly in the setting of organ transplantation, confers a significant degree of vulnerability to aggressive NMSC. Compared to the immunocompetent population, immunosuppressed patients are at 8 to 65 times increased risk for developing NMSC, with SCC predominating (rather than BCC). Although lesions appear 2 to 4 years after the beginning of immunosuppression, the risk of developing NMSC increases with each year of immunosuppression. Among immunosuppressed patients, the most virulent cutaneous malignancies have been described in cardiothoracic transplant recipients. In an Australian study, 26 of 629 cardiothoracic transplant patients developed aggressive NMSC, and 13 of these 26 succumbed to skin cancer. Ten of the 13 died of systemic disease.[52]

Immunosuppressed patients appear to experience greater mortality from smaller and less deeply invasive lesions than do immunocompetent patients. Martinez et al[73] identified a 3-year disease-specific survival of 56% among organ transplant recipients with metastatic cutaneous malignancies. The median lesion size was 12 mm and the median depth of invasion was 3.2 mm, substantially less than the size and depth standards for aggressive NMSC among immunocompetent patients.[73]

Although iatrogenic immunosuppression following organ transplantation is the classic setting for the development of aggressive NMSC, it is by no means the only immunocompromised state prone to cutaneous malignancy. Patients with AIDS and hematologic malignancies, specifically chronic lymphocytic leukemia, also are at a heightened risk for aggressive NMSC.[74] Unfortunately, in most cases, it is neither safe nor possible to reverse the state of immunosuppression. These patients must be managed and monitored with particular vigilance in order to eradicate existing disease and to diagnose recurrence at an early stage.

Management of Aggressive NMSC

Diagnosis and Staging

History and Physical Examination

As in all disease processes, comprehensive evaluation begins with a complete history and physical examination. In evaluating NMSC, the history should detail the progression of the lesion in question, specifically focusing on a change in the character or perception of a pre-existing cutaneous lesion. Personal history of cutaneous malignancy, sunburns, extensive exposure to ultraviolet light, history of immunosuppression, radiation exposure, or family history of cutaneous malignancy, particularly in the first 2 to 3 decades of life, should be noted. Patients with any of the above risk factors should undergo yearly cutaneous evaluation by both a head and neck surgeon and dermatologist. Early detection of cutaneous malignancies theoretically allows for less extensive treatments and improved functional and aesthetic outcomes.

Biopsy Techniques

Once a suspicious lesion has been identified and qualified by history and physical, a biopsy should be performed in order to obtain a histopathologic diagnosis. Although the clinical examination offers a reasonable estimation of the extent of spread in the superficial planes, the biopsy offers valuable information regarding the deep extent of the lesion. Punch/incisional or excisional biopsy are both acceptable methods for head and neck lesions. Specimens obtained via excisional biopsy should include 1- to 2-mm margins and should be marked to orient the pathologist and to facilitate further excision. Techniques such as shave biopsy and needle aspiration yield inadequate specimens because the depth of the lesion may not be assessed, and therefore do not have a place in the evaluation of cutaneous malignancy in the head and neck.[73]

Imaging

Nonmelanoma skin cancer (NMSC) mostly afflicts sun-exposed skin and can be easily seen, but identification of subtle invasive disease, nonpalpable lymphadenopathy, and early perineural spread can be challenging on initial clinical evaluation. Although computed tomography (CT) scan can identify the primary skin cancer site as a focus of increased soft tissue attenuation (Figs 8–2A and B), an ulceration (Fig 8–3A) or a polypoid mass (Fig 8–4A), small superficial dermal lesions (Fig 8–3B) potentially could be missed.

Nodal staging on initial imaging is performed by a CT neck scan with contrast. Abnormal appearance of lymph nodes is based on morphologic criteria such as enlargement, heterogeneous enhancement, necrosis, rounded contour and/or loss of fatty hilum. Imaging criteria for nodal enlargement of homogeneous-appearing lymph nodes vary based on whether one is using the maximal or minimal axial diameter. Maximal axial diameter of 1.5 cm for lymph nodes in level I and jugulodigastric level II constitutes the upper limits of normal; for the rest of the neck, the upper limit is 1 cm.[75] Studies utilizing the minimal axial diameter report 6 to 7 mm as being optimal.[76] Additional characterization of metastatic adenopathy, specifically macroscopic extracapsular

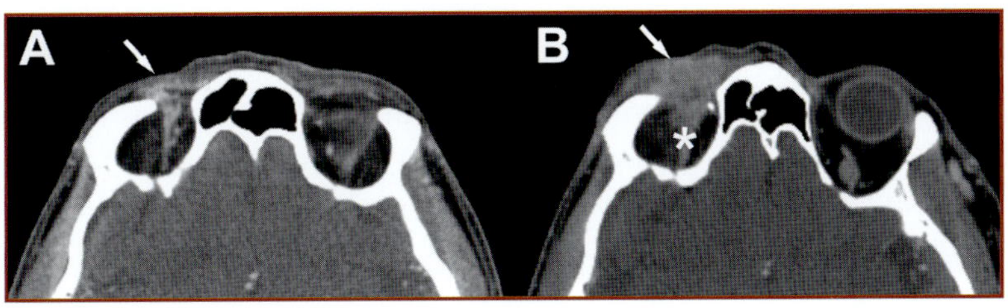

Figure 8–2. 79-year-old male with spindle cell carcinoma of the dermis. **A.** Initial postcontrast axial CT scan shows slight increased soft tissue density in the right supraorbital region, and **B.** follow-up scan at 2 months reveals an enhancing mass in the right supraorbital soft tissues with involvement of the supraorbital nerve (*asterisk in* ***B***).

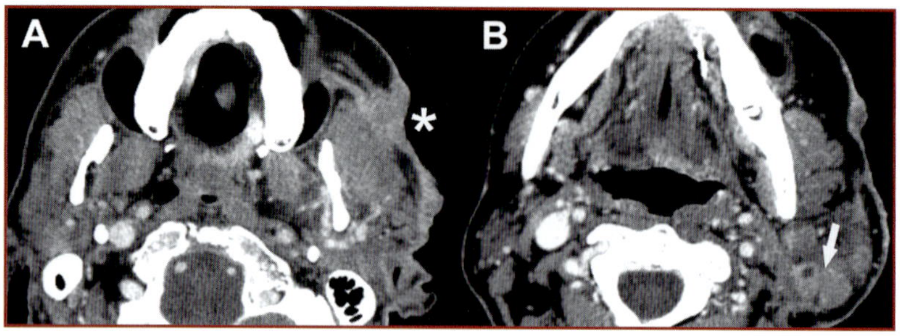

Figure 8–3. 84-year-old male with an ulcerated left cheek lesion. Axial postcontrast CT image demonstrates squamous cell carcinoma infiltrating into subdermal tissues including: **A.** left masseter muscle and **B.** heterogeneously enhancing metastatic lymph nodes.

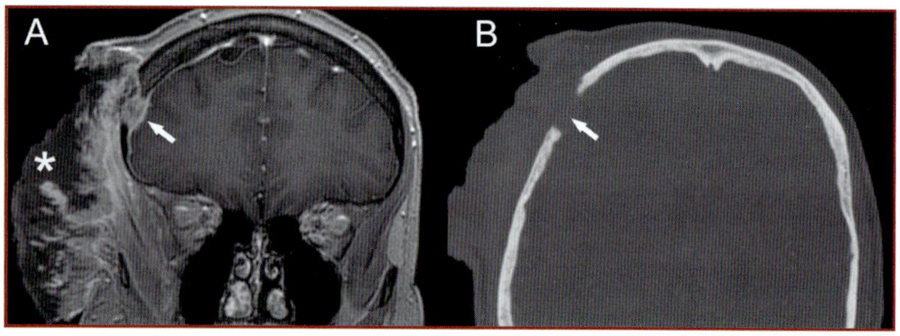

Figure 8–4. 63-year-old male with a large ulcerated, exophytic, right frontotemporal scalp squamous cell carcinoma. A heterogeneously enhancing mass is visualized on the coronal postcontrast T1-weighted MR image (*asterisk in* **A**) eroding through the calvarium (**B**), with an intracranial, epidural tumoral component (*arrow in **A***).

spread, number, and size also is important, because the presence of extracasupsular spread, multiple metastatic nodes, or nodes larger than 3 cm are linked to a worse prognosis.[77]

Acquisition of dedicated angled images through the oral cavity helps to decrease the streak artifact caused by dental amalgam, thereby aiding visualization of abnormal-appearing small parotid lymph nodes (Fig 8–5). Subdermal infiltration into the deeper tissues such as subcutaneous fat, fascia, salivary glands or muscle (see Fig 8–3A), erosion into the adjacent cartilage or bone (Figs 8-4B and 8–6B) are also evaluated on CT scans. Furthermore, complications of therapy such as abscess, soft tissue necrosis, fistulas, or osteoradionecrosis can be identified, and response to therapy of the primary and metastatic sites monitored on postcontrast CT scans.

Magnetic resonance imaging (MRI) also can detect abnormal skin lesions and metastatic lymph nodes. However, longer image acquisition time, degraded image quality due to inhomogeneous fat suppression, and artifacts (eg, motion, foreign body) can result in suboptimal evaluation. Metastatic nodes appear inhomogeneous on T2-weighted imaging, but are best visualized on fat suppressed, postcontrast T1-weighted images that reveal nodal necrosis.[75] Advances in MRI such as diffusion weighted imaging (DWI), and contrast imaging with ultra-small iron oxide particles may aid in improved characterization and detection of metastatic nodes on MRI.[78]

The present advantage of MRI lies primarily in detection and delineating extent of perineural spread (PNI), intraorbital and intracranial extension. Radiographic evidence of PNI frequently can

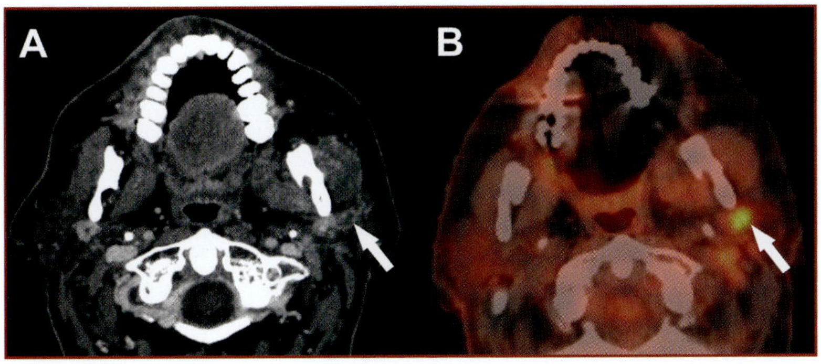

Figure 8–5. 59-year-old male with left preauricular skin cancer on axial postcontrast CT image identifying a rim-enhancing intraparotid lymph node, which also demonstrates increased uptake on FDG-PET imaging.

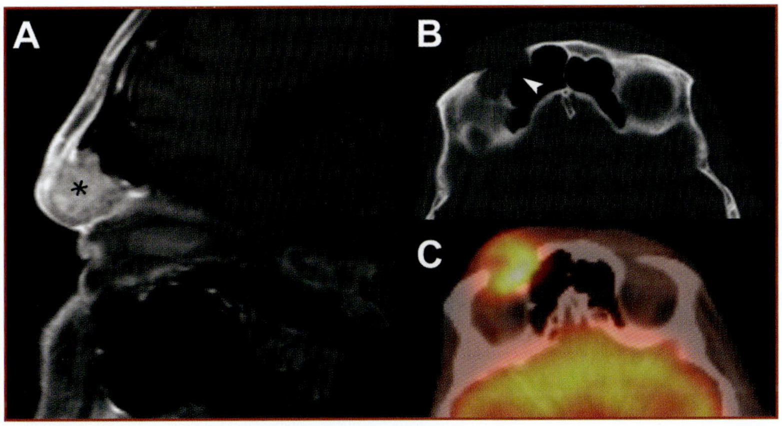

Figure 8–6. 64-year-old male presenting with squamous cell carcinoma of the right supraorbital skin (**A**), with subtle frontal bone erosion seen on axial CT image obtained with bone algorithm (**B**) and, increased FDG uptake on PET (**C**).

be appreciated earlier on an MRI than on a CT study.[79] PNI manifests as abnormal enhancement and thickening of the nerves (Fig 8–7A) or effacement and obliteration of fat planes surrounding the nerve. CT images obtained with bone algorithm demonstrate bone remodeling as widening of skull base foramina and expansion of the nerve canals (Fig 8–7B and 8–9). Patients with clinical signs and symptoms of PNI, but without corroborative findings on imaging, are reported to have a better prognosis following therapy than those with radiologic evidence.[80] Studies with semiquantitative grading of perineural disease on imaging have demonstrated that, although locoregional control was better achieved in patients with minimal to moderate peripheral disease, survival was the same as in patients with skull base involvement on initial pretreatment scans.[81]

Distant hematogenous metastases to lungs and bones in NMSC rarely are seen in aggressive basosquamous carcinoma or Merkel call carcinoma.[82,83] The impact of positron emission tomography (PET) on intended cancer management of NMSC during initial staging has been reported to be 10%, but its

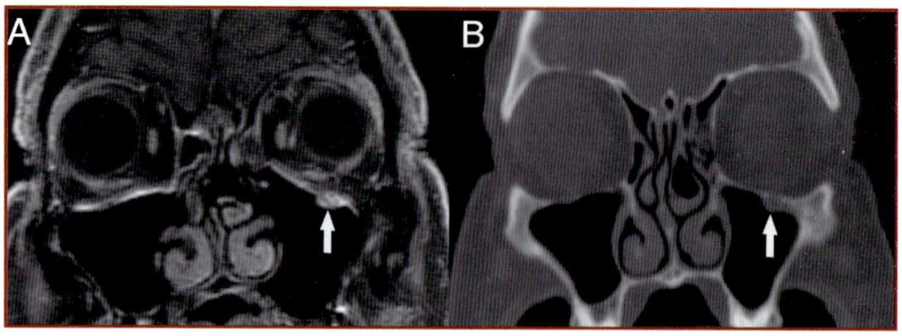

Figure 8–7. 75-year-old male with left cheek paresthesias exhibits (**A**) increased size and enhancement of the left infraorbital nerve on postcontrast, fat-supressed, T1-weighted coronal MRI; and (**B**) widening of the canal on the coronal CT with bone windows.

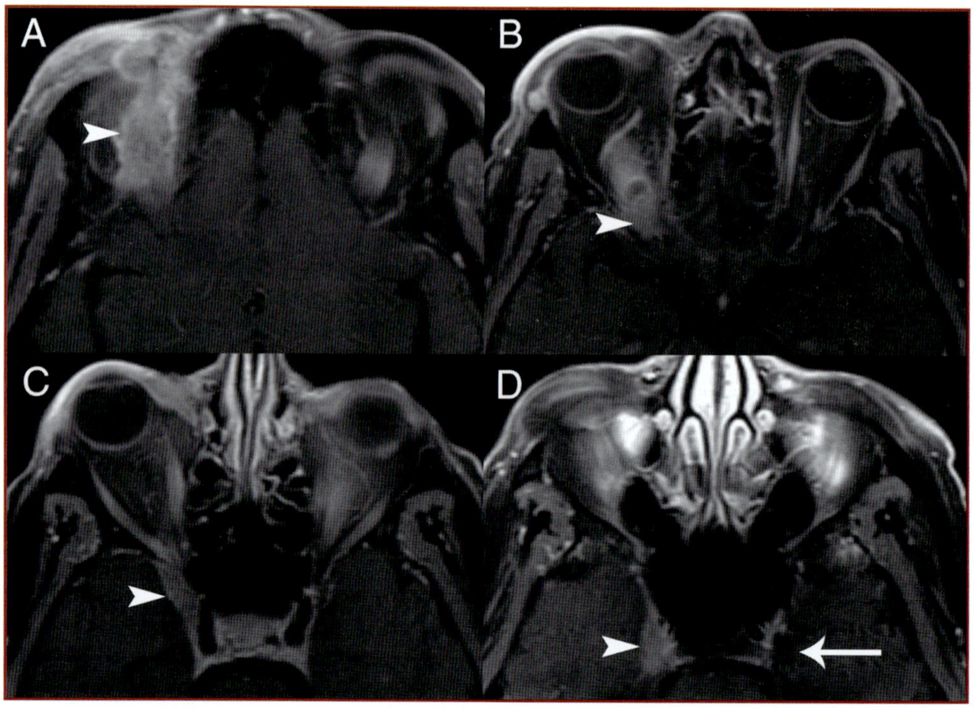

Figure 8–8. 66-year-old male with dull throbbing pain in the right forehead and eye with nontender fullness under the right eyebrow on examination. Postcontrast fat suppressed axial T1-weighted images demonstrate retrograde perineural tumor spread along the thickened enhancing right ophthalmic branch of the trigeminal nerve (*arrowhead in* **A**) extending up to the orbital apex (**B**), with asymmetric increased enhancement in the right cavernous sinus (**C**), and Meckel's cave (**D**); the contralateral Meckel's sinus reveals normal appearance (*arrowhead in* ***D***).

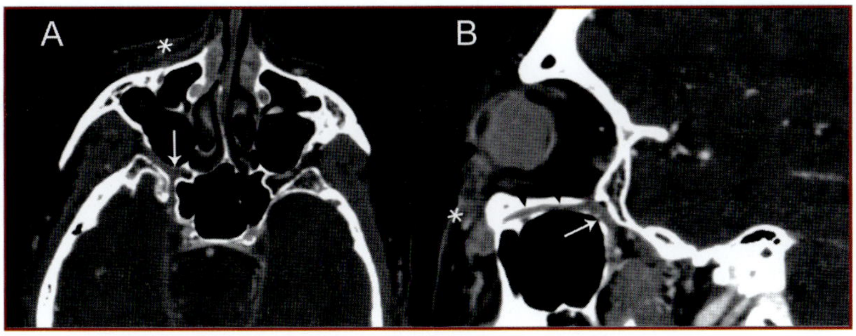

Figure 8–9. 65-year-old male presenting with a right malar erythematous lesion, and complaint of paresthesias in the mid-face. Axial postcontrast axial CT image (**A**) shows increased density in the right premaxillary region abutting the infraorbital nerve canal with loss of fat in the pterygopalatine fossa (*arrow in **A***) reflective of retrograde perineural tumor spread. Sagittal reconstruction (**B**) shows the infraorbital nerve canal along its length (*black arrowheads in **B***) with soft tissue density extending into the pterygopalatine fossa (*arrow in **B***).

application at the present time is limited.[84] The primary role of imaging in initial staging of NMSC lies in defining local and nodal disease extent, detecting clinically asymptomatic PNI, and determining PNI tumor volume. These goals are best achieved by MRI and CT scan of head and neck with contrast.

Staging

The AJCCC tumor, node, metastases (TNM) staging system serves as the universal language of cancer staging and fills a crucial role in treatment planning. The current staging system for NMSC is outlined in Table 8–2. This staging system focuses on the apparent dimensions of the primary lesion, its involvement with adjacent noncutaneous tissues, the status of the regional lymph nodes, and the presence or absence of distant metastases. Multiple shortcomings of the prior classification system were addressed in the 2010 staging system. The TNM staging system for cutaneous malignancies applies to NMSC arising from skin anywhere on the body, not only the head and neck.[85]

Although the TNM staging system serves as the basic rubric by which clinical decisions are made, it is an imperfect guide. However, recent amendments to the staging system have served to highlight important histopathologic findings and increased the focus on the status of the regional lymphatics. Due to significant contributions by multiple investigators, the current staging system the primary tumors of the skin takes into account depth of invasion, PNI, anatomic location, and degree of histologic differentiation.[86,87]

The description of cervical nodal disease has also been amended in the most recent staging system. In no small part due to the work of O'Brien and other investigators, the all-or-nothing N0 versus N1 characterization of the regional lymphatics has been replaced by the traditional N1-N3 system utilized in staging mucosal carcinomas of the upper aerodigestive tract. This new staging system offers a comprehensive description of these tumors by including, if not explicitly, the status of the parotid nodes in the evaluation of the regional lymphatics. Beyond the previous N0 versus N1 system, this new schema accounts for the possibility of the presence of multiple involved nodes of different sizes and adjusts the prognosis and stage of disease based on their presence.[71,72]

Table 8–2. 2010 AJCC Staging TNM Classification for Cutaneous Squamous and Basal Cell Carcinoma (excludes eyelid skin)

Primary Tumor (T)	Regional Lymph Nodes (N)
TX Primary tumor cannot be assessed	NX Regional lymph nodes cannot be assessed
T0 No evidence of primary tumor	N0 No regional lymph node metastases
Tis Carcinoma in situ	N1 Metastasis in a single ipsilateral lymph node, 3 cm or less in greatest dimension
T1 Tumor 2 cm in greatest dimension with less than two high-risk features*	N2a Metastasis in a single ipsilateral lymph node more than 3 cm but not more than 6 cm in greatest dimension
T2 Tumor greater than 2 cm in greatest dimension or tumor any size with two or more high-risk features	N2b Metastasis in multiple ipsilateral lymph nodes, none more than 6 cm in greatest dimension
T3 Tumor with invasion of maxilla, mandible, orbit, or temporal bone	N2c Metastasis in bilateral or contralateral lymph nodes, none more than 6 cm in greatest dimension
T4 Tumor with invasion of skeleton (axial or appendicular) or perineural invasion of the skull base	N3 Metastasis in a lymph node, more than 6 cm in greatest dimension

*High-risk features

Depth/invasion	>2 mm thickness
	Clark level IV or greater
	Perineural invasion
Anatomic Site	Primary site ear or nonhair-bearing lip
Differentiation	Poorly differentiated or undifferentiated

Distant Metastasis (M)	Staging			
M0 No distant metastases	Stage 0	Tis N0 M0	Stage IV	T1 N2 M0
M1 Distant metastases	Stage I	T1 N0 M0		T2 N2 M0
	Stage II	T2 N0 M0		T3 N2 M0
	Stage III	T3 N0 M0		T Any N3 M0
		T1 N1 M0		T4 N Any M0
		T2 N1 M0		T Any N Any M1
		T3 N1 M0		

Source: Used with the permission of the American Joint Committee on Cancer (AJCC), Chicago, Illinois. The original source for this material is the AJCC Cancer Staging Manual, Seventh Edition (2010) published by Springer Science and Business Media LLC, www.springer.com.

Treatment of Aggressive Nonmelanoma Skin Cancer

Treatment of the Primary Lesion

Although a number of different therapeutic modalities are utilized in the treatment of nonaggressive NMSC, the cornerstone of treatment for primary NMSC lesions is wide excision with appropriately sized margins. However, it is important to remember that the distinction between indolent and aggressive lesions often is nebulous, and standard dermatologic treatments, such as cryotherapy, topical therapy, and electrodessication and curettage, may be employed as a first-line therapy for undiagnosed aggressive NMSC. Furthermore, many patients will present to the multidisciplinary cutaneous malignancy team after undergoing one of these prior therapies, or with overt recurrence. Wide excision generally allows for an onocologically sound operation without compromising future reconstructive efforts. Although the primary objective of any operation to treat malignancy is the complete extirpation of tumor, the primacy of the head and neck as an aesthetic and functional center should always be kept in mind. To maximally preserve function and cosmesis, the smallest margin that does not compromise cure should be excised with the primary lesion. However, tissue sparing techniques and reconstructive considerations should never drive resection margins in aggressive cutaneous malignancy.

Surgical Margins

No consensus statement regarding the appropriate size of surgical margins in excision of aggressive NMSC exists. However, one should always remember that appropriate surgical margins for a lesion are those that, on histopathologic analysis, are free of disease. To ensure tumor extirpation, frozen section control with meticulous mapping of surgical margins should be used liberally.

With the emphasis on the use of frozen section control, it would seem that Mohs micrographic surgery represents an ideal treatment modality for NMSC. In lesions confined to the skin, Mohs surgery constitutes an outstanding treatment modality. Due to the presence of underlying neurovascular and musculoskeletal structures and because of the limited application of Mohs techniques in these tissues, Mohs surgery is not indicated in the treatment of NMSC that extends into the subcutaneous tissue. In these circumstances, Mohs techniques should be combined with traditional ablative techniques. Regardless of the therapeutic modality that ultimately is chosen, it is incumbent on any participating Mohs surgeon to detect the histopathologic features of aggressive NMSC so that the appropriate treatment may be rendered in concert with a multidisciplinary cutaneous oncology team.

Traditional recommendations for margin size have been quite variable for both BCC and SCC. BCC less than 2 cm in size requires a margin of at least 4 mm. Such margins in lesions less than 2 cm in greatest dimension have been shown to yield a 98% cure rate. Larger lesions, micronodular and infiltrative BCC, and SCC require larger margins. BCC lesions larger than 2 cm in greatest dimension, however, exhibit unpredictable subclinical spread.[88] This finding underscores the fact that negative margins are best ensured by frozen section evaluation at the time of the initial excision.

A recent prospective study examined patients with NMSC and sought to define the average distance of peripheral tumor spread and, consequently, ideal margin size. After analysis of 71 patients, the average microscopic tumor extent was determined to be 5.2 mm. This value was noted to be substantially greater in those with aggressive BCC and SCC larger than 2 cm in size. Ultimately, this study suggested a 95% chance of obtaining cure with a margin of 1 cm beyond the grossly visible lesion.[89]

Treatment of Regional Lymphatics

The N0 Neck

In "standard" cases of NMSC of the head and neck, the concern for metastases to the cervical lymphatics is quite low. In cases of aggressive NMSC, though, one must always be mindful of the potential development of regional disease. Multiple risk factors for regional metastases in NMSC exist and are enumerated in Table 8–1.

The management of the clinically negative neck in cases of NMSC remains a topic of considerable controversy. Generally, the incidence of nodal metastases in patients with cutaneous SCC is less than 5%. In certain instances of NMSC, though, the incidence of nodal disease may exceed 10 to 15%.[90–92] The characteristics classically associated with NMSC, such as large size, increased thickness, or depth of invasion, are suggestive of an increased risk of subclinical nodal disease. No single factor, however, is considered a strong enough predictor upon which a recommendation can be based. Several options exist for the management of the clinically negative neck in patients with aggressive NMSC.

Watchful Waiting. Historically, expectant management of the parotid and cervical lymphatics has been the standard of care for the clinically negative neck in NMSC. Analogous data from mucosal head and neck sites suggest that patients with high-risk lesions tend to develop nodal disease in spite of close follow-up.[93,94]

Elective Neck Dissection. There are advocates of elective neck dissection in patients with high-risk lesions. Because there is unexpected lymphatic drainage in nearly 30% of cases, preoperative lymphoscintigraphy may be of benefit in planning which nodal basins to incorporate in the elective neck dissection. Anatomic variations aside, lesions located on the face and scalp anterior to a line extending cephalad through the external auditory canal are best served with a superficial parotidectomy and dissection of levels II through IV.[95] Those with lesions posterior to this line should undergo a posterolateral neck dissection with removal of levels II through V along with the postauricular and occipital nodes. Finally, patients with lesions of the lips or midface are best served with, at least, a unilateral supraomohyoid neck dissection. In those with midface lesions, bilateral neck dissection should be considered.

The classic teaching regarding elective neck dissection for mucosal SCC advocates for elective neck dissection when the risk of occult malignancy exceeds 20%.[96,97] Although effective in the treatment of the regional lymphatics in mucosal SCC, elective neck dissection falls short in several aspects when applied to aggressive cutaneous malignancies. First, the cutaneous malignancies generally represent a significantly less aggressive spectrum of neoplasms when compared to mucosal SCC. Second, standard neck dissection techniques do not address the perifacial and parotid nodes that represent the first echelon of lymphatic drainage for much of the skin of the head and neck.[70,98] Considering that few prospective data exist to support the routine use of elective neck dissection in aggressive NMSC and that simple extrapolation of its use in high-risk mucosal SCC to the arena of aggressive NMSC is flawed, one must rely on clinical judgment to guide the management of the negative neck in patients with aggressive NMSC. Elective neck dissection should be given consideration in those with histologically aggressive lesions, in those in whom the primary lesion invades the neck or parotid, and in lesions that have failed primary radiation therapy and display aggressive features.

Sentinel Lymph Node Biopsy. Sentinel lymph node biopsy has long been regarded as a useful investigation in the evaluation of regional nodal basins in both malignant melanoma and breast carcinoma. The success of these applications has created enthusiasm for the potential use of sentinel lymph node biopsy in cases of aggressive NMSC. A paucity of data on the topic has historically prevented sentinel lymph node biopsy from emerging as the standard of care in NMSC patients with a clinically aggressive primary lesion and negative neck. However, some recent data reveal sentinel lymph node biopsy in the setting of NMSC to have a high negative predictive value. These studies are limited by small sample size and short mean follow-up times.[99–101] In spite of these promising findings, sentinel lymph node biopsy remains an option only in select cases managed by those experienced with the technique.

The N+ Neck

Patients presenting with NMSC metastatic to the cervical or parotid lymphatics are considered to be at heightened risk for a poor outcome. It has been shown that up to 80% of NMSC develop nodal metastases within 9 months following treatment of the primary lesion.[102] Both the parotid and cervical nodes represent the first echelon of lymphatic drainage of the skin of the face and scalp. Fortunately, it is a rare occurrence for patients to present with both nodal and distant metastases.[90]

NMSC metastatic to the parotid is not an uncommon scenario. In a retrospective study, Lai et al[54] presented indications for parotidectomy in the context of metastatic NMSC. Superficial parotidectomy alone is indicated in cases of parotid nodal disease or parotid capsular invasion with an intact facial nerve. There is no evidence to suggest that a total parotidectomy, when followed by adjuvant radiation therapy improves locoregional control when compared to a superficial parotidectomy with facial nerve dissection. In fact, recently published evidence suggests that a superficial parotidectomy with adjuvant radiotherapy may be adequate therapy in cases of cutaneous SCC metastatic to the parotid with microscopic residual disease involving the facial nerve and normal facial function.[103]

Weakness of the facial nerve or temporal bone invasion requires a radical parotidectomy with sacrifice of the involved branches of the nerve, potentially an appropriate reanimation procedure and, likely a lateral temporal bone resection.[54] Although a variant of temporal bone resection can be performed to follow perineural invasion in the facial nerve, there is no indication to proceed beyond the geniculate ganglion, or beyond the skull base foramina, for PNI. The prognosis for these patients is generally poor, and radiation therapy is often a reasonable option. Please see Chapter 12 for additional information on this topic.

One also should be mindful that a cervical lymphadenectomy, at least of the upper neck, should accompany a parotidectomy in patients with clinically negative necks due to the high risk of occult metastases to the upper cervical nodes.[104] NMSC patients with clinically operable nodal metastases should undergo a comprehensive neck dissection. The extent of neck dissection and the preservation or sacrifice of neurovascular structures should be tailored to the individual patient based on the location of the primary and the predicted lymphatic drainage patterns.[95] Unless adjuvant radiation is not possible, both patients with parotid metastases and a clinically negative neck and those with obvious cervical nodal disease should undergo postoperative radiotherapy.[71,72,98,103,105–111]

Considering the gestalt of regionally metastatic head and neck NMSC, Oddone and colleagues[112] set out to establish a prognostic scoring model for this group of patients. Immune status, treatment rendered to the primary lesion and regional lymphatics in the form of surgery or surgery with adjuvant radiotherapy, the presence of extranodal spread, and the status of the surgical margins were included as components of this scoring system. These four variables were used to calculate the so-called ITEM score, a quantitative measure of disease severity, for a cohort of 250 patients with regionally metastatic head and neck NMSC. This cohort was divided into low-, moderate-, and high-risk groups based on the ITEM score, with the highest risk group exhibiting a 56% risk of dying at 5-years after treatment compared to 24 and 6% risk, respectively, for the moderate and low-risk groups.

The ultimate conclusion of the ITEM score study is that those patients with regionally metastatic NMSC of the head and neck are best served with surgery followed by radiation therapy. Those exhibiting extranodal spread or positive surgical margins tend to experience poor outcomes and should be considered for enrollment in adjuvant chemoradiotherapy trials.[112] The evidence supporting the utilization of adjuvant therapies for NMSC is discussed next.

Adjuvant Therapies in NMSC

Radiation

Although primary radiation therapy does play a role in the treatment of low-risk NMSC, its role in the management of aggressive NMSC usually is limited to the adjuvant setting. Indications for adjuvant radiotherapy in the management of aggressive NMSC include the following: large (>4 cm) or recurrent tumors, aggressive histology of the primary lesion, and perineural invasion. The classic triad indicating radiation includes close or positive margins, multiple positive nodes, and extracapsular spread.

In cases of PNI, adjuvant radiotherapy has demonstrated benefit in improving local control, disease-specific survival and overall survival. Generally, asymptomatic patients with only pathologic evidence of PNI enjoy a better prognosis than those with clinical or radiographic evidence of PNI. These differences in oncologic outcome are attributed to the more advanced state of disease associated with clinical or radiographic manifestations of PNI compared to the incidental finding of PNI on histopathologic examination of a biopsy or surgical specimen from an asymptomatic patient.[113] A recent study from Australia corroborated this difference and suggested a high rate of local control when adjuvant radiotherapy was applied in cases of NMSC with PNI. Those with pathologic evidence of PNI exhibited 90% local control at 5 years whereas the local control rate for those with clinical or radiographic evidence of PNI was 57%. Interestingly, this study demonstrated significantly better local control in cases of BCC with PNI compared with SCC exhibiting PNI.[114] Although not performed in the above study, there is evidence to suggest that elective irradiation of the neck in those exhibiting PNI may serve to improve local control.[115–118]

The true bulk of radiation therapy is applied to cases in which surgical margins are grossly or microscopically positive, there is obvious metastatic disease in multiple regional nodes, or there is histopathologic evidence of extracapsular spread. In patients with nodal disease, data from multiple studies suggest that locoregional control is improved in those undergoing surgery followed by radiation when compared with those only undergoing surgery.[71,72,98,105–111] The work of Bron et al[111] underscored the vital role of adjuvant radiotherapy, suggesting that adjuvant radiation is the only factor that decreased locoregional recurrence in patients with parotid or neck metastases.

Cases in which parotid metastases are present but the remainder of the neck is clinically negative pose a unique clinical question. The current treatment recommendation is that these patients receive adjuvant radiotherapy to the entire ipsilateral neck in order to account for the high risk of subclinical disease.[98,105,119] There is no need to include the contralateral neck in the radiation field as the risk of contralateral subclinical disease is exceptionally low.

Chemotherapy

Combined chemotherapy/radiation therapy has been established as a useful tool in armamentarium of the clinician treating head and neck SCC of mucosal origin. Much like these patients with primary upper aerodigestive tract lesions, those with NMSC metastatic to the regional lymphatics may benefit from combined chemotherapy/radiation. NMSC patients with positive surgical margins, multiple positive nodes, or extracapsular spread should be considered candidates for adjuvant multimodality therapy. Two recent trials comparing upper aerodigestive tract squamous cell carcinoma patients treated with adjuvant chemotherapy/radiation versus radiation alone revealed a significant improvement in locoregional control, disease-free, progression-free, and overall survival in those treated with multimodality therapy.[120,121]

The future of systemic therapy for metastatic aggressive NMSC lies in biochemotherapy and targeted molecular therapy. Promising data regarding the use of combined interferon-α, cisplatin, and retinoic acid in NMSC patients with advanced locoregional and metastatic disease have been published.[122,123] A recent analysis of the topical application of the DNA repair enzyme OGG1 to SCC and BCC lesions in a mouse model revealed significant decreases in both tumor size and progression of SCC lesions.[124] A trial currently underway at The University of Texas MD Anderson Cancer Center is examining the role of ZD1839, an orally administered inhibitor of the intracellular tyrosine kinase domain of the epidermal growth factor receptor (EGFR), in combination with radiation therapy, and early reports have been favorable.[125] Isolated reports of cetuximab as a primary therapy for cutaneous SCC also exist in the head and neck literature.[126]

Prevention

Significant public health campaigns seeking to increase skin-protective behaviors have been executed in recent years. In spite of efforts promoting the use of sunscreen, avoiding the sun during the midday hours, and wearing protective clothing, the incidence of skin cancer continues to rise. Some evidence does exist that sunscreen, particularly older formulations that are limited in their protection against UVA, does not prevent skin cancer.[127] Although current preventive initiatives apparently are failing to decrease the incidence of cutaneous malignancy, additional time is necessary for longitudinal studies to determine if skin-protective behaviors initiated in childhood will serve to curtail the American skin cancer epidemic.

Interest in chemoprevention of NMSC using cyclooxygenase (COX) inhibitors, retinoids, and dietary modifications has increased recently.[128] Preliminary data regarding these chemopreventive strategies are promising, but further investigation is certainly required.

Conclusions

Although NMSC represents a common and generally well-tolerated malignancy, not all NMSC is created equal. Aggressive NMSC presents a therapeutic challenge with its propensity for local recurrence, regional spread, and distant metastases. The head and neck surgeon must be intimately familiar with the clinical and pathologic characteristics of aggressive NMSC and apply this knowledge in selecting an evidence-based therapeutic plan.

The cornerstone of treatment for aggressive NMSC remains surgical resection of the primary lesion with appropriately sized margins with either neck dissection or radiotherapy directed toward the regional lymphatics. The N0 neck presents a unique challenge in clinical decision making with little evidence to support the routine use of elective neck dissection or sentinel lymph node biopsy. In addressing the N+ neck, one must give careful consideration to the location of the primary tumor and include the predicted first echelon of drainage, namely, the perifacial, parotid, and/or external jugular nodes, in the lymphadenectomy specimen.

Currently adjuvant therapy in the form of radiotherapy with or without chemotherapy should be given consideration in those exhibiting perineural invasion, multiple positive nodes, or extracapsular spread. Although reports of cetuximab as a primary therapy for unresectable NMSC do exist, the horizons of biologic and targeted therapy are discussed in subsequent chapters.

References

1. Santimyire BR, Feldman SR, Fleischer AB Jr. Lifestyle high-risk behaviors and demographics may predict the level of participation in sun-protection behaviors and skin cancer primary prevention in the United States: results of the 1998 National Health Interview Survey. *Cancer.* 2001;92:1315–1324.
2. Alam M, Ratner D. Primary care: cutaneous squamous cell carcinoma. *N Engl J Med.* 2001;344:975–983.
3. Chen JG, Fleischer AB Jr, Smith ED, et al. Cost of non-melanoma skin cancer treatment in the United States. *Dermatol Surg.* 2001;27:1035–1038.
4. Christenson LJ, Borrowman TA, Vachon CM, et al. Incidence of basal cell and squamous cell carcinomas in a population younger than 40 years. *JAMA.* 2005;294: 681–690.
5. Leffell DJ, Headington JT, Wong DS, Swanson NA. Aggressive-growth basal cell carcinoma in young adults. *Arch Dermatol.* 1991;127:1663–1667.
6. Melnikova VO, Ananthaswamy HN. Cellular and molecular events leading to the development of skin cancer. *Mutat Res.* 2005;571:91–106.
7. Tilli CMLJ, Van Steese IMAM, Krekels GAM, et al. Molecular aetiology and pathogenesis of basal cell carcinoma. *Br J Dermatol.* 2005;152:108–112.
8. Tsao H. Update on familial cancer syndromes and the skin. *J Am Acad Dermatol.* 2000;42:939–969.
9. Bootsma D, Kraemer KH, Cleaver JE, et al. Nucleotide excision repair syndromes: xeroderma pigmentosum, Cockayne syndrome, and trichothiodystrophy. In: Vogelstein BV, Kinzler K, eds. *The Genetic Basis of Human Cancer.* New York, NY: McGraw-Hill; 1998: 245–274.
10. Williams C, Ponten F, Ahmadian A, et al. Clones of normal keratinocytes and a variety of simultaneously present epidermal neoplastic lesions contain a multitude of p53 gene mutations in a xeroderma pigmentosum patient. *Cancer Res.* 1998;58:2449–2455.
11. Giglia G, Dumaz N, Drougard C, et al. p53 mutations in skin and internal tumors of xeroderma pigmentosum patients belonging to the complementation group C. *Cancer Res.* 1998;58:4402–4409.
12. Daya-Grosjean L, Robert C, Drougard C, et al. High mutation frequency in ras genes of skin tumors isolated from DNA repair deficient xeroderma pigmentosum patients. *Cancer Res.* 1993;53:1625–1629.
13. Wicking C, Berkman J, Wainwright B, et al. Fine genetic mapping of the gene for nevoid basal cell carcinoma syndrome. *Genomics.* 1994;22:505–511.
14. Gailani MR, Bale SJ, Leffell DJ, et al. Developmental defects in Gorlin syndrome related to a putative tumor suppressor gene on chromosome 9. *Cell.* 1992;69:111–117.
15. Farndon PA, Del Maestro RG, Evans DG, et al. Location of gene for Gorlin syndrome. *Lancet.* 1992;339:581–582.
16. Reis A, Kuster W, Linss G, et al. Localisation of a gene for the naevoid basal cell carcinoma syndrome. *Lancet.* 1992;339:617.
17. Goldstein AM, Stewart C, Bale AE, et al. Localization of the gene for the nevoid basal cell carcinoma syndrome. *Am J Hum Genet.* 1994;54:765–773.
18. Johnson RL, Rothman AL, Xie J, et al. Human homolog of patched, a candidate gene for the basal cell nevus syndrome. *Science.* 1996;272:1668–1671.
19. Hahn W, Wicking C, Zahiropoulous PG, et al. Mutations of the human homolog of Drosophila patched in the nevoid basal cell carcinoma syndrome. *Cell.* 1996; 85:841–851.
20. Aszterbaum M, Rothman A, Johnson RL, et al. Identification of mutations in the human PATCHED gene in sporadic basal cell carcinomas and in patients with the basal cell nevus syndrome. *J Invest Dermatol.* 1998;110:885–888.
21. Wicking C, Shanley S, Smyth I, et al. Most germ-line mutations in the nevoid basal cell carcinoma syndrome lead to a premature termination of the PATCHED protein, and no genotype-phenotype correlations are evident. *Am J Hum Genet.* 1997;60:21–26.
22. Stone DM, Hynes M, Armanini M, et al. The tumour-suppressor gene patched encodes a candidate receptor for Sonic hedgehog. *Nature.* 1996;384:129–134.

23. Xie J, Johnson RL, Zhang X, et al. Mutations of the PATCHED gene in several types of sporadic extracutaneous tumors. *Cancer Res.* 1997;57:2369–2372.
24. Raffel C, Jenkins RB, Frederick L, et al. Sporadic medulloblastomas contain PTCH mutations. *Cancer Res.* 1997; 57:842–845.
25. Xie J, Murone M, Luoh SM, et al. Activating smoothened mutations in sporadic basal-cell carcinoma. *Nature.* 1998; 391:129–134.
26. Reifenberger J, Wolter M, Weber RG, et al. Missense mutations in SMOH in sporadic basal cell carcinomas of the skin and primitive neuroectodermal tumors of the central nervous system. *Cancer Res.* 1998;58:1798–1803.
27. Perry PK and Silverberg NB. Cutaneous malignancy in albinism. *Cutis.* 2001;67:427–430.
28. Ray K, Chaki M, Sengupta M. Tyrosinase and ocular diseases: some novel thoughts on the molecular basis of oculocutaneous albinism type 1. *Prog Retin Eye Res.* 2007;26(4):323–358.
29. Rooryck C, Morice-Picard F, Elcioglu NH, Lacombe D, Taieb A, Arveiler B. Molecular diagnosis of oculocutaneous albinism: new mutations in the OCA1-4 genes and practical aspects. *Pigment Cell Melanoma Res.* 2008; 21(5):583–587.
30. Zuhlke C, Criee C, Gemoll T, Schillinger T, Kaesmann-Kellner B. Polymorphisms in the genes for oculocutaneous albinism type 1 and type 4 in the German population. *Pigment Cell Res.* 2007;20(3):225–227.
31. Cohen PR, Kohn SR, Kurzrock R. Association of sebaceous gland tumors and internal malignancy: the Muir-Torre syndrome. *Am J Med.* 1991;90:606–613.
32. Vasen HF, Mecklin JP, Khan PM, et al. The International Collaborative Group on Hereditary Non-Polyposis Colorectal Cancer (ICG-HNPCC). *Dis Colon Rectum.* 1991; 34:424–425.
33. Rodriguez-Bigas MA, Boland CR, Hamilton SR, et al. A National Cancer Institute Workshop on Hereditary Nonpolyposis Colorectal Cancer Syndrome: meeting highlights and Bethesda guidelines. *J Nat Cancer Inst.* 1997;89:1758–1762.
34. Peltomaki P, Aaltonen LA, Sistonen P, et al. Genetic mapping of a locus predisposing to human colorectal cancer. *Science.* 1993;260:810–812.
35. Fishel R, Lescoe MK, Rao MR, et al. The human mutator gene homolog MSH2 and its association with hereditary nonpolyposis colon cancer. *Cell.* 1993;75:1027–1038.
36. Leach FS, Nicolaides NC, Papadopoulos N, et al. Mutations of a mutS homolog in hereditary nonpolyposis colorectal cancer. *Cell.* 1993;75:1215–1225.
37. Strand M, Prolla TA, Liskay RM, et al. Destabilization of tracts of simple repetitive DNA in yeast by mutations affecting DNA mismatch repair. *Nature.* 1993;365: 274–276.
38. Honchel R, Halling KC, Schaid DJ, et al. Microsatellite instability in Muir-Torre syndrome. *Cancer Res.* 1994;54: 1159–1163.
39. Halling KC, Honchel R, Pittelkow MR, et al. Microsatellite instability in keratoacanthoma. *Cancer.* 1995;76: 1765–1771.
40. Peris K, Onorati MT, Keller G, et al. Widespread microsatellite instability in sebaceous tumors of patients with the Muir-Torre syndrome. *Br J Dermatol.* 1997;137: 356–360.
41. Marci II, Stern RS. Risk of developing a subsequent nonmelanoma skin cancer in patients with a history of nonmelanoma skin cancer: a critical review of the literature and meta-analysis. *Arch Dermatol.* 2000;136: 1524–1530.
42. Lewaandowsky F, Lutz W. Ein Fall einer bischer nicht beschriebenen Hauterkrankung (Epidermodysplasia verruciformis). *Arch Dermatol.* 1922;14:193–203.
43. Majewski S, Jablonska S, Orth G. Epidermodysplasia verruciformis. Immunological and nonimmunological surveillance mechanisms: role in tumor progression. *Clin Dermatol.* 1997;15:321–334.
44. Pass F, Reissig M, Shah KV, et al. Identification of an immunologically distinct papillomavirus from lesions of epidermodysplasia verruciformis. *J Natl Cancer Inst.* 1977;59:1107–1112.
45. Orth G. Genetics of epidermodysplasia verruciformis: insights into host defense against papillomaviruses. *Semin Immunol.* 2006;18:362–374.
46. de Villiers EM, Fauquet C, Broker TR, et al. Classification of papillomaviruses. *Virology.* 2004;324:17–27.
47. Karagas MR, Nelson HH, Sehr P, et al. Human papillomavirus infection and incidence of squamous cell and basal cell carcinomas of the skin. *J Natl Cancer Inst.* 2006;98:389–395.
48. Harwood CA, Proby CM. Human papillomavirus and nonmelanoma skin cancer. *Curr Opin Infect Dis.* 2002;15: 101–114.
49. Pfistr H. Human papillomavirus and skin cancer. *J Natl Cancer Inst Monogr.* 2003;31:52–56.
50. Asgari MM, Kiviat NB, Critchlow CW, et al. Detection of human papillomavirus DNA in cutaneous squamous cell carcinoma among immunocompetent individuals. *J Invest Dermatol.* 2008;128:1409–1417.
51. Perkins JL, Liu Y, Mitby PA, et al. Nonmelanoma skin cancer in survivors of childhood and adolescent cancer: a report from the cancer survivor study. *J Clin Oncol.* 2005;23:3733–3741.
52. Veness MJ, Quinn DI, Ong CS, et al. Aggressive cutaneous malignancies following cardiothoracic transplantation: the Australian experience. *Cancer.* 1999;85:1758–1764.
53. Wong CSM, Strange RC, Lear JT. Basal cell carcinoma. *Br Med J.* 2003;327:794–798.
54. Lai SY, Weinstein GS, Chalian AA, et al. Parotidectomy in the treatment of aggressive cutaneous malignancies. *Arch Otolaryngol Head Neck Surg.* 2002;128:521–526.
55. Panje WR, Ceilley RI. The influence of the midface on the spread of epithelial malignancies. *Laryngoscope.* 1979;89:1914–1920.

56. Rudolph R, Zelac DE. Squamous cell carcinoma of the skin. *Plast Reconstr Surg*. 2004;114:82e–94e.
57. Breuninger H, Schaumberg-Lever G, Holzschuh J, Horny H-P. Desmoplastic squamous cell carcinoma of the skin and vermillion surface. *Cancer*. 1997;79:915–919.
58. Martin RCG II, Edwards MJ, Cawte TG, et al. Basosquamous carcinoma: analysis of prognostic factors influencing recurrence. *Cancer*. 2000;88:1365–1369.
59. Vico P, Fourez, Nemec E, et al. Aggressive basal cell carcinoma of the head and neck areas. *Eur J Surg Oncol*. 1995;21(5):490–497.
60. Rowe DE, Carroll RJ, Day CL Jr. Prognostic factors for local recurrence, metastasis, and survival rates in squamous cell carcinoma of the skin, ear, and lip. *J Am Acad Dermatol*. 1992;26(6):976–990.
61. Veness MJ, Palme CE, Morgan GJ. High-risk cutaneous squamous cell carcinoma of the head and neck: results from 266 treated patients with metastatic lymph node disease. *Cancer*. 2006;106:2389–2396.
62. Veness MJ. High-risk cutaneous squamous cell carcinoma of the head and neck. *J Biomed Biotechnol*. 2007; 2007(3):80572.
63. Clayman GL, Lee JJ, Holsinger FC, et al. Mortality risk from squamous cell skin cancer. *J Clin Oncol*. 2005;23: 759–765
64. Huang CC, Boyce SM. Surgical margins of excision for basal cell carcinoma and squamous cell carcinoma. *Sem Cut Med Surg*. 2004;23:167–173.
65. Grover R, Douglas RG, Shaw JHF. Carcinoma of the lip in Auckland, New Zealand, 1969–1987. *Head Neck*. 1989; 11:264–268.
66. Tavin E, Persky M. Metastatic cutaneous squamous cell carcinoma of the head and neck region. *Laryngoscope*. 1996;106:156–158.
67. Goepfert H, Dichtel WJ, Medina JE, et al. Perineural invasion in squamous cell skin carcinoma of the head and neck. *Am J Surg*. 1984;148:542–547.
68. Breuninger H, Black B, Rassner G. Brief scientific statement: microstaging of squamous cell carcinomas. *Am J Clin Pathol*. 1990;94:624–627.
69. Moore BA, Weber RS, Prieto V, et al. Perineural invasion in cutaneous squamous cell carcinoma of the head and neck. Paper presented at 6th International Conference on Head and Neck Oncology. Washington DC, August 10, 2004.
70. Netterville JL, Sinard RJ, Bryant GL, et al. Delayed regional metastasis from midfacial squamous carcinomas. *Head Neck*. 1998;20:328–333.
71. O'Brien CJ, McNeil EB, McMahon JD, et al. Significance of clinical stage, extent of surgery, and pathologic findings in metastatic cutaneous squamous carcinoma of the parotid gland. *Head Neck*. 2002;24:417–422.
72. Palme CE, O'Brien CJ, Veness MJ, et al. Extent of parotid disease influences outcome in patients with metastatic cutaneous squamous cell carcinoma. *Arch Otolaryngol Head Neck Surg*. 2003;129:750–753.
73. Martinez J-C, Clark CO, Stasko T, et al. Defining the clinical course of metastatic skin cancer in organ transplant recipients. *Arch Dermatol*. 2003;139:301–306.
74. Mehrany K, Weenig RH, Lee KK, et al. Increased metastasis from primary cutaneous squamous cell carcinoma in patients with chronic lymphocytic leukemia. *J Am Acad Dermatol*. 2005;53:1067–1071.
75. Gor DM, Langer JE, Loevner LA. Imaging of cervical lymph nodes in head and neck cancer: the basics. *Radiol Clin North Am*. 2006;44(1):101–110
76. Castelijns JA, van den Brekel MW. Imaging of lymphadenopathy in the neck. *Am J Neuroradiol*. 2002;23(10): 1618–1619.
77. Talmi YP. Problems in the current TNM staging of nonmelanoma skin cancer of the head and neck. *Head Neck*. 2007;29(6):525–527.
78. Nakamura T, Sumi M. Nodal imaging in the neck: recent advances in US, CT and MR imaging of metastatic nodes. *Eur Radiol*. 2007;17(5):1235–1241.
79. Ginsberg LE. MR imaging of perineural tumor spread. *Neuroimaging Clin North Am*. 2004;14(4):663–677.
80. Williams LS, Mancuso AA, Mendenhall WM. Perineural spread of cutaneous squamous and basal cell carcinoma: CT and MR detection and its impact on patient management and prognosis. *Int J Radiat Oncol Biol Phys*. 2001;49(4):1061–1069.
81. Galloway TJ, Morris CG, Mancuso AA, Amdur RJ, Mendenhall WM. Impact of radiographic findings on prognosis for skin carcinoma with clinical perineural invasion. *Cancer*. 2005;103(6):1254–1257.
82. Garcia C, Poletti E, Crowson AN. Basosquamous carcinoma. *J Am Acad Dermatol*. 2009;60(1):137–143.
83. Medina-Franco H, Urist MM, Fiveash J, Heslin MJ, Bland KI, Beenken SW. Multimodality treatment of Merkel cell carcinoma: case series and literature review of 1024 cases. *Ann Surg Oncol*. 2001;8(3):204–208.
84. Hillner BE, Siegel BA, Shields AF, Liu D, Gareen IF, Hunt E, Coleman RE. Relationship between cancer type and impact of PET and PET/CT on intended management: findings of the national oncologic PET registry. *J Nucl Med*. 2008;49(12):1928–1935.
85. Edge SB, Carducci M, Byrd DR, eds. *AJCC Cancer Staging Manual*. 7th ed. New York, NY: Springer-Verlag; 2009.
86. Silverman MK, Kopf AW, Grin CM, et al. Recurrence rates of treated basal cell carcinomas. Part 1: overview. *J Dermatol Surg Oncol*. 1991;17:713–718.
87. Silverman MK, Kopf AW, Grin CM, et al. Recurrence rates of treated basal cell carcinoma. Part 2: curettage-electrodessication. *J Dermatol Surg Oncol*. 1991;17: 720–726.
88. Wolf DJ, Zitelli JA. Surgical margins for basal cell carcinoma. *Arch Dermatol*. 1987;123:340–344.
89. Choo R, Woo T, Assaad D, et al. What is the microscopic tumor extent beyond clinically delineated gross tumor boundary in nonmelanoma skin cancers? *Int J Radiat Oncol Biol Phys*. 2005;62:1096–1099.

90. Veness MJ. Treatment recommendations in patients diagnosed with high-risk cutaneous squamous cell carcinoma. *Australasian Radiol.* 2005;49:365–376.
91. Cherpelis BS, Marcusen C, Lang PG. Prognostic factors for metastasis in squamous cell carcinoma of the skin. *Dermatol Surg.* 2002:28:268–273.
92. Afzelius LE, Gunnarsson M, Nordgren H. Guidelines for prophylactic radical lymph node dissection in cases of carcinoma of the external ear. *Head Neck Surg.* 1990;2:361–365.
93. Anderson PE, Cambronero E, Shaha AR, Shah JP. The extent of neck disease after regional failure during observation of the N0 neck. *Am J Surg.* 1996;172:689–691.
94. Kowalski LP. Results of salvage treatment of the neck in patients with oral cancer. *Arch Otolaryngol Head Neck Surg.* 2002;128:58–62.
95. Lentsch EJ, Myers JN. Melanoma of the head and neck: current concepts in diagnosis and management. *Laryngoscope.* 2001;111:1209–1222.
96. Weiss M, Harrison L, Isaacs R. Use of decision analysis in planning a management strategy for the stage N0 neck. *Arch Otolaryngol Head Neck Surg.* 1994;120:699–702.
97. Martinez J-C and Cook JL. High-risk cutaneous squamous cell carcinoma without palpable lymphadenopathy: is there a therapeutic role for elective neck dissection? *Dermatol Surg.* 2007;33:410–420.
98. Veness MJ, Palme CE, Smith M, et al. Cutaneous head and neck squamous cell carcinoma metastatic to cervical lymph nodes (nonparotid): a better outcome with surgery and adjuvant radiotherapy. *Laryngoscope.* 2003; 113:1827–1833.
99. Reschly MJ, Messina JL, Zaulyanov LL, et al. Utility of sentinel lymphadenectomy in the management of patients with high-risk cutaneous squamous cell carcinoma. *Dermatol Surg.* 2003;29:135–140.
100. Wagner JD, Evodkimow DZ, Weisberger E, et al. Sentinel node biopsy for high-risk nonmenlanoma cutaneous malignancy. *Arch Dermatol.* 2004;140:75–79.
101. Weisberg NK, Bertagnolli MM, Becker DS. Combined sentinel lymphadenectomy and Mohs micrographic surgery for high-risk cutaneous squamous cell carcinoma. *J Am Acad Dermatol.* 2000;43:483–488.
102. Chu A, Ogusthorpe JD. Nonmelanoma cutaneous malignancy with regional metastasis. *Otolaryngol Head Neck Surg.* 2003;128:663–673.
103. Iyer NG, Clark JR, Murali R, et al. Outcomes following parotidectomy for metastatic squamous cell carcinoma with microscopic residual disease: Implications for facial nerve preservation. *Head Neck.* 2009;31:21–27.
104. Moore BA, Weber RS, Prieto V, et al. Lymph node metastases from cutaneous squamous cell carcinoma of the head and neck. *Laryngoscope.* 2005;115:1561–1567.
105. Dona E, Veness MJ, Cakir B, et al. Metastatic cutaneous squamous cell carcinoma to the parotid: the role of surgery and adjuvant radiotherapy to achieve best outcome. *Aust N Z J Surg.* 2003;73:692–696.
106. Jol JAD, van Vethuysen MLF, Hilgers FJM, et al. Treatment results of regional metastasis from cutaneous head and neck squamous cell carcinoma. *Eur J Surg Oncol.* 2002;29:81–86.
107. Cassisi NJ, Dickerson DR, Million RR. Squamous cell carcinoma of the skin metastatic to parotid nodes. *Arch Otolaryngol.* 1978;104:136–139.
108. Mendenhall NP, Million RR, Cassisi NJ. Parotid area lymph node metastases from carcinoma of the skin. *Int J Radiat Oncol Biol Phys.* 1985;11:707–714.
109. Taylor BW, Brant TA, Mendenhall NP, et al. Carcinoma of the skin metastatic to parotid area lymph nodes. *Head Neck.* 1991;13:427–433.
110. delCharco JO, Mendenhall WM, Parsons JT, et al. Carcinoma of the skin metastatic to the parotid area lymph nodes. *Head Neck.* 1998;20:369–373.
111. Bron LP, Traynor SJ, McNeil EB, et al. Primary and metastatic cancer of the parotid: comparison of clinical behavior in 232 cases. *Laryngoscope.* 2003;113:1070–1075.
112. Oddone N, Morgan GJ, Palme CE et al. Metastatic cutaneous squamous cell carcinoma of the head and neck: The immunosuppression, treatment, extranodal spread, and margin status (ITEM) prognostic score to predict outcome and the need to improve survival. *Cancer.* 2009;115(9):1883–1891.
113. Mendenhall WM, Amdur RJ, Hinerman RW, et al. Skin cancer of the head and neck with perineural invasion. *Am J Clin Oncol.* 2007:30;93–96.
114. Jackson JE, Dickie GJ, Wiltshire KL, et al. Radiotherapy for perineural invasion in cutaneous head and neck carcinomas: toward a risk-adapted treatment approach. *Head Neck.* 2009;31:604–610.
115. Garcia-Serra A, Hinerman RW, Mendenhall WM, et al. Carcinoma of the skin with perineural invasion. *Head Neck.* 2003;25:1027–1033.
116. Mendenhall WM, Parsons JP, Mendenhall NP, et al. Carcinoma of the skin of the head and neck with perineural invasion. *Head Neck.* 1989;11:301–308.
117. Mendenhall WM, Amdur RJ, Williams LS, et al. Carcinoma of the skin of the head and neck with perineural invasion. *Head Neck.* 2002;24:78–83.
118. McCord MW, Mendenhall WM, Parsons JT, et al. Skin cancer of the head and neck with clinical perineural invasion. *Int J Radiat Oncol Biol Phys.* 2000;47:89–93.
119. Chua M, Veness MJ, Morgan G, et al. Parotid lymph node metastases from cutaneous squamous cell carcinomas: treatment outcome and prognostic factors following surgery and adjuvant radiotherapy. *Australas Radiol.* 2002;46:174–179.
120. Cooper JS, Pajak TF, Forastiere AA, et al. Postoperative concurrent radiotherapy and chemotherapy for high-risk squamous cell carcinoma of the head and neck. *N Engl J Med.* 2004;350:1937–1944.
121. Bernier J, Domenge C, Osahim M, et al. Postoperative irradiation with or without concomitant chemotherapy for locally advanced head and neck cancer. *N Engl J Med.* 2004;350:1945–1952.
122. Lippman SM, Parkinson DR, Itri LM, et al. 13-cis-retinoic acid and interferon-alpha-2a: effective combi-

nation therapy for advanced squamous cell carcinoma of the skin. *J Natl Cancer Inst.* 1992;84:235–241.

123. Shin DM, Glisson BS, Khuri F, et al. Phase II and biologic study of interferon alfa, retinoic acid, and cisplatin in advanced squamous skin cancer. *J Clin Oncol.* 2002; 20:364–370.
124. Wulff BC, Schick JS, Thomas-Ahner JM, et al. Topical treatment with OGG1 enzyme affects UVB-induced skin carcinogenesis. *Photochem Photobiol.* 2008;84:317–321.
125. Weber RS, Lustig R, Glisson D, et al. A phase II trial of ZD 1869 for advanced cutaneous squamous cell carcinoma of the head and neck. *J Clin Oncol.* 2007;25(18S): 6038.
126. Kim S, Eleff M, Nicolaou N. Cetuximab as primary treatment for cutaneous squamous cell carcinoma to the neck. *Head Neck.* 2010; epub ahead of print.
127. Autier P, Dore JF, Schifflers E, et al. Melanoma and the use of sunscreens: an EORTC case-control study in Germany, Belgium, and France. *Cancer.* 1995;61:749–755.
128. Chakrabarty A, Geisse JK. Medical therapies for nonmelanoma skin cancer. *Clin Dermatol.* 2004;22:1214–1218.

9

SURGICAL MANAGEMENT OF LOCOREGIONAL DISEASE

STEPHEN Y. LAI
RANDAL S. WEBER

Introduction

Surgical resection is the most common method for treatment of nonmelanoma skin cancer (NMSC) of the head and neck. The great majority of these lesions are squamous cell carcinoma (SCC) and basal cell carcinoma (BCC). Depending on the type and size of the tumor, overall patient status, and the availability and experience of specific practitioners, surgical options include cryosurgery, electrodessication, and curettage, Mohs micrographic surgery, and standard resection.

Multidisciplinary care for locoregionally advanced disease is likely to optimize oncologic and functional outcomes. Preoperative assessment (discussed in Chapters 2 and 8) is critical to assess specific cosmetic and functional deficits that may result from surgical resection. Additional reconstructive planning may be necessary for tumors near the eyes, ears, skull, or dura, and these unique situations merit discussion in subsequent chapters. Histologic diagnosis must be confirmed by biopsy, ideally with a full-thickness specimen that includes epidermis, dermis, and a portion of subcutaneous tissue. Imaging studies may be useful, especially in patients with lesions in high-risk areas, such as the preauricular region. Appropriate selection of the proper technique for a given lesion and patient results in comparable cure rates in most cases.

Cryosurgery and Curettage with Electrodessication

Cryosurgery involves the use of freezing temperatures to selectively destroy skin cancers. Liquid nitrogen is the most commonly applied cryogen and typically is applied by spray or metal probe. Following sharp curettage of a skin lesion, electrodessication uses heat to kill residual tumor cells. Both modalities have similar indications and limitations. Advantages include low cost, ease of treatment in the office, and comparable cure rates of 94 to 99%.[1] However, as these methods do not permit pathologic control of tumor margins, their use should be limited to nonmalignant lesions. Definitive treatment of true malignancies may be achieved with other modalities.

Mohs Micrographic Surgery

Given the sensitive cosmetic and function issues in the head and neck, Mohs micrographic surgery is frequently employed to maximize preservation of normal tissue. A complete description of this technique is provided in Chapter 30. Developed by Frederic E. Mohs when he was a medical student in the 1930s, the original technique involved preoperative application of a zinc chloride paste to "fix" the specimen in vivo.[2] Modern application of this technique utilizes frozen section analysis.

The Mohs surgeon, who is also the primary pathologist, outlines the tumor with 1- to 3-mm margins. After appropriate anesthesia has been given, the gross tumor is resected. A scalpel angled at 45 degrees is employed to excise the lesion along with 1 to 3 mm of the surrounding tissue. Small nicks are made on the specimen and on the remaining wound edge prior to final excision for orientation purposes. The operative specimen is divided and a map is created with the use of color and numeric coding. Horizontal frozen sections are prepared to facilitate histologic examination of the entire tumor margin. Areas of residual tumor can be removed from the surgical defect using the tumor map for reference. Ideally, this cycle of resection and pathological examination is repeated until the margins are tumor-free.[1,3] However, this procedure may be terminated if critical structures are encountered (eg, facial nerve).

Standard Surgical Excision

The most common technique used by head and neck surgeons is standard surgical excision for NMSC. This technique is ideal for wide local excision in areas with sufficient skin elasticity.[4] Cure rates of 90% to 95% are achieved for primary tumors.[5] Typically, early lesions are excised in the outpatient setting with local anesthesia (1% xylocaine) for patient comfort. Depending on the patient's cardiac status, epinephrine (1:100,000) may be used for vasoconstriction. The maximum tolerated dosage of xylocaine is 4 mg per kg, which is increased to 7 mg per kg when combined with epinephrine.

Intermediate size lesions may be removed in an ambulatory surgery center to permit sedation and monitored anesthesia care. Large and/or aggressive lesions should be removed under general anesthesia to facilitate en bloc resection and subsequent reconstruction. Unlike Mohs micrographic surgery, the initial resection is designed to remove the entire tumor with a clear margin. Special attention needs to be given to specimen orientation for pathologic analysis. We typically mark the specimen prior to complete removal to avoid potential errors. En bloc resection is critical for aggressive NMSC lesions as these tumors tend to deeply infiltrate the subcutaneous tissue and may involve muscle and peripheral nerves.

For patients with aggressive or recurrent NMSC lesions, optimal results are most likely to be achieved through multidisciplinary planning and management.[6] The multidisciplinary team is composed of the head and neck oncologic surgeon, Mohs micrographic surgeon, reconstructive plastic surgeon, dermatologist, radiation oncologist, neurosurgeon, dental prosthodontist, anaplastologist, and pathologist. With the developing role of targeted therapy for cutaneous lesions, input from medical oncologists also has become important, as discussed in Chapter 15. Patients with high-risk NMSC frequently are seen at large referral hospitals, including academic institutions after an initial biopsy or treatment. In such cases, the original pathology slides should be obtained and the pathology should be confirmed. A recent study demonstrated that a consequential number of patients (54 of 814) had changes in their pathologic diagnosis that resulted in major therapeutic and prognostic modifications when a secondary review of the specimen was performed.[7]

Patients typically are evaluated by the surgeon who performs the initial clinical staging of the disease and obtains the appropriate diagnostic imaging studies. In many centers, the Mohs surgeon and head and neck surgeon collaborate in the preoperative planning and surgical resection.[8–10] The radiation oncologist should evaluate the patient initially when definitive radiation therapy is considered as a possible therapeutic option, or when postoperative treatment may be necessary. Examination of the patient prior to surgical excision permits the radiation oncologist the opportunity to assess the extent of disease and plan the postsurgical treatment volume required. NMSC lesions that invade the calvarium, extend into the skull base from the paranasal sinuses, invade intracranially along nerves, or involve the temporal bone will require combined efforts with a neurosurgeon. Evaluation by the dental prosthodontist, anaplastologist, and reconstructive plastic surgeon provides the available options for cosmetic and functional rehabilitation.

Surgical Resection Margins

The most important principle in the management of NMSC is complete tumor excision. Failure to adequately account for the extent or aggressiveness of a skin lesion can lead to inadequate treatment and local recurrence. Few clinical scenarios are more difficult for the patient and physician than an uncontrollable skin cancer of the head and neck. Wentzell and Robinson[11] have suggested that surgeons frequently underestimate the depth of invasion of aggressive NMSC. Less aggressive excision of these lesions may be due to concerns regarding the potential cosmetic and functional consequences of surgical resection. Despite their importance, functional and cosmetic concerns must remain secondary to achieving local control.

Depending on the size and location of the tumor, proper surgical resection may require resection of surrounding critical structures and the use of rotational flaps and/or free flaps for reconstruction. Careful preoperative assessment, including diagnostic imaging and consultation with an experienced reconstructive surgeon, is essential in these cases. Separation of the tumor resection and reconstruction procedures also facilitates achieving optimal results. The ablative surgeon may focus on complete tumor resection without compromising the excision because of a specific reconstructive plan. The reconstructive surgeon can perform cosmetic and functional restoration with the assurance that surgical margins are clear. Delayed reconstruction may be preferred to confirm negative tumor margins by permanent histologic analysis.

Peripheral Margins

An adequate margin of resection is critical to ensure successful surgical treatment and reduce the possibility of local recurrence and uncontrollable disease. The "clinical margin" refers to the visible edge of the tumor, whereas the "surgical margin" refers to the normal tissue included in the lesion resection. Published recommendations of empirical surgical margins are simply guidelines based on the statistical probability of achieving a complete resection. For BCC and SCC, a margin of 4 mm will yield a more than 95% cure rate for lesions that have a low risk of subclinical extension.[12,13] Low-risk BCC lesions are well-defined, primary lesions, less than 2 cm in diameter, have nonaggressive histology, and are located in low- or intermediate-risk areas (cheeks, forehead, scalp, neck).[14] Larger margins are likely to yield minimal additional benefit. As the diameter of the primary lesion increases, the required surgical margin also must be increased to maximize the likelihood of achieving a complete excision. In a prospective study of BCC lesions, the margin required for a 95% 5-year tumor-free interval was determined to be 5 mm for a tumor less than 1 cm. This increased to 8 mm for tumors 1 to 2 cm in diameter and 12 mm for tumors larger than 2 cm in diameter.[15]

The amount of normal tissue to be excised along with the tumor ultimately depends on the histologic and clinical behavior of the individual tumor.[4,8,16,17] For example, a recurrent tumor may require a larger peripheral margin than a new primary lesion. SCC of the skin usually requires a larger margin than BCC of the same size. Wolf and Zitelli[13] determined that the maximum subclinical extension of BCC lesions ranged from 1 to 6 mm. Additionally, a noduloulcerative BCC requires a different margin than the morpheaform type, which tends to be more invasive and have indistinct margins. The average margin required to completely remove nodular BCC was 4.7 mm, as compared to 7.2 mm for infiltrative BCC in a retrospective study that matched lesions by tumor location and size, patient characteristics, and number of recurrences.[18]

Aggressive NMSC

Issues related to perineural extension and the presence of regional metastatic disease also are important. Perineural invasion is of concern in the infraorbital region, supraorbital area, and lower lip.[19,20] When peripheral nerve branches are involved, the main nerve trunk should be identified and followed in a retrograde fashion to obtain a clear margin. With cranial nerves, intracranial extension through the various foramina may be identified. In this situation, the nerve should be marked to facilitate subsequent neurosurgical resection or postoperative radiation therapy. Ultimately, although published standards of surgical margins are available, intraoperative margin control through frozen section analysis is necessary.

Management of Perineural Invasion

Aggressive lesions require wider local excision and should increase clinical suspicion for potential regional metastasis to the parotid gland and/or neck. Additionally, the potential for perineural invasion is increased. Rowe and associates identified several common features of aggressive NMSC that are listed in Table 9–1.[4] These lesions may be 2 cm or larger at presentation with a history of recurrence or rapid growth. Recurrent BCC lesions tend to remain at the primary site, whereas recurrent SCC lesions are more likely to metastasize. However, regional metastases also may be evident at presentation. Histologic features include poorly differentiated lesions, spindle cell SCC, and basosquamous or morpheaform BCC. These lesions commonly occur in the "H-zone," which includes the central midface and the lateral face from the temporal fossa to the mandibular angle (Fig 9–1).[8] Specific structural units within this area include the medial canthus, glabella, posterolateral nares, alar rims, nasolabial sulcus, columella-labial junction, and auricular regions such as the tragus and antitragus.[4]

Table 9–1. Characteristics of Aggressive Nonmelanoma Skin Cancer

Large lesion (>2 cm)
Rapid growth
Recurrent disease
Regional metastasis (parotid or neck)
Pathologic findings
Poorly differentiated
Spindle cell SCC
Basosquamous or morpheaform BCC
Midface "H-zone" involvement
Invasion of bone, cartilage, and/or muscle

NMSC may invade along nerves, and the critical functional and aesthetic structures in this region may lead to suboptimal resection in an attempt to preserve cosmetic and functional units. Careful judgment is required in these situations. Margins of up to 2 cm may be required, if possible. Garcia-Serra et al suggested that Mohs micrographic surgery should not be used for the excision of primary tumors with clinical evidence of perineural invasion, due to the extent of tumor infiltration and possible "skip" lesions.[21,22] Highly aggressive lesions, such as Merkel cell or dermatofibrosarcoma protuberant (DFSP) tumors, may require even more extensive resection, with margins of at least 2 to 3 cm.[23,24]

Deep Margins

Similar attention must be given regarding the deep margin of excision. A substantial amount of subcutaneous tissue should be included in the deep margin for superficial lesions. Invasive tumors may require inclusion of the underlying fascia or muscle in the deep margin. Resection of muscle and/or bone

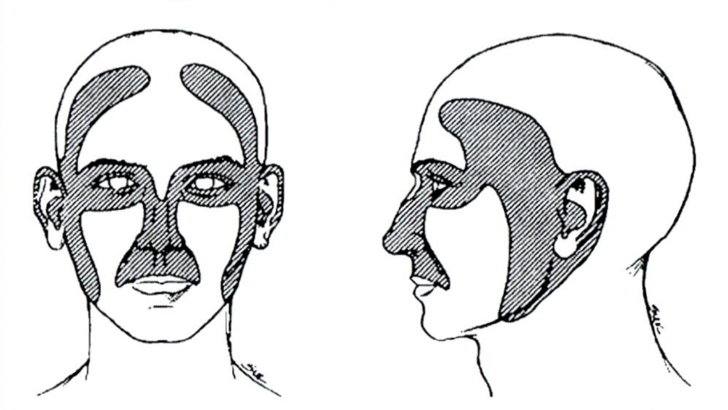

Figure 9–1. The H-zone encompasses the midface, extending from the lower eyelids horizontally to the preauricular region. This area includes the temple to the level of the angle of the mandible and includes the ear, postauricular sulcus, upper lip, nose, and medial canthus. (Reprinted with permission from Baker SR, Swanson NA, Grekin RC. An interdisciplinary approach to the management of basal cell carcinoma of the head and neck. *J Dermatol Surg Oncol.* 1987;13(10):1096.

may be necessary, depending on the extent of the tumor. With lesions that are fixed to the periosteum or create frank bone destruction, en bloc resection may include rhinectomy, maxillectomy, mandibulectomy, or craniectomy, depending on the lesion site. As such, preoperative diagnostic imaging and intraoperative palpation are critical in determining the appropriate deep margin.

Frozen Section Margin Assessment

In all cases, intraoperative frozen section margin assessment should be performed. The surgeon should carefully orient the specimen relative to the patient anatomy and the excision site (Fig 9–2). Ideally, this orientation is reviewed directly with the surgical pathologist. The method of sectioning used by the pathologist can significantly impact the efficacy of resection. Serial cross-sectioning ("bread-loafing") method of margin analysis is commonly used, but yields suboptimal results because the margin is only sampled rather than fully examined.[25,26]

To avoid improper sampling technique and to fully analyze the tumor margin, en face sections of the peripheral margin should be taken around the entire circumference of the specimen, including the entire deep margin. A specimen map should be created by the surgeon and pathologist so that, if a positive margin is identified, the location of the residual tumor can be precisely described to facilitate additional resection, in a manner similar to Mohs micrographic surgery, which is delineated elsewhere in this text. The accuracy of intraoperative frozen sections will vary by institution and the type of lesion being analyzed.[27] In addition to clear communication with regard to specimen origin, the surgeon and pathologist should clearly define terms such as "clear" and "close" with regard to tumor margins.

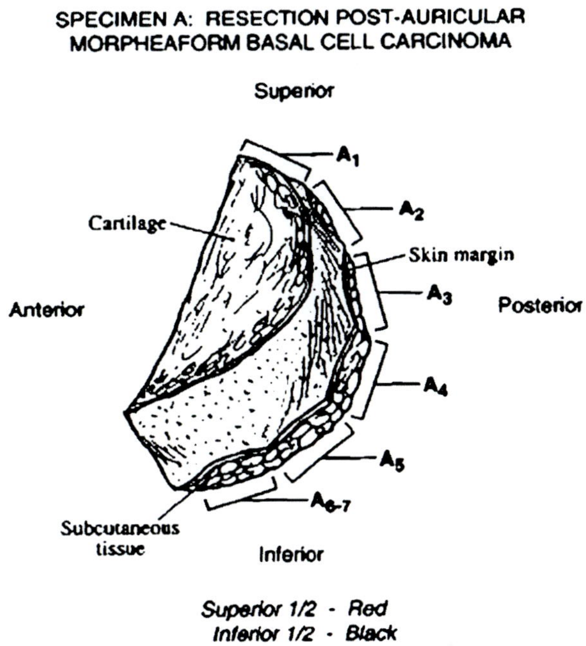

Figure 9–2. The tumor margin is carefully delineated so that sections submitted for frozen section pathologic analysis can be correlated with the original en bloc specimen. Positive margins can be precisely localized if additional margins must be obtained. The head and neck surgeon and pathologist should collaborate in creating a tumor map that specifically describes the surgical specimen and the structures resected. (Reprinted with permission from Weber, Randal S., Miller, Michael J., Goepfert, Helmuth: *Nasal and Squamous Cell Skin Cancers of the Head and Neck.* Williams & Wilkins, 1996.

Management of Regional Disease

Local and regional metastasis must be evaluated and treated appropriately when present. However, even in advanced cases, clinically evident lymph node metastasis is quite rare. When lymph nodes are palpable and/or clinical suspicion is high for metastatic tumor, diagnostic imaging should be obtained to assess the extent of regional disease. Fine-needle aspiration biopsy is useful for preoperative confirmation.

Sentinel Lymph Node Biopsy and Observation

Although commonly employed in the treatment of melanoma, sentinel lymph node biopsy is not routinely performed for NMSC.[28] Recent reports have explored sentinel node staging for the detection of occult regional lymph node metastasis in high-risk NMSC, but larger studies are needed to evaluate overall efficacy of this approach and the development of formal clinical practice guidelines.[29,30] Due to the low rates of regional metastases, elective neck dissection is not indicated for NMSC. When cervical metastatic disease is present, a regional neck dissection is performed at the time of the resection of the primary tumor. The intervening subdermal fat and underlying fascia between the lymph node groups and the primary disease should be removed to ensure removal of smaller nests of metastasizing tumor cells. Delayed metastases from cutaneous NMSC may occur many years following removal of the primary tumor, and the patient may have forgotten the initial lesion. The parotid, upper cervical, and facial lymph nodes are most often the sites of delayed metastases.

At-Risk Cervical Lymphatic Basins

For cutaneous lesions of the anterior and lateral face with cervical lymphadenopathy, neck dissection should comprise levels I to III. Particular attention needs to be paid to removal of the prevascular (facial) lymph nodes in the submandibular triangle. Cutaneous malignancies of the preauricular, anterior scalp, and temporal regions, neck dissection should include levels II, III, and VA. Lymph nodes lying adjacent to the external jugular vein should also be removed. Selective or posterolateral neck dissection, including levels II to V, postauricular and suboccipital nodal basins, is indicated for cutaneous lesions of the posterior scalp and upper neck that present with cervical lymphadenopathy.[31] The superior limit of dissection is the skull base anteriorly and the nuchal ridge posteriorly, with extension to the anterior border of the trapezius muscle at the posterolateral limit. Additionally, the upper portion of the attachment of the trapezius to the skull base should be divided to allow for complete exposure of the suboccipital nodes that lie along the occipital artery.

Parotid Metastases

Metastases to the parotid gland also must be carefully evaluated, as they are more commonly encountered for cutaneous lesions, than cervical metastases.[32] Malignant parotid masses often may be linked to an identifiable primary skin lesion.[33] The parotid gland serves as a watershed for lymphatics of the antero - parietal scalp, forehead, temple, eyelids, ear, and zygomatic region.[34]

O'Brien et al[35] described their experience in Australia with high-risk NMSC and demonstrated clinical neck involvement in 26% of patients with cutaneous disease metastatic to the parotid gland. Sixty to 80% of aggressive NMSC lesions involving the facial nerve may present asymptomatically.[22,32,36] In a multi-institutional retrospective study, the most common primary sites with regional metastasis were the cheek (22%), pinna (21%), temple (16%), and forehead (16%).[37] In this series, 80% of these patients had involvement of the parotid gland. Within histologically positive neck specimens, level II was the most commonly involved (80%).

Recent studies have demonstrated prognostic value in separately staging parotid involvement in cases of metastatic NMSC, prompting an update in staging of regional metastases from nonmelanoma skin cancer. Under the traditional TNM staging system from the American Joint Commission on Cancer (AJCC), the N1 staging classification applied equally to a patient with a single 2-cm parotid metastasis, a patient with facial nerve invasion related to parotid metastasis, or metastatic disease involving both the parotid gland and the neck.[38] Given the impact of parotid and cervical nodal metastatic burden on disease control and survival, the 2010 AJCC staging system, described in Chapters 7 and 8 of this text, has been expanded.[39,40]

Parotidectomy in the treatment of skin cancer should be performed when intraparotid metastasis is present or the lesion has directly invaded the parotid capsule (Fig 9–3). Parotidectomy may be necessary to ensure complete tumor resection and protection of the facial nerve.[41] Overt facial nerve invasion and/or temporal bone involvement requires similar intervention.[22,42] Typically, a superficial parotidectomy is sufficient if no facial nerve involvement is encountered, as most of the parotid lymph nodes are located lateral to the facial nerve.[33] The extent of parotid resection, including radical parotidectomy with nerve sacrifice in these situations, has not led to decreased recurrence or increased survival.[36,43]

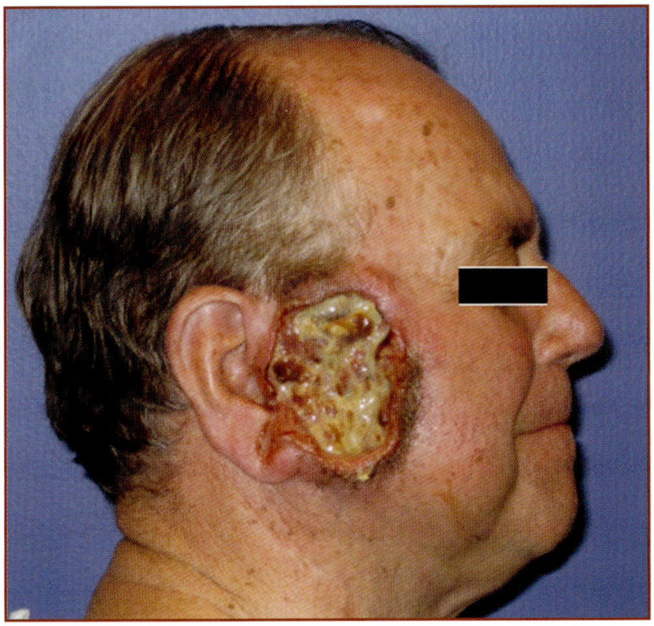
A

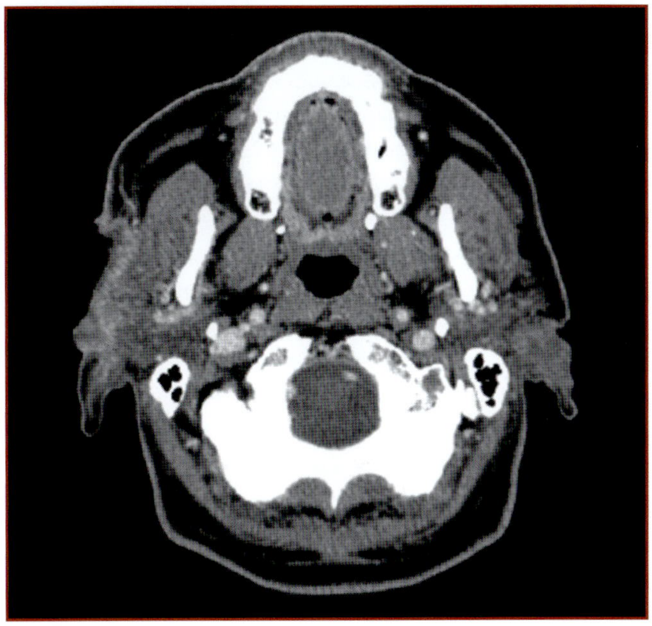
B

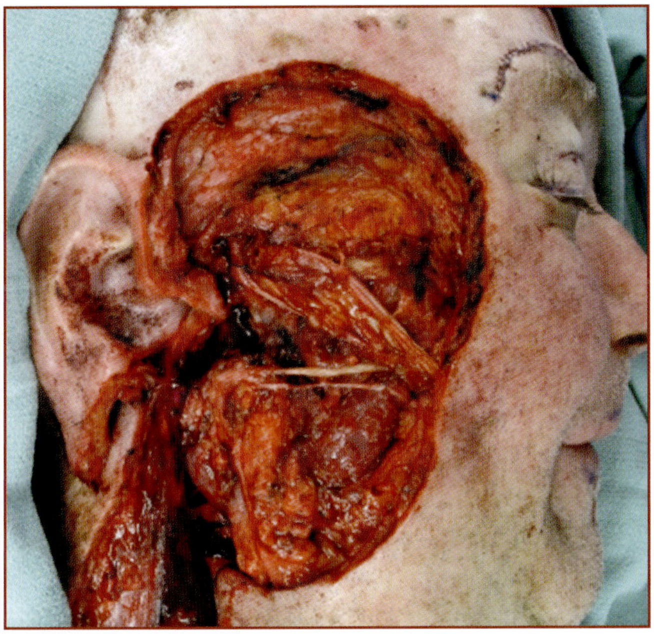
C

Figure 9–3. **A.** Patient presented with a large, ulcerated preauricular lesion and loss of upper division facial nerve function. **B.** CT scan axial image demonstrated direct invasion of the parotid gland. **C.** Resection included sacrifice of the upper division of the facial nerve which was reconstructed with a cable graft harvested from the cutaneous branch of the femoral nerve to the thigh.

With removal of the superficial lobe of the parotid gland, the primary echelon lymph nodes are also removed.[42,44] O'Brien et al[35] reported in their series that greater than 25% of patients with SCC involving the parotid gland had clinical involvement of cervical nodes and an additional 35% of those patients treated with elective neck dissections were found to have occult positive nodes. Occult neck disease in the presence of parotid metastasis may range from 20 to 44%.[43,45,46] Thus, a supraomohyoid neck dissection is recommended. Additionally, in the presence of cervical lymphadenopathy, an elective parotidectomy can be justified even if involvement is not clinically apparent, especially when the lymphatic drainage patterns cross the path of the parotid gland.[47] Elective parotidectomy for NMSC generally is not recommended.

Adjuvant external beam radiation therapy is indicated in the setting of parotid and/or cervical nodal metastases from NMSC. Taylor and colleagues[44] demonstrated the effectiveness of this combined approach. Ultimate control of disease in patients with parotid metastases from head and neck skin cancers was 62.5% with surgical treatment and 46% with radiation therapy, but improved to 89% when both forms of treatment were employed. The indications and role of external beam radiation therapy for NMSC treatment is covered in more detail in Chapter 13.

Reconstruction of the Surgical Defect

Reconstruction of the surgical defect after management of the primary disease and regional metastases can take many forms. The concept of the "reconstructive ladder" frequently applies in these cases. The primary concept is that reconstructive efforts should start with the safest and least invasive methods of closure, although special attention should be given to the cosmetic and functional consequences related to a selected approach, due to the primary of the head and neck. For smaller lesions, primary closure and healing by secondary intention are appropriate options. Intermediate defects may warrant a skin graft or local advancement of a rotational flap for adequate closure. Large defects may require regional or distant pedicled flaps and/or free-tissue transfer for reconstruction. Typically, the use of flaps that will cover areas with close or indistinct margins should be avoided so that recurrence may be more quickly diagnosed.

Delayed reconstruction may be advantageous, as tumor margins may be confirmed negative by permanent histologic analysis. In a staged procedure, the excision site is covered with a sterile dressing and expedited processing of the pathology is requested. Reconstruction usually is performed within 7 days of the initial resection when negative margins have been verified. This staged process also allows for additional margin resection if necessary. For high-risk lesions, a skin graft may be applied to facilitate surveillance of the site for recurrence. After pathologic confirmation of clear margins and perhaps even a period of observation, the skin graft may be removed and a more cosmetically acceptable method of reconstruction may be used.

Some situations may require immediate reconstruction. An SCC of the upper eyelid that requires complete lid resection should be reconstructed immediately to prevent corneal dessication and loss of the eye. Similarly, through-and-through defects into the oral cavity following resection of an advanced skin cancer of the cheek also should be reconstructed immediately with both internal lining and external coverage in order to restore oral competency. Lesions that invade the parotid gland or involve the facial nerve may require resection of the facial nerve, and initial surgical management should anticipate primary nerve grafting with possible eye protection via either temporary tarsorrhaphy or insertion of an upper eyelid gold weight.

The reconstructive considerations, and options for cutaneous wounds of the head and neck are quite extensive, and they are covered in great detail in the final section of this text (Chapters 32 to 39).

Special Anatomic Considerations

The management of NMSC requires special consideration in particular subsites of the head and neck. As previously stated, resection of aggressive lesions with attendant significant cosmetic and functional effects demands careful preoperative evaluation and planning. No precise description of surgical treatment for skin cancer in a particular site is possible, as resection is dictated by the extent of the specific lesion. However, treatment of these lesions requires proper assessment of tumor extent and a complete understanding of the factors influencing tumor resection and facial reconstruction. Periauricular lesions (Chapter 10), periorbital lesions (Chapter 11), and neurosurgical issues (Chapter 12) are covered elsewhere.

Forehead and Scalp

The skin of the forehead and scalp includes the temporal, supra-eyebrow, and glabellar regions. Most of this skin is thick and contains abundant vascular subcutaneous tissue, except the temporal skin, which is quite thin and has facial nerve branches directly under the surface. Lesions in this subsite may have "silent" microscopic extensions that require multidisciplinary management (Fig 9–4).[2,48]

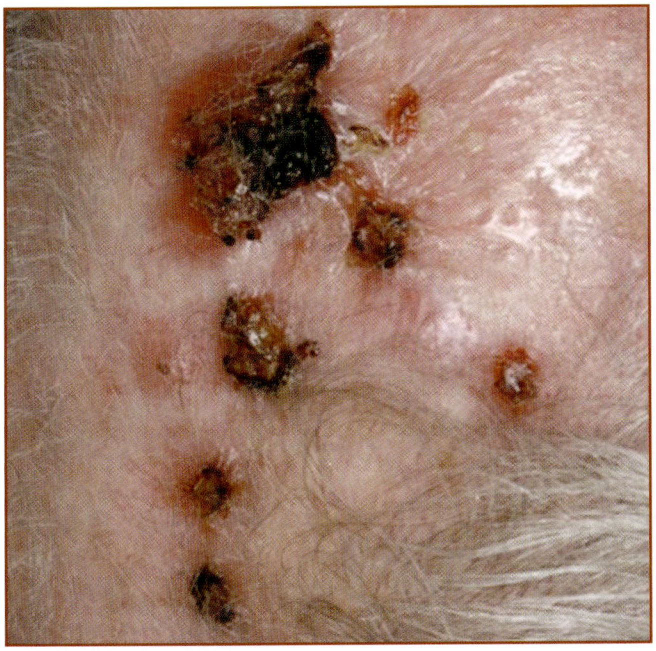

A

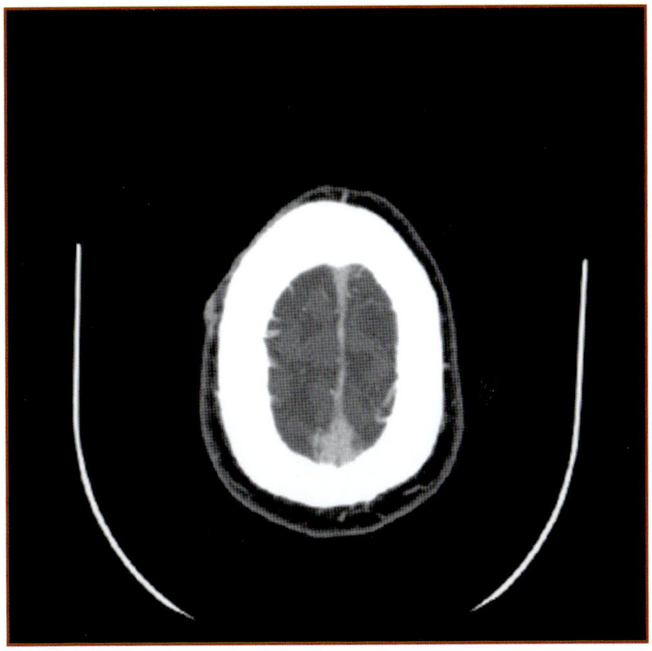

B

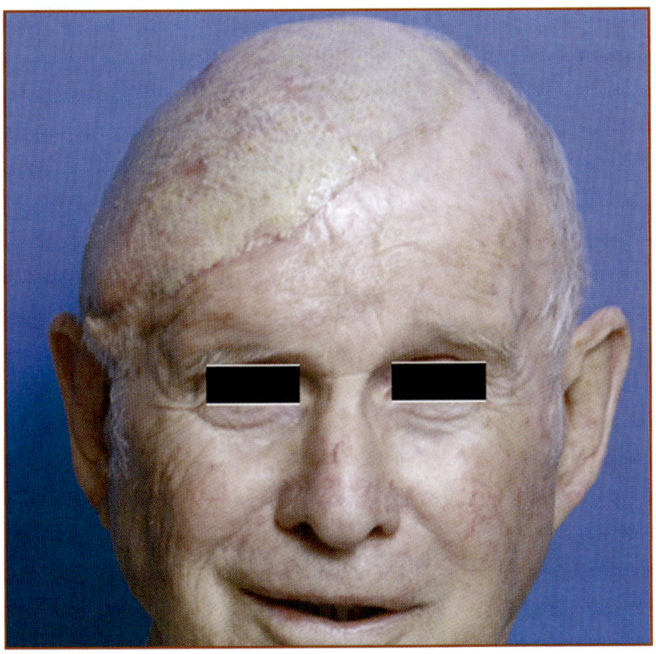

C

Figure 9–4. A. This patient had a recurrent, rapidly spreading atypical fibroxanthoma of the scalp after a Mohs microsurgical procedure. **B.** CT scan axial image demonstrated that the lesion was directly contiguous with the outer table of the skull. Intraoperative dissection demonstrated involvement of the outer table and a neurosurgeon performed a craniectomy with titanium mesh reconstruction. **C.** The excised scalp was reconstructed with a latissimus dorsi free flap and a skin graft.

A majority of nodular and nodular-ulcerative types of BCC can be controlled even when the lesions are quite extensive. Although the more aggressive infiltrating type of BCC represents only 10% of all BCC lesions, 32% of forehead and temple lesions are of this type.[9] BCC lesions rarely metastasize, but aggressive lesions of the ear and scalp that are deeply invasive or larger than 3 cm are more likely to metastasize than are lesions located in other head and neck sites. These lesions spread along lymphatics within the parotid gland and the jugulodigastric chain or to distant sites, including lung, bone, and skin.[49] Both aggressive BCC and SCC lesions of the scalp and forehead exhibit an increased potential for parotid gland involvement, with a resultant worse prognosis, especially if the facial nerve is involved.[22,42]

SCC lesions typically are well differentiated in the forehead and scalp. Aggressive lesions tend to occur in areas of previous radiation therapy, thermal injury, and chemical burn. These malignancies tend to be more invasive and are more likely to metastasize locally.[50] Additionally, perineural invasion by SCC in this area is of particular concern. In one study, 14% of lesions in the forehead and scalp demonstrated invasion into one or more major cranial nerve branches.[20] Lesions in the frontozygomatic region have an increased frequency of perineural invasion, often involving the supraorbital nerves. Most often, the facial and trigeminal nerves are involved. In the majority of cases, no signs or symptoms of nerve involvement are noted at initial presentation. Although treatment can provide appropriate local cancer control, overall survival of patients with perineural invasion by cutaneous SCC is quite poor; 5-year survival rates for patients treated with radiation therapy alone or with combined surgery and postoperative radiation therapy are about 30%.[20]

Local invasion of underlying bone by SCC in the forehead and scalp region can compromise excision and tumor control. Risks for involvement of the calvarium include large lesions, tumor fixation, CNS symptoms, and a history of previous radiation therapy. Careful physical examination and a contrast-enhanced CT scan are the primary means of determining the presence and extent of bone involvement. MRI studies can delineate intracranial tumor extention. The head and neck surgeon must be prepared to remove the outer table or full thickness of the calvarium if invasion is present at the time of resection, as depicted in Chapter 12.

Additionally, appropriate management of the frontal sinuses, including frontonasal duct preservation or even sinus obliteration, is necessary if the lesion extends into this space. Neurosurgical involvement is required when the tumor involves the full thickness of the skull. Full-thickness craniectomy is recommended given the possibility of bone invasion or extension of tumor along venous channels. Tumors involving the inner cortex of the cranium may require resection of the underlying dura. Violation of the inner dura may require coagulation and resection of adjacent brain tissue at the site of involvement. However, the likelihood of cure for patients with transdural involvement of cutaneous SCC is exceedingly low.

Midface (Nose and Upper Lip)

The "H-zone" encompasses the glabella, medial canthus, nasolabial sulcus, columella-labial junction, alar rim, and posterolateral nares.[4] NMSC in this region have higher rates of recurrence and are more challenging to treat surgically. Tumors in this area tend to grow more vertically, rather than laterally in a superficial plane, and this growth pattern may be related to the presence of facial embryologic fusion planes in this region. The use of Mohs micrographic treatment in this area may not be optimal and should be carefully evaluated, especially with recurrent lesions or tumors that may demonstrate perineural invasion.

The portion of the "H-zone" encompassing the nose and upper lip represents a difficult area for tumor resection and subsequent reconstruction in order to preserve cosmetic and functional attributes. Tumors adherent to the nasal cartilage or bone will require at least a partial rhinectomy. Intraoperative frozen section assessment of surgical margins is necessary to ensure complete tumor resection. Reconstruction is this region is challenging given the requirements of preserving as normal an appearance as possible and maintaining function through nasal airway patency and oral sphincter competence. The reconstructive options for nasal and lip defects, as well as prosthetic rehabilitation, are discussed in subsequent chapters.

Conclusions

The surgical management of locoregional disease for NMSC requires a multidisciplinary approach, especially when patients present with aggressive lesions that may pose significant functional and cosmetic challenges. The devastating potential outcomes of high-risk NMSC highlight the need for appropriate initial clinical assessment and comprehensive treatment based on detailed understanding of the disease behavior. En bloc resection of the tumor with intraoperative frozen section analysis of the entire tumor margin is critical. Unfortunately, therapy for NMSC does not end with treatment of the presenting lesion because almost 50% of patients with an NMSC lesion will develop another lesion within the next 5 years.[51]

References

1. Padgett JK, Hendrix JD Jr. Cutaneous malignancies and their management. *Otolaryngol Clin North Am.* 2001;34:523–553.
2. Mohs FE, Zitelli JA. Microscopically controlled surgery in the treatment of carcinoma of the scalp. *Arch Dermatol.* 1981;117:764–769.
3. Shriner DL, McCoy DK, Goldberg DJ, Wagner RF Jr. Mohs micrographic surgery. *J Am Acad Dermatol.* 1998;39:79–97.
4. Rowe DE, Carroll RJ, Day CL Jr. Prognostic factors for local recurrence, metastasis, and survival rates in squamous cell carcinoma of the skin, ear, and lip. Implications for treatment modality selection. *J Am Acad Dermatol.* 1992;26:976–990.
5. Rowe DE, Carroll RJ, Day CL Jr. Long-term recurrence rates in previously untreated (primary) basal cell carcinoma: implications for patient follow-up. *J Dermatol Surg Oncol.* 1989;15:315–328.
6. Weber RS. Multidisciplinary management of advanced basal and squamous cell skin cancer of the head and neck. In: Lucente F, ed. *Highlights of the Instructional Courses. Vol. 7.* St. Louis, MO: Mosby-Year Book; 1984:37–52.
7. Westra WH, Kronz JD, Eisele DW. The impact of second opinion surgical pathology on the practice of head and neck surgery: a decade experience at a large referral hospital. *Head Neck.* 2002;24:684–693.
8. Baker SR, Swanson NA, Grekin RC. Mohs surgical treatment and reconstruction of cutaneous malignancies of the nose. *Facial Plast Surg.* 1987;5:29–47.
9. Grekin RC, Schaler RE, Crumley RL. Cancer of the forehead and temple regions. *Dermatol Clin.* 1989;7:699–710.
10. Siegle RJ, Schuller DE. Multidisciplinary surgical approach to the treatment of perinasal nonmelanoma skin cancer. *Dermatol Clin.* 1989;7:711–731.
11. Wentzell JM, Robinson JK. Embryologic fusion planes and the spread of cutaneous carcinoma: a review and reassessment. *J Dermatol Surg Oncol.* 1990;16:1000–1006.
12. Brodland DG, Zitelli JA. Surgical margins for excision of primary cutaneous squamous cell carcinoma. *J Am Acad Dermatol.* 1992;27:241–248.
13. Wolf DJ, Zitelli JA. Surgical margins for basal cell carcinoma. *Arch Dermatol.* 1987;123:340–344.
14. Huang CC, Boyce SM. Surgical margins of excision for basal cell carcinoma and squamous cell carcinoma. *Sem Cut Med Surg.* 2004;23:167–173.
15. Breuninger H, Dietz K. Prediction of subclinical tumor infiltration in basal cell carcinoma. *J Dermatol Surg Oncol.* 1991;17:574–578.
16. Panje WR, Ceilley RI. The influence of embryology of the mid-face on the spread of epithelial malignancies. *Laryngoscope.* 1979;89:1914–1920.
17. Weber RS, Lippman SM, McNeese MD. Advanced basal and squamous cell carcinomas of the skin of the head and neck. *Cancer Treat Res.* 1990;52:61–81.
18. Hendrix JD Jr., Parlette HL. Duplicitous growth of infiltrative basal cell carcinoma: analysis of clinically undetected tumor extent in a paired case-control study. *Dermatol Surg.* 1996;22:535–539.
19. Ballantyne AJ, McCarten AB, Ibanez ML. The extension of cancer of the head and neck through peripheral nerves. *Am J Surg.* 1963;106:651–667.
20. Goepfert H, Dichtel WJ, Medina JE, et al. Perineural invasion in squamous cell skin carcinoma of the head and neck. *Am J Surg.* 1984;148:542–547.
21. Garcia-Serra A, Hinerman RW, Mendenhall WM, et al. Carcinoma of the skin with perineural invasion. *Head Neck.* 2003;25:1027–1033.
22. Lai SY, Weinstein GS, Chalian AA, et al. Parotidectomy in the treatment of aggressive cutaneous malignancies. *Arch Otolaryngol Head Neck Surg.* 2002;128:521–526.
23. Ratner D, Thomas CO, Johnson TM, et al. Mohs micrographic surgery for the treatment of dermatofibrosarcoma protuberans. Results of a multiinstitutional series with an analysis of the extent of microscopic spread. *J Am Acad Dermatol.* 1997;37:600–613.
24. Sandel HD, Day T, Richardson MS, et al. Merkel cell carcinoma: does tumor size or depth of invasion correlate

with recurrence, metastasis, or patient survival? *Laryngoscope.* 2006;116:791–795.
25. Gephardt GN, Zarbo RJ. Interinstitutional comparison of frozen section consultations. A College of American Pathologists Q-Probes study of 90,538 cases in 461 institutions. *Arch Pathol Lab Med.* 1996;120:804–809.
26. Kimyai-Asadi A, Goldberg LH, Jih MH. Accuracy of serial transverse cross-sections in detecting residual basal cell carcinoma at the surgical margins of an elliptical excision specimen. *J Am Acad Dermatol.* 2005;53:469–474.
27. Manstein ME, Manstein CH, Smith R. How accurate is frozen section for skin cancers? *Ann Plast Surg.* 2003;50:607–609.
28. Chao C, McMasters KM. Update on the use of sentinel node biopsy in patients with melanoma: who and how. *Curr Opin Oncol.* 2002;14:217–220.
29. Michl C, Starz H, Bachter D, Balda BR. Sentinel lymphonodectomy in nonmelanoma skin malignancies. *Br J Dermatol.* 2003;149:763–769.
30. Wagner JD, Evdokimow DZ, Weisberger E, et al. Sentinel node biopsy for high-risk nonmelanoma cutaneous malignancy. *Arch Dermatol.* 2004;140:75–79.
31. Goepfert H, Jesse RH, Ballantyne AJ. Posterolateral neck dissection. *Arch Otolaryngol.* 1980;106,:618–620.
32. Khurana VG, Mentis DH, O'Brien CJ, et al. Parotid and neck metastases from cutaneous squamous cell carcinoma of the head and neck. *Am J Surg.* 1995;170:446–450.
33. Hong TS, Kriesel KJ, Hartig GK, Harari PM. Parotid area lymph node metastases from cutaneous squamous cell carcinoma: implications for diagnosis, treatment, and prognosis. *Head Neck.* 2005;27:851–856.
34. Chu A, Osguthorpe JD. Nonmelanoma cutaneous malignancy with regional metastasis. *Otolaryngol Head Neck Surg.* 2003;128:663–673.
35. O'Brien CJ, McNeil EB, McMahon JD. Incidence of cervical node involvement in metastatic cutaneous malignancy involving the parotid gland. *Head Neck.* 2001;23:744–748.
36. Audet N, Palme CE, Gullane PJ, et al. Cutaneous metastatic squamous cell carcinoma to the parotid gland: analysis and outcome. *Head Neck.* 2004;26:727–732.
37. Vauterin TJ, Veness MJ, Morgan GJ, et al. Patterns of lymph node spread of cutaneous squamous cell carcinoma of the head and neck. *Head Neck.* 2006;28:785–791.
38. Andruchow JL, Veness MJ, Morgan GJ, et al. Implications for clinical staging of metastatic cutaneous squamous carcinoma of the head and neck based on a multicenter study of treatment outcomes. *Cancer.* 2006;106:1078–1083.
39. O'Brien CJ, McNeil EB, McMahon JD, et al. Significance of clinical stage, extent of surgery, and pathologic findings in metastatic cutaneous squamous carcinoma of the parotid gland. *Head Neck.* 2002;24:417–422.
40. Palme CE, O'Brien CJ, Veness MJ, et al. Extent of parotid disease influences outcome in patients with metastatic cutaneous squamous cell carcinoma. *Arch Otolaryngol Head Neck Surg.* 2003;129:750–753.
41. Talmi YP, Gal R, Finkelstein Y, et al. Squamous and basal cell cancers directly invading major salivary glands. *Ann Plast Surg.* 1991;26:483–487.
42. Jackson GL, Ballantyne AJ. Role of parotidectomy for skin cancer of the head and neck. *Am J Surg.* 1981;142:464–469.
43. Moore BA, Weber RS, Prieto V, et al. Lymph node metastases from cutaneous squamous cell carcinoma of the head and neck. *Laryngoscope.* 2005;115:1561–1567.
44. Taylor BW Jr., Brant TA, Mendenhall NP, et al. Carcinoma of the skin metastatic to parotid area lymph nodes. *Head Neck.* 1991;13:427–433.
45. Barzilai G, Greenberg E, Cohen-Kerem R, Doweck I. Pattern of regional metastases from cutaneous squamous cell carcinoma of the head and neck. *Otolaryngol Head Neck Surg.* 2005;132:852–856.
46. Ying YL, Johnson JT, Myers EN. Squamous cell carcinoma of the parotid gland. *Head Neck.* 2006;28:626–632.
47. Lee K, McKean ME, McGregor IA. Metastatic patterns of squamous carcinoma in the parotid lymph nodes. *Br J Plast Surg.* 1985;38:6–10.
48. Hanke CW, Weisberger EC, Lingeman RE. Cancer of the scalp. *Dermatol Clin.* 1989;7:797–814.
49. Snow SN, Sahl W, Lo JS, et al. Metastatic basal cell carcinoma: report of five cases. *Cancer.* 1994;73:328–335.
50. Stern HS, Haertsch P. Local recurrence and intracerebral spread of squamous cell carcinoma of the scalp. *Plast Reconstr Surg.* 1990;85:284–288.
51. Nguyen TH, Ho DQ. Nonmelanoma skin cancer. *Curr Treat Options Oncol.* 2002;3:193–203.

10

SPECIAL CONSIDERATIONS: PERIAURICULAR LESIONS

PAUL W. GIDLEY

Introduction

In the United States, over one million persons develop cutaneous malignancies every year.[1] The incidence of non-melanoma skin cancer is highest in Australia, with an annual occurrence of 1200 per 100,000 population.[2] In a population-based study, squamous cell carcinoma (SCC) was noted to occur on the ear as the site of first cancer in 12 per 100,000 men and 0.6 per 100,000 women.[3] Fortunately, the mortality rate of nonmelanoma skin cancer, regardless of site of origin, is low, amounting to roughly 0.44 per 100,000.[4]

Overwhelmingly, the leading cause of skin cancer is exposure to ultraviolet solar radiation.[5] In the sun-drenched parts of the United States, cancer of the external ears is a common clinical entity, likely because the prominent location of the external ear renders it very vulnerable to sun exposure. Radiotherapy also has been implicated as a risk factor for development of squamous cell carcinoma (SCC).[6] Cutaneous squamous cell carcinoma has also been identified on the ear in patients with burn chondritis and chronic scarring lupus erythematosus.[7]

Histology of Periauricular Cutaneous Lesions

Typically, basal cell carcinoma (BCC) is the most common skin malignancy. Basal and squamous cell carcinoma are the most common malignancies to affect the outer ear and its surrounding skin.[8] Carcinoma of the auricle and periauricular skin is estimated to account for approximately 6% of all skin tumors, and 5 to 10% of all skin cancers.[9–11] Within the head and neck, the external ear represents the second most common site of cutaneous squamous cell carcinoma.[12] Primary ear SCC accounts for the index lesion in 20% of the patients with documented regional metastases, a higher rate than both lip and cheek primaries.[13]

Unlike other head and neck cutaneous sites, the incidence of SCC of the external ear rivals that of BCC, although BCC is almost 4 times more common than SCC as a cutaneous malignancy.[14–16] Ahmad and Das Gupta[17] determined that the ratio of BCC:SCC for the external ear is nearly equal (1.3 BCC: 1 SCC). Similarly, Bumsted et al[18] analyzed 780 patients with external ear cancer and found that

55% had squamous cell carcinoma. In a review of the literature, SCC comprised 55 to 67% of malignancies of the outer ear, whereas BCC was identified in only 28 to 32%, and melanoma in 1 to 5%.[19]

Although most cutaneous SCCs have a low rate of metastatic spread to regional lymph nodes (range: 0.5 to 5%), auricular and periauricular SCC metastasizes at a much higher rate, ranging from 10 to 16%.[20–27] Likewise, the rate of metastatic spread to regional lymph nodes for melanoma is very high. Byers et al[28] noted an overall incidence of clinically positive nodes in 42 of 102 auricular melanoma patients, and regional metastases predicted worse survival.

Epidemiology and Prognosis

Generally speaking, external ear cancers occur in older, Caucasian men in their 6th and 7th decades of life.[11,18,22,25,27] Men are much more likely to be affected than women—cutaneous SCC is 17 times more common in men.[8,12,29] Although SCC of the outer ear makes up somewhere between 11% to 25% of skin cancers in men, SCC of the outer ear is found in only 0.2 to 3% of women, potentially due to a protective effect from long hair or hairstyles.[3,12,17,30]

When compared to primary lesions of other cutaneous sites, SCC of the auricle has the highest death rate, approaching 47% in one study.[4] Other groups estimate that auricular or pericauricular cancers are responsible for more than 25% of deaths caused by nongenital, nonmelanoma skin cancers.[31] Subsequently, location on the ear is considered a high-risk feature for BCC and SCC, potentially upstaging smaller tumors, as documented in the 2010 American Joint Cancer Committee (AJCC) Staging System and National Comprehensive Cancer Network (NCCN) Guidelines.[32]

Melanoma of the external ear is a unique disease, as the external ear is infrequently involved. In the United States, roughly 1% of the 48,000 new cases of melanoma involve the outer ear, although 20% of melanomas occur in the head and neck.[33,34] External ear melanoma accounts for approximately 7 to 15% of head and neck sites.[28,34] Of the four common subtypes of melanoma, superficial spreading and nodular melanoma are most commonly identified on the external ear.[28]

A recent review of the incidence of external ear cancers seen at the University of Texas MD Anderson Cancer Center is depicted in Table 10–1. In our patient population, basal cell carcinoma was slightly more common than squamous cell carcinoma and its variants. Our patient cohort has nearly as many malignant melanoma patients as SCC, probably

Table 10–1. Histologic Types of External Ear Cancer at the University of Texas MD Anderson Cancer Center (1990–2006).

Cancer Type	N, pts	%
Basal cell carcinoma	527	30.1%
Basosquamous carcinoma	70	4.0%
Squamous cell carcinoma	388	22.2%
Squamous cell carcinoma in situ	41	2.3%
Squamous cell carcinoma, adenoid variant	25	1.4%
Squamous cell carcinoma, spindle cell variant	5	0.3%
Carcinoma in situ, Bowen's disease	8	0.5%
Melanoma, malignant	386	22.1%
Melanoma arising in melanotic freckle	64	3.7%
Melanoma in situ	22	1.3%
Malignant neoplasm unclassifiable	158	9.0%
Carcinoma, NOS	20	1.1%
Merkel cell carcinoma	15	0.9%
Atypical fibrous histiocytoma	6	0.3%
Angiosarcoma	3	0.2%
Unusual tumors*	10	0.6%
Total	1748	100.0%

*Unusual tumors occurring in two or fewer patients during this time include: adnexal carcinoma (1), apocrine carcinoma (1), adenocarcinoma (1), adenoid cystic carcinoma (1), papillary squamous carcinoma (1), sarcomatoid carcinoma (1), sebaceous gland carcinoma (1), atypical fibroxanthoma (2), and angiomatoid fibrous histiocytoma (1).

Source: Used with permission, © Paul Gidley, MD, University of Texas MD Anderson Cancer Center, 2009.

attributable to the institution's location in the "sunbelt" in the southern United States and inherent referral bias as a comprehensive cancer institution.

Pertinent Anatomy

Embryologically, the auricle arises from the six hillocks of His that each give rise to one or more of the structures of the outer ear. The area in front of the ear, at the sideburn in men, marks an area of embryologic fusion planes.[35] These fusion planes are thought to play a role in the depth of invasion of tumors and, perhaps, contribute to the insidious and profound invasion that is a notorious hallmark for this anatomic site.[18] The embryologic compartments from each hillock may also explain why tumor spread is often limited in the early stages of the disease.[35]

Anatomically, the outer ear is described by its subunits: helix, antihelix, tragus, antitragus, lobule, concha, and scapha (Fig 10–1). The conchal bowl can be further subdivided into a concha cavum and a concha cymbum. The scapha is divided by branching of the antihelix, thus creating a fossa triangularis. The ear protrudes from the scalp creating a posterior, or medial, surface.

The skin of the anterior surface of the pinna is tightly bound to the underlying perichondrium and cartilage, whereas the skin of the posterior surface is thicker and contains more intervening soft tissue. The lymphatics occupy the space between the skin and perichondrium. Subsequently, the short vertical distance between the epidermis and the lymphatics may contribute to the increased metastatic rate to lymph nodes for external ear cancer.[36] This close apposition may account for the high incidence of regional metastases from both SCC and melanoma, despite their different cell of origin.[36]

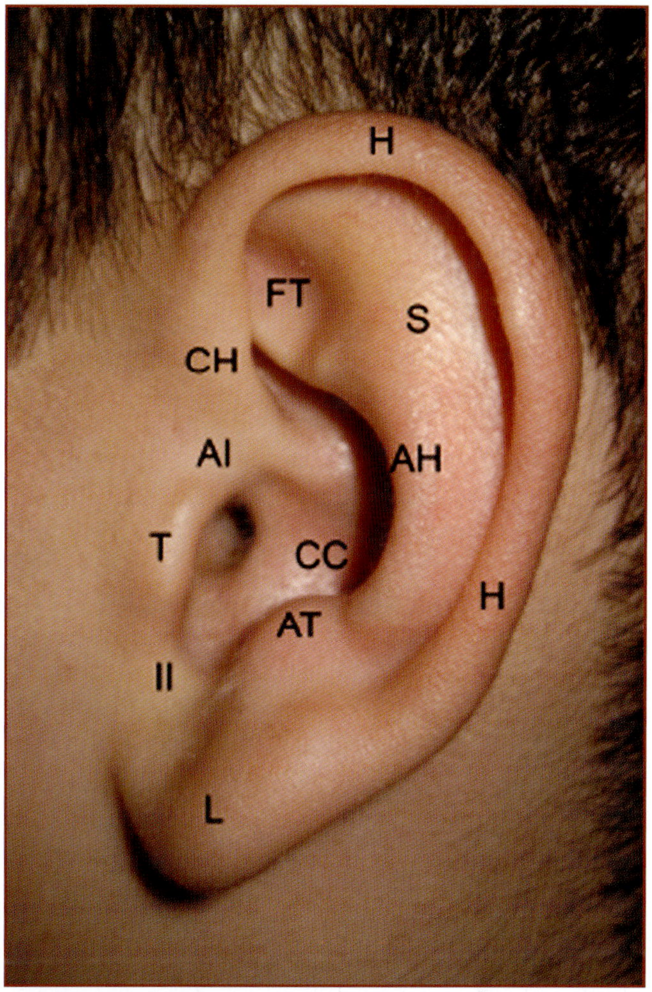

Figure 10–1. Anatomic subdivision of the external ear. Abbreviations: AH-antihelix, AI-anterior incisura, AT-antitragus, CC-conchal cavum, CH-crus of helix, FT-fossa triangularis, H-helix, II-intertragic incisures, L-lobule, S-scaphoid fossa, T-tragus.

Location of Auricular Tumors

The helix constitutes the most common site of auricular cancer, accounting for approximately 50% of tumors.[25,29] This observation is true across the three major histologic types: BCC, SCC, and melanoma (Table 10–2). The concha and scapha account for approximately 17 to 30% of tumors, the posterior surface is involved in 12 to 28% (Fig 10–2), and the lobule is affected in 2.7 to 8% of cases.[19,25,37–39] Interestingly, the triangular fossa and antihelix were not reported as involved by melanoma in two large series.[28,40]

The two sides are equally affected, with only minor differences seen in individual studies. Left

Table 10–2. Sites of External Ear Involvement from Squamous Cell Carcinoma (SCC), Basal Cell Carcinoma (BCC) and Melanoma

Anatomic Site	Bailin[35] BCC	Afzelius[24] SCC	Byers[25] SCC	Shockley[37] SCC	Silapunt[41] SCC	Byers[28] Melanoma	Cole[40] Melanoma
Helix	58%	51%	53%	44%	50.7%	58.8%	47%
Antihelix and triangular fossa	18.6%	15%	19%	14%	17.4%	0%	0%
Posterior pinna	18.6%	27%	14%	27%	16%	0%	11%
Lobule	2.3%	1.5%	5%	6%	6.2%	23.5%	21%
Concha	4.7%	4.5%	5%	6%	7.6%	5.9%	5%
Tragus	0%	0%	4%	3%	1.4%	11.8%	5%

Source: Used with permission, © Paul W. Gidley, MD, UT MD Anderson Cancer Center, 2009.

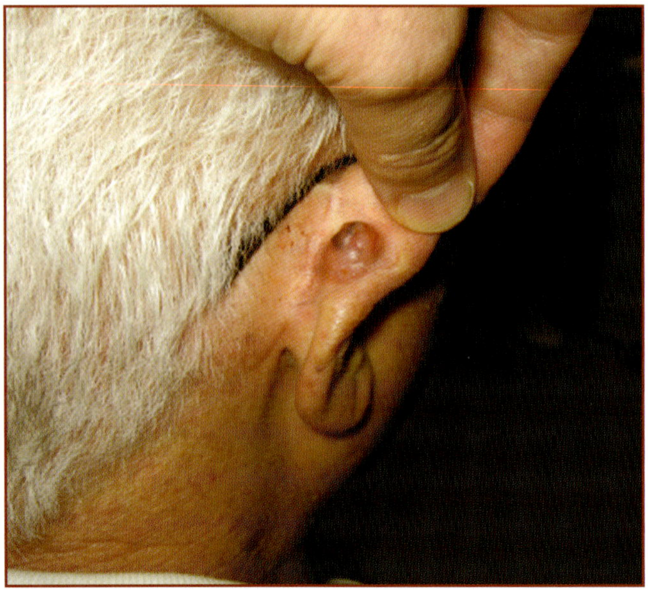

Figure 10–2. Basal cell carcinoma involving the posterior surface of the pinna.

sided primaries occur in 39.6% to 62% of patients, versus 38 to 60% on the right in various studies.[19,24,29,37,41] Bilateral disease occurs in roughly 10% of patients.[19] Of note, up to 18% of patients may develop either multiple lesions or bilateral lesions during their clinical course.[25] Subsite of origin may carry some prognostic significance, as centrally located tumors of the concha, tragus, and antitragus have a worse prognosis than more peripherally positioned tumors in melanoma, but this observation has not been confirmed in other studies.[42]

Staging

The external ear does not have a unique staging system. The staging systems for external ear cancer is based on fundamental histology and adheres to the same principles as cutaneous malignancies from other anatomic regions, excluding the eyelid. The 2010 AJCC Staging Systems address many of the weaknesses of prior versions.[32] For the first time, depth of invasion, primary site location, histology, and perineural invasion receive added focus as high-risk features in nonmelanoma skin cancer. Invasion of bone (including the temporal bone), muscle, or cartilage classify a T3 lesion, but perineural invasion at the skull base constitutes a T4 lesion.

Previously, many authors concluded that the TNM staging system poorly prognosticates the metastatic potential.[13,43] Tumor size is predictive of disease-specific survival, and tumors less than 4 cm in size have a significantly better survival than those larger than 4 cm ($p = 0.002$).[44] O'Brien championed modifications of the TNM system for nonmelanoma skin cancer of the head and neck to account for parotid and cervical node involvement, and many of his precepts were incorporated into the 2010 AJCC TNM system.[32,45]

Risk Factors for Nodal Metastasis in Periauricular Skin Cancer

Although indications for evaluation of regional lymphatics are well accepted in malignant melanoma (MM), risk factors for nodal metastasis and management philosophies continue to evolve from a historically reactive posture in nonmelanoma skin cancer (NMSC). Many risk factors were extrapolated from other body primary sites. Few have specifically examined auricular and periauricular issues, although this subsite exhibits some unique features regarding regional metastases.

Periauricular Lesions

In general, primary cutaneous malignancies of the ear and adjacent tissues are associated with an increased rate of lymphatic metastases in both NMSC and MM.[11,24,46,47] Rowe et al[47] reported a metastatic rate for ear lesions of 11.0%, versus 5.2% for other sun-exposed sites. Similarly, location on the ear was identified as a risk factor for metastatic spread in a multivariate analysis of 615 patients with cutaneous SCC.[46] However, not all reports support this association.[25,38,48,49] Veness et al[13] comment that any tumor in proximity to the parotid gland should be considered high-risk for metastatic spread.

Lateral Dimension Over 2 Cm

Horizontal size more than 2 cm, the cutoff between T1 and T2 lesions in the TNM system, has also been associated with regional metastases.[44,46,47,50] In an analysis of over 220 published reports, Rowe et al[47] determined that lesions under 2 cm in size had a metastatic rate of 9.1%, whereas lesions over 2 cm in size had a metastatic rate of 30.3%. Although this analysis includes ear SCC, the data are not specific for the ear as a subsite.

Increasing horizontal spread may be a hallmark of aggressive disease, as 50% of patients with an initial primary tumor size of larger than 3 cm manifest neck metastasis in a series of 160 patients with SCC of the pinna.[26] In this study, patients with metastatic disease exhibited a mean primary tumor size of 2.8 cm compared to 1.7 cm in patients without metastasis. Subsequent reports have supported this contention, with size larger than 2 cm indicating a greater likelihood of regional metastases.[8,13] However, there also is evidence to suggest that increasing lateral size may not be as important in auricular cancer.[25] Lee et al[11] studied 147 cases of SCC of the external ear and reported 14 patients with metastatic neck disease, all of whom had primary tumors less than 2 cm.

Increasing Tumor Thickness

Tumor thickness more than 4 mm has been found to be highly predictive for local recurrence and regional metastasis.[13,46,47,51] The risk of metastasis from skin lesions deeper than 8 mm is so great that prophylactic lymph node dissection or treatment has been advocated in NMSC.[47] Metastases have been documented in 4% of patients with tumors 2.1 to 6.0 mm in thickness and in 16% of patients with tumors thicker than 6.0 mm.[46] Thickness greater than 5 mm may be an important determinant of lymph node metastasis, as 17.5% of 509 patients with SCC developed nodal metastases within a mean follow-up of 5.3 years, versus 2.9% of lesions under 5 mm.[52] The depth threshold for lymphatic metastases may be even lower, as Veness et al[13] identified a majority (65%) of tumors with metastatic spread were larger than 4 mm in thickness.

Depth of Invasion

Afzelius et al[24] reported that tumors reaching Clark level V had a metastatic rate of 30.6%, whereas tumors reaching Clark level IV had only a 10% rate.

Although multiple studies have indicated that patients with metastasis were more likely to have deeper depth of growth, at least beyond Clark III, than patients without metastasis ($p < 0.01$), other authors were not able to reproduce this connection.[24,26,50] Tumor invasiveness has been correlated to incomplete surgical margins, and invasion beyond subcutaneous tissues has been described as an independent indicator of disease control and survival.[44,53]

Degree of Differentiation

Poorly differentiated or undifferentiated NMSC are more likely to recur and metastasize than well-differentiated lesions.[47,50,52,54] As with other surveys of risk factors for nodal disease, other authors have not been able to link histologic differentiation to regional spread.[24–26,46]

Immunosuppression

Although fewer than 5% of patients with cutaneous malignancy of the head and neck are immunosuppressed, immunosuppression, especially after solid organ transplantation, has been linked to the development of aggressive NMSC.[13,43] The chance of a patient developing a skin cancer after renal transplantation is roughly 66% within 24 years, and these patients manifest regional metastasis and disease-related death with smaller index lesions.[46,56]

Other Histopathologic Risk Factors

Positive margins, recurrent lesions, and desmoplastic SCC have each been identified as risk factors for regional metastases in auricular carcinoma.[26,46,47,52,54] Recurrent tumors exhibit up to a 45% incidence of lymph node metastasis.[47] Similarly, perineural invasion, which is identified in 5 to 10% of cutaneous SCC of the head and neck, is associated with nodal metastases and distant metastases.[13,50,57–60] Lymphovascular invasion often coexists with perineural invasion, indicating an aggressive phenotype that is prone to lymphatic spread.[60]

Incidence of Lymph Node Metastasis in Periauricular Skin Cancer

Several studies have examined the incidence of lymph node metastasis. The overall incidence of lymph node metastasis from SCC is 2 to 4%.[22,23,46] Lymph node metastasis represents a significant prognostic marker for both NMSC and MM. In the United States, 2,500 patients die annually from advanced skin cancer and invariably develop metastatic lymph nodes during their clinical course.[61]

Lewis[39] was the first to note the high metastatic rate of SCC of the outer ear; his landmark paper revealed a 15% metastatic rate. Although cutaneous SCC from other body areas have a low rate of metastatic spread to regional lymph nodes, ranging from 0.5 to 2%, SCC from the outer ear metastasizes at a much higher rate, ranging from 10 to 16%.[20,21,24–26] The nodal metastases often are frequently not apparent clinically and are often identified on pathologic analysis of surgical specimens.[25,36]

The rate of metastatic spread from auricular melanoma is even higher, perhaps as high as 40%.[62] Byers et al[28] noted an overall incidence of clinically positive nodes in 42 of 102 patients with melanoma of the outer ear, and the presence of metastatic neck disease is a significant correlate for survival.

The majority of patients who develop regional spread will do so within the first year following diagnosis. Clark and Soutar[36] found that lymph node metastasis occurred in 85% of patients within the first 12 months, and in 98% of patients within the first 24 months of diagnosis. Other authors support a median time to presentation with delayed metastases of 9 to 10 months from the index lesion.[8,63]

Mechanisms of Spread for Auricular Skin Cancer

Both SCC and BCC spread in the mesodermal plane of the auricle before spreading into cartilage or bone, and these tumors remain localized to the auricle until late in their clinical course.[35,64] Bailin et al[35] noted that tumors of the helix spread longitudinally before involving the antihelix or posterior surface of the ear, whereas conchal bowl and antihelical fold tumors evolve concentrically. Tumors that involve the lobule may further spread to directly invade the parotid gland, and those that arise in preauricular skin tend to grow toward the superior helix and tragus. Once the tragus is reached, tumors can spread along the tragal cartilage to involve the parotid, temporomandibular joint, and other deep structures.[35] Postauricular tumors tend to grow toward the helix and then spread along the length of the helix. Once the helix is involved, these tumors then spread to the antihelix and ear canal. Mohs et al[65] notes that these postauricular tumors are notorious for a high rate of recurrence, likely due to spread of disease in the dermis, perichondrium, periosteum, nerve sheaths, and embryologic fusion planes.

The lymphatics of the outer ear drain to preauricular, postauricular, parotid and upper cervical lymph nodes.[25,29,66] The parotid and upper jugular nodes are the most frequent site of involvement.[26,28,36,66] Turner et al noted that 70% of their patients had parotid involvement, 30% had cervical node involvement, and 14% had both.[8] The most common site of cervical lymph node involvement is levels II and III, and suboccipital nodes have not been found to be involved by periauricular primaries.[8,25]

Management of Auricular and Periauricular Skin Cancer

Surgical Margins

Consistent with all head and neck tumors, negative surgical margins are associated with superior disease-free and overall survival. Incompletely excised tumors are at high risk for local recurrence and neck metastasis, regardless of histology.[47,67] In a prospective study of BCC treated with Mohs micrographic surgery, Wolf and Zitelli[68] found than 4-mm margins were needed to eradicate 95% of BCC less than 2 cm in diameter. Such margins may be difficult to achieve on the ear without significant cosmetic deformity. Perhaps it is not surprising that numerous authors have shown that the rate of incomplete excision of SCC from the external ear is higher than all other skin sites (20.5% vs 4.8%, $p = 0.001$).[53,69] As a result, larger excision margins of 5 mm are recommended when feasible.[69] Positive margins may be a stronger predictor for disease control in NMSC than surgeon experience and training, tumor size, and patient factors such as gender and age.[53,69]

The most recent National Comprehensive Cancer Network guideline recommends a 4- to 6-mm surgical margin for SCC.[32] Similar support is found for margins of at least 4 mm in uncomplicated, primary BCC and SCC under 2 cm in lateral dimension.[67,68]

Margins for melanoma have been studied extensively. Narayan and Ariyan[70] did not observe any recurrences for auricular melanoma patients with 1-cm negative margins. Pockaj[71] reported that 80% of recurrences occurred in patients with a margin less than 1 cm. Most authors recommend a 1-cm margin for invasive ear melanoma.[70,72]

Essentially the same, if not slightly larger, margins should be taken for cutaneous malignancy of the auricle as for other body sites, despite the potential for cosmetic deformity. It remains unclear whether surgeon reticence to create morbidity or intrinsic features of auricular malignancy, or both, constitute the major contributor to positive margins and local recurrence. Although technically challenging, reconstruction or prosthetic rehabilitation of auricular defects may be readily accomplished and is discussed elsewhere in this text.

Surgical Techniques

Cryosurgery or Curettage and Electrodesiccation[73,74]

Both cryosurgery and electrodessication and curettage (ED&C) have been reported to be useful in previously untreated, nodular BCC.[73,74] In ED&C, the tumor is electrodesiccated and removed with a curette that allows the surgeon to distinguish between tumor and normal skin, based on subtle tactile differences between tumor and healthy tissue.[68] Although this author does not have experience with these techniques, the interested reader is referred to other sections in this text and key references.[75]

Recurrence rates for favorable basal cell carcinomas after cryosurgery or ED&C are generally low, but repeated treatments might be required.[75] Neither treatment is appropriate for tumors that are large, infiltrating, fibrosing, or recurrent, particularly on the ear, which has been identified as a high-risk area for recurrence when treated by such techniques.[76]

Mohs Micrographic Surgery (MMS)

For SCC, MMS has been shown to effective in complete excision of disease and superior in local tissue conservation.[77] In a cosmetically prominent area such as the external ear, conservation of local tissue is important. Multiple studies have shown low recurrence rates with this technique, usually less than 5%.[18,41,47,65,78–80] Primary wound closure, split thickness skin grafts, healing by secondary intention, and local flaps have all been described in the reconstruction of the resulting defect.[77,81]

Standard Excision

The goal of surgical excision is complete tumor removal with minimal cosmetic deformity.[25,26,82] As most tumors occur on the helix, simple wedge excision with primary closure can be achieved with good cosmetic results. However, resections should be performed in a comprehensive fashion, without biasing the reconstructive technique, as wedge resection and primary closure is not a panacea for helical lesions. Tumors of the conchal bowl can be excised and the site reconstructed with a skin graft. Local flaps may be employed in reconstructing helical, scapha, conchal bowl, and lobule defects, and these techniques are well described.[77,82–101]

Total Auriculectomy

Total auriculectomy is required only for tumors that occupy most of the pinna (Fig 10–3). It has been our experience that, in this circumstance, the tumor almost always extends into the ear canal, and complete excision will require a lateral temporal bone resection. Leaving the ear canal intact, while excising all of the external ear cartilage, risks canal stenosis and trapping of debris, with chronic otorrhea that may be compounded by postoperative radiotherapy.

Temporal Bone Considerations

Tumors that extend from the outer ear into the ear canal deserve special attention. Generally, tumors

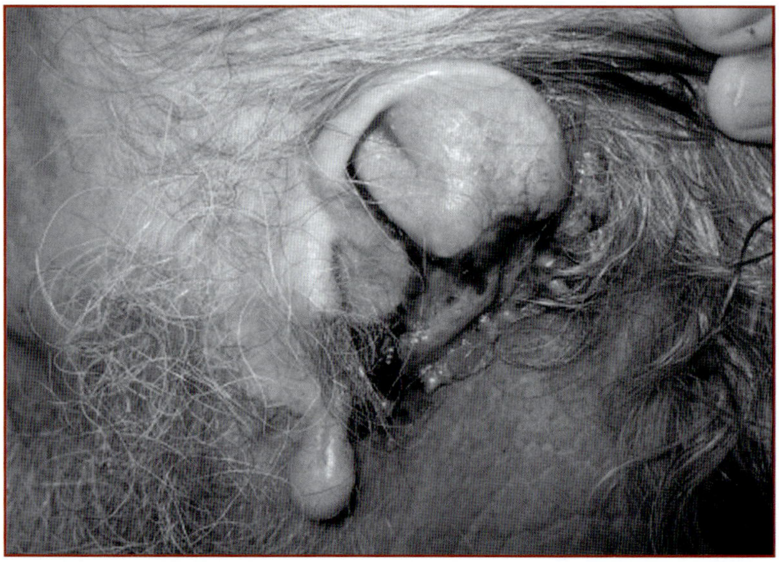

Figure 10–3. Neglected basal cell carcinoma involving the outer ear.

that do not extend past the bony-cartilaginous junction of the ear canal can be cleared with wide local excision of the lesion. In the cartilaginous canal, the cartilage provides an important deep margin and may be readily resected along with the overlying skin tumor. An incision between the tragus and root of the helix may improve visualization of the tumor margins. Excision is improved with dissection under the operative microscope. The defect can be adequately reconstructed with a skin graft.

However, when the tumor involves the bony ear canal, the tumor cannot be reliably cleared with local excision alone (Fig 10–4). In the bony canal, the skin is thin and directly overlies bone. Scraping the tumor off the bone does not provide an adequate surgical margin, and recurrence rates are high with this approach. For this circumstance, lateral temporal bone resection (LTBR) is required.

LTBR is performed through a postauricular mastoidectomy approach. The facial nerve is identified and preserved in the middle ear and mastoid. The bony canal is disarticulated from the petrous temporal bone, removing the tympanic membrane, malleus, and incus. Total auriculectomy is not a prerequisite for LTBR. Incisions can be designed that adequately excise the involved portions of the external ear with the ear canal, leaving the remainder of the outer ear intact.

Superficial parotidectomy usually will be required for tumors that involve the external auditory canal. If the tumor involves the temporomandibular joint (TMJ), then the TMJ can be resected concurrent with LTBR as an en bloc procedure.

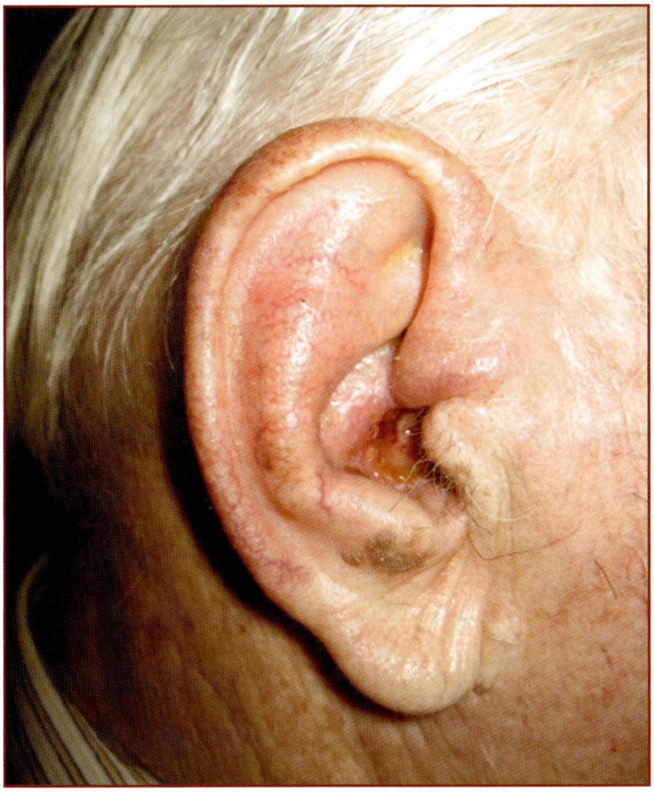

Figure 10–4. Squamous cell carcinoma of conchal bowl. The disease extends subcutaneously under the crus of the helix and into the external ear canal. Surgical excision required lateral temporal bone resection, parotidectomy, neck dissection, and reconstruction with an anterolateral thigh-free flap.

Role of Sentinel Lymph Node Biopsy

The role of sentinel lymph node biopsy (SLNB) has yet to be defined for auricular NMSC. The rationale for SLNB is to identify potential lymph nodes for sampling in the clinically N0 neck. SLNB has been shown to be effective at determining the rate of occult malignancies in melanoma and in some head and neck squamous cell carcinomas.[40,43,50,63,71,102–113] Sentinel lymph node biopsy has been reported in patients with melanoma of the external ear, although the indications are not unique for this anatomic site. Similar to other regions, negative SLNB results support an excellent prognosis.[40,71]

Pathak et al[104] studied lymphatic metastasis from head and neck melanoma, and including 20 patients with ear melanoma in their cohort of 169 patients. There was a 100% correlation between the predicted site of involvement and the clinical site of metastatic disease for the auricle, namely the parotid and cervical lymph node levels I through V. This finding represented a dramatic contradistinction from the reported 34% discordance between lymphoscintigraphic positive nodes and clinically suspected basins elsewhere. Even when lymphoscintigraphy suggests involvement of postauricular nodes, no metastases were documented in this basin from ear or periauricular melanomas.[114] This predilection for MM to drain to the parotid and upper cervical nodes, rather than occipital or posterior cervical nodes, has been corroborated by other authors.[107]

Shpitzer[111] studied SLNB in 15 patients with melanoma of the helix of the ear. Tumor thickness varied from 0.70 mm to 10 mm, with a mean of 1.2 mm and a median of 2.13 mm. Sentinel lymph nodes were found in level IIA in 13 of the 15 patients (87%) and in the parotid gland in 4 patients (27%). No lymph nodes were found in the retroauricular region. All examined lymph nodes examined free of metastatic deposits, and all patients remained tumor free during a short follow-up of 39 months.[111]

Parotidectomy and Neck Dissection

Nonmelanoma Skin Cancer

A persistent controversy in the discussion of SCC of the external ear is the role of elective parotidectomy and neck dissection. Although the parotid gland contains lymph nodes that can be the first echelon in metastatic spread from an external ear site, elective parotidectomy has not been endorsed.[29] Historically, authors have surmised that parotid involvement is infrequent, and therefore, parotidectomy was unwarranted unless clinically involved, but these discussions predominately occurred before the sentinel node era.[38]

In the presence of clinically apparent disease or a positive SLN biopsy, parotidectomy and upper neck dissection is warranted. The risks of parotidectomy are well known and include facial nerve injury, cosmetic deformity, and Frey's syndrome.[115] The incidence of temporary facial paralysis in this setting ranges from 5% to 43%, whereas permanent paralysis is usually less than 3%.[29,60,116–124]

As a principle, a working facial nerve should be spared unless overtly and macroscopically involved with tumor.[8] The patient with a past history of skin cancer, particularly in the temporoparietal region, who returns with a partial or total facial palsy should be viewed with caution. This patient likely has perineural spread along the facial nerve, with the resultant weakness. Occasionally, cancer from the sideburn area can travel along the auriculotemporal nerve, potentially involving both the facial and the trigeminal nerves (Fig 10–5).[125]

Rates of facial nerve sacrifice are difficult to compare. Byers[25] noted that 46 patients out his series of 486 required facial nerve sacrifice. The study by Moore et al[60] found that, in patients with aggressive cutaneous SCC, facial nerve preservation could be performed in only 70% of patients. The majority of patients benefit from superficial parotidectomy with preservation of the facial nerve to manage suspected metastatic disease within the parotid.[60] Radical parotidectomy with facial nerve sacrifice is indicated for macroscopic nerve involvement or preoperative facial nerve dysfunction. For the patient with a clinically involved parotid gland, cervical lymphadenectomy, minimally including levels II and III, should be also be performed, as a significant proportion of these clinically N0 necks will harbor occult metastatic disease (30 to 42%).[8,48,60]

The role of neck dissection in the clinically N0 neck remains a topic of discussion about a broad range of tumor types and locations within the head and neck. Historically, a 20% rate of occult neck metastasis represented the threshold of risk that justified neck dissection, but this threshold has been lowered to 15%.[126,127] Migration to selective neck dissection rather than radical neck dissection avoids many of complications of radical neck dissection and allows for this broadening of the indications. In the absence of SLNB in NMSC, elective neck dissection in the N0 neck promotes proper staging and determining the role of adjuvant therapy.[128,129]

In the report by Byers et al,[25] the constellation of initial ear cancer, histologically poorly differentiated tumor, and lesion over 3 cm merits a comprehensive supraomohyoid neck dissection, sparing the spinal accessory nerve, jugular vein, and sternocleidomastoid muscle. Nodal metastases frequently occur in concert with recurrent auricular lesions that also must be aggressively addressed, often with auriculectomy.[8,47] Surgical management of the parotid and regional lymphatics may strongly be considered in this scenario, particularly in patients who have been previously radiated.

Malignant Melanoma

As previously discussed, sentinel lymph node biopsy has supplanted elective nodal dissection in the management of malignant melanoma of the auricle and

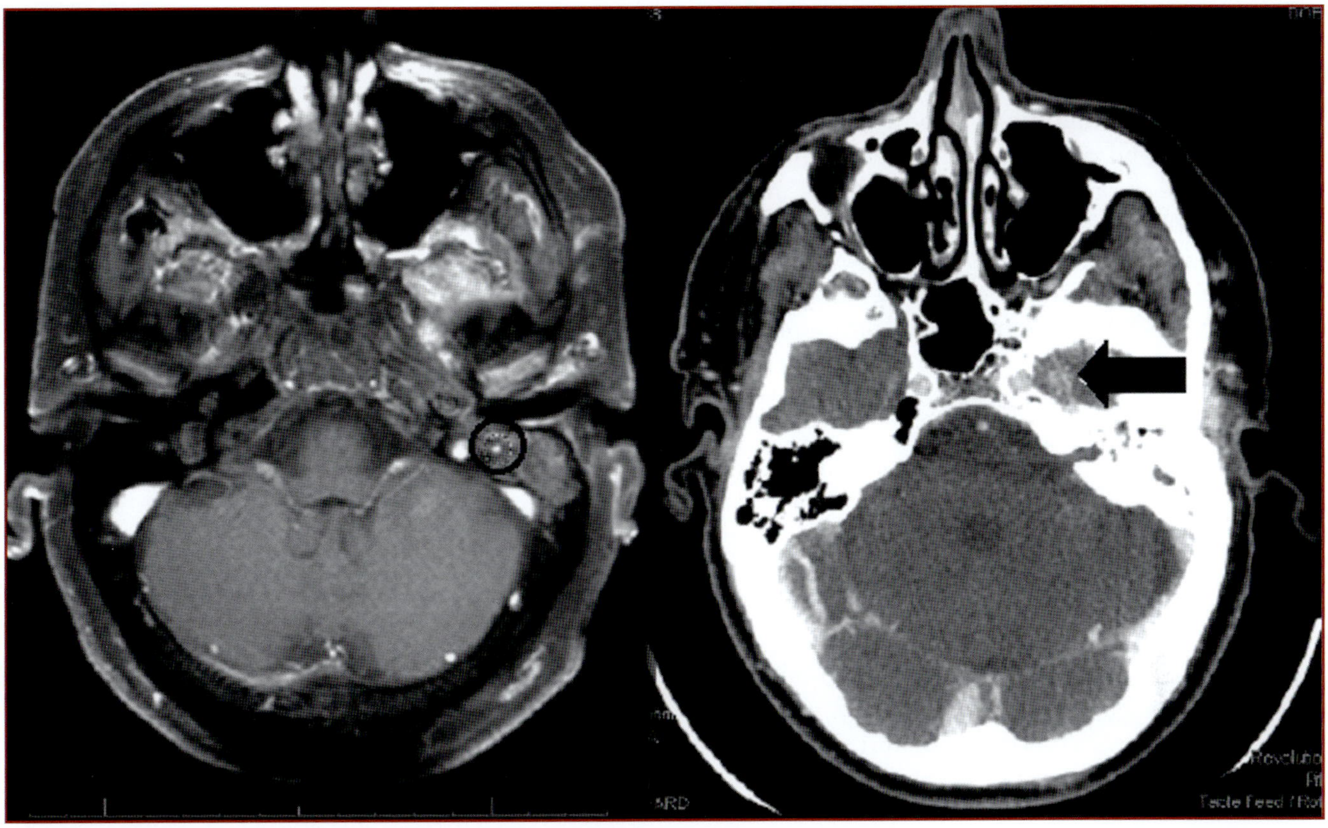

Figure 10–5. Perineural spread along the left facial and trigeminal nerves from an ear canal squamous cell carcinoma. **A.** Axial MRI showing enhancement of the mastoid portion of the left facial nerve (*circled*). **B.** Axial CT showing enhancement of the left trigeminal nerve as it enters Meckel's cave (*arrow*).

periauricular region. Multiple large, prospective, randomized trials failed to demonstrate a survival benefit for elective lymphadenectomy.[130–133] Although regional failure often portends a poor prognosis, Byers could not elucidate a survival difference between elective or salvage neck dissection in auricular melanoma.[28] Sentinel lymph node biopsy remains the standard for assessing subclinical regional metastases in MM, determining the need for therapeutic treatment of the regional lymphatics and systemic therapy. Logically, the applications of SLNB are extending into nonmelanoma skin cancer.

Radiotherapy

Radiotherapy has been used either as single modality therapy or as adjuvant therapy in the postoperative setting. Most multidisciplinary teams advocate primary surgical therapy for auricular and periauricular cutaneous malignancy, reserving radiotherapy for recurrences or locoregional failures.[25] Primary radiotherapy for auricular primaries lacks high level supporting evidence.[13] Adjuvant radiotherapy has been shown to increase local and regional control in aggressive SCC of the ear.[134]

Adjuvant Radiotherapy

The majority of patients will be managed successfully with wide local excision achieving negative margins. Postoperative radiotherapy (PORT) should be considered for the patient with key pathologic indicators: multiple positive lymph nodes, extracapsular spread, perineural invasion, involvement of a named nerve, lymphovascular invasion, and positive or "close" margins. Furthermore, PORT may be employed for extensive local disease requiring resection of the temporomandibular joint or ascending ramus of the mandible, or when temporal bone resection or total parotidectomy are required.[25]

The role of radiotherapy for external ear cancer and the clinical N0 neck has not been suggested or reported, although there has been proven benefit for other diseases with suspected micrometastasis.[135,136] Aggressive NMSC exhibiting the aforementioned features may benefit from adjuvant RT, with improvements in locoregional control and survival compared to single modality therapy.[45,137–141] Recent publications suggest 60 Gy in 2-Gy daily fractions as an acceptable dose for positive disease, along with 50 Gy to the undissected neck, if applicable.[43,60]

Survival and Recurrence Rates

The ear, anterior scalp, forehead, and temple are the most frequent sites of primary SCC in the head and neck.[43] Survival is overwhelmingly dependent on locoregional control. Most patients with SCC who experience a relapse will do so in the regional lymphatic basins. Logically, any treatment that improves locoregional control is likely to increase survival.

As previously stated, neck recurrences usually do not occur coincident with the primary lesion, but usually become apparent within 9 to 12 months.[142,143] Recurrence rates for SCC of the ear are higher than for other sun-exposed skin, reaching 18.7% in one study, compared to 7.9% for other body areas.[47] This discrepancy may reflect intrinsic characteristics of the ear or surgeon reticence to create significant disfigurement and morbidity.

Neck recurrence rates are also higher for external ear (11.0%) than for other body sites (5.2%), with a significant impact on overall survival.[47] Byers et al[25] noted that the 2-year and 5-year survival of patients with SCC of the external ear and neck disease was 65% and 46%, respectively. If two or more nodes were found, then survival rates dropped to 57% and 14%, respectively.[25] Interestingly, they found extracapsular spread (ECS) in 93% of patients; this was not a significant contributor on univariate analysis. Clearly, aggressive treatment is indicated for these patients, and multidisciplinary treatment is required, although locoregional failure may still occur in 10% to 38% of cases.[8,43,60,144]

Unfortunately, recurrence following multimodality therapy is often regional (70 to 80%), and often incurable.[144] Survival for the patient with recurrent squamous cell cancer following multimodality therapy is poor. Overall survival is 65% at 2 years and 46% at 5 years.[27] Lymph node metastasis is associated with lower 3-year disease-free survival, disease-specific survival, and overall survival.[60] A summary of outcomes in published studies of external ear SCC is presented in Table 10–3.

Conclusion

The auricle and periauricular region frequently are involved by cutaneous malignancy of the head and neck. Auricular skin cancer is associated with more aggressive disease, including recurrence, regional metastases, and disease-related mortality, compared to skin cancers of other sites. As such, aggressive therapy with wide local excision or Mohs micrographic surgery is required, achieving wide negative margins. Auriculectomy or lateral temporal bone resection may be required. Regional metastases involve the parotid gland and upper cervical lymphatics, and SLNB or elective dissection may be considered, depending on histology, for large, recurrent, deeply invasive, or otherwise aggressive malignancies. Both the upper cervical nodes and parotid should be surgically treated if one or the other is involved, and every effort should be made to save a functioning facial nerve in the absence of direct tumor invasion.

Patients with aggressive auricular and periauricular cutaneous malignancies demand similarly aggressive treatment, and these patients benefit from multidisciplinary evaluation and treatment.

Table 10–3. Compilation of Published Reports of SCC of the External Ear. Parotid and Neck Metastasis Rates Are at Presentation.

Authors	Year	Total No. Patients	Median Age, yrs (Range)	Parotid Metastasis Rate at Presentation	Neck Metastasis Rate at Presentation	Local Recurrence Rate	Regional Recurrence Rate	Distant Metastasis Rate	Overall Survival	Disease-Free Survival	Mean F/U, months
Silapunt et al[41]*	2005	117	71 (34–90 yrs)	NS	NS	3.4%	2.6%	NS	NS	NS	NS
Thomas and Matthews[19]	1994	44	76 (61–91 yrs)	NS	0%	14.8%	9.3%	NS	NS	NS	NS
Yoon et al[27]	1992	40	71 (43–93 yrs)	NS	10%	22.5%	20%	7.5%	70% at 5 years	NS	NS
Mohs et al[65]	1988	871	NS	NS	NS	NS	NS	NS	92.3% (5-yr cure rate)		
Shockley and Stucker[37]	1987	75	66 (range NS)	NS	NS	12.5%	10%	2.5%	93% (F/U NS)	NS	NS
Byers et al[25]	1983	486	68 (16–98 yrs)	NS	6%	14%	6%	1%	68% at 2 yrs 48% at 5 yrs		
Freedlander and Chung[26]	1983	160	72 yrs (range NS)	9.4%	11.3%	17%	13%	NS	93% (F/U more than 12 months)	NS	NS

*Mohs Micrographic surgery technique.

NS—not stated.

References

1. SEER Cancer Statistics Review, 1975–2003, National Cancer Institute. Bethesda, MD, based on November 2005 SEER data submission, posted to the SEER Web site, 2006. (Retrieved from http://seer.cancer.gov/csr/1975_2003/.)
2. Staples MP, Elwood M, Burton RC, Williams JL, Marks R, Giles GG. Non-melanoma skin cancer in Australia: the 2002 national survey and trends since 1985. *Med J Aust.* 2006;184(1):6–10.
3. Chuang TY, Popescu NA, Su WP, Chute CG. Squamous cell carcinoma. A population-based incidence study in Rochester, Minn. *Arch Dermatol.* 1990;126(2):185–188.
4. Weinstock MA, Bogaars HA, Ashley M, Litle V, Bilodeau E, Kimmel S. Nonmelanoma skin cancer mortality. A population-based study. *Arch Dermatol* 1991;127(8):1194–1197.
5. Ramirez CC, Federman DG, Kirsner RS. Skin cancer as an occupational disease: the effect of ultraviolet and other forms of radiation. *Int J Dermatol.* 2005;44(2):95–100.
6. Conley J, Schuller DE. Malignancies of the ear. *Laryngoscope.* 1976;86(8):1147–1163.
7. Levine H. Cutaneous carcinoma of the head and neck: management of massive and previously uncontrolled lesions. *Laryngoscope.* 1983;93(1):87–105.
8. Turner SJ, Morgan GJ, Palme CE, Veness MJ. Metastatic cutaneous squamous cell carcinoma of the external ear: a high-risk cutaneous subsite. *J Laryngol Otol.* 2009;1(1):1–6.
9. Pless J. Carcinoma of the external ear. *Scand J Plast Reconstr Surg.* 1976;10(2):147–151.
10. Gal TJ, Futran ND, Bartels LJ, Klotch DW. Auricular carcinoma with temporal bone invasion: outcome analysis. *Otolaryngol Head Neck Surg.* 1999;121(1):62–65.
11. Lee D, Nash M, Har-El G. Regional spread of auricular and periauricular cutaneous malignancies. *Laryngoscope.* 1996;106(8):998–1001.
12. Iversen T, Tretli S. Trends for invasive squamous cell neoplasia of the skin in Norway. *Br J Cancer.* 1999;81(3):528–531.
13. Veness MJ, Palme CE, Morgan GJ. High-risk cutaneous squamous cell carcinoma of the head and neck: results from 266 treated patients with metastatic lymph node disease. *Cancer.* 2006;106(11):2389–2396.
14. Mackie R. Epidermal skin tumours. In: Champion R, Burton D, Breathnach S, eds. *Text Book of Dermatology.* Oxford, UK: Blackwell Science, Ltd; 1998:1651–1658.
15. Buettner PG, Raasch BA. Incidence rates of skin cancer in Townsville, Australia. *Int J Cancer.* 1998;78(5):587–593.
16. Raasch B, Maclennan R, Wronski I, Robertson I. Body site specific incidence of basal and squamous cell carcinoma in an exposed population, Townsville, Australia. *Mutat Res.* 1998;422(1):101–106.
17. Ahmad I, Das Gupta AR. Epidemiology of basal cell carcinoma and squamous cell carcinoma of the pinna. *J Laryngol Otol.* 2001;115(2):85–86.
18. Bumsted RM, Ceilley RI, Panje WR, Crumley RL. Auricular malignant neoplasms. When is chemotherapy (Mohs' technique) necessary? *Arch Otolaryngol.* 1981;107(11):721–724.
19. Thomas SS, Matthews RN. Squamous cell carcinoma of the pinna: a 6–year study. *Br J Plast Surg.* 1994;47(2):81–85.
20. Lund HZ. Metastasis from sun-induced squamous-cell carcinoma of the skin: an uncommon event. *J Dermatol Surg Oncol.* 1984;10(3):169–170.
21. Katz AD, Urbach F, Lilienfeld AM. The frequency and risk of metastases in squamous-cell carcinoma of the skin. *Cancer.* 1957;10(6):1162–1166.
22. Czarnecki D, Staples M, Mar A, Giles G, Meehan C. Metastases from squamous cell carcinoma of the skin in southern Australia. *Dermatology.* 1994;189(1):52–54.
23. Joseph MG, Zulueta WP, Kennedy PJ. Squamous cell carcinoma of the skin of the trunk and limbs: the incidence of metastases and their outcome. *Aust N Z J Surg.* 1992;62(9):697–701.
24. Afzelius LE, Gunnarsson M, Nordgren H. Guidelines for prophylactic radical lymph node dissection in cases of carcinoma of the external ear. *Head Neck Surg.* 1980;2(5):361–365.
25. Byers R, Kesler K, Redmon B, Medina J, Schwarz B. Squamous carcinoma of the external ear. *Am J Surg.* 1983;146(4):447–450.
26. Freedlander E, Chung FF. Squamous cell carcinoma of the pinna. *Br J Plast Surg.* 1983;36(2):171–175.
27. Yoon M, Chougule P, Dufresne R, Wanebo HJ. Localized carcinoma of the external ear is an unrecognized aggressive disease with a high propensity for local regional recurrence. *Am J Surg.* 1992;164(6):574–577.
28. Byers RM, Smith JL, Russell N, Rosenberg V. Malignant melanoma of the external ear. Review of 102 cases. *Am J Surg.* 1980;140(4):518–521.
29. Osborne RF, Shaw T, Zandifar H, Kraus D. Elective parotidectomy in the management of advanced auricular malignancies. *Laryngoscope.* 2008;118(12):2139–2145.
30. Kaldor J, Shugg D, Young B, Dwyer T, Wang YG. Nonmelanoma skin cancer: ten years of cancer-registry-based surveillance. *Int J Cancer.* 1993;53(6):886–891.
31. Lewis KG, Weinstock MA. Nonmelanoma skin cancer mortality (1988–2000): the Rhode Island follow-back study. *Arch Dermatol.* 2004;140(7):837–842.
32. Basal cell and squamous cell skin cancers. v.1.2009. 2009. (Retrieved from http://www.nccn.org.)
33. Greenlee RT, Murray T, Bolden S, Wingo PA. Cancer statistics, 2000. *CA Cancer J Clin.* 2000;50(1):7–33.
34. Urist MM, Balch CM, Soong SJ, et al. Head and neck melanoma in 534 clinical Stage I patients. A prognostic factors analysis and results of surgical treatment. *Ann Surg.* 1984;200(6):769–775.

35. Bailin PL, Levine HL, Wood BG, Tucker HM. Cutaneous carcinoma of the auricular and periauricular region. *Arch Otolaryngol.* 1980;106(11):692–696.
36. Clark RR, Soutar DS. Lymph node metastases from auricular squamous cell carcinoma. A systematic review and meta-analysis. *J Plast Reconstr Aesthet Surg.* 2008;61(10):1140–1147.
37. Shockley WW, Stucker FJ Jr. Squamous cell carcinoma of the external ear: a review of 75 cases. *Otolaryngol Head Neck Surg.* 1987;97(3):308–312.
38. Blake GB, Wilson JS. Malignant tumours of the ear and their treatment. I. Tumours of the auricle. *Br J Plast Surg.* 1974;27(1):67–76.
39. Lewis JS. Cancer of the ear: a report of 150 cases. *Laryngoscope.* 1960;70:551–579.
40. Cole MD, Jakowatz J, Evans GR. Evaluation of nodal patterns for melanoma of the ear. *Plast Reconstr Surg.* 2003;112(1):50–56.
41. Silapunt S, Peterson SR, Goldberg LH. Squamous cell carcinoma of the auricle and Mohs micrographic surgery. *Dermatol Surg.* 2005;31(11 pt 1):1423–1427.
42. Sylven B, Hamberger CA. Malignant melanoma of the external ear. Report of 36 cases treated between 1928–1944. *Ann Otol Rhinol Laryngol.* 1950;59(3):631–647.
43. Veness MJ, Porceddu S, Palme CE, Morgan GJ. Cutaneous head and neck squamous cell carcinoma metastatic to parotid and cervical lymph nodes. *Head Neck.* 2007;29(7):621–631.
44. Clayman GL, Lee JJ, Holsinger FC, et al. Mortality risk from squamous cell skin cancer. *J Clin Oncol.* 2005;23(4):759–765.
45. O'Brien CJ, McNeil EB, McMahon JD, Pathak I, Lauer CS, Jackson MA. Significance of clinical stage, extent of surgery, and pathologic findings in metastatic cutaneous squamous carcinoma of the parotid gland. *Head Neck.* 2002;24(5):417–422.
46. Brantsch KD, Meisner C, Schonfisch B, et al. Analysis of risk factors determining prognosis of cutaneous squamous-cell carcinoma: a prospective study. *Lancet Oncol.* 2008;9(8):713–720.
47. Rowe DE, Carroll RJ, Day CL, Jr. Prognostic factors for local recurrence, metastasis, and survival rates in squamous cell carcinoma of the skin, ear, and lip. Implications for treatment modality selection. *J Am Acad Dermatol.* 1992;26(6):976–990.
48. O'Brien CJ. The parotid gland as a metastatic basin for cutaneous cancer. *Arch Otolaryngol Head Neck Surg.* 2005;131(7):551–555.
49. Afzelius LE, Ehnhage A, Nordgren H. Basal cell carcinoma in the head and neck. The importance of location and histological picture, studied with a new scoring system, in predicting recurrences. *Acta Pathol Microbiol Scand A.* 1980;88(1):5–9.
50. Cherpelis BS, Marcusen C, Lang PG. Prognostic factors for metastasis in squamous cell carcinoma of the skin. *Dermatol Surg.* 2002;28(3):268–273.
51. Kraus DH, Carew JF, Harrison LB. Regional lymph node metastasis from cutaneous squamous cell carcinoma. *Arch Otolaryngol Head Neck Surg.* 1998;124(5):582–587.
52. Breuninger H, Schaumburg-Lever G, Holzschuh J, Horny HP. Desmoplastic squamous cell carcinoma of skin and vermilion surface: a highly malignant subtype of skin cancer. *Cancer.* 1997;79(5):915–919.
53. Tan PY, Ek E, Su S, Giorlando F, Dieu T. Incomplete excision of squamous cell carcinoma of the skin: a prospective observational study. *Plast Reconstr Surg.* 2007;120(4):910–916.
54. Petter G, Haustein UF. Histologic subtyping and malignancy assessment of cutaneous squamous cell carcinoma. *Dermatol Surg.* 2000;26(6):521–530.
55. Sheil AG, Disney AP, Mathew TH, Amiss N. De novo malignancy emerges as a major cause of morbidity and late failure in renal transplantation. *Transplant Proc.* 1993;25(1 pt 2):1383–1384.
56. Martinez JC, Otley CC, Stasko T, et al. Defining the clinical course of metastatic skin cancer in organ transplant recipients: a multicenter collaborative study. *Arch Dermatol.* 2003;139(3):301–306.
57. Frierson HF, Jr., Cooper PH. Prognostic factors in squamous cell carcinoma of the lower lip. *Hum Pathol.* 1986;17(4):346–354.
58. Goepfert H, Dichtel WJ, Medina JE, Lindberg RD, Luna MD. Perineural invasion in squamous cell skin carcinoma of the head and neck. *Am J Surg.* 1984;148(4):542–547.
59. Garcia-Serra A, Hinerman RW, Mendenhall WM, et al. Carcinoma of the skin with perineural invasion. *Head Neck.* 2003;25(12):1027–1033.
60. Moore BA, Weber RS, Prieto V, et al. Lymph node metastases from cutaneous squamous cell carcinoma of the head and neck. *Laryngoscope.* 2005;115(9):1561–1567.
61. Silverberg E, Boring CC, Squires TS. Cancer statistics, 1990. *CA Cancer J Clin.* 1990;40(1):9–26.
62. Ravin AG, Pickett N, Johnson JL, Fisher SR, Levin LS, Seigler HF. Melanoma of the ear: treatment and survival probabilities based on 199 patients. *Ann Plast Surg.* 2006;57(1):70–76.
63. Chu A, Osguthorpe JD. Nonmelanoma cutaneous malignancy with regional metastasis. *Otolaryngol Head Neck Surg.* 2003;128(5):663–673.
64. Bryarly RC, Jr., Veach SR, Kornblut AD. Metastasizing auricular basal cell carcinoma. *Otolaryngol Head Neck Surg.* 1980;88(1):40–43.
65. Mohs F, Larson P, Iriondo M. Micrographic surgery for the microscopically controlled excision of carcinoma of the external ear. *J Am Acad Dermatol.* 1988;19(4):729–737.
66. Leferink VJ, Nicolai JP. Malignant tumors of the external ear. *Ann Plast Surg.* 1988;21(6):550–554.
67. Thomas DJ, King AR, Peat BG. Excision margins for nonmelanotic skin cancer. *Plast Reconstr Surg.* 2003;112(1):57–63.

68. Wolf DJ, Zitelli JA. Surgical margins for basal cell carcinoma. *Arch Dermatol.* 1987;123(3):340–344.
69. Talbot S, Hitchcock B. Incomplete primary excision of cutaneous basal and squamous cell carcinomas in the Bay of Plenty. *N Z Med J.* 2004;117(1192):U848.
70. Narayan D, Ariyan S. Surgical considerations in the management of malignant melanoma of the ear. *Plast Reconstr Surg.* 2001;107(1):20–24.
71. Pockaj BA, Jaroszewski DE, DiCaudo DJ, et al. Changing surgical therapy for melanoma of the external ear. *Ann Surg Oncol.* 2003;10(6):689–696.
72. Bono A, Bartoli C, Maurichi A, Moglia D, Tragni G. Melanoma of the external ear. *Tumori.* 1997;83(5):814–817.
73. Nordin P, Stenquist B. Five-year results of curettage-cryosurgery for 100 consecutive auricular non-melanoma skin cancers. *J Laryngol Otol.* 2002;116(11):893–898.
74. Nordin P. Curettage-cryosurgery for non-melanoma skin cancer of the external ear: excellent 5–year results. *Br J Dermatol.* 1999;140(2):291–293.
75. Rodriguez-Vigil T, Vazquez-Lopez F, Perez-Oliva N. Recurrence rates of primary basal cell carcinoma in facial risk areas treated with curettage and electrodesiccation. *J Am Acad Dermatol.* 2007;56(1):91–95.
76. Silverman MK, Kopf AW, Grin CM, Bart RS, Levenstein MJ. Recurrence rates of treated basal cell carcinomas. Part 2: curettage-electrodesiccation. *J Dermatol Surg Oncol.* 1991;17(9):720–726.
77. Bumsted RM, Ceilley RI. Auricular malignant neoplasms. Identification of high-risk lesions and selection of method of reconstruction. *Arch Otolaryngol.* 1982;108(4):225–231.
78. Niparko JK, Swanson NA, Baker SR, Telian SA, Sullivan MJ, Kemink JL. Local control of auricular, periauricular, and external canal cutaneous malignancies with Mohs surgery. *Laryngoscope.* 1990;100(10 pt 1):1047–1051.
79. Robins P, Nix M. Analysis of persistent disease on the ear following Mohs surgery. *Head Neck Surg.* 1984;6(6):998–1006.
80. Clark DP, Hanke CW. Neoplasms of the conchal bowl: treatment with Mohs micrographic surgery. *J Dermatol Surg Oncol.* 1988;14(11):1223–1228.
81. Levin BC, Adams LA, Becker GD. Healing by secondary intention of auricular defects after Mohs surgery. *Arch Otolaryngol Head Neck Surg.* 1996;122(1):59–66; discussion 67.
82. Ceilley RI, Bumsted RM, Smith WH. Malignancies on the external ear: methods of ablation and reconstruction of defects. *J Dermatol Surg Oncol.* 1979;5(10):762–767.
83. Butler CE. Reconstruction of marginal ear defects with modified chondrocutaneous helical rim advancement flaps. *Plast Reconstr Surg.* 2003;111(6):2009–2013.
84. Calhoun KH, Chase SP. Reconstruction of the auricle. *Facial Plast Surg Clin North Am.* 2005;13(2):231–241, vi.
85. Cook TA, Miller PJ. Auricular reconstruction. *Facial Plast Surg.* 1995;11(4):319–329.
86. Dessy LA, Figus A, Fioramonti P, Mazzocchi M, Scuderi N. Reconstruction of anterior auricular conchal defect after malignancy excision: revolving-door flap versus full-thickness skin graft. *J Plast Reconstr Aesthet Surg.* 2010;63(5):746–752.
87. Elsahy NI. Reconstruction of the ear after skin and cartilage loss. *Clin Plast Surg.* 2002;29(2):201–212, vi.
88. Fader DJ, Johnson TM. Ear reconstruction utilizing the subcutaneous island pedicle graft (flip-flop) flap. *Dermatol Surg.* 1999;25(2):94–96.
89. Finical SJ, Johnson CH. Reconstruction after extirpation of the auricle. *J Reconstr Microsurg.* 2001;17(5):325–329.
90. Fortier-Riberdy G, Gloster HM Jr. Reconstruction of the superior helical rim with a postauricular transposition flap. *Dermatol Surg.* 2005;31(1):99–101.
91. Hendi A, Brodland DG. Split-thickness skin graft in nonhelical ear reconstruction. *Dermatol Surg.* 2006;32(9):1171–1173.
92. Mahajan AL. Helix reconstruction with wedge resection in the right place. *J Plast Reconstr Aesthet Surg.* 2009;62(1):125–127.
93. Majumdar A, Townend J. Helix rim advancement for reconstruction of marginal defects of the pinna. *Br J Oral Maxillofac Surg.* 2000;38(1):3–7.
94. Mathews SS, Ninan S. Reconstruction of the conchal bowl and external auditory canal. *Ear Nose Throat J.* 2006;85(7):425.
95. Mazzocchi M, Bistoni G, Buccheri EM, Alfano C. Ear reconstruction after cancer excision. *Acta Chir Plast.* 2006;48(1):15–19.
96. Papadopoulos ON, Karypidis DK, Chrisostomidis CI, Konofaos PP, Frangoulis MB. One-stage reconstruction of the antihelix and concha using postauricular island flap. *Clin Exp Dermatol.* 2008;33(5):647–650.
97. Reddy LV, Zide MF. Reconstruction of skin cancer defects of the auricle. *J Oral Maxillofac Surg.* 2004;62(12):1457–1471.
98. Talmi YP, Wolf M, Horowitz Z, Bedrin L, Kronenberg J. "Second look" at auricular reconstruction with a postauricular island flap: "flip-flop flap." *Plast Reconstr Surg.* 2002;109(2):713–715.
99. Yotsuyanagi T, Nihei Y, Sawada Y. Reconstruction of defects involving the upper one-third of the auricle. *Plast Reconstr Surg.* 1998;102(4):988–992.
100. Yotsuyanagi T, Watanabe Y, Yamashita K, et al. Reconstruction of defects involving the middle third of the auricle with a full-thickness conchal chondrocutaneous flap. *Plast Reconstr Surg.* 2002;109(4):1366–1371.
101. Zenn MR. Helical advancement with a posterior auricular pull-through flap: a technique for reconstruction of combined helical and scaphal defects. *Aesthetic Plast Surg.* 1999;23(2):131–133.
102. TJ O-Lee, Rowe M. Auricular malignant melanoma of early childhood: the role of sentinel node biopsy. *Int J Pediatr Otorhinolaryngol.* 2004;68(10):1345–1348.
103. Wagner JD, Park HM, Coleman JJ 3rd, Love C, Hayes JT. Cervical sentinel lymph node biopsy for melanomas

of the head and neck and upper thorax. *Arch Otolaryngol Head Neck Surg.* 2000;126(3):313–321.
104. Pathak I, O'Brien CJ, Petersen-Schaeffer K, et al. Do nodal metastases from cutaneous melanoma of the head and neck follow a clinically predictable pattern? *Head Neck.* 2001;23(9):785–790.
105. Cordova A, Moschella F. Evaluation of nodal patterns for melanoma of the ear. *Plast Reconstr Surg.* 2004;113(5): 1528; author reply 1529.
106. Mondin V, Rinaldo A, Shaha AR, et al. Malignant melanoma of the auricle. *Acta Otolaryngol.* 2005;125(11): 1140–1144.
107. Carlson GW, Murray DR, Greenlee R, et al. Management of malignant melanoma of the head and neck using dynamic lymphoscintigraphy and gamma probe-guided sentinel lymph node biopsy. *Arch Otolaryngol Head Neck Surg.* 2000;126(3):433–437.
108. Jahn V, Breuninger H, Garbe C, Moehrle M. Melanoma of the ear: prognostic factors and surgical strategies. *Br J Dermatol.* 2006;154(2):310–318.
109. Carlson GW, Murray DR, Lyles RH, Hestley A, Cohen C. Sentinel lymph node biopsy in the management of cutaneous head and neck melanoma. *Plast Reconstr Surg.* 2005;115(3):721–728.
110. Wey PD, De La Cruz C, Goydos JS, Choi ML, Borah GL. Sentinel lymph node mapping in melanoma of the ear. *Ann Plast Surg.* 1998;40(5):506–509.
111. Shpitzer T, Gutman H, Barnea Y, et al. Sentinel node-guided evaluation of drainage patterns for melanoma of the helix of the ear. *Melanoma Res.* 2007;17(6): 365–369.
112. Wagner JD, Evdokimow DZ, Weisberger E, et al. Sentinel node biopsy for high-risk nonmelanoma cutaneous malignancy. *Arch Dermatol.* 2004;140(1):75–79.
113. Reschly MJ, Messina JL, Zaulyanov LL, Cruse W, Fenske NA. Utility of sentinel lymphadenectomy in the management of patients with high-risk cutaneous squamous cell carcinoma. *Dermatol Surg.* 2003;29(2): 135–140.
114. O'Brien CJ, Uren RF, Thompson JF, et al. Prediction of potential metastatic sites in cutaneous head and neck melanoma using lymphoscintigraphy. *Am J Surg.* 1995; 170(5):461–466.
115. Farrell ML, Kalnins IK. Frey's syndrome following parotid surgery. *Aust N Z J Surg.* 1991;61(4):295–301.
116. Bron LP, O'Brien CJ. Facial nerve function after parotidectomy. *Arch Otolaryngol Head Neck Surg.* 1997;123(10):1091–1096.
117. Ying YL, Johnson JT, Myers EN. Squamous cell carcinoma of the parotid gland. *Head Neck.* 2006;28(7):626–632.
118. Lai SY, Weinstein GS, Chalian AA, Rosenthal DI, Weber RS. Parotidectomy in the treatment of aggressive cutaneous malignancies. *Arch Otolaryngol Head Neck Surg.* 2002;128(5):521–526.
119. Ellingson TW, Cohen JI, Andersen P. The impact of malignant disease on facial nerve function after parotidectomy. *Laryngoscope.* 2003;113(8):1299–1303.
120. Nichols RD, Stine PH, Bartschi LR. Facial nerve function in 100 consecutive parotidectomies. *Laryngoscope.* 1979;89(12):1930–1934.
121. Audet N, Palme CE, Gullane PJ, et al. Cutaneous metastatic squamous cell carcinoma to the parotid gland: analysis and outcome. *Head Neck.* 2004;26(8):727–732.
122. Hong TS, Kriesel KJ, Hartig GK, Harari PM. Parotid area lymph node metastases from cutaneous squamous cell carcinoma: implications for diagnosis, treatment, and prognosis. *Head Neck.* 2005;27(10):851–856.
123. Dona E, Veness MJ, Cakir B, Morgan GJ. Metastatic cutaneous squamous cell carcinoma to the parotid: the role of surgery and adjuvant radiotherapy to achieve best outcome. *ANZ J Surg.* 2003;73(9):692–696.
124. Baker NJ, Webb AA, Macpherson D. Surgical management of cutaneous squamous cell carcinoma of the head and neck. *Br J Oral Maxillofac Surg.* 2001;39(2):87–90.
125. Ginsberg LE, Eicher SA. Great auricular nerve: anatomy and imaging in a case of perineural tumor spread. *AJNR Am J Neuroradiol.* 2000;21(3):568–571.
126. Lee JG, Krause CJ. Radical neck dissection: elective, therapeutic, and secondary. *Arch Otolaryngol.* 1975;101(11): 656–659.
127. Pitman KT, Johnson JT, Myers EN. Effectiveness of selective neck dissection for management of the clinically negative neck. *Arch Otolaryngol Head Neck Surg.* 1997;123(9):917–922.
128. Ferlito A, Rinaldo A, Silver CE, et al. Elective and therapeutic selective neck dissection. *Oral Oncol.* 2006;42(1): 14–25.
129. Tavin E, Persky M. Metastatic cutaneous squamous cell carcinoma of the head and neck region. *Laryngoscope.* 1996;106(2 pt 1):156–158.
130. Sim FH, Taylor WF, Ivins JC, Pritchard DJ, Soule EH. A prospective randomized study of the efficacy of routine elective lymphadenectomy in management of malignant melanoma. Preliminary results. *Cancer.* 1978; 41(3):948–956.
131. Balch CM, Soong SJ, Bartolucci AA, et al. Efficacy of an elective regional lymph node dissection of 1 to 4 mm thick melanomas for patients 60 years of age and younger. *Ann Surg.* 1996;224(3):255–263; discussion 63–66.
132. Veronesi U, Adamus J, Bandiera DC, et al. Stage I melanoma of the limbs. Immediate versus delayed node dissection. *Tumori.* 1980;66(3):373–396.
133. Cascinelli N, Morabito A, Santinami M, MacKie RM, Belli F. Immediate or delayed dissection of regional nodes in patients with melanoma of the trunk: a randomised trial. WHO Melanoma Programme. *Lancet* 1998;351(9105):793–796.
134. Kwan W, Wilson D, Moravan V. Radiotherapy for locally advanced basal cell and squamous cell carcinomas of the skin. *Int J Radiat Oncol Biol Phys.* 2004;60(2): 406–411.
135. Withers HR, Suwinski R. Radiation dose response for subclinical metastases. *Semin Radiat Oncol.* 1998;8(3): 224–228.

136. Mendenhall WM, Million RR. Elective neck irradiation for squamous cell carcinoma of the head and neck: analysis of time-dose factors and causes of failure. *Int J Radiat Oncol Biol Phys.* 1986;12(5):741–746.
137. Bron LP, Traynor SJ, McNeil EB, O'Brien CJ. Primary and metastatic cancer of the parotid: comparison of clinical behavior in 232 cases. *Laryngoscope.* 2003;113(6): 1070–1075.
138. delCharco JO, Mendenhall WM, Parsons JT, Stringer SP, Cassisi NJ, Mendenhall NP. Carcinoma of the skin metastatic to the parotid area lymph nodes. *Head Neck.* 1998;20(5):369–373.
139. Veness MJ, Palme CE, Smith M, Cakir B, Morgan GJ, Kalnins I. Cutaneous head and neck squamous cell carcinoma metastatic to cervical lymph nodes (non-parotid): a better outcome with surgery and adjuvant radiotherapy. *Laryngoscope.* 2003;113(10):1827–1833.
140. Barzilai G, Greenberg E, Cohen-Kerem R, Doweck I. Pattern of regional metastases from cutaneous squamous cell carcinoma of the head and neck. *Otolaryngol Head Neck Surg.* 2005;132(6):852–856.
141. Jol J, van Velthuysen M, Hilgers F, Keus R, Neering H, Balm A. Treatment results of regional metastasis from cutaneous head and neck squamous cell carcinoma. *Eur J Surg Oncol.* 2002;29:81–86.
142. Talmi YP, Horowitz Z, Wolf M, Kronenberg J. Delayed metastases in skin cancer of the head and neck: the case of the "known primary." *Ann Plast Surg.* 1999;42(3): 289–292.
143. Netterville JL, Sinard RJ, Bryant GL Jr. Burkey BB. Delayed regional metastasis from midfacial squamous carcinomas. *Head Neck.* 1998;20(4):328–333.
144. Veness MJ, Morgan GJ, Palme CE, Gebski V. Surgery and adjuvant radiotherapy in patients with cutaneous head and neck squamous cell carcinoma metastatic to lymph nodes: combined treatment should be considered best practice. *Laryngoscope.* 2005;115(5):870–875.

11

SPECIAL CONSIDERATIONS: PERIORBITAL AND OCULAR ADNEXAL CUTANEOUS LESIONS

BITA ESMAELI
AARON SAVAR

Introduction

The periorbital region is one of the areas within the head and neck most frequently affected by cutaneous malignancy.[1] A number of different histologic types of cutaneous tumors can occur in this area. Basal cell carcinoma (BCC) is the most common, followed by squamous cell carcinoma (SCC) and melanoma. Sebaceous carcinoma, although relatively rare, is also an important periorbital cutaneous malignancy. It is rarely seen elsewhere in the body and often is misdiagnosed because clinically it can resemble benign eyelid conditions. A number of other cancers can arise in the periocular region, including adnexal carcinomas, Merkel cell carcinoma, lymphoproliferative lesions, and sarcomas.

Periorbital skin cancers can be the source of significant morbidity and mortality. The majority of periocular skin cancers are primarily managed surgically. Chemotherapy, radiation therapy, and other modalities are used as adjuncts or as primary treatments in certain situations. Because of the delicate nature of the eye and associated adnexal structures, certain unique considerations must be taken into account when one deals with cutaneous malignancies in the periorbital region.

Anatomic Considerations

The complex nature of the anatomy of the periorbital region makes the management of skin cancers in this area particularly challenging. There are a number of structures in this area that can be either affected by cutaneous tumors or damaged by surgery.

The globe is protected by the upper and lower eyelids. Each eyelid is composed of two lamellae. The anterior lamella consists of the skin and the orbicularis oculi. The posterior lamella consists of the tarsus and conjunctiva (Fig 11–1). Both lamellae are important for normal functioning of the eyelid and protection of the ocular surface. On the medial aspect of each lid is a lacrimal punctum that opens into the canaliculus. The canaliculi drain tears into the lacrimal sac, which in turn drains into the inferior meatus of the nose via the nasolacrimal duct (Fig 11–2). These anatomic relationships become particularly important when one is removing medial canthal lesions.

There are seven extraocular muscles: the four rectus muscles, the two oblique muscles, and the levator palpebrae superioris. Resections involving the eyelid can affect the levator muscle, whereas those involving the conjunctiva can affect the rectus muscles.

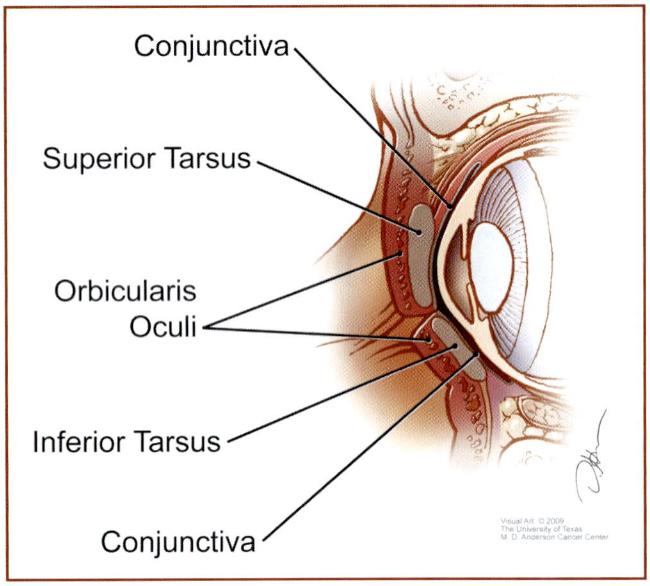

Figure 11–1. Cross-section of an eyelid demonstrates the anterior lamella, composed of skin and orbicularis muscle, and the posterior lamella, composed of tarsus and conjunctiva. (Visual Art: © 2010 The University of Texas MD Anderson Cancer Center)

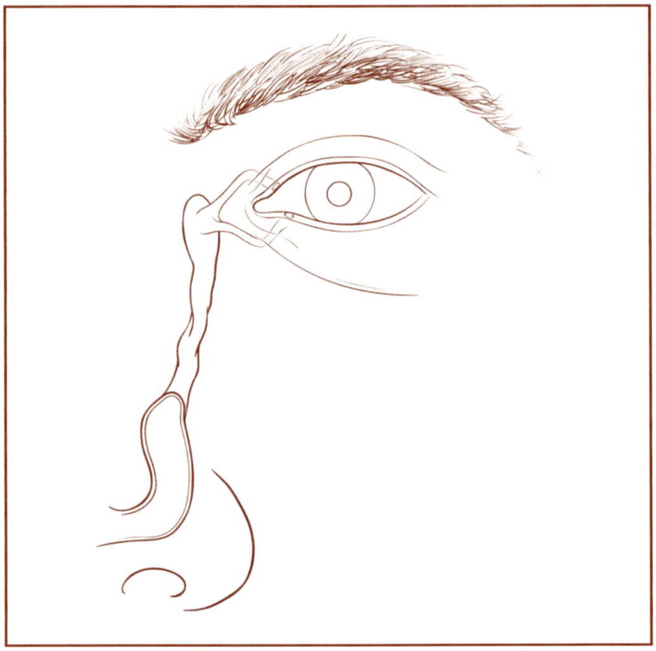

Figure 11–2. The components of the lacrimal drainage apparatus. (Visual Art: © 2010 The University of Texas MD Anderson Cancer Center)

Inadvertent injury to the levator muscle or its aponeurosis can cause blepharoptosis, whereas injury to any of the other extraocular muscles can result in diplopia. The inferior oblique muscle originates from the inferomedial aspect of the orbit and can be damaged during surgery in this area. The superior oblique muscle passes through the trochlea in the anterior, superonasal orbit and can be similarly damaged.

Several sensory nerves emanate from the orbit and can be affected by nearby tumors or damaged during surgical resections. These include the infraorbital nerve, which receives sensory input from the midface, and the supraorbital and supratrochlear nerves, which receive sensory input from the upper lid, forehead, and upper nose. Perineural invasion by a tumor can result in pain, numbness, paresthesia, or formication in the distribution of the nerve. Likewise, surgical damage to one of the sensory nerves can result in anesthesia.

The lacrimal gland is located in the superotemporal orbit, and the palpebral lobe of the gland protrudes anteriorly under the upper eyelid. Damage to either the palpebral or the orbital lobe of the lacrimal gland or the lacrimal ductules can result in a dry eye.

Preoperative Issues

In the evaluation of patients with periocular skin cancers, a complete ophthalmic examination is necessary. Because skin cancers affecting the eyelid can involve the palpebral or bulbar conjunctiva, it is important to perform an inspection of the entire conjunctival surface, including upper eyelid eversion. Although nodal metastasis is rare with BCC, it is more common with other cutaneous malignancies in the periocular region such as SCC, sebaceous carcinoma, and melanoma. Examination therefore should include palpation of preauricular, parotid, submandibular, and cervical lymph nodes.

Preoperative imaging of the orbit and the head and neck is done to evaluate the full extent of the tumor, particularly to rule out involvement of postseptal orbital soft tissues and to assess the regional lymph nodes. Laboratory assessment and systemic workup should be tailored to the type of tumor—for example, for melanomas of the conjunctiva and eyelid, chest radiograph and a baseline lactate dehydrogenase measurement are obtained. In addition, an ultrasound of the regional lymph nodes is obtained to rule out macroscopic involvement of the regional lymph nodes. In select cases of eyelid or conjunctival malignancy, consideration is given to sentinel lymph node biopsy to rule out microscopic metastasis in the regional lymph nodes.[2–5] For conjunctival and eyelid tumors, the nodal basins at risk include the parotid and submandibular nodes.

The unique considerations for eyelid carcinoma have been appreciated by the American Joint Committee on Cancer, as a novel staging system for eyelid carcinoma has been devised for the 2010 Cancer Staging Manual. The staging system takes into account the distinct anatomic structure of the eyelids including size considerations, as well as the proximity to vital ocular, orbital, or craniofacial structures. The staging system is described in Tables 11–1 and 11–2.[6]

Table 11–1. 2010 AJCC Carcinoma of the Eyelid TNM Staging System[6]

Stage of Primary Lesion	Features
Tx	Primary tumor cannot be assessed
T0	No evidence of primary tumor
Tis	Carcinoma in situ
T1	Tumor ≤5 mm in greatest dimension Not invading tarsal plate or lid margin
T2a	Tumor >5 mm, but not >10 mm in greatest dimension *Or*, any tumor invading tarsal plate or lid margin
T2b	Tumor >10 mm, but not >20 mm *Or*, involves full thickness of eyelid
T3a	Tumor >20 mm in greatest dimension *Or*, any tumor that invades adjacent ocular or orbital structures Any T with perineural invasion
T3b	Tumor complete resection requires enucleation, exenteration or bone resection
T4	Tumor is not resectable because of extensive invasion Invasion of ocular, orbital, craniofacial structures, *Or* brain
Stage of Regional Nodes	**Features**
Nx	Nodes cannot be assessed
N0	No clinical or radiographic evidence of nodal metastasis
N1	Regional lymph node metastasis
Stage of Distant Disease	**Features**
M0	No distant metastasis
M1	Distant metastasis

Source: Used with permission of the American Joint Committee on Cancer (AJCC) Chicago, Illinois. The original source for this material is the AJCC Cancer Staging Manual, Seventh Edition (2010) published by Springer Science and Business Media LLC, www.springer.com.

Table 11–2. 2010 AJCC Carcinoma of the Eyelid Stage Groupings[6]

Stage Group	T Stage	N Stage	M Stage
0	Tis	0	0
IA	T1	0	0
IB	T2a	0	0
IC	T2b	0	0
II	T3a	0	0
IIIA	T3b	0	0
IIIB	Any T	N1	0
IIIC	T4	Any N	0
IV	Any T	Any N	M1

Source: Used with permission of the American Joint Committee on Cancer (AJCC) Chicago, Illinois. The original source for this material is the AJCC Cancer Staging Manual, Seventh Edition (2010) published by Springer Science and Business Media LLC, www.springer.com.

Intraoperative Issues

Protection of Delicate Structures

Surgery for some cutaneous malignancies of the head may require exenteration of the orbit. When such radical surgery is not necessary, however, care must be taken in operating near the eye. Periocular surgery has the potential to interfere with the protection of the eye, with visual function, and with ocular motility. Simple precautions should be taken when operating around the globe to avoid ocular injury. The cornea should be protected with lubricating drops or ointment, a corneal shield, or a temporary tarsorrhaphy.

The delicate nature of the ocular adnexal tissues and the importance of eye as a sensory organ make it desirable to resect as little normal tissue as is safely possible, without compromising the oncologic goal of tumor clearance. Typically, resections of eyelid tumors are carried out with excision of narrower margins of normal tissue than would be obtained elsewhere on the body, depending on the tumor type.

Excision Margins

Historically, very wide margins were recommended for excision of cutaneous melanoma, as much as 4 cm. Over the past 20 years, however, recommendations have changed; the current recommendations are in many cases 1-cm margins for thin melanomas (≤2 mm thick) and 2-cm margins for thick melanomas (>2 mm thick).[7–9] However, margins of that size in the periocular region would necessitate removal of the eye in many cases and may not be necessary.

Recommendations for the appropriate margin of normal tissue to excise for melanoma in the eyelids vary.[10,11] The Collaborative Eyelid Skin Melanoma Group aimed to address this issue through a retrospective analysis of 44 periocular melanomas managed by 23 different surgeons. The group concluded that margins of 5 mm or more were appropriate for melanomas less than 1 mm thick in the periocular region. At The University of Texas MD Anderson Cancer Center, a margin of 5 mm of normal tissue usually is removed for tumors in the periocular area, and reconstruction is delayed until the margins are confirmed to be negative by evaluation of permanent (paraffin-embedded) sections.

For nonmelanoma skin cancers, smaller margins often are acceptable. In an Australian series of 485 periocular BCCs and SCCs, Nemet and associates[12] used excision margins of 3 mm for BCC and 5 mm for SCC. There is, however, no consensus on the appropriate clinical excision margin in the periocular region. In order to achieve complete excision, it is important to have negative margins on histologic evaluation. The issue of histologic safety margins for eyelid BCC was evaluated by Auw-Haedrich and associates.[13] They studied 101 periocular BCCs with a mean follow-up of 7 years. For nodular BCCs, they found no recurrences with histologic safety margins greater than 0 mm and a 20% recurrence rate if the margin was left positive. Among morpheaform, or infiltrative, BCCs, they found a 100% recurrence rate if the histologic safety margin was less than 0.2 mm and an 8% recurrence rate if the margin was greater than 0.2 mm. Clearly, a wider safety margin is needed for infiltrative BCC than for nodular basal BCC.

Surgical Options

Multiple options exist for excising periocular skin cancers. Both wide local excision with frozen section control of margins and Mohs micrographic surgery can be used for certain tumors. Because of the importance of removing as little tissue as is safe around the eye, Mohs micrographic surgery or a modified Mohs technique may be advantageous in selected tumors.[14] However, Mohs surgery is not appropriate for melanocytic lesions unless a "slow" Mohs technique is used, as traditional frozen sections are regarded as unreliable for evaluating such lesions.

Managing the Lid Margin

Lesions extending to the eyelid margin require a full-thickness excision of eyelid tissue, including the tarsal plate (Fig 11–3). When tarsal tissue is excised in such situations, it is necessary to excise the full vertical height of the tarsus. Failure to do so will result in eyelid contour abnormalities.

Managing the Medial Canthus

Lesions involving the medial canthus require special considerations. Tumors in this area, especially BCC, have a higher risk of orbital invasion.[15] Signs suggestive of orbital invasion include fixation of the tumor to underlying bone, ocular motility disturbance, and displacement of the globe.[15] The risk of incomplete excision is also higher in the medial canthal region.[12] Although preoperative imaging may not be necessary for many BCCs, it is recommended for those in the medial canthal region because of these risks. Because of the possibility of tumor spread to a variety of critical structures and in a variety of directions, especially in the medial canthal region, appropriate specimen labeling and careful evaluation of all margins on frozen section is mandatory.

Skin cancers near the medial canthus can be in very close proximity to, or can directly involve, the lacrimal drainage apparatus. For these lesions, intra-operative probing of the canaliculi can help identify these structures and determine if they have been violated by tumor or during surgical resection

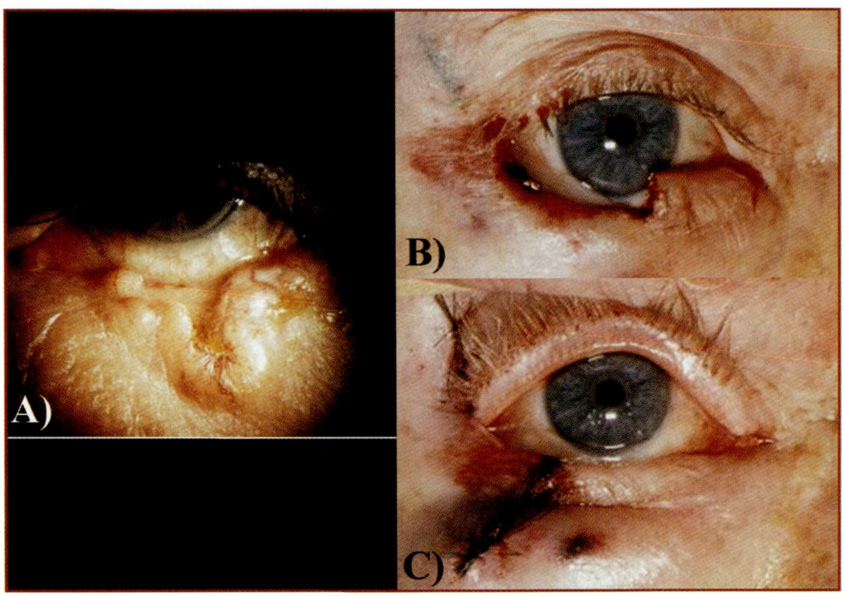

Figure 11–3. A. Basal cell carcinoma of eyelid involving the eyelid margin. **B.** The tumor was resected through a full-thickness pentagonal resection of eyelid, and **C.** the eyelid was reconstructed.

of obvious tumor. If there is obvious involvement of the lacrimal drainage system, it is necessary to excise part or all of it (Fig 11–4). Reconstruction of the lacrimal drainage system frequently will be required for symptomatic epiphora, but this can be performed in a delayed fashion because some patients will not be symptomatic.

Managing the Conjunctiva

Periorbital cutaneous cancers can spread to, or emanate from, the conjunctival surface. When one resects eyelid malignancies with involvement of the bulbar conjunctiva, the conjunctival edges and underlying sclera generally are treated with cryotherapy in a double freeze-thaw manner. In the case of SCC or melanoma, margins that are microscopically positive for in situ disease can be treated with topical chemotherapy such as topical mitomycin C or 5-fluorouracil. Surgical specimen handling is extremely important when the bulbar conjunctiva is involved, as the conjunctiva can easily become folded or heaped up, causing tangential sectioning and loss of the ability to accurately determine the depth of invasion of a melanoma.[16]

Management of Orbital Invasion

Invasion of the postseptal structures in the orbit, or invasion of the globe by a periocular cutaneous malignancy, are typically treated with orbital exenteration with or without adjuvant radiation therapy (Fig 11–5).[15] Eyelid malignancy is the most frequent indication for orbital exenteration, and BCC is the most common tumor type requiring this treatment.[17,18] Typically, involvement of postseptal orbital fat with

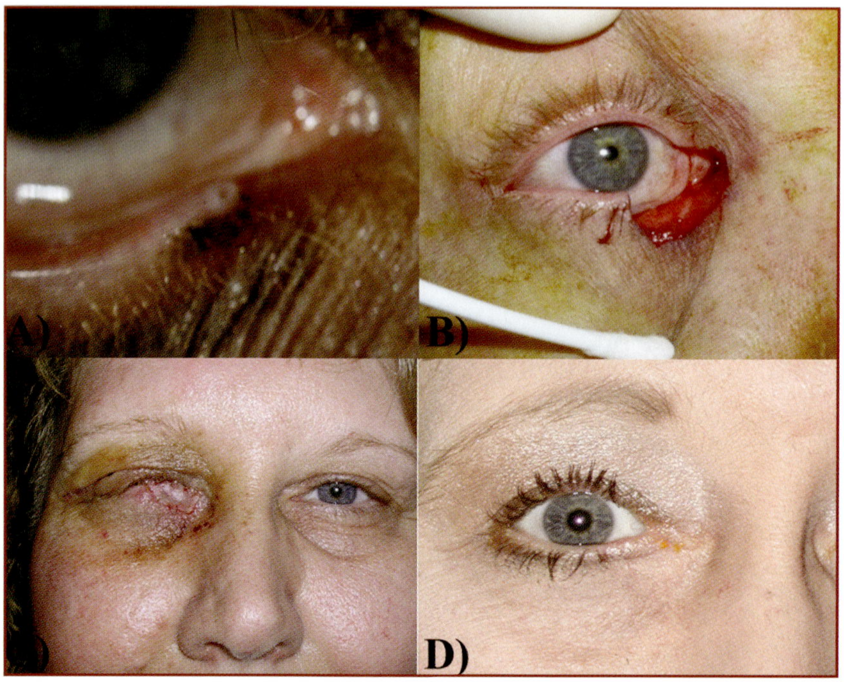

Figure 11–4. A. Melanoma of the eyelid margin involving the lower canalicular region. **B.** Full-thickness defect of the lower eyelid resulting from removal of the melanoma including removal of the entire lower canaliculus. **C.** Appearance after the first stage of a Hughes tarsoconjunctival flap procedure and **D.** final appearance after the second stage of the Hughes procedure. The patient was not bothered by epiphora and did not pursue lacrimal bypass surgery.

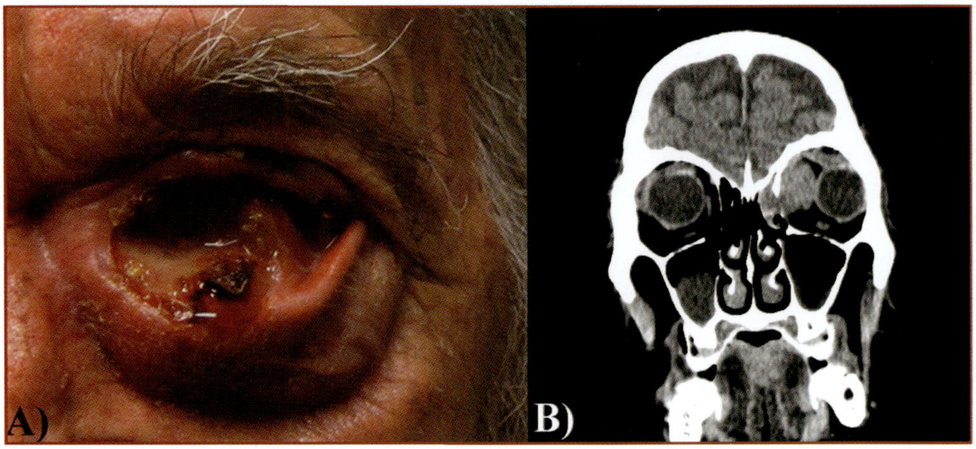

Figure 11–5. **A.** External photograph of a recurrent squamous cell carcinoma of the medial canthus with involvement of the globe surface and invasion of the postseptal orbital tissues. **B.** Computed tomography findings in the same patient demonstrating the postseptal extension of the tumor.

cancer necessitates an orbital exenteration. In some cases with only limited anterior orbital soft tissue involvement, particularly with cancers that have a limited potential for metastasis such as BCC, globe-sparing surgery can be considered in combination with adjuvant postoperative radiation therapy.[19]

Surgical Challenges: Risk of Eyelid Malposition

Although reconstructive procedures around the eyes are covered in a separate chapter in this book, it is important to stress that periocular surgery carries the risk of causing eyelid malposition. Cicatricial ectropion is the most common eyelid abnormality resulting from periocular surgery and most frequently results from vertical tension. This can be avoided by ensuring that there is minimal tension on the skin closure. Horizontal closure should be avoided in the lower eyelid when possible, and vertical tension should be displaced to the horizontal direction.

In addition to the obvious cosmetic problems, lower or upper eyelid ectropion can lead to exposure keratopathy. In most cases, this can be treated with topical lubricants. Patients with exposure keratopathy should be monitored closely, as this condition can result in corneal ulceration and even perforation in severe situations. Surgical correction of upper or lower eyelid ectropion can be accomplished with release of scar tissue, resuspension of the upper and lower eyelids to the lateral or medial canthus, and the use of full-thickness skin grafts.

Additional Considerations

Radiation Therapy

Radiation therapy is an important component of treatment for cutaneous malignancies of the head and neck. It can be used as a primary therapy, in the adjuvant setting, or for palliation of inoperable tumors. Periorbital radiation therapy requires special considerations because of concerns regarding ocular radiation toxicity. Hsu and associates[19] reviewed 20 cases of eyelid or conjunctival malignancies in which external-beam radiation therapy was used in the adjuvant setting. In that series, there were several different indications for radiation treatment.

The most common indication was concern about recurrence of an aggressive tumor variety, such as Merkel cell carcinoma, intermediate- to high-thickness melanoma, and myxoid sarcoma. Other indications for adjuvant radiation therapy included recurrent tumors, perineural invasion, lymph node metastases, positive surgical margins, and refusal of radical surgery by the patient. Although there was some variation in the regimen used and the timing of treatment, the median time from surgery to initiation of radiation therapy was 7 weeks. Radiation-related side effects included dry eyes, conjunctival keratinization, exposure keratopathy, blepharitis, retinopathy, and trichiasis.[19]

Eye shields typically are used to minimize these complications and have been shown to be effective in reducing the amount of radiation exposure to the globe.[20,21] It is important to monitor patients for ocular radiation side effects during the course of treatment and for some of the more severe side effects, such as radiation retinopathy, for several years after the completion of radiation therapy.

Reconstruction

Reconstruction of defects arising from the treatment of periorbital cutaneous malignancy is discussed elsewhere in this book. The choice of reconstructive procedure may be influenced by whether or not a patient has received, or will receive, radiation therapy. Because of the relative ischemia in irradiated areas, free grafts are used less frequently, and local flaps or vascularized free flaps are favored in patients who have undergone irradiation. In patients treated with eyelid-sharing procedures (eg, modified Hughes reconstruction or Cutler-Beard procedure), the flap or pedicle separation can be done either before or after postoperative radiation therapy has been administered. The advantages of separating the pedicle before radiation therapy include better definition of the tumor bed and easier insertion of a scleral shield to protect the globe. The disadvantage of separating the pedicle prior to radiation therapy is the increased risk of flap compromise and exposure keratopathy. The latter concern is more relevant to upper eyelid reconstruction and is not as much of an issue for lower eyelid reconstruction. We favor separation of the flap within 4 weeks of ablative surgery, to facilitate initiation of postoperative radiation therapy 2 weeks later with shielding of the globe (Fig 11–6).

Surveillance

As with cutaneous malignancies elsewhere in the head and neck, postoperative surveillance is necessary to identify local recurrences, metastases, and other problems that may arise after periocular surgery, such as eyelid malposition. At the MD Anderson Cancer Center Oculoplastics and Orbit Clinic, patients with eyelid and ocular adnexal cancers usually have follow-up examinations every 3 to 6 months during the first 2 years after resection, and then annually for 5 years.

Conclusion

The periorbital region is frequently involved by cutaneous malignancy of the head and neck. Because the thin, delicate tissues of the eyelids and ocular adnexa are very close to the critical structures of the orbit and globe, a comprehensive ophthalmologic examination is mandatory before starting treatment. Due the complexity of the surgical procedures and potential need for adjuvant therapy in aggressive lesions, multidisciplinary evaluation and treatment is paramount.

Accepted resection margins for both melanoma and NMSC are narrower than in other sites in the head and neck, and tissue-conserving techniques are particularly applicable in this area. Careful attention must be devoted to lesions of the lid margin, medial canthus, lacrimal apparatus, and conjunctiva, as special extirpative, tissue handling, and reconstructive techniques may be required. Surgeons should be attentive to the development of postoperative ectropion, and the entire multidisciplinary team should be attuned to the potential complications of primary or adjuvant radiotherapy.

As with other cutaneous malignancies of the head and neck, patients with periorbital lesions benefit

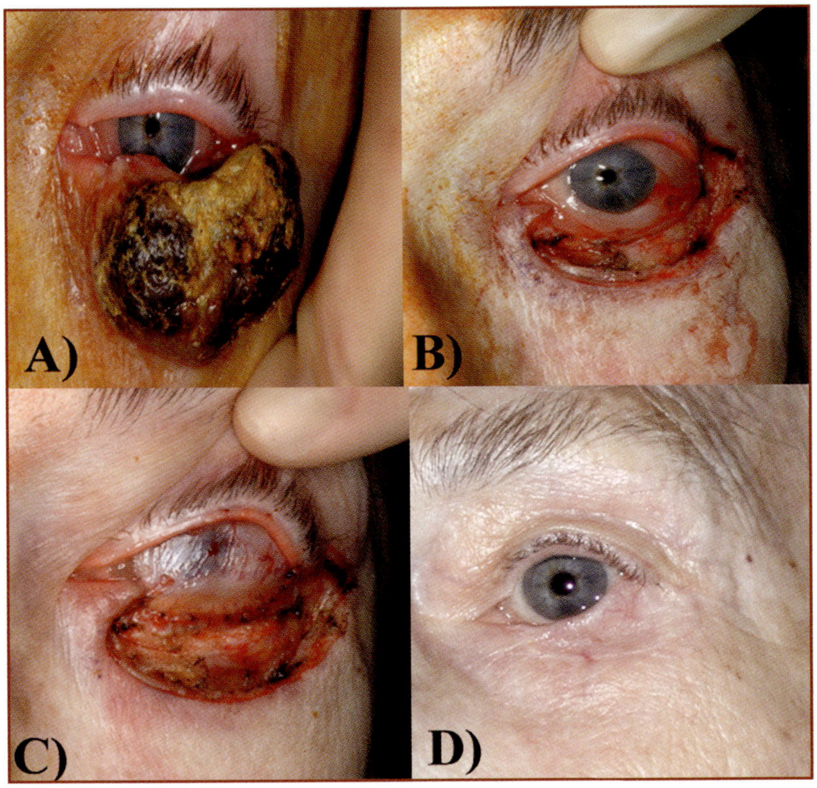

Figure 11–6. **A.** A mass lesion representing squamous cell carcinoma of the tarsal aspect of the lower eyelid. **B.** Surgical defect after removal of lesion with frozen section control of margins. **C.** The defect was closed with a tarsoconjunctival flap and a full-thickness skin graft. Postoperative radiation therapy was administered to the eyelid and the parotid area, because this lesion had already metastasized to the parotid regional nodes. The eye was shielded with a tungsten eye shield during radiation therapy. **D.** Final postoperative appearance after completion of radiation therapy.

from a multidisciplinary approach that fully leverages primary and adjuvant treatment modalities, as well as reconstruction and prosthetic rehabilitation.

References

1. Pearl DK, Scott EL. The anatomical distribution of skin cancers. *Int J Epidemiol.* 1986;15(4):502–506.
2. Esmaeli B, Reifler D, Prieto VG, Amir Ahmadi M, Hidaji L. Delpassand E, Ross MI. Conjunctival melanoma with a positive sentinel lymph node. *Arch Ophthalmol.* 2003; 121:1779–1783.
3. Esmaeli B, Naderi A, Hidaji L, Blumenschein G, Prieto VG. Merkel cell carcinoma of the eyelid with a positive sentinel node. *Arch Ophthalmol.* 2002;120(5):646–648.
4. Savar A, Ross MI, Prieto VG, Ivan D, Kim S, Esmaeli B. Sentinel lymph node biopsy for ocular adnexal melanoma: experience in 30 patients. *Ophthalmology.* 2009;116(11): 2217–2223.
5. Savar A, Oellers P, Myers J, Prieto V G, Torres-Cabala C, Frank S J, Ivan D, Esmaeli B. Positive sentinel node in sebaceous carcinoma of the eyelid. *Ophthal Plast Reconstr Surg.* Oct 2010 [Epub ahead of print].
6. American Joint Committee on Cancer. Edge SB, Byrd DR, Compton CC, et al, eds. *AJCC Cancer Staging Manual.* 7th ed. New York, NY: Springer, 2010.
7. Veronesi U, Cascinelli N, Adamus J, et al. Thin stage I primary cutaneous malignant melanoma. Comparison of

excision with margins of 1 or 3 cm. *N Engl J Med.* 1988; 318(18):1159–1162.
8. Cascinelli N. Margin of resection in the management of primary melanoma. *Semin Surg Oncol.* 1998;14(4):272–275.
9. Lens MB, Nathan P, Bataille V. Excision margins for primary cutaneous melanoma: updated pooled analysis of randomized controlled trials. *Arch Surg.* 2007;142(9): 885–891.
10. Esmaeli B, Youssef A, Naderi A, et al. Margins of excision for cutaneous melanoma of the eyelid skin: the Collaborative Eyelid Skin Melanoma Group Report. *Ophthal Plast Reconstr Surg.* 2003;19(2):96–101.
11. Chan FM, O'Donnell BA, Whitehead K, et al. Treatment and outcomes of malignant melanoma of the eyelid: a review of 29 cases in Australia. *Ophthalmology.* 2007; 114(1):187–192.
12. Nemet AY, Deckel Y, Martin PA, et al. Management of periocular basal and squamous cell carcinoma: a series of 485 cases. *Am J Ophthalmol.* 2006;142(2):293–297.
13. Auw-Haedrich C, Frick S, Boehringer D, Mittelviefhaus H. Histologic safety margin in basal cell carcinoma of the eyelid: correlation with recurrence rate. *Ophthalmology.* 2009;116(4):802–806.
14. Wong VA, Marshall JA, Whitehead KJ, et al. Management of periocular basal cell carcinoma with modified en face frozen section controlled excision. *Ophthal Plast Reconstr Surg.* 2002;18(6):430–435.
15. Leibovitch I, McNab A, Sullivan T, et al. Orbital invasion by periocular basal cell carcinoma. *Ophthalmology.* 2005; 112(4):717–723.
16. Esmaeli B, De Martelaere S, Ozkan Y, et al. Surgical specimen handling for conjunctival melanoma: implications for tumor thickness determination and sentinel lymph node biopsy. *Ophthal Plast Reconstr Surg.* 2006;22(3):238–239.
17. Rahman I, Cook AE, Leatherbarrow B. Orbital exenteration: a 13 year Manchester experience. *Br J Ophthalmol.* 2005;89(10):1335–1340.
18. Tyers AG. Orbital exenteration for invasive skin tumours. Eye. 2006;20(10):1165–1170.
19. Hsu A, Frank SJ, Ballo MT, et al. Postoperative adjuvant external-beam radiation therapy for cancers of the eyelid and conjunctiva. *Ophthal Plast Reconstr Surg.* 2008;24(6): 444–449.
20. Shiu AS, Tung SS, Gastorf RJ, et al. Dosimetric evaluation of lead and tungsten eye shields in electron beam treatment. *Int J Radiat Oncol Biol Phys.* 1996;35(3):599–604.
21. Weaver RD, Gerbi BJ, Dusenbery KE. Evaluation of eye shields made of tungsten and aluminum in high-energy electron beams. *Int J Radiat Oncol Biol Phys.* 1998;41(1): 233–237.

12

SPECIAL CONSIDERATIONS: NEUROSURGICAL MANAGEMENT

FRANCO DEMONTE

Introduction

Neurosurgical intervention for cutaneous malignancy of the head and neck is required under 2 specific circumstances: (1) when there is direct calvarial (or deeper) invasion of a cranial convexity tumor in which a craniectomy is required, and (2) when subcranial soft tissue extension (orbit, sinus, infratemporal fossa) that requires intracranial access for complete resection (craniofacial resection) is present.

Surgical considerations vary depending on whether the neoplastic involvement is of the calvarium or of the skull base, and these two circumstances are discussed separately.

Cranial Convexity Tumors

Cutaneous malignancy of the scalp may invade the calvarium, the dura, and, at times, the brain itself (Fig 12–1). The complete extirpation of such tumors may require wide excision of the soft tissues of the scalp, a craniectomy (partial or full thickness), dural resection, and even resection of brain tissue.[1–7] These complex resections typically require complex reconstruction with duroplasty, cranioplasty, and free tissue transfer.

En Bloc Resection

In certain circumstances, en bloc resection of the scalp neoplasm along with the calvarium, dura, and even brain can be performed. Once the circumferential scalp incision is made, the scalp edges are sutured up out of the way and a trough is cut in the

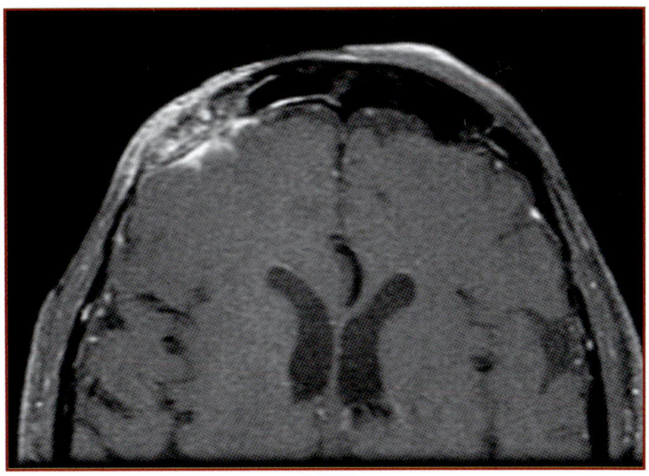

Figure 12–1. Axial T1-weighted, postcontrast MRI reveals intracranial extension of this recurrent right fronto-orbital SCC. (Used with permission of the Department of Neurosurgery, The University of Texas, MD Anderson Cancer Center.)

calvarium down to the dura. This can be accomplished using 2 parallel cuts with the craniotome or by placing a series of holes with the cranial perforator and removing residual intervening bone with rongeurs (Fig 12–2). Then the dura is incised circumferentially within the trough and the specimen is gently tipped up to inspect the brain surface. Arachnoidal adhesions are carefully divided and the specimen removed. In rare circumstances, partial venous sinus or involved cerebral tissue resec-

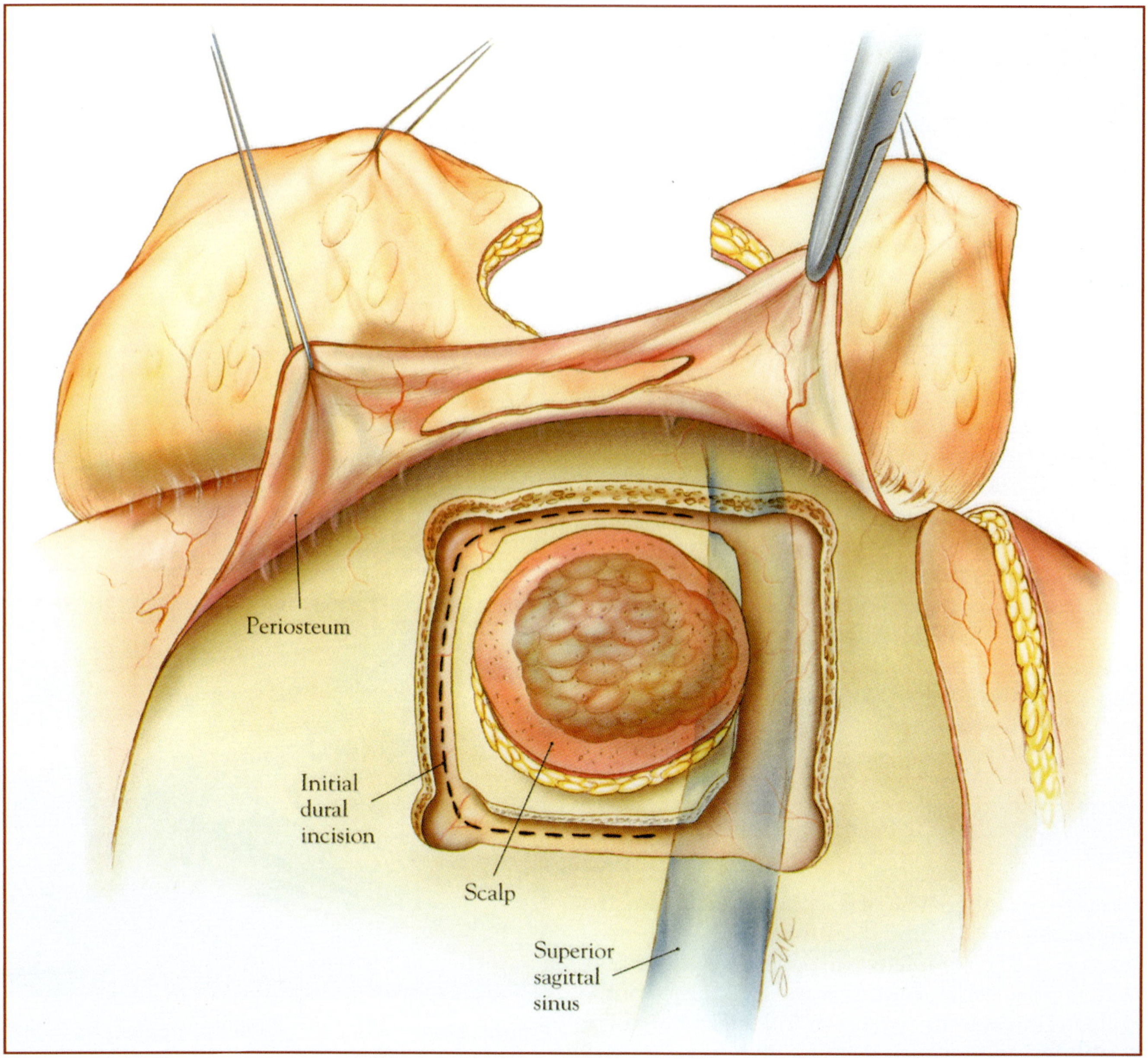

Figure 12–2. Artist's illustration of an en bloc resection of a scalp tumor. The bone troughs have been constructed and the dura is to be opened along the dotted line. (Used with permission of the Department of Neurosurgery, The University of Texas, MD Anderson Cancer Center.)

tion can be accomplished (Fig 12–3). Involvement of critical brain areas, large cortical veins, or the great sinuses behind the anterior third precludes the use of this technique.

Other Resection Techniques

Much more commonly, the involved tissues are removed layer by layer. A wide scalp excision is followed by craniotomy and then by any needed dural resection. A useful technique to judge the needed extent of calvarial resection is to subtotally circumscribe the scalp neoplasm, stain the areas of periosteal penetration with ink, and replace the flap in its original position thus "tattooing" the underlying, potentially involved calvarium prior to completing the scalp excision. The stained calvarium is then resected, as in Figure 12–4.

Management of Critical Vascular Structures

Special consideration needs to be given to neoplastic involvement of the great venous sinuses and adjacent cortical veins.[2,5,8] In most circumstances, neoplastic involvement of the anterior one-third of the superior sagittal sinus can be managed by sinus ligation and surgical resection. Ligation of the superior sagittal sinus behind its anterior third or of a solitary, highly dominant, or isolated transverse or

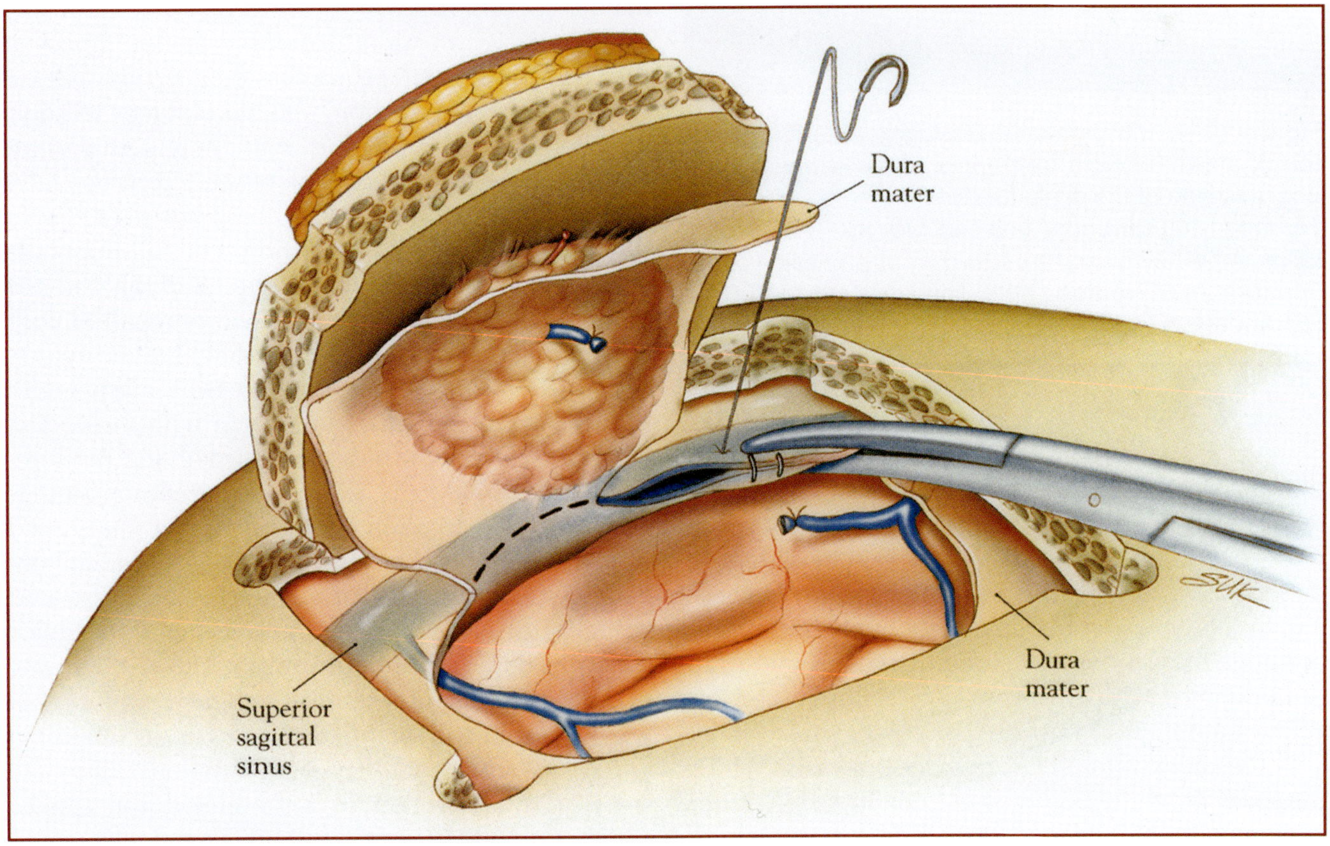

Figure 12–3. Artist's illustration of the en bloc resection of a scalp tumor. The dura has been opened and the lateral edge of the sagittal sinus is being resected. (Used with permission of the Department of Neurosurgery, The University of Texas, MD Anderson Cancer Center.)

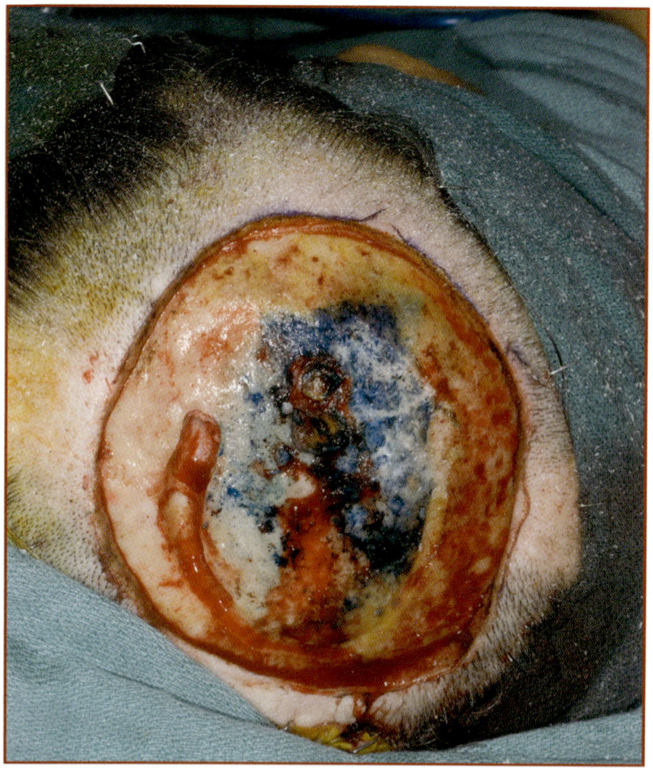

Figure 12–4. Intraoperative photograph during resection of a sarcomatoid carcinoma of the scalp. A wide local excision of the scalp has been accomplished and the underlying calvarium "tattooed" with ink. The affected calvarium is being excised. (Used with permission of the Department of Neurosurgery, The University of Texas, MD Anderson Cancer Center.)

sigmoid sinus can be associated with serious morbidity or mortality. If the dura is superficially involved, then the outer (periosteal) dura can be carefully dissected off of the underlying venous walls keeping the sinus patent. Conversely, if the neoplasm occludes the venous sinus, segmental resection can be performed with great care to preserve the cortical veins draining into the adjacent patent sinus.

The most difficult circumstance is one in which the sinus is deeply involved but not occluded. Management in this circumstance is controversial. Options include partial sinus resection with primary suture, resection of the sinus wall with patch grafting, or venous bypass and sinus resection. These maneuvers should be considered only when surgical cure is felt to be possible. These techniques are beyond the scope of this chapter and the reader is referred to standard neurosurgical texts. One unique circumstance is neoplastic involvement of the transverse-sigmoid sinus junction. In the author's opinion, this region is unresectable if it results in the isolation of the vein of Labbé due to the high risk of temporal lobe hemorrhagic infarction.

Reconstruction

Reconstruction begins with a watertight dural repair (Fig 12–5). Options for autologous tissue include uninvolved pericranium (periosteum + loose connective tissue layers adjacent to the galea), temporalis fascia, or fascia lata. Several commercially available allographs exist and are useful when the above tissues are not available or when their use is deemed suboptimal.

Similarly, multiple options exist for repair of the calvarium. Partial thickness defects typically do not require reconstruction, save for cosmetic reasons. The defect can be filled in with polymethylmeth-acrylate (PMMA) or one of several commercially available bone cements. Covering the defect with titanium mesh also is an option. For full-thickness defects, the reconstructive choice is based on the size of the defect. Small defects can be repaired with reconstruction plates or mesh alone. Larger defects are amenable to repair with PMMA alone, with PMMA and mesh, or bone cement with mesh. The largest defects, as well as those involving the forehead and orbital rims, may be repaired in a similar way, but consideration should be given to a staged reconstructive approach with the use of a custom patient-specific cranial implant, as is demonstrated in Figure 12–6.[9] Typically, it is not difficult to elevate the scalp flap or free flap from the dura at the time of the subsequent implant placement.

Repair of the scalp defect is by local rotational flap or by free tissue transfer. Rotational flaps are not usually sufficient for large effects but can be successful with careful patient and defect selection.[10] Managing complex defects of the scalp and calvarium is a technically demanding endeavor, and this topic is discussed in greater detail in Chapter 37.

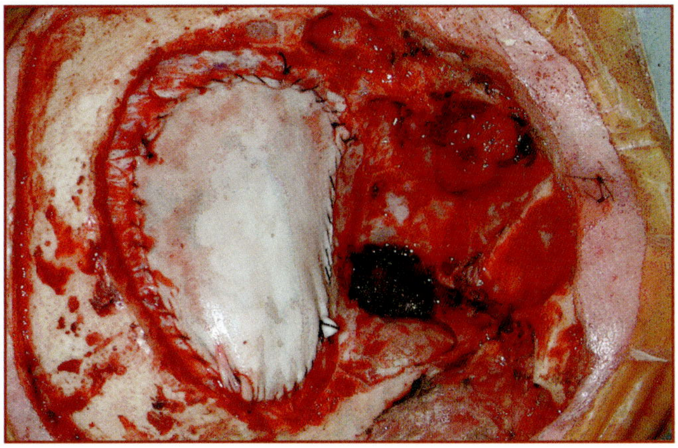

Figure 12–5. A watertight dural repair is the first step in the repair of a composite defect of the craniofacial skeleton. This intraoperative photograph is of the patient whose MRI is shown in Figure 12–1. In this case an allograft was utilized. (Used with permission of the Department of Neurosurgery, The University of Texas, MD Anderson Cancer Center.)

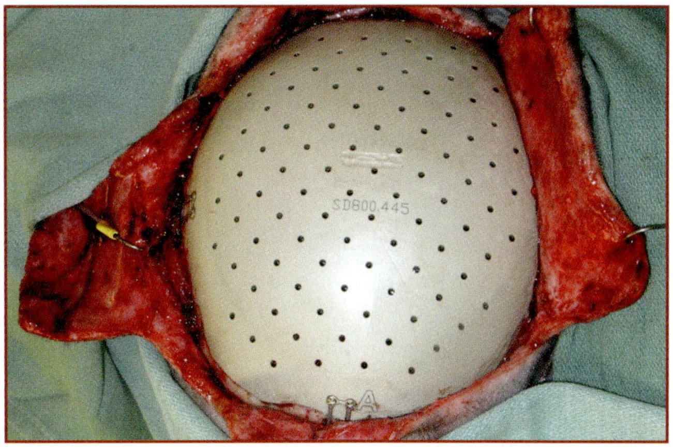

Figure 12–6. Intraoperative photograph after placement of a patient-specific cranial implant. Note the exact fit at each bone edge and of the overall favorable contour of the implant. (Used with permission of the Department of Neurosurgery, The University of Texas, MD Anderson Cancer Center.)

Prognosis

Few reports address the long-term outcome of patients with deeply invasive cutaneous malignancies that require neurosurgical intervention. Multidisciplinary treatment is required, as patients may benefit from adjuvant therapy, if possible. Soma et al[5] described 25 patients who manifest aggressive malignancies of the scalp with intracranial extension. Of the 25 patients treated, 22 were still alive 5 to 13 years later (mean = 7), whereas 3 patients had died of non-tumor-related causes. This report underscores the importance of comprehensive tumor extirpation in a multidisciplinary setting.

Skull Base and Subcranial Soft Tissue Extension

In rare circumstances, aggressive cutaneous malignancy can extend to the skull base or to the adjacent tissues of the orbit and infratemporal fossa, either directly or via perineural invasion. Tumor resection and reconstruction in these patients typically requires an experienced multidisciplinary team of experts skilled in craniofacial surgical techniques (Fig 12–7). Neurosurgical intervention may require orbitocranial, subtemporal-infratemporal, or transpetrosal approaches to access the anterior, anterolateral, lateral, posterolateral, or, rarely, the posterior skull base (Fig 12–8). Although en bloc resection is preferable, it should be abandoned if there is concern for neurologic compromise.

Perineural Invasion

Perineural invasion is common in aggressive cutaneous malignancy, particularly squamous cell carcinoma. Disease may spread centripetally or centrifugally along cranial nerves and ultimately involve the nerve at the skull base. Branches of cranial nerves V and VII most commonly are affected, and the nerve may be grossly involved proximally along its course.[11]

Although there is occasional debate about intracranial efforts to clear perineural invasion to the cranial nerve ganglion (at least for cranial nerve V), the prognosis in patients with extensive perineural

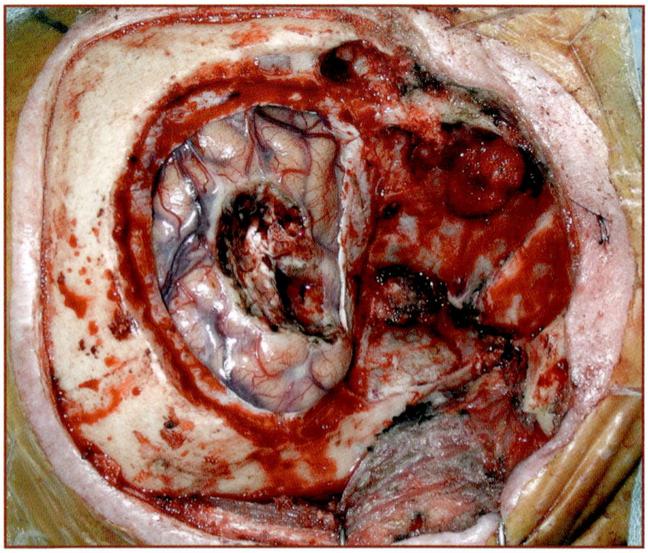

Figure 12–7. Extensive craniofacial resection of the patient whose MRI is shown in Figure 12–1. This patient with recurrent SCC underwent an en bloc-wide local excision of the scalp lesion with orbitectomy, craniectomy, dural resection, and focal brain resection. He remained locally controlled but developed nodal recurrence 2 years later. (Used with permission of the Department of Neurosurgery, The University of Texas, MD Anderson Cancer Center.)

invasion is poor. In our experience, the cranial nerve may be cleared to its foramen in the skull base, and only rarely do we pursue perineural invasion intracranially. Postoperative radiation, or chemoradiation, may be administered along the path of the cranial nerve or targeted to the involved ganglion in these cases. The techniques and benefits of radiation therapy for perineural invasion to the skull base are included in another chapter. Gross perineural involvement of the facial nerve may be followed into the mastoid, but does not usually merit lateral temporal bone resection. Management of the facial nerve within the temporal bone is discussed in Chapter 13.

Prognosis

The MD Anderson Cancer Center Skull Base Team has previously reported on 35 patients with aggressive basal cell carcinoma (BCC) or squamous cell carcinoma (SCC) who underwent craniofacial resection.[12] This was a heavily treated cohort of patients, with 20 patients having previously been irradiated and only four patients treated at initial disease pres-

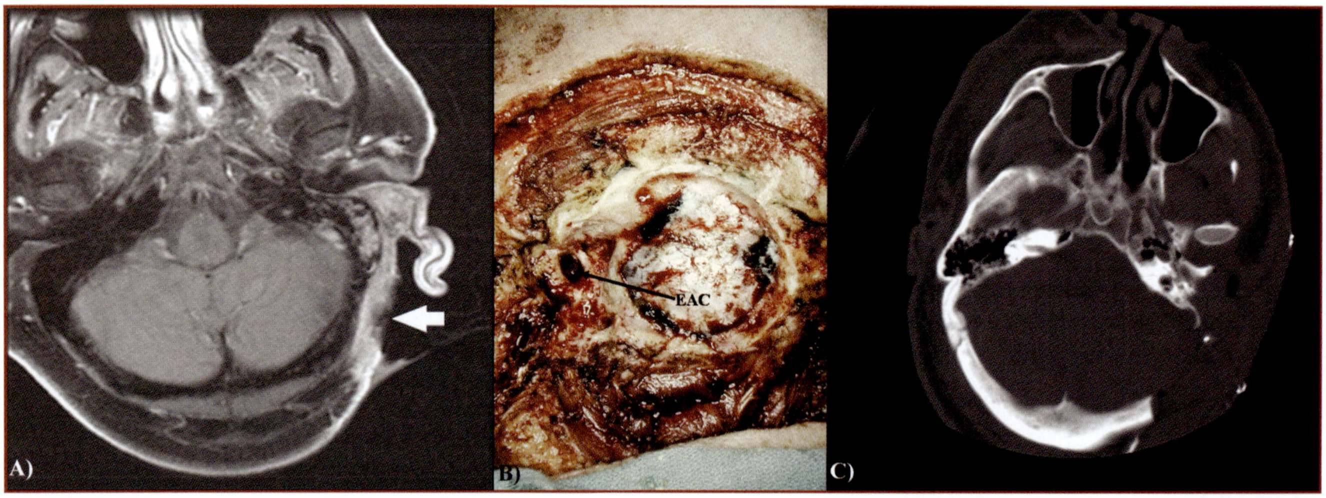

Figure 12–8. A. Preoperative axial postcontrast T1-weighted MRI identifies the depth of invasion of this retroauricular BCC. **B.** Intraoperative photograph depicts the extent of resection. The ear canal has been transected and the posterior temporal bone and occipital bone have been removed to expose the noninvolved posterior fossa dura. **C.** Postoperative CT quantifies the extent of bone resection performed. (Used with permission of the Department of Neurosurgery, The University of Texas, MD Anderson Cancer Center.)

entation. Disease-specific survival was significantly better in patients with BCC and was significantly decreased in patients with intracranial extension, regardless of tumor histology. Overall, disease-specific survival was only 20%, and the mean time from treatment to recurrence was 24.9 months. A trend toward improved local control was seen in patients who were able to receive postoperative radiotherapy and in patients with BCC.[12]

Since the publication of that report, 28 additional patients have undergone craniofacial resection of invasive cutaneous malignancy as part of a multimodal management plan with curative intent. Nine of these patients had a diagnosis of BCC and 19 patients had SCC. As with our prior cohort of patients, this group was heavily pretreated, as 12 patients previously underwent surgery and radiation therapy, 5 had at least one prior resection (range 1 to 4), and 4 patients had been extensively treated with surgery, radiation, and chemotherapy. Only 7 patients were treated at presentation, which is twice the percentage in the earlier report.

Postoperatively, 11 patients received radiation, 2 underwent chemoradiation, 2 were treated with radiosurgery, and 11 received chemotherapy alone. Eight patients did not receive adjuvant therapy, and information was unavailable for 4 patients. At the time of last follow-up, 12 patients were alive and free of disease (NED), 6 patients had died of causes unrelated to their treated cancer and were free of disease at death (DOC), 3 patients, all with SCC, died of their disease (DOD). One patient with BCC was alive 10 years following treatment, but disease status was uncertain. Another patient with SCC was alive with regional recurrence at 2 years but was subsequently lost to follow-up. There was 1 death within 30 days of surgery due to a myocardial infarction, and 4 patients were lost to follow-up.

The mean follow-up for living patients was 4.4 years, with a range 1.2 to 15 years and a median follow-up of 2.6 years. Four of 12 patients had follow-up of more than 5 years, and 5 of 12 had follow-up of more than 3 years. The mean follow-up time for patients who died of other causes was 5.2 years (range 1.75–10 yrs; median: 3.5 yr; 5/6 had follow-up >3 years). Patients who died of their disease had a mean time to death of only 11 months, and all of these patients succumbed to SCC.

Special Considerations

Invasive cutaneous malignancy requiring craniofacial resection is more common in the elderly population. In a study from our institution, one third of a cohort of patients older than 70 years of age undergoing craniofacial resection did so for invasive cutaneous malignancy.[13] These patients had a similar disease-specific survival to a cohort of younger patients (mean age 56 years), but as a group had almost 3 times the incidence of systemic complications, underscoring the need for meticulous perioperative care in this population.

Conclusions

The successful management of deeply invasive cutaneous malignancy reaching the calvarium, skull base, or intracranial contents clearly remains a challenging undertaking, although outcomes seem to be improving over time. In order to achieve optimal outcomes, patients with these tumors must be evaluated and treated by a multidisciplinary team of experts in the management of these aggressive malignancies. Disease control and survival rates are improved with such multidisciplinary care at the time of initial presentation, rather than at the time of recurrence. Consistent with other sites within the head and neck, patients with BCC fare better than those with SCC. Postoperative radiotherapy or chemoradiotherapy seem to be of benefit in these aggressive cases.

References

1. Hierner R, van Loon J, Goffin J, van Calenbergh F. Free latissimus dorsi flap transfer for subtotal scalp and cranium defect reconstruction: report of 7 cases. *Microsurgery.* 2007;27(5):425–428.
2. Mathieu D, Fortin D. Intracranial invasion of a basal cell carcinoma of the scalp. *Can J Neurol Sci.* 2005;32(4):546–548.
3. McCombe D, Donato R, Hofer S, Morrison W. Free flaps in the treatment of locally advanced malignancy of the scalp and forehead. *Ann Plast Surg.* 2002;48(6):600–605.

4. Sedira MA, Amin AA, Rifaat MA, El-Sebai HI, El-Badawy MAA, Kassem HAA. Locally advanced tumors of the scalp: the Egyptian National Cancer Institute experience. *J Egypt Nat Cancer Inst.* 2006;18(3):250–257.
5. Soma PF, Chibbaro S, Makiese O, et al. Aggressive scalp carcinoma with intracranial extension: a multidisciplinary experience of 25 patients with long-term follow-up. *J Clin Neurosci.* 2008;15(9):988–992.
6. Wang HT, Erdmann D, Olbrich KC, Friedman AH. Levin LS, Zenn MR. Free flap reconstruction of the scalp and calvaria of major neurosurgical resections in cancer patients: lessons learned closing large, difficult wounds of the dura and skull. *Plast Reconstr Surg.* 2007;119(3): 865–872.
7. Wax MK, Burkey BB, Bascom D, Rosenthal EL. The role of free tissue transfer in the reconstruction of massive neglected skin cancers of the head and neck. *Arch Facial Plast Surg.* 2003;5(6):479–482.
8. Michael CB, Gokaslan ZL, DeMonte F, McCutcheon IE, Sawaya R, Lang FF. Surgical resection of calvarial metastases overlying dural sinuses. *Neurosurgery.* 2001;48(4): 745–755.
9. Hanasono MM, Goel N, DeMonte F. Calvarial reconstruction with polyetheretherketone implants. *Ann Plast Surg.* 2009;62(6):653–655.
10. Chang DW, Langstein HN, Gupta A, DeMonte F, Do KA, Wang X, Robb G. Reconstructive management of cranial base defects after tumor ablation. *Plast Reconstr Surg.* 2000;107(6):1346–1355.
11. Goepfert H, Dichtel WJ, Medina JE, Lindberg RD, Luna MD. Perineural invasion in squamous cell carcinoma of the head and neck. *Am J Surg.* 1984;148(4):542–547.
12. Backous DD, DeMonte F, El-Naggar A, Wolf P, Weber RS. Craniofacial resection for nonmelanoma skin cancer of the head and neck. *Laryngoscope.* 2005;115(6):931–937.
13. Hentschel SJ, Nader R, Suki D, Dastgir A, Callender DL, DeMonte F. Craniofacial resections in the elderly: an outcome study. *J Neurosurg.* 2004;101(6):935–943.

13

RADIOTHERAPY FOR CUTANEOUS SQUAMOUS AND BASAL CELL CARCINOMA

WILLIAM M. MENDENHALL
ROBERT J. AMDUR
NANCY P. MENDENHALL

Introduction

Carcinoma of the skin may be successfully treated by a variety of modalities including surgery, radiotherapy (RT), electrofulguration and curettage, and cryotherapy. This chapter reviews the role of RT in the management of squamous and basal cell carcinomas of the skin of the head and neck, including metatypical basal cell carcinomas (basosquamous carcinomas). The goal of treatment is cure with preservation of function and cosmesis. In the management of skin cancer arising in the head and neck particularly, resection may compromise function and/or result in an unacceptable cosmetic deformity.

Patients are staged according to the 2010 American Joint Committee on Cancer (AJCC) staging system, which underwent significant revision from the 2002 version (Table 13–1).[1] Staging of the primary lesion depends on tumor diameter, anatomic location, the presence of certain high-risk features, and invasion of deeper structures such as the mandible, maxilla, orbit, and temporal bone. The high-risk features were identified for the first time, and they include thickness >2 mm, invasion to or beyond Clark level IV, perineural invasion, and poorly differentiated or undifferentiated histology. Additionally, the impact of tumor location on prognosis is stressed by the inclusion of primary lesions on the non-hair-bearing lip and ear as high-risk features. If tumors exhibit more than two high-risk features, they may be upstaged. The importance of anatomic site is further highlighted by a unique system for eyelid carcinoma (Table 13–2).[1] Parenthetically, when analyzing data, one should avoid comparing lesions that were clinically staged and those that were pathologically staged because clinical staging is more likely to underestimate the extent of the lesion and thus bias the comparison.

Although the probability of regional and/or distant metastasis is low, the risk increases with lesions that are extensive, poorly differentiated, and/or recurrent after prior treatment. Patients with squamous cell carcinoma (SCCA) and perineural invasion (PNI) exhibit an increased risk of regional metastases.[2] Lymph nodes most often involved are in the parotid and/or neck.[3–5] O'Brien and colleagues[6] proposed a modification of the staging system for patients with positive nodes in these sites (Table 13–3), and its impact has been validated by modifications of nodal staging in the 2010 AJCC system (see Table 13–1), reflecting the prognostic significance of increasing nodal burden.[1,5]

Table 13–1. The American Joint Committee on Cancer Definition of TNM[1]

Primary Tumor (T)	
TX	Primary tumor cannot be assessed
T0	No evidence of primary tumor
Tis	Carcinoma in situ
T1	Tumor 2 cm or less in greater dimension with less than 2 high-risk features*
T2	Tumor greater than 2 cm *or* Tumor any size with two or more high-risk features*
T3	Tumor with invasion of maxilla, mandible, orbit, or temporal bone
T4	Tumor with invasion of skeleton (axial or appendicular) or perineural invasion of skull base
Regional Lymph Nodes (N)	
NX	Regional lymph nodes cannot be assessed
N0	No regional lymph node metastasis
N1	Metastasis in a single ipsilateral lymph node, 3 cm or less in greatest dimension
N2a	Metastasis is a single ipsilateral lymph node, more than 3 cm but not more than 6 cm in greatest dimension;
N2b	Metastasis in multiple ipsilateral lymph nodes, none more than 6 cm in greatest dimension
N2c	Metastasis in bilateral or contralateral lymph nodes, none more than 6 cm in greatest dimension
N3	Metastasis in a lymph node, more than 6 cm in greatest dimension
Distant Metastasis (M)	
MX	Distant metastasis cannot be assessed
M0	No distant metastasis
M1	Distant metastasis

Note: In case of multiple simultaneous tumors, the tumor with the highest T category will be classified and the number of separate tumors will be indicated in parentheses.

*High risk features include depth of invasion >2 mm thickness or Clark level IV, perineural invasion, primary site on ear or hair-bearing lip, and poorly differentiated or undifferentiated histology.

Source: Used with permission of the American Joint Committee on Cancer (AJCC), Chicago, Illinois. The original source for this material is the AJCC Cancer Staging Manual, Seventh Edition (2010) published by Springer Science and Business Media, LLC, www.springer.com.

Selection of Treatment Modality

The likelihood of cure is similar after surgery or RT for early-stage basal cell carcinomas (BCCAs) and SCCAs.[7] Therefore, selection of one modality over another is based on other parameters such as function, cosmesis, age of the patient, convenience, cost, availability of appropriate RT equipment, and the wishes of the patient. Patients with advanced cancers often are best treated with surgery and adjuvant RT, if the cancer is resectable and the functional and cosmetic outcomes are acceptable.

Radiotherapy Alone

Small skin cancers located on "free skin," such as the cheek or forehead, may be excised easily with a good cosmetic result and minimal inconvenience;

Table 13–2. Carcinoma of the Eyelid by the American Joint Committee on Cancer[1]

Primary Tumor (T)	
TX	Primary tumor cannot be assessed
T0	No evidence of primary tumor
Tis	Carcinoma in situ
T1	Tumor 5 mm or less in greatest dimension. Not invading the tarsal plate or eyelid margin.
T2a	Tumor more than 5 mm, but not more than 10 mm, in greatest dimension. *or*, any tumor that invades the tarsal plate or eyelid margin
T2b	Tumor more than 10 mm, but not more than 20 mm in greatest dimension. *or*, involves full-thickness eyelid
T3a	Tumor more than 20 mm in greatest dimension. *or*, any tumor that invades adjacent ocular, or orbital structures Any tumor with perineural invasion
T3b	Tumor complete resection requires enucleation, exenteration, or bone resection
T4	Tumor is not resectable due to extensive invasion of ocular, orbital, craniofacial structures, or brain
Regional Lymph Nodes (N)	
NX	Regional lymph nodes cannot be assessed
N0	No regional lymph node metastasis based on clinical evaluation, imaging, or lymph node biopsy
N1	Regional lymph node metastasis
Distant Metastasis (M)	
MX	Distant metastasis cannot be assessed
M0	No distant metastasis
M1	Distant metastasis

Source: Used with permission of the American Joint Committee on Cancer (AJCC), Chicago, Illinois. The original source for this material is the AJCC Cancer Staging Manual, Seventh Edition (2010) published by Springer Science and Business Media, LLC, www.springer.com.

Table 13–3. Clinical Staging System for Metastatic Cutaneous Squamous Cell Carcinoma of the Parotid and/or Neck[6]

Parotid	
P0	No clinical disease in the parotid
P1	Metastatic node up to 3 cm in diameter
P2	Metastatic node >3 cm and up to 6 cm in diameter or multiple nodes
P3	Metastatic node >6 cm in diameter or disease involving the facial nerve or skull base
Neck	
N0	No clinical disease
N1	Single ipsilateral neck node up to 3 cm in diameter
N2	Single node >3 cm in diameter or multiple nodes or contralateral nodes

Source: O'Brien CJ, McNeil EB, McMahon JD, Pathak I, Lauer CS, Jackson MA. Significance of clinical stage, extent of surgery and pathological findings in metastatic cutaneous squamous cell carcinoma of the parotid gland. *Head Neck.* 2002;24:417–422.

therefore, surgery usually is the treatment of choice for such lesions. It also is desirable to avoid RT in young patients because the late effects of irradiation progress gradually with time and, with very long-term follow-up, may be associated with a suboptimal cosmetic result compared with resection and reconstruction. In contrast, resection of an early stage skin cancer of the eyelid, external ear, or nose may result in a significant cosmetic deformity and necessitate complex reconstruction that compares unfavorably with RT. This is particularly relevant in the case of older patients who have a limited life expectancy and who are at higher risk for a perioperative complication.

Patients with locally advanced skin cancers present a difficult problem. Although the likelihood of cure may be better with combined RT and surgery, in some situations, the cosmetic result is sometimes unacceptable. Patients receive postoperative RT if surgery is indicated and feasible. If surgery is not feasible, the patient is managed with RT alone. Although it might seem that the risk of bone and/or cartilage necrosis would be high after RT for a skin cancer invading these structures, the observed risk of complications is relatively low.[8,9] An exception is advanced cancers of the scalp and those overlying the anterior aspect of the tibia where there is little tissue between the skin surface and the bone. Following definitive RT, bone exposure is likely and may progress to an osteoradionecrosis (ORN) requiring surgical intervention.

Adjuvant Radiotherapy

Postoperative RT is added after surgery if pathologic examination of the surgical specimen reveals findings indicative of a high risk for local recurrence, such as close or positive margins and/or invasion of nerve, cartilage, or bone. A significant proportion of patients with positive margins after resection of an early-stage skin cancer may never develop a local recurrence. Postoperative RT may be withheld if the histologic subtype is BCCA, if the primary site is located on the "free skin," if the patient is reliable and will return for close follow-up, and if salvage treatment would have a high likelihood of eradicating recurrent tumor with a good cosmetic result. BCCAs of the nose, eyelid, or ear and lesions that would have immediate access to major nerve trunks usually are re-treated immediately when resection margins are positive. The risk of recurrence probably is greater than for lesions of the free skin, and the consequences of recurrence may be significant. Observation is particularly attractive for the elderly patient in poor medical condition who may not live to experience a local recurrence. Metatypical BCCAs behave more aggressively than BCCAs and those with positive margins after surgery should be re-excised and/or treated with postoperative RT.

The usual policy for patients with positive margins from squamous cell carcinoma is immediate retreatment by either re-excision, irradiation, or both, depending on the situation. There is evidence that this approach leads to a reduced risk of metastasis and reduced likelihood of death from cancer.[10–12]

Management of Regional Lymph Node Metastases

Carcinoma of the skin metastatic to the parotid lymph nodes is managed as a high-grade parotid neoplasm, usually with superficial or total parotidectomy followed by postoperative RT.[3–5] If only one node is involved and there is no extracapsular extension, it may be safe to withhold RT. However, if the tumor recurs in the parotid area after parotidectomy, the likelihood of salvage is remote.[3] Therefore, it has been our practice to use combined treatment in all patients. If the parotid lymph-node metastasis is fixed and thought to be incompletely resectable, the patient is treated with high-dose preoperative RT (6000–7000 cGy) followed by parotidectomy. RT alone is used only in patients who are inoperable because of tumor extent or poor medical condition.

Cervical lymph node metastases are managed just as they would be for other carcinomas of the head and neck. Neck dissection alone is adequate treatment if only one node is involved and there is no extracapsular extension. If two or more nodes contain tumor or if extracapsular extension is noted, neck dissection is followed by postoperative RT.

Radiation Therapy Techniques

Treatment techniques vary for primary lesions, and for parotid-area lymph-node metastases.

Primary Lesion

Radiation therapy of the primary lesion usually is accomplished using one of three basic external-beam techniques (orthovoltage RT, electron beam, and high energy x-rays or photons) or with an interstitial implant either alone or in combination with external-beam techniques. Most early skin cancers are managed with orthovoltage RT with beam energies of 100 to 250 KeV. The advantages of this technique, compared with electron beam, are that the maximum dose is at the skin surface; bolus is not required; there is less beam constriction both at the surface and at depth so that smaller fields can be used (Fig 13–1); shielding of the eye is easier and more effectively accomplished, particularly if electron energies of 10 MeV or higher are used (Table 13–4); it is less expensive; and the likelihood of tumor control may be higher, possibly as a result of increased radiobiologic effectiveness (RBE), but more likely because of technical problems that are difficult to overcome when using electrons alone.[13] The disadvantage of orthovoltage x-rays, compared with electron beam, is that a higher dose is delivered to deeper tissues and to underlying bone and cartilage. The latter problem can be largely eliminated by using heavily filtered orthovoltage beams for tumors involving or overlying cartilage or bone. Another significant problem associated with orthovoltage RT is that most radiation oncology departments do not have an orthovoltage machine and, thus, it is unavailable. Electron beam is usually used for lesions of the scalp to reduce the dose to the underlying brain; orthovoltage x-rays are used to treat most other skin cancers of the head and neck.

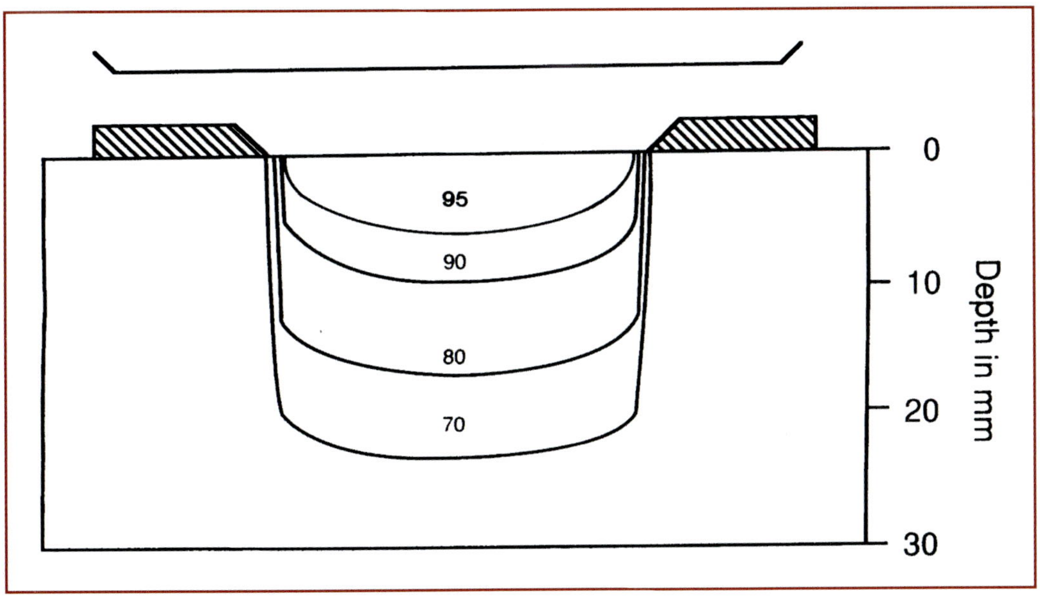

A

Figure 13–1. A. 250-kVp x-rays (HVL 1.4-mm Cu) with secondary collimation on the phantom surface, Source-to surface distance (SSD) = 50 cm. Iso dose %: 95, 90, 80, 70. *(continues)*

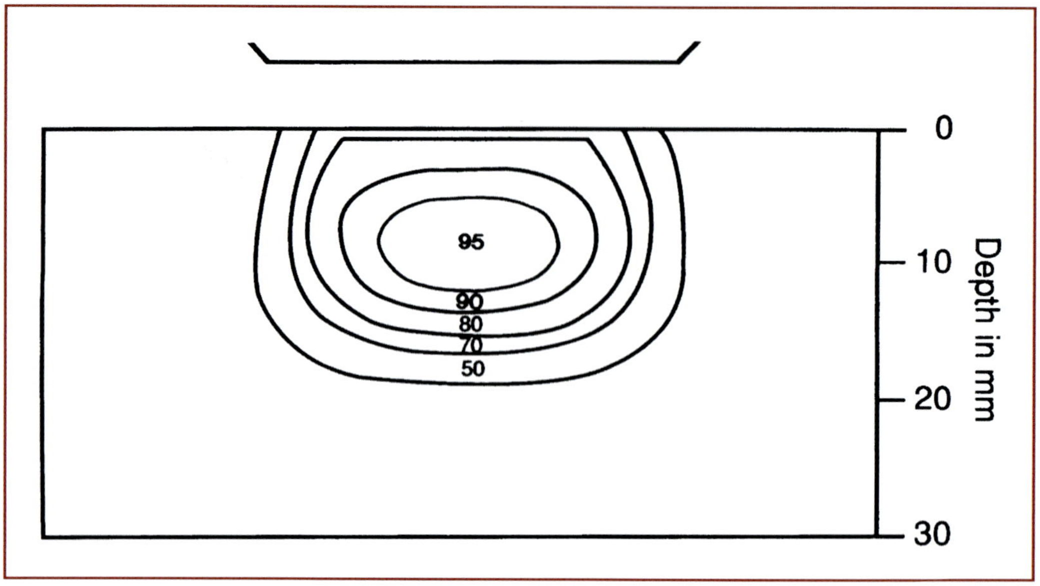

B

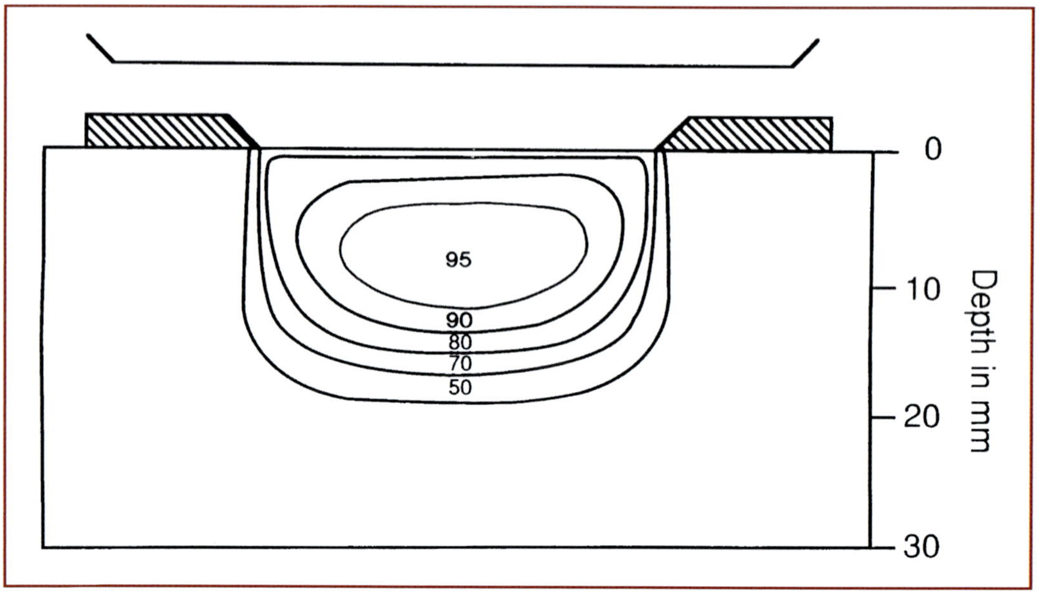

C

Figure 13–1. *(continued)* **B.** 6-MeV electron beam with secondary collimation 5 cm above the phantom surface (at the level of the electron cone). Source of collimator distance (SCD) = 95 cm. SSD = 100 cm. Isodose %: 95, 90, 80, 70, 50. **C.** 6-MeV electron beam with tertiary collimation on the phantom surface. SSD = SCD = 100 cm. isodose %: 95, 90, 80, 70, 50.

Before treatment with either electron-beam or orthovoltage x-rays, a customized lead mask is constructed to collimate the beam directly on the skin surface. A 1.0- to 1.5-cm margin is adequate for a well-defined T1 lesion treated with orthovoltage RT. An additional 1 cm is added to the margin when the electron beam is used to account for beam constriction. For larger and/or ill-defined tumors, a 2-cm margin usually is necessary. If the tumor is located near the eye, a gold-plated lead eye shield is placed directly on the anesthetized cornea to minimize the irradiation dose to underlying structures (Fig 13–2). The dose beneath the eye shield is depicted for orthovoltage x-rays and electron beams of various energies in Table 13–4. Isodose distributions for the two techniques are shown in Figure 13–1; note that the dose distribution is better for orthovoltage RT than for electron beam, particularly if a lead mask is not used with the electron beam.

Advanced skin cancers that are deeply invasive often are treated with high-energy photons in order to adequately cover the deep extent of the tumor. Bolus is used to ensure an adequate surface dose. Field arrangement varies with primary site: for example, a wedge pair technique may be used for lesions involving the external ear, whereas a three-field technique (similar to that used for paranasal sinus cancer) frequently is used for skin cancers with extension proximally along the second division of the fifth cranial nerve. The target volume includes the entire course of the involved nerve, which would include the Gasserian ganglion in this case, to the brainstem. Intensity-modulated radiotherapy (IMRT) may be used in some patients to produce a more conformal dose distribution to reduce the dose to surrounding normal structures. Proton beam also may be used to produce a very conformal dose distribution with steep dose gradients to limit the dose to the visual apparatus and the central nervous system (CNS).[14,15]

Table 13–4. Ocular Protection: Dose Beneath the Eye Shield[9]

Structure (Depth)	250 kVp x-ray (HVL 1.4-mm Cu)	Electron-Beam Energy (MeV)						
		6	8	10	12	14	17	20
Cornea (1 mm)	10%	18%	37%	64%	75%	93%	98%	102%
Lens (8 mm)	9%	9%	19%	36%	46%	61%	70%	87%
Retina (23 mm)	10%	19%	22%	22%	21%	23%	25%	29%

Note: Dose is expressed as a percentage of the dose to D_{max} (depth of maximum dose deposition).

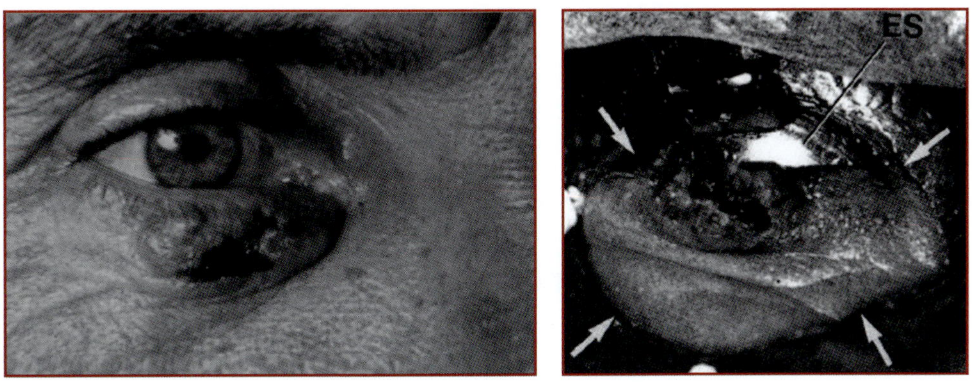

A. B.

Figure 13–2. A. 1 × 1-cm basal cell carcinoma of the midportion of the lower lid. **B.** Treatment setup that was used to irradiate the patient. ES = eye shield; arrows indicate the field edge.

The regional lymph nodes are electively irradiated if the suspected risk of subclinical disease exceeds 10 to 15%.[2,16]

Dose-fractionation schedules used for irradiation of skin cancers are outlined in Table 13–5. We recently have used twice-daily RT with megavoltage photons or protons at 1.2 Gy per fraction to doses of 74.4 Gy in a continuous course with a minimum 6-hour interfraction interval, for advanced lesions near radiosensitive structures.[15,17,18] The suggested maximum doses for short course orthovoltage RT are listed in Table 13–6.

Parotid-Area Lymph Node Metastases

The parotid gland and upper neck are treated with an en face mixed beam of 6-MV x-rays and high-energy electrons (usually 20 MeV), weighted 1.0 to 6.7 in favor of the electron beam. The electron-beam field is 1 cm larger than the x-ray field to account for the beam constriction of the electrons, except where the field abuts the low neck field (Fig 13–3). This field arrangement is treated to 4600 cGy in 23 fractions, specified at a depth of 4 to 5 cm from the skin surface. An anterior field is matched to the lateral mixed-beam field to treat the ipsilateral low neck and is irradiated to 5000 cGy in 25 fractions, specified at Dmax.

At 4600-cGy tumor dose, the primary field is reduced off of the spinal cord and the dose to the tumor bed is boosted with an anteriorly angled 20-MeV electron-beam field or an appositional mixed-beam field with an abutting posterior electron strip. The final dose for patients treated at 200 cGy per fraction is, with negative margins, 6000 cGy; with positive margins, 6600 cGy; and with gross residual disease, 7000 cGy. If the dose per fraction is reduced to 180 cGy, the total dose is increased by 500 cGy. An alternative to the mixed electron-photon beam is

Table 13–5. Guidelines for Selection of External-Beam Dose[7]

Orthovoltage Dose (cGy)[a]	Examples
6500 over 7 weeks	Large untreated lesion with bone/cartilage invasion or large recurrent tumor[b]
6000 over 7 weeks	Large untreated lesion with minimal or suspected bone/cartilage invasion[b]
5500 over 6 weeks	Moderate to large inner canthus, eyelid, nasal, or pinna lesions (20–30 cm^2 area)
5000 over 4 weeks	Small, thin lesion (less than 1.5 cm) around eye, nose, or ear (10 cm^2 area)
4500 over 3 weeks	Moderate-sized lesion on "free" skin or postoperative treatment of moderate sized cancer on "free" skin with positive margins
4000 over 2 weeks or 3000 over 1 week	Small lesions (1 cm) on "free" skin
The following schemes are used when the late cosmetic result is not important and travel for the patient is difficult:	
4000 in 10 fractions or 3000 in 5 fractions or 2000 in 1 fraction	Rapid fractionation schemes produce a high cure rate for small lesions but the cosmetic result may be less than optimal after 5 years.

"Free": Not involving ear, nose, eye, or eyelid.

[a]Add 10% to dose for supervoltage therapy.

[b]All or a portion of the therapy given with supervoltage photons and/or electrons.

Table 13–6. Suggested Maximum Skin Doses[a] for Palliation with 250-kVp x-Rays (Below Moist Desquamation Level for the Average Patient)

Field Size (Area in cm^2)	Total Dose (cGy) One Day (1 Exposure)	2 Days (2 Exposures)	4 Days (4 Exposures)	5 Days (5 Exposures)	2 Weeks (10 Exposures)	3 Weeks (15 Exposures)	5 Weeks (25 Exposures)
Small fields							
10	2,000	2,750	3,500	3,750	5,000	5,500	6,000
50	1,750	2,500	3,250	3,500	4,500	5,000	5,500
Medium fields							
100	1,500	2,000	2,500	2,750	3,750	4,250	5,000
150	1,250	1,750	2,250	2,500	3,250	3,750	4,500
Large fields							
200	1,000	1,500	2,000	2,250	3,000	3,500	4,250
300	NR	NR	NR	2,000	2,750	3,250	4,000

[a]The total dose listed is administered over a treatment course of the indicated length, divided into the indicated number of fractional treatments.

NR = Not recommended.

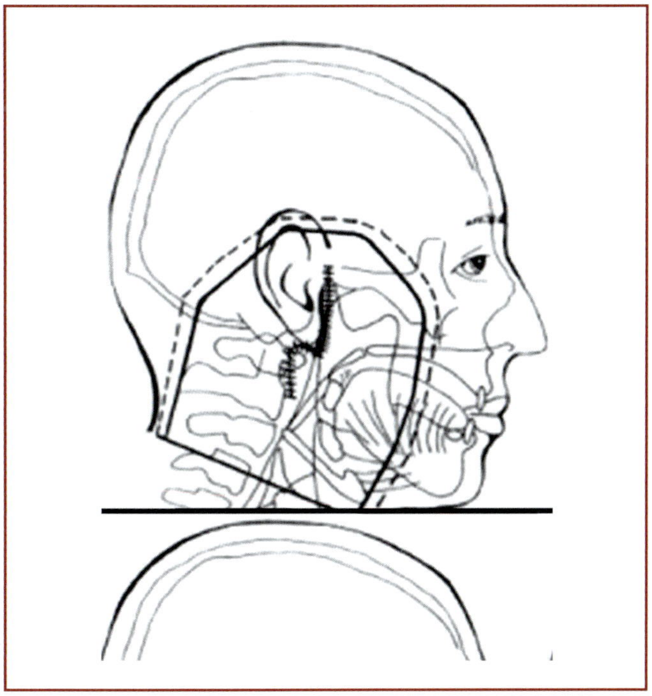

Figure 13–3. Typical en face mixed-beam field used in the treatment of parotid node metastases to encompass the entire parotid bed and surgical scar. Patients are treated supine with a face mask made of low-temperature thermal plastic (polycaprolactone) for immobilization, and a lead lollipop to decrease the dose to the contralateral salivary gland. A bolus of petrolatum-coated gauze is applied to all scars.

a wedge-pair technique using 4- to 6-MV photon beams. IMRT also may be considered to reduce the dose to the temporal lobe and cerebellum, particularly if the margins are positive and/or tumor involves the deep lobe of the parotid.

Surveillance and Management of Recurrent Disease

After RT, patients are evaluated every 2 to 3 months for the first 2 years, every 4 months for the 3rd year, every 6 months for the 4th and 5th years, and annually thereafter, in conjunction with the other members of the multidisciplinary team. Chest roentgenograms are obtained annually, and follow-up computed tomography or magnetic resonance imaging is obtained as needed for patients irradiated for advanced lesions. Thyroid function blood tests (thyroid stimulating hormone and free thyroxine) are obtained every 6 to 12 months if the entire thyroid gland is included in a low neck field.

Treatment of local-regional recurrences after RT alone or combined with surgery usually is resection. If a local recurrence is amenable to en bloc surgical resection with frozen section control of the margins, this may be preferable for selected cases. Local recurrences after RT may be significantly more extensive than is clinically apparent so that wide margins are preferred. Retreatment with RT rarely is indicated because of the high likelihood of complications. The most common scenario for recurrence in the neck nodes is failure in a solitary submandibular location; the success rate of salvage neck dissection is high in this circumstance.

Outcomes Following Radiation Therapy for Cutaneous Malignancy

Most series reporting the results of treatment for skin cancer contain a preponderance of early lesions and do not employ a staging system, making it difficult to compare various series and the relative efficacy of different treatment modalities.

Management of the Primary Lesion

The likelihood of local control after irradiation for skin carcinomas of various sizes managed at Mallinckrodt Institute of Radiology is outlined in Table 13–7.[19] The probability of local control is higher for smaller lesions, for BCCA compared with SCCA, and for previously untreated lesions compared with recurrent cancers. The results of RT using various beam energies are listed in Table 13–8; treatment with orthovoltage irradiation yields local control rates that are as good as, or better than, local control rates yielded by other treatment modalities.[16]

Table 13–7. Local Tumor Control with Radiotherapy According to Size, Cell Type, and Presentation

Size	Basal Cell, Previously Untreated	Basal Cell, Recurrent	Squamous Cell, Previously Untreated	Squamous Cell, Recurrent
≤1 cm	64/66 (97%)	22/23 (96%)	11/11 (100%)	10/12 (83%)
1.1 to 3 cm	71/75 (95%)	27/36 (75%)	19/21 (90%)	7/13 (54%)
3.1 to 5 cm	11/13 (85%)	7/9 (78%)	7/8 (88%)	6/9 (67%)
>5 cm	12/13 (92%)	1/2 (50%)	3/5 (60%)	6/11 (55%)
Size not specified	4/4 (100%)	1/1 (100%)	0/1 (0%)	4/6 (67%)
TOTAL	162/171 (95%)	58/71 (82%)	40/46 (87%)	33/51 (65%)

Source: Malinckrodt Institute of Radiology based on a total of 339 patients.

Table 13–8. Local Control Rates According to External-Beam Technique

	Size			
Modality	**≤1 cm (%)**	**1.1 to 5 cm (%)**	**>5 cm (%)**	**Not specified (%)**
Basal cell carcinoma				
Superficial x-ray	69/71 (97%)	84/90 (93%)	4/4 (100%)	3/3 (100%)
Electron beam	11/12 (92%)	16/22 (73%)	4/5 (80%)	1/1 (100%)
Combination	5/5 (100%)	13/16 (81%)	5/6 (83%)	0/0
Photons (1.2 to 4 MV)	1/1 (100%)	3/5 (60%)	0/0	1/1 (100%)
Squamous cell carcinoma				
Superficial x-ray	12/12 (100%)	10/11 (91%)	1/1 (100%)	0/0
Electron beam	3/4 (75%)	7/10 (70%)	3/4 (75%)	0/1 (0%)
Combination	4/5 (80%)	19/26 (73%)	4/8 (50%)	2/4 (50%)
Photons (1.2 to 4 MV)	2/2 (100%)	3/4 (75%)	1/3 (33%)	2/2 (100%)

Significance levels: basal cell carcinoma, 1.1 to 5 cm, superficial x-ray (84/90) vs. electron beam/combination (29/38), $p = .013$; squamous cell carcinoma, ≤1 cm, superficial x-ray (12/12) vs. electron beam/combination (7/9), $p = .17$; squamous cell carcinoma 1.1 to 5 cm, superficial x-ray (10/11) vs. electron beam/combination (26/36), $p = .41$.

Source: Data from Mallinckrodt Institute of Radiology based on 339 patients.[12]

Schulte and co-workers[20] reported on 1,113 patients treated with orthovoltage RT for 1,267 skin cancers and followed for a median of 82 months (Table 13–9). Patients were usually treated at 5 Gy per fraction. The incidence of soft-tissue necrosis was 6.3%; 83% healed with conservative treatment.

Al-Othman et al[21] reported on 85 patients with 88 clinical T4 SCCAs (37), BCCAs (41), and metatypical BCCAs (10) treated with definitive RT at the University of Florida between 1964 and 1997. Forty-three lesions were previously untreated and 45 cancers were recurrent after prior surgery. The 5-year outcomes were as follows: local control, 53%; ultimate local control, 90%; regional control, 93%; ultimate regional control, 100%; distant metastasis-free survival, 95%; cause-specific survival, 76%; and overall survival, 56%. Thirteen (15%) of 85 patients developed a severe treatment-related complication.

Another paper from the University of Florida by Garcia-Serra and co-workers[2] reported on 135 patients with skin carcinomas that exhibited incidental (59 patients) or clinical (76 patients) PNI; minimum follow-up was 2 years. One-hundred five patients (78%) had SCCAs and the remainder had BCCAs or metatypical BCCAs. Patients with incidental PNI were treated with surgery and postoperative RT (55 patients), preoperative RT and surgery (2 patients), and RT alone (2 patients). Nine of 59 patients (15%) presented with clinically positive nodes. The outcomes for patients treated with incidental PNI are depicted in Table 13–10. Six of 59 patients (10%) developed treatment complications. Patients with clinical PNI were treated with surgery and postoperative RT (40 patients), preoperative RT and surgery (1 patients), or RT alone (35 patients). Twelve of 76 patients (16%) presented with clinically positive nodes. The outcomes for patients treated for clinical PNI are depicted in Table 13–11. Cranial neuropathies improved after treatment in 7% of patients. Ninety percent of recurrences were observed within 4 years of treatment. Twenty-five of 76 patients (33%) developed treatment complications.

Galloway et al[22] reported on a subset of these patients and compared their outcomes with radiographic extent of PNI and found that extent of PNI was inversely related to the likelihood of local control and survival (Table 13–12).

Table 13–9. Raw and Cumulative Recurrence Rates of BCCs and SCCs After Soft x-Ray Therapy[13]

		Recurrence Rates (%)			
			Cumulative After		
Tumor	Number	Raw	5 yr	10 yr	15 yr
BCCs and SCCs, total[a]	1267	5.1	4.7	6.9	7.4
BCCs, total	1019	4.5	4.2	6.1	6.1
T1[b]	615	2.4[c]	3.9	4.7	4.7
T2[b]	366	5.2[c]	4.2	8.6	8.6
T3[b]	22	9.1[c]	11.4	11.4	
Previously untreated (primary)	964	4.4	4.2	5.7	5.7
Previously treated and recurrent	55	7.3	4.3	13.2	13.2
SCCs, total	245	6.9	6.0	10.5	12.8
Tis[b]	13	7.7[d]	11.1		
T1[b]	79	1.3[d]	1.7	1.7	1.7
T2[b]	138	8.7[d]	7.4	14.2	19.0
T3[b]	14	21.4[d]	25.9	25.9	
Previously untreated (primary)	233	6.4	5.8	9.6	12.0
Previously untreated and recurrent	12	16.7	30.0	30.0	

BCC = basal cell carcinoma.
SCC = squamous cell carcinoma.
[a]Including 3 patients with combinations of BCCs and SCCs.
[b]Multiple (>1) tumors in same irradiated field were excluded.
[c]Difference of the raw recurrence rate of BCCS Tis-T3 were statistically significant (X^2, 6.99; $p < .05$).
[d]Differences of the raw recurrence rate of SCCs Tis-T3 were statistically significant (X^2, 9.13; $p < .05$).

Table 13–10. Outcomes After Treatment for Skin Carcinoma with Incidental Perineural Invasion (59 Patients)[2]

Parameter	5-Year Outcome
Local control	87%
Ultimate local control	87%
Local-regional control	72%
Ultimate local-regional control	80%
Cause-specific survival	65%
Overall survival	50%

Table 13–11. Outcomes After Treatment for Skin Carcinoma with Clinical Perineural Invasion (76 Patients)[2]

Parameter	5-Year Outcome
Local control	55%
Ultimate local control	57%
Local-regional control	50%
Ultimate local-regional control	56%
Cause-specific survival	59%
Overall survival	55%

Table 13–12. Clinical Perineural Invasion: 5-Year Outcome Versus Pretreatment Radiographic Findings (45 Patients)[15]

	Radiographic Findings			
5-Year Outcome	Imaging Negative (n = 10)	Minimal or Moderate Peripheral PNI (n = 14)	Central and/or Macroscopic PNI (n = 21)	p
Local control	76%	57%	25%	0.2027
Cause-specific survival	100%	56%	61%	0.0206
Overall survival	90%	50%	58%	0.0817

PNI = perineural invasion.

Management of Regional Disease

Veness and colleagues[3] reported on 167 patients treated at Westmead Hospital (Sydney, Australia) between 1980 and 2000 for cutaneous SCCAs metastatic to the parotid and/or cervical nodes. Twenty-one patients (13%) were treated with surgery alone and the remainder received surgery and adjuvant RT. The median time to recurrence after treatment was 8 months. The 5-year local-regional recurrence and disease-free survival rates were as follows: surgery and RT, 20% and 73%; and surgery alone, 43% and 54%, respectively. Multivariate analysis revealed that multiple positive nodes and treatment with surgery alone were significantly associated with decreased survival.

Hinerman et al[4] reported on 117 patients with 121 clinically positive parotids treated at the University of Florida between 1969 and 2005. Patients were treated with preoperative RT and surgery (17 parotids), surgery and postoperative RT (87 parotids), and RT alone (17 parotids). The 5-year outcomes were as follows: local (parotid) control, 78%; local-regional control, 74%; distant metastasis-free survival, 92%; disease-free survival, 70%; and overall survival, 54%. The 5-year local-regional control rate was 83% after surgery and postoperative RT versus 47% after preoperative RT and surgery or RT alone. Three (3%) patients developed severe complications.

Conclusion

Radiation therapy is an effective modality for the primary treatment of skin cancer, as well as in the adjuvant setting. It is used to treat the primary skin lesion when resection would result in an unacceptable functional and/or cosmetic outcome, as well as in the patient who is medically unsuitable for, or who declines, surgery. Adjuvant RT usually is indicated after surgery for close or positive margins, perineural invasion, bone and/or cartilage involvement, metastatic parotid-area lymph nodes, multiple lymph-node metastases, and extracapsular extension. The addition of radiation therapy to aggressive surgery improves outcomes in patients with high-risk features such as perineural invasion and nodal metastases.[6,12]

References

1. American Joint Committee on Cancer. Edge SB, Byrd D, Compton CC, Fritz AG, Greene FL, Trotti A, eds. . *AJCC Cancer Staging Handbook.* 7th ed. New York, NY: Springer; 2010.
2. Garcia-Serra A, Hinerman RW, Mendenhall WM, et al. Carcinoma of the skin with perineural invasion. *Head Neck.* 2003;25:1027–1033.

3. Veness MJ, Morgan GJ, Palme CE, Gebski V. Surgery and adjuvant radiotherapy in patients with cutaneous head and neck squamous cell carcinoma metastatic to lymph nodes: combined treatment should be considered best practice. *Laryngoscope.* 2005;115:870–875.
4. Hinerman RW, Amdur RJ, Morris CG, et al. Cutaneous squamous cell carcinoma metastatic to parotid-area lymph nodes. *Laryngoscope.* 2008;118:1989–1996.
5. Andruchow JL, Veness MJ, Morgan GJ, et al. Implications for clinical staging of metastatic cutaneous squamous carcinoma of the head and neck based on a multicenter study of treatment outcomes. *Cancer.* 2006; 106:1078–1083.
6. O'Brien CJ, McNeil EB, McMahon JD, Pathak I, Lauer CS, Jackson MA. Significance of clinical stage, extent of surgery and pathological findings in metastatic cutaneous squamous cell carcinoma of the parotid gland. *Head Neck.* 2002;24:417–422.
7. Mendenhall WM, Million RR, Mancuso AA, Cassisi NJ, Flowers FP. Carcinoma of the skin. In: Million RR, Cassisi NJ, eds. *Management of Head and Neck Cancer: A Multidisciplinary Approach.* 2nd ed. Philadelphia, PA: J.B. Lippincott Company; 1994:643–691.
8. Million RR. The myth regarding bone or cartilage involvement by cancer and the likelihood of cure by radiotherapy. *Head Neck.* 1989;11:30–40.
9. Mendenhall WM, Parsons JT, Mendenhall NP, Million RR. T2-T4 carcinoma of the skin of the head and neck treated with radical irradiation. *Int J Radiat Oncol Biol Phys.* 1987;13:975–981.
10. Glass RL, Perez-Mesa CM. Management of inadequately excised epidermoid carcinoma. *Arch Surg.* 1974;108:50–51.
11. Glass RL, Spratt JS, Jr., Perezmesa C. The fate of inadequately excised epidermoid carcinoma of the skin. *Surg Gynecol. Obstet.* 1966;122:245–248.
12. Gooding CA, White G, Yatsuhashi M. Significance of marginal extension in excised basal-cell carcinoma. *N Engl J Med.* 1965;273:923–924.
13. Amdur RJ, Kalbaugh KJ, Ewald LM, et al. Radiation therapy for skin cancer near the eye: kilovoltage x-rays versus electrons. *Int J Radiat Oncol Biol Phys.* 1992;23: 769–779.
14. Bhandare N, Kennedy L, Malyapa RS, Morris CG, Mendenhall WM. Hypopituitarism after radiotherapy for extracranial head and neck cancers. *Head Neck.* 2008;30:1182–1192.
15. Monroe AT, Bhandare N, Morris CG, Mendenhall WM. Preventing radiation retinopathy with hyperfractionation. *Int J Radiat Oncol Biol Phys.* 2005;61:856–864.
16. Mendenhall WM, Amdur RJ, Hinerman RW, Cognetta AB, Mendenhall NP. Radiotherapy for cutaneous squamous and basal cell carcinomas of the head and neck. *Laryngoscope.* 2009;119:1994–1999.
17. Mendenhall WM, Riggs CE, Vaysberg M, Amdur RJ, Werning JW. Altered fractionation and adjuvant chemotherapy for head and neck squamous cell carcinoma. *Head Neck.* 2010;32:939–945.
18. Bhandare N, Monroe AT, Morris CG, Bhatti MT, Mendenhall WM. Does altered fractionation influence the risk of radiation-induced optic neuropathy? *Int J Radiat Oncol Biol Phys.* 2005;62:1070–1077.
19. Lovett RD, Perez CA, Shapiro DL, Garcia DM. External irradiation of epithelial skin cancer. *Int J Radiat Oncol Biol Phys.* 1990;19:235–242.
20. Schulte KW, Lippold A, Auras C, et al. Soft x-ray therapy for cutaneous basal cell and squamous cell carcinomas. *J Am Acad Dermatol.* 2005;53:993–1001.
21. Al-Othman MOF, Mendenhall WM, Amdur RJ. Radiotherapy alone for clinical T4 skin carcinoma of the head and neck with surgery reserved for salvage. *Am J Otolaryngol.* 2001;22:387–390.
22. Galloway TJ, Morris CG, Mancuso AA, Amdur RJ, Mendenhall WM. Impact of radiographic findings on prognosis for skin carcinoma with clinical perineural invasion. *Cancer.* 2005;103:1254–1257.

14

PHOTODYNAMIC THERAPY FOR NONMELANOMA SKIN CANCER

JOSEPH P. HOUSEL
NATHALIE C. ZEITOUNI

Introduction and History of Photodynamic Therapy

Photodynamic therapy (PDT), also referred to as photoradiation, or photochemotherapy, involves the administration of a photosensitizing drug, molecular oxygen, and light to cause selective destruction of tumor cells.[1,2] Using light to cure disease is not a modern concept, as writings from ancient Greece, Egypt, and India have shown us.[3]

Unfortunately, the practice was lost for many centuries and was finally revived in modern times by a German medical student, Oscar Raab, in 1900. Raab showed that the combination of acridine orange and light caused the death of paramecium and correctly postulated that it was the fluorescence of the acridine that led to the destruction of the paramecia.[4] Raab's mentor, Herman Von Tappeiner, continued with this work along with Jesionek, and in 1903 showed that topical or intralesional eosin plus light could be used successfully to treat nonmelanoma skin cancer (NMSC), along with other cutaneous lesions.[3,5,6] Hausmann subsequently developed an iron-free preparation of blood with which he successfully photosensitized mice.[7] Friedrich Meyer-Betz, a German scientist, tested this iron-free preparation of blood developed on himself—the resulting photosensitivity lasted longer than 2 months.[8]

Although PDT was first developed around the turn of the 20th century, it was not until the 1960s that any rigorous research was performed.[3,9–11] In 1924, Policard[12] observed that tumors fluoresced more than uninvolved tissue. Using this knowledge, Lipson and Schwartz[1] of the Mayo Clinic injected a preparation of hematoporphyrin and showed neoplasms fluorescing during surgical procedures. To optimize the hematoporphyrin used for tumor localization, Schwartz combined hematoporphyrin along with acetic acid and sulfuric acid to form what he called hematoporphyrin derivative (HPD). Thomas Dougherty from Roswell Park Cancer Institute took the next big step in PDT and attempted to treat various malignancies with HPD and later, a purified form of HPD named porfimer sodium (Photofrin®).[10] Porfimer sodium was the first photosensitizer approved by the FDA in the United States in 1995 for the treatment of Barrett's esophagus and esophageal cancer, and then in 1998 for early and late-stage lung cancers.

Newer systemic agents have become available, along with topical prophotosensitizers such as 5-aminolevulinic acid (5-ALA) and methyl aminolevulinic acid (MAL). Topical PDT offers the advantage of tissue preservation with little to no scarring and good cosmesis compared to well-established treatments for NMSC such as surgery, electrodessication and curettage, and radiotherapy. There is growing evidence that both 5-ALA and MAL PDT should be considered as valuable therapeutic options for precancerous lesions, as well as other conditions including extramammary Paget's disease, acne, localized scleroderma, granuloma annulare, and photoaging.[13–18]

Mechanism of Action

PDT involves the administration of a photosensitizing agent either topically or systemically along with light, and oxygen.[1] The photosensitizer preferentially accumulates in tumor cells and is then exposed to a specific wavelength of light that matches the absorption peak of the photosensitizer.[1,2] Following the absorption of light by the photosensitizer, energy is then transferred to molecular oxygen, yielding singlet oxygen, along with other reactive oxygen species.[9,19–21] Singlet oxygen is a highly reactive form of oxygen and is one of the most potent oxidants, which, when formed, is capable of oxidizing the cellular components necessary for cell survival. Direct cellular death occurs by necrosis and apoptosis, vascular compromise, and local damage by inflammatory and immune mediators including tumor necrosis factor-α, interleukin 1 and 6, along with neutrophils, lymphocytes, and macrophages.[2,9,19,20]

Photosensitizers

Three photosensitizing agents or prophotosensitizers have been used to treat NMSC. These are systemic porfimer sodium, topical 5-ALA, and topical MAL. Photosensitizers can be administered to patients in a number of forms (intravenous, oral, intralesional, or topical) that are chosen by the physician based on tumor characteristics.[1] Systemic forms are preformed lipophilic macrocyclic photoactive porphyrins. In contrast, topical forms are prophotosensitizers that, when absorbed into the skin, are converted to photoactive porphyrins.[1]

Porfimer Sodium

Porfimer sodium is FDA approved to treat Barrett's esophagus, esophageal cancer, and early and late-stage lung cancer. In addition, it has been used successfully off-label for NMSC, bladder, brain, thoracic, gynecologic, oral, head, and neck carcinomas, as well as breast metastases.[1–3,9–11]

The disadvantages of Porfimer sodium are high cost, systemic administration, possible disfiguring scars, and a prolonged photosensitivity of up to 6 weeks. New systemic photosensitizers are being developed in an attempt to decrease the photosensitivity period. One compound, HPPH (2[1-hexyloxyethyl]-2 devinyl pyropheophorbide, or photochlor), a second-generation photosensitizer, has shown promise for early and late-stage lung cancer, esophageal cancer and Barrett's esophagus. Several authors have demonstrated that patients being treated for endobronchial lung cancer, when given HPPH, experience only mild irritation when exposed to direct sunlight following a 24-hour administration.[22,23]

5-Aminolevulinic Acid (5-ALA)

In 1990, a topical alternative to the systemic photosensitizing agents was devised.[24] Aminolevulinic acid (ALA), a naturally occurring lipophilic prophotosensitizer, is formed by the conversion of succinyl CoA and glycine by ALA-synthetase, an enzyme that constitutes the rate-limiting step in the heme biosynthetic pathway found in all human cells. Through a series of steps, ALA forms heme, and with the addition of iron, becomes protoporphyrin IX (PpIX), an endogenous photosensitizer. When 5-ALA is absorbed into the skin, the normal rate-limiting step is bypassed, allowing for the accumulation of PpIX.[25–27] Tumor cells preferentially accumulate PpIX due to enhanced conversion of ALA to PpIX, decreased heme formation, and increased absorption of 5-ALA.[24,25,27] Eventually PpIX is converted to heme over a period of 1 to 2 days.[26]

5-ALA was approved by the US FDA in 1999 for nonhyperkeratotic actinic keratoses as Levulan Kerastick (DUSA Pharmaceuticals Inc, Wilmington, MA) in a 20% solution of 5-ALA in an alcohol-water-surfactant vehicle to be used with blue fluorescent light (Blu U, 417 nm).[13,25] Other formulations utilizing topical 20% 5-ALA mixed with an oil-in-water vehicle have been used for research purposes.[28]

Methyl Aminolevulinic Acid (MAL)

MAL is similar in structure to 5-ALA, except for the addition of a methyl group. MAL is marketed as Metvixia (Galderma Pharmaceuticals, Fort Worth, TX) in the United States, and as Metvix in Europe, New Zealand, and Australia. Once absorbed into the skin, MAL is demethylated by esterases to form ALA. With the addition of the methyl group, which renders the compound lipophilic, MAL has been shown in some studies to offer improved penetration into tissues compared to 5-ALA, which is hydrophilic.[29] Recent studies have shown that the difference in efficacy is negligible between 5-ALA and MAL.[30,31] The importance of the lipophilic nature and potentially increased penetration is unknown at this point. Further research is needed to assess whether MAL's improved penetration offers other benefits. MAL, like 5-ALA, tends to accumulate preferentially in neoplastic cells, thereby decreasing the destruction of normal surrounding tissue.[29]

For the treatment of NMSC and actinic keratoses, both 5-ALA and MAL need to be applied for several hours prior to starting the procedure to allow absorption of the drug into the tissues and then conversion into the photoactive PpIX. A number of incubation times have been studied. For MAL, the FDA approved incubation time is 2.5 to 4 hours. Conversely, for 5-ALA the FDA approved incubation time is 14 to 18 hours, based on peak accumulation of PpIX at 12 hours after ALA application. 5-ALA subsequently dissipates after 40 hours. Other incubation times of 1 to 2 hours have been attempted, but shorter intervals failed to show similar benefits.[32]

Light Sources and Dosimetry

Since the inception of PDT, a variety of light sources have been utilized. The most common are continuous-wave (nonpulsed) monochromatic coherent light sources, along with broad band, incoherent light sources, and light emitting diodes (LED).[1–3,10,33] Lasers such as the argon pumped-dye laser can be set to very specific wavelengths of light at high power or irradiance, thus shortening the treatment times necessary to achieve maximum efficacy. Another important innovation developed at Roswell Park Cancer Institute was the introduction of fiberoptics and beam splitting for PDT. This allows for the simultaneous treatment of multiple cutaneous lesions or internal malignancies. Less expensive, light-emitting diodes with narrowband spectral output are now commercially available and have been approved for use in the United States.

The choice of light source depends on two key elements: absorption peak of the photosensitizer and depth of light penetration. Photosensitizers have various absorption peaks. PpIX has 5 main absorption or photoactivation peaks from about 410 to 630 nm, with the two most commonly utilized being 410 nm (Soret band, blue) and 630 nm (Q-band, red) bands.

Penetration of light into skin depends on its wavelength. Longer wavelengths have deeper skin penetration, up to about 800 nm. Below 400 nm, there is limited tissue penetration, but more importantly, there is the theoretical risk that ultraviolet radiation may induce cutaneous carcinoma.[34] Melanin and hemoglobin in the vasculature of the dermis impede wavelengths of light below 600 nm, thus limiting penetration. Because of this, blue light exciting the 410-nm band of PpIX should be used for only superficial lesions that lie above the dermis. When deeper penetration into the lesion is required, red light exciting the 630 nm peak of PpIX should be used.

Fluence and irradiance are two other important factors in the choice of the excitation light. Fluence, or light dose, is the number of photons per unit area delivered in joules per square centimeter (J per cm^2). Power is the number of photons delivered per unit time (watts). The irradiance, or power per unit area, is given as watts per cm^2. Exposure time can be calculated using the relationship: time = fluence/irradiance. Practically speaking, absorption, rather than the amount of light delivered, is the critical consideration. For PpIX, there is almost double the absorption of light at the 410-nm absorption peak versus the 630-nm peak. This means that 10 J per cm^2 at 410 nm is equal to approximately 150 J per cm^2 at 635 nm.

Auto-oxidation, or photobleaching, is another important consideration for treatment planning. As

PpIX is photoactivated, singlet oxygen is produced, as described earlier. This singlet oxygen acts on and consumes the PpIX, limiting the amount of damage possible with PDT. Oxygen consumed too rapidly during the PDT process will cause the reaction to cease. To ensure appropriate levels of oxygen, lower irradiance levels should be utilized to prevent the total consumption of oxygen. As described by Zilberstein,[35] fractionation of light with alternating short light and dark periods may allow for tissue reoxygenation, thereby minimizing the risk of oxygen overconsumption and photobleaching.

Indications for PDT

Topical PDT currently is used to treat a number of cutaneous lesions, including actinic keratoses and NMSC. Skin is easily accessible to both topical medications and an external light source, making PDT an excellent treatment option for some patients. NMSC is the most common malignancy in fair skinned individuals, comprising more than 30% of adult cancers in the United States. A recent study estimated that 900,000 to 1,200,000 new cases of NMSC are diagnosed per year, with rates increasing worldwide between 3 to 8% per year.[36,37] The total cost of NMSC was estimated to be $426 million in 2001, and this does not include the lost wages from missed work.[38] NMSCs have a favorable prognosis if diagnosed and treated early in the disease process.

Basal cell carcinomas rarely metastasize, but can be locally destructive. Squamous cell carcinomas have the potential to metastasize and also to invade locally. Actinic keratoses (AK) are precancerous lesions that may develop into SCCs.[39,40] A volume of literature exists that compares topical PDT to established treatments for AK, SCC in situ (Bowen's disease), BCC, and invasive SCC, and PDT compares favorably to other accepted treatments.

Actinic Keratoses

Actinic keratoses most commonly occur on the face, scalp, forearms, and hands.[39,40] AKs can be cosmetically displeasing to patients, but their potential for malignant transformation to invasive SCC requires that they be treated appropriately, and in a timely manner. The estimated risk of malignant transformation is 5 to 20% over a 10- to 25-year period.[39,40]

Topical PDT has been very successful in treating AK's. Multiple well-designed, randomized, controlled studies have compared either ALA or MAL to cryotherapy or 5-fluorouracil (5-FU). Two phase III ALA-PDT studies and four MAL-PDT studies have been performed.[41–46] In one study, Morton et al[41] showed significantly higher lesion reduction with MAL-PDT versus cryotherapy (86.9% vs 76.2%). Two other well-designed studies demonstrated that one PDT session was comparable to one cryotherapy session but two PDT sessions showed superior efficacy.[42,43] Kurwa's group[47] treated 17 patients with both ALA-PDT and 5-FU, with each patient serving as his or her own control. The right and left hands were randomized to receive either a 3-week course of topical 5-FU applied twice per day, or a single treatment of ALA-PDT. No statistical differences for lesion resolution were identified between the two treatments. Patient satisfaction and cosmetic outcome were similar, or better than both 5-FU and cryotherapy in each of these studies.[41–47]

Additionally, ALA-PDT may be most effective when used to treat AKs on the head, compared to those on the extremities.[48,49] Although the reasons behind this observation remain unproven, several hypotheses have evolved: the skin on the head is thinner, lesions tend to be less hyperkeratotic, and the skin may be more permeable, allowing for better drug absorption. Outcomes of PDT with AK may improve with longer application times, higher absorbed light doses, and removal of the hyperkeratotic areas.[48,49]

Topical PDT using either 5-ALA or MAL has been shown to be highly effective in the treatment of AK, with response rates comparable to cryotherapy and 5-FU. Topical PDT is well tolerated by patients, with excellent cosmetic results. Because patients with AKs often have large numbers of lesions grouped together, the introduction of LEDs that can treat multiple lesions has added to the convenience of this treatment and improved outcomes for patients. When lesions are refractory to aggressive treatment, a biopsy must be performed to rule out SCC.

Squamous Cell Carcinoma in Situ (SCCIS)

Squamous cell carcinoma in situ, also referred to as Bowen's disease (BD), typically arises on sun-exposed skin in elderly individuals and often occurs in the head and neck. Lesions typically manifest as an erythematous, scaly papule or thin plaque. The risk of transformation into invasive SCC is approximately 3%.[50] Arsenic-induced SCCIS differs slightly, in that it arises as clusters in non-sun-exposed areas.

Several studies utilizing systemic PDT for SCCIS have been performed, with complete response ranging from 95% to 100% at standard light doses.[51,52]

ALA-PDT has been the most widely studied agent for SCCIS, and it is associated with complete response rates ranging from 88% to 100%. MAL-PDT has shown similar efficacy.[15,48–52,58] Five-year recurrence rates for ALA-PDT are comparable to standard therapies, with a 17% recurrence rate for lesions originally classified as having a complete response, compared to 34% local failure with cryotherapy and 19% with curettage.[59,60] A large, 24-center, Phase III randomized, placebo-controlled study compared MAL-PDT to both cryotherapy and 5-FU demonstrated a complete response rate of 93% with MAL-PDT.[58] Recurrence rates for MAL-PDT, cryotherapy, and 5-FU were 15%, 21%, and 17%, respectively, at 1 year.[60] MAL-PDT was better tolerated by patients and was considered to deliver superior early cosmetic outcomes, compared to cryotherapy and topical 5-FU.[60] Although the appearance of the treated area improved over time for all treatment modalities, PDT was still deemed superior compared to cryotherapy at 12 months.[60] Additionally, MAL-PDT was reported to be less painful than cryotherapy, without the prolonged period of localized erythema, crusting, and ulceration associated with topical 5-FU.

Based on these studies, topical ALA/MAL-PDT is regarded as efficacious for the treatment of SCCIS and is well tolerated by patients. Furthermore, PDT can treat large areas or multiple lesions in a single session, potentially increasing patient compliance.

Basal Cell Carcinoma (BCC)

Basal cell carcinoma is the most common cutaneous malignancy in humans. It rarely metastasizes, but it can be locally aggressive and cause significant morbidity.[61,62] BCCs make up approximately 75% to 80% of NMSC and are subdivided into at least 26 different types, the most common of which are superficial (sBCC) and nodular (nBCC) basal cell carcinomas. Nodular BCCs are the most common subtype, accounting for approximately 60% of BCCs, and they present as translucent nodules or pearly papules with rolled borders and telangiectasias. Nodular BCCs have a tendency to develop on the face, but can be located in other areas. Superficial BCC presents as an erythematous macule or thin scaly plaque on the head, neck, trunk, or extremities (Fig 14–1).

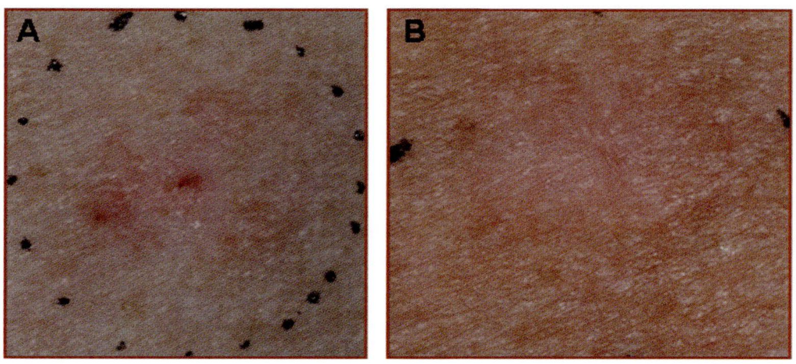

Figure 14–1. A. Superficial basal cell carcinoma on the scalp prior to ALA-PDT. **B.** Resolution of the same lesion 18 months following ALA-PDT.

Multiple BCCs in certain individuals may be associated with a rare autosomal dominant disorder, basal cell carcinoma syndrome/Gorlin-Goltz syndrome. Patients with NBCCS can develop up to hundreds of BCCs each year, usually in sun-exposed areas. These individuals often undergo multiple surgical procedures that can result in significant scars. Nevoid basal cell carcinoma syndrome has been traced to a mutation in the PTCH gene on chromosome 9Q22.3.[63]

Mal-PDT and ALA-PDT have both been shown to be effective in the treatment of sBCC, with initial clearance rates ranging from 80% to 100% for sBCC.[24,64–70] MAL-PDT has shown long-term disease control rates comparable to standard therapies such as cryotherapy.[67–69] A large multicenter, randomized study of 219 sBCCs compared MAL-PDT to cryotherapy and found similar 48-month recurrence rates in both groups (22% MAL-PDT vs 19% cryotherapy).[68,69] Recurrence rates of only 6% were found in patients with sBCCs less than 1 cm treated by MAL-PDT. Conversely, long-term efficacy of ALA-PDT has shown less promise, with recurrence rates of 38% for ALA vs 7% for cryotherapy at 12 months.[70]

Nodular BCC can be effectively treated with MAL-PDT. Typically, nBCCs are thicker lesions that demand increased depth of penetration of drug, making them more appropriate for MAL due to its lipophilic nature.[14] In a comparative study with surgery, MAL-PDT exhibited an initial response rate of 91%, compared to 98% with surgery, as well as a 5-year recurrence rate of 14% versus 4%, respectively.[71] Other studies utilizing MAL-PDT for nBCC have been performed that reveal complete response rates of 73% to 94%, with only a 14% 5-year recurrence rate.[66,68,71,72] Conversely, another study examining ALA for nBCC exhibited local failure in 33% of cases at 29 months, potentially related to the limited depth of penetration of ALA.[64]

PDT for both nBCC and sBCC generally is a well-tolerated procedure. Common side effects include erythema and mild to moderate pain, which can be managed effectively with oral analgesics or intralesional anesthesia. The erythema typically resolves over a 24- to 48-hour period following the procedure. Subjectively acceptable cosmetic outcomes following PDT have been shown to be superior to cryotherapy (89% PDT vs 50% cryotherapy) and surgery (92% PDT vs 33% surgery) in some studies.[67,68,71]

Topical ALA/MAL-PDT has been shown to be efficacious, and it can be recommended for the treatment of sBCC. MAL-PDT may be recommended for the treatment of select, low-risk nBCC. Individuals with genetic conditions such as NBCCS who develop hundreds of BCCs, or patients with particularly large or multiple BCCs, may also benefit from PDT and its tissue-sparing technique. However, it is not indicated for recurrent lesions, larger lesions, or those without histologic confirmation, due to the lack of securing pathologic data from treatment.

Squamous Cell Carcinoma (SCC)

Several studies detail the use of PDT for invasive SCC.[73–75] The results to date have been less than satisfactory when compared to surgical excision with intraoperative margin control. The largest PDT studies involving SCCs demonstrate recurrence rates over 50%, making it poorly suited for the majority of these neoplasms.[73–75] Although the tissue-sparing nature of PDT seems intuitively appropriate for patients who are immunosuppressed following organ transplantation and are at greatly increased risk for developing cutaneous SCC, the results to date have been disappointing, with only a 50% response achieved at 6 and 14 months in several case reports.[64] Given the high recurrence rates, potential for aggressive disease based on key histopathologic findings, and increased risk for metastasis, PDT should be reserved as an adjunctive therapy in cutaneous SCC, or as an option in patients when surgery is contraindicated.[64,76]

Conclusions

Photodynamic therapy is an evolving treatment option not only for NMSC, but also in other disease from oncology to cardiology. PDT is ideally suited for the head and neck, where NMSC tends to develop and where aesthetic concerns are especially important. Topical 5-ALA and MAL are suitable for AKs, both superficial and nodular BCC, and SCC in situ.

Evidence suggests that MAL may be more applicable to nodular BCC than ALA, due to its increased depth of penetration. PDT may be used independently or as an adjunct to surgery, particularly Mohs micrographic surgery.

Systemic porfimer sodium and similar agents are suitable for thicker lesions or those that have been unresponsive to topical PDT treatments. However, systemic photosensitizers are rarely indicated for routine use because patients may experience up to 4 to 6 weeks of photosensitivity. HPPH may emerge as a viable alternative treatment option in the future because it exhibits similar effectiveness to porfimer sodium with a shorter photosensitivity period. Photodynamic therapy constitutes a minimally invasive treatment option for select premalignant and malignant lesions of the head and neck, and it is a valuable component of a multidisciplinary approach to cutaneous malignancy of the head and neck.

References

1. Dougherty TJ, Gomer CJ, Henderson BW, et al. Photodynamic therapy. *J Natl Cancer Inst.* 1998;90:889–905.
2. Henderson BW, Dougherty TJ. How does photodynamic therapy work? *Photochem Photobiol.* 1992;55:145–157.
3. Daniell MD, Hill JS. A history of photodynamic therapy. *Aust N Z J Surg.* 1991;61(5):340–348.
4. Raab O. Ueber die wirkyng Fluoreszierender stoffe auf infusorien. *Z boil.* 1900;39:524–546.
5. Tappeiner H, Jesionek A. therapeutische versuche mit fluoreszier enden stoffe. *Muench Med Wochschr.* 1904;1: 2042–2044.
6. Jesionek A, Tappeiner H. Zur behandlung der haufcarcinome mit fluorescierenden stiffen. *Deut Arch Kling Med.* 1904;82:223–227.
7. Hausmann W. Die sensibilisierende wirkung des hematoporphyrins. *Biochem Z.* 1911;30:276.
8. Meyer-Betz F. Untersuchungen uber die biologische (photodyanmische) Wirkung des Hamatoporphyrins und ander Derivate des Blut-und Gallenfarbstoffs. *Dtsch Arch Klin Med.* 1913;112:476–503.
9. Garcia-Zuazaga J, Cooper KD, Baron ED. Photodynamic therapy in dermatology: current concepts in the treatment of skin cancer. *Exper Rev Anticancer Ther.* 2005; 5(5):791–800.
10. Dougherty TJ. A brief history of clinical photodynamic therapy development at Roswell Park Cancer Institute. *J Clin Laser Med Surg.* 1996;14(5):219–222.
11. Ackroyd R, Kelty C. Brown N, Reed M. The history of photodetection and photodynamic therapy. *Photochem Photobiol.* 2001;74(5):656–669.
12. Policard A. Etudes sur les aspects oferts par des tumeurs experimentales examinee a la lumiere de Woods. *Comp Rend Soc Biol.*1924;91:1423–1424.
13. Babilas P, Karrer S, Sidoroff A, Landthaler M, Szeimies RM. Photodynamic therapy in dermatology—an update. *Phodermatol Photoimmunol Photomed.* 2005;21(3):142–149.
14. Jeffes EW. Levulan: The first approved photosensitizer for the treatment of actinic keratosis. *J Dermatolog Treat.* 2002;13(suppl1):S19–S23.
15. Varma S, Wilson H, Kura HA, et al. Bowen's disease, solar keratoses and superficial basal cell carcinoma treated by photodynamic therapy using a large-field incoherent light source. *Br J Dermatol.* 2001;144(3):567–574.
16. Clayton TH, Tait J, Whitehurst C, Yates VM. Photodynamic therapy for superficial basal cell carcinoma and Bowen's disease. *Eur J Dermatol.* 2006(1);16:39–41.
17. Kurwa HA, Barlow RJ. The role of photodynamic therapy in dermatology. *Clin Exp Dermatol.* 1992;24(3):143–148.
18. Dover JS, Bhatia AC, Stewart B, Arndt KA. Topical 5-aminolevulinic acid combined with intense pulsed light in the treatment of photoaging. *Arch Dermatol.* 2005; 141(10):1247–1252.
19. Gollnick SO, Liu X, Owczarczak B, Musser DA, Henderson BW. Altered expression of interleukin 6 and interleukin 10 as a result of photodynamic therapy in vivo. *Cancer Res.* 1997;57(18):3904–3909.
20. Oseroff AR. PDT as a cytotoxic agent and biological response modifier: implications for cancer prevention and treatment in immunosuppressed and immunocompetent patients. *J Invest Dermatol.* 2006;126(3):542–544.
21. Dougherty TJ, Kaufman JE, Goldfarb A. et al. Photoradiation therapy for the treatment of malignant tumors. *Cancer Res.* 1978;38(8):2628–2635.
22. Loewen GM, Pandey R, Bellnier D, Henderson B, Dougherty TJ. Endobronchial photodynamic therapy for lung cancer. *Lasers Surg Med.* 2006;38(5):364–370.
23. Bellnier DA, Greco WR, Nava H, Loewen GM, Oseroff AR, Dougherty TJ. Mild skin photosensitivity in cancer patients following injection of Photochlor (2-[1-hexyloxyethyl]-2-devinyl pyropheophorbide-a; HPPH) for photodynamic therapy. *Cancer Chemother Pharmacol.* 2006;57(1):40–45.
24. Kennedy JC, Pottier RH, Pross DC, Photodynamic therapy with endogenous protoporphyrin IX: basic principles and present clinical experience. *J Photochem Photobiol B.* 1990;6(1–2):143–148.
25. Kormeili T, Yamauchi PS, Lowe NJ. Topical photodynamic therapy in clinical dermatology. *Br J Dermatol.* 2004;150(6):1061–1069.
26. Morton CA. Photodynamic therapy for nonmelanoma skin cancer and more? *Arch Dermatol.* 2004;140(1):116–120.
27. Rittenhouse-Diakun K, Van Leengoed H, Morgan J, Hryhorenko E, et al. The role of transferrin receptor (CD71) in

photodynamic therapy of activated and malignant lymphocytes using the heme precursor delta-aminolevulinic acid (ALA). *Photochem Photobiol.* 1995;61(5):523–528.
28. Oseroff AR, Shieh S, Frawley NP, et al. Treatment of diffuse basal cell carcinomas and basaloid follicular hamartomas in nevoid basal cell carcinoma syndrome by wide-area 5-aminolevulinic acid photodynamic therapy. *Arch Dermatol.* 2005;141(1):60–67.
29. Peng Q, Soler AM, Warloe T, Nesland JM, Giereksky KE. Selective distribution of porphyrins in skin thick basal cell carcinoma after topical applications of methyl 5-aminolevulinate. *J Photochem Photobiol B.* 2001;62(3): 140–145.
30. Kuijpers DI, Thissen MR, Thissen CA, Neumann MH. Similar effectiveness of methyl aminolevulinate and 5-aminolevulinate in topical photodynamic therapy for nodular basal cell carcinoma. *J Drugs Dermatol.* 2006;5(7): 642–645.
31. Krammer B, Verwanger T. Photodynamic therapy with aminolevulinic acid or its methyl ester: which one is superior? *Med Laser Appl.* 2009;24(4):221–226.
32. Redbord KP, Hanke DW. Topical photodynamic therapy for dermatologic disorders: results and complications. *J Drugs Dermatol.* 2007;6(12):1197–1202.
33. Blume JE, Oseroff AR. Aminolevulinic acid photodynamic therapy for skin cancers. *Dermatol Clin.* 2007;25(1): 5–14.
34. Runger TM, Role of UVA in the pathogenesis of melanoma and non-melanoma skin cancer. A short review. *Photodermatol Photoimmunol Photomed.* 1999;15(6):212–216.
35. Zilberstein, J, Bromberg A, Frantz A, et al. Light-dependent oxygen consumption in bacteriochlorophyll-serine treated melanoma tumors: online determination using a tissue-inserted oxygen microsensor. *Photochem Photobiol.* 1997;65(6):1012–1019.
36. Miller DL, Weinstock MA. Nonmelanoma skin cancer in the United States: incidence. *J Am Acad Dermatol.* 1994; 30(5 pt 1):774–778.
37. Green A. Changing patterns in incidence of non-melanoma skin cancer. *Epithelial Cell Biol.* 1992;1(1): 47–51.
38. Chen JG, Fleischer AB Jr., Smith ED, et al. Cost of non-melanoma skin cancer in the United States. *Dermatol Surg.* 2001;27(12):1035–1038.
39. Marks R, Rennie G, Selwood TS. Malignant transformation of solar keratoses to squamous cell carcinoma. *Lancet.* 1988;1(8589):795–797.
40. Dodson JM, DeSpain J, Jewett JE, Clark DP. Malignant potential of actinic keratoses and the controversy over treatment. A patient-oriented perspective. *Arch Dermatol.* 1991;127(7):1029–1031.
41. Morton C, Campbell S, Gupta G, et al. Intraindividual right-left comparison of topical methyl aminolaevulinate-photodynamic therapy and cryotherapy in subjects with actinic keratoses: a multicentre, randomized controlled study. *Br J Dermatol.* 2006;155(5):1029–1036.
42. Szeimies RM, Karrer S, Radakovic-Fijan S, et al. Photodynamic therapy using topical methyl 5-aminolevulinate compared with cryotherapy for actinic keratosis: a prospective, randomized study. *J Am Acad Dermatol.* 2002;47(2):258–262.
43. Freeman M, Vinciullo C, Francis D, et al. A comparison of photodynamic therapy using topical methyl aminolevulinate (Metvix®) with single cycle cryotherapy in patients with actinic keratosis: a prospective, randomized study. *J Dermatolog Treat.* 2003;14(2):99–106.
44. Piacquadio DJ, Chen DM, Farber HF, et al. Photodynamic therapy with aminolevulinic acid topical solution and visible blue light in the treatment of multiple actinic keratoses of the face and scalp: investigator blinded, phase 3, multicenter trials. *Arch Dermatol.* 2004;140(1):41–46.
45. Tarstedt M, Rosdahl I, Berne B, et al. A randomized multicenter study to compare two treatment regimens of topical methyl aminolevulinate (Metvix®)-PDT in actinic keratosis of the face and scalp. *Acta Derm Venereol.* 2005; 85(5): 424–428.
46. Pariser DM, Lowe NJ, Stewart DM, et al. Photodynamic therapy with topical methyl aminolevulinate for actinic keratoses: results of a prospective randomized multicenter trial. *J Am Acad Dermatol.* 2003;48(2):227–232.
47. Kurwa HA, Yong-Gee SA, Seed PT, et al. A randomized paired comparison of photodynamic therapy and topical 5-fluorouracil in the treatment of actinic keratoses. *J Am Acad Dermatol.* 1999;41(3 pt 1):414–418.
48. Alexiades-Armenakas MR, Geronemus RG. Laser-mediated photodynamic therapy of actinic keratoses. *Arch Dermatol.* 2003;139(10):1313–1320.
49. Itoh Y, Ninomiya Y, Henta T, et al. Topical delta-aminolevulinic acid-based photodynamic therapy for Japanese actinic keratoses. *J Dermatol.* 2000;27(8):513–518.
50. Cox NH, Eedy DJ, Morton CA. Guidelines for management of Bowen's disease. British Association of Dermatologists, *Br J Dermatol.* 1999;141(4):633–641.
51. Jones CM, Mang T, Cooper TM, et al. Photodynamic therapy in the treatment of Bowen's disease. *J Am Acad Dermatol.* 1992;27(6 pt 1):979–982.
52. Lui H, Hobbs L, Tope WD, et al. Photodynamic therapy of multiple nonmelanoma skin cancers with verteporfin and red light-emitting diodes: two-year results evaluating tumor response and cosmetic outcomes. *Arch Dermatol.* 2004;140(1):26–32.
53. Morton C, Horn M, Lehman J, et al. A 24-month update of a placebo controlled European study comparing MAL-PDT with cryotherapy and 5-fluorouracil in patients with Bowen's disease. *J Eur Acad Dermatol Venereol.* 2005;19 (suppl 2):237–238.
54. Morton CA, Whitehurst C, Moseley H, et al. Comparison of photodynamic therapy with cryotherapy in the treatment of Bowen's disease. *Br J Dermatol.* 1996;135(5): 766–771.
55. Morton CA, Whitehurst C, Moore JV, MacKie RM. Comparison of red and green light in the treatment of

Bowen's disease by photodynamic therapy. *Br J Dermatol.* 2000;143(4):767–772.

56. Salim A, Leman JA, McColl H, et al. Randomized comparison of photodynamic therapy with topical 5-fluorouracil in Bowen's disease. *Br J Dermatol.* 2003;148(3):539–543.
57. Morton CA, Whitehurst C, McColl JH, et al. Photodynamic therapy for large or multiple patches of Bowen disease and basal cell carcinoma. *Arch Dermatol.* 2001; 137(3):319–324.
58. Morton C.A., Horn M., Leman J, et al. A randomized, placebo-controlled, European study comparing MAL-PDT with cryotherapy and 5-fluoracil in subjects with Bowen's disease. *J Eur Acad Dermatol Venereol.* 2004; 18(suppl 2):415.
59. Leman A, Mackie RM and Morton CA. Recurrence rates following aminolaevulinic acid- photodynamic therapy for intra-epidermal squamous cell carcinoma compare favourably with outcome following conventional modalities. *Br J Dermatol.* 2002;147 (suppl 62):35.
60. Thestrup-Pedersen K, Ravnborg L, Reymann F. Morbus Bowen: a description of the disease in 617 patients. *Acta Derm Venereol.* 1988;68(3):236–239.
61. Lo JS, Snow SN, Reizner GT, et al. Metastatic basal cell carcinoma: report of twelve cases with a review of the literature. *J Am Acad Dermatol.* 1991;24(5 pt 1):715–719.
62. Ting PT, Kasper R, Arlette JP. Metastatic basal cell carcinoma: report of two cases and literature review. *J Cutan Med Surg.* 2005;9(1):10–15.
63. Johnson RL, Rothman AL, Xie J, et al. Human homolog of patched, a candidate gene for the basal cell nevus syndrome. *Science.* 1996;272(5268):1668–1671.
64. Calzavara-Pinton PG. Repetitive photodynamic therapy with topical delta-aminolaevulinic acid as an appropriate approach to the routine treatment of superficial nonmelanoma skin tumours, *J Photochem Photobiol B.* 1995; 29(1):53–57.
65. Fink-Puches R, Soyer HP, Hofer A, et al. Long-term follow-up and histological changes of superficial nonmelanoma skin cancers treated with topical delta-aminolevulinic acid photodynamic therapy. *Arch Dermatol.* 1998;134(7):821–826.
66. Horn M, Wolf P, Wulf HC, Warloe T, et al. Topical methyl aminolevulinate photodynamic therapy in patients with basal cell carcinoma prone to complications and poor cosmetic outcome with conventional therapy. *Br J Dermatol.* 2003;149(6):1242–1249.
67. Foley P, Freeman M, Siller G, Gebauer K, et al. *MAL-PDT or placebo cream in nodular basal cell carcinoma: results of an Australian double-blind randomised multicenter study.* Poster presented at the International Skin Cancer Conference 2004, Zurich July 22–24, 2004.
68. Basset-Seguin N, Ibbotson S, Emtestam L, et al. MAL-PDT versus cryotherapy in primary sBCC: results of 36 months follow-up. *J Eur Acad Dermatol Venereol.* 2004; 18(suppl 2):412.
69. Basset-Seguin N, Ibbotson S, Emtestam L, et al. MAL-PDT vs. cryotherapy in primary sBCC: results of 48-month follow up. *J Eur Acad Dermatol Venereol.* 2005;19(suppl 2):237.
70. Wang I, Bendsoe N, Klinteberg CA, et al. Photodynamic therapy vs. cryosurgery of basal cell carcinomas: results of a phase III clinical trial. *Br J Dermatol.* 2001;144(4): 832–840.
71. Thissen MR, Schroeter CA, Neumann HA. Photodynamic therapy with delta-aminolaevulinic acid for nodular basal cell carcinomas using a prior debulking technique. *Br J Dermatol.* 2000;142(2):338–339.
72. Tope WD, Menter A, El-Azhary RA, et al. Comparison of topical methyl aminolevulinate photodynamic therapy versus placebo photodynamic therapy in nodular BCC. *J Eur Acad Dermatol Venereol.* 2004;18(suppl 2):413–414.
73. Petrelli NJ, Cebollero JA, Rodriguez-Bigas M, Mang T. Photodynamic therapy in the management of neoplasms of the perianal skin. *Arch Surg.* 1992;127(12):1436–1438.
74. Kubler AC, Haase T, Staff C, et al. Photodynamic therapy of primary nonmelanomatous skin tumours of the head and neck. *Lasers Surg Med.* 1999;25(1):60–68.
75. Gross DJ, Waner M, Schosser RH, Dinehart SM. Squamous cell carcinoma of the lower lip involving a large cutaneous surface. *Arch Dermatol.* 1990;126(9):1148–1150.
76. Pennington DG, Waner M, Knox A. Photodynamic therapy for multiple skin cancers. *Plast Reconstr Surg.* 1988; 82(6):1067–1071.

15

THERAPEUTIC HORIZONS FOR CUTANEOUS MALIGNANCIES

MICHAEL E. KUPFERMAN
RANDAL S. WEBER
EBEN L. ROSENTHAL

Introduction

Over the last two decades, there has been an exponential increase in our understanding of the fundamental molecular alterations that result in human malignancy. These advances have created opportunities for molecular-based targeting of many cancers, including both solid and hematological cancers. Cancer-inducing genetic mutations and signaling dysregulation can be now addressed at the cellular level with a number of clinically approved small molecule inhibitors and humanized antibodies, some of which have led to profound improvements in patient outcomes. However, the impact of these novel agents has been infrequently explored in skin cancer. This chapter reviews the current status of targeted therapy and describes novel targets for future therapeutic strategies for nonmelanoma cutaneous malignancy.

Use of Adjuvant Therapy in Cutaneous SCC

Advanced cancers involving peripheral nerves or invading deep structures (T3-T4 lesions) are treated with wide local excision and the removal of lymph nodes in the regional lymphatic drainage basin, which in the head and neck is usually the superficial parotid and/or internal jugular lymphatics.[1,2] Attempts to improve outcomes have focused on the addition of postoperative radiotherapy and more aggressive surgical procedures aimed at obtaining negative margins.[3] Both of these approaches have become more popular, and more possible, with improvements in defect reconstruction over the past several decades.[4,5]

Identification and exploitation of molecular pathways that promote tumor growth have defined new developments in chemotherapeutic agents. Unlike conventional chemotherapeutic agents, targeted inhibition of unregulated cell proliferation or signaling results in less systemic toxicity and spares bone marrow regeneration. Targeted therapy promises to enhance therapeutic response without overlapping toxicities when used in combination with chemotherapies that induce cell death in rapidly dividing cells. Although targeted agents have been used successfully in the clinic, results in solid tumor types suggest that single agent responses are low, and that the agents work best when delivered with radiotherapy or conventional chemotherapeutic agents.

Target Patient Population for Targeted Therapy

Patients at high risk for recurrence are most likely to benefit from the added toxicity and cost associated with targeted therapy. Indications for addition of targeted therapy have mirrored indications for adjuvant radiotherapy. Although radiotherapy has been used in the primary treatment of cutaneous SCC, it often is applied as adjuvant therapy after surgical resection of advanced lesions.

Current National Comprehensive Cancer Network (NCCN) guidelines recommend postoperative adjuvant radiotherapy for positive margins, perineural involvement, or regional lymphatic involvement. These treatment recommendations are class 2A (nonuniform NCCN consensus, based on lower level evidence including clinical experience). The most widely accepted indication for adjuvant therapy includes regional metastatic disease, positive margins after surgical resection, and perineural invasion of named nerves. There are some data to support these guidelines, although it is based largely on retrospective studies. Patients with regional lymph node involvement (N+) are at high risk for recurrence, and the success of radiotherapy in disease control is well established.[6-8] Adjuvant radiotherapy has been the only factor that improved local control in metastatic cutaneous SCC in retrospective studies.[9,10]

Perineural invasion is present in approximately 10% of cases and is defined as pathological evidence of tumor cell invasion into the sheath of peripheral nerves.[11,12] These cases represent more aggressive disease with a worse prognosis and, therefore, commonly are treated with adjuvant radiotherapy.[13] Pathologic perineural invasion results in a 20% recurrence rate with surgery plus radiotherapy; whereas symptomatic perineural invasion is associated with a 55% recurrence rate.[12] NCCN guidelines (v.2.2005) consider large nerve perineural invasion as a high-risk feature requiring adjuvant radiotherapy (category 2A recommendation).

Positive margins after surgical resection results also are associated with recurrence.[14,15] NCCN guidelines (v.2.2005) consider positive margins as a high-risk feature requiring adjuvant radiotherapy (category 2A recommendation). Positive margins that require postoperative radiotherapy in the head and neck are due to involvement of unresectable structures including the skull base, carotid artery, brain parenchyma, or deep cervical fascia. SCC that invade extradermal structures (T3-T4 lesions) also are considered to be high-risk lesions requiring adjuvant radiotherapy.[1-3] Extradermal structures commonly involved in the head and neck include cartilage (most commonly external auditory canal or auricular cartilage), skeletal muscle, and bone such as the temporal bone or calvarium.

Adjuvant Chemotherapy

Although the benefit of systemic platinum-based regimens in the treatment of high-risk head and neck mucosal SCC in the postoperative setting recently has been demonstrated, little investigation into systemic chemotherapeutics has been applied to cutaneous SCC.[16,17] In part, this is because the rates of regional and systemic disease are comparatively low and partly because this disease often affects elderly patients. Aggressive platinum-based treatments are poorly tolerated in this patient population. Although topical applications of 5-FU have been found to be valuable in some cutaneous lesions, systemic cytotoxic therapies have not been found to have any benefit in cutaneous SCC.[18,19]

Applications of targeted chemotherapy to aggressive cutaneous malignancies have been based largely on results from therapies shown to be effective in head and neck mucosal squamous cell carcinoma. Based on histologic features, cutaneous and mucosal metastatic squamous cell are indistinguishable. This has led to the assumption that the two diseases will behave similarly to novel treatment modalities. The success of anti-epidermal growth factor receptor (EGFR) therapies alone, and in combination with other agents, represents the most productive area of active investigation.

EGFR Pathway as a Molecular Target in SCC

EGFR Blockade

There are preclinical and clinical data to suggest that EGFR targeted therapy could improve patient outcomes in cutaneous SCC. Ligand stimulation of

EGFR in cutaneous SCC has been associated with cellular dedifferentiation and angiogenesis. Furthermore, EGFR overexpression in cutaneous SCC correlates positively with metastasis.[20,21] Data to support the use of EGFR targeted therapy in cutaneous SCC are based largely on preclinical and clinical studies of these agents in mucosal head and neck SCC. Cetuximab has gained widespread acceptance in the treatment of mucosal SCC of the head and neck in conjunction with radiotherapy, and there are sporadic recent reports on the clinical utility of these agents in aggressive cutaneous SCC.[22,23]

Mucosal head and neck cancers are derived from the epithelial surfaces of the oral cavity, and they are histologically similar to cutaneous lesions, as both are derived from contiguous embryologic ectoderm. Clinically, cutaneous SCC that arise on the face and, especially, the auricle behave more like mucosal SCC than cutaneous SCC derived from the trunk or extremities.[12,24] Head and neck squamous cell carcinomas are widely known to have greater than 95% EGFR expression, whereas most other epithelial malignancies have between 20 to 80% EGFR expression.[24] EGFR is a logical target for inhibition in cutaneous SCC for the reasons summarized in Table 15–1.[25–27]

Tyrosine Kinase Inhibitors

Tyrosine kinase inhibitors represent the most clinically efficient molecules to study, as they are delivered orally, side effects are dose related, and they are relatively inexpensive. There have been no published trials using EGFR targeted agents in cutaneous SCC; therefore, most data available for the potential role of EGFR blockade in SCC are derived from the results of clinical trials in head and neck mucosal cancers. Gefitinib has been found to have single agent activity (response rate of 10.6% and disease control rate of 53%) when evaluated in phase II trial against recurrent or metastatic head and neck SCC.[28] The primary side effect was a skin rash that correlated positively with improved response to therapy.

Early applications of gefitinib to cutaneous SCC of the head and neck appear promising. In a Phase II dose-escalation trial of induction gefitinib prior to surgery and/or radiotherapy, 68.2% of 22 evaluable patients demonstrated a response to induction therapy, including 3 patients with a complete response to gefitinib alone. These promising results have prompted further investigations into the role of gefitinib (and other tyrosine kinase inhibitors) in the management of aggressive cutaneous SCC.[29]

Erlotinib (Tarceva or OSI-774) is an orally administered, reversible, ATP-competitive inhibitor of tyrosine phosphorylation that results in G1 arrest, reduced proliferation, and increased apoptosis.[30] Erlotinib as a single agent at 150 mg per day is well tolerated, although higher doses resulted in severe diarrhea or rash that is considered to be a result of EGFR expression in the intestinal mucosa and skin.[31,32] Erlotinib inhibits head and neck carcinoma growth in preclinical studies, but demonstrates limited efficacy in previously treated head and neck cancer patients as single agent therapy. In vitro, the antiproliferative activity of erlotinib is linked to the increased expression of cell cycle regulatory proteins and the induction of apoptosis.[30] Erlotinib inhibits head and neck tumor xenograft growth in nude mice.[33]

Erlotinib has been assessed as a single agent therapy in a multicenter phase II trial in recurrent head and neck SCC using doses of 150 mg daily.[34] Disease stabilization occurred in 38% of patients for a median duration of 16 weeks. At this dose, skin reactions (79%) and diarrhea (37%) were the most common toxicities, which were classified as mild to moderate in most cases.

Combination of anti-EGFR therapy with other targeted agents has been promoted in multiple tumor types, including cutaneous SCC. A case report demonstrated the successful combination of anti-EGFR therapy (cetuximab) and COX-2 inhibitor (celecoxib) in treating advanced stage, unresectable, cutaneous

Table 15–1. Rationale for EGFR Targeted Therapy in Cutaneous SCC

- Ligand and receptor expression correlate with patient outcome[25]
- EGFR stimulation accelerates oncogenic signaling in vivo and in vitro[26]
- EGFR is highly overexpressed in SCC[24]

SCC after failure of radiotherapy.[35] Combined anti-EGFR therapy and COX-2 inhibition has a clear rationale. Because EGFR stimulation results in upregulation of COX-2, which in turn promotes phosphorylation of the EGFR receptor by production of prostaglandin E2, a cycle of activation is established.

Radiotherapy Combined with EGFR Inhibition

The combination of radiotherapy with targeted EGFR therapy has a strong biological rationale.[36] Although combinations with Erlotinib have not been investigated in the clinical setting, molecular studies have shown that down-regulation of EGFR by erlotinib potentiates the effects of radiotherapy in head and neck squamous cell carcinoma cell lines in vivo.[37] A significant amount of in vitro and in vivo data has demonstrated that radiotherapy for SCC increases EGFR expression.[36] Combination radiotherapy with anti-EGFR monoclonal antibody therapy (C225, Erbitux, or cetuximab) improves cell cytotoxicity.[38,39] Interestingly, the level of EGFR expression does not correlate with response to treatment in this setting. It has been demonstrated that head and neck SCC patients treated with radiotherapy combined with cetuximab had double the median overall survival and statistically significant improvement in locoregional control.[22] However, how these results compare with the use of traditional cytotoxic therapy in combination with radiotherapy remains unclear. Ongoing trials in advanced stage cutaneous SCC using erlotinib in combination with radiotherapy as postoperative adjuvant therapy suggest that erlotinib (150 mg dose) is well tolerated with a toxicity profile similar to radiation alone (Rosenthal, unpublished data).

Other Molecular Targets

mTOR

One of the more promising targets that has been identified in solid malignancies is the mammalian target of rapamycin (mTOR), a signal transduction molecule that induces cellular proliferation when activated by upstream pathways, which may result from genetic mutations or RTK activation.[40] mTOR is a central regulator of protein translation and transcription, and it responds to diverse nutritional and environmental stimuli.[41] Its dysregulation in cancer has been long established, and mTOR can be inhibited by rapamycin or many of its analogs ("rapalogs").[42,43]

Selected clinical trials have identified the efficacy of mTOR inhibition, particularly for renal cell carcinoma, but the impact of this approach in SCC has only been identified in preclinical models.[44–47] Preclinical studies suggest that mTOR may be a promising target for cutaneous SCC, and given the antitumoral effects of mTOR inhibition in other tumors, this approach likely will gain traction in the near future.[48] One population at particularly elevated risk for aggressive skin cancers is the solid-organ transplant community, and this group comprises a logical starting point for investigations of rapalogs in cutaneous SCC.[49] Interestingly, rapalogs initially were utilized in the solid organ transplant population for immunosuppression. Currently, clinical trials are underway to assess the impact of these agents in preventing cutaneous malignancies in the post-transplant population.

Hedgehog Pathway

Due to the defined genetic mutations seen in basal cell carcinoma (BCC), the Hedgehog pathway is a unique target for therapy in skin cancer. Hedgehog pathway genes play key roles in embryogenesis and are usually inactive in adult skin.[50] However, Hedgehog signaling can be activated by either gain-of-function mutations in the smoothened (SMO) gene or loss of function mutations in the patched homologue 1 (PTCH1) gene.[51]

Basal cell carcinomas are characterized by frequent mutations in PTCH1, leading to constitutive Hedgehog signaling and unrestrained basal cell proliferation and resultant aggressive skin cancers.[52] A recently identified inhibitor of the Hedgehog pathway has been studied in patients with aggressive basal cell cancers and was found to be active in advanced or metastatic BCC.[53] Whether these results will be durable and, ultimately, translatable to SCC is unclear at present.

Summary

Currently, little is known about the potential of targeted therapy in advanced stage cutaneous SCC. Most of the supporting data is derived from use of these agents in mucosal head and neck cancer, which shares many similarities with aggressive cutaneous disease. This has led investigators to consider use of anti-EGFR based therapies alone and in combination with radiation therapy. Incorporation of targeted therapy into the clinical treatment for advanced stage cutaneous SCC is limited by several factors. First, the anatomic location of the tumor impacts biology and treatment options, but is not well accounted for in the clinical staging system, which makes comparison of results between patients difficult. Second, the biology of advanced cutaneous SCC is poorly understood and there are a limited number of model systems for preclinical assessment. Third, clinical trials with targeted agents often require large number of patients to pick up small differences or identify cancers with a major response. Because of the limited number of patients with advanced disease, enrollment is difficult even for a multi-institutional trial, potentially limiting industry support. Other promising molecular targets currently are under study in a variety of settings; ultimately, these may be incorporated into the care of patients with nonmelanoma cutaneous malignancies of the head and neck.

References

1. Johnson TM, Rowe DE, Nelson BR, Swanson NA. Squamous cell carcinoma of the skin (excluding lip and oral mucosa). *J Am Acad Dermatol.* 1992;26:467–484.
2. Motley R, Kersey P, Lawrence C. Multiprofessional guidelines for the management of the patient with primary cutaneous squamous cell carcinoma. *Br J Plast Surg.* 2003;56:85–91.
3. Wax MK, Burkey BB, Bascom D, Rosenthal EL. The role of free tissue transfer in the reconstruction of massive neglected skin cancers of the head and neck. *Arch Facial Plast Surg.* 2003;5:479–482.
4. Chaturvedi P, Pai PS, Pathak KA, et al. Simultaneous reconstruction of large skin and mucosal defect following head and neck surgery with a single skin paddle pectoralis major myocutaneous flap. *J Laryngol Otol.* 2005; 119:303–305.
5. Rosenthal E, Carroll W, Dobbs M, et al. Simplifying head and neck microvascular reconstruction. *Head Neck.* 2004;26:930–936.
6. Dona E, Veness MJ, Cakir B, Morgan GJ. Metastatic cutaneous squamous cell carcinoma to the parotid: the role of surgery and adjuvant radiotherapy to achieve best outcome. *ANZ J Surg.* 2003;73:692–696.
7. Veness M. Treatment recommendations in patients diagnosed with high-risk cutaneous squamous cell carcinoma. *Australas Radiol.* 2005;49:365–376.
8. Chu A, Osguthorpe JD. Nonmelanoma cutaneous malignancy with regional metastasis. *Otolaryngol Head Neck Surg.* 2003;128:663–673.
9. Bron LP, Traynor SJ, McNeil EB, O'Brien CJ. Primary and metastatic cancer of the parotid: comparison of clinical behavior in 232 cases. *Laryngoscope.* 2003;113: 1070–1075.
10. Veness MJ, Palme CE, Smith M, et al. Cutaneous head and neck squamous cell carcinoma metastatic to cervical lymph nodes (nonparotid): a better outcome with surgery and adjuvant radiotherapy. *Laryngoscope.* 2003;113: 1827–1833.
11. Garcia-Serra A, Hinerman RW, Mendenhall WM, et al. Carcinoma of the skin with perineural invasion. *Head Neck.* 2003;25:1027–1033.
12. Mendenhall WM, Amdur RJ, Williams LS, et al. Carcinoma of the skin of the head and neck with perineural invasion. *Head Neck.* 2002;24:78–83.
13. McCord MW, Mendenhall WM, Parsons JT, et al. Skin cancer of the head and neck with clinical perineural invasion. *Int J Radiat Oncol Biol Phys.* 2000;47:89–93.
14. Spratt JS, Jr. Cancer mortality after nonmelanoma skin cancer. *JAMA.* 1999;281:325.
15. Glass RL, Spratt JS, Jr., Perezmesa C. The fate of inadequately excised epidermoid carcinoma of the skin. *Surg Gynecol Obstet.* 1966;22:245–248.
16. Bernier J, Cooper JS, Pajak TF, et al. Defining risk levels in locally advanced head and neck cancers: a comparative analysis of concurrent postoperative radiation plus chemotherapy trials of the EORTC (#22931) and RTOG (#9501). *Head Neck.* 2005;27:843–850.
17. Cooper JS, Pajak TF, Forastiere AA, et al. Postoperative concurrent radiotherapy and chemotherapy for high-risk squamous-cell carcinoma of the head and neck. *N Engl J Med.* 2004;350:1937–1944.
18. Kraus S, Miller BH, Swinehart JM, et al. Intratumoral chemotherapy with fluorouracil/epinephrine injectable

gel: a nonsurgical treatment of cutaneous squamous cell carcinoma. *J Am Acad Dermatol.* 1998;38:438–442.
19. Smith KJ, Germain M, Skelton H. Squamous cell carcinoma in situ (Bowen's disease) in renal transplant patients treated with 5% imiquimod and 5% 5-fluorouracil therapy. *Dermatol Surg.* 2001;27:561–564.
20. Shimizu T, Izumi H, Oga A, et al. Epidermal growth factor receptor overexpression and genetic aberrations in metastatic squamous-cell carcinoma of the skin. *Dermatology.* 2001;202:203–206.
21. Casanova ML, Larcher F, Casanova B, et al. A critical role for ras-mediated, epidermal growth factor receptor-dependent angiogenesis in mouse skin carcinogenesis. *Cancer Res.* 2002;62:3402–3407.
22. Bonner JA, Harari PM, Giralt J, et al. Radiotherapy plus cetuximab for squamous-cell carcinoma of the head and neck. *N Engl J Med.* 2006;354:567–578.
23. Kim S, Eleff M, Nicolaou N. Cetuximab as primary treatment for cutaneous squamous cell carcinoma to the parotid gland. *Head Neck.* 2010 (Epub 2009 1 Dec).
24. Audet N, Palme CE, Gullane PJ, et al. Cutaneous metastatic squamous cell carcinoma to the parotid gland: analysis and outcome. *Head Neck.* 2004;26: 727–732.
25. Ritter CA, Arteaga CL. The epidermal growth factor receptor-tyrosine kinase: a promising therapeutic target in solid tumors. *Semin Oncol.* 2003;30:3–11.
26. He Y, Zeng Q, Drenning SD, Melhem MF, et al. Inhibition of human squamous cell carcinoma growth in vivo by epidermal growth factor receptor antisense RNA transcribed from the U6 promoter. *J Natl Cancer Inst.* 1998;90: 1080–1087.
27. Grandis JR, Sok JC. Signaling through the epidermal growth factor receptor during the development of malignancy. *Pharmacol Ther.* 2004;102:37–46.
28. Cohen EE, Rosen F, Stadler WM, et al. Phase II trial of ZD1839 in recurrent or metastatic squamous cell carcinoma of the head and neck. *J Clin Oncol.* 2003;21: 1980–1987.
29. Glisson B, Kim E, Kies M, et al. Phase II study of gefitinib in patients with metastatic/recurrent squamous cell carcinoma of the skin. *J Clin Oncol.* 2006;24:Abstract 5531.
30. Moyer JD, Barbacci EG, Iwata KK, et al. Induction of apoptosis and cell cycle arrest by CP-358,774, an inhibitor of epidermal growth factor receptor tyrosine kinase. *Cancer Res.* 1997;57:4838–4848.
31. Hidalgo M. Erlotinib: preclinical investigations. *Oncology (Williston Park).* 2003;17:11–16.
32. Grunwald V, Hidalgo M. Development of the epidermal growth factor receptor inhibitor OSI-774. *Semin Oncol.* 2003;30:23–31.
33. Pollack VA, Savage DM, Baker DA, et al. Inhibition of epidermal growth factor receptor-associated tyrosine phosphorylation in human carcinomas with CP-358,774: dynamics of receptor inhibition in situ and antitumor effects in athymic mice. *J Pharmacol Exp Ther.* 1999;291: 739–748.
34. Soulieres D, Senzer NN, Vokes EE, et al. Multicenter phase II study of erlotinib, an oral epidermal growth factor receptor tyrosine kinase inhibitor, in patients with recurrent or metastatic squamous cell cancer of the head and neck. *J Clin Oncol.* 2004;22:77–85.
35. Jalili A, Pinc A, Pieczkowski F, et al. Combination of an EGFR blocker and a COX-2 inhibitor for the treatment of advanced cutaneous squamous cell carcinoma. *J Dtsch Dermatol Ges.* 2008;6:1066–1069.
36. Baumann M, Krause M. Targeting the epidermal growth factor receptor in radiotherapy: radiobiological mechanisms, preclinical and clinical results. *Radiother Oncol.* 2004;72:257–266.
37. Chinnaiyan P, Huang S, Vallabhaneni G, et al. Mechanisms of enhanced radiation response following epidermal growth factor receptor signaling inhibition by erlotinib (Tarceva). *Cancer Res.* 2005;65:3328–3335.
38. Safavy A, Georg GI, Vander Velde D, et al. Site-specifically traced drug release and biodistribution of a paclitaxel-antibody conjugate toward improvement of the linker structure. *Bioconjug Chem.* 2004;15:1264–1274.
39. Bonner JA, Raisch KP, Trummell HQ, et al. Enhanced apoptosis with combination C225/radiation treatment serves as the impetus for clinical investigation in head and neck cancers. *J Clin Oncol.* 2000;18:47S–53S.
40. Engelman JA. Targeting PI3K signaling in cancer: opportunities, challenges and limitations. *Nat Rev Cancer.* 2009;9:550–562.
41. Bjornsti M-A, Houghton PJ. The tor pathway: a target for cancer therapy. *Nat Rev Cancer.* 2004;4:335–348.
42. Gibbons JJ, Abraham RT, Yu K. Mammalian target of rapamycin: discovery of rapamycin reveals a signaling pathway important for normal and cancer cell growth. *Semin Oncol.* 2009;36:S3–S17.
43. Easton JB, Houghton PJ. mTOR and cancer therapy. *Oncogene.* 2006;25:6436–6446.
44. Dancey JE, Curiel R, Purvis J. Evaluating temsirolimus activity in multiple tumors: a review of clinical trials. *Semin Oncol.* 2009;36:S46–S58.
45. Hudes G, Carducci M, Tomczak P, et al. Temsirolimus, interferon alfa, or both for advanced renal-cell carcinoma. *N Engl J Med.* 2007;356:2271–2281.
46. Nathan C-AO, Amirghahari N, Rong X, et al. Mammalian target of rapamycin inhibitors as possible adjuvant therapy for microscopic residual disease in head and neck squamous cell cancer. *Cancer Res.* 2007;67:2160–2168.
47. Czerninski R, Amornphimoltham P, Patel V, Molinolo AA, Gutkind JS. Targeting mammalian target of rapamycin by rapamycin prevents tumor progression in an oral-specific chemical carcinogenesis model. *Cancer Prev Res.* 2009;2:27–36.
48. Amornphimoltham P, Leelahavanichkul K, Molinolo A, Patel V, Gutkind JS. Inhibition of mammalian target of rapamycin by rapamycin causes the regression of car-

cinogen-induced skin tumor lesions. *Clinl Cancer Res.* 2008;14:8094–8101.
49. Vajdic CM, McDonald SP, McCredie MRE, et al. Cancer incidence before and after kidney transplantation. *JAMA.* 2006;296:2823–2831.
50. Varjosalo M, Taipale J. Hedgehog: functions and mechanisms. *Genes Devel.* 2008;22:2454–2472.
51. Rubin LL, de Sauvage FJ. Targeting the Hedgehog pathway in cancer. *Nat Rev Drug Discov.* 2006;5:1026–1033.
52. Theunissen J-W, de Sauvage FJ. Paracrine Hedgehog signaling in cancer. *Cancer Res.* 2009;69:6007–6010.
53. Von Hoff DD, LoRusso PM, Rudin CM, et al. Inhibition of the Hedgehog pathway in advanced basal-cell carcinoma. *N Engl J Med.* 2009;361:1164–1172.

16

ADNEXAL TUMORS

AMY C. HESSEL

Introduction

Adnexal tumors of the head and neck are very rare neoplasms that arise in the appendages of the skin. The majority of these lesions affect the sweat glands as well as the pilosebaceous unit, which includes the hair shaft, hair follicle, and the erector pili muscle. Although uncommon, adnexal tumors encompass a wide spectrum of benign and malignant lesions. Adnexal tumors are characterized by their morphologic differentiation: follicular, eccrine, apocrine, sebaceous, or mixed. This chapter discusses the normal anatomy and the histologic classification of these tumors, and identifies the most common adnexal tumors seen in the head and neck. Furthermore, the chapter stresses contemporary multidisciplinary treatment and outcomes for these very rare neoplasms.

Anatomy of Skin Appendages

Embryology

The skin contains specialized structures such as hair follicles with the attached sebaceous gland, eccrine glands, and apocrine glands. Skin appendages arise from the ectoderm around the 8th week of embryologic development. As the epithelial cells invaginate into mesenchyme, the follicle structure begins to form as dermal papillae. Around the 13th to 16th week, the follicular cells that eventually will develop into the sebaceous gland can be seen as a bulge on the side of the follicle.[1] As the sebaceous gland develops, it will connect directly to the shaft, making it considered to be hair-follicle dependent.

At the same time, the arrector pili muscle begins to anchor to the same area, developing independently along the shaft. As the epithelial cells push into the dermis, a bulb forms at the distal end. This eventually creates a dermal papilla that is destined to become the hair fiber itself. The hair follicle will be completely developed by the 24th to 28th week of gestation.[1]

The apocrine glands also form along the developing hair follicle, arising from a bulge in the follicle shaft. These glands are seen primarily in the axilla, groin, pubic, and perineal regions. Like sebaceous glands, apocrine glands drain directly into the hair follicle through a wide lumen duct. Conversely, eccrine glands develop separately from the pilosebaceous unit. These sweat glands can be found all over the skin and are created from independent epithelial rests that protrude into the dermis.

Histology

In normal skin, sebaceous glands, apocrine glands, and eccrine glands are all histologically distinct. The pilosebaceous unit contains basophilic cells in the epidermis surrounded by mesenchymal cells. Given its ectodermal origins, the hair shaft is highly keratinized. The sebaceous gland is made up of multiple lobules of round sebocytes that converge into a short duct that dumps into the hair follicle. The cells that make up the apocrine glands along the hair follicle are cuboidal, with apical snouts, which likely allow for secretion, and they often express androgen receptors.[1] Eccrine sweat glands have ductal systems that contain a secretory coil made up of pyramidal cells that is deep in the dermis. The excretory part of the eccrine duct is lined with cuboidal cells and contains a straight intradermal component and a spiral intraepidermal component.[2]

Classification of Adnexal Tumors

Older classification schemes for adnexal tumors were based on the morphological differences of the tumors as apocrine versus eccrine. However, as pathologists have become more familiar with histologic appearance of these tumors and the normal cells from which they arise, it was discovered that many of these tumors contain cells with more than one line of differentiation, including both apocrine and eccrine features. Contemporary classification is based on the structure of origin: hair follicle, sebaceous gland, or sweat gland. Meticulous examination of hair-bearing skin allows differentiation of adnexal tumors arising from the follicular-sebaceous-apocrine unit and those developing from the more isolated eccrine unit.[3]

Patient and Tumor Evaluation

Clinical Features

Because adnexal tumors demonstrate many similar pathologic features, the clinical history should augment the histopathologic assessment to facilitate an accurate diagnosis. Clinical information such as patient age and gender, as well as known inherited or systemic diseases, can assist in the diagnosis. Tumor location, growth rate, size, color, and specific details such as whether it was solitary or multiple, smooth or ulcerated, and nodular or plaquelike constitute pertinent details from the history and physical examination.

Histopathologic Assessment

The rarity of these tumors highlights the importance of an established multidisciplinary cutaneous oncology team. An experienced dermatopathologist will be able to find features on routine hematoxylin and eosin (H&E) staining that may be consistent with sebaceous differentiation (vacuolated cytoplasm and starry nuclei) or follicular differentiation (basaloid proliferation, peripheral nuclear palisading, and papillary mesenchymal cells). Apocrine differentiation is suggested by eosinophilic cytoplasm and eccentric, basally located nuclei.[2]

Benign adnexal tumors typically are characterized by smooth borders and symmetry. Usually, there is no necrosis, atypia, or mitoses. However, malignant processes are more likely to demonstrate asymmetric growth, infiltrative borders, and irregular neoplastic cells, as well as increased cellular atypia and mitotic activity. The use of immunohistochemical stains may be helpful in specific neoplasms, and is discussed in greater detail in the following sections.[2]

Benign Adnexal Tumors

Tumors of Hair Follicle Origin

Proliferating Trichilemmal Cyst (Pilar Tumor)

This is a benign solitary lesion found in elderly female patients, primarily on the scalp. These can grow quite large. These tumors consist of well-defined lobulated, solid, or cystic masses of proliferating squamous epithelium that involve the deep dermis and subcutaneous tissues. Long-standing lesions can become multiloculated, making complete resection difficult and increasing the risk of recurrence.

Malignant transformation is rare, but should be considered in very large lesions or those that experience rapid growth.[2]

Pilomatricoma

This benign dermal or subcutaneous lesion characteristically is found in young adolescents. It is a solitary, firm nodule that arises on the head and neck and may be associated with other conditions such as myotonic dystrophy, Turner syndrome, or Rubinstein-Taybi syndrome.[2,3]

Histologically, the characteristic ghost cells infiltrate the subcutaneous tissues in islands, with central calcification (Fig 16–1).

Tumors of Sebaceous Gland Origin

Sebaceous Adenoma

This is a benign skin lesion that presents as a lobulated, yellow papule on the cheek or forehead of middle-aged and elderly patients. Histologically, it is a well-circumscribed dermal nodule that is composed of mature sebaceous cells and aggregates of basaloid cells. Because of the basaloid appearance, it can be confused with basal cell carcinoma with sebaceous differentiation.[2]

Tumors of Sweat Gland Origin

Hidradenoma

This tumor is a benign dermal tumor that occurs primarily in women. Its other names include solid-cystic hidradenoma, eccrine acrospiroma, clear cell hidradenoma, and acrospiroma. Although it appears benign, long-standing lesions may devolve into malignant lesions, and if not completely excised, they demonstrate a high incidence of recurrence.[4]

Syringoma

Syringomas arise from the straight segment of intradermal eccrine sweat ducts. This tumor presents primarily around the eyelid in middle-aged adults. The tumor consists of well-circumscribed nodules within the dermis that lack an epidermal connection. Clasically, syringomas are described as containing nests that display a comma or tadpole shape.[3]

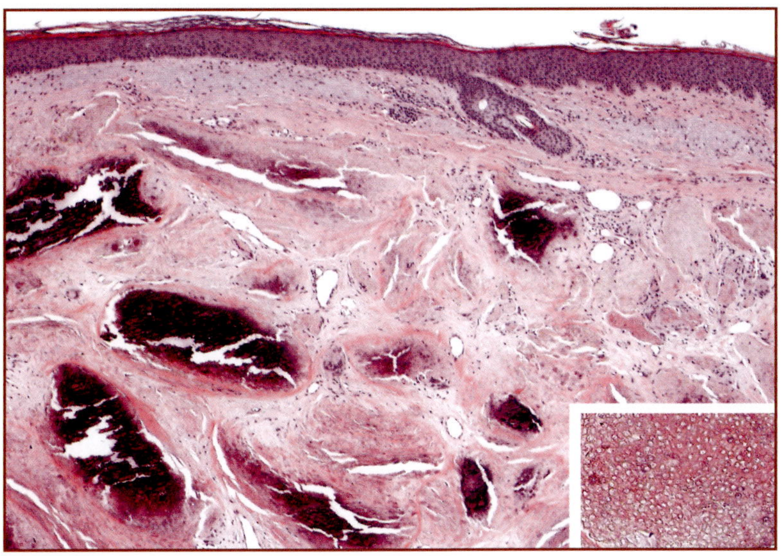

Figure 16–1. Pilomatricoma. The subcutaneous tissue is replaced by pale islands composed of ghost cells with absent nuclei (*inset*) and central calcification. (40× and 100×)

Cylindroma

This benign tumor is seen primarily on the scalp or face of women. The lesions can be solitary, but they also may form a disfiguring, coalescent mass. It is associated with a genetic mutation that leads familial cylindromatosis. Histologically, the tumor may arise from the coiled part of the eccrine duct (but it may be apocrine origin). Tumors are composed of islands of epithelial cells with a thick, "jigsaw puzzle" pattern of basement membrane.[3]

Malignant Adnexal Tumors

Tumors of Hair Follicle Origin

Pilomatrix Carcinoma

This rare malignancy is the counterpoint to a pilomatrixoma that exhibits asymmetry and cellular atypia. It commonly occurs in the head and neck, upper limbs, and buttocks, primarily in men, with a 5:1 male to female ratio. Affected patients are older, with an average age of 61 years.[6] Clinically, the tumors appear as subcutaneous or dermal nodules, which range in size from 0.5 cm to 20 cm, with an average of 4.0 cm. Lesions are poorly circumscribed and may infiltrate into the adjacent tissues.

Gross examination may reveal a cyst filled with chalky material. Histologically, these tumors contain 2 cell types: basaloid cells and shadow, or ghost, cells. Basaloid cells are formed in sheets, bands, or solid nests with a high mitotic rate. Shadow cells demonstrate eosinophilic cytoplasm and no nuclei. Tumor nests are surrounded by a dense, fibrous stroma, and lymphovascular and perineural invasion are common.[6]

Pilomatrix carcinoma can be locally aggressive, plus it can metastasize to regional lymphatics in up to 16% of cases, or even spread distantly.[2] Simple resection has resulted in local recurrences in up to 50%. Therefore, wide local excision with clear margins on frozen section, or Mohs micrographic surgery, is indicated, although there is no consensus as to size of margins.[6] Radiation therapy to the primary site has been used successfully, but there is no clear benefit to adjuvant radiation after complete resection.

Tumors of Sebaceous Gland Origin

Sebaceous Carcinoma

Sebaceous carcinoma also is rare, with fewer than 200 patients described in the literature. Most of these tumors are located in the head and neck, primarily on the eyelid. Because the meibomian glands are modified sebaceous glands, sebaceous carcinoma constitutes the fourth most common neoplasm of the eyelid.[2] Risk factors for this tumor include advanced age, Asian heritage, female gender, and prior radiation exposure. The median age of diagnosis is 72 years old, and up to 85% of afflicted patients are Caucasian.[7]

Clinically, this tumor presents as a slowly enlarging, firm nodule that is often mistaken for common dermatologic diseases. Gross examination reveals a dermally based lobule or cord that travels intraepithelially. Histologically, there is cytoplasmic lipid and the characteristic sebaceous cell, which is characterized by vacuolated cytoplasm and a scalloped appearing nucleus (Fig 16–2).[8] There also are undifferentiated germinative cells within the tumor and undifferentiated basaloid cells along the periphery, mimicking a palisading basal cell carcinoma.

Sebaceous carcinoma is characterized by local recurrence and distant metastases. Although the regional metastatic potential is only about 1.5%, detection of cervical lymphadenopathy is associated with mortality in up to 50 to 67% of cases.[7] Patients are treated primarily with surgery, particularly Mohs micrographic surgery, although radiation has been used in a minority of patients. Overall survival is around 79%.[7]

Tumors of Sweat Gland Origin

Hidradenocarcinoma

Hidradenocarcinoma is extremely rare and can be mistaken for benign disease.[4] The malignant version of the hidradenoma can occur either sponta-

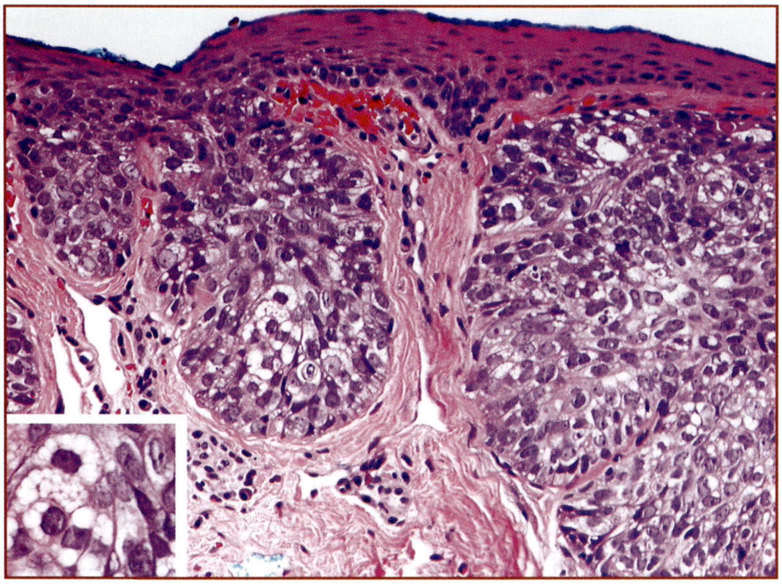

Figure 16–2. Sebaceous carcinoma. Epithelial proliferation is present with marked clearing and vacuolization leading to scalloping of the nuclei is characteristic of sebaceous differentiation (*inset*). (100× and 200×)

neously or from a pre-existing lesion. Occasionally, the only way to determine that it is a malignancy is after recurrence or metastasis. Clinically, these tumors are nonspecific with a single, firm, nontender nodule that may be multilobulated. The overlying skin may be normal appearing, or it may be discolored. It is most often seen in the head and neck and can range from 1 to 4 cm in lateral dimension.[4]

On histopatholgic assessment, hidradenocarcinoma is a multinodular, solid neoplasm that contains ductal structures, areas of necrosis, and cytonuclear atypia with increased mitotic activity. These tumors can show apocrine differentiation and may stain positive for epithelial membrane antigen (EMA) and carcinoembryonic antigen (CEA). These lesions resemble mucoepidermoid carcinoma of the skin and often are referred to by other names, including malignant nodular/clear cell hidradenoma, malignant clear cell acropiroma, and clear cell eccrine carcinoma. Furthermore, hidradenocarcinoma may be difficult to differentiate from metastatic clear cell carcinomas such as thyroid, lung, or renal cell carcinomas.[5]

Surgical resection with wide margins is the most common therapy, although Mohs micrographic surgery has demonstrated success in local control. Simple removal can lead to recurrences in 10 to 50% of cases.[4] Tumors may metastasize to the regional lymphatics in up to 60% of cases. Distant metastases are also encountered, and as many as 40% of patients will succumb to disease.[4] Adjuvant radiation is commonly recommended for positive surgical margins, perineural invasion, and involved cervical lymph nodes, but the paucity of this condition precludes meaningful assessment of the efficacy of adjuvant therapy.

Syringoid Eccrine Carcinoma

Syringoid eccrine carcinoma is the very rare malignant variant of syringoma, and these tumors often are mistaken for microcystic adnexal carcinoma. It demonstrates aggressive histologic features including cytonuclear atypia, mitotic activity, and lymphovascular or perineural invasion. These tumors are very invasive, with extension into the deep dermis and subcutaneous tissues.[5]

Malignant Cylindroma

This very rare tumor arises from a pre-existing, benign cylindroma. Malignant transformation is characterized by rapid growth, ulceration, or bleeding. This lesion has a predilection for recurrence and may even metastasize distantly.[5]

Microcystic Adnexal Carcinoma

Perhaps the best-known adnexal tumor, microcystic adnexal carcinoma (MAC) is an uncommon eccrine-derived neoplasm that exhibits keratinous cysts. In addition, lesions also demonstrate apocrine and sebaceous differentiation, suggesting a mixed lineage. Microcystic adnexal carcinoma is very rare, with an incidence of 1.6 per 100,000.[12] Other names for this tumor include sclerosing sweat gland duct carcinoma, malignant syringoma, sweat gland carcinoma with syringomatous features, aggressive trichofolliculoma, and combined adnexal tumor of the skin.[9] Patients usually are Caucasian (90%), although it occurs in African-Americans in up to 3% of cases.[12] The African-American population may present with lesions in unusual locations such as the scalp.[14] Affected patients range in age from 30 to 70 years old, and the tumor occurs equally in men and women.[12]

Most (85%) of these tumors occur in the head and neck, primarily in the central face or T-zone, and they also have a predilection to arise on the lips. Risk factors include sun exposure, immunosuppression, and prior radiation therapy.[3,9] Among patients who had prior radiation exposure, 8% of MAC occurred 30 to 40 years after radiation.[11] Clinically, MAC presents as a smooth, nonulcerated, yellowish nodule, papule, plaque, or cyst. It grows gradually but may have a period of rapid growth. Most are asymptomatic but, occasionally, patients will complain of numbness, paresthesias, burning or discomfort—all features suggestive of perineural invasion.

Histologically, the tumor demonstrates significant subclinical extension, with a proliferation of epithelial neoplastic cells that infiltrate the dermis and subcutaneous tissues (Fig 16–3). The cell of origin is thought to be a pluripotent adnexal keratinocyte that is capable of differentiating into pilar

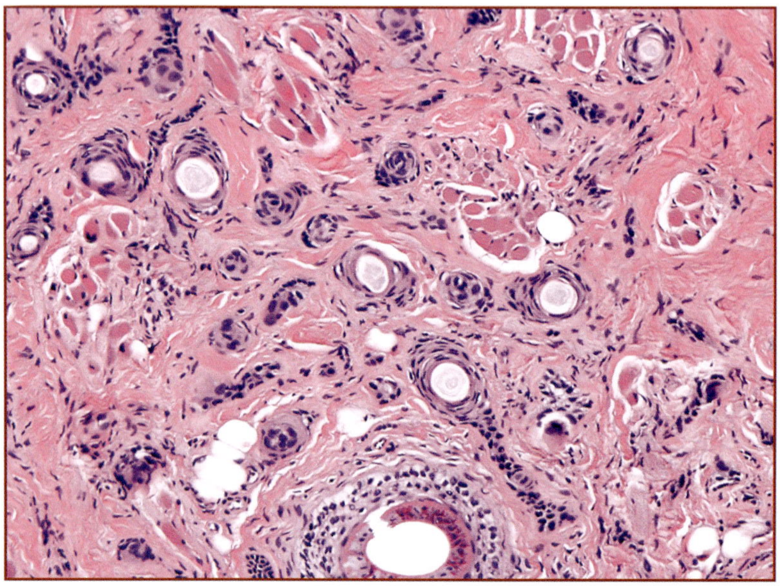

Figure 16–3. Microcystic adnexal carcinoma. Small bland nests of tumor cells form cystic spaces and infiltrate through the fibromuscular tissue. (100× magnification)

or sweat ducts.[9–11] The tumor is usually stratified with keratin horns and epithelial nests in the superficial dermis and desmoplastic stroma and rudimentary ductal structures in the deeper dermis. Mitotic figures and cellular atypia are rare.[9,10] As previously noted, perineural invasion is common. Superficially, this tumor can be mistaken for benign lesions such as syringoma, desmoplastic trichoepithelioma, sclerosing/morpheaform basal cell carcinoma, and papillary eccrine adenoma, leading to misdiagnosis in up to 30% of cases.[3,9,13] Therefore, a deep biopsy that includes the base of the lesion is required to clarify the diagnosis. These tumors tend to stain positive for CEA, cytokeratin, and EMA, facilitating differentiation from other adnexal neoplasms.[9]

Microcystic adnexal carcinoma behaves aggressively, with perineural invasion or deep extension to muscle, vascular adventitia, perichondrium, periosteum, and bone marrow. Because of its aggressive behavior and subclinical extension, MAC demonstrates a relatively high potential for local recurrence, but the regional metastasis rate is low (1–2.1%).[9,10,12] Distant metastases are possible, but rare.

Treatment of MAC includes complete surgical resection, and the lesions frequently are amenable to Mohs micrographic surgery because of its ability to map and excise the significant subclinical extension. In 30% of patients undergoing standard wide local excision, a second procedure was needed to clear the margins.[9,13] Therefore, many authors support the use of Mohs micrographic surgery.[9,11] Recurrence rates seem to vary widely and are likely related to the ability to clear the surgical margins: standard excision 40 to 60% and Mohs 0 to 12%.[9,11,13] Recurrent lesions typically manifest within the first 2 to 3 years after initial therapy.

Radiation therapy has been used as adjuvant therapy as well as primary treatment, but this experience is primarily limited to case reports. Radiation was frequently employed in cosmetically sensitive locations or in the adjuvant setting for advanced tumors, with mixed results. Radiation does not seem to affect overall survival for this tumor, but probably should be considered in patients who have aggressive and adverse features on histology.[9,12] Despite this heterogeneity in treatment protocols, SEER data reveal 10-year survival rates of 86%.[12]

Primary Cutaneous Mucinous Carcinoma

Primary cutaneous mucinous carcinoma (PCMC) is a rare, low-grade malignancy that occurs on the head and neck of elderly adults, frequently around the eyelids. Characteristically, these lesions are well-circumscribed, lobulated dermal masses that resemble mammary glandular tumors. In fact, it is difficult to differentiate this tumor from metastatic breast cancer. However, metastatic breast cancer is more likely to present on the chest wall, breast, and axilla; whereas the PCMC tumors primarily are on the face.[4]

Ductopapillary Apocrine Carcinoma

Around 50 cases of this rare variant of sebaceous carcinoma have been reported in the literature.[15] It behaves aggressively and presents with regional metastasis in over 50% of cases. Most commonly seen in middle-aged women, it is located in apocrine-rich skin such as the axilla, but can be seen in the eyelid, ear, and scalp. Clinically, these appear as asymmetric, poorly demarcated tumors with tubular and ductal structures on histologic examination.[3]

Treatment of Adnexal Tumors

This diverse collection of very rare skin neoplasms constitutes a very small percentage of all head and neck cutaneous tumors. They are inconspicuous in their clinical appearance and often are mistaken for other more benign lesions. Because adnexal tumors are so rare, the treatment experience with them is not well documented.

Surgery with negative margins constitutes the definitive treatment for adnexal tumors, but there is no agreement on margin size. Preoperative planning should consider potentially wide margins, and plastic and reconstructive surgical consultation should be pursued in the event of a possible complex defect.[4,6] Because some of these tumors, particularly microcystic adnexal carcinoma, have indistinct margins and can be deeply invasive, Mohs micrographic surgery has been advocated to ensure complete surgical removal and 100% margin assessment.[4,11,13]

The majority of these carcinomas have a very low regional metastasis rate, so elective management of the neck is not warranted. Sentinel lymph node mapping and biopsy have not been widely applied to these rare neoplasms, but the technique may be applicable in certain pathologies. Regardless, meticulous clinical evaluation and radiographic imaging of the cervical lymphatics with computed tomography (CT) scans may be helpful in identifying metastases. Enlarged lymph nodes in the draining lymphatics should be investigated with fine needle aspiration biopsy, and an appropriate parotidectomy and/or neck dissection pursued for documented regional metastases

The role of radiation therapy is not well described in the literature. Most reports do not demonstrate any benefit of using radiation as a primary therapy, even in lesions that are surgically challenging, because disease control may not be durable.[9] However, palliative radiation may play a role in disease stabilization and symptom control in unresectable or widely metastatic tumors, despite a lack of evidence.

Similarly, there is very limited experience with adjuvant radiotherapy for adnexal tumors. Although MAC and hidradenocarcinoma commonly exhibit pathologic features that normally constitute indications for radiation such as perineural invasion, deep infiltration, and initial positive margins, there is no clearcut evidence that radiation will improve disease control.[4,9,12] Until there are more data on the role of radiation therapy in adnexal tumors, it probably is wise to use the familiar indications for adjuvant therapy as seen in the more common head and neck cancers: close or positive margins, deep invasion of critical structures, perineural invasion, multiple recurrences, and lymph node involvement.[4,7,9]

Outcomes

Overall survival rates in this heterogeneous mix of adnexal tumors seem to be very good, especially in those lesions associated with a low metastasis rate. Sebaceous carcinoma has a 10-year overall survival of 91%, whereas microcystic adnexal carcinoma demonstrates a 10-year overall survival rate of 86%.[7,8,12] The more aggressive adnexal tumors such as hidradenocarcinoma and ductopapillary apocrine carcinoma seem to metastasize early, and, therefore, most likely carry a poor prognosis. Unfortunately, most descriptions of these tumors are limited to case series and reports, precluding meaningful survival analysis.

Conclusions

The adnexal apparatus including the hair follicle with its attached sebaceous gland constitutes a fundamental component of the skin. The pilosebaceous unit also contains apocrine sweat glands in certain anatomic locations and eccrine sweat glands. Although the structures are ubiquitous, tumors of the cutaneous adnexal structures are rare; they require a multidisciplinary approach among dermatologists, Mohs micrographic surgeons, head and neck surgeons, radiation oncologists, and reconstructive surgeons.

Adnexal tumors generally are characterized by the structure of origin: either hair follicle or sweat gland. It often is difficult to differentiate between eccrine and apocrine sweat gland tumors because these neoplasms often contain histologic features of both. There are many benign and malignant tumors of the adnexa; however, not all are found in the head and neck. Within the head and neck, adnexal tumors are very rare and are often misdiagnosed as the more common skin lesions such as basal cell carcinoma. In addition, the differences between these tumors often are small and only can be delineated histologically by a skilled and knowledgeable dermatopathologist. Because many of these lesions present as inconspicuous nodules, the index of suspicion is low for malignancy, thus leading to long delays in diagnosis or superficial biopsies that may miss the deeper portions of the tumor that are essential to accurate diagnosis.

Of this heterogeneous array of tumors, the most commonly seen include pilomatrix carcinoma arising from a hair follicle, sebaceous carcinoma from sebaceous glands, and microcystic adnexal carcinoma arising from sweat glands. Although generally low grade in nature, these tumors may exhibit dramatic subclinical extension. Regional metastases are uncommon, although pilomatrix carcinoma and sebaceous carcinoma can behave aggressively with distant metastasis over time.

Microcystic adnexal carcinoma is a locally invasive process with a very low potential for metastasis. Mohs micrographic surgery has emerged as a successful treatment method for these tumors, and the interested reader is referred to Chapter 30 of this text for a more thorough discussion of this technique and its contemporary indications. The role of radiation is not clearly defined, but generally is not recommended as an alternative for surgical resection. The benefit of adjuvant postoperative radiation also is not well understood, but is recommended for tumors that exhibit adverse pathologic features that are traditionally associated with poor prognosis.

Overall survival with adnexal tumors is very good, provided that local control is achieved. However, as with most rare cancers, there are reports of highly aggressive behavior and widely metastatic distant disease. Long-term follow-up is needed due to reports of late recurrences.

References

1. Paus R, Cotsarelis G. The biology of hair follicles. *New Engl J Med.* 1999;341:491–497.
2. Alsaad KO, Obaidat NA, Ghazarian D. Skin adnexal neoplasms—part 1: an approach to tumors of the pilosebaceous unit. *J Clin Pathol.* 2007;60:129–141.
3. Cassiarino DS. Cutaneous adnexal neoplasms: classification and a practical diagnostic approach. Presentation at the American Society for Clinical Pathology Annual Meeting; New Orleans, LA; September 2007.
4. Yavel R, Hinshaw M, Rao V, Hartig GK, et al. Hidradenomas and a hidradenocarcinoma of the scalp managed using Mohs micrographic surgery and a multidisciplinary approach: case reports and review of the literature. *Dermatol Surg.* 2009;35:273–281.
5. Obaidat NA, Alsaad KO, Ghazarian D. Skin adnexal neoplasms—part 2: an approach to tumours of cutaneous sweat glands. *J Clin Pathol.* 2007;60:145–159.
6. Hardisson D, Linarea MD, Cuevas-Santos J, Contreras F. Pilomatrix carcinoma—a clinicopathologic study of six cases and review of the literature. *Am J Dermpathol.* 2001;23:394–401.
7. Dasgupta T, Willson LD, Yu JB. A retrospective review of 1349 cases of sebaceous carcinoma. *Cancer.* 2009;115: 158–165.
8. Dowd MB, Kumar RJ, Sharma R, Murali R. Diagnosis and management of sebaceous carcinoma: an Australian experience. *ANZ J Surg.* 2008;78:158–163.
9. Wetter R, Goldstein GD. Microcystic adnexal carcinoma: a diagnostic and therapeutic challenge. *Dermatol Ther.* 2008;21:452–458.
10. Kirkland PM, Solomons NB, Ratcliffe NA. Microcystic adnexal carcinoma. *J Laryngol Otol.* 1997;111:674–675.
11. Friedman PM, Fiedman RH, Jiang SB, et al. Microcystic adnexal carcinoma: collaborative series review and update. *J Am Acad Dermatol.* 1999;41:225–231.
12. Yu JB, Blitzblau RC, Patel SC, et al. Surveillance, epidemiology, and end results (SEER) database analysis of microcystic adnexal carcinoma (sclerosing sweat duct carcinoma) of the skin. *Am J Clin Oncol.* 2010;33:125–127.
13. Chiller K, Fassaro D, Scheullar M, et al. Microcystic adnexal carcinoma: 48 cases, their treatment, and their outcome. *Arch Dermatol.* 2000;136:1355–1359.
14. Nadiminti H, Nadiminti U, Washington C. Microcystic adnexal carcinoma in African-Americans. *Dermatol Surg.* 2007;33:1384–1387.
15. Akhtar I, Ispas CL, Flowers R, et al. Ductopapillary apocrine carcinoma of the eyelid metastatic to the parotid gland: report of a case diagnosed by fine-needle aspiration biopsy. *Diagn Cytopathol.* 2009;37:91–95.

17

MERKEL CELL CARCINOMA

CECELIA E. SCHMALBACH

Introduction

Merkel cell carcinoma (MCC) represents a rare and exceedingly aggressive malignancy of presumed neuroendocrine origin.[1] Although it is an uncommon tumor, the head and neck (H&N) region is the most common site involved, accounting for 50% of all lesions.[2] Although the overall incidence of MCC is rare compared to other cutaneous malignancies, an increasing trend in cases is reported as the population continues to age and life expectancy increases. Unfortunately, MCC combines the local recurrence rates of nonmelanoma skin cancer with the regional and distant metastatic rate of advanced stage melanoma.[3] MCC remains both a diagnostic and therapeutic challenge. The low incidence of cases precludes high-level, evidence-based recommendations stemming from large clinical trials. For this reason, an ongoing debate continues with respect to the optimal treatment. Significant variability among institutions is found with respect to surgical technique, sentinel lymph node biopsy, postoperative radiotherapy to primary tumor and regional sites, and adjuvant chemotherapy.

Epidemiology

Since its original description in 1972, approximately 2,000 MCC cases have been reported in the literature.[1,4] The overall incidence of MCC tripled from 1986 to 2001, increasing from 0.15 per 100,000 to 0.44 per 100,000, respectively.[5] This change represents an annual 8% increase, compared to an annual increase of only 3% in cutaneous melanoma.[6] The rising incidence of MCC is attributed to increasing awareness, improved biomarkers, better diagnostic capabilities, greater number of immunosuppressed patients, increasing sun exposure, as well as the overall aging patient population.[4,6,7] About 1,500 new cases of MCC are diagnosed annually.[8]

MCC is recognized as a disease of the elderly. An individual over the age of 65 years is 24 times more likely to develop MCC compared to his younger counterpart.[5] Only 5% of MCC cases are diagnosed in patients less than the age of 50 years. The Caucasian population has the highest incidence of MCC, accounting for 95% of all cases, with an incidence 11 times greater than in the black community.[4] A slight male predominance consistently has been reported in the literature.[4,6,9]

Tumor Biology

Merkel cells were first described in 1875 when Friedrich S. Merkel identified large "clear cells" associated with nerve endings in the epidermal layer of the skin.[10] These cells now are recognized as type I mechanoreceptors, with a known neural crest origin.[11] Although Merkel cells are dispersed throughout the skin, they often cluster in sensitive locations such as the lips and face, or around hair follicles.[12]

In 1972, Toker identified electron-dense neurosecretory granules in the cytoplasm of what he termed "*trabecular cell carcinoma.*"[1] These neurosecretory granules are common in Merkel cells and neuroendocrine cells. For this reason, the terms *cutaneous neuroendocrine carcinoma* and *Merkel cell carcinoma* were suggested.[13] Although it generally is accepted that MCC originates from neuroendocrine cells of the basal layer of the epidermis, some controversy remains because other scientists attribute epidermal cells, specifically keratinocytes, as the tumor origin.[4] For this reason, alternative names for MCC have been proposed including: *small cell carcinoma of the skin, small cell undifferentiated carcinoma, cutaneous small cell tumor, and anaplastic cancer of the skin.*

Anatomic Distribution

The head and neck region remains the most common site for MCC diagnosis, accounting for approximately 50% of all cases.[2] The second most common site is the upper extremity (21%) followed by the lower extremity (14%), trunk (12%), and other sites (7%).[14] Up to 19% of patients are diagnosed with MCC of unknown tumor origin.[15]

Although MCC is most often found on a sun-exposed area of the skin, review of the Surveillance, Epidemiology, and End Results (SEER) Program reveals that 4.5% of cases arise in mucosal anatomic sites.[8] Cases involving the nasal cavity, oral tongue, upper lip, lower lip, pharynx, and larynx all have been described in the literature.[8,16] Common risk factors for this subset of patients includes tobacco and alcohol exposure, as well as mucosal trauma.

Etiology/Risk Factors/Pathogenesis

The pathogenesis of MCC remains unknown and is speculated to be multifactorial. A causative role of ultraviolet (UV) radiation is strongly supported within the literature. The majority of MCCs are found on sun-exposed regions of the body, and it is not uncommon for the lesion to be diagnosed in the setting of known cutaneous squamous cell carcinoma. SEER demographics report a correlation between solar UVB indices and regional differences in MCC incidence.[17] UVB specific mutations in the *p53* and *Haras* genes are common findings in MCC tumors.[6] Furthermore, psoriasis patients undergoing treatment with UVA and methoxsalen carry a 100-fold increased risk for developing MCC.[18]

An increased incidence of MCC also is reported among immunocompromised patients. The mean age of MCC diagnosis is 10 years younger for organ transplant recipients.[19] In fact, 29% of cases are diagnosed before the age of 50 years in transplant patients, a stark contrast to the 5% rate of new diagnoses among the general population in this age group. Several case reports have described MCC development in patients with human immunodeficiency virus and acquired immunodeficiency syndrome, as well as patients suffering from chronic lymphocytic leukemia, multiple myeloma, non-Hodgkin's lymphoma, and melanoma.[4,6,20] Unfortunately, when MCC develops in the setting of immunosuppression, the cancer is more aggressive, with over 60% of patients developing regional spread and 56% of patients eventually dying of their disease.[19] Finally, chronic arsenic exposure also has been implicated as a potential cause for MCC.[21]

At the molecular level, several chromosomal abnormalities have been identified in MCC tumors and associated cell lines. 40% of patients were found to have structural aberrations involving the short arm of chromosome 1 (1p36).[22] Loss of heterozygosity at this location led scientists to speculate that tumor suppressor genes on 1p may play a role in the development of MCC. Increased expression of the *bcl-2* proto-oncogene, which is responsible for inhibiting apoptosis, thereby promoting cell survival and tumor growth, was identified in 50% of MCC patients studied by Kennedy et al.[23] Interestingly, the *BRAF* oncogene mutations previously reported in the setting of melanoma have not been observed in MCC tumors.[24] Other chromosomal abnormalities that have been linked to the development of MCC include loss of portions of 3p, 4, 5q, 7, 10, and 13, as well as duplication of 1, 3q, 5p, and 6. In particular, loss of *Rb*1 and amplification of *L-Myc* have been identified frequently in MCC.[25]

The recent discovery of a novel polyomavirus identified as MCPyV in the MCC tumor genome has raised the possibility that infection with this double-stranded DNA virus may play a role in tumorigenesis.[26] The potential association between the polyomavirus and MCC triggered a workshop cosponsored by the National Institutes of Health Office of Rare Diseases and the National Cancer Institute to discuss and promote further investigation into this relationship.[27]

Clinical Presentation

MCC usually presents as a solitary, firm, pink, purple, or red nodule involving sun-exposed cutaneous areas of elderly Caucasians. These common characteristics are demonstrated in Figure 17–1. It is not uncommon to see telangiectasias on the surface of the lesion, as well as ulceration.[2] Up to 63% of patients report a period of rapid, painless growth.[28] The lesion can mimic other cutaneous neoplasms, and diagnosis is further complicated by the rarity of the lesion and subsequent provider unfamiliarity with its appearance. Consequently, a median delay from lesion appearance to biopsy is 3 months, and the cancer often is not on the differential diagnosis list until after the pathology report returns.[15,28] Heath and colleagues[28] conducted a cohort study of 195 MCC patients to define clinical characteristics. They summarized the most significant features using the acronym *AEIOU*: *A*symptomatic/lack of tenderness; *E*xpanding rapidly; *I*mmune suppression; *O*lder than 50 years; and Ultraviolet-exposed site on a fair skinned person.

Diagnostic Workup

History and Physical Exam

The workup of MCC begins with a thorough history, including previous skin biopsies, previous skin cancers, sun exposure, occupation, immunosuppression, and radiation exposure. As previously stated, MCC diagnosis can be challenging. In addition, cases of spontaneous regression of the primary tumor have been reported following biopsy.[29,30] For these reasons, pathology slides from previous biopsies or "mole" excisions should be rereviewed, whenever possible, by an experienced dermatopathologist. All patients

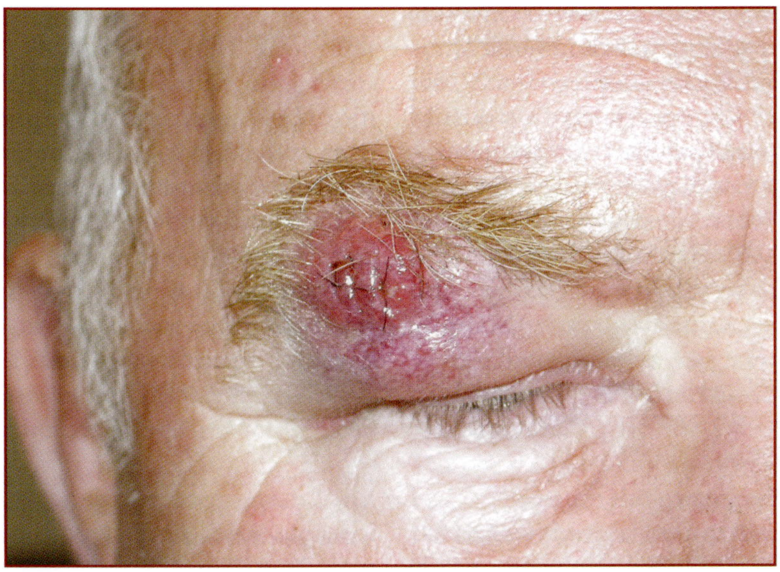

Figure 17–1. Merkel cell carcinoma of the brow. Note the classic features including a red-pink nodule located on the sun-exposed skin of an elderly Caucasian.

presenting with a suspicious cutaneous lesion warrant a full body evaluation of the skin and draining nodal basins by a physician well versed in cutaneous cancers.

Biopsy

All suspicious lesions demand histologic evaluation via a biopsy that should be considered as a distinct, two-staged process. The first step involves biopsy for tissue diagnosis. Ideally, a complete excisional biopsy, with narrow 1- to 2-mm clinical margins of surrounding skin is performed. Some lesions simply are not amenable to excisional biopsy due to large size or anatomic location. In such cases, punch biopsy or incisional biopsy through the thickest portion of the neoplasm is recommended. Unfortunately, punch and incisional biopsies are subject to sampling error, and a repeat biopsy may be necessary.

Biopsy results obtained during the first stage then serve as the guide for the second stage, which entails wide local excision (WLE) using a 1- to 3-cm margin of normal surrounding tissue, with or without sentinel lymph node mapping and biopsy (SLNB). Obtaining wider margins at the time of the initial biopsy may seem both cost and time effective. However, this practice is highly discouraged because clinical accuracy is uncertain, and removal of significant amounts of skin surrounding the lesion may preclude accurate regional staging using lymphoscintigraphy and SLNB technique.[3] Therefore, initial biopsy with narrow margins, with a planned second stage for wide local excision and potential SLNB, is advocated.

Similarly, any patient presenting with a palpable lymph node, which, by definition represents clinically N-positive disease, warrants fine needle aspiration (FNA) of the node. The specific MCC immunohistochemical analysis outlined below is required. If the FNA is nondiagnostic, current National Cancer Comprehensive Network (NCCN) guidelines recommend open biopsy.[3]

Histologic Workup

Histologic features characteristic for MCC include the following: neuroendocrine granules, intercellular junctions, rigid spinous processes, and paranuclear collection of intermediate filaments.[4,16] MCC has three presenting patterns: trabecular, intermediate, and small cell. The latter two subtypes are considered more aggressive.[31]

On hematoxylin and eosin (H& E) staining, MCC appears as small blue cells with intense basophilic staining (Fig 17–2).[31] It is this appearance that makes micrometastatic disease, especially at the tumor margin, difficult to diagnose because the small blue cells carry an appearance similar to the inflammatory response, which can also be present. This diagnostic challenge is depicted in Figure 17–2.

The differential diagnosis for a small blue cell neoplasm is broad and listed in Table 17–1.[16] Due to the heterogeneity of these tumors, specific immunohistochemical (IHC) markers are required to render the diagnosis of MCC and exclude other small blue cell neoplasms such as lymphoma and melanoma.[4] As demonstrated in Figure 17–3, cytokeratin-20 (CK-20) is specific to MCC, particularly in a para-

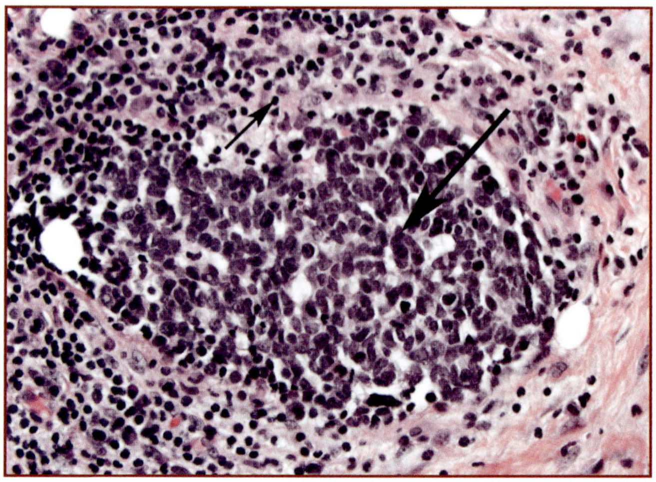

Figure 17–2. Hematoxylin and eosin staining (*H&E*) demonstrating the small round blue cell appearance of Merkel cell carcinoma (*MCC*). Common histologic features include: neuroendocrine granules, intercellular junctions, rigid spinous processes, and paranuclear collection of intermediate filaments.[4,14] Note the similarity in appearance been the MCC small round blue cells (*large arrow*) and surrounding lymphocytes (*small arrow*), which can lead to diagnostic difficulties at the tumor margin.

Table 17–1. Differential Diagnosis of Small Blue Cell Tumors

Merkel Cell Carcinoma
Melanoma
Lymphoma
Neuroblastoma
Carcinoid
Metastatic Small Cell Carcinoma of the Lung
Rhabdomyosarcoma
Extraskeletal Ewing's Sarcoma
Primitive Neuroectodermal Tumor (PNET)

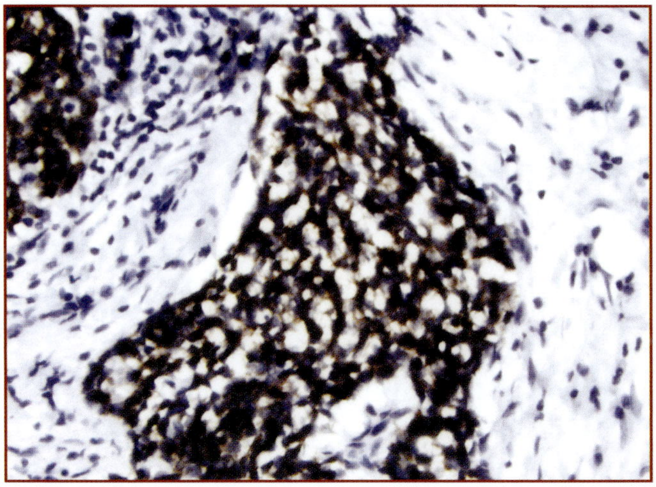

Figure 17–3. Intense Cytokeratin-20 (CK)-20 staining for Merkel cell carcinoma. This antibody is recognized as highly specific for MCC and is used to differentiate the carcinoma from other small blue cell neoplasms.

nuclear staining pattern.[27] If a tumor is negative for this antibody, a different diagnosis should be sought. The majority of MCC tumors will also stain positive for neuroendocrine markers such as neuron-specific enolase, synaptophysin, chromogranin, and neurofilament protein.[15] CD 117 (c-kit receptor), S-100 protein, leukocyte common antigen (CD45), and pancytokeratin (panCK) are other nonspecific IHC markers common to MCC.[3,16] Negative IHC staining is equally important because positive staining for thyroid transcription factor 1 (TTF-1) is specific to small cell lung cancer and is used to exclude MCC from the diagnosis.[3]

Radiographic Workup

Once the diagnosis of MCC is rendered, multidisciplinary tumor board consultation is recommended and further metastatic workup is required.[3] A constrasted CT scan of the neck to assess cervical lymphadenopathy should be accomplished. Additional radiographic studies may be warranted depending on the patient's history and symptoms. Specifically, additional imaging with CT, MRI, or PET-CT may be required to rule out the possibility of skin metastasis from a noncutaneous primary neuroendocrine carcinoma, such as small cell carcinoma of the lung, especially in CK-20 negative cases.[3] A thorough review of systems will serve as a guide for additional studies such as a CT of the abdomen or MRI of the brain to rule out distant metastasis. CT-PET scanning may be helpful in working up a case of metastatic MCC of unknown primary origin and for restaging patients with recurrent disease.[14]

Prognostic Factors and Staging

Similar to other head and neck malignancies, the most important predictor of MCC survival is the initial stage at presentation, with advanced stage portending a poor prognosis.[32] Additional poor prognostic factors include advanced age, male gender, tumor size greater than 2 cm, and tumor location involving the head, neck, or trunk.[32] Analysis of the SEER database indicated that female sex, tumor presentation on the limbs, localized stage I disease, and young age at diagnosis were positive predictors for survival. Additionally, lymphatic invasion, vascular invasion, and small-cell variant are prognostic features specifically related to the primary lesion that indicate aggressive tumor biology.[33]

Until the publication of the 7th edition of the American Joint Commission on Cancer staging manual in 2010, a single, standardized staging system for MCC did not exist.[34] Previously, the most common system cited was published by the Memorial

Sloan Kettering Cancer Center (MSKCC) in 1999, but in clinical practice, up to four other systems were employed.[35–39] The development of the AJCC system was driven by a need to improve physician communication and compare patient information and data. The system is similar to that employed in other cutaneous malignancies, with clinical and pathologic staging and subsequent significant implications for patient prognosis. Based on review of published data and analysis of over 4,700 patients in the National Cancer Database, patient age at presentation, tumor size, the pathologic status of lymph nodes (determined by sentinel lymph node biopsy or lymphadenectomy), and immunosuppression are important determinants of survival.[34] The specific TNM criteria in the 2010 AJCC staging system are summarized in Tables 17–2 and 17–3.

The AJCC identified key pathologic features that should be collected on each patient. Much of this information is obtained from the biopsy: mea-

Table 17–2. American Joint Commission on Cancer Staging System for Merkel Cell Carcinoma (modified from reference 34)

Primary Tumor Stage	Features
Tx	Tumor cannot be assessed
T0	No evidence of primary tumor
Tis	In situ primary tumor
T1	Tumor ≤2 cm in maximum dimension
T2	Tumor >2 cm but ≤5 cm in maximum dimension
T3	Tumor >5 cm in maximum dimension
T4	Tumor invades extracutaneous structures
Regional Lymph Nodes	
Nx	Nodes cannot be assessed
cN0	No regional lymph nodes on clinical or radiographic exam
pN0	No regional lymph node metastases on pathologic exam
N1a	Micrometastasis
N1b	Macrometastasis
N2	In transit metastasis
Distant Metastases	
M0	No distant metastasis
M1a	Metastasis to skin, subcutaneous tissues, or distant lymph nodes
M1b	Metastasis to lung
M2b	Metastasis to all other visceral sites

Source: Used with permission of the American Joint Committee on Cancer (AJCC), Chicago, Illinois. The original source for this material is the AJCC Cancer Staging Manual, Seventh Edition (2010) published by Springer Science and Business Media, LLC, www.springer.com.

Table 17–3. Stage Grouping for Merkel Cell Carcinoma[34]

Stage	Tumor	Nodal Status	Metastasis
0	Tis	N0	M0
IA	T1	pN0	M0
IB	T1	cN0	M0
IIA	T2/3	pN0	M0
IIB	T2/3	cN0	M0
IIC	T4	N0	M0
IIIA	Any T	N1a	M0
IIIB	Any T	N1b/N2	M0
IV	Any T	Any N	M1

Source: Used with permission of the American Joint Committee on Cancer (AJCC), Chicago, Illinois. The original source for this material is the AJCC Cancer Staging Manual, Seventh Edition (2010) published by Springer Science and Business Media, LLC, www.springer.com.

sured tumor thickness, margin status, the presence of tumor infiltrating lymphocytes, and the growth pattern. When lymph nodes from either sentinel lymph node biopsy or lymphadenectomy are evaluated, the presence of isolated tumor cells in the nodes, the size of tumor nests within the nodes, and the presence of extracapsular extension should be documented. Because of the disparity in prognosis between patients with uncertain nodal status and those with confirmed negative nodes, stage groupings for early MCC are divided into A and B subdivisions, based on clinical assessment (B) or histopathologic evaluation (A). Similarly, the extent of nodal disease is associated with worsened prognosis, and this is reflected by separation of stage III into A and B divisions based on the presence of micrometastatic nodal disease (A) and macroscopic nodal disease or in-transit metastases (B).[34]

Approximately 70% of MCC patients present with localized (stage I and II) disease.[6,14] An additional 25% present with regional, or stage III, disease. Five to 10% of patients initially present with distant stage IV disease, and stage IV MCC is far more common in the setting of recurrence.

Management of the Primary Tumor

Wide Local Excision and Surgical Margins

Surgical excision remains the gold standard for treatment of primary MCC. Given the propensity for local recurrence, wide local excision (WLE) to achieve clear pathologic margins is recommended whenever feasible. Specifically, a 1- to 3-cm margin to the depth of muscle fascia, perichondrium or pericranium is recommended.[3]

Achieving wide margins in the head and neck region can be challenging from the standpoint of both cosmesis and function. One small series reported 0 cases of local recurrence following surgical excision with a margin of greater than 2 cm; whereas 30% (7 of 24) patients excised with a margin of equal to or less than 2 cm relapsed.[40] However, a difference in overall survival was not reported. Similarly, a significant difference in locoregional recurrence was reported in patients achieving a margin 2.5 cm or larger compared to narrow excision (27% vs 89%; p <0.01). At 2 year follow-up, the survival rate was also significantly different (86% vs 28%; $p = 0.03$).[41] For this reason, adjuvant radiation to the primary site should be considered if only a narrow margin is obtainable (see below). When possible, the surgical site can be closed immediately following resection. However, in the event that surgical margins remain questionable and require additional immunohistochemical analysis, extensive undermining and local flaps should be delayed until the margins are cleared.[3]

Mohs Micrographic Surgery

Although complete surgical excision with 1- to 3-cm margins is recognized as the gold standard for MCC treatment, small studies support the application of Mohs micrographic surgery (MMS) for treatment of this aggressive cancer. Proponents of MMS argue that the technique offers a more thorough evaluation by the pathologist, with 100% histologic assessment of both superficial and deep margins. Conversely, traditional margins, which entail vertically oriented sections to sample the tumor specimen, provide the pathologist with less than 0.1% of the true tumor margin for analysis.[42]

Although MMS is recognized as a superior technique to traditional WLE for treatment of basal cell and cutaneous squamous cell carcinoma, its role in MCC is yet to be fully defined. O'Connor et al[43] retrospectively reviewed 86 patients treated for local stage I disease. At a mean follow-up of 60 months, 32% of MCC patients undergoing traditional WLE developed recurrent disease at the primary site, and 49% of patients in this group developed regional metastasis. In comparison, a smaller subset of patients underwent Mohs surgery for treatment of their localized MCC. Only 8% of patients developed recurrent disease at the primary site, with a regional failure rate of 33%. For this reason, the authors conclude that Mohs surgery compares favorably with traditional WLE for treatment of MCC. Similar local and regional control rates following the application of the Mohs technique have been reported by other investigators treating MCC.[42,44]

Current NCCN recommendations include the use of Mohs surgery to ensure complete removal of the cancer with clear margins.[3] However, it is important to recognize that tissue sparing capabilities in this setting is considered secondary to complete disease eradication. In addition, the guidelines suggest the possible application of a modified Mohs technique in which Mohs evaluation is used to fully evaluate and clear all margins, with an additional final margin removed specifically for permanent section assessment. As previously noted, the application of IHC analysis for CK-20 may augment traditional or frozen section margin assessment.

Radiotherapy

Merkel cell carcinoma is recognized as a radiosensitive small cell tumor. Anecdotal reports in the literature demonstrate some success with the use of definitive radiation in the treatment of MCC.[14] However, surgical excision remains the standard of care for localized disease, and primary radiation should be reserved for patients who are medically unfit for surgery or who have advanced localized disease in which excision would leave them functionally crippled.

Although some institutions still advocate surgery alone for treatment of localized disease, evidence is mounting to suggest improved locoregional control and disease-free survival with multimodality treatment in which adjuvant radiotherapy is administered after surgery.[14,15] Lewis et al[45] performed a meta-analysis of 1,254 patients to determine the effect of adjuvant local irradiation on both disease recurrence and overall survival. Patients treated with combined surgery and radiation had a significantly reduced local recurrence rate (Hazard ratio [*HR*] = 0.27; $p < 0.001$) and regional recurrence rate (*HR* = 0.34; $p < 0.001$) compared to individuals treated with surgery alone. However, the difference in overall and cause-specific survival failed to reach significance, and the impact on overall survival remains to be determined.

Adjuvant radiation to the primary site should be considered if only a narrow margin is achieved or for stage II tumors measuring greater than 2 cm in diameter.[6] When negative surgical margins are achieved, 50 to 56 gray (Gy) is administered in 2 Gy per day standard fractions. Microscopically positive margins require 56 to 60 Gy, and grossly positive margins 60 to 66 Gy.[3]

Management of Regional Disease

Clinically Positive Lymph Nodes

Therapeutic Lymph Node Dissection

Similar to the primary lesion, surgical treatment remains the standard of care for known regional metastasis. The therapeutic lymph node dissection (TLND) must include all draining nodal basins as well as the intervening lymphatics between the primary tumor and the site of regional disease. In the absence of gross tumor involvement or disruption from open biopsy/previous surgical dissection, concerted efforts should be made to preserve the spinal accessory nerve, internal jugular vein, and sternocleidomastoid muscle during the TLND.

The location of the primary tumor dictates the specific type of TLND, as well as the need for a superficial parotidectomy. MCC involving the anterolateral scalp, temple, lateral forehead, lateral cheek, and ear, arising anterior to an imaginary coronal plane through the external auditory canals (EACs), drain via the parotid nodal basin to the jugular lymph node chain, and, therefore, warrant a superficial parotidectomy along with a modified radical neck dissection (MRND). If the MCC arises in a more inferior location, such as the chin or neck, a superficial parotidectomy is not warranted. MCC of the scalp and occiput, posterior to the imaginary coronal plane through the EACs, can drain to postauricular, suboccipital, and posterior triangle lymph nodes. These nodal basins are not addressed during routine MRND. In this situation, a posterolateral neck dissection, which extends to the midline of the posterior neck, is required. In the event that a patient is medically unfit to undergo a TLND, primary irradiation (60 to 66 Gy) to the draining nodal basins may be considered as an alternative, second-line treatment.[3,6]

Adjuvant Regional Radiotherapy

Traditionally, the benefits of adjuvant radiotherapy for MCC have been mixed. However, increasing support has emerged for improved locoregional control in this setting, and multimodality treatment has gained considerable popularity.[3,6,15] Retrospective analysis of 1,665 MCC cases recorded in the SEER database (1973 to 2002) identified a median survival rate of 63 months for those individuals receiving adjuvant radiation compared to only 45 months for patients treated with surgery alone. This survival advantage was noted for all tumor sizes, but the improvement with the addition of adjuvant radiation was particularly evident for patients with tumors larger than 2 cm in diameter.[46] Similarly, Clark et al[38] reported significant improvement in local control ($p = 0.009$), regional control ($p = 0.006$) and disease-free survival ($p = 0.013$) with multimodality treatment involving surgery and postoperative radiation compared to surgery alone. Although the current MCC NCCN guidelines identify radiation as a potential treatment option for all stages, adjuvant radiation to the nodal basins should be highly considered for patients with regional metastasis, especially in the setting of bulky disease or extracapsular spread.[3] Following TLND, 50 to 60 Gy is administered to the nodal basins in 2 Gy per day standard fractionation.

Adjuvant Chemotherapy

Although most institutions reserve chemotherapy for advanced stage IV disease (see below), some clinicians offer this additional modality for select stage III cases involving regional disease. Combination treatment with either etoposide and cisplatin or carboplatin, or cyclophosphamide, doxorubicin, and vincristine is recommended in this setting.[3] However, the current literature fails to demonstrate prolonged survival even with the addition of chemotherapy.[3,6] Given the significant comorbidities associated with chemotherapy, and the advanced age of most MCC patients, adjuvant chemotherapy does not have an established role for localized (stage I, II) or regional disease (stage III).

Sentinel Lymph Node Biopsy in the Clinically N0 Neck

As mentioned above, the most important predictor for survival remains the presence of nodal disease, which decreases 5-year survival rates from 88% to 48%.[47] Accurate staging of MCC remains challenging. Although 75% of patients present with clinically localized disease, a high incidence of occult nodal metastasis is presumed because 40% of these individuals eventually develop regional disease. Identification of micrometastatic MCC is exceedingly challenging. The small aggregate of metastatic Merkel cells are often difficult to differentiate from background lymphocytic tissues (see Fig 17–2); and 40% of patients harboring disease will be missed if pathologic evaluation is limited to standard H&E staining.[47]

Advocates of sentinel lymph node biopsy (SLNB) argue that it is the most sensitive means for achieving MCC regional staging.[6,47] SLNB is a minimally invasive, cost effective, and highly accurate means to evaluate the nodes most likely harboring occult disease. This staging modality allows for identification of patients with stage III disease who then may benefit from TLND and adjuvant radiotherapy. At the same time, the technique spares the remaining patients without regional disease, many of whom are elderly, the additional morbidity associated with such treatments.

SLNB involves preoperative lymphoscintigraphy performed 2 to 4 hours prior to surgery using techniques previously described.[47] In brief, 2 to 4 μCi of technetium sulfur colloid (CIS-US, Inc, Bedford, MA) is injected intradermally into the four quadrants surrounding the primary MCC lesion, and planar imaging is performed 15 to 30 minutes following injection. Lymphoscintigraphy serves as an intraoperative guide to surgeons as it identifies the number, location, and laterality of nodal basins at risk for metastatic disease. SPECT CT, which provides increased resolution of tissue landmarks, also can be applied in conjunction with lymphoscintigraphy to further define the location of SLNs.

After induction of general anesthesia, intraoperative lymphatic mapping is achieved by injecting approximately 1 mL of blue dye into the intradermal layer surrounding the MCC lesion. Following wide local excision of the primary lesion with 1- to 3-cm margins, nodal basins are evaluated for increased radioactivity using a hand held gamma probe (Navigator GPS, RMD Instruments, Watertown, MA). A 1- to 3-cm incision is then made overlying the areas of increased radioactivity. A preauricular incision is employed for SLNB in the parotid region.

Sentinel lymph nodes are identified using a combination of gamma probe and visual cues from the blue dye. Each SLN is individually dissected from surrounding tissue. Facial nerve monitoring is recommended for SLNB within the parotid nodal basin. The staging procedure is considered complete when all nodal basins demonstrate minimal background radioactivity relative to the primary lesion and SLNs.

All SLNs are sent for histologic evaluation using formalin-fixed permanent sections. The evaluation should include serial sectioning at 2- to 3-mm intervals and H&E staining. Immunochemical staining with CK-20 is required for all SLNs that are negative on initial H&E examination.

Patients with a positive SLN for MCC should be counseled on the role of TLND and adjuvant radiation therapy. Ideally, the patient returns to the operating room within 2 weeks of the SLNB. The remaining patients with a negative SLN biopsy do not require a TLND or nodal radiation and are followed clinically.

It is imperative to appreciate that SLNB is a team effort involving experienced surgeons, nuclear medicine staff, and pathologists. The experience and technical skill of the surgeon is vital and may account for some of the variability of SLN failures reported in the literature.[47] The most recent Multicenter Selective Lymphadenectomy Trial (MSLT-1) identified a 55-case learning curve in order to achieve at least 95% accuracy for melanoma SLNM; a similar learning curve is presumed in MCC.[48] In addition, nuclear medicine staff well versed in SLNB are necessary because inappropriate administration of the radioactive tracer can lead to "shine through," which renders the hand-held gamma probe useless in the operating room. Communication with the nuclear medicine team is critical not only in interpreting the lymphoscintigram, but also in ensuring that the appropriate lesion is mapped as patients with MCC often present with significant solar skin changes.

Investigators at the University of Michigan demonstrated that SLNB is a safe and reliable means of regional staging for head and neck MCC patients presenting with localized disease.[47] A cohort of 10 patients underwent SLNB and CK-20 immunostaining. At least 1 SLN was identified in every patient. 79% of SLNs were identified within neck nodal basins, and 21% were harvested from the parotid nodal bed. No cranial nerve complications were reported. The occult MCC nodal metastatic rate was 20% (2 of 10 patients). It is important to note that both positive nodes were negative for metastatic disease on H&E staining and only identified following CK-20 immunostaining. At a mean follow-up of 34.5 months, only 1 (12%) of 8 SLN-negative patients developed regional disease in the setting of a previously mapped nodal basin. This false negative rate of 12% is deemed acceptable given the previously high reported failure rates of 63 to 75% in the untreated neck.[47]

More recently, the Dana Farber group published their experience of 30 MCC patients staged with SLNB, along with a meta-analysis of an additional 92 SLNB patient reported in the literature.[49] One third of patients were found to harbor occult nodal metastasis despite clinically and radiographically negative examinations. At 3 years follow-up, patients with a positive SLN had a 60% recurrence rate, which was 3 times higher than their negative SLNB counterparts who experienced only a 20% recurrence rate ($p = 0.03$). In addition, the 26 SLNB-positive patients who underwent adjuvant nodal therapy (TLND, radiation, or chemotherapy) demonstrated a relapse-free survival rate of 60%. In contrast, 3 SLNB-positive patients who did not pursue adjuvant nodal treatment had a 0% relapse-free survival rate. This survival difference was significant ($p < 0.01$) and led the authors to conclude that adjuvant therapy provides a significant benefit to positive SLNB MCC patients. In contrast, patient with a negative SLNB did not demonstrate a significant difference in relapse-free survival from those treated with and without adjuvant therapy (90% versus 70% respectively; $p = 0.26$). However, a trend of increased relapse-free survival was noted in the setting of the adjuvant regional therapy.

SLNB currently is recognized as an important component for MCC staging and subsequent treatment.[47,48] All participating NCCN institutions routinely implement SLNB in staging of MCC patients.[3] Every healthy patient presenting with disease limited to the primary site (stage I and II) should be offered sentinel lymph node biopsy. A recent retrospective review of 346 MCC patients, 63% of whom had head and neck primary tumors, supported the use of SLNB in patients with lesions larger than 1cm in diameter.[7] In this study, only 2 patients (4%) with a tumor ≤ 1cm in diameter had regional lymph node metastasis, compared to 51(24%) of patients with larger tumors ($p < 0.0001$). Similar to cutaneous melanoma, SLNB is ideally performed before definitive excision of the primary tumor. However, in the event that a MCC patient presents after WLE, SLNB still may be offered as long as the patient understands that the biopsy results may be less accurate due to scarring and/or lymphatic disruption.[3]

Management of Stage IV Disease

Up to 10% of patients present with distant metastasis, usually involving visceral organs or bones.[14] Furthermore, 40% of patients presenting with recurrent MCC will have distant sites involved. Unfortunately, these patients have an exceedingly grave prognosis, with a mean survival of only 3 to 6 months.

Numerous chemotherapeutic regimens have been used to treat patients with distant and/or inoperable disease, often in the setting of clinical trials. MCC is recognized as a chemosensitive tumor, with initial 60 to 70% overall response rates reported for distant disease; however, the median duration of response is only 8 months.[6] Although chemotherapy is unlikely to prolong survival beyond a few months, it may provide stage IV patients with symptomatic relief and, therefore, a better quality of life.

Patients demonstrating a good performance status should be considered for combination chemotherapy of cisplatin or carboplatin plus etoposide. Associated toxicities include myelosuppression, skin desquamation, and tumor lysis syndrome with acute renal failure requiring dialyses.[6] Chemotherapeutic toxicity during MCC treatment is substantial, with a toxic death rate of 7.7%.[50] In contrast, a toxic death rate of only 0.6% is reported for patients undergoing chemotherapy treatment for non-MCC malignancies. Given the advanced age and often frail status of many MCC patients, reasonable second-line options include single-agent topotecan, oral etoposide, irinotecan, taxanes, or gemcitabine.[6]

Patients with solitary distant disease may benefit from surgical intervention to reduce pain and improve quality of life. When considering surgery, the patient and family must understand that the intervention is palliative in nature. An alternative treatment, especially for patients with poor performance status, is palliative radiation. Symptomatic sites are radiated with 20 to 25 Gy administered in four to five fractions.[15]

Follow-Up and Surveillance

MCC is recognized as an aggressive cancer with a propensity for nodal metastasis, usually within the first 12 months of diagnosis.[47] An overall recurrence rate of 37% is reported in the literature. Local recurrence rates range from 20 to 75%.[2] Thirteen percent of patients fail regionally, 50% of whom will be locoregional failures. Distant disease accounts for 40% of recurrent cases.[14]

Overall cancer-specific death from MCC falls between 25 and 50%.[15] For this reason close follow-up and patient education is imperative. All patients, regardless of clinical stage, should undergo routine examination of the skin and mucosa, with particular attention paid to the original MCC site and associated draining nodal basins. Photodocumentation may be helpful in monitoring change in patients who have a significant number of nevi and associated solar changes. The current schedule set forth by the NCCN is every 1 to 3 months for the first year following MCC diagnosis, every 3 to 6 months during the second year, and annually thereafter.[3]

The high rate of MCC recurrence and its association with other cutaneous carcinomas highlight the importance of patient education. Each follow-up office visit should be viewed as an opportunity to re-educate patients on MCC warning signs and the importance of monthly skin self-examination. Sun education including the use of sunscreen, avoidance of peak sun hours, shade seeking, sun-protective clothing, and the potential risks of tanning booths all should be emphasized.

Conclusions

Merkel cell carcinoma (MCC) is a rare, aggressive cutaneous carcinoma of neuroendocrine origin, which has a propensity to involve the head and neck region. Although the paucity of MCC cases limits the ability to conduct large, prospective clinical trials, current literature provides increasing support for multimodality treatment combining surgery with adjuvant radiation in order to achieve maximal loco-regional control.[3] The most important prognostic feature is tumor stage at initial presentation. For this reason it is imperative that physicians consider MCC in the differential diagnosis whenever evaluating an elderly, Caucasian patient presenting with an asymptomatic, red, pink or purple cutaneous nodule involving sun-exposed areas of the H&N, especially in the setting of rapid growth. The recent introduction of a staging system by the AJCC for MCC should improve communication about patient care, prognosis, and research endeavors that may also shed light on the pathogenesis of this rare cutaneous neoplasm. One hopes increased physician and patient awareness will lead to earlier diagnosis, prompt treatment, and, ultimately, improved survival in Merkel cell carcinoma.

References

1. Toker C. Trabecular carcinoma of the skin. *Arch Dermatol.* 1972;105:107–110.
2. Padgett JK. Cutaneous lesions: benign and malignant. *Facial Plast Surg Clin North Am.* 2005;13:195–202.
3. National Comprehensive Cancer Network, Inc. NCCN Clinical Practice Guidelines in Oncology, v.1.2009. Retrieved October 26, 2009 from http://www.nccn.org/physician_gls/f_guidelines.html .
4. Dinh V, Feun L, Elgart G, Savaraj N. Merkel cell carcinoma. *Hematol Oncol Clin North Am.* 2007;21:527–544.
5. Hodgson NC. Merkel cell carcinoma: changing incidence trends. *J Surg Oncol.* 2005;89:1–4.
6. Bichakjian CK, Lowe L, Lao CD, et al. Merkel cell carcinoma: critical review with guidelines for multidisciplinary management. *Cancer.* 2007;110:1–12.
7. Stokes JB, Graw KS, Dengel LT, et al. Patients with Merkel cell carcinoma tumors ≤ 1.0 cm in diameter are unlikely to harbor regional lymph node metastasis. *J Clin Oncol.* 2009;27:3772–3777.
8. Lemos B, Nghiem P. Merkel cell carcinoma: more deaths but still no pathway to blame. *J Invest Dermatol.* 2007;127:2100–2103.
9. Agelli M, Clegg LX. Epidemiology of primary Merkel cell carcinoma in the United States. *J Am Acad Dermatol.* 2003;49:832–841.
10. Moll I, Roessler M, Brandner JM, et al. Human Merkel cells- aspects of cell biology, distribution and fundtions. *Eur J Cell Biol.* 2005;84:259–271.
11. Winkelmann RK, Breathnach AS. The Merkel cell. *J Invest Dermatol.* 1972;60:2–15.
12. Lacour JP, Dubois D, Pisani A, et al. Anatomical mapping of Merkel cells in normal human adult epidermis. *Br J Dermatol.* 1991;125:535–542.

13. De Wolff Peeters C, Marien K, Mebis J, et al. A cutaneous APUDoma or Merkel cell tumor? A morphologically recognizable tumor with a biological and histological malignant aspect in contrast with its clinical behavior. *Cancer.* 1980;46:1810–1816.
14. Veness MJ. Merkel cell carcinoma (primary cutaneous neuroendocrine carcinoma): an overview on management. *Austral J Dermatol.* 2006; 47:160–165.
15. Veness MJ, Palme CE, Morgan GJ. Merkel cell carcinoma: a review of management. *Curr Opin Otolaryngol Head Neck Surg.* 2008;16:170–174.
16. Yom SS, Rosenthal DI, El-Naggar AK, Kies MS, Hessel AC. Merkel cell carcinoma of the tongue and head and neck oral mucosal sites. *Oral Surg Oral Med Oral Pathol Oral Radiol Endod.* 2006;101:761–768.
17. Miller RW, Rabkin CS. Merkel cell carcinoma and melanoma: etiological similarities and differences. *Cancer Epidemiol Biomarkers Prev.* 1999;8:153–258.
18. Lunder EJ, Stern RS. Merkel-cell carcinomas in patients treated with methoxsalen and ultraviolet A radiation. *N Engl J Med.* 1998;339:1247–1248.
19. Penn I, First MR. Merkel's cell carcinoma in organ recipients: report of 41 cases. *Transplantation.* 1999;68:1717–1721.
20. An KP, Ratner D. Merkel cell carcinoma in the setting of HIV infection. *J Am Acad Dermatol.* 2001;45:309–312.
21. Ho SY, Tsai YC, Lee MC, Guo HR. Merkel cell carcinoma in patients with long-term ingestion of arsenic. *J Occup Health.* 2005;47:188–192.
22. Leonard JH, Cook AL, Nancarrow D, et al. Deletion mapping on the short arm of chromosome 1 in Merkel cell carcinoma. *Cancer Detect Prev.* 2000;24:620–627.
23. Kennedy MM, Blessing K, King G, Kerr KM. Expression of bcl-2 and p53 in Merkel cell carcinoma. An immunohistochemical study. *Am J Dermatopathol.* 1996;18:273–277.
24. Houben R, Michel B, Better-Kauczok CS, et al. Absence of classical MAP kinase pathway signaling in Merkel cell carcinoma. *J Invest Dermatol.* 2006;126:1135–1142.
25. Paulson KG, Lemos BD, Feng B, et al. Array-CGH reveals recurrent genomic changes in Merkel cell carcinoma including amplification of L-myc. *J Invest Dermatol.* 2009;129:1547–1555.
26. Feng H, Shuda M, Chang Y, et al. Clonal integration of a polyomavirus in human Merkel cell carcinoma. *Science.* 2008;319:1096–1100.
27. Goedert JJ and the Rockville Merkel Cell Carcinoma Group. Merkel cell carcinoma: recent progress and current priorities on etiology, pathogenesis, and clinical management. *J Clin Oncol.* 2009;27:4021–4026.
28. Heath M, Jaimes N, Lemos B, et al. Clinical characteristics of Merkel cell carcinoma at diagnosis in 195 patients: the AEIOU features. *J Am Acad Dermatol.* 2008;58:375–381.
29. Huber GF. Merkel cell carcinoma with solitary parotid metastasis: diagnostic dilemma in the absence of a primary site. *J Otolaryngol Head Neck Surg.* 2008;37:19–25.
30. Torroni A, Lore' B, Iannetti G. The importance of the head and neck region in regression of advanced MCC: a clinical report. *J Craniofac Surg.* 2007;18:1173–1176.
31. McGuire JF, Ge NN. Nonmelanoma skin cancer of the head and neck I: histopathology and clinical behavior. *Am J Otolarynogl Head Neck Med Surg.* 2009;20:121–133.
32. Eich HT, Eich D, Staar S, et al. Role of postoperative radiotherapy in the management of Merkel cell carcinoma. *Am J Clin Oncol.* 2002;25:50–56.
33. Tai P. Merkel cell cancer: update on biology and treatment. *Curr Opin Oncol.* 2008; 20:196–200.
34. Merkel cell carcinoma. In: *American Joint Committee on Cancer: AJCC Cancer Staging Manual.* 7th ed. New York, NY: Springer; 2010: 315–319.
35. Allen PJ, Zhang ZF, Coit DG. Surgical management of Merkel cell carcinoma. *Ann Surg.* 1999;229:97–105.
36. Allen PJ, Bowne WB, Jaques DP, et al. Merkel cell carcinoma: prognosis and treatment of patients from a single institution. *J Clin Oncol.* 2005;23:2300–2309.
37. American Joint Committee on Cancer. *AJCC Cancer Staging Manual.* 6th ed. New York, NY: Springer; 2002.
38. Clark JR, Veness KJ, Gilber R, et al. Merkel cell carcinoma of the head and neck: is adjuvant radiotherapy necessary? *Head Neck.* 2007;29:249–257.
39. Yiengpruksawan A, Coit DG, Thaler HT, et al. Merkel cell carcinoma: prognosis and management. *Arch Surg.* 1991;126:1514–1519.
40. Ott MJ, Tanabe KK, Gadd MA, et al. Multimodality management of Merkel cell carcinoma. *Arch Surg.* 1999;134: 288–393.
41. Kokoshka ER, Kokoska MS, Collins BT, Stapleton DR, Wade TP. Early aggressive treatment for Merkel cell carcinoma improves outcome. *Am J Surg.* 1997;174:688–693.
42. Boyer JD, Zitelli JA, Brodland DG, D'Angelo G. Local control of primary Merkel cell carcinoma: review of 45 cases treated with Mohs micrographic surgery with and without adjuvant radiation. *J Am Acad Dermatol.* 2002;47: 885–892.
43. O'Connor WJ, Roenigk RK, Broadland DG. Merkel cell carcinoma-comparison of Mohs micrographic surgery and wide local excision in eighty-six patients. *Dermatol Surg.* 1997;23:929–933.
44. Pennington BE, Leffell DJ. Mohs micrographic surgery: established uses and emerging trends. *Oncology.* 2005;19: 1165–1171.
45. Lewis KG, Weinstock MA, Weaver AL, Otley CC. Adjuvant local irradiation for Merkel cell carcinoma. *Arch Dermatol.* 2006;142:693–700.
46. Mojica P, Smith D, Ellenhorn JDI. Adjuvant radiation therapy is associated with improved survival in Merkel cell carcinoma of the skin. *J Clin Oncol.* 2007;27:1043–1047.
47. Schmalbach CE, Lowe L, Teknos TN, Johnson TM, Bradford CR. Reliability of sentinel lymph node biopsy for regional staging of head and neck Merkel cell carcinoma. *Arch Otolaryngol Head Neck Surg.* 2005;131:610–614.
48. Morton DL, Cochran AJ, Thompson JF, et al. Sentinel node biopsy for early-stage melanoma accuracy and morbidity in MSLT-I, an international multicenter trial. *Ann Surg.* 2005;242:302–313.

49. Gupta SG, Wang LC, Penas PF, et al. Sentinel lymph node biopsy for evaluation and treatment of patients with Merkel cell carcinoma. *Arch Dermatol.* 2006;142:685–690.

50. Voog E, Biron P, Martin JP, Blay JY. Chemotherapy for patients with locally advanced or metastatic Merkel cell carcinoma. *Cancer.* 1999;85:2589–2595.

18

DERMATOFIBROSARCOMA PROTUBERANS

THOMAS D. SHELLENBERGER
ERICH M. STURGIS

Introduction

Dermatofibrosarcoma protuberans (DFSP) is an uncommon form of sarcoma arising in the dermis and underlying subcutaneous tissue that differentiates along the lines of fibroblasts or myofibroblasts. A low-grade sarcoma, DFSP is characterized by indolent clinical behavior with a progressive, locally infiltrative growth pattern and rare metastases. The pattern of growth for DFSP is characterized by irregular shapes and microscopic fingerlike projections of tumor that extend well beyond the clinical extent of disease.[1,2]

Because of this irregular growth pattern, incomplete excision and subsequent recurrence commonly occur. The local recurrence rate for DFSP ranges from 0% to 60%, whereas the rate of regional or distant metastatic disease is only 1% and 4%, respectively.[3] Although DFSP is rare, both among sarcomas and among malignant tumors of the head and neck, occurrence at head and neck sites can account for significant morbidity and mortality. Initial misdiagnosis, prolonged time to accurate diagnosis, and large tumor size at the time of diagnosis all are common for DFSP. An understanding of the clinical presentation, evaluation, and multidisciplinary management is requisite for optimal care of the patient with DFSP of the head and neck.

Epidemiology

Although rare among sarcomas, accounting for between 2 and 6% of soft tissue sarcomas in adults, DFSP is the most common sarcoma of skin.[4,5] The incidence of DFSP in the United States is approximately 4 cases per million per year, and approximately 15% of DFSP occur in the head and neck.[6] DFSP also is rare among head and neck malignancies, accounting for far fewer than 0.1% of all malignancies arising in the head and neck region. In fact, only a small proportion of sarcomas arising in the head and neck region are DFSP.

Only 5% of almost 1,200 incident sarcomas of the head and neck region evaluated at The University of Texas M.D. Anderson Cancer Center Houston between 1970 and 2004 were DFSP, with approximately 80% occurring in the scalp/face and all others arising within the parotid/neck.[7] DFSP develops predominantly in adults between 30 and 50 years of age, but it may arise in childhood or even congenitally.[6,8,9] There is no apparent sex disparity, but a higher incidence has been suggested in African-Americans as compared to Caucasians.[6,8–10] No clear risk factors for DFSP have been identified.

Clinical Presentation

The clinical presentation of patients with DFSP is quite variable. On one hand, patients may present with nonspecific features such as asymptomatic, plaquelike areas of cutaneous thickening or small nodular lesions. On the other hand, presentation later in the course of disease may be characterized by the multinodular, protruberant masses for which DFSP was named (Fig 18–1).

Primary Disease

The head and neck region is the site of disease in 10 to 20% of patients with DFSP.[6,8,9,11,12] Among tumors arising in the head and neck, the most frequent subsites include the scalp and face, accounting for more than three-quarter of cases, followed by the parotid and neck.[7] An indurated, firm lesion with infiltrative and locally destructive growth is typical. The overlying skin is often brownish-yellow or red-tinged with atrophic, telangiectatic, or sclerodermiform changes. Nodules may be fixed to the overlying epidermis but move freely over the deeper tissues.

DFSP may remain indolent, slowly enlarging over a long period that may range from months to decades. Approximately 90% of patients have the classic form of DFSP, a low-grade malignancy.[13] However, accelerated growth may result in ulceration, bleeding, and pain. Fixation to deep structures by tumor invasion of underlying fascia, muscle, or bone accompanies a more advanced stage of disease. Rarely, DFSP can transform into a fibrosarcomatous form with more aggressive clinical behavior and greater metastatic potential. The risk of fibrosarcomatous transformation increases for DFSP that recur repeatedly and thus require more intense treatment approaches.[8]

Although the prognosis generally is good and patients rarely die from DFSP, significant morbidity can occur as a consequence of disease at the primary site. The infiltrative growth pattern for DFSP accounts for a high rate of local recurrence after initial surgery, as high as 80% in some series.[10] A risk

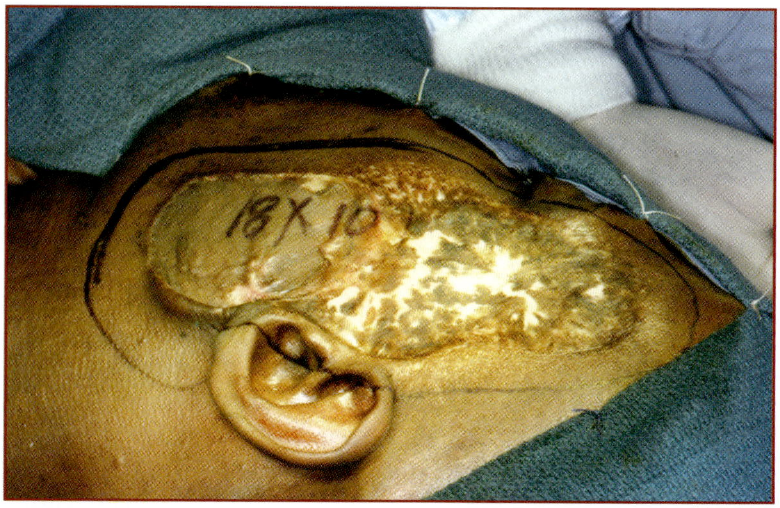

Figure 18–1. Clinical picture of DFSP of preauricular cheek and upper neck skin.

factor for recurrence appears to be age greater than 50, although tumor size may not have as clear an influence on recurrence rates as one might assume.[11,13]

Metastatic Disease

DFSP generally manifests as locally restricted disease. However, there is a low, but significant, potential for metastasis. The reported rate of distant metastasis of 5% is accounted for mostly by aggressive variants of DFSP. Conversely, the reported rate of distant metastasis for the classic form of DFSP is only 0.5%.[14] The most frequent sites of distant hematogenous metastasis are the lungs followed by the brain, bone, and other soft tissues.[15,16] Metastasis to lymph nodes is even rarer, with only a few individual cases reported in the literature. Regardless, the development of metastasis is an ominous sign; most patients die within 2 years from uncontrolled disease.

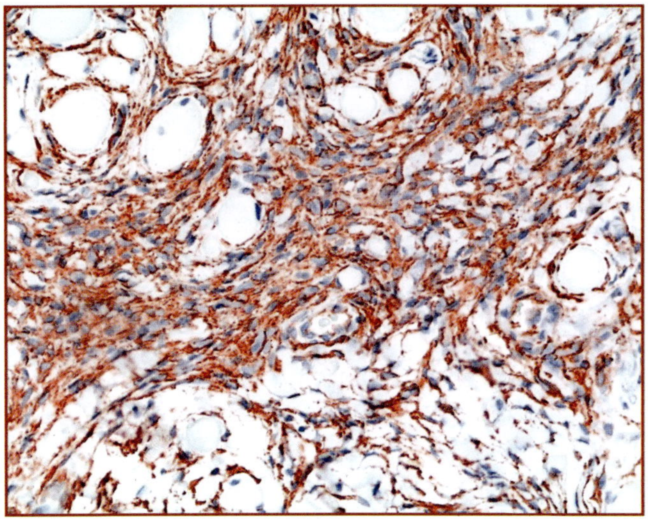

Figure 18–2. Immunohistochemical analysis of DFSP. Tumor cells strongly and diffusely express CD34. (×20; Anti-CD34, aminoethylcarbazol and light hematoxylin as counterstain).

Pathology

DFSP is characterized histologically by a monomorphous proliferation of cytologically bland spindle cells with whorled, storiform, or rush matlike architecture and low mitotic activity with deep, honeycomb infiltration into the subcutaneous adipose tissue.[1,11,13] Irregular, fingerlike projections of neoplastic cells can diffusely infiltrate the surrounding dermis and subcutis to deeply invade fascia and muscle. The result is microscopic spread of disease far beyond that appreciated clinically. Moreover, tumor cells of the fingerlike projections may be so bland that the border of the tumor is difficult to determine even microscopically.

The characteristic appearance of DFSP on light-microscopy is diagnostic in most cases. Occasionally, it may be difficult to differentiate DFSP from other neoplasms such as dermatofibroma, dermatomyofibroma, fibrosarcoma, pleomorphic sarcoma, leiomyosarcoma, and atypical fibroxantoma.[10] DFSP generally stains positively for CD34 (Fig 18–2) and vimentin, but negatively for factor XIIIa.[1]

In up to 15% of patients with DFSP, the tumor contains a high-grade fibrosarcomatous component that typically occupies between 20 and 80% of the tumor mass.[10] The cells in these areas usually show a higher rate of mitotic activity, increased cellularity, and focal loss of CD34 staining, along with marked nuclear pleomorphism in relation to the areas of classic DFSP. Fibrosarcomatous change in DFSP appears to be a form of tumor progression that heralds a worse prognosis.

Molecular Biology and Genetics of DFSP

In more than 90% of DFSP tumors, a supernumerary ring chromosome is found and represents a unique translocation that fuses the strongly expressed collagen type I alpha 1 gene (*COL1A1*) on chromosome 17 with the platelet-derive growth factor B-chain gene (*PDGFβ*) on chromosome 22, t(17;22). *PDGFβ* encodes the B-chain of PDGF, a ligand for the cell-surface tyrosine kinase PDGF receptor and a growth factor with potent mitogen activity for connective tissue cells. The resulting fusion protein expressed by the fusion gene *COL1A1-PDGFβ* is processed into mature PDGFβ in cells of DFSP and leads to autocrine stimulation of PDGF receptors on the DFSP cell surface and, therefore, constant generation and proliferation of tumor cells.[10] This molecular alteration is thought to be fundamental to the pathogenesis of DFSP. The ring chromosome can be shown by fluorescence in situ hybridization whereas the mRNA coding for the fusion protein COL1A1-PDGFβ can be detected by reverse transcriptase polymerase chain reaction.

Diagnosis and Staging

Physical Examination

The correct and timely diagnosis of DFSP is requisite to optimal management and to prevent morbidity and mortality from complications of treatment or progression of disease. Evaluation of a patient with cutaneous malignancy of the head and neck begins with physical examination to determine the character and extent of disease. Owing to the often indolent pattern of growth, the variability in presentation, and the frequent lack of specific signs or symptoms in a patient with DFSP, a clinical diagnosis is rarely of any certainty. Nonetheless, for an indurated, firm lesion with characteristic changes in the overlying skin and with infiltrative or locally destructive growth, the differential diagnosis should include DFSP.

Although offering insight to the pathologic diagnosis of the lesion, physical examination findings suggest the degree of involvement of local and regional anatomic structures by disease on which to base further evaluation and selection of treatment. Fixation or immobility of the lesion implies extension to deeper structures such as fascia, muscle, and bone and a more advanced stage of disease at the primary site. Multiple lesions of similar appearance suggest diffuse disease manifest as dermal metastasis. Paresis or paralysis in the distribution of a facial nerve branch suggests local involvement of a peripheral branch, whereas dysfunction in the distribution of the upper division, the lower division, or the main trunk implies parotid gland invasion and more proximal involvement. Palpable adenopathy in a regional basin, although extremely rare, suggests lymphatic metastasis. In addition to the complete history and physical examination, evaluation should include a complete skin evaluation for any synchronous or second primary lesions.

Biopsy

In any patient with a lesion suspicious for cutaneous malignancy, an accurate diagnosis is crucial for optimal management and depends on acquisition of sufficient tissue for histologic evaluation. Therefore, excisional or incisional/punch biopsy should be performed to confirm the clinical suspicion, as morphologic diagnosis based on microscopic examination of histologic sections remains the gold standard in diagnosis of DFSP. When the clinician's suspicion for DFSP persists despite an initial negative biopsy, repeat biopsy is recommended. DFSP is frequently misdiagnosed, and multiple nonsupportive or equivocal biopsies before a definitive diagnosis are common in the clinical history.

The primary goal of any technique in biopsy of a lesion is to obtain an adequate specimen from which a definitive pathologic diagnosis can be established. At the same time, the technique should be easily incorporated into any future treatment strategies without compromising further management. As DFSP typically are superficial, an incisional biopsy can be performed in most cases and thus leave the majority of the lesion in situ for evaluation by the treating surgeon and other consultants prior to definitive treatment. Excisional biopsies should be reserved for the smallest of lesions in which complete resection is possible without dissection into uninvolved tissue planes and without compromise to adjacent anatomic structures.

The incision for a biopsy should be designed to easily incorporate into any definitive surgical approaches that might follow. Core or fine-needle aspiration biopsies can be useful in previously treated patients in which recurrence is suspected or for deep/less accessible incident tumors. The clinical features should be reviewed with the evaluating pathologist, preferably one experienced in dermatopathology and sarcoma subtyping. Specimens should be handled with consideration for special staining and cytogenetic studies as supplements to routine processing to clinch a definitive diagnosis. Although evaluation of hematoxylin and eosin-stained specimens by light microscopy results in unequivocal diagnosis in most cases, differentiation of DFSP from dermatofibroma may be difficult. In such instances, immunostaining with CD34, factor XIIIa, metallothioneins, tenascin, and stromelysin-3 may be useful.[3,16–19] Therefore, appropriate and confirmatory immunostaining should be performed in all cases of suspected DFSP.

Additionally, it is unclear whether the histologic features of a high mitotic rate or evidence of fibrosarcomatous change (typically in more than 5% of the surgical specimen) have prognostic significance in DFSP, since published studies both support and refute this notion.[8,13,14,20] However, both features should be documented in any DFSP pathology report. As few centers have extensive experience in the evaluation of tumors as rare as DFSP, review of a specimen by a second pathologist often can help resolve any diagnostic dilemmas, and repeat biopsy should be considered whenever specimen adequacy is in question.

Imaging

Diagnostic imaging augments the physical examination to more accurately assess the extent of disease at the primary site, as well as any sites of regional or distant metastasis. Computed tomography (CT) by high-resolution technique with intravenous contrast is readily available, rapid, and highly sensitive in detecting underlying soft-tissue and bony involvement by primary tumor in relation to adjacent structures. CT additionally offers superior evaluation of the neck and chest to complete initial pretreatment staging. Routine imaging by CT is crucial to assess for the possibility of metastatic disease prior to initial treatment and to serve as baseline imaging for comparison during the subsequent surveillance after treatment.

Magnetic resonance imaging (MRI) often can complement the evaluation by CT, especially for tumors of the skull base or paraspinal regions (Fig 18–3). MRI can be accomplished without iodinated contrast material in patients with allergy or impaired renal function. No cross-sectional imaging technique

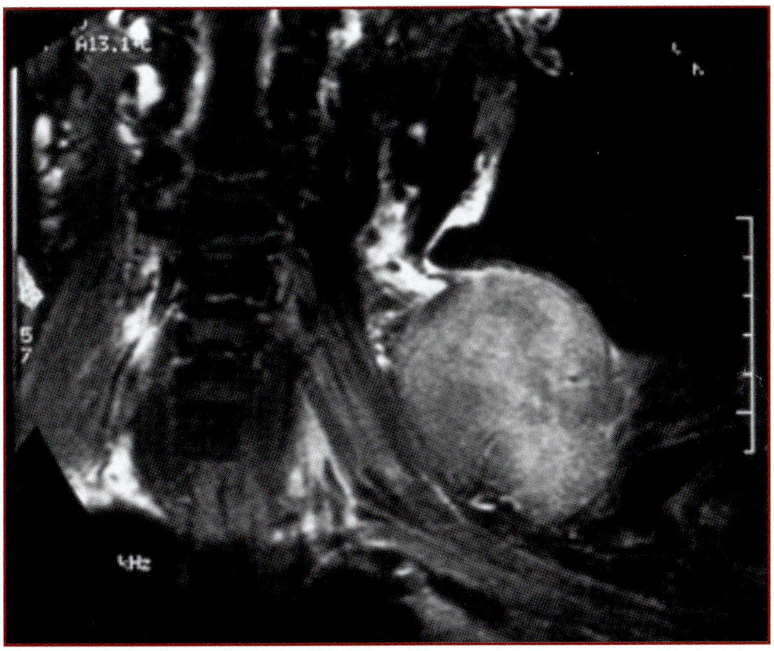

Figure 18–3. MRI of recurrent DFSP of posterior triangle with nonspecific imaging characteristics including involvement of the skin and abutting deep neck musculature.

is sufficiently sensitive to detect the subclinical extension of disease by microscopic fingerlike projections characteristic of DFSP. Ultrasonography also is useful in selected cases where core or fine-needle aspiration biopsy can be accomplished. Because lymphatic and hematogenous dissemination of DFSP is rare, more exhaustive investigation for disease is not routinely recommended and should be based only on specific signs or symptoms that warrant further evaluation or adverse prognostic/histologic features.

Staging

A definitive staging system for DFSP has not been developed. Although the current American Joint Committee of Cancer (AJCC) staging system for soft-tissue sarcomas is optimally designed for staging extremity tumors, a major limitation is the lack of consideration for the anatomic and histologic heterogeneity among soft-tissue sarcomas. These limitations are most notable for sarcomas of the head and neck region and for DFSP in particular. For instance, the AJCC staging system for soft tissue sarcomas would classify virtually all DFSP as stage I, with the rare exceptions of a high-grade DFSP (stage II or III) or the presence of metastases (stage IV). Thus, it is readily apparent that a system with accurate prognostication and stage discrimination for DFSP remains lacking.

Treatment

The treatment goals for DFSP of the head and neck region are determined by the anatomic location, histology, and stage of disease, along with consideration for the age and performance status of the patient. The intent should be curative with surgery whenever the probability for cure is realistic and the risks of treatment are acceptable. The optimal management of DFSP of the head and neck relies on a multidisciplinary approach to patient evaluation and treatment. In order to optimize outcomes, all potential modes of therapy, reconstructive strategies, and rehabilitation needs should be fully anticipated and considered prior to initiating treatment. Because of the rarity of DFSP, high-level evidence from randomized controlled trials on which to base treatment recommendations for DFSP is lacking. Nonetheless, there is sufficient lower level evidence (category 2A) to reach uniform consensus guidelines by the Nonmelanoma Skin Cancer Panel of the National Comprehensive Cancer Network.[21,22]

Surgery

Wide Local Excision

Surgery is the mainstay in the initial treatment of patients with DFSP, and the foremost goal of surgery is complete removal at the initial operation with every effort made to achieve clear surgical margins.[21] The conduct of surgery should be based on sound oncologic principles and an understanding of the growth pattern of long, irregular, and deep subclinical fingerlike tumor projections. Hence, the surgical approach should be planned carefully. The size and location of the tumor along with the implications on form and function dictate the appropriate surgical procedure. Two- to four-centimeter margins to investing fascia of muscle or pericranium with clear pathologic margins should be achieved whenever clinically feasible and subsequently verified by traditional pathologic assessment.[12,23]

The tumor should be removed by three-dimensional en bloc resection along with skin, underlying subcutaneous tissue and fascia. In areas of suspected bone invasion, periosteum and the underlying partial or full thickness of bone should be included. Complete circumferential and peripheral deep-margin assessment should be performed routinely. Additional surgery should be considered whenever margins are positive or close to positive. Unfortunately, generous margins are not always practical for tumors of the head and neck region, particularly when the lesion is located near critical facial structures. Accordingly, high recurrence rates after traditional surgery, up to 75%, have been reported for DFSP at head and neck sites.[24]

In most cases, the risks of morbidity and mortality from uncontrolled local disease with invasion of vital structures should outweigh reluctance to resect tumor with wide margins. The pathologic report should include the site, depth of tumor, size of tumor, extent of necrosis, status of margins and lymph nodes, as well as any additional tumor features such as mitotic rate, vascular invasion, character of the tumor margin, and inflammatory infiltrate. The results of ancillary studies with immunohistochemistry and cytogenetics should be clearly documented.

Mohs Micrographic Surgery

As an alternative to traditional wide local excision, Mohs micrographic surgery, or a modified Mohs technique, have been proposed in the surgical management of DFSP.[8,9,11,23,25–31] Mohs technique is used primarily to ensure complete removal and clear margins, and secondarily for its tissue sparing capabilities. In modified Mohs, an additional final margin is obtained for permanent section assessment. In contrast to wide local excision, which uses representative vertical sectioning, Mohs micrographic surgery requires continuous, sequential horizontal sectioning (5–7 μm) during the resection with immediate microscopic examination of the resected tissue by frozen section until a clear margin is obtained.[10] The intention is to detect the microscopic extensions of tumor and enable complete excision with greater accuracy, while maximally conserving uninvolved normal tissue.

Mohs thus may offer an advantage in patients with tumors in particularly challenging anatomic sites within the head and neck. Although some reports suggest a higher local control rates with Mohs compared to wide local excision, caution should be exercised.[9,10] The meticulous analysis of large lesions can be elaborate, time-consuming, and labor-intensive. Moreover, the pathologic analysis can be inaccurate because of the difficult in clearly differentiating minimal residual DFSP cells from scattered spindle cells in normal dermis or connective tissue. Additionally, techniques that rely on CD34 immunohistochemistry for margin control can suffer from high variability in the staining technique.

Reconstruction

Only after complete histologic assessment has assured negative margins should reconstruction of the defect follow resection of DFSP. It is preferable to delay reconstruction involving extensive undermining or flaps until negative margins are assessed and certified pathologically clear. If there is concern that the surgical margin may not be completely clear, skin grafting can be used to avoid tissue rearrangement and allow monitoring for recurrence. However, immediate reconstruction can be performed in the majority of cases, but the reconstructive approach is determined by the size and complexity of the defect.

Options vary from simple primary closure to more advanced techniques such as microvascular free-tissue transfer. The primary reconstructive goals are to restore form while providing coverage of exposed bone underlying soft tissue to prevent radiotherapy-associated complications. Additional goals include restoration of eyelid function, oral competence, and a patent nasal airway. Well-executed reconstruction is critical to maximizing form, function, and quality of life. Primary closure with local rotation or advancement flaps is often adequate for facial soft tissue defects, whereas scalp defects more commonly require skin graft coverage. For defects widely exposing cortical bone, removal of the outer table can provide a well-vascularized medullary bone surface capable of supporting a skin graft. Larger defects resulting from resection of facial bones and underlying soft tissue are best addressed by microvascular free flap reconstruction. Reconstruction of defects arising from resection of cutaneous malignancy of the head and neck is discussed in great detail elsewhere in this text.

Chemotherapy

As discussed, DFSP is characterized by a translocation between chromosome 17 and 22 [t(17:22)] resulting in overstimulation of the PDGF receptor.[32–34] These findings suggest that targeting PDGF receptors may lead to the development of new therapeutic options for DFSP. In recently published results, imatinib mesylate, a protein tyrosine kinase inhibitor, has shown clinical activity against localized and metastatic DFSP tumors containing the t(17:22).[22,35–38] Imatinib mesylate recently has been approved by the FDA for the treatment of unresectable, recurrent and/or metastatic DFSP in adult patients.[39] Because tumors lacking the t(17:22) translocation may not respond to imatinib mesylate, molecular analysis of a tumor by cytogenetics may be useful prior to the institution of therapy with imatinib mesylate. The impact of targeted therapy on the clinical treatment of DFSP awaits the outcome of several clinical trials currently underway investigating imatinib mesylate. Early reports indicate response rates of up to 50% in DFSP treated with either 400 mg daily or twice daily of imatinib mesylate.[40]

Radiotherapy

Radiotherapy occasionally has been used as a primary therapeutic modality for DFSP, but it is more commonly used as postoperative adjuvant therapy.[41–44] Postoperative radiation therapy (or possibly imatinib mesylate) should be considered for positive surgical margins following re-resection or if further resection is not feasible (unresectable disease). Postoperative radiation doses of 5,000 to 6,000 cGy typically are given for positive or close-to-positive margins in 1.8 to 2.0-cGy fractions per day. Fields should extend widely beyond surgical margins by 3 to 5 cm when clinically feasible.

For patients with recurrent disease, surgery alone can be effective for isolated recurrences. For those with more advanced and/or multifocal recurrences, multimodal therapy such as preoperative radiation therapy (and/or imatinib mesylate) followed by surgery should be considered. Definitive radiation therapy, if not given previously (or imatinib mesylate), should be used for isolated recurrences if additional resection would lead to unacceptable outcomes in form or function. When feasible under specific clinical situations or under the aegis of clinical trials, imatinib mesylate, radiation therapy or re-resection should all be considered in the rare event of metastatic disease.

Follow-Up and Surveillance

Given the historically high rates of local recurrence for DFSP, ongoing clinical follow-up of the primary site every 6 to 12 months for at least 5 years is indicated. Biopsy should be considered for any lesions suspicious for recurrence. Although metastatic disease is rare, a guided history and physical exam should be performed as well, with additional imaging studies as indicated. Patients should be educated about signs and symptoms that might suggest recurrence, as well as the importance of regular self-examination.

Summary

DFSP are extremely rare tumors, yet 15% of these lesions will occur in the head and neck region, typically in the skin of the scalp and face. Typically, these are low-grade malignancies that rarely metastasize but exhibit an aggressive, locally infiltrative pattern of growth and high local recurrence rates. The standard treatment is surgical resection with careful pathologic control of margins and postoperative radiation given for positive margins. A promising nonsurgical treatment appears to be the PDGF-receptor inhibitor, imatinib mesylate, which ultimately may have a role as a surgical adjuvant or as a primary treatment for recurrent or unresectable tumors.

References

1. Haycox CL, Odland PB, Olbricht SM, Casey B. Dermatofibrosarcoma protuberans (DFSP): growth characteristics based on tumor modeling and a review of cases treated with Mohs micrographic surgery. *Ann Plast Surg*. 1997; 38(3):246–251.
2. Ratner D, Thomas CO, Johnson TM, et al. Mohs micrographic surgery for the treatment of dermatofibrosarcoma protuberans. Results of a multiinstitutional series with an analysis of the extent of microscopic spread. *J Am Acad Dermatol*. 1997;37(4):600–613.
3. Vidimos AT, Helm TN., Papay FA. Dermatofibrosarcoma protuberans. In: Miller SJ, Maloney ME, eds. *Cutaneous Oncology: Pathophysiology, Diagnosis, and Management*. Malden, MA: Blackwell Sceintific; 1998:822–831.
4. Chang CK, Jacobs IA, Salti GI. Outcomes of surgery for dermatofibrosarcoma protuberans. *Eur J Surg Oncol*. 2004; 30(3):341–345.
5. Kransdorf MJ. Malignant soft-tissue tumors in a large referral population: distribution of diagnoses by age, sex, and location. *AJR Am J Roentgenol*. 1995;164(1):129–134.

6. Criscione VD, Weinstock MA. Descriptive epidemiology of dermatofibrosarcoma protuberans in the United States, 1973 to 2002. *J Am Acad Dermatol.* 2007;56(6):968–973.
7. Shellenberger TD, Sturgis EM. Sarcomas of the head and neck region. *Curr Oncol Rep.* 2009;11(2):135–142.
8. Fiore M, Miceli R, Mussi C, et al. Dermatofibrosarcoma protuberans treated at a single institution: a surgical disease with a high cure rate. *J Clin Oncol.* 2005;23(30):7669–7675.
9. Paradisi A, Abeni D, Rusciani A, et al. Dermatofibrosarcoma protuberans: wide local excision vs. Mohs micrographic surgery. *Ca Treat Rev.* 2008; 34(8):728–736.
10. Lemm D, Mugge LO, Mentzel T, Hoffken K. Current treatment options in dermatofibrosarcoma protuberans. *J Cancer Res Clin Oncol.* 2009;135(5):653–665.
11. Gloster HM, Jr., Harris KR, Roenigk RK. A comparison between Mohs micrographic surgery and wide surgical excision for the treatment of dermatofibrosarcoma protuberans. *J Am Acad Dermatol.* 1996;35(1):82–87.
12. Stojadinovic A, Karpoff HM, Antonescu CR, et al. Dermatofibrosarcoma protuberans of the head and neck. *Ann Surg Oncol.* 2000;7(9):696–704.
13. Bowne WB, Antonescu CR, Leung DH, et al. Dermatofibrosarcoma protuberans: a clinicopathologic analysis of patients treated and followed at a single institution. *Cancer.* 2000;88(12):2711–2720.
14. Mentzel T, Beham A, Katenkamp D, Dei Tos AP, Fletcher CD. Fibrosarcomatous ("high-grade") dermatofibrosarcoma protuberans: clinicopathologic and immunohistochemical study of a series of 41 cases with emphasis on prognostic significance. *Am J Surg Pathol.* 1998;22(5): 576–587.
15. Rutgers EJ, Kroon BB, Albus-Lutter CE, Gortzak E. Dermatofibrosarcoma protuberans: treatment and prognosis. *Eur J Surg Oncol.* 1992;18(3):241–248.
16. Cribier B, Noacco G, Peltre B, Grosshans E. Stromelysin 3 expression: a useful marker for the differential diagnosis dermatofibroma versus dermatofibrosarcoma protuberans. *J Am Acad Dermatol.* 2002;46(3):408–413.
17. Kahn HJ, Fekete E, From L. Tenascin differentiates dermatofibroma from dermatofibrosarcoma protuberans: comparison with CD34 and factor XIIIa. *Hum Pathol.* 2001;32(1):50–56.
18. Kim HJ, Lee JY, Kim SH, et al. Stromelysin-3 expression in the differential diagnosis of dermatofibroma and dermatofibrosarcoma protuberans: comparison with factor XIIIa and CD34. *Br J Dermatol.* 2007;157(2):319–324.
19. Zelger BW, Ofner D, Zelger BG. Atrophic variants of dermatofibroma and dermatofibrosarcoma protuberans. *Histopathology.* 1995;26(6):519–527.
20. Goldblum JR, Reith JD, Weiss SW. Sarcomas arising in dermatofibrosarcoma protuberans: a reappraisal of biologic behavior in eighteen cases treated by wide local excision with extended clinical follow up. *Am J Surg Pathol.* 2000;24(8):1125–1130.
21. Miller SJ. NCCN *Clinical Practice Guidelines in Oncology: Dermatofibrosarcoma Protuberans.* V.1.2009. 2009. http://www.nccn.org/professionals/physician_gls/f_guidelines.asp
22. *NCCN Updates Dermatofibrosarcoma Protuberans Guidelines.* Retrieved 9-11-2007 from http://www.nccn.org/professionals/physician_gls/f_guidelines.asp
23. DuBay D, Cimmino V, Lowe L, Johnson TM, Sondak VK. Low recurrence rate after surgery for dermatofibrosarcoma protuberans: a multidisciplinary approach from a single institution. *Cancer.* 2004;100(5):1008–1016.
24. Barnes L, Coleman JA, Jr., Johnson JT. Dermatofibrosarcoma protuberans of the head and neck. *Arch Otolaryngol.* 1984;110(6):398–404.
25. Kimmel Z, Ratner D, Kim JY, Wayne JD, Rademaker AW, Alam M. Peripheral excision margins for dermatofibrosarcoma protuberans: a meta-analysis of spatial data. *Ann Surg Oncol.* 2007;14(7):2113–2120.
26. Dawes KW, Hanke CW. Dermatofibrosarcoma protuberans treated with Mohs micrographic surgery: cure rates and surgical margins. *Dermatol Surg.* 1996;22(6):530–534.
27. Haas AF, Sykes JM. Multispecialty approach to complex dermatofibrosarcoma protuberans of the forehead. *Arch Otolaryngol Head Neck Surg.* 1998;124(3):324–327.
28. Snow SN, Gordon EM, Larson PO, Bagheri MM, Bentz ML, Sable DB. Dermatofibrosarcoma protuberans: a report on 29 patients treated by Mohs micrographic surgery with long-term follow-up and review of the literature. *Cancer.* 2004;101(1):28–38.
29. Sondak VK, Cimmino VM, Lowe LM, Dubay DA, Johnson TM. Dermatofibrosarcoma protuberans: what is the best surgical approach? *Surg Oncol.* 1999;8(4):183–189.
30. Huether MJ, Zitelli JA, Brodland DG. Mohs micrographic surgery for the treatment of spindle cell tumors of the skin. *J Am Acad Dermatol.* 2001;44(4):656–659.
31. Pennington BE, Leffell DJ. Mohs micrographic surgery: established uses and emerging trends. *Oncology (Williston Park).* 2005;19(9):1165–1171.
32. McArthur G. Molecularly targeted treatment for dermatofibrosarcoma protuberans. *Semin Oncol.* 2004;31(2 suppl 6):30–36.
33. Mendenhall WM, Zlotecki RA, Scarborough MT. Dermatofibrosarcoma protuberans. *Cancer.* 2004;101(11): 2503–2508.
34. Sjoblom T, Shimizu A, O'Brien KP et al. Growth inhibition of dermatofibrosarcoma protuberans tumors by the platelet-derived growth factor receptor antagonist STI571 through induction of apoptosis. *Cancer Res.* 2001;61(15): 5778–5783.
35. Labropoulos SV, Fletcher JA, Oliveira AM, Papadopoulos S, Razis ED. Sustained complete remission of metastatic dermatofibrosarcoma protuberans with imatinib mesylate. *Anticancer Drugs.* 2005;16(4):461–466.
36. McArthur GA, Demetri GD, van OA, et al. Molecular and clinical analysis of locally advanced dermatofibrosarcoma protuberans treated with imatinib: Imatinib Target Exploration Consortium Study B2225. *J Clin Oncol.* 2005; 23(4):866–873.

37. Rubin BP, Schuetze SM, Eary JF, et al. Molecular targeting of platelet-derived growth factor B by imatinib mesylate in a patient with metastatic dermatofibrosarcoma protuberans. *J Clin Oncol.* 2002;20(17):3586–3591.
38. Ugurel S, Utikal J, Mohr P et al. Imatinib in locally advanced dermatofibromasarcoma protuberans (DFSP): a phase II trial of the Dermatologic Cooperative Oncology Group (DeCOG). *J Clin Oncol.* 2006;24:9561.
39. McArthur GA. Molecular targeting of dermatofibrosarcoma protuberans: a new approach to a surgical disease. *J Natl Compr Canc Netw.* 2007;5(5):557–562.
40. Rutkowski P, Van Glabbeke M, Rankin CJ, et al. Imatinib mesylate in advanced dermatofibrosarcoma protuberans: pooled analysis of two phase II clinical trials. *J Clin Oncol.* 2010;28(10):1772–1779.
41. Suit H, Spiro I, Mankin HJ, Efird J, Rosenberg AE. Radiation in management of patients with dermatofibrosarcoma protuberans. *J Clin Oncol.* 1996;14(8):2365–2369.
42. Ballo MT, Zagars GK, Pisters P, Pollack A. The role of radiation therapy in the management of dermatofibrosarcoma protuberans. *Int J Radiat Oncol Biol Phys.* 1998;40(4):823–827.
43. Dagan R, Morris CG, Zlotecki RA, Scarborough MT, Mendenhall WM. Radiotherapy in the treatment of dermatofibrosarcoma protuberans. *Am J Clin Oncol.* 2005;28(6):537–539.
44. Sun LM, Wang CJ, Huang CC, et al. Dermatofibrosarcoma protuberans: treatment results of 35 cases. *Radiother Oncol.* 2000;57(2):175–181.

19

ANGIOSARCOMA

AMY C. HESSEL
BRIAN A. MOORE
ERICH M. STURGIS

Introduction

Malignant vasoformative tumors are uncommon lesions in the head and neck. Batsakis et al[1] classifies malignant vascular lesions into two groups: those arising from endothelial cells (angiosarcoma and possibly Kaposi's sarcoma) and those arising from the perithelial pericyte (hemangiopericytoma). Although angiosarcoma (AS) is a rare soft tissue sarcoma that accounts for less than 0.1% of all head and neck malignancies, two-thirds arise in the skin, and approximately 50% of angiosarcomas occur in the head and neck. Other sites for angiosarcoma include the breast or chest wall, liver, and heart.[2] Because angiosarcoma is rare, treatment recommendations are based largely on single institution case series and retrospective analyses of small cohorts. A multidisciplinary approach that incorporates head and neck surgeons, radiation oncologists, medical oncologists, reconstructive surgeons, dermatologists, and pathologists (preferably with sarcoma experience) therefore is paramount to maximize treatment outcomes in cutaneous angiosarcoma of the head and neck.

Traditionally, treatment for cutaneous AS of the head and neck included radical surgical excision, often leading to both functional and cosmetic deformity. Although surgical excision remains a central component of therapy, advances in radiation therapy, chemotherapy, and reconstruction have solidified combined modality therapy to optimize disease control and survival in localized disease.[3] Unfortunately, in many cases, the propensity of AS for recurrence and metastasis continues to defy this aggressive approach. Five-year survival rarely exceeds 50%, despite multimodality therapy.[2–8] Early identification of suspicious lesions, comprehensive surgical resection of localized disease, adjuvant radiation, and appropriate use of radiation therapy and chemotherapy comprise the best chance for disease control. Investigation continues into the evolving targets and modalities for both neoadjuvant and adjuvant molecular therapy, as well as applications of traditional neoadjuvant chemotherapy to decrease tumor burden and the resultant resection volume and surgical morbidity, in cutaneous AS of the head and neck.[8–10] Radical resection with clear microscopic margins is rarely feasible, making aggressive use of neoadjuvant chemotherapy and adjuvant radiation (with or without additional agents) preferable to massive resections chasing an elusive negative margin.

Clinical Characteristics

Demographics

Cutaneous angiosarcoma of the head and neck commonly afflicts males in the sixth through eighth decades, with a mean age of 61 to 68 reported in numerous studies.[2–15] The disease is not restricted to older males, as patients as young as 15 have been reported in institutional series.[3,8] Almost all patients are Caucasian, but there are isolated reports of persons from other racial backgrounds who develop AS of the head and neck.[12,16]

Risk Factors

The cause of angiosarcoma remains unclear, although there are reported associations with chronic lymphedema and prior radiation therapy. Regardless, most cases of cutaneous AS of the head and neck arise spontaneously.[8] The linkage between lymphedema and AS is more pertinent in the extremities, particularly in the setting of chronic venous stasis, but this relationship has not been reported in the head and neck.[12] Angiosarcoma also has been described in several conditions, such as bilateral retinoblastoma, Maffucci's syndrome, neurofibromatosis, Ollier's disease, nevoid nasal cell carcinoma syndrome, and xeroderma pigmentosum, although it is not pathognomonic for any particular disorder.[17,18]

Prior radiation therapy has also been reported as a potential risk factor for cutaneous AS in several studies, but the mechanism for this association is unknown.[12,19] In a recently published, single institution experience, 25% of AS patients had received prior radiation therapy, with reported intervals from conclusion of XRT to the development of AS of 60 to 78 months.[8,18] Other potential exposure risks include polyvinyl chloride, thorium dioxide, and ultraviolet light.[3] The association between sun exposure and AS of the head and neck, although logical in light of the commonly affected demographic (an elderly Caucasian male with significant lifetime sun exposure and a history of metachronous skin cancer), is challenged by the rare presentation of a patient with concurrent AS and other nonmelanoma skin cancers.[2] Similarly, trauma has also been implicated in the development of cutaneous AS, but it is more likely that incidental trauma brings a pre-existing lesion into view.[14]

Pathogenesis

Whether spontaneous or secondary to an exposure noted previously, numerous cellular mechanisms have been theorized to go awry in the development of cutaneous AS, although the discrete molecular events leading to angiosarcoma remained undefined. The rarity of angiosarcoma forces researches to evaluate the cutaneous, soft tissue, and visceral lesions together, although there may be distinct developmental pathways.[10]

As endothelial tumors, abnormalities in angiogenesis comprise one of the prevailing theories in the pathogenesis of AS. Overexpression of subtypes of vascular endothelial growth factor (VEGF) is detected frequently, particularly VEGF-A and VEGF-C.[8,10] Conversely, loss of VEGF-2 expression has been associated with poor prognosis.[20] Animal studies suggest that spontaneous AS may be related to the tumor suppressor gene *TP53*, although more investigation is required.[2] Invasion and metastasis of AS may depend on metalloproteinases, and lesions may be associated with an inflammatory response often containing mast cells.[10] Other oncogenic pathways that have been implicated in the development of angiosarcoma include cKIT, activated AKT, p-4EBP1, and eIF4E.[8] These pathways may comprise potential targets for molecular therapeutics, although the low expression of epidermal growth factor receptor by AS renders anti-EGFR therapy of limited value in angiosarcoma.[8]

Clinical Presentation

Angiosarcoma is an insidious lesion characterized by a subtle, often asymptomatic presentation. Most lesions are described as an enlarging bruise-like macule, with the color ranging from red to blue to purple (Fig 19–1).[4] The tumor may appear as a flat plaque or a raised nodule, and it is generally soft

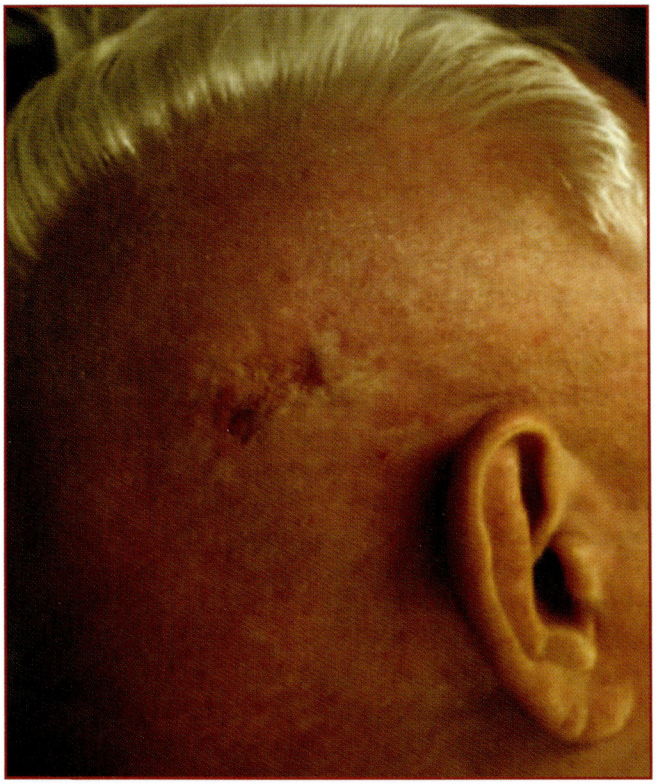

Figure 19–1. Cutaneous angiosarcoma on the scalp of a 74-year-old male. Note the innocuous appearance of the lesion as an erythematous plaque hidden in the hairline.

and compressible. Cutaneous AS enlarges by centrifugal infiltration of the surrounding skin, with pain, ulceration, and bleeding occurring in advanced lesions.[5,21] Because of the innocuous appearance of early AS, they are often misdiagnosed as bruises, other benign entities, or even more indolent nonmelanoma skin cancers; for instance, AS of the eyelid often can be mistaken for a stye.[22] Because of the subtle clinical features of AS, there often is a delay between the onset of symptoms and diagnosis that may exceed 12 months, with a median interval of just over 5 months.[5,7]

Head and neck AS typically occurs on the scalp, with at least 50% of lesions located behind the hairline.[21] Other sites include the upper face, eyelid, lower face, and neck.[3,4,5,22] The tumor often presents as a large lesion, with size distributions similar to that noted by Holden et al,[4] as most patients present with advanced disease (>10 cm in maximum dimension, versus <5 cm or 5–10 cm). Angiosarcoma exhibits a predilection to travel horizontally through the dermis and subcutaneous tissues, often with extensive subclinical spread.[17] The tumor may be surrounded by an area of induration and erythema, with an ill-defined border that blends into normal skin.[4] Tumors are not encapsulated and poorly circumscribed, often with significant subclinical spread and satellitosis.[5,8,13]

Despite the interval from onset of symptoms to diagnosis, most patients present with localized disease, although AS may be multicentric in up to 15% of cases.[3,8] Cervical adenopathy is uncommon at presentation, with reported rates of 7% to 23%.[3,8,11,13] Twenty to 45% of patients will present with metastatic disease, most commonly to the lung and bones.[8,10]

Patient Evaluation

History and Physical Examination

As with all disease processes, the evaluation of a patient with suspected cutaneous AS of the head and neck begins with a thorough history and physical, focusing on risk factors such as prior radiotherapy. Visible disease should be measured carefully, and clinical photographs often are valuable for planning or monitoring response to therapy.[6] Tumor margins, and even subclinical or multifocal disease, may be highlighted by having the patient perform a "head-tilt" maneuver, in which the head is lowered between the knees, for several seconds. This may increase the engorgement and violaceous color of the lesion during clinical assessment.[23] The parotid glands and regional lymphatics should be scrutinized for evidence of enlargement or nodularity, and cranial nerve integrity assessed.

Diagnostic Tests

Biopsy

The diagnosis of cutaneous angiosarcoma of the head and neck is predicated on a tissue exam, which is accomplished via incisional or punch biopsy.[17]

Because most lesions are quite large at presentation, excisional biopsy is unlikely to be possible. However, given the propensity for subclinical spread, "scouting" biopsies may facilitate an accurate determination of tumor extension. The differential diagnosis includes capillary hemangiomas, atypical postradiation vascular lesions, Kaposi's sarcoma, hemangiopericytomas, and epithelioid hemangioendotheliomas, among other vascular lesions.[9] Additional considerations include other high-grade sarcomas and spindle cell lesions such as malignant fibrous histiocytoma or pleomorphic/undifferentiated sarcoma, sarcomatoid-carcinoma, and desmoplastic melanoma. Misdiagnosis is common, and an experienced pathologist and/or tertiary pathology consultation is essential.

Imaging Studies

Due to the high risk of regional and distant metastases, it is imperative to attempt to determine the true extent of disease as part of the multidisciplinary evaluation. Although a contrasted computed tomography (CT) scan may provide some evidence on the extent of the primary lesion, cranial invasion, and the presence of regional metastases, magnetic resonance imaging (MRI) scanning with gadolinium contrast has demonstrated value in delineating the primary tumor extent because of its superior soft-tissue resolution. On MRI scans, angiosarcoma appears as an area of thickened scalp that enhances after the administration of contrast and is less intense than fat on T1-weighted images; AS is high intensity on T2 images, with prolonged T1 and T2 relaxation times. Invasion of the subcutaneous fat and galea may be apparent on both T2-weighted images with fat saturation and post-gadolinium T1 images, potentially revealing subclinical spread.[24] Given the high rate of metastases and the aggressive nature of cutaneous AS of the head and neck, a PET-CT may be beneficial in the initial patient evaluation to detect distant metastases. Routine chest radiography with CT scan also may be helpful to rule out pulmonary metastases.

Other Tests

There are no diagnostic blood tests for angiosarcoma, although several potential markers have recently emerged that merit further validation. Serum vascular endothelial growth factor-D (VEGF-D) and angiopoeitin-2 have been found to be elevated in angiosarcoma patients compared to healthy controls, with the highest levels of VEGF-D noted in advanced disease.[25,26] Currently, basic laboratory studies such as a complete blood count and comprehensive metabolic panel can be useful in the initial evaluation of AS patients, although no standards have been promulgated.

Histopathology

Angiosarcoma is a malignant vascular tumor whose pathogenesis remains undefined, and it is unclear whether AS arises from a malignant change in blood vessels, lymphatic vessels, or both.[13] Despite this controversy, angiosarcoma is diagnosed by its pathologic features. Grossly, there are 3 presentations: ulcerating, diffuse or superficial spreading, and nodular.[1] Macular lesions are more diffuse with an ill-defined dermal infiltrate, whereas nodular lesions are more defined. As angiosarcoma enlarges, malignant cells may occupy the entire dermis, potentially leading to ulceration.

On light microscopy, tumor cells reside primarily in the dermis with extension into the deeper tissues, generally sparing the epidermis. Tumor cells are pleomorphic, abnormal-appearing endothelial cells that may appear round, polygonal, fusiform, or epithelioid.[10] However, as the tumor enlarges, the epidermis becomes atrophic and eventually ulcerates. Tumor cells are seen at the base of the ulcer, but do not directly invade the epidermis, thus maintaining the "grenz zone."[27] Angiosarcoma exhibits three patterns of growth that facilitate histologic grading. While AS may be graded as low- or high-grade based on the predominant features, these are heterogeneous malignancies, with multiple growth patterns existing in one tumor. Although histologic grading is discussed frequently, its prognostic significance remains a matter of debate.[8,9,21]

The angiomatous pattern is a low-grade lesion characterized by the formation of dilated dermal channels with frequent anastomoses, creating a network of thin-walled neoplastic vessels that dissect dermal collagen and surround adnexal structures. Malignant endothelial cells push into the lumen of the abnormal vessels, forming "tufts" or "intraluminal buds." Vascular spaces far from the main tumor mass commonly exhibit a papillary arrangement of proliferated endothelium that represents the earliest signs of neoplastic transformation. Normal capillaries intermingle with neoplastic vessels, sparing the medium sized arteries and veins of the deep dermis.[27]

In the spindle cell pattern, tumor cells do not form recognizable vascular channels. Instead, the cells are arranged in compact bundles that invade the dermis and spare the adnexa. The spindle cells are oval or plump, and form clefts and cytoplasmic vacuoles, resulting in a loose, sponge-like network. The spindle cell variant is less circumscribed, and exhibits bundles of tumor streaming into neighboring tissues at the periphery.[27]

Undifferentiated, or high-grade, angiosarcoma consists of a solid mass of polygonal shaped cells with large nuclei, hyperchromasia, and abundant cytoplasm. Mitoses are abundant and cellular pleomorphism is prominent.[27] Malignant endothelial cells may form sheets with an epithelioid appearance—these epithelioid features have been associated with a greater risk of recurrence and metastasis in recent studies.[8] Again, the tumor cells grow through the dermis without invading the epidermis or the skin adnexa.[27]

If the diagnosis is still uncertain, electron microscopy may further characterize the lesion. As a vascular neoplasm, the endothelial cells demonstrate numerous pinocytotic vesicles and thin cytoplasmic processes projecting into the lumen. As the lesion becomes more undifferentiated, the endothelial cells are larger, polygonal, and several layers thick. The basal lamina is intact in the angiomatous patterns; however, as the tumor becomes more undifferentiated, the basal lamina frequently is absent. Pinocytotic vesicles are less common, but primitive lumen formation is still evident.[1]

Immunohistochemistry is increasingly valuable in diagnosing angiosarcoma.[10] Reflecting the endothelial origin of the lesion, the majority of tumors will stain positively for CD-31 and/or D2-40.[8] CD-31 may be the most sensitive and specific immunohistochemical marker of angiosarcoma.[28] Other stains, such as reticulin, von Willebrand factor, VEGF, factor VIII, CD-34, also may be employed to further define AS. Angiosarcoma does not stain for HHV-8, which is commonly seen in Kaposi's sarcoma, or with typical melanoma markers such as S100, HMB-45, and melanoma antigen.[10,29]

Staging

No unique staging system for cutaneous angiosarcoma of the head and neck exists. Lesions may be staged as either soft tissue sarcoma (STS) or nonmelanoma skin cancer.[17,30] Contemporary staging of nonmelanoma skin cancer is depicted elsewhere in this text (please see Chapters 7 and 8 for complete details). Because nonmelanoma skin cancer staging is devised primarily for squamous cell carcinoma, with the greatest prognostic stratification driven by nodal metastases or bone invasion (both of which are rare in AS at initial presentation), soft tissue sarcoma staging would seem more relevant. Unfortunately, soft tissue sarcoma staging is based on tumor grade (Table 19–1), limiting the prognostic import of the STS staging system because virtually all patients present with stage III or stage IV angiosarcoma.

Treatment

Managing Localized Disease

With its ability to spread throughout the dermis and known propensity for multifocal disease, the treatment of angiosarcoma remains challenging. Surgery with postoperative radiation therapy has been described as the "optimal" therapy; however, there is a growing experience with chemotherapy, including targeted molecular therapy, in either the adjuvant or neoadjuvant setting.[6,17] Because angiosarcoma is an extremely rare malignancy, patients with this disease benefit from a multidisciplinary evaluation and treatment approach, as well as participation in clinic trials whenever possible.[8,9]

Historically, outcomes for localized angiosarcoma of the head and neck are poor, with local recurrence rates in excess of 66% after either surgery or external beam radiation therapy (RT) alone.[5,13,27]

Table 19–1. Staging of Soft Tissue Sarcoma

Tumor		Nodes		Distant Metastasis	
Tx	Primary tumor cannot be assessed	**Nx**	Regional lymph nodes cannot be assessed	**M0**	No distant metastasis
T0	No evidence of primary tumor	**N0**	No regional lymph node metastasis	**M1**	Distant metastasis
T1	Tumor ≤5 cm in greatest dimension	**N1**	Regional lymph node metastasis		
T1a	Superficial tumor				
T1b	Deep tumor				
T2	Tumor >5 cm in greatest dimension				
T2a	Superficial tumor				
T2b	Deep tumor				

Stage	Tumor	Nodes	Metastasis	Grade
Stage IA	T1a	N0	M0	G1, GX
	T1b	N0	M0	G1, GX
Stage IB	T2a	N0	M0	G1, GX
	T2b	N0	M0	G1, GX
Stage IIA	T1a	N0	M0	G2, G3
	T1b	N0	M0	G2, G3
Stage IIB	T2a	N0	M0	G2
	T2b	N0	M0	G2
Stage III	T2a, T2b	N0	M0	G3
	Any T	N1	M0	Any G
Stage IV	Any T	Any N	M1	Any G

G = Grade. Grading of soft tissue sarcoma is based on three factors, with a point value assigned and higher scores indicating more aggressive disease: differentiation (1–3 points), mitotic count (1–3 points), and tumor necrosis (0–2 points). GX = tumor cannot be assessed. G1 = total score of 2–3; G2 = total score of 4–5; G3 = total score of 6 or higher.

Source: Used with permission of the American Joint Committee on Cancer (AJCC), Chcago, Illinois. The original source for this material is the AJCC Cancer Staging Manual, Seventh Edition (2010) published by Springer Science and Business Media, LLC, http://www.springer.com.

Not only did these earlier reports reflect the difficulty in achieving negative margins with surgical resection, but also the importance of radiation dosimetry in optimizing outcomes. Holden et al[4] demonstrated the limitations and potential benefits of definitive RT in a retrospective analysis. Patients who survived longer than 2 years (29% of patients) were more likely to have smaller lesions, particularly under 5 cm, and to receive higher radiation doses (54 Gy versus 44 Gy, average) than patients who did not survive longer than 2 years, supporting higher RT doses for cutaneous angiosarcoma. Multiple investigators have documented improved local control with surgery and adjuvant radiation therapy, even in the setting of positive margins or gross residual disease, compared to either modality in isolation.[2,3,6,7,11] This experience supports the contention that surgery followed by RT is the best available approach for cutaneous AS of the head and neck.[17] However, the extent of surgery remains a matter of limited debate.

Cutaneous AS of the head and neck presents a surgical challenge due to its propensity for extensive subclinical spread, rendering negative margins (R0 resection) difficult to achieve. Although surgical margins ranging from 2 to 5 cm have been recommended, positive margins are still encountered in at least 50% of cases.[6,8,21] The high rate of positive margins and the known risk of local and regional recurrence have prompted some groups to advocate an aggressive surgical approach for scalp AS, with 5-cm margins, resection of the outer table of the calvarium, parotidectomy, and free flap reconstruction of the scalp defect. This aggressive approach facilitated negative surgical margins in a limited retrospective series of patients, with 100% disease free survival (DFS) at 18 months, although the impact of adjuvant radiation therapy may minimize the impact of such radical surgery.[31]

Conversely, microscopically positive margins have repeatedly not been associated with compromised disease control and survival in patients treated with both surgery and RT in numerous studies, questioning the benefits of this philosophy in view of the added surgical morbidity from wider margins.[6,7] Although an R0 resection is an excellent surgical goal, an R1 resection, with microscopically positive margins, has not been shown to compromise local control or survival, when adjuvant RT is used.[6,8] Recently, some authors have suggested that the surgical goal should be gross tumor resection (accepting microscopically positive margins), termed an R1 resection, such that the resultant defect may be managed by primary closure or local flaps, rather than free tissue transfer, potentially hastening the recovery from surgery and initiation of wide-field postoperative RT.[6] Intraoperative frozen section assessment is of limited benefit, as its negative predictive value has been reported to be only 33.3%.[7] The inability to impact disease control by chasing frozen section margins, and the poor negative predictive value of frozen sections together suggest that Mohs micrographic surgery is contraindicated in cutaneous angiosarcoma. As discussed below, neoadjuvant chemotherapy is often advocated in an attempt to improve the chances for a complete, yet conservative, resection.

Because local recurrence still occurs more commonly than distant metastases and portends an equally poor prognosis, intensive local therapy with a gross total resection (R1 resection) or complete R0 resection (if it will not create significant morbidity) followed by wide field RT, often to 60 Gy in 30 fractions and encompassing known tumor and extremely wide margins, constitutes a standard recommendation for cutaneous AS of the head and neck (Fig 19–2).[6,7,21] Recent advances in chemotherapy (both adjuvant and neoadjuvant) and targeted molecular therapy are emerging to augment surgery and RT in an attempt to improve disease-specific survival (DSS) and overall survival (OS).

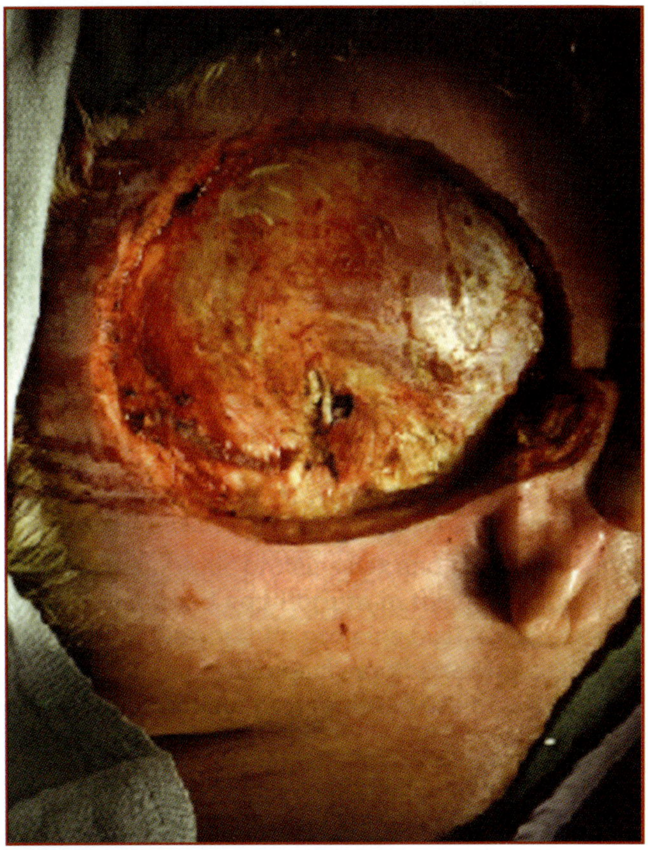

Figure 19–2. Wide local excision of the tumor depicted in Figure 19–1, with 2-cm margins in order to resect all gross disease. The defect was reconstructed with a split-thickness skin graft.

Chemotherapy

Systemic therapy constitutes the primary modality used in the treatment of disseminated disease, and there is an increasing experience with chemotherapy in the neoadjuvant setting. Unfortunately, the rarity and heterogeneity of the disease render randomized, controlled studies difficult to accomplish. Nevertheless, cutaneous angiosarcoma of the head and neck has been the object of novel applications and recent innovations in both traditional cytotoxic chemotherapy and targeted molecular therapy.

Traditionally, chemotherapy in cutaneous AS of the head and neck has been based on doxorubicin with or without ifosfamide, with brief progression-free survival (PFS) rates of less than 6 months in a minority of patients.[9,32,33] There has been recent interest in pegylated liposomal doxorubicin in advanced or metastatic AS due to the improved tissue targeting and decreased risk of cardiotoxicity.[34] Improved response rates, if not significantly different durations, have been noted with the taxanes—paclitaxel and docetaxel.[35,36] By inhibiting microtubule depolymerization and through attendant anti-angiogenic effects, the taxanes have garnered increased attention in AS and other vascular malignancies, like Kaposi's sarcoma. Some authors[35,36] hypothesize that docetaxel may even suppress lung metastases from AS, which is a common precursor to death from disease. Common toxicities of taxanes-based therapy include neutropenia and peripheral neuropathy.[36]

Adjuvant Chemotherapy

There is often a desire to add chemotherapy to the treatment plan for AS, particularly for recurrent disease. While there is no clear choice to the drugs employed, paclitaxel, doxorubicin, 5-fluorouracil, interferon alfa-2b, cyclophosphamide, cisplatin, eto - poside, mensa, and ifosfamide have all been reported.[7] Data supporting a benefit of adjuvant chemotherapy alone or concurrent to postoperative radiation therapy versus radiation alone does not exist.[6]

Neoadjuvant Chemotherapy

Given the difficulty in achieving negative margins, even with radical surgery, and the cosmetic and functional consequences of radical resection in the head and neck, there is significant interest in the use of neoadjuvant chemotherapy in AS of the head and neck to improve the chances of an R0 resection and potentially minimize postoperative morbidity. In a small series of patients with periorbital AS from a tertiary cancer center,[37] 14 of 15 patients manifest a clinical complete response to a heterogeneous mix of neoadjuvant chemotherapy, and some patients avoided radical eyelid resection. Although this approach did not translate to improved survival, it did prolong their median disease-free interval.[37]

Building on the work of Fata and colleagues[35] who demonstrated objective responses of patients to paclitaxel, other authors have employed taxane-based chemotherapy prior to surgical resection or radiation therapy with reasonable results. Neoadjuvant taxane-based chemotherapy followed by gross tumor resection of residual disease and postoperative RT constitutes the current approach to cutaneous AS of the head and neck at The University of Texas-MD Anderson Cancer Center.[6]

Managing Advanced or Disseminated Disease

The agents employed in the neoadjuvant or adjuvant setting for localized AS of the head and neck are also the main agents used for disseminated AS. Although sporadic reports of long-term survival of patients with unresectable or disseminated disease exist, virtually all such patients die.[38] Single agent docetaxel has been associated with long-term survival of over 40 months in at least one case of metastatic AS,[38] and paclitaxel has even demonstrated activity as a second-line agent after failure of pegylated doxorubicin and radiation therapy.[39] A recent Phase II clinical trial of paclitaxel in unresectable AS (ANGIOTAX) reported a median time to progression of 4 months and median overall survival of 8 months, with a toxicity profile consisting mainly of anemia and fatigue.[40]

Targeted Molecular Therapy

Given the poor prognosis and the relatively low response rate to chemotherapy, there is also keen interest in targeted molecular therapy for angiosarcoma. The monoclonal antibody imatinib inhibits tyrosine kinase proteins such as KIT and platelet-derived growth factor receptors (PDGFR). Up to 56% of cutaneous AS exhibit mutations in the c-KIT proto-oncogene, supporting a potential benefit of imatinib, and investigations are ongoing.[41] A recent phase II trial of imatinib (600 mg/day) in 185 patients with advanced or metastatic sarcoma (<10% AS) documented a response rate of 12% (2/16 AS), with a PFS of 20% at 3 months.[42]

Responses to sorafenib, a multikinase inhibitor that targets the VEGFR, PDGFR, and raf pathways, appear slightly more promising in another phase II trial, with an overall response rate of 13% but a non-progression rate of 65% at 3 months in a heterogeneous population of 147 patients with soft tissue sarcomas (27% AS).[43] Given the vascular origins of AS and the high rate of VEGF overexpression, there is obvious interest in antiangiogenic targeted therapy with bevacizumab, a monoclonal antibody targeting VEGF, used alone or in combination with other agents.[9,41] Because the AKT pathway also has been implicated in the pathogenesis of AS, there is interest in rapamycin, a potent mTOR inhibitor, in the treatment of angiosarcoma.[8,44] The use of targeted therapy in conjunction with more traditional approaches against AS constitutes an area of ongoing, intense research, and the potential for thoughtful clinical trials.[40]

Other Therapies

In addition to the approaches outlined above, a multitude of other approaches have been described in anecdotal cases of AS, including scalp perfusion with pegylated doxorubicin,[45] local injection of OK-432 and Interleukin-2,[46] and neoadjuvant bevacizumab with preoperative RT.[47] Clearly, more clinical trials and larger studies are required to define the optimum treatment for all presentations of cutaneous AS of the head and neck.

Treatment Outcomes

Despite advances in neoadjuvant chemotherapy and RT for cutaneous AS, the prognosis remains grim, with reported 5-year overall survival ranging from 10% to 53%.[2,4,6,8] Local recurrence occurs more commonly than regional or distant metastases as the first site of failure,[6,7] but the gravity of an initial local recurrence appears as poor as initial distant metastases.[6] The lung is the most common site of distant metastases, and the development of distant metastases is a common harbinger of death.[9]

Prognostic Factors

Because AS has such a poor outcome, numerous studies have attempted to identify factors that predict its prognosis. The most consistent prognostic factor for head and neck angiosarcoma is the size of the lesion. Holden et al[4] demonstrated that the smaller (<10-cm tumors) had an improved probability of survival better than the larger tumors (>10 cm) ($p < 0.001$), but the difference between 5 and 10 cm was not significant. Other authors have corroborated the association between lesion size over 10 cm and poor outcome.[2] TNM staging of soft tissue sarcomas uses 5 cm to stratify tumors, and several authors have confirmed improved locoregional control for AS under 5 cm and decreased disease-specific survival beyond this threshold.[3,8,12] A recent study reveals that increasing tumor size analyzed as a continuous variable correlates with worsened outcomes as a continuous variable.[6]

Unifocal disease or localized disease restricted to the eyelid (rather than eyelid involement by a larger facial lesion) is less likely to recur than multifocal disease.[7,22,48] Some reports document worsened prognosis in patients with a scalp primary versus other sites.[6] In addition, unlike other soft tissue sarcomas, histologic grade has not been a clear predictor of survival, although the presence of an epithelioid component or more than 3 mitoses per high powered field (HPF) may portend more aggressive disease.[2,7,8] Conversely, patients younger than 70 years at presentation, pathologic stage T1 disease, and the presence of a moderate to severe lymphocytic infiltrate may predict better survival.[7,8]

Treatment can impact prognosis in localized disease, as patients who receive a single modality (either radiation alone or surgery alone) are more likely to suffer recurrence and disease-related mortality than patients treated with surgery and radiation therapy (Fig 19–3).[6,7] As previously noted, microscopic margin status (R0 versus R1) does not appear to be associated with outcome, but residual gross disease following attempted surgical resection has been noted to worsen survival.[6–8]

Conclusions

Cutaneous angiosarcoma of the head and neck is an aggressive disease, prone to local recurrence and metastases, with reported overall survival rarely exceeding 50% at 5 years. Lesions often present insidiously as a bruise or erythematous macule, typically on the scalp, in older white males. Delays in diagnosis are common, but metastases are infrequent at presentation. After establishing the diagnosis with an incisional biopsy, multidisciplinary treatment is paramount in optimizing outcomes. Although no standard protocol exists, there is evidence that neoadjuvant chemotherapy, often with paclitaxel or docetaxel, may facilitate a gross total resection of disease. Surgery followed by wide-field radiation therapy provides the best chance for cure, although research continues into chemotherapeutics and targeted molecular agents.

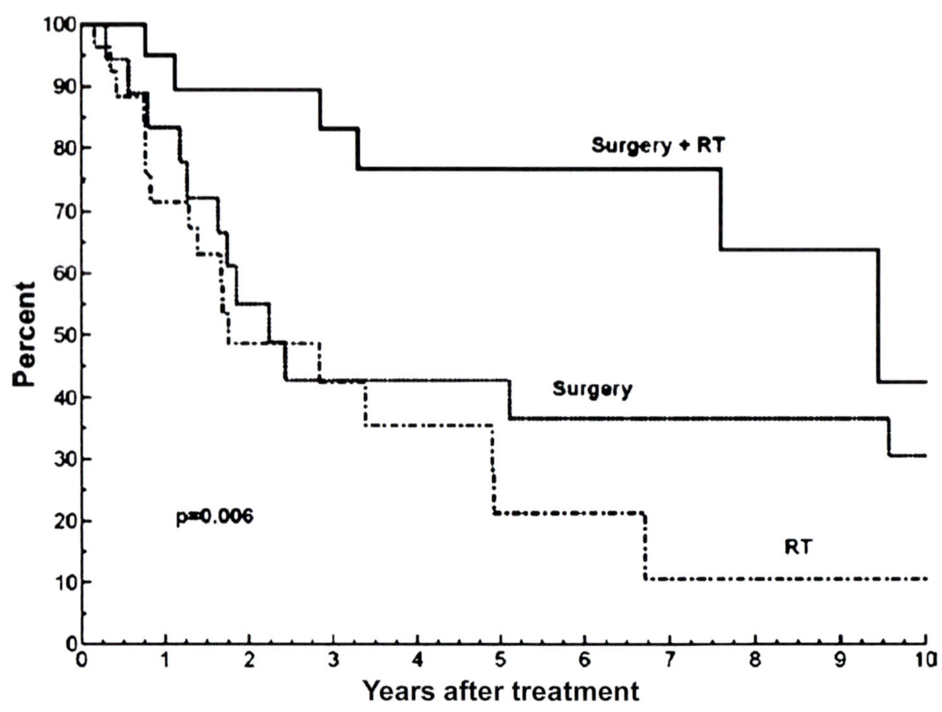

Figure 19–3. Disease-specific survival (DSS) curves based on local therapy for head and neck angiosarcoma. There is a statistically significant improvement in DSS with combined surgery and radiation therapy, versus either modality alone. Reprinted with permission from Guadagnolo BA, Zagars GK, Araujo D, et al. Outcomes after definitive treatment for cutaneous angiosarcoma of the face and scalp. *Head Neck.* 2010. Epub 19 Oct 2010.

References

1. Batsakis JG, Rice DH. The pathology of head and neck tumors: vasoformative tumors, Part 9B. *Head Neck Surg.* 1981;3:231–239.
2. Lydiatt WM, Shaha AR, Shah JP. Angiosarcoma of the head and neck. *Am J Surg.* 1994;168:451–454.
3. Mark RJ, Tran LM, Sercarz J, et al. Angiosarcoma of the head and neck—the UCLA experience 1955 through 1990. *Arch Otolarygol Head Neck Surg.* 1993;119: 973–978.
4. Holden CA, Spittle MF, Jones EW. Angiosarcoma of the face and scalp: prognosis and treatment. *Cancer.* 1987; 59:1046–1057.
5. Panje WR, Moran WJ, Bostwick DG, Kitt VV. Angiosarcoma of the head and neck: review of 11 cases. *Laryngoscope.* 1986;96:1381–1384.
6. Guadagnolo BA, Zagars GK, Araujo D, et al. Outcomes after definitive treatment for cutaneous angiosarcoma of the face and scalp. *Head Neck.* 2010;Epub 19 Oct 2010.
7. Pawlik TM, Paulino AF, Mcginn CJ, et al. Cutaneous angiosarcoma of the scalp: a multidisciplinary approach. *Cancer.* 2003;98:1716–1726.
8. Lahat G, Dhuka AR, Hallevi H, et al. Angiosarcoma: clinical and molecular insights. *Ann Surg.* 2010;251: 1098–1106.
9. Penel N, Marreaud S, Robin Y-M, Hohenberger P. Angiosarcoma: state of the art and perspectives. *Crit Rev Oncol Hematol.* 2010; Epub 3 Nov 2010.
10. Young RJ, Brown NJ, Reed MW, et al. Angiosarcoma. *Lancet Oncol.* 2010;11:983–991.
11. Morrison WH, Byers RM, Garden AS, et al. Cutaneous angiosarcoma of the head and neck—a therapeutic dilemma. *Cancer.* 1995;76: 319–327.
12. Maddox JC, Evans HL. Angiosarcoma of skin and soft tissue: a study of forty-four cases. *Cancer.* 1981;48: 1907–1921.
13. Hodgkinson DJ, Soule EH, Woods JE. Cutaneous angiosarcoma of the head and neck. *Cancer.* 1979;44:1106–1113.
14. Cocharan JH, Fee WE. Angiosarcoma of the head and neck. *Otolaryngol Head Neck Surg.* 1979;87:409–416.
15. Cooper PH. Angiosarcomas of the skin. *Semin Diagn Pathol.* 1987;4:2–17.
16. Rajinikanth J, Gaikwad P, Raj JP, et al. Angiosarcoma of the scalp. *Otolaryngol Head Neck Surg.* 2008;138:255–256.
17. Mendenhall WM, Mendenhall CM, Werning JW, et al. Cutaneous angiosarcoma. *Am J Clin Oncol.* 2006;29: 524–528.
18. Penel N, Robin Y-M, Mallet Y et al. Association head and neck angiosarcoma and nevoid basal cell carcinoma syndrome (Gorlin syndrome). *Oral Oncol.* 2005;41:289–291.
19. Gagnon PJ, Galderisi C, Page BR, Holland JM. Angiosarcoma developing after curative induction chemotherapy and radiotherapy for locally advanced squamous cell carcinoma of the head and neck. *Head Neck.* 2009;31:829–832.
20. Itakura E, Yamamoto H, Oda Y, Tsuneyoshi M. Detection and characterization of vascular endothelial growth factors and their receptors in a series of angiosarcomas. *J Surg Oncol.* 2008;97:74–81.
21. Kohler HF, Neves RI, Brechtbuhl ER, et al. Cutaneous angiosarcoma of the head and neck: report of 23 cases from a single institution. *Otolaryngol Head Neck Surg.* 2008;139:519–524.
22. Papalas JA, Manavi CK, Woodward JA, et al. Angiosarcoma of the eyelid: a clinicopathologic comparison between isolated unilateral tumors and tumors demonstrating extrapalpebral involvement. *Am J Dermatopathol.* 2010;32:694–699.
23. Asgari MM, Cockerell CJ, Weitzul S. The head-tilt maneuver: a clinical aid in recognizing head and neck angiosarcoma. *Arch Dermatol.* 2007;143:75–77.
24. Isoda H, Imai M, Inagawa S, et al. Magnetic resonance imaging findings of angiosarcoma of the scalp. *J Comput Assist Tomogr.* 2005;29:858–862.
25. Amo Y, Masuzawa M, Hamada Y, et al. Serum concentrations of vascular endothelial growth factor-D in angiosarcoma patients. *Br J Dermatol.* 2004;150:160–161.
26. Amo Y, Masuzawa M, Hamada Y, et al. Observations on angiopoietin 2 in patients with angiosarcoma. *Br J Dermatol.* 2004;150:1028–1029.
27. Rosai J, Sumner HW, Kostianovsky M, Perez-Mesa C. Angiosarcoma of the skin—a clinicopathologic and fine structural study. *Hum Pathol.* 1979;7:83–108.
28. Yang XJ, Zheng JW, Zhou Q, et al. Angiosarcomas of the head and neck: a clinico-immunohistochemical study of 8 consecutive patients. *Int J Oral Maxillofac Surg.* 2010;39: 568–572.
29. Schmid H, Zietz C. Human herpes virus 8 and angiosarcoma: analysis of 40 cases and review of the literature. *Pathology.* 2005;37:284–287.
30. Edge SB, Carducci M, Byrd DR, eds. *AJCC Cancer Staging Manual.* 7th ed. New York, NY: Springer-Verlag; 2009.
31. Lim SY, Pyon JK, Mun GH, et al. Surgical treatment of angiosarcoma of the scalp with superficial parotidectomy. *Ann Plast Surg.* 2010;64:180–182.
32. Fury MG, Antonescu CR, Van Zee KJ, et al. A 14-year retrospective review of angiosarcoma: clinical characteristics, prognostic factors, and treatment outcomes with surgery and chemotherapy. *Cancer J.* 2005;11:241–247.
33. Fayette J, Martin E, Piperno-Neumann S, et al. Angiosarcomas, a heterogeneous group of sarcomas with specific behavior depending on primary site: a retrospective study of 161 cases. *Ann Oncol.* 2007;18:2030–2036.
34. Holloway CL, Turner AR, Dundas GS. Cutaneous angiosarcoma of the scalp: a case report of sustained complete response following liposomal doxorubicin and radiation therapy. *Sarcoma.* 2005;9:29–31.
35. Fata F, O'Reilly E, Ilson D, et al. Paclitaxel in the treatment of patients with angiosarcoma of the scalp or face. *Cancer.* 1999;86:2034–2037.

36. Nagano T, Yamada Y, Ikeda T, et al. Docetaxel: a therapeutic option in the treatment of cutaneous angiosarcoma—report of 9 patients. *Cancer.* 2007;110:648–651.
37. DeMartelaere SL, Roberts D, Burgess M, et al. Neoadjuvant chemotherapy-specific and overall treatment outcomes in patients with cutaneous angiosarcoma of the face with periorbital involvement. *Head Neck.* 2008;30:639–646.
38. Nakamura Y, Nakamura Y, Hori E, et al. Complete long-term response of angiosarcoma of the scalp with cervical lymph node metastases treated with a combination of weekly and monthly docetaxel. *Br J Dermatol.* 2010;163:1357–1358.
39. Hofmann UB, Wobser M, Kneitz H, et al. Major response to paclitaxel combined with irradiation as second-line therapy in metastatic angiosarcoma of the face and scalp. *Br J Dermatol.* 2008;160:456–458.
40. Penel N, Bui BN, Bay JO, et al. Phase II trial of weekly paclitaxel for unresectable angiosarcoma: the ANGIOTAX study. *J Clin Oncol.* 2008;26:5269–5274.
41. Gonzalez MJ, Koehler MM, Satter EK. Angiosarcoma of the scalp : a case report and review of the current and novel therapeutic regimens. *Derm Surg.* 2009;35:679–684.
42. Chugh R, Wathen JK, Maki RG, et al. Phase II multicenter trial of imatinib in 10 histologic subtypes of sarcoma using a Bayesian hierarchical statistical model. *J Clin Oncol.* 2009;27:3148–3153.
43. Maki RG, D'Adamo DR, Keohan ML, et al. Phase II study of sorafenib in patients with recurrent or metastatic sarcomas. *J Clin Oncol.* 2009;27:3133–3140.
44. Bundscherer A, Vogt T, Kohl G, et al. Antiproliferative effects of rapamycin and celecoxib in angiosarcoma cell lines. *Anticancer Res.* 2010;30:4017–4023.
45. Bong AB, Bonnekoh B, Schon MP, et al. Treatment of scalp angiosarcoma by controlled perfusion of A. carotis externa with pegylated liposomal doxorubicin and intralesional application of pegylated interferon-alpha. *J Am Acad Dermatol.* 2005;52(2 suppl 1):20–23.
46. Miura H, Inui S, Sakai H, et al. Angiosarcoma of the scalp treated with OK-432 and rIL-2. *Int J Dermatol.* 2002;41:286–288.
47. Koontz BF, Miles EF, Rubio MAD, et al. Preoperative radiotherapy and bevacizumab for angiosarcoma of the head and neck: two case studies. *Head Neck.* 2008;2:262–266.
48. Espat NS, Lewis JJ, Woodruff JM, et al. Confirmed angiosarcoma: prognostic factors and outcome in 50 prospectively followed patients. *Sarcoma.* 2000;4:173–177.

20

MELANOMA: EPIDEMIOLOGY, STAGING, AND PROGNOSIS

AUDREY B. ERMAN
CAROL R. BRADFORD

Introduction

Melanoma has been researched extensively in the past few decades, with minimal advances in treatment and survival. Most survival gains have been in identifying earlier staged tumors for which a surgical cure is still attainable, rather than advances in treatment for metastatic disease.

Head and neck melanoma differs from melanoma at other sites in risk factor assessment, age of patient at diagnosis, ultraviolet radiation exposure history, and prognosis, leading some to believe that head and neck melanoma should be considered a separate entity. The narrow anatomic field and complex lymphatic system of the head and neck add further complexity to the natural history and treatment of the disease.

This chapter reviews the incidence and mortality, risk factors, and current American Joint Committee on Cancer (AJCC) staging system for cutaneous melanoma as it pertains to the head and neck.

Incidence

The incidence of cutaneous melanoma has been consistently rising in countries with Caucasian populations by 3% to 7% annually, and is the most rapidly increasing cancer in white populations[1–3]. Australia and New Zealand have the highest melanoma rates in the world, where incidence rates are up to 60 cases per 100,000 population.[4]

In the United States, cutaneous melanoma is currently the fifth most common cancer in men and the sixth in women.[5] The lifetime risk of developing invasive melanoma has been steadily increasing.[6] One in 1,500 individuals born in 1935 will develop malignant melanoma, and individuals born in 2010 have a lifetime probability of developing melanoma that is 1 in 39 for men and 1 in 58 for women.[5] Trends in overall cancer rates have declined in the United States, but melanoma remains one of the few that is increasing in frequency.[5] In recent years, however, this trend is stabilizing in some countries.[7–9] The cause for this is unknown, although the plateau may be due to primary prevention efforts.

Melanoma incidence is dependent on race, age, and gender. Caucasians have the highest rates globally, and in the United States, men have higher rates than women.[7,10] Incidence rises with age, and at a faster rate in men. In the United States, women have a slightly higher risk prior to the age of 40, after which men have a higher incidence. For men, the risk rises dramatically during life, eclipsing women at age 40 and doubling that of women by age 85.[11]

Reasons for the increasing incidence of melanoma are unclear. Intrinsic changes in attitudes toward tanning and extrinsic changes in the environment may cause increased ultraviolet (UV) exposure. Climate change and ozone depletion have been implicated in rising rates. Projected increases in melanoma for Scandinavian regions estimated a 10% ozone depletion associated with a 19% increase in melanoma in men and a 32% increase in melanoma in women.[12] Other models suggest that, without control measures for ozone depletion, the United States can expect 223 million more cases of skin cancer due to ozone depletion alone by 2030.[13] This, in addition to changing behavioral patterns relating to sun exposure and indoor tanning, may result in considerable increases in environmental UV radiation exposure.[14,15]

Others postulate that the observed increase in incidence is not a biological change, but rather is due to improved screening and diagnosis of the disease.[16,17] Increased screening for melanoma may lead to the detection of thinner, less aggressive lesions.[17] One analysis in the United States found that melanoma from all stages increased from 1988 to 1997, although thin lesions accounted for the greatest number of new cases.[7] A more recent study revealed an increasing incidence of melanoma of all thicknesses among all socioeconomic levels. Furthermore, the greatest increase in incidence was among those of the lowest socioeconomic status, who theoretically have the lowest access to screening services. The study suggests that the increase of melanoma screening is not the sole factor responsible for increasing incidence.[18]

Increasing numbers of skin biopsies and variability in histologic interpretation may falsely elevate incidence rates.[19] Levell[20] argues the dramatic increase is due to "diagnostic drift," in which lesions previously described as benign melanocytic nevi are reclassified as early stage I melanoma, although these findings do not explain increases in mortality.[2]

Mortality

Melanoma is the most deadly of all skin cancers. Although it comprises only 4% of all cutaneous malignancies, it is responsible for over 70% of deaths related to skin cancer.[5,10] Despite public health campaigns aimed at early detection and screening programs, the mortality rate of melanoma has continued to rise over the last few decades.[1] Peaking in the early 1990s, melanoma mortality has recently leveled off in some European countries, especially in young adults.[21] This may be attributable to early detection of thinner melanomas with a chance at surgical cure.[22] Conversely, mortality rates in the elderly, especially men, have remained stable.[3]

Risk Factors for Cutaneous Melanoma

A variety of environmental and genetic factors determine the risk of developing malignant melanoma, including the amount of sun exposure and the patient's inherent susceptibility to UV radiation. Identifying high-risk individuals is important in tailoring public health efforts. Risk factors are summarized in Table 20–1.

Table 20–1. Risk Factors for Cutaneous Melanoma

Risk Factors for Melanoma
Genetic characteristics
Susceptibility genes: CDKN2A,[27] CDK4,[85] MC1R[86]
Family history: 1st degree relative with melanoma,[87] atypical mole syndrome
Previous personal history of melanoma
Phenotypic characteristics
Fair skin with inability to tan[88]
Light or blue eyes[88]
Red or blond hair[34]
Nevi
Giant congenital nevus: >5% of total body surface area[89]
Common nevi: >100 (any size)[37,90]
More than 3 dysplastic nevi[88]
Environmental factors
Solar UV radiation[43]
Artificial UV radiation (tanning beds)[91]

Genetic Factors

Familial Atypical Mole—Melanoma Syndrome

Approximately 5% of all cutaneous melanomas arise in patients with a family history of melanoma, indicating a strong genetic tendency for some individuals to develop this deadly disease. The nomenclature has evolved over the years to accurately describe families with a higher than normal incidence of melanoma. First described by Clark[23] as the "B-K mole syndrome," it is now referred to as familial atypical mole-melanoma syndrome (FAM-M), or simply the dysplastic nevus or atypical mole syndrome.[23,24] The syndrome is inherited in an autosomal dominant fashion, and family members have multiple large moles that may vary in size and color. Patients have a lifetime cumulative incidence of melanoma of nearly 100%.[25] The most common mutation associated with familial melanoma occurs in CDKN2A, or p16, an important regulator of cell cycle entry.[26] Several other chromosomal mutations have been identified in families prone to melanoma, although most families with cutaneous melanoma remain without a specific genetic diagnosis.[27]

Xeroderma Pigmentosa

Xeroderma pigmentosa (XP) is an autosomal recessive disease in which fibroblasts have a limited ability to repair DNA damaged by ultraviolet radiation.[28] Patients with XP develop multiple cutaneous malignancies including melanoma, basal cell carcinoma, and squamous cell carcinoma. Many patients are diagnosed with their first skin cancer before adolescence, and die from the disease at a young age.[29]

Pigment Characteristics and Nevi

A patient's inherent susceptibility to the sun may be more important than sun exposure and is correlated with endogenous pigment. Melanin is a highly conjugated molecule produced by melanosomes in the basal layer of the dermis. Variation in skin color is based on the distribution of melanin within keratinocytes rather than the absolute number of melanosomes.[30] Melanin acts as an endogenous sunscreen, located in supranuclear "caps" over surrounding keratinocytes.[31] Pigmentary characteristics of the skin have long been associated with melanoma risk, with light skin color and high freckle density as significant risk factors.[32] Studying multiethnic populations in a single environment, melanoma rates are 5- to 10-fold higher in non-Hispanic whites than in Hispanic whites, and Hispanic whites have twice the risk as blacks.[33] Hair and eye color are also noted as independent risk factors and are considered markers for skin phenotypes.[34,35]

Benign appearing nevi are sometimes precursor lesions to malignant melanoma, although the risk is low. The lifetime risk of transformation of any selected mole into melanoma is 0.03% for men and 0.009% for women.[36] More often, benign nevi are used as a surrogate marker for UV-induced skin damage.

Although the risk of transformation of benign appearing nevi is low, the absolute number of benign appearing nevi is an important predictive factor in determining melanoma risk. Patients with 50 to 100 nevi are at increased risk of developing melanoma, with a relative risk of 5 to 17.[37] Interestingly, an increased number of nevi may not be a reliable risk factor in the development of head and neck melanoma. A pooled analysis of case-control studies showed increasing numbers of nevi associated with trunk and extremity melanoma but not melanoma of the head and neck.[38]

Differing sun exposure patterns and association with nevi have prompted some to consider head and neck melanoma as a separate entity. Whiteman hypothesized two divergent pathways to melanoma.[39] Individuals with large numbers of nevi may require less UV radiation to induce carcinogenesis in melanocytes, and will develop melanomas on less sun-exposed sites like the trunk or legs. Individuals without large numbers of nevi are hypothesized to require more UV-induced injury before developing melanoma, and will do so only on sun-exposed sites such as the head and neck. Pigmentary characteristics, such as skin, hair, or eye color, do not differ among different body sites, further supporting this hypothesis.[39,40]

UV Exposure

The evidence that UV radiation causes cutaneous malignant melanoma in humans is based on a substantial body of epidemiologic evidence, and is strongly supported by animal models of UV radiation induced melanoma.[33,41] The dose-response curve, however, remains unclear.

Studying populations living at different latitudes gives information on the effect of cumulative doses of UV radiation. The incidence of melanoma is highest in equatorial areas, decreasing proportionately with distance from the equator.[42] Using latitude as a surrogate marker for ambient solar radiation, studies consistently show increased rates of melanoma across a latitude gradient among different populations.[33] Exposure early in life is particularly important, demonstrated by migration studies and the incidence of melanoma in Australia. In those who migrated to Australia before the age of 10, skin cancer rates equaled those of native Australians. Immigration after the age of 10 reduced the incidence by threefold.[33]

In addition to the cumulative dose of UV radiation, the pattern of exposure also is important. Both occupational (chronic) and recreational (intense or intermittent) sun exposure are important factors in melanoma development. Elwood et al[43] systematically reviewed the major case-controlled studies evaluating the incidence of melanoma and sun exposure. A history of multiple severe sunburns was a strong predictor of melanoma risk, especially on parts of the body with only sporadic sun exposure such as the legs or trunk.[44] This study also revealed a small but significant reduction in risk of melanoma associated with high amounts of occupational exposure, although this may be confounded by high intermittent sun exposure in the "low" occupational group. Chang et al[45] found occupational exposure to be positively associated with the development of head and neck melanoma, especially at low latitudes, but had no effect on melanoma at other sites.

Prevention

Sunscreen use has been shown to reduce the risk of nonmelanoma skin cancers; some estimate regular sunscreen use will decrease the risk by 78%.[46] However, the relationship between sunscreen use and melanoma is less clear. Several reports indicate that there was no protection from melanoma with sunscreen use and, in fact, sunscreen use may be positively associated with melanoma development as an independent risk factor.[47,48] Unfortunately, these studies are challenging to conduct, as patients tend to be poor historians when reporting prior sunscreen use.[49] Furthermore, these studies were conducted with earlier sunscreens with low SPF and no UVA coverage.[47] A recent meta-analysis examined 18 case-control studies and found no good evidence for increased risk of melanoma with use of sunscreen, citing failure of many studies to control for "bias by indication," in that sunscreen users are inherently more sun sensitive.[50]

Studies also are confounded by behavioral factors promoted by sunscreen use. The phenomenon of the "sunscreen abuser" has recently been described in the literature, referring to individuals reapplying sunscreen to increase total time spent in the sun.[51] Sunscreen prevents erythematous change from UVB rays, and by delaying sunburn, the "sunscreen abuser" has a false sense of security that UV radiation is not damaging the skin. Autier proposes the use of a personal UV dosimeter as a more accurate measure of UV exposure.[51]

Although the relationship between melanoma and sunscreen use remains unclear, Gallagher[52] explored the relationship between sunscreen use and new nevi development in school-age children. A randomized controlled trial showed that regular use of sunscreen during the summer months decreased the appearance of new nevi, which has been associated with increased risk for developing melanoma.

Sunscreen use is but one way to decrease solar radiation, and the American Academy of Dermatology encourages patients to practice overall reduction in UV exposure. The AAD currently recommends multiple strategies for skin cancer prevention: general sun protection including protective clothing, regular use of broad-spectrum high sun protection factor (SPF) sunscreen, and the avoidance of midday sun and intentional sunbathing. Active prevention campaigns and public response may be resulting in a decreased incidence of melanoma in some populations.[53]

Staging and Prognosis

Accurate staging systems are crucial in anticipating prognosis, counseling patients, and designing clinical trials. The AJCC analyzes large databases of patients presenting with newly diagnosed cutaneous melanoma, allowing for correlation of clinical and pathologic features with long-term outcomes. As we learn more about the natural history of melanoma, staging systems are continually updated to reflect current diagnostic trends.

The most recent version of the AJCC staging system was published in October 2009, an update from the previous system in 2001. [54,55] The new staging system is based off of a markedly expanded data set (from 17,600 patients in 2001 to 30,946 in 2009) from patients treated at 17 centers. Mitotic rate of the primary tumor proved to be a powerful indicator of survival, replacing level of invasion for defining T1b melanoma. Increasing acceptance and use of sentinel lymph node biopsy warranted verification of previous criteria for stage III disease. Lastly, a five-fold increase in patients with stage IV disease provided information about the prognostic value of serum lactate dehydrogenase (LDH) level as an independent marker. An overview of the current staging system may be found in Table 20–2.

AJCC System

The AJCC divides prognostic groups into four stages and is based on evaluations of the primary tumor (T), involvement of regional lymph nodes (N), and distant metastases (M). Staging for melanoma mirrors staging for other types of cancers: patients with localized disease are classified as stage I or II, involvement of regional lymph nodes are stage III, and distant metastatic disease is stage IV.

Stages I and II: Localized Melanoma

More than 27,000 patients with localized melanoma are included in the current staging system. Primary tumor thickness, the presence of ulceration, and the primary tumor mitotic rate are the most powerful predictors of survival in localized melanoma. Tumor thickness was originally described by Breslow[56] and remains an important prognostic factor in localized melanoma. Modified now as even integers of 1.0, 2.0, and 4.0 mm in depth, the T category thresholds remain unchanged from the previous staging system.[55,56]

Tumor ulceration is defined as the histologic absence of intact epithelium over the melanoma.

Table 20–2. AJCC 2009 TNM and Staging Classification

Tumor Classification (T)		
T	**Tumor Thickness (mm)**	**Ulceration or Mitoses**
Tis	Melanoma in situ	n/a
T1	≤1.00	a: without ulceration and mitoses <1/mm^2 b: with ulceration or mitoses ≥1/mm^2
T2	1.01–2.00	a: without ulceration b: with ulceration
T3	2.01–4.00	a: without ulceration b: with ulceration
T4	>4.00	a: without ulceration b: with ulceration

continues

Table 20–2. *continued*

Node Classification (N)		
N	**Number of Metastatic Nodes**	**Nodal Metastatic Burden**
N0	0	n/a
N1	1	a: micrometastasis b: macrometastasis
N2	2–3	a: micrometastasis b: macrometastasis c: In transit metastases/satellites without metastatic nodes
N3	4+, or matted nodes, or in transit metastases/satellites with metastatic nodes	

Metastatic Classification (M)		
M	**Site**	**Serum LDH**
M0	No distant metastases	n/a
$M1_a$	Distant skin, subcutaneous, or nodal metastases	normal
$M1_b$	Lung metastases	normal
$M1_c$	All other visceral metastases	normal
	Any distant metastsis	elevated

Staging for Cutaneous Melanoma							
	Clinical Staging				**Pathologic Staging**		
	T	**N**	**M**		**T**	**N**	**M**
0	Tis	N0	M0	0	Tis	N0	M0
IA	T1a	N0	M0	IA	T1a	N0	M0
IB	T1b, T2a	N0	M0	IB	T1b, T2a	N0	M0
IIA	T2b, T3a	N0	M0	IIA	T2b, T3a	N0	M0
IIB	T3b, T4a	N0	M0	IIB	T3b, T4a	N0	M0
IIC	T4b	N0	M0	IIC	T4b	N0	M0
III	Any T	N> N0	M0	IIIA	T1-4a	N1a, N2a	M0
				IIIB	T1-4b	N1a, N2a	M0
					T1-4a	N1b, N2b, N2c	M0
				IIIC	T1-4b	N1b, N2b, N2c	M0
					Any T	N3	M0
IV	Any T	Any N	M1	IV	Any T	Any N	M1

Source: Used with the permission of the American Joint Committee on Cancer (AJCC), Chicago, Illinois. The original source for this material is the AJCC Cancer Staging Manual, Seventh Edition (2010) published by Springer Science and Business Media LLC, www.springer.com..

Ulceration remains an indicator of a biologically aggressive tumor, and is considered one of the most reproducible histologic findings.[57,58] An ulcerative lesion has similar survival rates as nonulcerated lesions of the next highest T category and is staged accordingly. Primary tumor ulceration has also been shown to retain its prognostic value in patients with lymphatic involvement.[59]

A growing body of evidence points to mitotic rate as an important prognostic feature, prompting evaluation by the AJCC for inclusion in the current staging system.[60–62] A multifactorial analysis of 10,233 patients with stage I or II melanoma identified mitotic rate of the primary tumor as the second most powerful predictor of survival, after tumor thickness.[54] In fact, after including mitotic rate and ulceration in evaluation of T1 tumors, level of invasion was no longer statistically significant in predicting survival. Mitotic rate now replaces level of invasion in defining T1a and T1b categories, except in rare cases when mitotic rate is unavailable. First described by Clark in 1969,[63] the tumor's level of invasion has played an important role in melanoma risk stratification. The inclusion of mitotic rate in statistical analyses effectively antiquates Clark's levels of invasion, after 40 years of a prominent role in melanoma staging.[54,63]

Stage III: Regional Metastatic Melanoma

Sentinel lymph node biopsy has become standard in staging the regional nodal basin in patients with occult metastasis. Since its introduction by Morton in 1992,[64] it has been met with controversy, namely that immediate lymphadenectomy may not offer patients a significant overall survival benefit. Discourse has been especially loud regarding its use in the head and neck, where complex lymphatic drainage patterns and difficult anatomy are often cited as barriers.[65,66] Despite some dispute, there is increasing agreement that sentinel lymph node biopsy accurately stages regional nodal basins at risk for metastases, and identifies patients who may benefit from regional lymphadenectomy. In contrast to previous staging systems, the majority of patients now included as stage III were identified as having micrometastasis in a sentinel lymph node. The AJCC Melanoma Staging Committee sought to reevaluate if the stage III inclusion criteria remained appropriate in this setting.

The most predictive independent factors for survival of patients with stage III disease included the number of tumor-bearing nodes, tumor burden, and presence or absence of primary tumor ulceration.[54] These are unchanged from staging guidelines in 2001.[55] Patients with intralymphatic metastasis continue to have prognoses similar to those with frank nodal metastasis, and are included in stage III disease. Five-year survival rates vary widely, from 70% for patients with a thin melanoma with micrometastasis to one lymph node to 39% for patients with four or more involved lymph nodes. Patients identified with occult regional metastasis may have a survival benefit with immediate lymphadenectomy.[67]

Metastatic disease to a regional node is the single most important prognostic indicator in early-stage melanoma, as both the primary predictor of disease recurrence and melanoma-specific death.[59,67] Given the drastic prognostic implications, accurate histologic staging of the sentinel lymph node is of paramount importance. Immunohistochemical (IHC) markers differ in sensitivity and specificity, and their use varies widely across institutions.[68] To define a positive specimen based on IHC alone, the AJCC Melanoma Staging Committee recommends at least one melanoma-associated marker in the presence of other malignant morphologic features.[54]

Patients with a positive sentinel lymph node will then undergo completion lymphadenectomy. Multiple studies have demonstrated considerably decreased prognosis in patients with additional positive nonsentinel lymph nodes.[69–71] Prognostic implications of the number of involved lymph nodes were originally introduced in the 2001 AJCC revision, replacing size of lymph nodes as a predictor of mortality.

Stage IV: Distant Metastatic Melanoma

The site of distant metastases and the serum levels of LDH define the three categories of stage IV disease. Patients with metastasis in the skin, subcutaneous tissue, or distant lymph nodes have a one-year survival rate of 62% and are categorized as M1a. Patients with lung metastasis are categorized as M1b with a one-year survival rate of 53%. Distant metastasis to any other visceral organ is classified as M1c and has a dismal prognosis of 33% survival rate at one year.[54]

Significantly increased patient numbers with stage IV disease made it possible to recognize elevated serum LDH as an independent and significant predictor of survival. Serum LDH should be measured at the first sign of distant metastatic disease and, if elevated, delineates patients to the M1c category, regardless of metastatic site.

Other Prognostic Indicators

Other prognostic factors have been identified as independent predictors of outcome, but are not included in the current staging system. Older age confers a poorer prognosis for melanoma survival. Although older patients present with thicker primary tumors, the negative impact remains even after correcting for tumor thickness.[59] Male sex has also been recognized as an independent risk for worse overall survival in some studies, but not others.[59,72]

Significantly, melanomas of the head and neck have a worse overall survival than those arising on the extremeties.[59,60,73] This is true for both patients with and without regional metastasis, although the site of the tumor was less important than other staging criteria.[59] Head and neck cutaneous melanoma also has a high local recurrence rate, possibly due to the surgeon's reluctance to violate critical structures in a narrow anatomic field.[74,75]

Gene expression profiling holds much promise for development of novel prognostic indicators. Current research suggests overexpression of the NCOA3 gene and osteopontin as useful markers for involvement of the sentinel lymph node.[76,77] Future analysis of gene expression in tissue and serum samples may identify further prognostic indicators as we continue to improve our understanding of melanoma at a molecular level.

Approach to Staging Patients with Newly Diagnosed Melanoma

To accurately stage the primary tumor, patients with newly diagnosed melanoma should undergo complete excisional biopsy of the melanoma with narrow margins.[78] Pathologic examination will determine tumor depth, mitotic rate, and the presence of ulceration. Large lesions may warrant an incisional biopsy, though sampling error may affect staging. Shave biopsies are discouraged, as they obfuscate tumor thickness evaluation.[79]

In patients with clinically negative lymph nodes, sentinel lymph node biopsy should be recommended for T2-T4 melanomas.[54] Sentinel lymph node biopsy also may be considered in patients with melanoma less than 1 mm in thickness but with worrisome pathologic findings such as ulceration, extensive regression, or high mitotic rate.[80]

Most patients present without symptoms of distant metastasis. For localized melanoma, no routine screening tests for metastatic disease are required, though the clinician may order specific tests based on patient history and physical exam.

Imaging is also optional for patients with occult nodal metastasis after a positive sentinel lymph node biopsy, although this may become important as a baseline for staging. Patients with clinically evident stage III disease with nodal or intralymphatic metastasis are at significant risk for distant metastasis. Fine needle aspiration of the node in question can confirm regional spread.[81] A chest x-ray and serum LDH should be ordered for all patients with macrometastatic regional disease. Further testing such as a computed tomography (CT) or magnetic resonance imaging (MRI) scan may be clinically warranted if patients have specific symptoms.

All patients with stage IV disease need evaluation for systemic disease to guide palliative treatment therapies. Further clinical guidelines for staging newly diagnosed melanoma are maintained by the National Comprehensive Cancer Network, and can be found at http://www.nccn.org.[82] A brief algorithm based on our institution's staging practice may be found in Table 20–3.[80]

Unknown Primary Melanoma

Patients presenting with nodal disease in the absence of a primary tumor may be assumed to have regional metastatic disease. Local metastases to the skin or subcutaneous tissues should also be considered as

Table 20–3. University of Michigan Guidelines for Initial Head and Neck Melanoma Evaluation

Stage	Evaluation
Stage 0	History and physical examination, no other tests
Stage I	History and physical examination, consider SLNB for patients with ulceration, high mitotic rate, or other aggressive pathologic features
Stage I–II	History and physical examination, SLNB, CXR, and LDH optional
Stage III	History and physical examination, FNA neck mass, CXR, LDH, consider other clinically relevant imaging studies
Stage IV	History and physical examination, CXR, LDH, consider head, chest, abdomen, pelvis CT/MRI if symptomatic

SLNB Sentinel lymph node biopsy; LDH, lactate dehydrogenase; CXR, chest radiograph; FNA, fine needle aspiration; CT, computed tomography; MRI, magnetic resonance imaging.

Source: Adapted from Johnson TM, Bradford CR, Gruber SB, et al: Staging workup, sentinel node biopsy, and follow-up tests for melanoma: update of current concepts. *Arch Dermatol.* 2004;140:107–113.

regional stage III disease. Survival of patients is similar to or slightly better compared to those with known primary tumors of the same stage.[83,84]

Conclusion

Head and neck melanoma presents a unique challenge because of the complex lymphatic drainage and a narrow anatomic field. Patients present with a distinct set of risk factors from those with melanoma of the trunk and extremities. Regardless of site, melanoma is considered a preventable disease, and the vast difference in survival between early melanoma and advanced disease underscores the importance of early detection by physicians and patients. Aggressive public health efforts aimed at primary prevention and early detection have already slowed the incidence in some countries.[7,9] Despite extensive clinical and biologic research, the mortality from melanoma has not improved. Adequate staging will remain important in counseling patients and designing future clinical trials to further elucidate better treatment plans.

References

1. Geller AC, Miller DR, Annas GD, et al. Melanoma incidence and mortality among US whites, 1969–1999. *JAMA.* 2002;288(14):1719–1720.
2. de Vries E, Bray FI, Coebergh JW, et al. Changing epidemiology of malignant cutaneous melanoma in Europe 1953–1997: rising trends in incidence and mortality but recent stabilizations in western Europe and decreases in Scandinavia. *Int J Cancer.* 2003;107(1): 119–126.
3. Garbe C, Leiter U. Melanoma epidemiology and trends. *Clin Dermatol.* 2009;27(1):3–9.
4. MacLennan R, Green AC, McLeod GR, et al. Increasing incidence of cutaneous melanoma in Queensland, Australia. *J Natl Cancer Inst.* 1992;84(18):1427–1432.
5. Jemal A, Siegel R, Ward E, et al. Cancer statistics, 2009. *CA Cancer J Clin.* 2009;59(4):225–249.
6. Rigel DS, Carucci JA. Malignant melanoma: prevention, early detection, and treatment in the 21st century. *CA Cancer J Clin.* 2000;50(4):215–236; quiz 237–240.
7. Jemal A, Devesa SS, Hartge P, et al. Recent trends in cutaneous melanoma incidence among whites in the United States. *J Natl Cancer Inst.* 2001;93(9):678–683.
8. Dennis LK. Analysis of the melanoma epidemic, both apparent and real: data from the 1973 through 1994 surveillance, epidemiology, and end results program registry. *Arch Dermatol.* 1999;135(3):275–280.

9. Marrett LD, Nguyen HL, Armstrong BK. Trends in the incidence of cutaneous malignant melanoma in New South Wales, 1983–1996. *Int J Cancer.* 2001;92(3):457–462.
10. Surveillance, Epidemiology and End Results, 2009 (http://www.seer.cancer.gov/)
11. Beddingfield FC 3rd. The melanoma epidemic: res ipsa loquitur. *Oncologist.* 2003 8(5):459–465.
12. Moan J, Dahlback A. The relationship between skin cancers, solar radiation and ozone depletion. *Br J Cancer.* 1992;65(6):916–921.
13. Slaper H, Velders GJ, Daniel JS, et al. Estimates of ozone depletion and skin cancer incidence to examine the Vienna Convention achievements. *Nature.* 1996;384(6606):256–258.
14. Robinson JK, Rigel DS, Amonette RA. Trends in sun exposure knowledge, attitudes, and behaviors: 1986 to 1996. *J Am Acad Dermatol.* 1997;37(2 pt 1):179–186.
15. Robinson JK, Kim J, Rosenbaum S, et al. Indoor tanning knowledge, attitudes, and behavior among young adults from 1988–2007. *Arch Dermatol.* 2008;144(4):484–488.
16. Lamberg L. "Epidemic" of malignant melanoma: true increase or better detection? *JAMA.* 2002;287(17):2201.
17. Swerlick RA, Chen S. The melanoma epidemic. Is increased surveillance the solution or the problem? *Arch Dermatol.* 1996;132(8):881–884.
18. Linos E, Swetter SM, Cockburn MG, et al. Increasing burden of melanoma in the United States. *J Invest Dermatol.* 2009;129(7):1666–1674.
19. Welch HG, Woloshin S, Schwartz LM. Skin biopsy rates and incidence of melanoma: population based ecological study. *Br Med J.* 2005;331(7515):481.
20. Levell NJ, Beattie CC, Shuster S, et al. Melanoma epidemic: a midsummer night's dream? *Br J Dermatol.* 2009;161(3):630–634.
21. Bosetti C, La Vecchia C, Naldi L, et al. Mortality from cutaneous malignant melanoma in Europe. Has the epidemic levelled off? *Melanoma Res.* 2004;14(4):301–309.
22. Crocetti E, Carli P. Changes from mid-1980s to late 1990s among clinical and demographic correlates of melanoma thickness. *Eur J Dermatol.* 2003;13(1):72–75.
23. Clark WH, Jr., Reimer RR, Greene M, et al. Origin of familial malignant melanomas from heritable melanocytic lesions. "The B-K mole syndrome." *Arch Dermatol.* 1978;114(5):732–738.
24. Lynch HT, Frichot BC, 3rd, Lynch JF. Familial atypical multiple mole-melanoma syndrome. *J Med Genet.* 1978;15(5):352–356.
25. Goldstein AM, Fraser MC, Clark WH, Jr., et al. Age at diagnosis and transmission of invasive melanoma in 23 families with cutaneous malignant melanoma/dysplastic nevi. *J Natl Cancer Inst.* 1994;86(18):1385–1390.
26. Kamb A, Gruis NA, Weaver-Feldhaus J, et al. A cell cycle regulator potentially involved in genesis of many tumor types. *Science.* 1994;264(5157):436–440.
27. Pho L, Grossman D, Leachman SA. Melanoma genetics: a review of genetic factors and clinical phenotypes in familial melanoma. *Curr Opin Oncol.* 2006;18(2):173–179.
28. Cleaver JE. Defective repair replication of DNA in xeroderma pigmentosum. *Nature.* 1968;218(5142):652–656.
29. Kraemer KH, Levy DD, Parris CN, et al. Xeroderma pigmentosum and related disorders: examining the linkage between defective DNA repair and cancer. *J Invest Dermatol.* 1994;103:96S–101S.
30. Freedberg IM, Eisen AZ, Wolff K, Austen KF, Goldsmith LA, & Katz SI, eds. *Fitzpatrick's Dermatology in General Medicine.* 6th ed. New York, NY: McGraw-Hill Professional Publishing; 2003.
31. Kobayashi N, Muramatsu T, Yamashina Y, et al. Melanin reduces ultraviolet-induced DNA damage formation and killing rate in cultured human melanoma cells. *J Invest Dermatol.* 1993;101(5):685–689.
32. Holman CD, Armstrong BK. Pigmentary traits, ethnic origin, benign nevi, and family history as risk factors for cutaneous malignant melanoma. *J Natl Cancer Inst.* 1984;72(2):257–266.
33. Armstrong BK, Kricker A. The epidemiology of UV induced skin cancer. *J Photochem Photobiol B.* 2001;63(1):8–18.
34. Bliss JM, Ford D, Swerdlow AJ, et al. Risk of cutaneous melanoma associated with pigmentation characteristics and freckling: systematic overview of 10 case-control studies. The International Melanoma Analysis Group (IMAGE). *Int J Cancer.* 1995;62(4):367–376.
35. Cho E, Rosner BA, Feskanich D, et al. Risk factors and individual probabilities of melanoma for whites. *J Clin Oncol.* 2005;23(12):2669–2675.
36. Tsao H, Bevona C, Goggins W, et al. The transformation rate of moles (melanocytic nevi) into cutaneous melanoma: a population-based estimate. *Arch Dermatol.* 2003;139(3):282–288.
37. Bataille V, Bishop JA, Sasieni P, et al. Risk of cutaneous melanoma in relation to the numbers, types and sites of naevi: a case-control study. *Br J Cancer.* 1996;73(12):1605–1611.
38. Olsen CM, Zens MS, Stukel TA, et al. Nevus density and melanoma risk in women: a pooled analysis to test the divergent pathway hypothesis. *Int J Cancer.* 2009;124(4):937–944.
39. Whiteman DC, Watt P, Purdie DM, et al. Melanocytic nevi, solar keratoses, and divergent pathways to cutaneous melanoma. *J Natl Cancer Inst.* 2003;95(11):806–812.
40. Cho E, Rosner BA, Colditz GA. Risk factors for melanoma by body site. *Cancer Epidemiol Biomarkers Prev.* 2005;14(5):1241–1244.
41. Ha L, Noonan FP, De Fabo EC, et al. Animal models of melanoma. *J Investig Dermatol Symp Proc.* 2005;10(2):86–88.
42. Bulliard JL, Cox B, Elwood JM. Latitude gradients in melanoma incidence and mortality in the non-Maori population of New Zealand. *Cancer Causes Control.* 1994;5(3):234–240.
43. Elwood JM, Jopson J. Melanoma and sun exposure: an overview of published studies. *Int J Cancer.* 1997;73(2):198–203.

44. Elwood JM, Gallagher RP. Body site distribution of cutaneous malignant melanoma in relationship to patterns of sun exposure. *Int J Cancer.* 1998;78(3):276–280.
45. Chang YM, Barrett JH, Bishop DT, et al. Sun exposure and melanoma risk at different latitudes: a pooled analysis of 5700 cases and 7216 controls. *Int J Epidemiol.* 2009;38(3):814–830.
46. Stern RS, Weinstein MC, Baker SG. Risk reduction for nonmelanoma skin cancer with childhood sunscreen use. *Arch Dermatol.* 1986;122(5):537–545.
47. Westerdahl J, Ingvar C, Masback A, et al. Sunscreen use and malignant melanoma. *Int J Cancer.* 2000;87(1):145–150.
48. Wolf P, Quehenberger F, Mullegger R, et al. Phenotypic markers, sunlight-related factors and sunscreen use in patients with cutaneous melanoma: an Austrian case-control study. *Melanoma Res.* 1998;8(4):370–378.
49. Rigel DS. The effect of sunscreen on melanoma risk. *Dermatol Clin.* 2002;20(4):601–606.
50. Dennis LK, Beane Freeman LE, VanBeek MJ. Sunscreen use and the risk for melanoma: a quantitative review. *Ann Intern Med.* 2003;139(12):966–978.
51. Autier P. Sunscreen abuse for intentional sun exposure. *Br J Dermatol.* 2009;161 (suppl 3):40–45.
52. Gallagher RP, Rivers JK, Lee TK, et al. Broad-spectrum sunscreen use and the development of new nevi in white children: a randomized controlled trial. *JAMA.* 2000;283(22):2955–2960.
53. Rigel DS, Naylor M, Robinson J. What is the evidence for a sunscreen and melanoma controversy? *Arch Dermatol.* 2000;136(12):1447–1449.
54. Balch CM, Gershenwald JE, Soong SJ, et al. Final version of 2009 AJCC melanoma staging and classification. *J Clin Oncol.* 2009;27(36):6199–6206.
55. Balch CM, Buzaid AC, Soong SJ, et al. Final version of the American Joint Committee on Cancer staging system for cutaneous melanoma. *J Clin Oncol.* 2001;19(16):3635–3648.
56. Breslow A. Thickness, cross-sectional areas and depth of invasion in the prognosis of cutaneous melanoma. *Ann Surg.* 1970;172(5):902–908.
57. Eigentler TK, Buettner PG, Leiter U, et al. Impact of ulceration in stages I to III cutaneous melanoma as staged by the American Joint Committee on Cancer Staging System: an analysis of the German Central Malignant Melanoma Registry. *J Clin Oncol.* 2004;22(21):4376–4383.
58. Corona R, Mele A, Amini M, et al. Interobserver variability on the histopathologic diagnosis of cutaneous melanoma and other pigmented skin lesions. *J Clin Oncol.* 1996;14(4):1218–1223.
59. Balch CM, Soong SJ, Gershenwald JE, et al. Prognostic factors analysis of 17,600 melanoma patients: validation of the American Joint Committee on Cancer melanoma staging system. *J Clin Oncol.* 2001;19(16):3622–3634.
60. Paek SC, Griffith KA, Johnson TM, et al. The impact of factors beyond Breslow depth on predicting sentinel lymph node positivity in melanoma. *Cancer.* 2007;109(1):100–108.
61. Sondak VK, Taylor JM, Sabel MS, et al. Mitotic rate and younger age are predictors of sentinel lymph node positivity: lessons learned from the generation of a probabilistic model. *Ann Surg Oncol.* 2004;11(3):247–258.
62. Azzola MF, Shaw HM, Thompson JF, et al. Tumor mitotic rate is a more powerful prognostic indicator than ulceration in patients with primary cutaneous melanoma: an analysis of 3661 patients from a single center. *Cancer.* 2003;97(6):1488–1498.
63. Clark WH, Jr., From L, Bernardino EA, et al. The histogenesis and biologic behavior of primary human malignant melanomas of the skin. *Cancer Res.* 1969;29(3):705–727.
64. Morton DL, Wen DR, Wong JH, et al. Technical details of intraoperative lymphatic mapping for early stage melanoma. *Arch Surg.* 1992;127(4):392–399.
65. Chao C, Wong SL, Edwards MJ, et al. Sentinel lymph node biopsy for head and neck melanomas. *Ann Surg Oncol.* 2003;10(1):21–26.
66. O'Brien CJ, Uren RF, Thompson JF, et al. Prediction of potential metastatic sites in cutaneous head and neck melanoma using lymphoscintigraphy. *Am J Surg.* 1995;170(5):461–466.
67. Morton DL, Thompson JF, Cochran AJ, et al. Sentinel-node biopsy or nodal observation in melanoma. *N Engl J Med.* 2006;355(13):1307–1317.
68. Ohsie SJ, Sarantopoulos GP, Cochran AJ, et al. Immunohistochemical characteristics of melanoma. *J Cutan Pathol.* 2008;35(5):433–444.
69. Roka F, Mastan P, Binder M, et al. Prediction of non-sentinel node status and outcome in sentinel node-positive melanoma patients. *Eur J Surg Oncol.* 2008;34(1):82–88.
70. Cascinelli N, Bombardieri E, Bufalino R, et al. Sentinel and nonsentinel node status in stage IB and II melanoma patients: two-step prognostic indicators of survival. *J Clin Oncol.* 2006;24(27):4464–4471.
71. Ariyan C, Brady MS, Gonen M, et al. Positive nonsentinel node status predicts mortality in patients with cutaneous melanoma. *Ann Surg Oncol.* 2009;16(1):186–190.
72. Scoggins CR, Ross MI, Reintgen DS, et al. Gender-related differences in outcome for melanoma patients. *Ann Surg.* 2006;243(5):693–698; discussion 698–700.
73. Lachiewicz AM, Berwick M, Wiggins CL, et al. Survival differences between patients with scalp or neck melanoma and those with melanoma of other sites in the Surveillance, Epidemiology, and End Results (SEER) program. *Arch Dermatol.* 2008;144(4):515–521.
74. Fisher SR. Cutaneous malignant melanoma of the head and neck. *Laryngoscope.* 1989;99(8 pt 1):822–836.
75. Fisher SR, Seigler HF, George SL. Therapeutic and prognostic considerations of head and neck melanoma. *Ann Plast Surg.* 1992;28(1):78–80.
76. Haqq C, Nosrati M, Sudilovsky D, et al. The gene expression signatures of melanoma progression. *Proc Natl Acad Sci U S A.* 2005;102(17):6092–6097.

77. Rangel J, Nosrati M, Torabian S, et al. Osteopontin as a molecular prognostic marker for melanoma. *Cancer.* 2008;112(1):144–150.
78. Sober AJ, Chuang TY, Duvic M, et al. Guidelines of care for primary cutaneous melanoma. *J Am Acad Dermatol.* 2001;45(4):579–586.
79. Stell VH, Norton HJ, Smith KS, et al. Method of biopsy and incidence of positive margins in primary melanoma. *Ann Surg Oncol.* 2007;14(2):893–898.
80. Johnson TM, Bradford CR, Gruber SB, et al. Staging workup, sentinel node biopsy, and follow-up tests for melanoma: update of current concepts. *Arch Dermatol.* 2004;140(1):107–113.
81. Basler GC, Fader DJ, Yahanda A, et al. The utility of fine needle aspiration in the diagnosis of melanoma metastatic to lymph nodes. *J Am Acad Dermatol.* 1997;36(3 pt 1): 403–408.
82. National Comprehensive Cancer Network Clinical Practice Guidelines in Oncology, v.1.2010, 2010 (http://www.nccn.org)
83. Cormier JN, Xing Y, Feng L, et al. Metastatic melanoma to lymph nodes in patients with unknown primary sites. *Cancer.* 2006;106(9):2012–2020.
84. Lee CC, Faries MB, Wanek LA, et al. Improved survival after lymphadenectomy for nodal metastasis from an unknown primary melanoma. *J Clin Oncol.* 2008;26(4):535–541.
85. Soufir N, Ollivaud L, Bertrand G, et al. A French CDK4-positive melanoma family with a co-inherited EDNRB mutation. *J Dermatol Sci.* 2007;46(1):61–64.
86. Box NF, Duffy DL, Chen W, et al. MC1R genotype modifies risk of melanoma in families segregating CDKN2A mutations. *Am J Hum Genet.* 2001;69(4):765–773.
87. Duggleby WF, Stoll H, Priore RL, et al. A genetic analysis of melanoma—polygenic inheritance as a threshold trait. *Am J Epidemiol.* 1981;114(1):63–72.
88. Rhodes AR, Weinstock MA, Fitzpatrick TB, et al. Risk factors for cutaneous melanoma. A practical method of recognizing predisposed individuals. *JAMA.* 1987; 258(21):3146–3154.
89. Swerdlow AJ, English JS, Qiao Z. The risk of melanoma in patients with congenital nevi: a cohort study. *J Am Acad Dermatol.* 1995;32(4):595–599.
90. Grob JJ, Gouvernet J, Aymar D, et al. Count of benign melanocytic nevi as a major indicator of risk for non-familial nodular and superficial spreading melanoma. *Cancer.* 1990;66(2):387–395.
91. International Agency for Research on Cancer Working Group on artifical ultraviolet (UV) light and skin cancer. The association of use of sunbeds with cutaneous malignant melanoma and other skin cancers: a systematic review. *Int J Cancer.* 2007;120(5):1116–1122.

21

MOLECULAR BIOLOGY AND GENETICS OF MELANOMA/ MECHANISMS OF SPREAD

HELMUT SCHAIDER
SUSAN E. ZABIEROWSKI
MEENHARD HERLYN

Introduction

In the last few years, progress has been made in identifying and understanding molecular and genetic signatures in melanoma development. Based on the initial idea of a "de-differentiation" process, in which primary melanocytes pass through a cascade of a benign nevus, dysplastic nevus, radial growth phase melanoma, vertical growth phase melanoma, and finally metastatic melanoma, new concepts of melanoma development have emerged. These models account for the clinical observation that the majority of melanomas do not evolve from pre-existing nevi, but rather appear in normal-appearing skin. Acquisition of genetic changes in melanocytes as well as in melanocytic precursors leads to unlimited proliferation, but additional events are necessary to attain full transforming capabilities, independence of contact inhibition, and invasive properties. Along with these changes, melanoma cells become resistant to apoptosis and are able to manipulate the tumor microenvironment for their purposes. The last, but most life-threatening, step in melanoma genesis, however, dissemination of highly malignant tumor cells with incredible plasticity and propensity to lie dormant for decades, still remains enigmatic and a challenge to clinicians and researchers alike.

This chapter focuses on genetic alterations harbored by melanocytic lesions, the survival mechanisms developed to restrain apoptotic stimuli, the prerequisite to adapt cell communications with progression, the pathways involved in unlimited proliferation, and the advent of melanocytic stem cells. Understanding each step at the genetic and molecular level will allow the identification of new therapeutic targets for an individualized treatment approach and will increase the pipeline for new therapeutic compounds.

Genetic Alterations and Proliferation in Melanocytic Lesions

For the last two decades, genes that are the driving force behind the initiation and progression of melanoma development have been elucidated. This has occurred primarily through the perception that the acquisition of somatic mutations in key regulatory pathways is crucial at the very beginning of melanoma genesis. In principle, some of the most common cellular pathways have been investigated in much detail.

The RAS-RAF-MEK-ERK Pathway

One of the most heavily scrutinized pathways is the RAS-RAF-MEK-ERK cascade. In response to various stimuli including the activation of receptor tyrosine kinases (RTKs), RAS is activated in a GTP-bound state and recruits RAF to the cell membrane. A consequent phosphorylation occurs, which drives signaling events along the MEK-ERK axis. Phosphorylated ERK translocates into the nucleus, where it activates transcription factors important for cell proliferation, including microphthalmia inducing transcription factor (MITF) (Fig 21–1).

NRAS

Several components of this pathway are proto-oncogenes, which remain in an activated state through mutations or amplifications. In fact, the first gene found to be specifically altered in a subset of melanomas was NRAS.[1] Approximately 15% to 25% of melanoma cell lines and primary tumors of

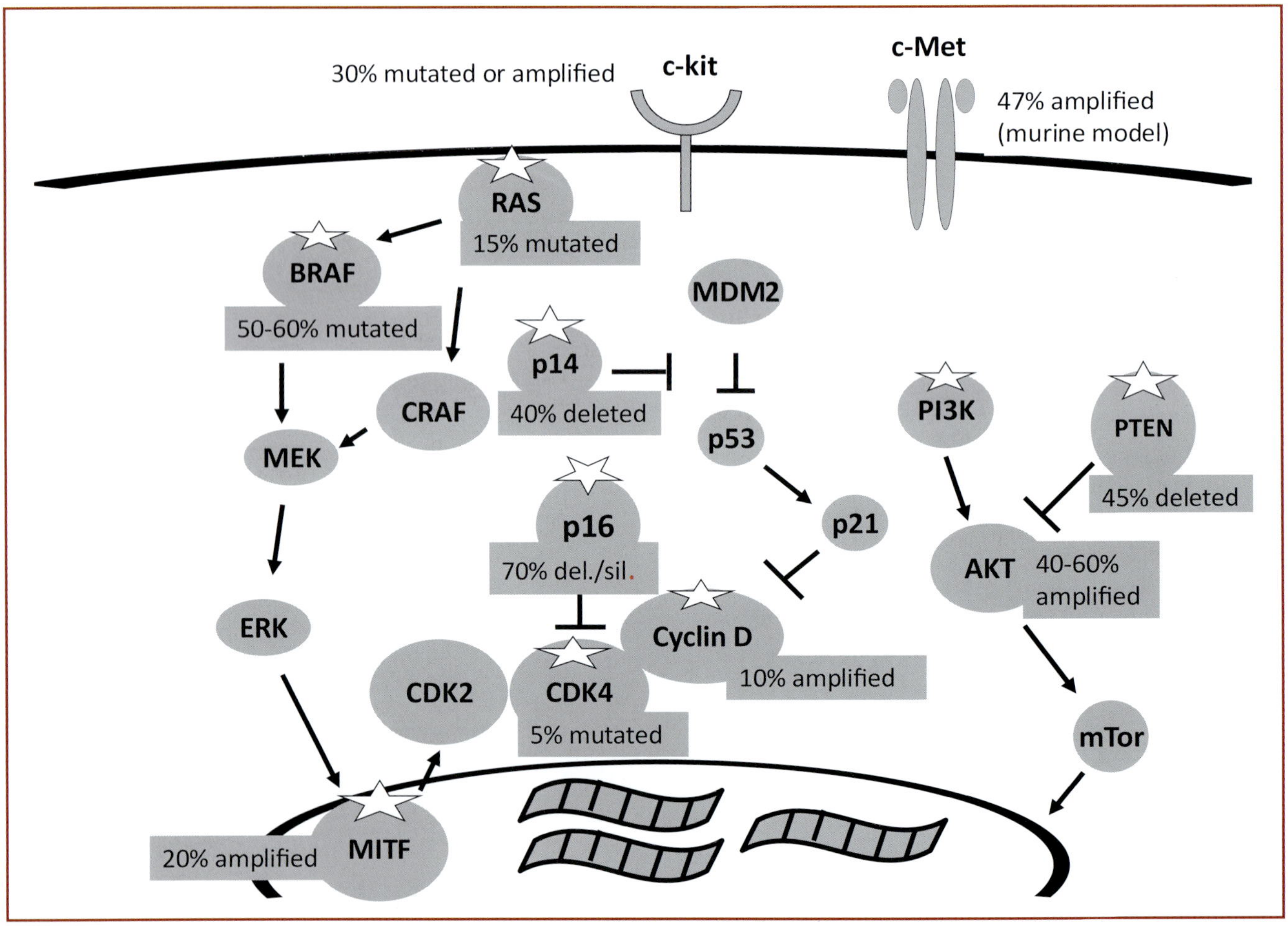

Figure 21–1. Summary of genetic alterations in cutaneous melanoma. Genes that are altered by mutation, deletion, or amplification are depicted by an asterisk (*), except for the two receptor tyrosine kinases c-Kit and c-Met. The frequency of alterations is given in %.

all sites show mutations in NRAS; it is mutated in congenital nevi even up to 56% of cases. Q61R is the most frequent mutation in NRAS, which leads to an activation of the protein. Mutations in KRAS and HRAS, two other variants of RAS, although often found in a variety of other human cancers, are rare in melanoma.

BRAF^{V600E}

A downstream signaling molecule of RAS, the RAF serine-threonine-specific protein kinase that activates MEK, has the highest reported frequency of alteration in melanoma (see Fig 21–1). Of the three RAF genes, ARAF, BRAF, and CRAF, mutations occur only in BRAF in about 50% to 70% of cases.[2] One specific mutation, a substitution of valine with glutamic acid at residue 600 (V600E), accounts for almost more than 90% of all BRAF mutations. This mutation causes a conformational change to constitutive activation of the protein, thereby increasing the basal kinase activity.

Surprisingly, BRAF^{V600E} mutations have been found not only in melanomas but also in benign and dysplastic nevi at frequencies of up to 80% of tumors. This suggests that the mutation represents an early, but crucial, event in melanocytic lesions, but is not sufficient for melanocytic cells to achieve fully malignant transformation. Mutations in BRAF are found in nonchronic sun-damaged skin in up to 50% of cases.

Mutations in BRAF and NRAS occur almost exclusively, and the coincidence of mutations in both genes is a rare event. This suggests that both are efficient in activating the RAS-MEK-ERK pathway.[3] Indeed, knocking down BRAF or NRAS by RNAi results in reduced signaling and finally cell death. To maintain signaling through the pathway, melanoma cell lines with NRAS-activating mutations alone switch their signaling from BRAF to CRAF (see Fig 21–1). This switch in signaling via CRAF in NRAS-mutated melanomas may have important implications for therapeutic interventions. Because BRAF and NRAS mutations occur in 80% to 90% of all melanomas, it seems that activation of the RAS-MEK-ERK pathway constitutes an obligatory event, making it an obvious therapeutic target. A number of potent chemical inhibitors of components in this pathway have been proven efficient in vitro but, so far, have shown only modest clinical responses in patients. This experience reflects a common problem in specifically targeting single pathways, whereupon other pathways and mechanisms for survival are then activated.

GNAQ^{Q209L}

A fraction of melanomas that do not carry mutations in BRAF and NRAS was recently identified with acquired mutations in GNAQ, the heterotrimeric Gq- protein α-subunit.[4] Blue nevi, an entity of congenital or acquired melanocytic proliferations which present as patches or moles in bluish colors, and uveal melanoma, arising from melanocytes within the choroidal plexus of the eye, show mutations in GNAQ in about 83% and 46% of tumors, respectively. These mutations exclusively occur at codon 209 (GNAQ^{Q209L}), resulting in constitutive activation of the protein.

As G protein α-subunits mediate signals between G-protein-coupled receptors (GPCRs) and multiple downstream signaling effectors including the RAS-RAF-MEK-ERK pathway, the mutation leads to increased levels of phosphorylated ERK. As has been demonstrated for BRAF and NRAS mutations, the genetic alteration in GNAQ occurs early in melanocytic lesions and thus additional genetic hits are necessary for a full progression to melanoma. Blue nevi are benign, genetically stable lesions, which rarely develop into malignant blue nevi. Thus, it remains to be determined whether mutations in GNAQ are potential targets for therapy.

Receptor Tyrosine Kinases

Growth factors, including hepatocyte growth factor (HGF), stem cell factor (SCF), basic fibroblast growth factor (bFGF), and the endothelins (ET1-3), promote melanocyte proliferation, survival, and differentiation. They bind to the extracellular domain of receptor tyrosine kinases (RTKs). Upon binding, receptor dimerization is mediated, followed by activation of intrinsic tyrosine kinase activity and autophosphorylation. Stimulated RTKs trigger a cascade of events, including the activation of the RAS-RAF-MEK-ERK pathway or the PI3K-AKT pathway (see

Fig 21–1). In mouse experiments, it was demonstrated that a combination of three different growth factors (bFGF, SCF and ET3) can indeed induce melanomas.[5] However, these lesions regress after withdrawal of the growth factors, suggesting that only genetic alterations in RTKs account for stable transformation and immortalization.

cKIT

cKIT encodes a RTK, which is activated by its ligand SCF. It belongs to the platelet-derived growth factor family of RTKs and has been described as a proto-oncogene for melanoma (see Fig 21–1). Signaling by cKIT is indispensable for melanocyte development. Inactivating mutations that prevent kinase activity of the receptor result in amelanotic congenital patches of white skin and are associated with human piebaldism.[6] Recent studies have demonstrated activating cKIT mutations in those melanomas that do not carry mutations in NRAS or BRAF.[7]

Likewise, as previously mentioned for NRAS and BRAF mutations, the constitutive activation of cKIT may result in an activation of the RAS-RAF-MEK-ERK pathway. Whereas mutations in NRAS and BRAF occur at a high frequency in nonchronic sun-damaged skin, cKIT activating mutations and/or gene amplifications have been found in melanomas arising in chronic sun-damaged skin (28%), melanomas occurring on mucosal membranes (39%), and melanomas on palms, soles, and subungual sites (acral melanomas, 36%). Therefore, identifying a subpopulation of melanoma patients with cKIT activating mutations may be part of a strategy of individualized therapy with tyrosine kinase inhibitors.

c-Met

Investigations into genetic alterations in RTKs led to the recent identification of amplifications in c-Met, the receptor for hepatocyte growth factor (HGF) (see Fig 21–1). Genomic amplifications of MET have been found in 47% of melanomas in a murine model.[8] In human tumor tissue sample analysis, a novel mutation in exon 14 was discovered.[9] The signaling of c-Met feeds into multiple pathways, such as the RAS-RAF-MEK-ERK, the phosphatidyl-inositol 3′kinase (PI3K) and Janus kinase-signal transducer and activator of transcription (Jak/STAT) pathway. The coincidence of MET amplifications with genetic alterations in one of these pathways accelerates the transformation process, revealing c-Met function as a proto-oncogene.

Melanoma Susceptibility Genes

The high frequency of activating mutations in the RAS-RAF-MEK-ERK pathway in benign nevi points to their role as initiators in melanoma genesis. However, it became clear that such activating mutations are not sufficient for malignant transformation into melanomas. In particular, $BRAF^{V600E}$ mutations trigger a cellular senescence response in nevi, which is a hindrance for successful transformation. Senescence is characterized by irreversible loss of division capacity and constitutes a mechanism against unlimited cell proliferation. It is a barrier against cancer development, which has to be disrupted. Cancer susceptibility genes are key elements that facilitate the bypassing of senescence. Four predisposing genes have been identified in melanoma, which present as germline mutations in familial melanoma but also occur as somatic mutations in sporadic melanomas. There are three high- and one low-penetrance genes.

Cyclin-Dependent Kinase Inhibitor 2A (CDKN2A)

Cyclin-dependent kinase inhibitor 2A (*CDKN2A*) is the best-characterized high-penetrance gene. It is a tumor suppressor gene located on chromosome 9p21, and it encodes two distinct melanoma-predisposing genes, p16 and p14. P16 and p14 are two splice variants of different reading frames, and the protein products are INK4A ($p16^{INK4A}$) and ARF ($p14^{ARF}$), respectively. $P16^{INK4A}$ is central to the regulation of the cell cycle, as it is an inhibitor of the G1 cyclin-dependent kinases (CDK) CDK4 and CDK6, which stimulate passage through the G1 phase of the cell cycle. It additionally keeps the tumor suppressor retinoblastoma protein (RB) in an activated, hypophosphorylated state. Inactivating mutations of $p16^{INK4A}$ lead to hyperphosphorylation of RB, and subsequent unopposed activity of CDK4, thereby releasing transcription factor E2F and allowing for S phase entry.

Somatic loss of p16^{INK4A} occurs via mutation, deletion, or promoter hypermethylation in 30% to 70% of sporadic melanomas (see Fig 21–1).[10] In familial melanoma, mutations in CDKN2A have been identified in 25% to 40% of cases.[11] The inactivation of p16^{INK4A} increases the susceptibility to melanoma by breaking cellular senescence in melanocytes, which otherwise are growth arrested in G1, and this inactivation is accompanied by increased tumor protein p53 DNA binding activity and an upregulation of p16^{INK4A}.

The second alternative spliced variant of CDKN2A, p14^{ARF}, is involved in controlling p53 (TP53) protein levels (see Fig 21–1). It sequesters and thus inactivates the MDM2 protein, which normally triggers the ubiquitinylation and, subsequently, proteosomal-targeted degradation of p53 (TP53). Inactivation of MDM2 leads to accumulation of TP53, causing cell cycle arrest in G2-M phase. Unlike p16^{INK4A}, germline mutations in p14^{ARF} have not yet been linked to melanoma susceptibility in familial melanoma. Its presumptive importance for melanomagenesis is related to its regulatory properties of TP53.

However, somatic modifications in metastases have been recently identified at a rate of 43%, and in many cases (30%), the alterations occurred in the presence of wild-type p16.[12] ARF inactivation was related to hemizygous deletions with or without promoter methylations. Inactivation of p16 was observed in 5%, whereas inactivation of p14 in 25%. Therefore, it seems that the p14 locus is a more frequent target of inactivation than p16 itself.

CDK4

The importance of the p16^{INK4A}-CDK4-RB axis is further strengthened by the fact that even in cells with wild type INK4A, activating mutations in CDK4 (the third high penetrant melanoma-predisposing gene) allow cells to bypass the G1/S cell-cycle checkpoint, resulting in uncontrolled cell proliferation. CDK4 mutations in familial melanoma are a rare but recurrent event, occurring in about 5% of cases and predominately affect arginine at codon 24, making CDK4 proteins insensitive to inhibition by p16^{INK4A} (see Fig 21–1).[13] Somatic changes have been described in some acral and mucosal sporadic melanomas via amplification, without alterations in p16^{INK4A} and p14^{ARF}.

Melanocortin-1 Receptor (MC1R)

The fourth gene implicated in melanomagenesis is the melanocortin-1 receptor (*MC1R*), and, unlike the others, is low-penetrance. MC1R encodes a seven-transmembrane G protein-coupled receptor (GPCR) expressed on epidermal melanocytes. The ligand of MC1R, α-MSH (melanocyte-stimulating hormone) stimulates intracellular adenylyl cyclase via MC1R and leads to generation of cyclic adenosine monophosphate (cAMP). cAMP in turn phosphorylates cAMP-responsive element (CREB), resulting in transcription of the melanocytic lineage gene microphthalmia transcription factor (MITF). Seventy-five allelic variants in MC1R have been described, which determine skin phenotypes and pigmentation in humans.

Whereas no gain-of-function mutations have been reported for MC1R, polymorphisms have been associated with melanoma.[14] In particular, the coincidence of MC1R variants and mutations in p16^{INK4A} in familial melanoma predisposes patients to present with melanoma at an earlier age. Families who carry p16^{INK4A} mutations but show a consensus sequence in MC1R develop melanomas later on.

Microphthalmia Transcription Factor (MITF)

MITF encodes a master determinant of melanocyte lineage commitment, a basic helix-loop-helix leucine zipper, dimeric transcription factor that is implicated in the development and survival of melanocytes. It is a key transcription factor for regulating the expression of major melanogenic proteins, like tyrosinase (TRY). The effects of MITF are not restricted to the induction of melanogenic proteins, but cover a broad range of genes, including the upregulation of the major antiapoptotic protein, B cell lymphoma-2 (Bcl-2), or the modulation of CDK2, p21, and p16INK4A. MITF levels are tightly regulated, which is important for proliferation of melanocytes and melanoma cells alike. Aberrant levels, which are too low or too high, lead to cell cycle arrest. MITF is amplified in 10% of primary and 15% to 20% of metastatic melanomas at high copy numbers (4 to 13 gene copies), suggesting that it may represent a 'lineage-survival oncogene' in melanoma (see Fig 21–1).[15] One possible explanation for the selective amplification of MITF during melanoma development could be the maintenance of MITF levels within certain limits required for continued growth.

Cyclin D1

In early to mid-G1 phase, cyclin D1 serves as a mediator and sensor of extracellular signals. It confers CDK binding properties and is involved, as a regulatory subunit of CDK4 and 6, in the phosphorylation of pRB. Indirectly, it activates cyclinE/CDK2, which in turn is regulated by MITF and functions as a collaborative oncogene that enhances oncogenic transformations of other oncogenes (see Fig 21–1). Cyclin D1 is overexpressed and/or amplified in a substantial proportion of different human tumors, and its changes occur early in tumorigenesis. In melanoma, frequent amplifications of cyclin D1 are observed in acral melanomas (44.4%), occasional amplifications in lentigo maligna melanoma (10.5%) and superficial spreading melanoma (5.6%). Cyclin D1 is overexpressed in all cases with amplifications and in an additional 20% of cases without amplification.[16] This observation is of clinical relevance, as it has been shown that increased levels of cyclin D1, resulting from additional gene copies, contribute to the resistance of BRAF inhibitors in melanomas harboring $BRAF^{V600E}$ mutations.

Survival Mechanisms and Progression

Mutations in the RAS-RAF-MEK-ERK pathway set the pace to acquire self-maintenance and proliferation in melanocytes. The senescence programs turned on in lesions with constitutive activation of BRAF, however, limit unrestricted proliferation. Second genetic hits are necessary and enhance the probability of bypassing the senescence response. This is mainly accomplished by the acquisition of apoptosis resistance and/or the downregulation of tumor suppressor mechanisms and gene amplifications (Figs 21–1, 21–2, and 21–3).

Apoptosis Resistance

Melanoma is notorious for its drug resistance. Drug resistance molecules confer inadequate tradeoffs as elements of resistance to classical approaches of melanoma therapy like chemotherapy and irradiation. Specifically, apoptosis resistance is a hallmark for many solid tumors, especially melanoma, and new insights may lead to the development of new treatment approaches based on the activation of the apoptotic pathways.

Traditionally, two principal pathways to apoptosis have been recognized: the transmembrane "extrinsic" pathway and the mitochondrial "intrinsic" pathway (see Fig 21–2). Both depend on the activation of cysteine proteases that cleave at aspartate residues (caspases). Irrespective of whether apoptosis is initiated by the intrinsic or the extrinsic pathway, changes in mitochondria play a central role. In response to cell damage signals, mitochondria release cytochrome c and other aptogenic proteins such as Omi or Smac/DIABLO. Cytochrome c translocates from the inner mitochondrion membrane to the cytoplasm, where it binds to apoptotic protease activating factor-1 (Apaf-1). This complex, called the apoptosome, activates caspase 9, culminating in cell death. Members of the B cell lymphoma protein (Bcl)-2 family are critical regulators of the mitochondrial pathway to apoptosis and are representatives of the extrinsic pathway (see Fig 21–2).

Bcl-2 Family

Some members of the Bcl-2 family inhibit apoptosis (eg, Bcl-2, Bcl-xl, Mcl-1, Bcl-w and AL), whereas others promote cell death (eg, Bax, Bak, Bok, Bcl-xs, Bid, Bad, Bik, Bim, Bmf, Puma, Noxa, and Hrf). The activity of the anti-apoptotic members of the Bcl-2 family can be inhibited by heterodimerization with some pro-apoptotic members (see Fig 21–2). Bcl-2 is expressed in both normal melanocytes and cuta-

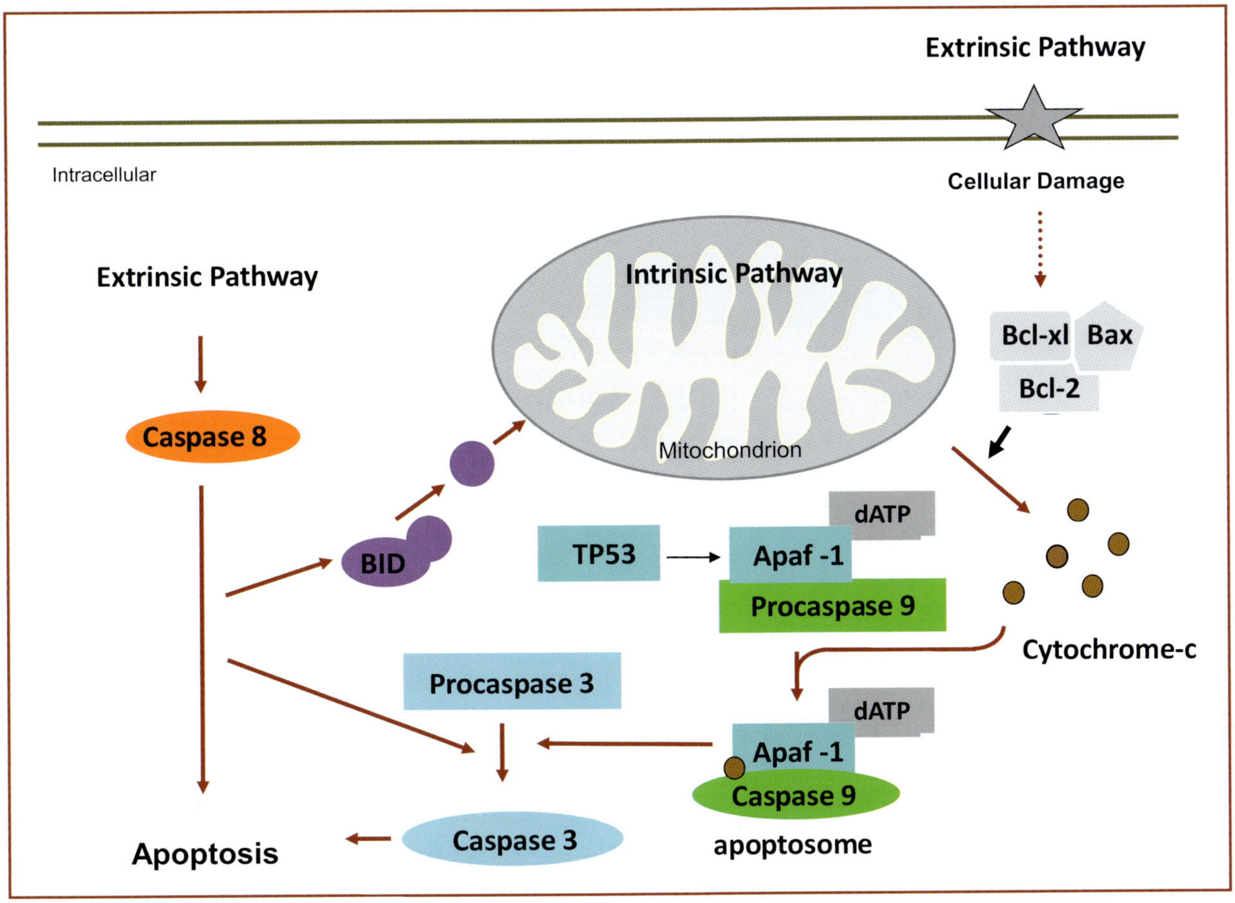

Figure 21–2. Regulation of apoptosis in melanoma. In response to cell damage signals, the extrinsic pathway is activated. B cell lymphoma-2 (Bcl-2) induces cytochrome c translocation from the inner mitochondrion membrane to the cytoplasm. Apoptosis protease-activating factor 1 (Apaf-1) interacts with cytochrome c and caspase 9, the apoptosome, to initiate activation of the classic caspase pathway, culminating in cell death. *TP53* (p53) upregulates *Apaf-1*. Apoptosis is also initiated through caspase 8 by the extrinsic pathway.

neous melanoma. High expression levels of Bcl-2, due to gene amplifications, have been found in up to 90% of primary malignant melanomas, and upregulation of Bcl-2 and Bcl-xl was demonstrated in melanoma cell lines.[17]

In many metastatic melanomas, however, Bcl-2 levels are low or even absent. In contrast to Bcl-2, the Mcl-1 protein, another anti-apoptotic protein, is increased in metastatic melanoma compared with primary melanoma. Poor prognosis in patients with stage IIa (Breslow-thickness 1.5 to 4.0 mm) cutaneous melanoma is associated with downregulation of the proapoptotic proteins Bax and Bak. These findings of disturbed equilibrium in the composition of pro- and anti-apoptotic proteins facilitate resistance to conventional cytotoxic chemotherapy, as damaged cells cannot initiate programmed cell death.

TP53

The p53 (TP53) tumor suppressor is mutated or otherwise inactivated in a wide range of human cancers (see Fig 21–1). In melanoma, however, the importance of the pathogenic significance of changes in

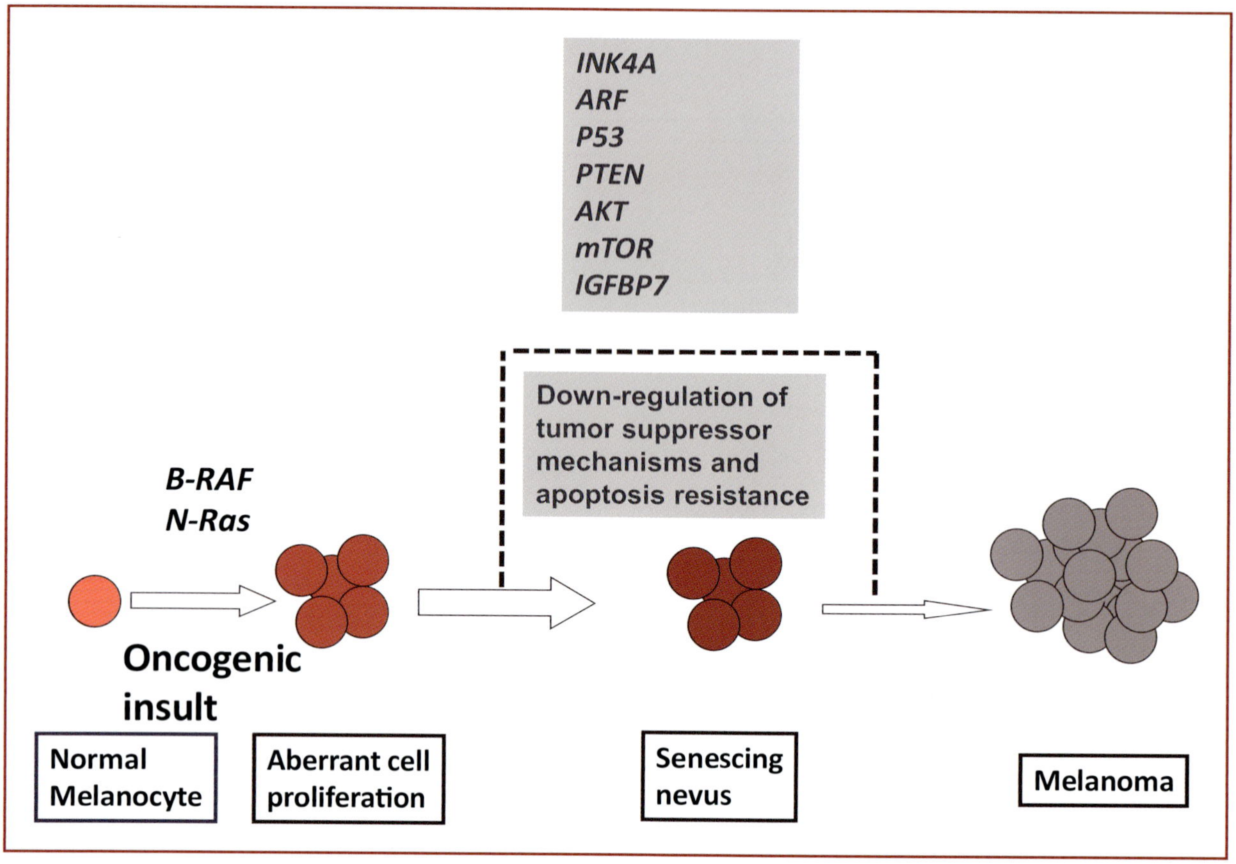

Figure 21–3. Concept of tumor initiation and progression in melanoma based on genetic hits. Normal melanocytes acquiring mutations in BRAF or NRAS exert aberrant cell proliferation. Constitutive activation, however, limits unrestricted proliferation due to induction of senescence. Second genetic hits are necessary and enhance the probability to bypass the senescence response. This is mainly accomplished by the acquisition of apoptosis resistance and/or the downregulation of tumor suppressor mechanisms.

p53 is poorly understood. Gene alterations in TP53 in melanocytic tumors are rare, ranging from 1% to 5% in primary and 11% to 25% in metastatic melanoma.[18] However, p53 is overexpressed at a highly variable rate in tissue of cutaneous melanoma (0 to 66%). Therefore, it seems that p53 is more commonly overexpressed, rather than mutated, in melanoma.

Apaf-1

Another regulator of apoptosis and member of the intrinsic pathway, Apaf-1, displays low protein levels in 52% of metastatic melanoma cell lines and in 42% of melanoma specimens.[19] Because Apaf-1 is a downstream effect of p53 in DNA damage-induced apoptosis and binds cytochrome c for execution of caspase mediated cell death, its efficacy in inducing apoptosis is dramatically reduced (see Fig 21–2). Inactivation of Apaf-1 occurs via loss of heterozygosity (LOH) or methylation of CpG islands. LOH is significantly more prevalent in metastatic melanoma than in primary melanoma, suggesting that loss of Apaf-1 is more important in progression than initiation of melanoma. Silencing of Apaf-1 through methylation of CpG islands is related to resistance to chemotherapeutic agents like doxorubicin. Individualized therapy will help in identifying patients with particular alterations in pro- or anti-apoptotic proteins.

Toward Progression and Metastasis

Besides acquisition of apoptosis resistance, the downregulation of tumor suppressive mechanisms and amplification of signaling proteins are key events in driving transformation and progression (see Fig 21–3). As outlined above, inactivation of p16^{INK4A} and p14^{ARF} are ways to circumvent the senescence barrier, and this is depicted graphically in Figures 21–1 and 21–3.

Phosphatidylinositol-3-Kinase (PI3K)-AKT Pathway

Mutations in the phosphatidylinositol-3-kinase (PI3K)-AKT pathway, a pathway implicated in cell proliferation, cell cycle progression, and angiogenesis through activation by growth signals enable unlimited proliferation, survival, and metastasis of immortalized melanocytes (see Fig 21–1). RTKs, like c-kit, signal through RAS, activating PI3K.

PTEN

A main element of the PI3K-AKT signal transduction pathway is the tumor suppressor, phosphatase and tensin homolog (PTEN). PTEN was identified from a region in chromosome 10 (10q23-24) that is frequently lost in melanomas. The lipid and protein phosphatase negatively regulates extracellular growth signals that are transmitted via the PI3K-AKT pathway. PI3K phosphorylates phosphoinositides in the plasma membrane and PTEN antagonizes PI3K activity by dephosphorylating phosphatidylinositol triphosphate.

Almost all benign and dysplastic nevi express PTEN, and approximately 30% to 45% of melanoma cell lines and 5% to 15% of uncultured tumor material carry homozygous deletions or inactivating PTEN mutations.[20] Interestingly, NRAS and PTEN mutations are mutually exclusive in melanoma specimens, similar to what is observed for NRAS and BRAF mutations. Conversely, BRAF and PTEN mutations coexist in more than 20% of the tumors. Activation of both the ERK and AKT pathways by RAS explains the occurrence of single mutations of NRAS, but combined mutations of BRAF and PTEN downstream of RAS.

Loss of PTEN activity leaves the PI3K-AKT pathway without threshold, resulting in increased signaling through the phosphoinositol-AKT axis (see Fig 21–1). There are three isoforms of AKT, and DNA copy gains at the AKT3 locus are instrumental for increased AKT activity. Forty to 60% of melanomas show amplifications of AKT3. Higher activity of AKT3 is responsible for progression to a more aggressive tumor.[21] Introduction of AKT into radial growth melanoma cells results in transformation to vertical growth melanoma. Finally, phosphorylated AKT increases dramatically with progression and is inversely correlated with patient survival.

mTOR

Downstream of AKT lies mammalian target of rapamycin (mTOR), which is named for being the cellular target of rapamycin. mTOR controls protein translation, and is therefore involved in the regulation of proliferation, angiogenesis, and cell-cycle progression (see Figs 21–1 and 21–3). Executive signals in the PI3K-Akt pathway rely on the subsequent activation of mTOR and explain its implications for melanoma progression. Additionally, up to 70% of human melanoma cell lines show activated mTOR.[22]

Impact of IGFBP7

BRAF^{V600E}-mediated senescence is a critical step that prevents normal melanocytes form proceeding to fully transformed cells. The nonuniform expression of genetically altered p16^{INK4A}, which otherwise would prevent BRAF-mutated melanocytes to senesce, demanded an explanation regarding mechanisms of senescence induction in BRAF activated melanocytes (see Fig 21–3). Insulin growth factor binding protein 7 (IGFBP7), a secreted protein with some homology to insulin growth factor binding proteins, has been identified as a senescence and apoptosis-inducing factor required for BRAF^{V600E}-mediated senescence (see Fig 21–3).[23] Nevi harboring BRAF^{V600E} mutations express high levels of IGFBP7. Because

IGFBP7 is a secreted protein, neighboring cells are also protected by its tumor suppressing effect. Unlike nevi, BRAFV600E-positive melanomas do not express IGFBP7, allowing escape from senescence. Loss of IGFBP7 in those melanomas results from epigenetic silencing involving promoter hypermethylation.

Changes in Cell-Cell Communication

Under normal physiologic conditions, melanocytes and keratinocytes form the epidermal melanin unit in the epidermis. The pigment producing melanocytes are interspersed among every 5 to 10 basal keratinocytes. Despite the dynamic nature of epidermal shedding, involving constant growth, differentiation, and vertical migration of keratinocytes, proliferation of melanocytes is strictly controlled and rarely observed under physiologic conditions. The undifferentiated keratinocytes of the basal layer regulate melanocyte growth, number of dendrites, and expression of cell surface molecules, providing evidence that this highly ordered organizational pattern serves as the structural basis for intercellular regulation. Based on these biological observations, it can be suggested that the dynamic changes in cell-cell communication play a critical role in cell growth and invasion during transformation.

Cadherins

Adherens junctions are contacts between adjacent epithelial cells and are anchored to the cytoskeleton. Cadherins traverse the membrane, associating with cadherins on adjacent cells in a calcium-dependent manner (Fig 21–4). On the cytoplasmic side, β-catenin connects to the cadherin tail and associates with α-catenin, which in turn binds to actin. Loss or alteration of these components leads to premalignant phenotypes and tumorigenesis. Of these components, E-cadherin has been a particular target of study, as this molecule is lost in many types of tumors.

E-cadherin serves as the major adhesion mediator between epidermal melanocytes and keratinocytes. Melanocytes, but not nevus cells or melanoma cells, express E-cadherin. Loss of E-cadherin is one of the critical steps in progression of melanoma, triggering the release of cancer cells from the primary site.[24] Significant downregulation of E-cadherin is observed frequently in melanoma cell lines but does not involve mutations in the E-cadherin gene. Released melanocytic cells escape from neighboring keratinocytes to invade the dermis. In the dermis, melanocytic cells acquire expression of N-cadherin, which allows for easier dissemination and communication with N-cadherin expressing fibroblasts. The cadherin switch from E-cadherin to N-cadherin represents a main event in melanoma progression.

Beta-Catenin

Beta-catenin is a key component of the canonical Wnt signaling transduction pathway. Signaling through this pathway controls a wide range of cellular functions. In the absence of a Wnt signal, free β-catenin binds to a destruction complex with the proteins adenomatous polyposis coli (APC), Axin, protein phosphatase 2A (PP2A), and glycogen synthase kinase 3b (GSK3b), as depicted in Figure 21–4.

GSK3b-mediated phosphorylation of specific regulatory sites at the N-terminus of β-catenin marks the protein for ubiquitylation and subsequent proteasomal degradation. Upon binding of an appropriate Wnt factor to its receptor, the activity of GSK-3b is inhibited, and β-catenin accumulates in the cytoplasm. Beta-catenin shuttles to the nucleus where it acts as an essential transcriptional co-activator of proteins of the T-cell factor (Tcf)/lymphoid enhancer factor (Lef) family. Nuclear and/or cytoplasmic localization of β-catenin is a potential indicator of Wnt pathway activation and has been found in approximately one third of melanoma specimens. In an early report, mutations in the β-catenin gene (*CTNNB1*) were found in 6 of 26 melanoma cell lines (23%).[25]

These mutations all affected phosphorylation sites (Ser33, Ser37, Thr41, and Ser45) at the N-terminal domain of β-catenin, rendering the protein resistant to degradation by the ubiquitin-proteasome pathway. However, several later studies have shown significantly lower mutation rates (2 to 8%) in primary

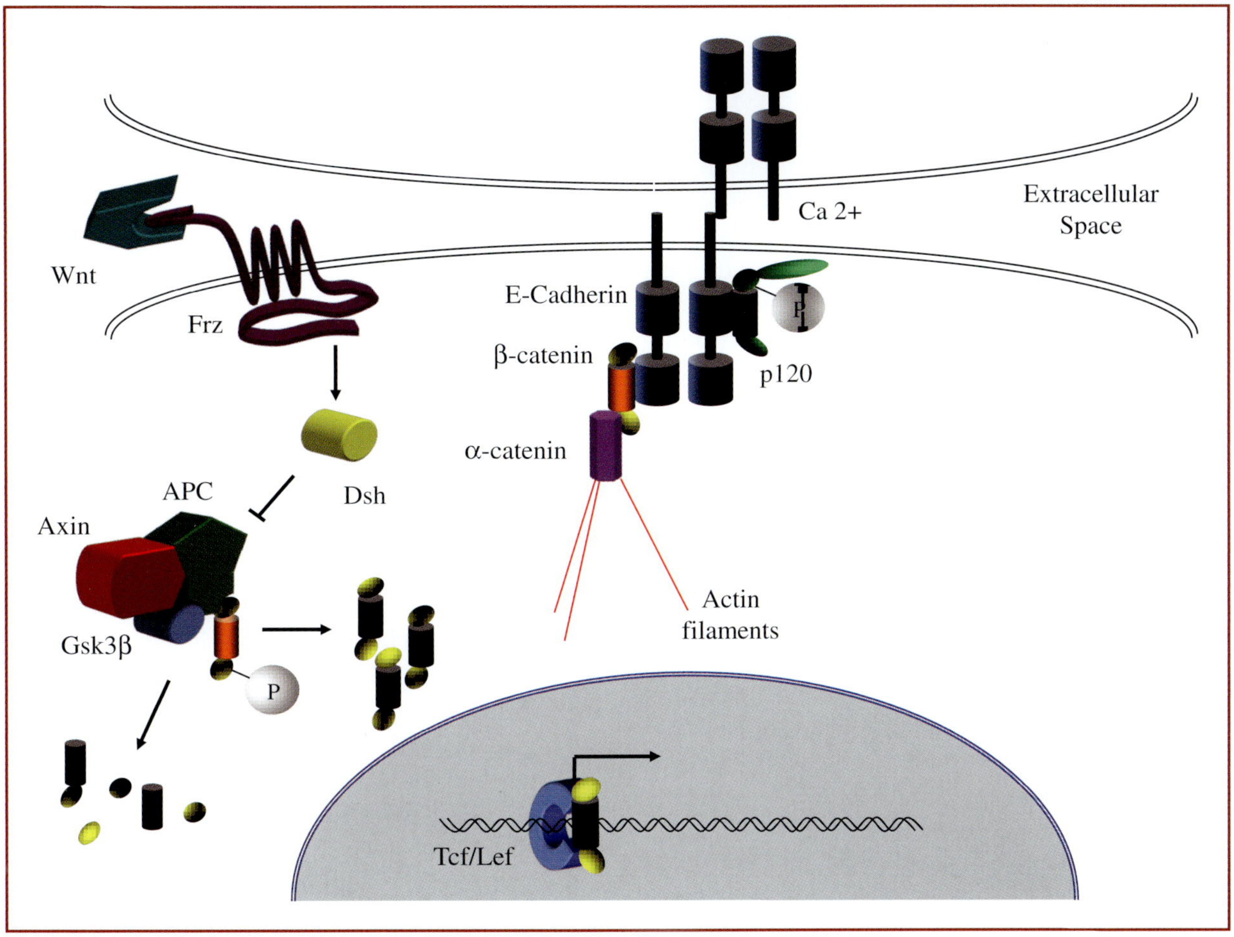

Figure 21–4. The β-catenin pathway. Signals from Wnt proteins are transmitted via G-protein-coupled receptors (Frizzled, Frz), leading to inactivation of GSK3 and accumulation of β-catenin, which then translocates to the nucleus where it increases the expression of several genes important for cell proliferation. E-cadherin is the essential part of an adherens junction. In the cytoplasm β-catenin binds to E-cadherin and to α-catenin.

melanomas, metastases, and cell lines, suggesting that activating mutation of *CTNNB1* is a rare cause of dysregulated β-catenin signaling in melanoma.[26,27] In the remaining cases, dysregulation might be caused by mutations in other components of the canonical Wnt signaling pathway, including *APC*.

Germline *APC* mutations segregate in families with adenomatous polyposis, and truncating *APC* mutations have been found in a large fraction of sporadic colorectal cancers. In a systematic analysis of the entire coding region of *APC* in melanoma cell lines, truncating mutations in this gene were found to be rare. On the other hand, hypermethylation of *APC* promoter 1A was present in 15% of melanoma biopsies and cell lines.[28] Interestingly, although melanoma cells carrying a truncating *APC* mutation showed highly increased expression from endogenous and ectopic β-catenin/Tcf-responsive target genes, similar to cell lines with *CTNNB1* mutations, cell lines harboring *APC* hypermethylation showed no evidence of increased Wnt signaling. The genetic basis for dysregulated β-catenin signaling in melanomas without activating *CTNNB1* or truncating *APC* mutations remains unknown.

Notch-1

Notch genes are evolutionarily conserved transmembrane receptors. Signaling is initiated on binding of membrane-bound ligands on the sending cell to one of four Notch receptors (1–4) on the receiving cell. Notch receptors are composed of two subunits, which are linked through calcium-dependent, noncovalent interactions in the cell membrane. On ligand binding, two proteolytic events occur to liberate the active intracellular Notch. The intracellular Notch protein is targeted to the nucleus by its nuclear localization sequence. Within the nucleus, Notch assembles into a transcriptional activation complex that targets a broad range of genes implicated in cell cycle regulation and lineage-specificity.

In melanoma cell lines and tissue, Notch1 signaling is elevated. Notch1 expression is controlled by both the PI3K/AKT pathway and by tissue hypoxia through HIF-1a.[29] Transformation of melanocytes through Akt is Notch1-dependent and Notch1 constitutes a driving event in melanocyte transformation. Furthermore, Notch1 pathway activation leads to increased signaling through the RAS-RAF-MEK-ERK pathway as well as PI3K/AKT pathway and upregulation of N-cadherin expression.[30] These events lead to higher aggressiveness of melanoma cells shifting toward metastatic capability.

Epithelial-Mesenchymal Transcriptional Regulators

Repression of *CDH1*, the gene encoding E-cadherin, is a crucial and initial step in dissociation and migration of melanoma cells from the primary site of tumor development. Signaling factors govern the continuous repression of E-cadherin to facilitate tumor progression. This is accomplished through transcription factors, such as the Snail and basic helix-loop-helix (bHLH) families, which strongly repress *CDH1* and other genes that encode integrins, cytokeratins and occludin, among others. These often are cited as epithelial-mesenchymal transcriptional regulators (EMTRs), and known representatives include Snail and Slug of the Snail family and Twist of the bHLH family. Sequence-specific DNA-binding domains that recognize consensus E2-box type elements exist in all three EMTRs.

Besides other genes containing "E-boxes," cadherins are supposedly regulated by specific binding of EMTRs to such "E-boxes." This has been demonstrated for mouse Snail that binds to the promoter and represses expression of CDH1. Following expression of Snail in epithelial cell lines, E-cadherin is downregulated and the cells become mesenchymal and migratory. Likewise, transient transfection of a Snail expression plasmid into human primary melanocytes led to significant down-regulation of E-cadherin.[31] Increasing evidence indicates that Snail family proteins are upregulated in invasive melanoma and that this is functionally important for the invasive and metastatic potential of the disease.

Snail proteins are able to decrease E-cadherin, occludin, and claudin expression while elevating N-cadherin levels, thereby favoring the interaction of melanoma cells with stromal cells and not keratinocytes. Furthermore, Snail coordinately regulates the expression of cell motility genes, including MMP-2, SPARC, TIMP-1, and RhoA. The increased activity of Snail family proteins in invasive melanoma mimics the activation of these factors during the migration of melanocyte precursor neural crest cells during development. Expression of the Snail-related factor, Slug, in melanocytes has been proposed as a reason why it is easier to generate metastatic tumors from melanocytes than other nontransformed cells using defined genetic lesions.[32]

The Melanocytic Stem Cell

The linear melanoma progression model does not account for the fact that more than half of all cutaneous melanomas arise from normal-appearing skin. A distinct cell population with stem cell properties residing within the dermis may acquire mutations that convert them to atypical melanocytic cells. Such a subpopulation may not follow the classical progression of melanoma development, but rather emerges to a specific stage without progressing through intermediates. Those cells are characterized by the expression of stem-cell markers and may represent cancer stem cells, which are self-renewing and tumor initiating. With support from the tumor microenvironment, melanoma stem cells show high tumorigenicity and are able to metastasize.

Four subpopulations of melanoma-initiating cells have been identified thus far: CD20⁺, CD133⁺, side-population cells and label-retaining cells (Fig 21–5). Whether these are distinct or overlapping populations and represent the true tumor-initiating cells remains to be determined. Classification of each subpopulation for the expression of cell-surface molecules will allow determining their usefulness as prognostic indicators. Furthermore, because of their drug resistance and slow-cycling status, therapeutic strategies aiming to destroy these cells are at high demand to conquer the disease.

CD20

Melanoma spheres generated from melanoma cells in embryonic stem cell-based media show remarkable capacity to differentiate into multiple mesenchymal lineages, including adipocytes, chondrocytes, and osteoblasts.[33] A subpopulation of melanoma spheres was found to consistently express CD20, although still maintaining melanoma-associated markers like MCAM and b3 integrin. CD20 is a cell surface marker expressed on B cells. CD20⁺ sphere cells can rapidly

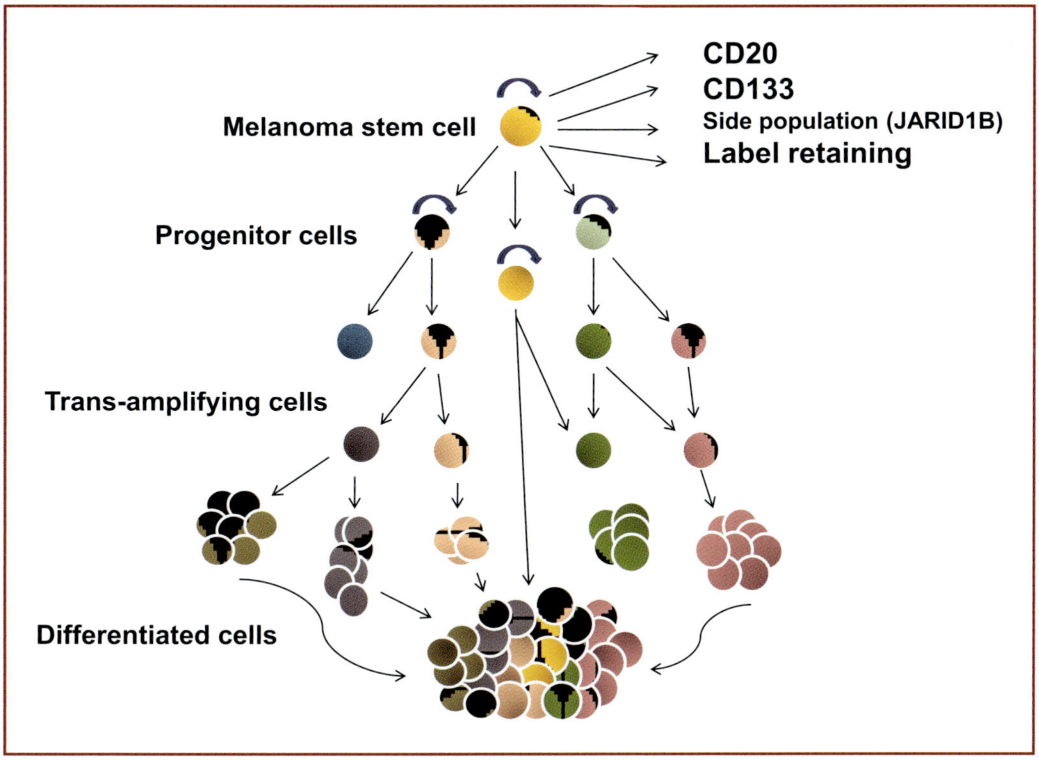

Figure 21–5. Tumor heterogeneity is supported by melanoma stem cells. Known and novel stem-cell markers such as CD20 or CD133 and stem-cell characteristics, including side-population (JARID1B) and label-retaining cells that have been distinguished in melanoma. Self-renewing melanoma stem cells sustain the stem-cell population while giving rise to progenitor cells that may or may not attain the capacity to self-renew. These progenitor and trans-amplifying cells can give rise to differentiating clones of varying dominance that contribute to the overall tumor heterogeneity found in melanomas.

proliferate, preserve their differentiating potential into mesenchymal lineages, and may be found in melanoma tissue.

CD133

CD133, a transmembrane glycoprotein, is expressed on undifferentiated cells like hematopoietic stem cells, fetal brainstem cells, and endothelial progenitor cells. In certain solid tumors like brain, prostate, and pancreatic cancers, CD133 has been exploited to identify cancer stem cells, and it appears that both normal and cancer stem cells are marked by the protein. Primary human melanocytes and melanomas express CD133 cells in about 0.2% to 2% of samples, respectively, thereby identifying a distinct subset of cells with this stem-cell marker.[34] In vivo, only the CD133+ fraction induces tumors, whereas CD133– cells fail to produce tumors.

Side-Population Cells

Like in hematopoietic stem cells, a fraction of melanoma cells, so called side-population (SP) cells, have been identified. In melanomas, a population of cells that show higher efflux of the fluorescent vital DNA binding dye, Hoechst 33342, than the other cells represents this subpopulation.[35] The SP phenotype is characterized by the expression of ABC transporters, which mediate drug resistance. In primary human melanocytes, melanomas, and cisplatin-resistant melanoma cells, ABC transporters are co-expressed with CD133, indicating that $ABC^{+}/CD133^{+}$ marks a subpopulation of melanoma cells that may harbor properties of cancer stem cells.

Label-Retaining Cells

Stem cells are undifferentiated, infrequently dividing cells that normally remain quiescent. Slow-cycling, label-retaining cells have defined the location of stem cells from tissues. In cultured melanoma cells utilizing the fluorescent dye CTO as a label to segregate and monitor proliferation, a subset of cells can be identified that also shows high efflux activities. These combined properties are useful to identify cells that not only are resistant to chemotherapeutic agents but also unaffected by drugs that block proliferation pathways.

Recently, JARID1B, a member of histone 3K4 (H3K4) demethylases, was identified in a small subpopulation of slow-cycling label-retaining melanoma cells.[36] Silencing of JARID1B in this subpopulation led to a steady decline of melanoma growth after several passages in immunodeficient mice indicating that the JARID1B-positive subpopulation is essential for continuous tumor growth. Moreover, the expression of JARID1B is dynamically regulated, because JARID1B-negative melanoma cells can become JARID1B-positive, suggesting a new model of melanoma heterogeneity in which temporarily distinct subpopulations determine tumor maintenance.

Conclusions

Our understanding of the molecular mechanisms in the pathogenesis of melanoma has increased tremendously over the last few years. This is based primarily on the fact that new techniques have allowed the identification of genetic fingerprints at the level of primary melanomas and early metastases more quickly. The future holds great promise in that more melanoma-associated mRNA alterations may be discovered through global studies of transcript structure. Genetic alterations as surrogate markers for disease progression are fueling the pipeline for new agents, which may be useful as a target for molecular therapy. However, we are far from a complete perception of the biology underlying the multiple genetic hits, as well as the clinical significance of these findings. To this end, combined efforts of basic and clinical researchers are necessary to gain comprehensive insights into melanomagenesis.

References

1. Demunter A, Stas M, Degreef H, De Wolf-Peeters C, Van Den Oord JJ. Analysis of N- and K-ras mutations in the

distinctive tumor progression of melanoma. *J Invest Dermatol.* 2001;117(6):1483–1489.

2. Pollock PM, Meltzer PS. A genome-based strategy uncovers frequent BRAF mutations in melanoma. *Cancer Cell.* 2002;2(1):5–7.
3. Goel VK, Lazar AJ, Warneke CL, Redston MS, Haluska FG. Examination of mutations in BRAF, NRAS, and PTEN in primary cutaneous melanoma. *J Invest Dermatol.* 2006;126(1):154–160.
4. Van Raamsdonk CD, Bezrookove V, Green G, et al. Frequent somatic mutations of GNAQ in uveal melanoma and blue naevi. *Nature.* 2009;457(7229):599–602.
5. Berking C, Takemoto R, Satyamoorthy K, et al. Induction of melanoma phenotype in human skin by growth factors and ultraviolet B. *Cancer Res.* 2004;64(3):807–811.
6. Spritz RA, Giebel LB, Holmes SA. Dominant negative and loss of function mutations of the c-kit (mast/stem cell growth factor receptor) proto-oncogene in human piebaldism. *Am J Hum Genet.* 1992;50(2):261–269.
7. Curtin JA, Busam K, Pinkel D, Bastian BC. Somatic activation of KIT in distinct subtypes of melanoma. *J Clin Oncol.* 2006;24(26):4340–4346.
8. Vanbrocklin MW, Robinson JP, Whitwam T, et al. Met amplification and tumor progression in Cdkn2a-deficient melanocytes. *Pigment Cell Melanoma Res.* 2009;22(4):454–460.
9. Puri N, Ahmed S, Janamanchi V, et al. c-Met is a potentially new therapeutic target for treatment of human melanoma. *Clin Cancer Res.* 2007;13(7):2246–2253.
10. Sharpless E, Chin L. The INK4a/ARF locus and melanoma. *Oncogene.* 2003;22(20):3092–3098.
11. Holland EA, Schmid H, Kefford RF, Mann GJ. CDKN2A [P16(INK4a)] and CDK4 mutation analysis in 131 Australian melanoma probands: effect of family history and multiple primary melanomas. *Genes Chromosom Cancer.* 1999;25(4):339–348.
12. Freedberg DE, Rigas SH, Russak J, et al. Frequent p16-independent inactivation of $p14^{ARF}$ in human melanoma. *J Natl Cancer Inst.* 2008;100(11):784–795.
13. Molven A, Grimstvedt MB, Steine SJ, et al. A large Norwegian family with inherited malignant melanomas, multiple atypical nevi, and CDK4 mutation. *Genes Chromosom Cancer.* 2005;44(1):10–18.
14. Stratigos AJ, Dimisianos G, Nikolaou V, et al. Melanocortin receptor-1 gene polymorphisms and the risk of cutaneous melanoma in a low-risk southern European population. *J Invest Dermatol.* 2006;126(8):1842–1849.
15. Garraway LA, Widlund HR, Rubin MA, et al. Integrative genomic analyses identify MITF as a lineage survival oncogene amplified in malignant melanoma. *Nature.* 2005;436(7047):117–122.
16. Sauter ER, Yeo UC, von Stemm A, et al. Cyclin D1 is a candidate oncogene in cutaneous melanoma. *Cancer Res.* 2002;62(11):3200–3206.
17. Jansen B, Schlagbauer-Wadl H, Brown BD, et al. BCL-2 antisense therapy chemosensitizes human melanoma in SCID mice. *Nat Med.* 1998;4(2):232–243.
18. Akslen IA, Monstad SE, Larsen B, Straume O, Ogreid D. Frequent mutations of the p53 gene in cutaneous melanoma of the nodular type. *Int J Cancer.* 1998;79(1):91–95.
19. Soengas MS, Capodieci P, Polsky D, et al. Inactivation of the apoptosis effector Apaf-1 in malignant melanoma. *Nature.* 2001;409(6817):207–211.
20. Tsao H, Zhang X, Benoit E, Haluska FG. Identification of PTEN/MMAC1 alterations in uncultured melanomas and melanoma cell lines. *Oncogene.* 1998;16(26):3397–3402.
21. Stahl JM, Sharma A, Cheung M, et al. Deregulated Akt3 activity promotes development of malignant melanoma. *Cancer Res.* 2004;64(19):7002–7010.
22. Karbowniczek M, Spittle CS, Morrison T, Wu H, Henske EP. mTOR is activated in the majority of malignant melanomas. *J Invest Dermatol.* 2008;128(4):980–987.
23. Waiapeyee N, Serra RW, Zhu X, Mahalingam M, Green MR. Oncogenic BRAF induces senescence and apoptosis through pathways mediated by the secreted protein IGFBP7. *Cell.* 2008;132(3):363–374.
24. Li G, Schaider H, Satyamoorthy K, Hanakawa J, Hashimoto K, Herlyn M. Downregulation of E-cadherin and Desmoglein 1 by autocrine hepatocyte growth factor during melanoma development. *Oncogene.* 2001;20(56): 8125–8135.
25. Rubinfeld B, Robbins P, El-Gamil M, Albert I, Porfiri E, Polakis P. Stabilization of beta-catenin by genetic defects in melanoma cell lines. *Science.* 1997;275(5307):1790–1792.
26. Rimm DL, Caca K, Hu G, Harrison FB, Fearon ER. Frequent nuclear/cytoplasmic localization of beta-catenin without exon 3 mutations in malignant melanoma. *Am J Pathol.* 1999;154(2):325–329.
27. Omholt K, Platz A, Ringborg U, Hansson J. Cytoplasmic and nuclear accumulation of beta-catenin is rarely caused by CTNNB1 exon 3 mutations in cutaneous malignant melanoma. *Int J Cancer.* 2001;92(6):839–842.
28. Worm J, Christensen C, Gronbaek K, Tulchinsky EM, Guldberg P. Genetic and epigenetic alterations of the APC gene in malignant melanoma. *Oncogene.* 2004;23(30): 5215–5226.
29. Bedogni B, Warneke JA, Nickoloff BJ, Giaccia AJ, Broome Powell M. Notch 1 is an effector of Akt and hypoxia in melanoma development. *J Clin Invest.* 2008;118(11): 3660–3670.
30. Liu Z-J, Xiao M, Balint K, et al. Notch 1 signaling promotes primary melanoma progression by activating mitogen-activated protein kinase/phosphatidylinositol 3-kinase-Akt pathways and up-regulating N-cadherin expression. *Cancer Res.* 2006;66(8):4182–4190.
31. Poser I, Dominquez D, de Herreros AG, Varnai A, Buettner R, Bosserhoff AK. Loss of E-cadherin expression in melanoma cells involves up-regulation of the transcriptional repressor Snail. *J Biol Chem.* 2001;276(27):24661–24666.
32. Gupta PB, Kuperwasser C, Brunet JP, et al. The melanocyte differentiation program predisposes to metastasis after neoplastic transformation. *Nat Genet.* 2005;37(10): 1047–1054.

33. Fang D, Nguyen TK, Leishear K, et al. A tumorigenic subpopulation with stem cell properties in melanomas. *Cancer Res.* 2005;65(20):9328–9337.
34. Frank NY, Margaryan A, Huang Y, et al. ABCB5-mediated doxorubicin transport and chemoresistance in human malignant melanoma. *Cancer Res.* 2005;65(10): 4320–4333.
35. Grichnik JM, Burch JA, Schulteis RD, et al. Melanoma, a tumor based on a mutant stem cell? *J Invest Dermatol.* 2006;126(1):142–153.
36. Roesch A, Fukunaga-Kalabis M, Schmidt EC, et al. A temporarily distinct subpopulation of slow-cycling melanoma cells is required for continuous tumor growth. *Cell.* 2010;141:583–594.

22

IMMUNOBIOLOGY AND IMMUNOTHERAPY OF MELANOMA

LAUREN L. LEVY
JOHNNY KAO
ANDREW G. SIKORA

Introduction

Activating the immune system to fight cancer is not a new idea. In the late 1800s, William Coley, a prominent New York surgeon, began a clinical investigation following the observation that cancer remission was sometimes associated with high fevers.[1] He administered killed bacterial pathogens to cancer patients and observed tumor regression in some patients. Following this discovery, "Coley's toxin" was administered to several hundreds of cancer patients and a cure rate of 10% was claimed. Coley's intriguing blend of science, showmanship, and controversy proved a fitting start to the modern science of immunotherapy. Although immunotherapy has been studied as a treatment for many cancers, melanoma is probably the best known model for immunotherapy due to the tumor's notorious resistance to both chemotherapy and radiation therapy, and the tumor's expression of well-characterized produce antigens that can be recognized by the immune system.

Immunosurveillance and the Immune System's Response to Cancer

The immune system responds to foreign pathogens both to protect the host from the development of pathology, and to eliminate the pathogens from the host. An important component of this response is the ability of T cells to recognize the foreign pathogens and subsequently initiate a cellular response that either directly eliminates the pathogen or activates other cells to assist in this process. In addition to recognition of these unique pathogen-specific antigens as "foreign" by the specific antigen receptors of T and B lymphocytes, the immune system also recognizes and responds to more broadly expressed molecules known as pathogen-associated molecular patterns (PAMPS) expressed by viruses, bacteria, and other microorganisms. Recognition of these molecules is by germ line-encoded pattern-recognition receptors, the most well-known being the toll-like receptor (TLR) family.[2] Because, by these criteria, the majority of human tumors that are not of viral origin are neither "foreign" nor "dangerous," it is not surprising that the role of the immune system in preventing and treating cancer often has been mysterious, controversial, or misunderstood, as is depicted in Table 22–1.

In a manner analogous to recognition of foreign microbial antigens, T cells recognize unique, mutated, or developmentally restricted tumor-associated antigens (TAAs) expressed on tumors.[3] The theory of immune surveillance suggests that the immune system, through recognition of TAAs, controls the development and progression of spontaneous tumors by constantly surveying the host and by mounting an antitumor response sufficient to halt progression to clinically apparent disease.[4] In fact, there is evidence from both clinical studies and mouse models that the immune system is activated during the development of cancer. Immunodeficient animals have a higher rate of tumor formation than immunocompetent animals, as do "knockout" mice lacking specific immune-stimulating cytokines.[5,6] Similarly, patients who are immunosuppressed due to AIDS or antirejection therapy after solid organ transplantation have a higher (although not equally higher) rate of both virally induced and nonviral cancers, suggesting the importance of the immune system in suppressing the development of cancer.[7]

Once cancers become established, many elicit tumor-infiltrating lymphocytes (TILs), T cells that enter the tumor and have the potential to act as antitumor effector cells via direct cytotoxicity or activa-

Table 22–1. Immunology Terms

Allogeneic Vaccination	Vaccine derived from tumor cell lysates or killed tumor cells, other than patient's own tumor.
Antigen Presenting Cell (APC)	Cells that present peptides to lymphocytes initiating an immune response. Includes macrophages and dendritic cells
Autologous Vaccination	Individualized vaccines created from the patient's own tumor
CD4+ "Helper" T Cells	Cytokine producing T-lymphocytes that help coordinate the immune response
CD8+ Cytotoxic T Cells (CTL)	Cytotoxic T-lymphocytes that can have an antitumor effect
Costimulatory Molecules	Cell surface molecules that provide a "second signal" needed for T cell activation after stimulation of the TCR
Cytokines	Small soluble signaling molecules released by immune cells to coordinate the immune response
Regulatory T-cells (Tregs)	CD4+CD25+FOXP3+cells that downregulate the immune response and provide a checkpoint to prevent overactivation and autoimmunity
Toll-like Receptors (TLRs)	Pattern recognition receptors on APCs that are activated by microbial "danger" signals
Tumor Associated Antigen(TAA)	Protein expressed by the tumor that is recognized and processed by the immune system
Tumor Infiltrating Lymphocytes (TILs)	T-lymphocytes located in the tumor microenvironment

tion of other immunocytes.[8] However, the majority of established tumors continue to progress, even in the face of a brisk TIL response. Analyses of TILs often reveal dysfunctional signaling, activation, and effector function due to tumor-mediated immunosuppression.[9]

Tumor cells secrete inhibitory cytokines, soluble products that suppress the actions of the effector cells and activate regulatory immunocytes that ultimately suppress the immune response.[10] For example, immunosuppressive regulatory T cells (Tregs) are found in increased numbers in cancer patients, suggesting that these cells act to disrupt the antitumor immune response.[11,12] Additionally, tumor cells have the ability to downregulate the antigen-presentation machinery (such as major histocompatability complex (MHC) and antigen-processing proteins) used to present tumor antigens to effector T cells. Tumor cells can even induce lymphoctytes to undergo apoptosis to evade the immune system.[13] This ongoing battle between immune recognition/activation and tumor-mediated immunosuppression is crucial to understanding how the immune system can be manipulated to provide a potent and specific treatment for cancer.

Immunobiology and Melanoma

Melanoma is one of the most studied models for understanding the immunobiology and immunotherapy of cancer. Both clinical and laboratory studies demonstrate that melanoma is an immunogenic tumor and that the immune system interacts significantly with melanoma during tumor development. It has been estimated that about 10% to 20% of small melanomas undergo complete regression, suggesting a role of the immune system in thwarting tumor growth and development.[14] There is evidence of immune activation, including increased numbers of activated T lymphocytes, in tumors that do undergo clinically apparent regression.[14] The fact that approximately 2% to 5% of melanoma cases have an unknown primary site is further clinical evidence of the immune system's role in melanoma.[15] Although theoretically it is possible that unknown primary tumors originate in the lymph node, it is more likely that the primary melanoma has undergone complete spontaneous regression.[16,17] Additionally, the degree of lymphocytic infiltration is a marker for improved survival of a subset of patients.[18,19] The development of vitiligo, an autoimmune response to pigmented melanocytes, in some patients with melanoma provides further support for the role of the immune system, as this is evidence of destruction of normal melanocytes as "bystanders" in the process of eradicating malignant cells.[20–22] Several studies have reported that the appearance of vitiligo during melanoma immunotherapy predicts a better prognosis.[23–26]

Approaches to Immunotherapy

Despite the apparent immunogenicity of melanoma, numerous clinical trials directed at manipulating the immune system to cause tumor regression have had only limited success. "Success" of immunotherapy during a clinical trial generally is evaluated by the objective clinical response to therapy: the regression of existing lesions without the growth of any prior lesion or the appearance of new lesions.[27] Other criteria for evaluating the efficacy of immunotherapy—various measures of overall and progression-free survival—have been proposed to be of equal or greater significance, but are less well accepted. In the absence of compelling clinical results, many trials focus on immunologic endpoints, such as elevated numbers of tumor-specific T cells, or enhanced T cell activation. However, these endpoints serve only as proof of principle and benchmarks for improvement, as they often fail to correlate with clinical effect. The different approaches to stimulating an immune response with the intention to treat melanoma are discussed in conjunction with results from relevant clinical trials for each of the approaches. Refer to Table 22–2 and Figure 22–1 for an overview of these approaches to immunotherapy.

Vaccination

The ultimate goal of cancer vaccination is to stimulate the patient's own immune system to eradicate the tumor or retard its progression. Cancer vaccination

Table 22–2. Immunotherapeutic Strategies

Target	Mechanism of Action	Example
CD40	Stimulate APCs	CD40 monoclonal antibody
4-1BB	Amplifies T-cell response	4-1BB monoclonal antibody
Granulocyte-Macrophage Colony Stimulating Factor (GM-CSF)	Stimulates maturation of dendritic cells	Administration of the growth factor
Interferon-alpha (IFN-α)	Immune stimulation	Administered either independently or as a vaccine adjuvant
Interleukin-2 (IL-2)	T-cell growth factor	Administered independently or as a vaccine adjuvant
Interleukin-12 (IL-12)	Stimulates numerous immune cells	Administered either independently or as a vaccine adjuvant
TLR-7 TLR-9	Stimulates cytokine release; enhances APC function/activation	Imiquimod CpG DNA
CTLA-4	Immune checkpoint blockade	CTLA-4 monoclonal antibody (Tremelimumab, Ipilimumab)
Treg	Immune checkpoint blockade	Ontak

has been a source of both great hope and great disappointment for the creation of new therapeutics because therapeutic cancer vaccines differ from standard microbiologic vaccinations in that they do not prevent disease but rather stimulate the immune system with the intention of treating established disease. Vaccination as a treatment modality is attractive due to the ease of delivery and limited side effects. Despite the great enthusiasm and solid theoretical rationale supporting cancer vaccination for melanoma, numerous melanoma trials have produced only a small number of patients with solid tumors who have undergone objective cancer regression (for one commonly used approach, peptide vaccination, the response rate has been calculated to be 2.6%).[27]

Cancer vaccination requires the processing and presentation of tumor antigens by an antigen presenting cell (APC). APCs must *mature* to present an antigen to a T cell. The maturation process is induced by numerous costimulatory molecules, including TLR ligands and other PAMPS, acting through receptors on the APC. The APC presents the antigen and other necessary stimulatory molecules to cytotoxic effector CD8+ T cells (CTL). As T cells are activated and proliferate, a repertoire of effector cells that specifically respond to the tumor antigen is created. The total number of tumor-specific T cells generated is one method of quantifying the results of a clinical cancer vaccine trial. The use of numerous costimulatory molecules as vaccine adjuvants has been extensively studied and is discussed further below.

Tumor Cell-Based Melanoma Vaccines

The earliest melanoma vaccines used either allogeneic (other-derived) or autologous (self-derived) killed melanoma cells or cell lysates to induce an immune response. After taking up antigens released by the melanoma cells, APCs can present certain epitopes (antigenic determinants) of the tumor cell or lysate and initiate a T cell response.[28] The use of Canvaxin, a polyvalent whole tumor cell vaccine created from three melanoma cell lines, is one of the

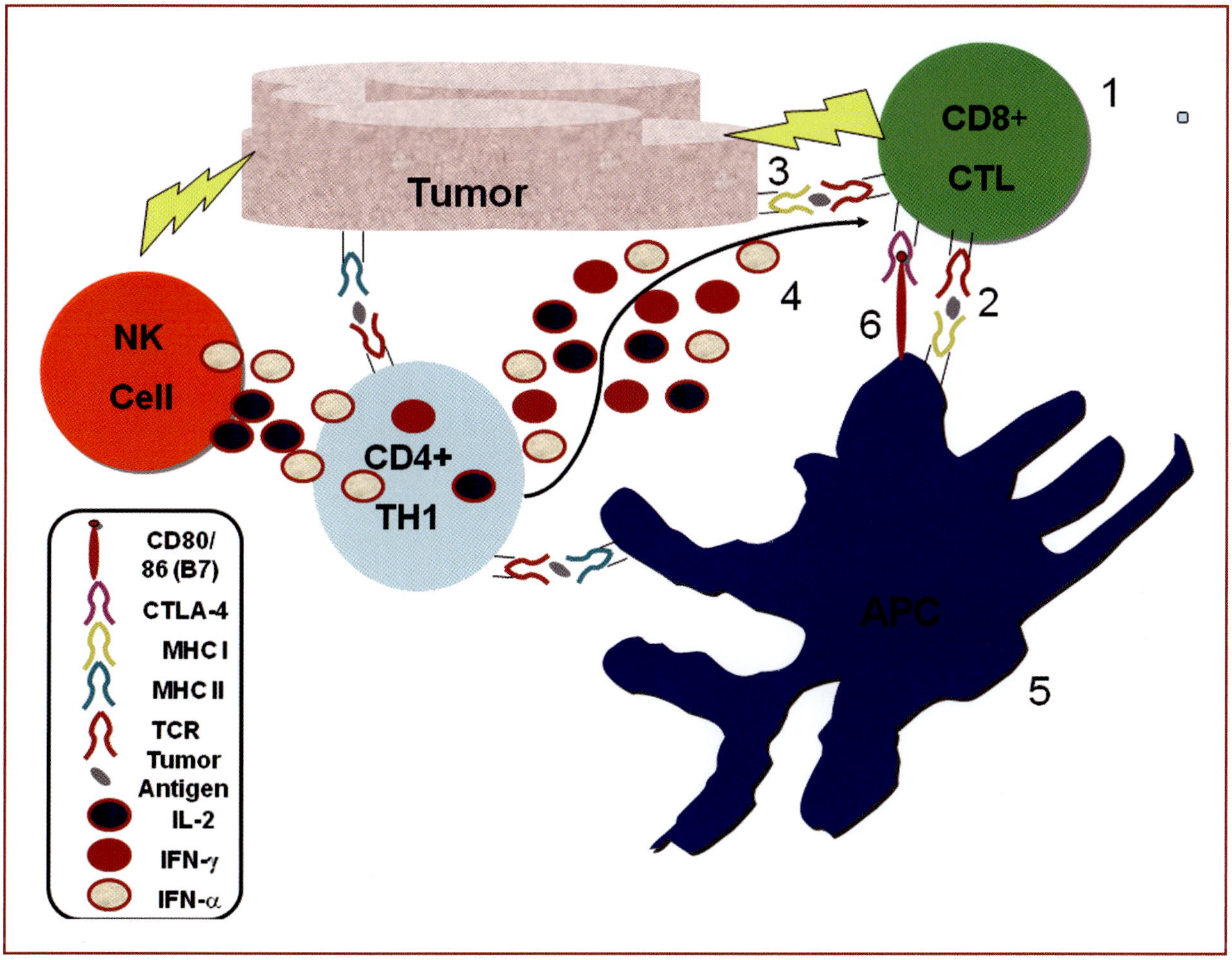

Figure 22–1. Immunotherapy sites of action at the tumor immune interface. **1.** Adoptive cytotoxic T lymphocyte cell transfer. **2.** Anti-tumor vaccination **3.** Interferon-α upregulation of MHC I-mediated antigen presentation **4.** Cytokine therapy **5.** Dendritic cell vaccination **6.** Immune checkpoint blockade. CD8+CTL-cytotoxic T lymphocyte; CD4+TH1-"helper" T cell; APC-antigen presenting cell; lightning bolt-cytolysis.

earliest whole cell vaccination clinical trials.[29] Although early studies with Canvaxin showed a modest immune response, a Phase III multicenter clinical trial demonstrated no benefit of vaccination when compared to patients receiving placebo.[30] A clinical trial using Melacine, another allogeneic whole cell vaccine, also showed no advantage over placebo.[31] The success of some whole-cell vaccines may be limited by the secretion of immunosuppressive molecules by tumor cells and the induction of tolerance.

Autologous tumor vaccines are individualized vaccines made from a patient's own tumor. Theoretically, they are more advantageous than allogeneic vaccines because they have greater specificity and may include unique mutated antigens that are not present in the standard melanoma cell lines. The creation of an autologous tumor vaccine requires a large amount of tumor tissue, which in practice may limit the use of these vaccines to patients with advanced disease.[32] The introduction of genes encoding immunostimulatory cytokines, (GM-CSF, IL-2, IL-12, IFN-α, and other cytokines) into autologous tumor cell vaccines to enhance the immune response during the processing and presentation of antigens is another area of active research.[33–35]

Melanoma-Associated Antigens

There are many well-characterized melanoma-associated peptide antigens that are processed by APCs and recognized by T cells (Table 22–3). Melanoma-associated antigens are classified as shared, present in many different tumors; or unique to a single melanoma. Shared melanoma antigens are further classified into three subgroups: differentiation antigens (expression restricted to certain cell types, such as melanocytes), tumor specific antigens (mutated or otherwise unique forms expressed only in tumors), and overexpressed antigens (expressed at higher levels in tumors compared to untransformed cells).

One of the first discovered melanoma antigens was Tyrosinase, a differentiation antigen present in all melanocytes, which catalyses the rate limiting step of melanin biosynthesis.[36] The discovery of Tyrosinase led to the identification of other differentiation antigens, proteins that are present in all melanocytes that can stimulate an immune response against melanoma. Other differentiation antigens include gp100, a core structural component of the melanosomes, and MART1/Melan-A, another melanosome protein.[37,38] Like Tyrosinase, both of these proteins can induce a T cell mediated antitumor response.

The second subgroup of melanoma-associated antigens, tumor-specific antigens, are expressed in melanoma or other cancerous cells but not in normal tissue. These antigens include mutated proteins involved in the transformation of melanocytes. These proteins potentially can be recognized as non-self by the immune system because of alterations to the normal gene. A subset of tumor-specific antigens termed cancer-testis antigens are expressed by melanoma cells and by the immune-privileged testis. MAGE-1 was the first antigen identified in this group and is present in approximately 40% of melanomas.[39]

Vaccination with mutated antigens or cancer-testis antigens is attractive as a therapeutic agent because these peptides are expressed in a large percentage of tumors without being present in normal tissue, lessening the theoretical risk of the vaccination causing autoimmunity. The last group of melanoma associated antigens is peptides overexpressed in melanoma and other cancers, but still expressed in normal tissue. Antigens in this category include CDK-4 and β-catenin, proteins involved in cellular proliferation. Developing a vaccine targeting this group of antigens is theoretically more challenging because the expression in normal tissue creates the possibility of autoimmune sequelae following vaccination.

Antigen Delivery

There are numerous strategies for introducing tumor antigens into the host with the goal of stimulating an antitumor response. One strategy is to provide peptides derived from common melanoma cell antigens, because the peptide is ultimately the "antigenic unit" recognized by T cells. In a natural immune response, antigenic proteins are degraded into smaller peptides (8–11 amino acids) by the APC. The APC then presents the peptide on a major histocompatability complex (MHC) molecule to the T cell for recognition by the T cell receptor. Tumor antigen peptides are presented on MHC class I molecules to CD8+ T cells (which generally have a

Table 22–3. Melanoma-Associated Antigens

Differentiation Antigens	Expression restricted to melanocytes or melanoma	Tyrosinase, gp100, MART-1/ Melan A, TRP-1, TRP-2, MAGE-1, MAGE-2
Tumor-Specific Antigens	Expressed only in tumors (or germ cells)	Cancer-testis antigens, MAGE 1
Overexpressed Antigens	Expressed in higher levels in transformed cells, but still present in untransformed cells	CDK-4, β-catenin,

cytotoxic function, thus are known as CTL = cytotoxic lymphocytes); or they are presented on MHC class II molecules to CD4+ T cells (most commonly, cytokine-secreting "helper" T cells). In peptide vaccination, antigenic peptides or "long" precursor peptides are provided to host cells, which either directly present them on cell-surface MHC molecules or internalize and process "long" peptides for presentation on the cell surface.

Dendritic cells are the body's most effective antigen presenting cells, and have a unique ability to potently activate and expand T cells. Because only "professional" APCs such as dendritic cells are thought to be capable of proper processing and presentation of the long peptides on the cell surface, this is one strategy for avoiding presentation by nonprofessional (and thus potentially tolerogenic APC).[40] Although immune responses to peptide vaccination are often seen, clinical trials using peptide vaccines have shown that immunologic response does not predict clinical objective response to vaccination.[41,42] Vaccination seems to be most successful in patients with melanoma confined to the skin or in the lymph nodes, rather than disseminated disease.[27] Another disadvantage of peptide vaccination is that MHC restriction limits the use of individual peptides to patients with a compatible MHC haplotype.

Another approach to antigen delivery, dendritic cell (DC) vaccination, involves differentiating DCs ex vivo from the patient's own blood precursor cells, activating them and pulsing with tumor antigens ex vivo, and re-infusing the patient's own stimulated DCs as a vaccine. Autologous dendritic cells may also be genetically engineered to express tumor antigens; genetic engineering can also be used to introduce immune-stimulating molecules to increase its ability to activate T cells.[43] Although dendritic cell vaccines are safe and produce few side effects, clinical responses are not frequently observed with vaccine administration, despite a typically robust immunologic response.[44,45] The overall clinical response rate of dendritic cell vaccine clinical trials is under 5%.

DNA vaccination is another method of antigen delivery, in which antigen-encoding DNA is cloned into a plasmid and administered to the patient. Following administration, dendritic cells and other APCs take up the DNA and present the antigen to T cells resulting in an immune response. DNA vaccination is relatively simple because DNA can be easily purified in large quantities. Additionally, the delivery of full length protein-encoding DNA produces many potential antigens that can be presented to the T cells, which avoids MHC restriction. Lastly, the DNA vectors typically contain unmethylated CpG motifs that act as immune stimulators via stimulation of TLR9.[46]

Despite the many theoretical advantages of DNA vaccination, clinical trials have produced limited success. However, there has been a report of immune response and increased survival after DNA vaccination for the tyrosinase antigen after DNA vaccination delivered to lymph nodes, rather than the skin.[47] However, a more recent trial using an intranodal DNA vaccination for a combination of three melanoma associated antigens, Melan-A, MART1, and Tyrosinase, resulted in an immune response to Melan-A, but without any evidence of clinical regression.[48]

Another approach is to utilize heat shock proteins (HSPs), which are produced by tumor cells in response to stress and contain a "snapshot" of antigenic tumor peptides. Loaded HSPs can be extracted from tumor cells and delivered into the body where they are taken up by dendritic cells for presentation of these antigens. Studies using vaccination with HSPs have concluded that vaccination is safe and well tolerated and can induce both clinical and immunogenic responses in some patients.[49,50]

The low rate of clinical efficacy of vaccination approaches, despite a high rate of immunologic response, is attributed to the active suppression of the immune system by the tumor, which ultimately renders this response ineffective and prevents tumor regression. The fact that, in a small subset of patients, clinical responses can be impressive and even lead to complete remission suggests that antitumor vaccination may be effective and that the tumor-induced immunosuppression can be reversed. In order to overcome tumor-induced immune suppression, immune stimulators have been administered, both in combination with vaccines and alone as therapeutic agents to induce tumor regression via stimulation of endogenous immunity.

Immune Stimulation

Due to the ever-present risk of autoimmunity, the immune system is regulated by many checks and balances, and multiple signals are generally required for immune activation. For example, in order for a T cell to become activated by an APC, two signals are needed: one from the antigen itself and one from a costimulatory molecule, such as the cell surface molecule B7. In the absence of a second signal, stimulation through the TCR renders a T cell anergic, or unresponsive, rather than triggering activation. Thus, manipulation of molecules responsible for up- or downregulating immune activation for the treatment of melanoma is a very active area of research.

Dendritic cells and other antigen presenting cells can be stimulated through engagement of the cell surface molecule CD40 by its natural ligand expressed on T cells, or by monoclonal antibodies, making them "mature" or "activated," and better at presenting antigens to T cells. The first clinical trial using a CD40 monoclonal antibody for patients with melanoma resulted in a partial response rate of 27%, which was attributed to immune stimulation.[51] Additionally, CD40 is expressed on some human melanoma cell surfaces and the stimulation of this receptor may indirectly result in tumor immunity through the induction of apoptosis and release of tumor antigens.[52]

The interaction between 4-1BB (CD137) and 4-1BB ligand serves as another costimulatory pathway, which helps to activate and amplify the T cell response. 4-1BB is expressed on T cells, natural killer cells, and dendritic cells and other antigen presenting cells.[53] Activation of this pathway leads to an increase in the Th1 cytokine response, increased IL-2 production, increased numbers of cytotoxic T cells, and elevated levels of T cell effector molecules, such as perforin.[54,55] Preclinical murine studies demonstrate that delivering monoclonal antibodies to the 4-1BB receptor can result in tumor regression.[56] Subsequently, an antibody to the CD137 receptor (BMS-663513) has been created, and preliminary clinical studies suggest that the antibody is well tolerated and capable of inducing both immunologic and clinical responses, with toxicity limited to mild autoimmune events.[57] Based on these results, a Phase II trial using this monoclonal antibody has been initiated.[58]

Toll-like receptors (TLRs), plus receptors for other PAMPs, provide another class of targets for immune-stimulating agents and represent the modern-day legacy of Coley's experiments with unfractionated pathogens. The TLRs most studied for cancer applications are TLR9 and TLR7. TLR 9 is expressed on antigen presenting cells such as dendritic cells and, when stimulated, increases cytokine production and enhances the ability of dendritic cells to activate T cells via increased expression of costimulatory molecules. TLR9 is activated by unmethylated CpG DNA located in bacteria or in plasmids of bacterial origin. However, CpG DNA can also be directly administered as an immune adjuvant to enhance the immune response. CPG7909 is a synthetic oligo - nucelotide that stimulates the TLR9 receptor. This approach has been studied alone, and in combination with peptide vaccination and has shown both immunologic and some limited clinical efficacy.[59] Imiquimod, a topical TLR7 agonist, has also been used to treat malignant melanoma in situ in patients presenting with lesions on the head and neck.[60]

Immunostimulatory Cytokines

Cytokines, small signaling molecules that coordinate immune responses, also can be used as therapeutic agents. In fact, the only two FDA-approved immunotherapeutic agents in the United States, Interleukin-2 (IL-2) and Interferon-α (IFN-α) are both cytokines. In a manner similar to costimulatory molecules, cytokines can be administered either as a monotherapy or in combination with vaccines to obtain a greater immune response.

Interferon-α

IFN-α was the first cytokine to demonstrate antitumor activity against melanoma. IFN-α has both direct antitumor effects and indirect effects through stimulation of the immune system by promoting the growth, differentiation, and effector function of various immunocytes.[61] Interferon activates effector cells of the immune system by increasing the numbers of natural killer cells, activating macrophages, and stimulating the activation and differentiation of anti-tumor T cells. The ability of lymphocytes to recognize and kill melanoma cells also is enhanced by IFN-α due to upregulation of the MHC I receptor and adhesion molecules on tumor cells. IFN-α also has antiangiogenic properties, thus adding to its direct antitumor effect.[62]

Clinical trials showing an increase in relapse free survival following treatment with high dose IFN-α prompted US FDA approval of the drug as adjuvant therapy for high-risk melanoma.[63] However, the benefits of IFN-α are both modest and unpedictable, and side effects can be considerable and sometimes fatal.[64] The first clinical trials using a long-term low dose regimen of IFN-α showed a lower incidence of relapse during treatment that equilibrated to the relapse incidence of the controls on discontinuation.[65] Further studies with low dose regimens indicated that patients with a worse prognosis responded better to IFN-α.[66]

However, it was the results from a high dose regimen trial that lead to the approval of IFN-α by the FDA. This randomized, controlled trial performed by the Eastern Cooperative Oncology Group (ECOG) administered the maximum tolerated dose of interferon for one month followed by a smaller dose for 48 weeks in patients with stage IIB/III melanoma following resection.[63] Patients who received the treatment had an increased relapse-free survival and overall survival, providing evidence that IFN-α could be a beneficial therapeutic. Further trials that compared differing doses of interferon with observation confirmed that high dose interferon results in increased disease-free survival, but failed to show an overall survival benefit.[67] Pooled analyses of the approximately 2000 patients who have participated in high dose trials using IFN-α as an adjuvant therapy following resection concluded that there is strong evidence that this treatment regimen improves recurrence-free survival and modestly improves overall survival.[68]

The positive results of these clinical trials for a subset of patients have challenged researchers to understand how to predict which patients will respond to therapy, as side effects include severe flulike symptoms, fatigue, hepatotoxicity, and psychiatric symptoms.[69,70] One predictor of the success of IFN-α therapy is the development of an auto-immune response, including thyroid dysfunction, vitiligo, or the presence of autoantibodies.[25,71] Unfortunately, because autoimmunity develops after the treatment begins, the phenomenon cannot be used to identify potential responders prior to treatment initiation. Another study of serum biomarkers after IFN-α therapy demonstrated decreased levels of immunosuppressive cytokines and tumor angiogenic growth factors and an increase in antiangiogenic factors in responders. Additionally, patients who had a significant increase in recurrence-free survival following high dose interferon intervention had higher pretreatment levels of proinflammatory cytokines IL-6, IL-1, and TNF, thus suggesting that proinflammatory cytokines are a potential predictor of favorable prognostic outcome following immunotherapy.[72,73]

The success of IFN-α as a single therapeutic agent prompted trials of its use in conjunction with vaccination. A randomized trial that administered a ganglioside vaccine either alone or in combination with high-dose IFN-α showed comparable antibody response among all groups, but a trend towards better relapse-free survival for patients receiving IFN-α.[74] Another study administered IFN- α to patients with metastatic melanoma who had previously failed to respond to vaccination wit Melacine. Five patients had a complete response and three other patients had a partial response. There was an increase in T cell response in the patients who had undergone complete regression, suggesting that IFN-α augments the initial response begun by vaccination.[75] The combination of IFN-α with melanoma peptides gp100 and Melan-A for patients with metastatic melanoma resulted in increased numbers of T cells recognizing these peptides, and some patients had a prolonged disease-free survival.[76] Thus, trials using interferon alpha-2b in combination with various vaccination regimens have shown promising results, but further studies are needed to validate the proper dose of the interferon and the best vaccination strategy that should be used for this therapy.

Interleukin-2

Interleukin-2 (IL-2) is a growth factor that supports T cell proliferation and has shown antitumor activity. IL-2 administered exogenously has clinical efficacy for patients with metastatic melanoma and is the only agent FDA-approved for patients with nonresectable metastatic melanoma. The pooled data of IL-2 administration shows an objective response rate of 16%, with 6% of patients having a complete response and 10% of patients having a partial response.[77] Additionally, 44% of responders remained alive with most having disease and progression free survival after follow-up at 6 years. IL-2 is thought to cure a selected subgroup of patients because some patients undergo immune-mediated eradication of disease.

IL-2 efficacy is dose dependent, and higher doses are associated with better response rate and longer duration of response. However, severe dose-limiting side effects of therapy include hypotension, cardiac arrhythmias, pulmonary edema, and fever. IL-2 toxicity resembles bacterial sepsis due to the release of numerous proinflammatory cytokines, thus administration must occur under physician supervision usually in a hospital. IL-2 therapy is recommended only for patients who have maintained good organ function.

Predicting which patients will have a favorable prognosis following treatment with IL-2 is a confusing yet important subject of research.[77] The development of autoimmune dysfunction during treatment, such as vitiligo or thyroid dysfunction may be a predictor of a favorable outcome.[78] A recent clinical study shows that elevated serum levels of VEGF predict lack of clinical response to IL-2 therapy, thus suggesting that inflammatory/angiogenic biomarkers may have some value in predicting therapeutic success.[79] Gene expression profiles of melanoma tumors have also been examined to understand whether the genetic composition of different tumors influences treatment efficacy.[80,81]

As IL-2 is a potent immune stimulator, it has been used as an adjuvant in numerous melanoma vaccine clinical trials with mixed results.[82–85] Despite many disappointing outcomes, a recent phase III trial from MD Anderson Cancer Center found that patients treated with IL-2 and a peptide vaccine, gp100:209–217, had a response rate of 22.9% and progression-free survival of 2.9 months compared to a response rate of 9.6% and 1.6 month progression-free survival in the group receiving only IL-2, thus supporting continued research on the combination of vaccination with IL-2 therapy.[86]

Granulocyte-Macrophage Colony Stimulating Factor (GM-CSF)

Granulocyte-macrophage colony stimulating factor (GM-CSF) increases the number of dendritic cells and aids in the maturation of these cells, making this molecule a potent activator of the immune system. GM-CSF in combination with cancer vaccines has been the subject of numerous clinical trials, with mixed results.[87,88] Overall, studies suggest that GM-CSF enhances the immunogenicity of vaccines because patients receiving vaccines with GM-CSF had increased numbers of lymphocytes infiltrating tumor sites and distant metastases.[87] However, there is evidence that high-dose GM-CSF can actually be immunosuppressive, possibly by increasing the number of myeloid-derived suppressor cells.[89] Further investigation of vaccine combinations with GM-CSF is required to determine the optimum regimen to maximize immunologic and clinical responses.

Interleukin-12 (IL-12)

Another powerful immune-stimulating cytokine is Interleukin-12. Produced by dendritic cells, IL-12 stimulates natural killer cells, and induces helper T cells to differentiate to Th1 cells. Murine models have shown that IL-12 has potent antitumor effects against melanoma as well as other cancers.[90] IL-12 increases the production of interferon-γ (IFN-γ) which enhances the cytotoxic effect of T cells.[91] IL-12 also induces the production of anti-angiogenic factors and inducible nitric oxide synthase (iNOS) and tumoricidal concentrations of nitric oxide (NO) production by macrophages.[92,93] The first phase I trial of IL-12 in human subjects enrolled 12 patients with metastatic melanoma, one of which had a complete response lasting for four weeks.[94] Following administration of IL-12, increases in IFN-γ levels were noted and tumor progression was retarded.[95] Another phase I trial combining IL-12 with IL-2 showed an increase in IFN-γ and a clinical response was reported in the group receiving IL-2 in addition to IL-12.[96]

IL-12 has also been investigated as an adjuvant for melanoma vaccination.[97] One of the first trials testing IL-12 as an adjuvant demonstrated that patients receiving a low dose of IL-12 in conjunction with peptide-pulsed dendritic cells developed increased numbers of antigen specific T cells, as well as six objective clinical responses.[98] Other studies evaluating the efficacy of IL-12 with peptide vaccination also have demonstrated consistent immunologic and varied clinical responses.[99,100]

Inhibiting the Inhibitors

Many, if not all, tumors acquire the ability to "hijack" host immunoregulatory pathways that evolved for the prevention of autoimmunity through multiple mechanisms of tumor-mediated immunosuppression. Tumor cells can suppress the immune system directly by expression of immunoregulatory cytokines or cell surface molecules that inactivate or kill effector T cells; or indirectly by inducing immunosuppressive host cells such as regulatory T cells (Treg) and myeloid-derived suppressor cells (MDSC). Treg are CD4+ T cells that suppress CD4 and CD8 T cells by both contact dependent and soluble pathways.[101] MDSC are immature myeloid cells which infiltrate tumors and suppress T cell activation by the production of reactive oxygen intermediates, nitric oxide, and the arginine-depleting enzyme arginase.[102] These immunoregulatory pathways are the subject of numerous completed and ongoing clinical trials which seek to blockade so called "immune checkpoints," which must be overcome for an immune response to move forward.

Cytotoxic T Lymphocyte-Associated Antigen 4 (CTLA-4)

Among the most studied of this class of immunomodulators are antibodies targeting the cell surface molecule cytotoxic T lymphocyte-associated antigen 4 (CTLA-4). Stimulation of the CD28 receptor on T cells by the B7 (CD80) molecule expressed on APCs is required for T cell activation. However, continued B7 expression leads to simulation of the inhibitory CTLA4 receptor on T cells once the CTLA4 receptor is upregulated 2 to 3 days after T cell activation. This mechanism restores immune homeostasis by inhibiting further T cell activation and proliferation.[103] Mechanisms of antitumor activity of CTLA-4 blockade include enhanced T cell activation/proliferation, interferon-γ production, increased tumor cell apoptosis, upregulation of antigen presentation, and decreased angiogenesis, and possibly inhibition of T reg cells.[104,105]

Because CTLA-4 blockade can positively affect T cell function, there is substantial interest in targeting the CTLA-4 molecule for the treatment of melanoma. Tremelimumab and ipilimumab are two humanized anti-CTLA-4 monoclonal antibodies that have been used in melanoma clinical trials. Tremelimumab and ipilimumab have half lives of 22 and 14 days, respectively, and both are administered intravenously in an outpatient setting. Both antibodies have been studied as single therapeutic agents and in combination with tumor vaccination.[106]

Studies of tremelimumab as a monotherapy have demonstrated acceptable toxicity and a 7% to 9% overall response rate.[107,108] Common side-effects of treatment with tremelimumab are immune-related adverse events (IRAEs), such as dermatitis, diarrhea, and thyroid dysfunction. The development of an IRAE may predict therapeutic efficacy of tremilimumab and other CTLA-4 blocking agents.[109] Another anti-CTLA4 antibody, ipilimumab, has also been well studied in several phase I and phase II clinical trials.[48,110] As with tremelimumab, IRAES were associated with greater response.[111,112] Recent trials have provided evidence that ipilimumab can potentially prolong survival for patients with advanced melanoma.[113,114]

The positive results of anti-CTLA4 antibodies as a single agent have led to studies evaluating the benefit of combining ipilimumab with other treatment modalities such as cytokines or vaccination. One study of ipilimumab with high dose IL-2 therapy in patients with metastatic melanoma reported a 22% objective response rate and increased numbers of tumor specific T cells.[115] The use of ipilimumab in combination with cancer vaccination also has been extensively studied and has produced some positive clinical results. In one trial, 14 patients with stage IV melanoma were treated with 3 mg/kg ipilimumab and vaccination with two gp100 peptides, resulting in three objective responses; however, responses were associated with grade III/IV autoimmune toxicities including hepatitis, colitis, hypophysitis, and dermatitis.[111] A similar study administered ipilimumab with gp100 peptide vaccine and obtained an overall objective response rate of 13%; again, autoimmunity was associated with clinical response.[112] Although clinical responses were seen in these studies, treatment with CTLA-4 antibody did not increase the magnitude of the immune response. Other studies have evaluated ipilimumab treatment in patients who had received prior vaccination with GVAX or various melanoma peptides, with an overall clinical response rate of 29%.[116,117]

Anti-CTLA-4 therapy also has been directly compared to chemotherapy and administered in combination with chemotherapy in several clinical trials. Tremelimumab therapy did not improve overall survival when compared to patients administered dacarbazide or temozolomide.[118] A phase II trial which administered ipilimumab as monotherapy or ipilimumab combined with dacarbazine found an overall response rate of 14.3% in the combination group compared to 5% in the monotherapy group.[119] Ongoing phase III trials continue to evaluate ipilimumab for melanoma.

Regulatory T cells (Tregs)

Regulatory T cells (Tregs) provide another checkpoint that can prevent both undesirable autoimmunity and the desired anti-tumor response. Tregs are CD4+CD25+ cells that classically express high levels of the IL-2 receptor (CD25) and the transcription factor FoxP3. Tregs mediate T cell responses directly through both contact dependent mechanisms and the secretion of inhibitory cytokines, such as IL-10 and TGF-β; and indirectly by decreasing the ability of APCs to activate T cells.[120] Although necessary for immune homeostasis, Treg induction is an important mechanism of tumor-mediated immunosuppression. Please refer to Table 22–4 for other mechanisms of tumor induced immune suppression. Studies have found that patients suffering from a variety of cancers, including melanoma, have increased number of Tregs.[121] Additionally, the tumors themselves can produce inhibitory cytokines that further augment the effects of the regulatory T cells.[122] Tregs also express CTLA-4, which then can act as a negative costimulator of T cells.[123] In the tumor microenvironment, Tregs also have been shown to induce apoptosis of tumor-infiltrating T cells, which further suppresses the immune response.[124]

It is clear that Tregs are a major barrier to the immune system's effort to halt tumor progression, as well as the success of immunotherapy, and thus are an active area of research. Ontak (denileukin difitox) is an IL-2/diphtheria toxin fusion protein

Table 22–4. Mechanisms of Tumor-Induced Immunosuppression

Expression of Self-Antigens	T-lymphocytes become tolerized to self-antigen and activation becomes less likely
Downregulation of class I MHC or antigen-processing molecules	Reduces the ability of CD8+ CTL to recognize and kill tumor cells
Induction of T-cell Tolerance	Failure of the tumor or APC to express costimulatory molecules resulting in T-cell anergy after stimulation of the TCR.
Secretion of Inhibitory Cytokines	Tumor secretion of Il-10, TGF-β, and VEGF which induce Treg and MDSC infiltration and inhibit effector T cell responses
Recruitment of Tregs to Tumor Microenvironment	Inhibits anti-tumor T cell responses, and induces apoptosis of lymphocytes
Recruitment of MDSC to Tumor Microenvironment	Inhibit T cell activation and proliferation; may cause T cell apoptosis; may enhance tumor angiogenesis
Altered Tumor-Associated Antigens	Inability of the T-cells to recognized the mutated tumor-associated antigens

that binds to the IL-2 receptor located on CD25+ T cells and kills them. Ontak is currently approved for the treatment of cutaneous T cell lymphoma, as it is cytotoxic to a subset of T cells in this disease.[125] Although results are variable, there have been numerous reports of Treg depletion following Ontak administration in patients with ovarian, lung, breast, and pancreatic cancer, and melanoma.[126,127] Ontak also has been combined with melanoma vaccination, with favorable decreases in Treg levels and increases in CTL response.[128,129]

Cyclophosphamide (CTX) is an alkylating cytotoxic chemotherapy agent with immunomodulatory effects. The exact mechanism of CTX's antitumor ability is poorly understood; however, CTX has been shown to deplete Tregs, increase levels of stimulatory cytokines, and decrease levels of inhibitory cytokines.[130,131] Cyclophosphamide has been tested in combination with numerous immunotherapy regimens in the hopes of increasing their efficacy. Early studies combining low dose cyclophosphamide with low dose IL-12 in patients with melanoma observed notable clinical responses, including regression of metastases.[132] Another early study compared CTX administration prior to autologous melanoma vaccination with vaccine alone in patients with metastatic melanoma. Patients who received combination treatment had a significant antitumor response and displayed a stronger T cell response to the vaccination.[133] More recent studies examining the efficacy of cyclophosphamide in combination with dendritic cell vaccination and results suggest that CTX may augment DC vaccination by inducing tumor death, leading to an increase in presentation of tumor antigens to lymphocytes.[131,134,135]

Adoptive Immunotherapy

Although they work through a variety of mechanisms, all immunotherapeutic approaches have the ultimate goal of expanding T cells that recognize tumor antigens and ultimately have the ability to eliminate them. Although vaccination expands the T cell repertoire in vivo, it is also possible to activate and expand tumor-specific T cells ex vivo and then return them to the patient. In a manner analogous to the genetic engineering of autologous tumor cells, T cells also can be genetically modified, for example, to express T cell receptors that recognize tumor antigens.

The earliest studies of adoptive immunotherapy used lymphocyte activated killer cells (LAKs). LAKs are cytotoxic cells that can be generated from the patient's peripheral blood following IL-2 administration either in vivo or ex vivo. These cells develop the ability to selectively lyse malignant cells.[136,137]

Currently, a more common approach is the use of the patient's own tumor infiltrating lymphocytes (TILs), which are extracted from the tumor after surgical resection. TILs have theoretical advantages over LAKs because they presumably have a high frequency of recognition of tumor antigens. Initial reports of infusing autologous TILs with concomitant IL-2 describes a response rate of 40%.[138] TILs cannot be generated from tumors that fail to induce a brisk lymphocyte infiltrate, thus limiting the application of this therapy. However, adoptive therapy with autologous TILs remains an active area of research, constituting the foundation of second generation techniques utilizing genetic engineering, pre-treatment lymphodepletion, and other strategies for enhancing the efficacy of TIL therapy.

Among the most successful strategies for adoptive immunotherapy are based on transfer of autologous T cells following systemic lymphodepletion.[139,140] Although it may seem counterintuitive that depletion of T cells would result in an increase in antitumor activity, ablation of the host's (primarily non-tumor-specific) T cell repertoire makes room for homeostatic proliferation of the adoptively transferred tumor-specific T cells. These cells require stimulatory cytokines to proliferate and, with decreased numbers of competing T cells present in the environment, the transferred T cells are efficiently stimulated and expanded.[141] Following depletion, the patient's APCs also become better at presenting tumor antigens to T cells, possibly due to activation of TLRs or a massive release of proinflammatory cytokines following radiation.[142,143] Additionally, during the depletion process, Tregs are also eliminated, and the proliferation of the autologous transferred cells can occur prior to their reconstitution.[144] Autologous T cell transfer into lymphodepleted hosts has seen significant success in clinical trials, with response rates of up to 50% to 70%.

Despite these results, adoptive cell transfer cannot yet be widely applied to patients with metastatic melanoma. The procedure is cumbersome and expensive and requires a highly trained team to perform successfully. Also, tumor-specific T cells cannot be expanded from all patients. In order to extend the application of adoptive cell transfer to these patients, genetic engineering of lymphocytes obtained from peripheral blood has been proposed as a treatment modality by using a retrovirus encoding T cell receptors for melanoma antigens inserted into a peripheral lymphocytes.[145–147] Molecules other than T cell receptors can also be introduced to lymphocytes through genetic engineering: T cells genetically engineered to secrete IL-2 have been administered to patients in the effort to prolong the survival of the transferred cells. Following administration of these transduced lymphocytes, one participant had a partial response, and the IL-2 secreting T cells were highly persistent in other patients.[148] Based on this preliminary success, further evaluation of other cytokines and costimulatory molecules to be engineered into adoptively transferred lymphocytes is warranted.

The Potential Role of Radiotherapy

There is increasing interest in combining immune therapy with conventional cancer therapeutics, such as radiotherapy. Although radiation is currently indicated for only a relatively small percentage of patients diagnosed with melanoma, contemporary trials refute the outdated concept that melanoma is resistant to radiation.[149] Although total body irradiation is immunosuppressive, numerous in vivo studies have demonstrated that tumor-directed RT enhances the effectiveness of different forms of immunotherapy, including dendritic cell vaccines with tumor associated antigens, cytokine-based viral gene therapy, and adoptive transfer of cytotoxic T cells.[150]

For instance, in one preclinical model, the combination of adoptive transfer of activated T cells and RT eradicated tumors in the majority of immune competent mice, whereas tumors re-grew in mice treated with either treatment alone. The enhancement of antitumor responses following RT was attributed to the ability of RT to alter the tumor microenvironment and enhance cross priming by stromal cells.[151] In a recent preclinical study using the well-established B16 murine melanoma model, doses of ablative RT (20 Gy $\times$ 1) increased T-cell priming in draining lymph nodes, contributing to control of distant metastases in a T cell-dependent fashion.[152] Interestingly, this effect was abrogated by either chemotherapy or the use of conventionally fractionated radiation (5 Gy $\times$ 4). It remains to be seen whether the effectiveness of these mechanisms can be demonstrated clinically and whether the resultant antitumor immunity can improve both local and systemic tumor control in patients. However, given these compelling clinical and preclinical data, the combination of radiation and immune therapy should be rigorously studied with regard to both clinical and immune endpoints in melanoma and other solid tumors.[153]

The Future of Immunotherapy

To date, with the exception of high-dose interferon-alpha treatment (which provides modest benefit at best), no immunotherapeutic approach to melanoma has been shown to consistently provide patient benefit. Despite this, results from the thousands of patients who have participated in clinical immunotherapy trials have revealed that there is certainly a small subset of patients that responds very well to immunotherapy. One of the most important unanswered questions is how to identify who will respond to immunotherapy prior to treatment initiation. Continued identification of genetic or molecular markers that predict therapeutic response will make this task easier.

Adoptive cell transfer following lymphodepletion has shown great potential for inducing a clinical and immunological response following treatment. The creation of lymphocytes that can respond to multiple antigens and persist in the blood of cancer patients also is an area of future research. By creating lymphocytes that can remain active for long periods of time, it may be possible to induce tumor regression without recurrence or induce stable disease in a larger subset of patients. The responses of patients who have undergone tumor regression following immunotherapy is often short lived, thus great benefits may be obtained in the understanding of how an immune response can be sustained in order to halt progression or prevent recurrence.

Another promising area of continued research is the development of strategies that specifically target molecular and cellular mechanisms of immunosuppression. Specific agents that ablate or inactivate immunoregulatory Treg and MDSC cells, or reverse the immunosuppressive tumor microenvironment, may be combined with other immunotherapeutic approaches to unmask the patient's endogenous antitumor response. Improved genetic methods for determining a tumor's molecular "fingerprint" may allow identification of immunosuppressive pathways to be blocked, and unique antigens to be targeted, to provide personalized immunotherapy for patients with melanoma. Finally, it is critical to continue moving toward testing combinations of agents that target multiple mechanisms of immune stimulation and reversal of tumor-mediated immunosuppression simultaneously. With continued clinical trials of new agents, new combinations of agents, and better identification of patient and tumor characteristics predictive of response to treatment, immunotherapy for cutaneous melanoma is poised to move from promise to reality.

Acknowledgments. We would like to acknowledge Racine Levy for help with preparation of Figure 22–1.

References

1. Parish CR. Cancer immunotherapy: the past, the present and the future. *Immunol Cell Biol.* 2003;81:106–113.
2. Aderem A, Ulevitch RJ. Toll-like receptors in the induction of the innate immune response. *Nature.* 2000;406: 782–787.
3. Shiku H, Takahashi T, Oettgen HF. Cell surface antigens of human malignant melanoma. II. serological typing with immune adherence assays and definition of two new surface antigens. *J Exp Med.* 1976;144:873–881.
4. Burnet FM. The concept of immunological surveillance. *Prog Exp Tumor Res.* 1970;13:1–27.
5. Kaplan DH, Shankaran V, Dighe AS, et al. Demonstration of an interferon gamma-dependent tumor surveillance system in immunocompetent mice. *Proc Natl Acad Sci U S A.* 1998;95:7556–7561.
6. Shankaran V, Ikeda H, Bruce AT, et al. IFN gamma and lymphocytes prevent primary tumour development and shape tumour immunogenicity. *Nature.* 2001;410: 1107–1111.
7. Schulz TF. Cancer and viral infections in immunocompromised individuals. *Int J Cancer.* 2009;125:1755–1763.
8. Oble DA, Loewe R, Yu P, Mihm MC Jr. Focus on TILs: prognostic significance of tumor infiltrating lymphocytes in human melanoma. *Cancer Immun.* 2009;9:3.
9. Frey AB, Monu N. Signaling defects in anti-tumor T cells. *Immunol Rev.* 2008;222:192–205.
10. Tada T, Ohzeki S, Utsumi K, et al. Transforming growth factor-beta-induced inhibition of T cell function, susceptibility difference in T cells of various phenotypes and functions and its relevance to immunosuppression in the tumor-bearing state. *J Immunol.* 1991;146: 1077–1082.
11. Liyanage UK, Moore TT, Joo HG, et al. Prevalence of regulatory T cells is increased in peripheral blood and tumor microenvironment of patients with pancreas or breast adenocarcinoma. *J Immunol.* 2002;169:2756–2761.
12. Beyer M, Schultze JL. Regulatory T cells in cancer. *Blood.* 2006;108:804–811.
13. Strand S, Hofmann WJ, Hug H, et al. Lymphocyte apoptosis induced by CD95 (APO-1/Fas) ligand-expressing tumor cells—a mechanism of immune evasion? *Nat Med.* 1996;2:1361–1366.
14. Printz C. Spontaneous regression of melanoma may offer insight into cancer immunology. *J Natl Cancer Inst.* 2001;93:1047–1048.
15. Chang AE, Karnell LH, Menck HR. The national cancer data base report on cutaneous and noncutaneous melanoma: a summary of 84,836 cases from the past decade. the American College of Surgeons Commission on Cancer and the American Cancer Society. *Cancer.* 1998;83:1 664–1678.
16. Bulkley GB, Cohen MH, Banks PM, Char DH, Ketcham AS. Long-term spontaneous regression of malignant melanoma with visceral metastases. report of a case with immunologic profile. *Cancer.* 1975;36:485–494.
17. Nathanson. Spontaneous regression of malignant melanoma: a review of the literature on incidence, clinical features, and possible mechanisms. *Natl Cancer Inst Monogr.* 1976;44:67–76.
18. Clark WH Jr, Elder DE, Guerry D 4th, et al. Model predicting survival in stage I melanoma based on tumor progression. *J Natl Cancer Inst.* 1989;81:1893–1904.
19. Clemente CG, Mihm MC Jr, Bufalino R, Zurrida S, Collini P, Cascinelli N. Prognostic value of tumor infiltrating lymphocytes in the vertical growth phase of primary cutaneous melanoma. *Cancer.* 1996;77:1303–1310.
20. Uchi H, Stan R, Turk MJ, et al. Unraveling the complex relationship between cancer immunity and autoimmunity: lessons from melanoma and vitiligo. *Adv Immunol.* 2006;90:215–241.

21. Le Gal FA, Avril MF, Bosq J, et al. Direct evidence to support the role of antigen-specific CD8(+) T cells in melanoma-associated vitiligo. *J Invest Dermatol.* 2001; 117:1464–1470.
22. Nordlund JJ, Kirkwood JM, Forget BM, Milton G, Albert DM, Lerner AB. Vitiligo in patients with metastatic melanoma: a good prognostic sign. *J Am Acad Dermatol.* 1983;9:689–696.
23. Yee C, Thompson JA, Roche P, et al. Melanocyte destruction after antigen-specific immunotherapy of melanoma: Direct evidence of t cell-mediated vitiligo. *J Exp Med.* 2000;192:1637–1644.
24. Dudley ME, Yang JC, Sherry R, et al. Adoptive cell therapy for patients with metastatic melanoma: evaluation of intensive myeloablative chemoradiation preparative regimens. *J Clin Oncol.* 2008;26:5233–5239.
25. Gogas H, Ioannovich J, Dafni U, et al. Prognostic significance of autoimmunity during treatment of melanoma with interferon. *N Engl J Med.* 2006;354:709–718.
26. Fujita M, High WA, Asgari S, Lewis KD, Gonzalez R. Development of vitiligo during melanoma treatment with a novel surviving inhibitor: a case report and review of the literature. *Int J Dermatol.* 2009;48:426–430.
27. Rosenberg SA, Yang JC, Restifo NP. Cancer immunotherapy: moving beyond current vaccines. *Nat Med.* 2004;10:909–915.
28. Riker AI, Radfar S, Liu S, Wang Y, Khong HT. Immunotherapy of melanoma: a critical review of current concepts and future strategies. *Expert Opin Biol Ther.* 2007; 7:345–358.
29. Van Epps D. Characterization of polyvalent allogeneic vaccines. *Dev Biol (Basel).* 2004;116:79–90; discussion 133–143.
30. Hsueh EC, Morton DL. Antigen-based immunotherapy of melanoma: canvaxin therapeutic polyvalent cancer vaccine. *Semin Cancer Biol.* 2003;13:401–407.
31. Sondak VK, Liu PY, Tuthill RJ, et al. Adjuvant immunotherapy of resected, intermediate-thickness, node-negative melanoma with an allogeneic tumor vaccine: overall results of a randomized trial of the Southwest Oncology Group. *J Clin Oncol.* 2002;20:2058–2066.
32. Chapman PB, Wolchock JD. Melanoma antigens: Vaccines and monoclonal antibodies. In: Borden EC, ed. *Melanoma: Biologically Targeted Therapeutics.* Totowa, NJ: Humana Press Inc; 2002:95.
33. Berinstein NL. Enhancing cancer vaccines with immu - nomodulators. *Vaccine.* 2007;25(suppl 2):B72–B88.
34. Dranoff G. GM-CSF-based cancer vaccines. *Immunol Rev.* 2002;188:147–154.
35. Astsaturov I, Petrella T, Bagriacik EU, et al. Amplification of virus-induced antimelanoma T-cell reactivity by high-dose interferon-alpha2b: implications for cancer vaccines. *Clin Cancer Res.* 2003;9:4347–4355.
36. Brichard V, Van Pel A, Wolfel T, et al. The tyrosinase gene codes for an antigen recognized by autologous cytolytic T lymphocytes on HLA-A2 melanomas. *J Exp Med.* 1993;178:489–495.
37. Bakker AB, Schreurs MW, de Boer AJ, et al. Melanocyte lineage-specific antigen gp100 is recognized by melanoma-derived tumor-infiltrating lymphocytes. *J Exp Med.* 1994;179:1005–1009.
38. Kawakami Y, Eliyahu S, Delgado CH, et al. Cloning of the gene coding for a shared human melanoma antigen recognized by autologous T cells infiltrating into tumor. *Proc Natl Acad Sci U S A.* 1994;91:3515–3519.
39. van der Bruggen P, Traversari C, Chomez P, et al. A gene encoding an antigen recognized by cytolytic T lymphocytes on a human melanoma. *J Immunol.* 2007;178: 2617–2621.
40. Melief CJ, van der Burg SH. Immunotherapy of established (pre)malignant disease by synthetic long peptide vaccines. *Nat Rev Cancer.* 2008;8:351–360.
41. Vujanovic L, Butterfield LH. Melanoma cancer vaccines and anti-tumor T cell responses. *J Cell Biochem.* 2007; 102:301–310.
42. Rosenberg SA, Yang JC, Schwartzentruber DJ, et al. Immunologic and therapeutic evaluation of a synthetic peptide vaccine for the treatment of patients with metastatic melanoma. *Nat Med.* 1998;4:321–327.
43. Onaitis M, Kalady MF, Pruitt S, Tyler DS. Dendritic cell gene therapy. *Surg Oncol Clin North Am.* 2002;11: 645–660.
44. Aarntzen EH, Figdor CG, Adema GJ, Punt CJ, de Vries IJ. Dendritic cell vaccination and immune monitoring. *Cancer Immunol Immunother.* 2008;57:1559–1568.
45. Tuettenberg A, Schmitt E, Knop J, Jonuleit H. Dendritic cell-based immunotherapy of malignant melanoma: success and limitations. *J Dtsch Dermatol Ges.* 2007;5: 190–196.
46. Schneeberger A, Wagner C, Zemann A, et al. CpG motifs are efficient adjuvants for DNA cancer vaccines. *J Invest Dermatol.* 2004;123:371–379.
47. Tagawa ST, Lee P, Snively J, et al. Phase I study of intranodal delivery of a plasmid DNA vaccine for patients with stage IV melanoma. *Cancer.* 2003;98:144–154.
48. Weber J, Boswell W, Smith J, et al. Phase 1 trial of intranodal injection of a melan-A/MART-1 DNA plasmid vaccine in patients with stage IV melanoma. *J Immunother.* 2008;31:215–223.
49. Belli F, Testori A, Rivoltini L, et al. Vaccination of metastatic melanoma patients with autologous tumor-derived heat shock protein gp96-peptide complexes: clinical and immunologic findings. *J Clin Oncol.* 2002;20:4169–4180.
50. Eton O, Ross MI, East MJ, et al. Autologous tumor-derived heat-shock protein peptide complex-96 (HSPPC-96) in patients with metastatic melanoma. *J Transl Med.* 2010;8:9.
51. Vonderheide RH, Flaherty KT, Khalil M, et al. Clinical activity and immune modulation in cancer patients treated with CP-870,893, a novel CD40 agonist monoclonal antibody. *J Clin Oncol.* 2007;25:876–883.
52. von Leoprechting A, van der Bruggen P, Pahl HL, Aruffo A, Simon JC. Stimulation of CD40 on immunogenic human malignant melanomas augments their

cytotoxic T lymphocyte-mediated lysis and induces apoptosis. *Cancer Res.* 1999;59:1287–1294.
53. Cheuk AT, Mufti GJ, Guinn BA. Role of 4-1BB:4-1BB ligand in cancer immunotherapy. *Cancer Gene Ther.* 2004; 11:215–226.
54. Wen T, Bukczynski J, Watts TH. 4-1BB ligand-mediated costimulation of human T cells induces CD4 and CD8 T cell expansion, cytokine production, and the development of cytolytic effector function. *J Immunol.* 2002;168: 4897–4906.
55. Bukczynski J, Wen T, Ellefsen K, Gauldie J, Watts TH. Costimulatory ligand 4-1BBL (CD137L) as an efficient adjuvant for human antiviral cytotoxic T cell responses. *Proc Natl Acad Sci U S A.* 2004;101:1291–1296.
56. Melero I, Shuford WW, Newby SA, et al. Monoclonal antibodies against the 4-1BB T-cell activation molecule eradicate established tumors. *Nat Med.* 1997;3:682–685.
57. Sznol M. Phase I study of BMS-663513, a fully human anti-CD137 agonist monoclonal antibody, in patients (pts) with advanced cancer (CA). *J Clin Oncol.* 2008; 26:3007.
58. Molckovsky A, Siu LL. First-in-class, first-in-human phase I results of targeted agents: highlights of the 2008 American Society of Clinical Oncology meeting. *J Hematol Oncol.* 2008;1:20.
59. Pashenkov M, Goess G, Wagner C, et al. Phase II trial of a toll-like receptor 9–activating oligonucleotide in patients with metastatic melanoma. *J Clin Oncol.* 2006; 24:5716–5724.
60. Ray CM, Kluk M, Grin CM, Grant-Kels JM. Successful treatment of malignant melanoma in situ with topical 5% imiquimod cream. *Int J Dermatol.* 2005;44:428–434.
61. Pfeffer LM, Dinarello CA, Herberman RB, et al. Biological properties of recombinant alpha-interferons: 40th anniversary of the discovery of interferons. *Cancer Res.* 1998;58:2489–2499.
62. Herberman RB. Effect of alpha-interferons on immune function. *Semin Oncol.* 1997;24:S978–S980.
63. Kirkwood JM, Strawderman MH, Ernstoff MS, Smith TJ, Borden EC, Blum RH. Interferon alfa-2b adjuvant therapy of high-risk resected cutaneous melanoma: the eastern cooperative oncology group trial EST 1684. *J Clin Oncol.* 1996;14:7–17.
64. Sabel MS, Sondak VK. Is there a role for adjuvant high-dose interferon-alpha-2b in the management of melanoma? *Drugs.* 2003;63:1053–1058.
65. Kokoschka EM, Trautinger F, Knobler RM, Pohl-Markl H, Micksche M. Long-term adjuvant therapy of high-risk malignant melanoma with interferon alpha 2b. *J Invest Dermatol.* 1990;95:193S-197S.
66. Rusciani L, Petraglia S, Alotto M, Calvieri S, Vezzoni G. Postsurgical adjuvant therapy for melanoma. Evaluation of a 3-year randomized trial with recombinant interferon-alpha after 3 and 5 years of follow-up. *Cancer.* 1997;79: 2354–2360.
67. Kirkwood JM, Ibrahim JG, Sondak VK, et al. High- and low-dose interferon alfa-2b in high-risk melanoma: first analysis of intergroup trial E1690/S9111/C9190. *J Clin Oncol.* 2000;18:2444–2458.
68. Kirkwood JM, Manola J, Ibrahim J, et al. A pooled analysis of Eastern Cooperative Oncology Group and intergroup trials of adjuvant high-dose interferon for melanoma. *Clin Cancer Res.* 2004;10:1670–1677.
69. Ponce R. Adverse consequences of immunostimulation. *J Immunotoxicol.* 2008;5:33–41.
70. Greenberg DB, Jonasch E, Gadd MA, et al. Adjuvant therapy of melanoma with interferon-alpha-2b is associated with mania and bipolar syndromes. *Cancer.* 2000; 89:356–362.
71. Satzger I, Meier A, Schenck F, Kapp A, Hauschild A, Gutzmer R. Autoimmunity as a prognostic factor in melanoma patients treated with adjuvant low-dose interferon alpha. *Int J Cancer.* 2007;121:2562–2566.
72. Kirkwood JM, Tarhini AA. Biomarkers of therapeutic response in melanoma and renal cell carcinoma: potential inroads to improved immunotherapy. *J Clin Oncol.* 2009;27:2583–2585.
73. Yurkovetsky ZR, Kirkwood JM, Edington HD, et al. Multiplex analysis of serum cytokines in melanoma patients treated with interferon-alpha2b. *Clin Cancer Res.* 2007;13:2422–2428.
74. Kirkwood JM, Ibrahim J, Lawson DH, et al. High-dose interferon alfa-2b does not diminish antibody response to GM2 vaccination in patients with resected melanoma: results of the multicenter eastern cooperative oncology group phase II trial E2696. *J Clin Oncol.* 2001; 19:1430–1436.
75. Mitchell MS, Jakowatz J, Harel W, et al. Increased effectiveness of interferon alfa-2b following active specific immunotherapy for melanoma. *J Clin Oncol.* 1994;12: 402–411.
76. Di Pucchio T, Pilla L, Capone I, et al. Immunization of stage IV melanoma patients with melan-A/MART-1 and gp100 peptides plus IFN-alpha results in the activation of specific CD8(+) T cells and monocyte/dendritic cell precursors. *Cancer Res.* 2006;66:4943–4951.
77. Atkins MB, Lotze MT, Dutcher JP, et al. High-dose recombinant interleukin 2 therapy for patients with metastatic melanoma: analysis of 270 patients treated between 1985 and 1993. *J Clin Oncol.* 1999;17:2105–2116.
78. Phan GQ, Attia P, Steinberg SM, White DE, Rosenberg SA. Factors associated with response to high-dose interleukin-2 in patients with metastatic melanoma. *J Clin Oncol.* 2001;19:3477–3482.
79. Sabatino M, Kim-Schulze S, Panelli MC, et al. Serum vascular endothelial growth factor and fibronectin predict clinical response to high-dose interleukin-2 therapy. *J Clin Oncol.* 2009;27:2645–2652.
80. Wang E, Marincola FM. cDNA arrays and the enigma of melanoma immune responsiveness. *Cancer J.* 2001;7:16–24.
81. Wang E, Miller LD, Ohnmacht GA, et al. Prospective molecular profiling of melanoma metastases suggests classifiers of immune responsiveness. *Cancer Res.* 2002; 62:3581–3586.

82. Roberts JD, Niedzwiecki D, Carson WE, et al. Phase 2 study of the g209–2M melanoma peptide vaccine and low-dose interleukin-2 in advanced melanoma: cancer and leukemia group B 509901. *J Immunother.* 2006;29: 95–101.
83. Slingluff CL,Jr, Petroni GR, Yamshchikov GV, et al. Immunologic and clinical outcomes of vaccination with a multiepitope melanoma peptide vaccine plus low-dose interleukin-2 administered either concurrently or on a delayed schedule. *J Clin Oncol.* 2004;22:4474–4485.
84. Escobar A, Lopez M, Serrano A, et al. Dendritic cell immunizations alone or combined with low doses of interleukin-2 induce specific immune responses in mela - noma patients. *Clin Exp Immunol.* 2005;142:555–568.
85. Lindsey KR, Gritz L, Sherry R, et al. Evaluation of prime/boost regimens using recombinant poxvirus/ tyrosinase vaccines for the treatment of patients with metastatic melanoma. *Clin Cancer Res.* 2006;12:2526–2537.
86. University of Texas M. D. Anderson Cancer Center. Vaccine shows therapeutic promise against advanced melanoma. *Science Daily* 2009. Retrieved June 1, 2009 from: http://www.sciencedaily.com/releases/2009/06/090601092239.html .
87. Dranoff G. GM-CSF-secreting melanoma vaccines. *Oncogene.* 2003;22:3188–3192.
88. Soiffer R, Lynch T, Mihm M, et al. Vaccination with irradiated autologous melanoma cells engineered to secrete human granulocyte-macrophage colony-stimulating factor generates potent antitumor immunity in patients with metastatic melanoma. *Proc Natl Acad Sci U S A.* 1998;95:13141–13146.
89. Serafini P, Carbley R, Noonan KA, Tan G, Bronte V, Borrello I. High-dose granulocyte-macrophage colony-stimulating factor-producing vaccines impair the immune response through the recruitment of myeloid suppressor cells. *Cancer Res.* 2004;64:6337–6343.
90. Brunda MJ, Luistro L, Rumennik L, et al. Interleukin-12: murine models of a potent antitumor agent. *Ann N Y Acad Sci.* 1996;795:266–274.
91. Brunda MJ, Luistro L, Hendrzak JA, Fountoulakis M, Garotta G, Gately MK. Role of interferon-gamma in mediating the antitumor efficacy of interleukin-12. *J Immunother Emphasis Tumor Immunol.* 1995;17:71–77.
92. Albini A, Fassina G, Nicolo M, et al. Inhibition of a vascular ocular tumor growth by IL-12 gene transfer. *Clin Exp Metastasis.* 2007;24:485–493.
93. Wigginton JM, Kuhns DB, Back TC, Brunda MJ, Wil - trout RH, Cox GW. Interleukin 12 primes macrophages for nitric oxide production in vivo and restores depressed nitric oxide production by macrophages from tumor-bearing mice: implications for the antitumor activity of interleukin 12 and/or interleukin 2. *Cancer Res.* 1996; 56:1131–1136.
94. Atkins MB, Robertson MJ, Gordon M, et al. Phase I evaluation of intravenous recombinant human interleukin 12 in patients with advanced malignancies. *Clin Cancer Res.* 1997;3:409–417.
95. Gollob JA, Mier JW, Veenstra K, et al. Phase I trial of twice-weekly intravenous interleukin 12 in patients with metastatic renal cell cancer or malignant melanoma: ability to maintain IFN-gamma induction is associated with clinical response. *Clin Cancer Res* 2000;6:1678–1692.
96. Gollob JA, Veenstra KG, Parker RA, et al. Phase I trial of concurrent twice-weekly recombinant human interleukin-12 plus low-dose IL-2 in patients with melanoma or renal cell carcinoma. *J Clin Oncol.* 2003;21: 2564–2573.
97. Portielje JE, Gratama JW, van Ojik HH, Stoter G, Kruit WH. IL-12: A promising adjuvant for cancer vaccination. *Cancer Immunol Immunother.* 2003;52:133–144.
98. Gajewski TF, Fallarino F, Ashikari A, Sherman M. Immunization of HLA-A2+ melanoma patients with MAGE-3 or MelanA peptide-pulsed autologous peripheral blood mononuclear cells plus recombinant human interleukin 12. *Clin Cancer Res.* 2001;7:895s-901s.
99. Peterson AC, Harlin H, Gajewski TF. Immunization with melan-A peptide-pulsed peripheral blood mono - nuclear cells plus recombinant human interleukin-12 induces clinical activity and T-cell responses in advanced melanoma. *J Clin Oncol.* 2003;21:2342–2348.
100. Lee P, Wang F, Kuniyoshi J, et al. Effects of interleukin-12 on the immune response to a multipeptide vaccine for resected metastatic melanoma. *J Clin Oncol.* 2001;19: 3836–3847.
101. Whiteside TL. The tumor microenvironment and its role in promoting tumor growth. *Oncogene.* 2008;27:5904–5912.
102. Ugel S, Delpozzo F, Desantis G, et al. Therapeutic targeting of myeloid-derived suppressor cells. *Curr Opin Pharmacol.* 2009;9:470–481.
103. Walunas TL, Lenschow DJ, Bakker CY, et al. CTLA-4 can function as a negative regulator of T cell activation. *Immunity.* 1994;1:405–413.
104. Paradis TJ, Floyd E, Burkwit J, et al. The anti-tumor activity of anti-CTLA-4 is mediated through its induction of IFN gamma. *Cancer Immunol Immunother.* 2001; 50:125–133.
105. Kirkwood JM, Tarhini AA, Panelli MC, et al. Next generation of immunotherapy for melanoma. *J Clin Oncol.* 2008;26:3445–3455.
106. Sarnaik AA, Weber JS. Recent advances using anti-CTLA-4 for the treatment of melanoma. *Cancer J.* 2009; 15:169–173.
107. Ribas A, Camacho LH, Lopez-Berestein G, et al. Antitumor activity in melanoma and anti-self responses in a phase I trial with the anti-cytotoxic T lymphocyte-associated antigen 4 monoclonal antibody CP-675,206. *J Clin Oncol.* 2005;23:8968–8977.
108. Camacho LH, Antonia S, Sosman J, et al. Phase I/II trial of tremelimumab in patients with metastatic melanoma. *J Clin Oncol.* 2009;27:1075–1081.
109. Downey SG, Klapper JA, Smith FO, et al. Prognostic factors related to clinical response in patients with metastatic melanoma treated by CTL-associated antigen-4 blockade. *Clin Cancer Res.* 2007;13:6681–6688.

110. O'Day SJ, Hamid O, Urba WJ. Targeting cytotoxic T-lymphocyte antigen-4 (CTLA-4): a novel strategy for the treatment of melanoma and other malignancies. *Cancer.* 2007;110:2614–2627.
111. Phan GQ, Yang JC, Sherry RM, et al. Cancer regression and autoimmunity induced by cytotoxic T lymphocyte-associated antigen 4 blockade in patients with metastatic melanoma. *Proc Natl Acad Sci U S A.* 2003;100: 8372–8377.
112. Attia P, Phan GQ, Maker AV, et al. Autoimmunity correlates with tumor regression in patients with metastatic melanoma treated with anti-cytotoxic T-lymphocyte antigen-4. *J Clin Oncol.* 2005;23:6043–6053.
113. Urba WJ, Weber JS, O'Day SJ, et al. Long-term survival of patients with advanced melanoma who received ipilimumab administered at 10 mg/kg every 3 weeks for 4 doses (induction dosing). *J Clin Oncol (Meeting Abstracts).* 2008;26:3018.
114. Hamid O, Chin K, Li J, et al. Dose effect of ipilimumab in patients with advanced melanoma: results from a phase II, randomized, dose-ranging study. *J Clin Oncol (Meeting Abstracts).* 2008;26:9025.
115. Maker AV, Phan GQ, Attia P, et al. Tumor regression and autoimmunity in patients treated with cytotoxic T lymphocyte-associated antigen 4 blockade and interleukin 2: a phase I/II study. *Ann Surg Oncol.* 2005;12: 1005–1016.
116. Hodi FS, Mihm MC, Soiffer RJ, et al. Biologic activity of cytotoxic T lymphocyte-associated antigen 4 antibody blockade in previously vaccinated metastatic melanoma and ovarian carcinoma patients. *Proc Natl Acad Sci U S A.* 2003;100:4712–4717.
117. Hodi FS, Butler M, Oble DA, et al. Immunologic and clinical effects of antibody blockade of cytotoxic T lymphocyte-associated antigen 4 in previously vaccinated cancer patients. *Proc Natl Acad Sci U S A.* 2008;105: 3005–3010.
118. Ribas A, Hauschild A, Kefford R, Gomez-Navarro J, Pavlov D, Marshall MA. Phase III, open-label, randomized, comparative study of tremelimumab (CP-675,206) and chemotherapy (temozolomide [TMZ] or dacarbazine [DTIC]) in patients with advanced melanoma. *J Clin Oncol (Meeting Abstracts).* 2008;26:LBA9011.
119. Hersh EM, O'Day SJ, Powderly J, et al. A phase II multicenter study of ipilimumab with or without dacarbazine in chemotherapy-naive patients with advanced melanoma. *Invest New Drugs.* 2010 (epub ahead of print).
120. Vignali DA, Collison LW, Workman CJ. How regulatory T cells work. *Nat Rev Immunol.* 2008;8:523–532.
121. Viguier M, Lemaitre F, Verola O, et al. Foxp3 expressing CD4+CD25(high) regulatory T cells are overrepresented in human metastatic melanoma lymph nodes and inhibit the function of infiltrating T cells. *J Immunol.* 2004;173:1444–1453.
122. Workman CJ, Szymczak-Workman AL, Collison LW, Pillai MR, Vignali DA. The development and function of regulatory T cells. *Cell Mol Life Sci.* 2009;66:2603–2622.
123. Wing K, Onishi Y, Prieto-Martin P, et al. CTLA-4 control over Foxp3+ regulatory T cell function. *Science.* 2008; 322:271–275.
124. Gondek DC, Lu LF, Quezada SA, Sakaguchi S, Noelle RJ. Cutting edge: contact-mediated suppression by CD4+ CD25+ regulatory cells involves a granzyme B-dependent, perforin-independent mechanism. *J Immunol.* 2005;174: 1783–1786.
125. Kaminetzky D, Hymes KB. Denileukin diftitox for the treatment of cutaneous T-cell lymphoma. *Biologics.* 2008; 2:717–724.
126. Attia P, Maker AV, Haworth LR, Rogers-Freezer L, Rosenberg SA. Inability of a fusion protein of IL-2 and diphtheria toxin (denileukin diftitox, DAB389IL-2, ONTAK) to eliminate regulatory T lymphocytes in patients with melanoma. *J Immunother.* 2005;28:582–592.
127. Curiel TJ. Tregs and rethinking cancer immunotherapy. *J Clin Invest.* 2007;117:1167–1174.
128. Mahnke K, Schonfeld K, Fondel S, et al. Depletion of CD4+CD25+ human regulatory T cells in vivo: kinetics of treg depletion and alterations in immune functions in vivo and in vitro. *Int J Cancer.* 2007;120:2723–2733.
129. Dannull J, Su Z, Rizzieri D, et al. Enhancement of vaccine-mediated antitumor immunity in cancer patients after depletion of regulatory T cells. *J Clin Invest.* 2005; 115:3623–3633.
130. Ghiringhelli F, Larmonier N, Schmitt E, et al. CD4+ CD25+ regulatory T cells suppress tumor immunity but are sensitive to cyclophosphamide which allows immunotherapy of established tumors to be curative. *Eur J Immunol.* 2004;34:336–344.
131. Liu JY, Wu Y, Zhang XS, et al. Single administration of low dose cyclophosphamide augments the antitumor effect of dendritic cell vaccine. *Cancer Immunol Immunother.* 2007;56:1597–1604.
132. Mitchell MS, Kempf RA, Harel W, et al. Effectiveness and tolerability of low-dose cyclophosphamide and low-dose intravenous interleukin-2 in disseminated melanoma [Corrected]. *J Clin Oncol.* 1988;6:409–424.
133. Berd D, Maguire HC Jr, Mastrangelo MJ. Induction of cell-mediated immunity to autologous melanoma cells and regression of metastases after treatment with a melanoma cell vaccine preceded by cyclophosphamide. *Cancer Res.* 1986;46:2572–2577.
134. Tong Y, Song W, Crystal RG. Combined intratumoral injection of bone marrow-derived dendritic cells and systemic chemotherapy to treat pre-existing murine tumors. *Cancer Res.* 2001;61:7530–7535.
135. Holtl L, Ramoner R, Zelle-Rieser C, et al. Allogeneic dendritic cell vaccination against metastatic renal cell carcinoma with or without cyclophosphamide. *Cancer Immunol Immunother.* 2005;54:663–670.
136. Rosenberg SA, Lotze MT, Muul LM, et al. A progress report on the treatment of 157 patients with advanced cancer using lymphokine-activated killer cells and interleukin-2 or high-dose interleukin-2 alone. *N Engl J Med.* 1987;316:889–897.

137. Rosenberg SA, Lotze MT, Yang JC, et al. Prospective randomized trial of high-dose interleukin-2 alone or in conjunction with lymphokine-activated killer cells for the treatment of patients with advanced cancer. *J Natl Cancer Inst.* 1993;85:622–632.
138. Rosenberg SA, Yannelli JR, Yang JC, et al. Treatment of patients with metastatic melanoma with autologous tumor-infiltrating lymphocytes and interleukin 2. *J Natl Cancer Inst.* 1994;86:1159–1166.
139. Dudley ME, Wunderlich JR, Robbins PF, et al. Cancer regression and autoimmunity in patients after clonal repopulation with antitumor lymphocytes. *Science.* 2002; 298:850–854.
140. Rosenberg SA, Yang JC, Robbins PF, et al. Cell transfer therapy for cancer: lessons from sequential treatments of a patient with metastatic melanoma. *J Immunother.* 2003;26:385–393.
141. Klebanoff CA, Khong HT, Antony PA, Palmer DC, Restifo NP. Sinks, suppressors and antigen presenters: how lymphodepletion enhances T cell-mediated tumor immunotherapy. *Trends Immunol.* 2005;26:111–117.
142. Sherman ML, Datta R, Hallahan DE, Weichselbaum RR, Kufe DW. Regulation of tumor necrosis factor gene expression by ionizing radiation in human myeloid leukemia cells and peripheral blood monocytes. *J Clin Invest.* 1991;87:1794–1797.
143. Hill GR, Crawford JM, Cooke KR, Brinson YS, Pan L, Ferrara JL. Total body irradiation and acute graft-versus-host disease: the role of gastrointestinal damage and inflammatory cytokines. *Blood.* 1997;90:3204–3213.
144. Gattinoni L, Powell DJ Jr, Rosenberg SA, Restifo NP. Adoptive immunotherapy for cancer: building on success. *Nat Rev Immunol.* 2006;6:383–393.
145. Clay TM, Custer MC, Spiess PJ, Nishimura MI. Potential use of T cell receptor genes to modify hematopoietic stem cells for the gene therapy of cancer. *Pathol Oncol Res.* 1999;5:3–15.
146. Morgan RA, Dudley ME, Wunderlich JR, et al. Cancer regression in patients after transfer of genetically engineered lymphocytes. *Science.* 2006;314:126–129.
147. Morgan RA, Dudley ME, Yu YY, et al. High efficiency TCR gene transfer into primary human lymphocytes affords avid recognition of melanoma tumor antigen glycoprotein 100 and does not alter the recognition of autologous melanoma antigens. *J Immunol.* 2003;171: 3287–3295.
148. Heemskerk B, Liu K, Dudley ME, et al. Adoptive cell therapy for patients with melanoma, using tumor-infiltrating lymphocytes genetically engineered to secrete interleukin-2. *Hum Gene Ther.* 2008;19:496–510.
149. Mathieu D, Kondziolka D, Cooper PB, et al. Gamma knife radiosurgery for malignant melanoma brain metastases. *Clin Neurosurg.* 2007;54:241–247.
150. Demaria S, Bhardwaj N, McBride WH, Formenti SC. Combining radiotherapy and immunotherapy: a revived partnership. *Int J Radiat Oncol Biol Phys.* 2005;63:655–666.
151. Zhang B, Bowerman NA, Salama JK, et al. Induced sensitization of tumor stroma leads to eradication of established cancer by T cells. *J Exp Med.* 2007;204:49–55.
152. Lee Y, Auh SL, Wang Y, et al. Therapeutic effects of ablative radiation on local tumor require CD8+ T cells: changing strategies for cancer treatment. *Blood.* 2009; 114:589–595.
153. Vu HL, Sikora AG, Fu S, Kao J. HPV-induced oropharyngeal cancer, immune response and response to therapy. *Cancer Lett.* 2010;288:149–155.

23

HISTOLOGY OF MELANOMA AND PRECURSOR LESIONS

A. HAFEEZ DIWAN
DOINA IVAN
VICTOR G. PRIETO

Introduction

Melanoma and its precursors can cause considerable diagnostic confusion. The main reason for this is that many of the precursor lesions may mimic or simulate melanoma (and vice versa). Therefore, appropriate diagnosis needs careful consideration of the histologic features of both melanoma and its precursor lesions.

In this chapter, we discuss the histologic appearance of benign and malignant melanocytic lesions. Also discussed are the ancillary immunohistochemical techniques that may help elucidate the diagnosis.

Melanocytic Nevi

Benign nevi may be regarded as precursor lesions of melanoma in the following two ways: patients with multiple benign melanocytic nevi (more than a hundred) are at a greater risk for developing melanoma, and giant melanocytic congenital nevi (>20 cm in size) exhibit a risk for development of melanoma within the lesion itself.[1–5]

Benign Melanocytic Nevi

Benign nevi are proliferations of nevus cells that are confined mostly to the epidermis (junctional nevi), mostly confined to the dermis (intradermal nevi), or are found in both the dermis and epidermis (compound nevi).

Junctional Nevi

These are composed of very bland nevus cells, arrayed in nests as well as single cells, along the dermal epidermal junction. The nevus cells typically are round. Cytologic atypia, manifest as hyperchromatic, large nuclei with or without nucleoli, is not prominent. Also, pagetoid or intraepidermal scatter is not usually seen—this histologic feature refers to the presence of melanocytic nevus cells at levels above the basal epidermal layer. It should be noted that, in situations where a lesion has been rubbed or traumatized, it may develop focal pagetoid spread. However, other features of rubbing also may be seen in this situation, including parakeratosis, serum crust, and epidermal acanthosis.

A variant of junctional nevi is the lentiginous junctional nevus.[6,7] This refers to a predominance of single nevus cells along the dermal epidermal junction, without other features of a dysplastic nevus, as discussed below.

Intradermal Nevi (Fig 23–1)

An intradermal nevus is composed of nests of bland nevus cells with abundant cytoplasm and is located closer to the epidermis and adnexa (Type A cells). Below this are smaller cells with less cytoplasm and smaller nuclei called Type B cells. The deepest cells are spindled and narrow, similar to Schwann cells and are referred to as Type C cells.[8] Not all cell types are present in all cases, but a gradual decrease in size of the nevus cells is expected from the top to the bottom of the lesion; this phenomenon is known as maturation.[9] The absence of maturation, in fact, is a feature of melanoma.

It is important to realize that some intradermal nevi might have the larger Type A type cells in nests lower down in the lesion, giving the appearance of lack of maturation. However, these lesions, known as inverted Type A or clonal nevi, have other features of nevi, and importantly, lack the features of melanoma.[10,11] Basically, these lesions resemble Type A cells stuck in middle of a benign nevus. Some nevi may have a very prominent Type C component, with areas that appear very neural (neurotized nevi). On occasion, almost no rounded nevus cells are present, and the lesion may resemble a neurofibroma. Immunohistochemical evaluation with markers such as MART1/Melan-A will decorate the nevus but not the neurofibroma, allowing an easy distinction to be made.

Other lesions may have nevus cells with very clear cytoplasm, giving rise to a morphological variant known as balloon cell nevi, as the clear cells have a ballooned appearance.[12] The ballooning is the result of dilated, vacuolated melanosomes; therefore, these cells are S-100/MART1/Melan-A/HMB45 positive, but are negative for glycogen.

Other features commonly seen in nevi that do not necessarily denote malignancy, include multinucleated nevus cells, vascular invasion, and perineural invasion.

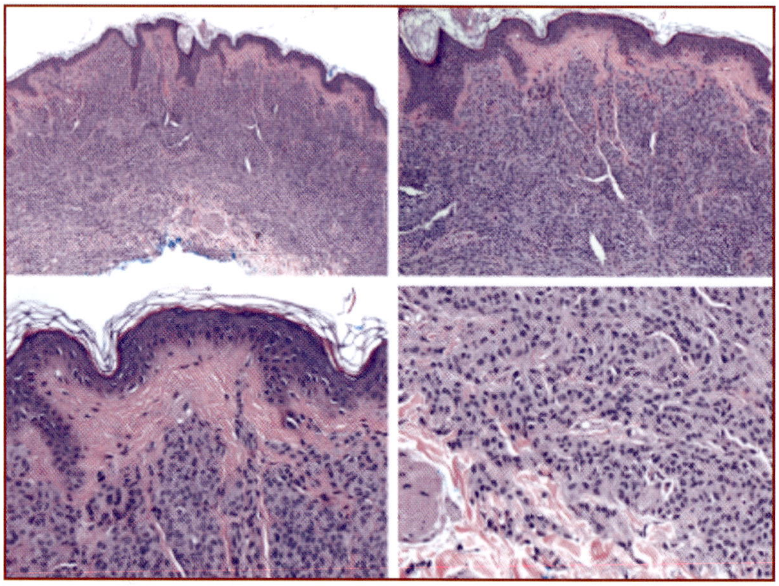

Figure 23–1. Intradermal nevus. Top left and right panels show low power images (20× and 40×, respectively). The bottom left panel is a higher power image (100×) showing the top of the lesion. The bottom right panel shows the lower half of the lesion at the same magnification (100×). Note the lack of cytologic atypia and the decrease in size from top to bottom (ie, maturation).

Compound Nevi

The word "compound" refers to the presence of both junctional and dermal components. This lesion is aptly named, as the histopathologic findings represent a composite of the findings for both junctional and intradermal nevi.

Halo Nevi

These nevi have a prominent inflammatory component composed of lymphocytes and macrophages. Inflammation may obscure the melanocytic component partially or completely. The halo phenomenon is a clinical descriptor, referring to a zone of hypopigmentation surrounding a pigmented lesion. Both benign junctional/intradermal/compound nevi and dysplastic nevi may be heavily inflamed and exhibit the halo phenomenon.

So-Called Nevi of Special Sites

Some anatomic areas, such as breast, groin, axilla, and ear, have been included in a loosely defined group of nevi called "of special sites." These lesions demonstrate architectural disorder, presenting as bridging, confluence of nests, and even focal pagetoid upward migration, but lack significant cytologic atypia or inflammatory response, features typical of dysplastic nevi.

Blue Nevus

Malignant transformation of a benign blue nevus is very rare, although we have seen sporadic cases of melanoma arising in association with blue nevi. The histologic features of blue nevi are important, because a subset of primary and metastatic melanomas may have a blue nevus-like morphology.[13,14] Also, blue nevi may arise in patients with prior melanoma.

Blue nevi are composed of spindled, pigmented cells with dendritic processes. Sometimes the lesions exhibit considerable fibrosis and are referred to as desmoplastic blue nevi. Mitotic figures or prominent nuclear atypia are not features of blue nevi.

Cellular Blue Nevus

Cellular blue nevi occasionally may undergo malignant transformation, with melanoma arising in association with a cellular blue nevus.[15] These nevi have two components: bundles of hypopigmented, spindled, or epithelioid cells interspersed with pigmented dendritic melanocytes. Melanophages (macrophages with melanin) also may be evident. Numerous or atypical mitotic figures, cellular atypia, and necrosis are not seen.

Atypical cellular blue nevi may have mild cytologic atypia and scattered mitotic figures, but atypical mitotic figures and necrosis are not seen.[16] The only situation in which focal necrosis may be seen in blue nevi is after previous trauma such as a prior punch biopsy.

Immunohistochemical studies may be helpful in difficult cases. These nevi are diffusely HMB45-positive, in contrast to possible patchy positivity in melanoma, and show a low proliferative rate when labeled for Ki-67.[17]

Combined Nevus

As the name suggests, these nevi combine the features of two types of nevi, most often blue nevus and compound/intradermal/junctional nevus.[18,19] However, other combinations may be present, such as combined dysplastic and blue nevus, or combined Spitz and intradermal nevus.

Spitz Nevi

Spitz nevi are not regarded as precursor lesions of melanoma.[20,21] However, they frequently pose diagnostic difficulties and share features with melanomas that have "spitzoid morphology." In addition, there is a gray zone of lesions with spitzoid morphology that cannot be classified histologically and that may metastasize and prove fatal. For these reasons, it is important to be aware of the histologic features of this entity.

Spitz nevi have spindled and epithelioid cells in the epidermis and dermis.[22] The epidermal nests are composed vertically oriented cells, creating the popular comparison to "bunches of bananas." There are pink, eosinophilic, globular deposits in the epidermis called Kamino bodies which may also be present in melanoma.[23] Pagetoid spread may be present in the center of the lesion. The dermal component shows maturation similar to other nevi, with diminution in size with descent in the dermis. Cytologic atypia may be present, but it should not be extreme. Mitotic figures may be present, but these are never atypical, nor are they present in the deeper portion or lower half of the lesion. Variants of Spitz nevi with increased dermal fibrosis are also recognized. These are called desmoplastic Spitz nevi.

Pigmented spindle cell nevus of Reed is a variant of Spitz nevus usually seen in the lower extremities, with heavily pigmented spindled cells.[22,24] These lesions are present in the epidermis and upper dermis. As with Spitz nevi, pagetoid spread, if present, is seen only in the center of the lesion.

Immunohistochemical studies may be very helpful in diagnosing or differentiating these lesions. Spitz nevi, like other nevi, may demonstrate maturation with HMB45.[25] This refers to the fact that the epidermal and upper portions of the lesion are labeled with HMB45, but there is loss of immunoreactivity with progressive descent in the dermis (alternatively, these lesions may be diffusely and uniformly labeled with HMB45). Nuclear Ki-67 labeling shows the same pattern, with an overall low proliferation rate that has been variously determined to be between 2% to 5%.[26]

Congenital Nevi

Congenital nevi exhibit the features of compound and intradermal nevi described above. In addition, they show aggregations of nevus cells around adnexal structures such as hair follicles and eccrine glands, as well as vessels.[27] It is important to note that these features are not pathognomonic of congenital nevi.[28] Some diagnosticians, therefore, refer to nevi having these histologic features as "nevi with features suggestive of congenital onset."

Congenital nevi may extend very deep into the subcutaneous tissue, with infiltration of fat lobules and even around nerves, thus mimicking perineural invasion. Such infiltration should not be regarded as a malignant feature, in the absence of other findings. The overlying intraepidermal component may exhibit plump melanocytic cells with architectural atypia, that is, crowded single and nested cells. However, pagetoid spread, especially at the periphery of the lesion, usually is not seen.

Significant cytologic atypia or extensive pagetoid spread in the epidermal component may be an indicator of melanoma in situ arising in a congenital nevus. Giant congenital nevi, defined as being larger than 20 cm in lateral dimension, have an increased incidence of melanoma developing within them. Melanomas arising within congenital nevi are characterized by cytologic atypia, increased mitoses (including atypical ones), necrosis, and possibly destruction of adnexal structures. The zone of melanoma usually is distinct from the surrounding nevus, in contrast to proliferative nodules. Benign proliferative nodules arising within congenital nevi show a gradation of cellular features from the nodule to the nevus around them. Furthermore, they do not show the obviously atypical features of melanoma listed above.[29]

Congenital leptomeningeal melanocytic proliferations may similarly transform into melanoma.[2,3,30] The benign lesions exhibit the features of nevus, with a lack of atypia, mitoses, or necrosis. Obviously, no epidermal component will be seen in this location, as nevus cells exist within soft tissue.

Dysplastic Nevi (Fig 23–2)

Dysplastic nevi constitute a contentious issue in dermatopathology, with various disagreements about their classification.[31,32] A recent review of dysplastic nevi was appropriately titled "Dysplastic Nevus: The Eye of the Hurricane," reflecting the lack of consensus on this topic.[33]

An NIH consensus conference in 1992 recommended the term "nevus with architectural disorder and melanocytic atypia."[34] This term neatly captures the two features common to all dysplastic nevi: these nevi exhibit both architectural disorder and cytologic atypia of the melanocytes. Moreover, "nevus with architectural disorder and melanocytic

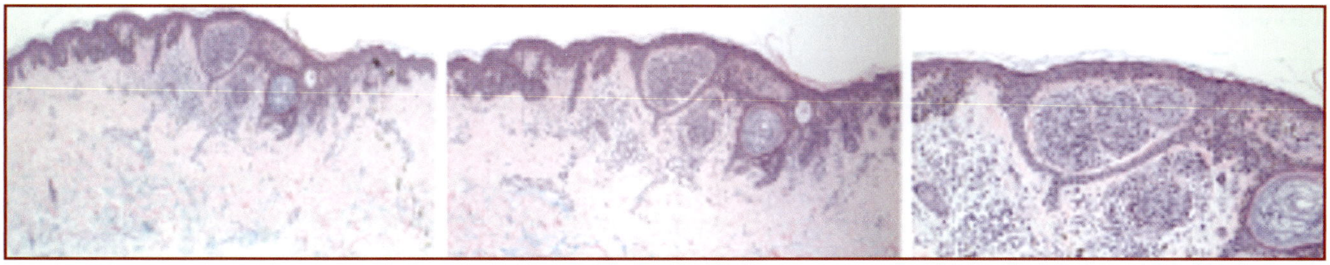

Figure 23–2. Dysplastic nevus. The left panel is a low power (20×) image of a dysplastic nevus. The middle panel (40×) shows bridging, extension of the epidermal component beyond the dermal ("shoulder"), dermal fibrosis, and a lymphocytic infiltrate. These features are more easily appreciated in the right panel (100×).

atypia" is understood by the many dermatologists and other clinicians who deal with these lesions. Therefore, the term, in our opinion is useful, so we recommend using it. Others call these lesions "nevus with architectural disorder" or NAD.

Shea et al[35] further subclassified both the architectural disorder and cytologic atypia into mild, moderate and severe categories, and this classification system is depicted in Table 23–1.

Interestingly, there is a direct correlation between architectural disorder and cytologic atypia. For example, a lesion with severe architectural disorder is also more likely to have severe cytologic atypia.[35] In our practice, we have found that often the two features differ just by one grade difference (eg, a nevus with moderate architectural disorder may have mild cytologic atypia). On the other hand, we recently described one instance of nevi which occur on the lower legs with severe architectural disorder but which have only mild cytologic atypia.[36] Such cases may represent early dysplastic nevi that later become more nested and thus will show a lesser degree of architectural disorder.[37]

Another system of classification was similarly based on the degree of architectural features of circumscription, symmetry, distortion of the rete ridges, pagetoid spread, and involvement of the zone between rete ridges (the suprapapillary plate), as well as cytologic factors of nuclear size, nucleolar size, and type of chromatin: euchromatic or hyperchromatic (dark).[38] In this system, mildly atypical nevi are circumscribed, symmetric, and involve only the tips of the rete ridges. The nuclei are not oval, are not larger than basal keratinocytes, and have a small nucleolus. Moderately atypical NADs are not well circumscribed (although they are symmetric), have distorted rete ridges with nevus cells at the tips and sides, tend to focally involve the suprapapillary plates, and may have a little pagetoid spread in the center of the lesion. The nuclei are at least as big as keratinocytes. Finally, severely atypical NADs are not symmetrical but are circumscribed, have considerable rete ridge distortion with prominent dermal fibrosis and nests that are at the tips and sides of rete ridges, with fusion of nests across rete ridges, with greater involvement of the suprapapillary plates. Cytologically, the nuclei are larger than keratinocytes with larger nucleoli.[38]

It should be noted that these systems are not used universally, and that there is, as yet, no agreement among dermatopathologists about which system to use, or whether any system should be used at all. Some simply use the term dysplastic nevus, whereas others advocate a two-tier system of low and high grade.

Does it make sense to classify nevi as exhibiting mild, moderate, or severe dysplasia? Arumi-Uria and coworkers[38] found that individuals with NAD with severe atypia had a 4 times greater risk of developing melanoma as compared to those with mild atypia, and nearly 3 times the risk as compared to patients who had NAD with moderate atypia. Clearly, there is a difference in the degree to which dysplastic nevi may act as precursors to melanoma, depending on whether they are mild, moderate, or severe. Many clinicians, moreover, treat severely dysplastic nevi as melanoma in situ, with a 5-mm margin of resection. Mildly dysplastic nevi are usually not re-excised

Table 23–1. Classification System for Dysplastic Nevi as per Shea et al[35]

Component	Definition	Scoring
Architectural Disorder		
Circumscription	Lesion ends with nests on both sides	0: Circumscribed 1: Absent nest on one or both sides
Symmetry	The two halves of the lesion are approximately similar, based on the following: 1. extension of the junctional or epidermal component beyond the dermal component (if present) 2. the kind of dermal fibrosis present (dysplastic nevi have a characteristic concentric fibrosis below the epidermis, called lamellar fibrosis); 3. The presence of lymphocytes (the amount of lymphocytic infiltrate should appear similar in both sides of the lesion).	0: Symmetric 1: Asymmetry is present
Cohesion of Nests	50% of nests are compact (not fragmented)	0: Present 1: Absent
Suprabasal melanocytes	Prominent or present on edge of lesion	0: Absent 1: Present
Confluence	Predominantly single confluent ((ie, next to each other) or as nests bridging rete ridges, in more than half the lesion	0: Absent 1: Present
Single cell proliferation	Predominantly single melanocytes vs. nests in more than 20% of the lesion	0: Absent 1: Present
Cytologic Atypia		
Nuclear features		0: Round/oval, not dark (ie, euchromatic) 1: The features above are not present
Nucleoli		0: Absent in >50% of cells 1: Present >50% of cells
Nuclear size		0: Not significantly enlarged 1: Melanocyte size >2× as big as basal keratinocytes
Cell size		0: Not significantly enlarged 1: Cytoplasm size >2× as big as basal keratinocytes

Based on this system, a score of 0–1 equals mild architectural disorder, 2–3 equals moderate architectural disorder, and 4–6 equals severe architectural disorder. Simlarly, a cytologic atypia score of 0–1 equals mild atypia, 2 equals moderate atypia, and 3–4 equals severe atypia.

and moderately dysplastic nevi are re-excised by some if they are present at the margins. At the University of Texas MD Anderson Cancer Center, we currently use a three-tier system of mild, moderate, and severe dysplasia and indicate in the report if the lesion has been completely excised or not.

Melanoma

There are 4 major types of melanoma. These are lentigo maligna type, superficial spreading type, acral-lentiginous-mucosal type, and nodular type. These 4 types describe not only morphologic groups but are also characterized by different genetic signatures.[39–42] Lentigo maligna type usually has KIT mutations (but not B-RAF) and other abnormalities associated with UV damage. Acral-lentiginous (and mucosal) melanomas also show KIT mutations. Superficial spreading melanomas and nodular melanomas exhibit BRAF and NRAS mutations.

In addition to these 4 main types, there are other subtypes including desmoplastic, nevoid, Spitzoid, and small cell. All types of melanoma may have associated benign or dysplastic nevi. These nevi may represent the precursor nevus from which the melanoma arose, but at present, there is no direct proof that this is indeed the case.

Histologic Features of Melanoma

The most important prognostic variable is Breslow thickness. Thickness is measured from the granular layer, when present, or the top of epithelium in mucosal melanoma, or, if there is an ulcer, from the base of the ulcer.[43,44] Melanoma in situ has the best prognosis. Invasive melanoma is stratified into 4 categories (T1-T4) as follows: T1 less than or equal to 1 mm, T2 between 1.01 and 2 mm, T3 between 2.01 and 4 mm, and T4 larger than 4 mm. Clark levels represent another method of describing thickness, and they are noted in Table 23–2.

Table 23–2. Clark Levels of Melanoma Thickness

Clark I	– in situ lesions
Clark II	– melanoma invading papillary dermis, without filling and expanding it
Clark III	– melanoma filling and expanding papillary dermis
Clark IV	– melanoma involving reticular dermis
Clark V	– melanoma invasive into subcutaneous fat

Vertical growth phase is defined as a dermal nest larger than an epidermal nest, or the presence of mitotic figure(s) in the dermal component.[45] Either criterion suffices for vertical growth phase. Vertical growth phase can be further subdivided into mitogenic, with dermal mitotic figures, or nonmitogenic when the lesion lacks mitotic figures. A mitogenic vertical growth phase constitutes a worse prognostic indicator and currently it is used to recommend sentinel lymph node examination.[46,47] Radial growth phase refers to extension of the epidermal component three rete ridges away from the dermal component.[45]

Ulceration of the primary melanoma may be present. The presence of ulceration upstages the melanoma to the next stage.[48]

Another feature that may be seen is partial regression, which refers to dermal fibrosis with vascular proliferation, inflammation and melanophages —melanoma cells are not seen in such zone of regression in the dermis. If partial regression is present in more than half the lesion, we regard it as extensive regression. Complete regression occurs when melanoma is absent from both the epidermis and dermis.

The dermal component may be composed of epithelioid, spindled or melanocytes exhibiting variable morphology. The dermal component can be classified as desmoplastic when there are spindled, atypical melanoma cells with intervening dermal fibrosis. When the desmoplastic component constitutes more than 90% of the lesion, the melanoma can be subclassified as a desmoplastic melanoma. If there are other components, such as more standard spindled or epithelioid components, that comprise greater than 10% of the lesion, then the tumor is regarded as mixed. These behave differently clinically, with a greater incidence of lymph node involvement than traditional desmoplastic melanoma.[49,50] It is important to note that in nearly half of desmoplastic melanomas, there is no obvious intraepidermal component.

Perineural invasion is quite common in both the spindled and desmoplastic variants. When prominent, the melanoma may be additionally classified as neurotropic.[51,52] Although some authors consider neurotropic melanoma equal to desmoplastic melanoma, we prefer not to use this term as it only describes a melanoma with prominent perineural spread.

An important consideration is the absence of maturation, which is the orderly decrease in size of melanocytic cytoplasm and nuclei with descent in the dermis.[53] This also should be evident with the help of HMB45 and Ki67 immunolabeling, both of which should be erratic, patchily reactive, without any evidence of orderly decrease in labeling from the top to lower portions (Figs 23–3 and 23–4).[54] Numerous Ki67 positive cells, indicative of increased proliferation, are expected in melanoma.

Microscopic satellitosis refers to the presence of intervening normal dermis or subcutaneous tissue between the main body of the lesion and the satellite focus. The presence of satellitosis confers poorer prognosis, similar to the presence of lymphatic metastases.[48,55,56]

Additionally, tumor-infiltrating lymphocytes may be present. When brisk, they are present throughout the tumor, and may confer a better prognosis, suggesting a heightened immune response to the neoplasm. [57,58] The immunology of melanoma and prospects for immunotherapy are discussed elsewhere in this text.

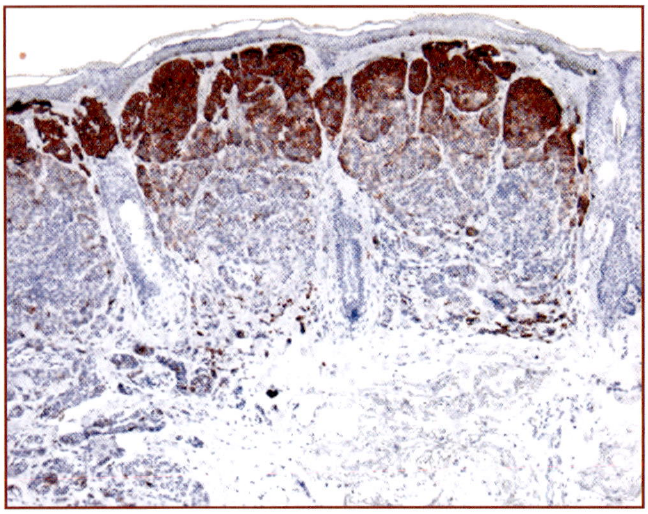

Figure 23–3. Eyelid melanoma labeled with HMB45 (40×). Note that, although the top portion is more intensely decorated, there is still patchy immunoreactivity in the lower portion of the lesion, evidence of lack of maturation.

Table 23–3 shows the parameters we incorporate into our melanoma reports.

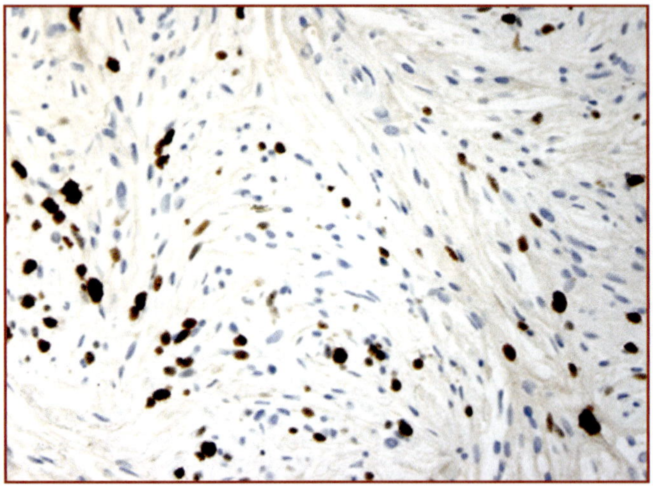

Figure 23–4. Dermal component of melanoma (100×) exhibiting brisk labeling with the Mib-1 antibody for Ki-67, indicative of high proliferation.

Table 23–3. Parameters included in pathology reports of melanoma at the University of Texas MD Anderson Cancer Center and Baylor College of Medicine

Type of melanoma
Depth of invasion (in mm)
Clark level
Ulceration
Dermal mitotic figures per mm^2
Vertical growth phase
Radial growth phase
Regression
Microscopic satellitosis
Tumor infiltrating lymphocytes
Perineural invasion
Vascular invasion
Associated nevus (if any)
Predominant cytology
Surgical margins

Lentigo Maligna Type (Fig 23–5)

This type is related to chronic sun damage and occurs mostly in the head and neck region. There is epidermal atrophy, with solar elastosis indicative of solar damage. There are atypical melanocytes in nests or as single cells. These are confluent lesions, meaning they have no or few intervening keratinocytes. Some pagetoid spread may be present. The melanocytes are atypical, being large and hyperchromatic, and they may be spindle-shaped or epithelioid. Melanocytes grow down hair follicles and other adnexal structures. If the proliferation is confined to the epidermis, the lesion is a melanoma in situ, lentigo maligna type. Presence of malignant cells in the dermis is invasive melanoma, lentigo maligna type.

Lentigo maligna melanoma in situ should be distinguished from atypical intraepidermal melanocytic proliferations. These arise in a background of sun damage, and the distinguishing features from melanoma in situ are the absence of intraepidermal confluence and nests. Cytologic atypia may be present, but usually is less marked. This consideration is very important when assessing the margins of excision, since atypical proliferations may extend close to or up to the margins—this is interpreted as a "field" effect of melanocytic atypia.[59]

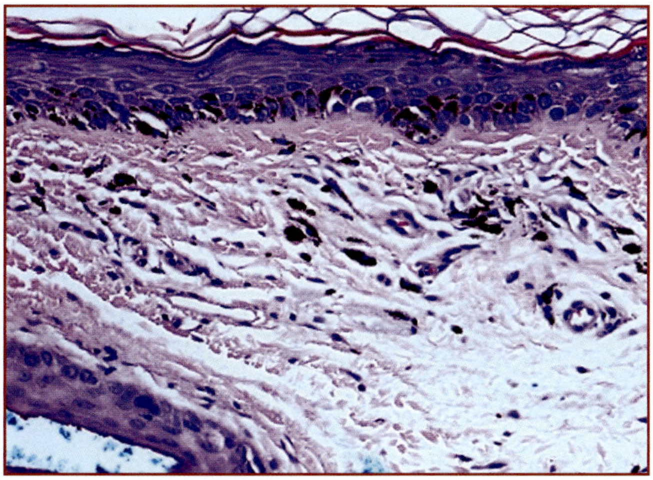

Figure 23–5. Lentigo maligna melanoma in situ (200×). Cytologically atypical melanocytes, confined to the lower epidermis, exhibiting confluence. There are melanophages in the upper dermis.

Superficial Spreading Melanoma (Fig 23–6)

This type is related to intermittent sun exposure, and often occurs on the legs of women and backs of

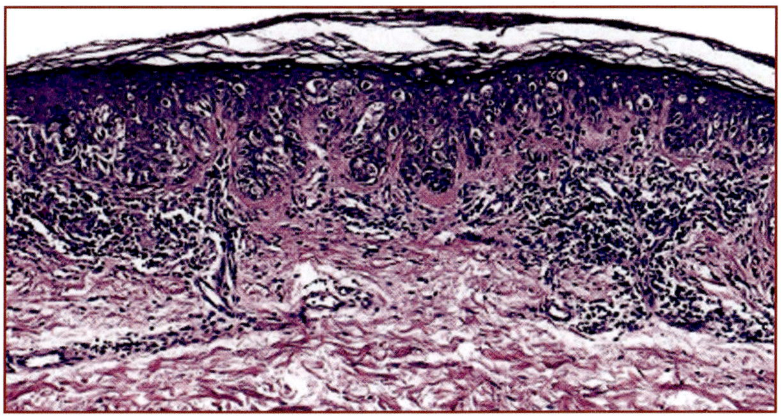

Figure 23–6. Melanoma in situ (100×). Contrast this with Figure 23–5. Here is melanoma in situ, with very atypical melanocytes, showing pagetoid spread. Had a dermal component been present, this would have been classified as a superficial spreading melanoma (which shows pagetoid spread).

men. They are composed of single and nested, cytologically atypical spindled or epithelioid melanocytes that are hyperchromatic or large, with prominent nuclei. Notably, the degree of pagetoid spread is very marked and much greater than in lentigo maligna melanoma. By definition, all superficial spreading melanomas have radial growth phase. The criteria for a vertical growth phase, regression, satellitosis, and lack of maturation are the same as given above. The invasive component may be spindled, epithelioid, nevoid, or composed of small cells. It is usually not desmoplastic. These lesions may or may not be ulcerated.

Acral Lentiginous Melanoma (Including Mucosal Melanoma)

Acral lentiginous melanoma does not only occur on the acral location, but is a category that also includes mucosal melanomas. This type is characterized by a prominent intraepidermal confluent, lentiginous proliferation of atypical melanocytes with prominent pagetoid spread. The stratum corneum contains irregularly arrayed pigment, but in mucosal sites, stratum corneum may not be seen. The dermal component and the characteristics that apply to it are similar to those described above for lentigo maligna melanoma and superficial spreading melanoma.

Nodular Melanoma

By definition, these melanomas do not have radial growth phase in that there is no extension of the epidermal component more than 3 rete ridges away from the dermal component. Otherwise, the features are otherwise the same as those described above for the other types of melanoma. In the differential diagnosis, we should consider metastatic melanoma.

Nevoid Melanoma

Nevoid melanomas can be missed very easily. As the name suggests these melanomas are composed of atypical cells that resemble nevus cells, making it possible for diagnostic inaccuracy to occur, especially at low power examination.[60–63]

Many regard nevoid melanoma as a nodular melanoma; others use the term to include melanomas with nevoid morphology and radial growth phase, like superficial spreading melanoma with nevoid melanoma cells. However it is defined, the important point is to appreciate that the nevoid morphology is associated with malignant behavior.

Higher power examination reveals that the cells, albeit nevoid, are large, with at least mild nuclear pleomorphism and atypia, manifest as dark nuclei with irregular nuclear contours. Nucleoli may also be present, and the cells usually are very crowded. Another key feature is that the cells do not decrease in size with descent in the dermis, which is to say that maturation is absent. It should be emphasized that the absence of maturation is not always readily apparent, and pseudomaturation is a well-recognized phenomenon. But, even when the cells apparently decrease in size, the nuclei might still be quite similar even in the deeper portion of the tumor, allowing one to make an estimation of apparent or pseudo-maturation. Dermal mitotic figures must be sought for and are almost always found.

Immunohistochemical evaluation for HMB45 and Ki-67 usually fail to show maturation; these lesions may show patchy labeling with HMB45 and more than 5% proliferation rate with anti-Ki-67.

Desmoplastic Melanoma (Fig 23–7)

Desmoplastic melanoma has already been discussed above in the section on the histologic features of melanoma. In desmoplastic melanoma, the malignant cells are cytologically atypical and spindled with considerable fibrosis (desmoplasia). Purely desmoplastic melanomas have more than 90% of this component. Perineural invasion and clusters of lymphocytes are quite common, and an overlying intraepidermal component is present in only half the cases.

A "scar" that looks too cellular may be a desmoplastic melanoma (which has been referred to as the "lawsuit melanoma" because it can be very easily missed). An important clue to the diagnosis is the presence of a lymphocytic infiltrate. Immunohistochemical studies may be helpful. The tumor cells are S-100 positive and may also show spotty gp100 (with HMB45)/MelanA/tyrosinase labeling.

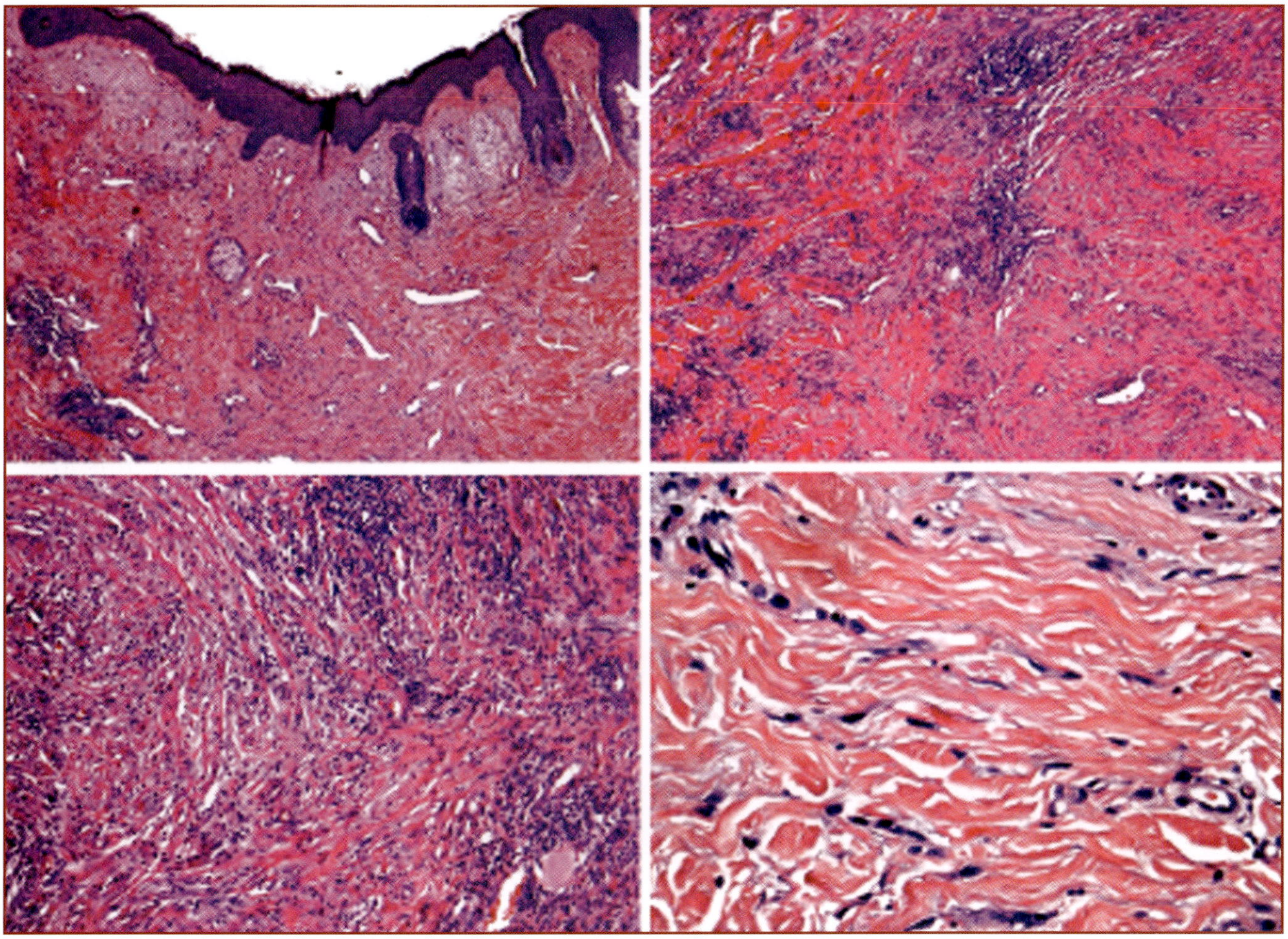

Figure 23–7. Desmoplastic melanoma. The top left panel (40×) shows the lack of an epidermal component. In the top right panel (40×), note that the lesions looks very cellular, with a lymphocytic infiltrate, and these features are seen at a higher power (100×) in the bottom right panel. The bottom left panel shows severely cytologically atypical spindle cells (200×)

Distinguishing a desmoplastic melanoma from desmoplastic nevus usually is easy, but in difficult cases, Ki-67 labeling is very helpful. On Ki-67 labeling, desmoplastic melanoma demonstrates more than 20 positive cells per mm^2, versus only rare cells in desmoplastic nevus.[64]

Spitzoid Melanoma and Atypical Spitzoid Lesions

Spitzoid melanomas are composed of spindled and epithelioid cells, similar to those seen in Spitz nevi. In contrast to Spitz nevi, several atypical features may be present: asymmetry, poorly circumscribed lesions that do not end with nests, pagetoid spread at the periphery (Spitz nevi may have central pagetoid spread), epidermal consumption, a lack of maturation (also seen on HMB45 and anti-Ki-67 immunohistochemical studies), mitotic figures (even atypical ones) in all parts of the tumor, marked cytologic atypia with extreme nuclear pleomorphism, and an absence of a wedge-shaped contour typically seen in Spitz nevi.

Epidermal consumption present in Spitzoid melanoma refers to the separation of the epidermis and dermis because of the proliferation of dermal-epidermal melanoma cells. This feature is not exclusive to Spitzoid melanoma, but may be present in other melanomas, as well as in some Spitz nevi. Finally, the tumor borders may be infiltrative, with satellitosis evident. It is important to realize that not all these features may be present, but the presence of several is a strong indication that the lesion may very well be a melanoma.

It is not at all clear how poorly these patients fare. There have been several studies on this issue, the largest of which evaluated the course of 38 patients diagnosed with Spitzoid melanoma. This study concluded that patients older than 11 years with Spitzoid melanoma fared worse, with an increased rate of metastases and death.[65]

Between the lesions classified as Spitz nevi and Spitzoid melanoma are those that are difficult to fit into either category.[66] They may lack peripheral circumscription, or have mild cytologic atypia or greater than expected pagetoid spread at the periphery. The findings may be difficult or impossible to categorize. In this situation, some diagnose these lesions as "atypical Spitz tumors," indicating that the biologic behavior or malignant potential of these lesions cannot be predicted.

Miscellaneous Melanoma Subtypes

Melanoma may display many morphologic features. They may be polypoid in silhouette (polypoid melanomas), have balloon cells, or have a verrucous architecture with keratinocytes exhibiting papillomatosis and hyperkeratosis (verrucous melanoma).[67–69] Other variants may have signet ring cells or demonstrate myxoid or chondrosarcomatous differentiation.[70–72]

Some melanomas have very prominent pigmentation and are stuffed with melanophages. The pigmentation may be so pronounced that the cytologic atypia of melanoma cells may not be appreciated unless the slide is bleached to remove the melanin. These melanomas variously have been referred to as "animal-type" melanomas (a term we do not prefer) or pigmented epithelioid melanocytoma.[73] These melanomas may behave less aggressively than other melanomas.[74]

Melanomas arising in cellular blue nevi have been previously described.[75–77] Some of these are alternatively called malignant blue nevi, and they exhibit severe cytologic atypia, mitotic figures (including atypical forms), and necrosis.[75,77] An epidermal component is typically not seen in malignant blue nevi. Some of these lesions have mutation of the GNAQ gene.

Small cell melanoma is composed of very atypical, small, blue cells, resembling neuroblastoma cells. Small cells may be seen in any melanoma subtype, and some may also have morphological features of nevoid melanomas.[78] Small cell melanoma may arise in younger patients and demonstrate very aggressive behavior.[79]

Metastatic Melanoma

Metastatic melanoma is typically intradermal, but there may be an intraepidermal component. Exclusively intraepidermal metastatic melanomas are uncommon.[80–81] The differential diagnosis for metastatic melanoma includes nodular melanoma, and it may be impossible to distinguish the two histologically. Clinical history is critical in making this determination.

Metastatic melanomas that appear to be blue nevi have also been documented, but the presence of severe cytologic atypia, lymphocytic infiltrate, and mitoses, along with clinical history are very useful.[13,14,82] Ki-67 labeling is expected to be high in metastatic melanoma, unlike blue nevi. HMB45 labeling may be patchy in many cases, in contrast with the strong and diffuse labeling of blue nevus, and this can be a valuable clue as well.

Clear Cell Sarcoma (Melanoma of Soft Parts)

Clear cell sarcoma is characterized by nests and fascicles of tumor cells, many of which may have clear cytoplasm. The tumor is labeled with melanocytic markers. The diagnosis is considered when a deep-seated, tendinous lesion is present, particularly when there is no history of prior melanoma. Because this is a deep lesion, without epidermal or even dermal involvement in many cases, the main concern in the differential diagnosis is metastatic melanoma. These lesions have also been described in the head and neck region, and a majority of them have a characteristic translocation involving chromosomes 12 and 22.[83–85]

Conclusion

This chapter reviewed several melanocytic lesions, including melanoma. The histopathologic diagnosis of melanoma may be challenging at times, and may require immunohistochemical studies.[86] Therefore, an experienced dermatopathologist can play an integral part in the multidisciplinary assessment and management of cutaneous melanocytic lesions of the head and neck.

References

1. Gandini S, Sera F, Cattaruzza MS, et al. Meta-analysis of risk factors for cutaneous melanoma: I. common and atypical naevi. *Eur J Cancer.* 2005;41(1):28–44.
2. Bittencourt FV, Marghoob AA, Kopf AW, Koenig KL, Bart RS. Large congenital melanocytic nevi and the risk for development of malignant melanoma and neurocutaneous melanocytosis. *Pediatrics.* 2000;106(4):736–741.
3. Hale EK, Stein J, Ben-Porat L, et al. Association of mela - noma and neurocutaneous melanocytosis with large congenital melanocytic naevi—results from the NYU-LCMN registry. *Br J Dermatol.* 2005;152(3):512–517.
4. Ruiz-Maldonado R, Tamayo L, Laterza AM, Duran C. Giant pigmented nevi: clinical, histopathologic, and therapeutic considerations. *J Pediatr.* 1992;120(6):906–911.
5. Swerdlow AJ, Green A. Melanocytic naevi and mela - noma: an epidemiological perspective. *Br J Dermatol.* 1987;117(2):137–146.
6. Marchesi L, Naldi L, Di Landro A, Cavalieri d'Oro L, Brevi A, Cainelli T. Segmental lentiginosis with "jentigo" histologic pattern. *Am J Dermatopathol.* 1992;14(4):323–327.
7. Stewart DM, Altman J, Mehregan AH. Speckled lentiginous nevus. *Arch Dermatol.* 1978;114(6):895–896.
8. Masson P. My conception of cellular nevi. *Cancer.* 1951; 4(1):9–38.
9. Goovaerts G, Buyssens N. Nevus cell maturation or atrophy? *Am J Dermatopathol.* 1988;10(1):20–27.
10. Ball NJ, Golitz LE. Melanocytic nevi with focal atypical epithelioid cell components: a review of seventy-three cases. *J Am Acad Dermatol.* 1994;30(5 pt 1):724–729.
11. Huynh PM, Glusac EJ, Bolognia JL. The clinical appearance of clonal nevi (inverted type A nevi). *Int J Dermatol.* 2004;43(12):882–885.
12. Martinez-Casimiro L, Sanchez Carazo JL, Alegre V. Balloon cell naevus. *J Eur Acad Dermatol Venereol.* 2009;23(2):236–237.
13. Busam KJ. Metastatic melanoma to the skin simulating blue nevus. *Am J Surg Pathol.* 1999;23(3):276–282.
14. Wieselthier JS, White WL. Cutaneous metastasis of ocular malignant melanoma. An unusual presentation simulating blue nevi. *Am J Dermatopathol.* 1996;18(3):289–295.
15. Temple-Camp CR, Saxe N, King H. Benign and malignant cellular blue nevus. A clinicopathological study of 30 cases. *Am J Dermatopathol.* 1988;10(4):289–296.
16. Barnhill RL, Argenyi Z, Berwick M, et al. Atypical cellular blue nevi (cellular blue nevi with atypical features): lack of consensus for diagnosis and distinction from cellular blue nevi and malignant melanoma ("malignant blue nevus"). *Am J Surg Pathol.* 2008;32(1):36–44.
17. Wang Q, Prieto V, Esmaeli B, et al. Cellular blue nevi of the eyelid: a possible diagnostic pitfall. *J Am Acad Dermatol.* 2008;58(2):257–260.
18. Leopold JG, Richards DB. The interrelationship of blue and common naevi. *J Pathol Bacteriol.* 1968;95(1):37–46.
19. Pulitzer DR, Martin PC, Cohen AP, Reed RJ. Histologic classification of the combined nevus. Analysis of the variable expression of melanocytic nevi. *Am J Surg Pathol.* 1991;15(12):1111–1122.
20. Spitz S. Melanomas of childhood. *Am J Pathol.* 1948;24(3): 591–609.
21. Dal Pozzo V, Benelli C, Restano L, Gianotti R, Cesana BM. Clinical review of 247 case records of Spitz nevus (epithelioid cell and/or spindle cell nevus). *Dermatology.* 1997;194(1):20–25.
22. Paniago-Pereira C, Maize JC, Ackerman AB. Nevus of large spindle and/or epithelioid cells (Spitz's nevus). *Arch Dermatol.* 1978;114(12):1811–1823.
23. Kamino H, Misheloff E, Ackerman AB, Flotte TJ, Greco MA. Eosinophilic globules in Spitz's nevi: new findings and a diagnostic sign. *Am J Dermatopathol.* 1979;1(4): 323–324.
24. Reed RJ, Ichinose H, Clark WH, Jr., Mihm MC, Jr. Common and uncommon melanocytic nevi and borderline melanomas. *Semin Oncol.* 1975;2(2):119–147.
25. Lazzaro B, Elder DE, Rebers A, et al. Immunophenotyping of compound and Spitz nevi and vertical growth-phase melanomas using a panel of monoclonal antibodies reactive in paraffin sections. *J Investigat Dermatol.* 1993; 100(3):313S–317S.
26. Vollmer RT. Use of Bayes rule and MIB-1 proliferation index to discriminate Spitz nevus from malignant melanoma. *Am J Clin Pathol.* 2004;122(4):499–505.

27. Mark GJ, Mihm MC, Liteplo MG, Reed RJ, Clark WH. Congenital melanocytic nevi of the small and garment type. clinical, histologic, and ultrastructural studies. *Hum Pathol.* 1973;4(3):395–418.
28. Rhodes AR, Silverman RA, Harrist TJ, Melski JW. A histologic comparison of congenital and acquired nevomelanocytic nevi. *Arch Dermatol.* 1985;121(10):1266–1273.
29. Xu X, Bellucci KS, Elenitsas R, Elder DE. Cellular nodules in congenital pattern nevi. *J Cutan Pathol.* 2004;31(2): 153–159.
30. Chang CS, Hsieh PF, Chia LG, et al. Leptomeningeal malignant melanoma arising in neurocutaneous melanocytosis: a case report. *Zhonghua yi xue za zhi.* 1997;60(6): 316–320.
31. Ackerman AB. What naevus is dysplastic, a syndrome and the commonest precursor of malignant melanoma? A riddle and an answer. *Histopathol.* 1988;13(3):241–256.
32. Ackerman AB, Mihara I. Dysplasia, dysplastic melanocytes, dysplastic nevi, the dysplastic nevus syndrome, and the relation between dysplastic nevi and malignant melanomas. *Hum Pathol.* 1985;16(1):87–91.
33. Arumi-Uria M. Dysplastic nevus: the eye of the hurricane. *J Cutan Pathol.* 2008;35 (suppl 2):16–19.
34. NIH Consensus Conference. Diagnosis and treatment of early melanoma. *JAMA.* 1992;268(10):1314–1319.
35. Shea CR, Vollmer RT, Prieto VG. Correlating architectural disorder and cytologic atypia in Clark (dysplastic) melanocytic nevi. *Hum Pathol.* 1999;30(5):500–505.
36. Khalifeh I, Taraif S, Reed JA, Lazar AF, Diwan AH, Prieto VG. A subgroup of melanocytic nevi on the distal lower extremity (ankle) shares features of acral nevi, dysplastic nevi, and melanoma in situ: a potential misdiagnosis of melanoma in situ. *Am J Surg Pathol.* 2007; 31(7):1130–1136.
37. Torres-Cabala CA, Plaza JA, Diwan AH, Prieto VG. Severe architectural disorder is a potential pitfall in the diagnosis of small melanocytic lesions. *J Cutan Pathol.* 2010;37(8):860–865..
38. Arumi-Uria M, McNutt NS, Finnerty B. Grading of atypia in nevi: correlation with melanoma risk. *Mod Pathol.* 2003;16(8):764–771.
39. Curtin JA, Busam K, Pinkel D, Bastian BC. Somatic activation of KIT in distinct subtypes of melanoma. *J Clin Oncol.* 2006;24(26):4340–4346.
40. Curtin JA, Fridlyand J, Kageshita T, et al. Distinct sets of genetic alterations in melanoma. *N Engl J Med.* 2005; 353(20):2135–2147.
41. Satzger I, Schaefer T, Kuettler U, et al. Analysis of c-KIT expression and KIT gene mutation in human mucosal melanomas. *Br J Cancer.* 2008;99(12):2065–2069.
42. Ohashi A, Funasaka Y, Ueda M, Ichihashi M. c-KIT receptor expression in cutaneous malignant melanoma and benign melanotic naevi. *Melanoma Res.* 1996;6(1):25–30.
43. Breslow A. Problems in the measurement of tumor thickness and level of invasion in cutaneous melanoma. *Hum Pathol.* 1977;8(1):1–2.
44. Breslow A. Tumor thickness, level of invasion and node dissection in stage I cutaneous melanoma. *Ann Surg.* 1975;182(5):572–575.
45. Elder DE, Guerry Dt, Epstein MN, et al. Invasive malignant melanomas lacking competence for metastasis. *Am J Dermatopathol.* 1984;(6 suppl):55–61.
46. Elder DE. Pathology of melanoma. *Clin Cancer Res.* 2006; 12(7 pt 2):2308s–2311s.
47. Gimotty PA, Guerry D, Ming ME, et al. Thin primary cutaneous malignant melanoma: a prognostic tree for 10-year metastasis is more accurate than American Joint Committee on Cancer staging. *J Clin Oncol.* 2004;22(18): 3668–3676.
48. Balch CM, Soong SJ, Gershenwald JE, et al. Prognostic factors analysis of 17,600 melanoma patients: validation of the American Joint Committee on Cancer melanoma staging system. *J Clin Oncol.* 2001;19(16):3622–3634.
49. Pawlik TM, Ross MI, Prieto VG, et al. Assessment of the role of sentinel lymph node biopsy for primary cutaneous desmoplastic melanoma. *Cancer.* 2006;106(4):900–906.
50. George E, McClain SE, Slingluff CL, Polissar NL, Patterson JW. Subclassification of desmoplastic melanoma: pure and mixed variants have significantly different capacities for lymph node metastasis. *J Cutan Pathol.* 2009;36(4): 425–432.
51. Quinn MJ, Crotty KA, Thompson JF, Coates AS, O'Brien CJ, McCarthy WH. Desmoplastic and desmoplastic neurotropic melanoma: experience with 280 patients. *Cancer.* 1998;83(6):1128–1135.
52. Carlson JA, Dickersin GR, Sober AJ, Barnhill RL. Desmoplastic neurotropic melanoma. A clinicopathologic analysis of 28 cases. *Cancer.* 1995;75(2):478–494.
53. Li LX, Crotty KA, Palmer AA, et al. Differentiating benign nevi from malignant melanoma using DNA microdensitometry and karyometry and maturation: a zonal comparison, correlation and multivariate analysis. *Analytical Quant Cytol Histol. International Academy of Cytology [and] American Society of Cytology.* 2002;24(4):234–243.
54. Li LX, Crotty KA, McCarthy SW, Palmer AA, Kril JJ. A zonal comparison of MIB1-Ki67 immunoreactivity in benign and malignant melanocytic lesions. *Am J Dermatopathol.* 2000;22(6):489–495.
55. Day CL, Jr., Harrist TJ, Gorstein F, et al. Malignant melanoma. Prognostic significance of "microscopic satellites" in the reticular dermis and subcutaneous fat. *Ann Surg.* 1981;194(1):108–112.
56. Harrist TJ, Rigel DS, Day CL Jr, et al. "Microscopic satellites" are more highly associated with regional lymph node metastases than is primary melanoma thickness. *Cancer.* 1984;53(10):2183–2187.
57. Masback A, Olsson H, Westerdahl J, Ingvar C, Jonsson N. Prognostic factors in invasive cutaneous malignant melanoma: a population-based study and review. *Melanoma Res.* 2001;11(5):435–445.
58. Tuthill RJ, Unger JM, Liu PY, Flaherty LE, Sondak VK. Risk assessment in localized primary cutaneous mela-

noma: a Southwest Oncology Group study evaluating nine factors and a test of the Clark logistic regression prediction model. *Am J Clin Pathol.* 2002;118(4):504–511.
59. Fallowfield ME, Cook MG. Epidermal melanocytes adjacent to melanoma and the field change effect. *Histopathol.* 1990;17(5):397–400.
60. Schmoeckel C, Castro CE, Braun-Falco O. Nevoid malignant melanoma. *Arch Dermatol Res.* 1985;277(5):362–369.
61. McNutt NS, Urmacher C, Hakimian J, Hoss DM, Lugo J. Nevoid malignant melanoma: morphologic patterns and immunohistochemical reactivity. *J Cutan Pathol.* 1995; 22(6):502–517.
62. Zembowicz A, McCusker M, Chiarelli C, et al. Morphological analysis of nevoid melanoma: a study of 20 cases with a review of the literature. *Am J Dermatopathol.* 2001; 23(3):167–175.
63. Massi G. Melanocytic nevi simulant of melanoma with medicolegal relevance. *Virchows Arch.* 2007;451(3):623–647.
64. Harris GR, Shea CR, Horenstein MG, Reed JA, Burchette JL, Jr., Prieto VG. Desmoplastic (sclerotic) nevus: an underrecognized entity that resembles dermatofibroma and desmoplastic melanoma. *Am J Surg Pathol.* 1999;23(7): 786–794.
65. Paradela S, Fonseca E, Pita S, Kantrow SM, Goncharuk VN, Diwan H et al. Spitzoid melanoma in children: clinicopathological study and application of immunohistochemistry as an adjunct diagnostic tool. *J Cutan Pathol.* 2009;36(7):740–752.
66. Barnhill RL. The Spitzoid lesion: rethinking Spitz tumors, atypical variants, 'Spitzoid melanoma' and risk assessment. *Mod Pathol.* 2006;19 (suppl 2):S21–S33.
67. Kiene P, Petres-Dunsche C, Folster-Holst R. Pigmented pedunculated malignant melanoma. A rare variant of nodular melanoma. *Br J Dermatol.* 1995;133(2):300–302.
68. Kao GF, Helwig EB, Graham JH. Balloon cell malignant melanoma of the skin. A clinicopathologic study of 34 cases with histochemical, immunohistochemical, and ultrastructural observations. *Cancer.* 1992;69(12):2942–2952.
69. Kuehnl-Petzoldt C, Berger H, Wiebelt H. Verrucous-keratotic variations of malignant melanoma: a clinicopathological study. *Am J Dermatopathol.* 1982;4(5):403–410.
70. Sheibani K, Battifora H. Signet-ring cell melanoma. A rare morphologic variant of malignant melanoma. *Am J Surg Pathol.* 1988;12(1):28–34.
71. Hitchcock MG, McCalmont TH, White WL. Cutaneous melanoma with myxoid features: twelve cases with differential diagnosis. *Am J Surg Pathol.* 1999;23(12): 1506–1513.
72. Ackley CD, Prieto VG, Bentley RC, Horenstein MG, Seigler HF, Shea CR. Primary chondroid melanoma. *J Cutan Pathol.* 2001;28(9):482–485.
73. Crowson AN, Magro CM, Mihm MC, Jr. Malignant melanoma with prominent pigment synthesis: "animal type" melanoma—a clinical and histological study of six cases with a consideration of other melanocytic neoplasms with prominent pigment synthesis. *Hum Pathol.* 1999;30(5):543–550.
74. Antony FC, Sanclemente G, Shaikh H, Trelles AS, Calonje E. Pigment synthesizing melanoma (so-called animal type melanoma): a clinicopathological study of 14 cases of a poorly known distinctive variant of melanoma. *Histopathol.* 2006;48(6):754–762.
75. Merkow LP, Burt RC, Hayeslip DW, Newton FJ, Slifkin M, Pardo M. A cellular and malignant blue nevus: a light and electron microscopic study. *Cancer.* 1969;24(5): 888–896.
76. Granter SR, McKee PH, Calonje E, Mihm MC, Jr., Busam K. Melanoma associated with blue nevus and melanoma mimicking cellular blue nevus: a clinicopathologic study of 10 cases on the spectrum of so-called 'malignant blue nevus'. *Am J Surg Pathol.* 2001;25(3):316–323.
77. Hernandez FJ. Malignant blue nevus. A light and electron microscopic study. *Arch Dermatol.* 1973;107(5): 741–744.
78. Blessing K, Grant JJ, Sanders DS, Kennedy MM, Husain A, Coburn P. Small cell malignant melanoma: a variant of naevoid melanoma. Clinicopathological features and histological differential diagnosis. *J Clin Pathol.* 2000; 53(8):591–595.
79. Barnhill RL, Flotte TJ, Fleischli M, Perez-Atayde A. Cutaneous melanoma and atypical Spitz tumors in childhood. *Cancer.* 1995;76(10):1833–1845.
80. Abernethy JL, Soyer HP, Kerl H, Jorizzo JL, White WL. Epidermotropic metastatic malignant melanoma simulating melanoma in situ. A report of 10 examples from two patients. *Am J Surg Pathol.* 1994;18(11):1140–1149.
81. White WL, Hitchcock MG. Dying dogma: the pathological diagnosis of epidermotropic metastatic malignant melanoma. *Semin Diag Pathol.* 1998;15(3):176–188.
82. Pouryazdanparast P, Newman M, Mafee M, Haghighat Z, Guitart J, Gerami P. Distinguishing epithelioid blue nevus from blue nevus-like cutaneous melanoma metastasis using fluorescence in situ hybridization. *Am J Surg Pathol.* 2009;33(9):1396–1400.
83. Bisceglia M, Carosi I, Lelli G, Pasquinelli G, Martinelli GN. [Clear cell sarcoma of soft tissues. Clinico-pathological and ultrastructural analysis of a case in the head-neck region and a literature review]. *Pathologica.* 1998;90(4): 391–396.
84. Hicks MJ, Saldivar VA, Chintagumpala MM, et al. Malignant melanoma of soft parts involving the head and neck region: review of literature and case report. *Ultrastr Pathol.* 1995;19(5):395–400.
85. Wang WL, Mayordomo E, Zhang W, et al. Detection and characterization of EWSR1/ATF1 and EWSR1/CREB1 chimeric transcripts in clear cell sarcoma (melanoma of soft parts). *Mod Pathol.* 2009;22(9):1201–1209.
86. Prieto VG, Shea CR. Use of immunohistochemistry in melanocytic lesions. *J Cutan Pathol.* 2008;35(suppl. 2): 1–10.

24

LOCAL MANAGEMENT OF MELANOMA

BENJAMIN L. JUDSON
DENNIS H. KRAUS

Introduction

The local treatment of malignant melanoma typically occurs in two stages. The first step involves a biopsy to determine the diagnosis and thorough histologic evaluation of the tumor. As discussed in the previous chapter, histologic characteristics such as tumor thickness provide prognostic information and are critically important in guiding subsequent treatment decisions. The second step generally is wide local excision of the tumor with the primary aim to completely remove gross or residual disease in order to achieve durable local control. Resection of an adequate margin around the lesion also removes skin potentially harboring clinically occult tumor cells in the cutaneous lymphatics capable of regional or distant spread.[1] The question of how much surrounding normal tissue to take during excision of a malignant melanoma in order to accomplish these aims, while avoiding unnecessary removal of adjacent structures, has been studied in several large prospective randomized trials. None of the clinical trials investigating adequacy of surgical margins specifically evaluated melanomas of the head and neck, focusing instead on melanomas of the trunk and extremity, so the question of adequate margin width remains a topic of debate. It is an important question, though, because tumors in the head and neck may have a higher risk of local recurrence compared to those in the trunk and extremity.

Biopsy

Patients frequently are referred for multidisciplinary management of melanoma after a diagnosis already has been obtained by some form of biopsy. Optimally, a full thickness biopsy has been performed so that the true depth of the lesion can be assessed. Patients referred for evaluation of a suspicious lesion that has not yet been biopsied should be assessed using the "ABCDE" criteria. These criteria include asymmetry, border irregularity, color variegation, diameter greater than 6 mm, and evolving (increasing) size or color. Lesions that meet any of these criteria or are symptomatic should be biopsied.

Biopsy of suspicious lesions may be accomplished via narrow margin excision (1 to 3 mm) at the closest edge. For medium or smaller lesions, primary closure usually is possible after narrow margin excisional biopsy. In some circumstances, small lesions can be left to close by secondary intention following excisional biopsy. Closure other than primary closure or closure by secondary intention should be avoided after biopsy, as this may contaminate a larger area prior to definitive treatment of the primary tumor. Design of the biopsy incisions should take into account skin tension lines to minimize the visibility of the resulting scar and to accommodate a wider excision, if required.

Lesions not amenable to excisional biopsy and primary closure because of their location or large size should undergo punch or incisional full thickness biopsy in the thickest area of the lesion. Analysis of data from a large prospective melanoma trial reveals that choice of an incisional biopsy versus an excisional biopsy did not affect local, regional, or distant outcomes.[2] A retrospective analysis of patients with melanoma specifically of the head and neck also shows no difference in local or regional outcomes between patients undergoing the two types of biopsy. Although the study did show a difference in overall survival, this difference is likely due to tumor characteristics that lead to selection of one biopsy type over another.[3]

Shave biopsy should be avoided, as it does not allow assessment of tumor depth in a majority of cases and therefore prevents adequate local staging of patients.[4] Management of patients referred after a shave biopsy is discussed in a following section. Likewise, needle biopsy of the primary tumor is discouraged, as it does not allow for assessment of tumor depth or histologic features. In most patients, biopsy can be performed in the office using local anesthetic.

Radiographic Assessment of the Primary Tumor

Generally, imaging of the primary melanoma is not indicated. However, there are situations when, based on physical exam findings, radiographic assessment is indicated to plan surgical excision. When a tumor appears to have invaded into subcutaneous and deeper structures as suggested by palpation or fixation to underlying structures, imaging should be performed to assess the extent of invasion and involvement of surrounding structures.

If the tumor is adherent to an underlying soft tissue structure such as a muscle, MRI is moderately accurate at evaluating the extent of invasion.[5] Melanotic tumors demonstrate hyperintensity on T1-weighted images and hypointensity on T2-weighted images; whereas amelanotic lesions are hypointense or isointense on T1-weighted images and hyperintense or isointense on T2-weighted images.[6] If the tumor is adherent to or directly adjacent to bone, then CT may be useful for detecting osseous invasion.

If a sensory or motor neurologic deficit is present in an area attributable to a cranial nerve, imaging should be performed to evaluate for evidence of perineural invasion. For example, loss of sensation in any of the divisions of the trigeminal nerve, facial nerve weakness, or ophthalmoplegia warrants imaging (Fig 24–1). Treatment of neurotropic melanoma and of tumors invading or approaching structures beyond the subcutaneous tissue layer will be dis-

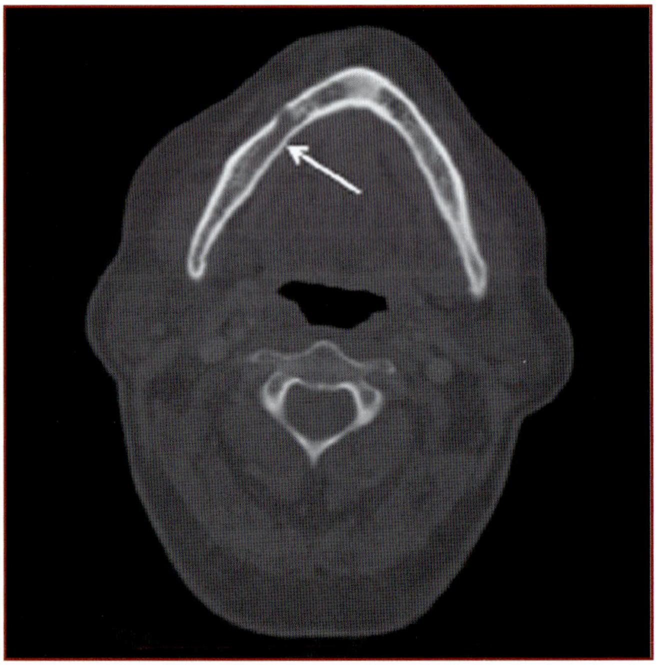

Figure 24–1. This patient with a desmoplastic melanoma reported right lower lip numbness 3 years after wide local excision of a tumor from the chin. CT imaging revealed widening of the mental nerve canal representing perineural invasion and recurrent disease.

cussed in subsequent sections. When assessing for perineural invasion, an MRI with and without gadolinium contrast is the best study to show abnormal enhancement or enlargement of the nerve. Computed tomographic scans may show enlargement of the bony passage through which the nerve traverses. In all cases, the results of radiologic evaluation should be considered in conjunction with physical examination findings in guiding management decisions.

Wide Local Excision

Numerous studies have demonstrated that local recurrence of melanoma is affected by tumor thickness and the presence or absence of ulceration. More recent studies have shown the impact of mitotic index and anatomic location on disease control and prognosis.[7,8] In a large series of almost one thousand patients with melanoma of the head and neck treated at the Sydney Melanoma Unit, overall local recurrence was 13% and local recurrence of tumors greater than 4 mm in thickness was 24%.[9] A multi-institutional series of patients with melanoma at all sites demonstrated a local recurrence rate for tumors in the head and neck of 4.4%, which was higher than the recurrence rate at other body sites in the study.[10] A subsequent prospective study of 740 patients revealed a local recurrence rate in the head and neck of 9.4%, compared to 1.1%, 3.1%, and 5.3% for tumors of the proximal extremity, trunk, and distal extremity, respectively.[11] Although reported local recurrence rates in the head and neck vary across different series, head and neck local failure is more common than that reported in other body locations, and still depends on tumor depth and other adverse features (Table 24–1).

Management of the Prior Biopsy Site

Patients referred after either an incisional biopsy or an excisional biopsy with narrow margins should have any remaining tumor and the biopsy site re-excised with a margin of normal appearing tissue. Any tissue that is violated during the biopsy or closure of the biopsy should be considered potentially contaminated with tumor cells. The size of the appropriate margin of normal-appearing tissue around the tumor or previous biopsy site is determined by the tumor thickness, as well as functional and aesthetic considerations given the tumor location.

Patients referred following a shave biopsy can present a management dilemma. The biopsy slides should be carefully reviewed by a pathologist at the treating institution with special attention paid to determine the maximum thickness of the tumor seen in the biopsy specimen. Because positive deep margins are frequent with shave biopsy, an accurate assessment of tumor thickness may be difficult. Careful examination of the biopsy site for any visible residual tumor also is important prior to wide local excision. The size of the margins should be determined according to the surgeon's judgment, using available data from the biopsy about tumor depth.

Except for very small lesions, wide local excision usually is best accomplished under monitored sedation or general anesthesia. In all cases, consideration

Table 24–1. Local Recurrence and Tumor Depth in Head and Neck Melanomas

Tumor Thickness	O'Brien et al[9]	Urist et al[32]	Fischer et al[33]
≤0.75 mm	2% (6/296)	1% (1/76)	8% (9/113)
0.76–1.49 mm	5% (10/207)	2% (2/100)	5% (154/308)
1.50–3.99 mm	15% (46/305)	5% (8/156)	9% (40/441)
≥4.0 mm	20% (32/158)	12% (7/57)	2% (4/174)

also should be given to addressing the regional lymphatics, either with lymph node dissection or sentinel lymph node biopsy if indicated, under the same anesthetic (Fig 24–2).

Margin Size

The question of how much of a normal tissue margin around a melanoma needs to be obtained during excision in order to achieve local and distant control has been the subject of six large prospective randomized trials (Table 24–2). In all of these trials, patients were enrolled based on the thickness of their tumor and then randomly assigned to excision with either narrow or wide margins. None of the trials detected a statistically significant difference between the narrow or wide margins in terms of survival. Therefore, smaller margins have been recommended for treatment of patients with the corresponding thickness of tumor.

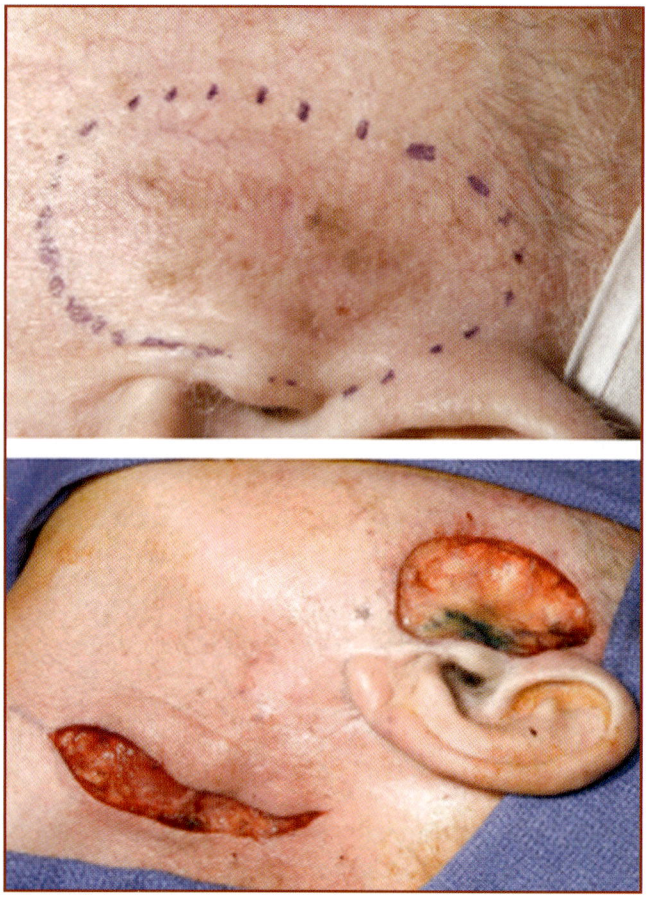

Figure 24–2. This medium thickness melanoma and adjacent lentigo maligna was excised with 2-cm margins around the melanoma and 1-cm margin around the areas of lentigo. Because the tumor was medium thickness, a sentinel lymph node biopsy was performed under the same anesthetic.

Three trials evaluated margins around tumors less than 2 mm thick (WHO, French Cooperative Group, and Swedish Melanoma Group trials).[12–14] The WHO trial compared 1-cm and 3-cm margins; the other two compared 2-cm and 5-cm margins. None of these three trials detected a statistically significant difference in overall survival or local recurrence. The United States Intergroup trial randomized intermediate thickness tumors between 1.0 and 4.0 mm in thickness to 2-cm versus 4-cm margins.[11,15] There was no difference in survival or local recurrence. Both the United Kingdom trial and the Swedish Melanoma Trial Group enrolled patients with tumors thicker than 2 mm.[16,17] Patients in the United Kingdom trial were randomized to either 1-cm or 3-cm margins. Patients in the Swedish Melanoma Trial Group trial were randomized to either 2 cm or 4 cm. The United Kingdom trial reported similar overall survival in the two groups; however, there was a statistically high rate of locoregional recurrence (p = 0.05, *HR* 1.26) in patients treated with 1-cm margins. Although the final results of the Swedish trial have not been reported, preliminary reports found no difference in overall survival or disease-free survival.

Based on the results of these trials, recommendations for margin size are shown in Table 24–3. Tumors thicker than 2 mm should be excised with 2-cm margins. Tumors less than 2 mm thick can safely be excised with 1-cm margins. There are no prospective trials looking specifically at margins for lesions between 1.0 and 2.0-mm thick. Similarly, there are no trials evaluating margins for melanoma in situ or lentigo maligna, although it is generally recommended to employ 0.5-cm margins.

Despite the extensive work done evaluating margins for excision of melanoma, none of these trials look at melanoma in the head and neck. Some excluded patients with melanoma in this location altogether, whereas others had relatively small

Table 24–2. Randomized Trials of Excision Margins and Local Recurrence

Trial	No. of Patients	Year	Tumor Thickness	Margins	Local Recurrence	
					Narrow	Wide
WHO-10	612	1988	<2.0 mm	1 vs 3 cm	2.6%	0.98%
French Group of Research	336	2004	<2.1 mm	2 vs 5 cm	0.62%	2.4%
Swedish Melanoma Group	989	2000	0.8–2.0 mm	2 vs 5 cm	0.6%	1%
US Intergroup Trial	740	2001	1.0–4.0 mm	2 vs 4 cm	2.1%	2.6%
United Kingdom	900	2004	>2.0 mm	1 vs 3 cm	3.3%	2.8%
Swedish Melanoma Trial Group	1000	2005	>2.0 mm	2 vs 4 cm	Not yet reported	Not yet reported

Table 24–3. Recommended Margins for Primary Melanoma Excision Based on Tumor Thickness

Tumor Thickness	Excision Margin
In situ	0.5 cm
<2.0 mm	1.0 cm
>2.0 mm	2.0 cm

numbers of head and neck patients.[13] The aesthetic and functional consequences of excision in the head and neck, as well as the complex and dense anatomy, make obtaining adequate margins challenging in many cases. Even if margins of 2 cm or more for intermediate thickness and thick melanomas produce slightly lower local recurrence rates, this potential benefit must be weighed against the increased morbidity and disfigurement associated with larger margins in some head and neck melanoma patients.

Excision of difficult to reconstruct structures such as the eyelid, parts of the nose, and face is clearly indicated if necessary to remove the tumor, but is less certain when a slightly smaller margin of normal appearing skin would spare this morbidity. Occasional compromise on margins is thus a reasonable approach when attempting to optimize local control versus the high cost in terms of morbidity or disfigurement. Obviously, this decision must be made very carefully, given the cost of potential local recurrence and subsequent significant risk for loss of life from recurrent melanoma.[18]

The recommended margin should be taken from the edge of the melanotic lesion. Any contiguous or adjacent melanotic skin should be included in the excision with an appropriate margin. Particularly in chronically sun-exposed skin there can be melanoma in situ adjacent to an invasive melanoma, and this should be excised along with the primary tumor (see Fig 24–2). The excision should be marked and oriented by the surgeon at the time of removal so that the pathologist is able to correctly assess the margin status histologically on permanent section. Frozen section margins should be taken from the edges of the excision, although the accuracy of frozen section margin analysis remains somewhat controversial.

If a margin is unexpectedly positive on permanent or frozen section, an additional margin of normal appearing tissue at least as large as the original margin should be obtained around the positive site. In chronically sun-damaged skin and when melanoma arises in a background of lentigo maligna, margins can be difficult to assess both clinically and histologically. In these cases, a staged margin control approach, in which the team waits for the results of permanent pathologic evaluation of all margins to determine the adequacy of resection before proceeding to reconstruction, can be useful. Wet-to-dry dressing is used on the wound until the pathologic status of the margins is known. This approach is especially useful when margins are close to delicate anatomic structures or when the lesion involves a large or difficult to reconstruct area of the face.[19]

Management of Deeply Invasive Tumors

It is necessary to obtain an adequate deep margin of normal tissue as well as circumferential skin margins. Most melanomas are confined to the skin. These can be excised by elevating the layer of subcutaneous fat down to the fascia of the underlying muscle. Some locally advanced tumors invade into the subcutaneous tissues and occasionally into underlying structures, although this is uncommon. Head and neck melanoma is unique compared to other body sites, in that tumors frequently have a shorter distance to invade before they encounter underlying muscle, bone, cartilage, and soft tissue structures. When tumor grossly invades these structures, every effort should be made to resect them en bloc with the tumor in order to achieve local control. When a tumor approaches, but does not clearly invade, bone or cartilage, it is important to consider resecting at least periosteum or perichondrium (if not the actual structure) to obtain a negative deep margin. The functional or aesthetic consequences to such key resections also must be considered. However, resection alone has little likelihood of obtaining local control if there are close or microscopically positive margins; adjuvant radiation should be considered in these cases.

A careful evaluation for regional and distant metastasis should be conducted in patients with deeply invasive tumors. Resection of the primary tumor in these advanced cases should be pursued after considering the morbidity of the planned resection and the benefit of local control in the context of each patient. Tumors of the scalp that extend to, but do not grossly invade, the skull can be treated with full thickness excision and removal of the outer cortex of the skull with a drill in order to obtain a deep margin free of disease. This has the added benefit of allowing skin grafting to the marrow space (if pericranium is absent) to provide physiologic support to the graft.

In the neck, the platysma can be excised as a deep margin around tumors invading into subcutaneous tissues. In the face, full thickness excision including the underlying mimetic muscles should be performed and the appropriate reconstruction undertaken to address the expected facial dysfunction. Preauricular lesions over the parotid gland that invade through subcutaneous tissues merit en bloc resection in conjunction with a formal superficial parotidectomy with identification and preservation of the facial nerve. This will include the first echelon lymph nodes with the primary tumor excision, although it does not obviate the need for a sentinel lymph procedure or therapeutic neck dissection as warranted by clinical evaluation.

Perineural Invasion

Melanoma is prone to neurotropic invasion, particularly desmoplastic melanoma and larger tumors. Desmoplastic melanoma exhibits perineural invasion in 17% to 78% of patients, regardless of size of the primary lesion, and more than half of the cases occur in the head and neck.[20–22] These tumors can be difficult to diagnose, both clinically and histologically, because of their innocuous appearance and the frequency of amelanosis, which ranges from 46% to 93%. Desmoplastic melanoma has a high rate of local recurrence and a low rate of regional metastasis compared to other cutaneous melanomas. Analysis of pooled data on 703 patients with desmoplastic melanoma found a local recurrence rate of 27.2% and a regional metastasis rate of only 7.1%.[20] Local recurrence will occur if there is neurotropic invasion and inadequate excision of tumor that may spread along either small cutaneous nerves or large sensory or motor nerves. Treatment of desmoplastic melanoma demonstrating perineural spread should include wide local excision with excision of the involved nerve. Similar to other melanomas of the head and neck, standard margin widths have not been established for these tumors.

Invasion of cranial nerves near the skull base is uncommon, but can occur with desmoplastic as well as other neurotropic melanomas. The most frequently involved nerves are the facial and trigeminal nerves. There is no consensus in how to best treat these patients, but, when there are no other sites of disease, surgical resection of extradural gross disease should be considered. Postoperative radiation should be administered along the entire course of the nerve to its origin at the skull base. When tumor has spread to the cavernous sinus, trigeminal ganglion/Meckel's cave, or other generally unresectable locations, primary radiation therapy should be considered. Several small series report acceptable local control with radiation of intracranial extension, although the long-term sequelae of high dose radiation to the skull base is significant.[23]

Satellite Lesions

Melanoma can become clinically apparent as tumor nodules discrete from the primary tumor that travel through local dermal lymphatics en route to regional lymph nodes. Various terms have been used to describe this phenomenon: in-transit metastasis, satellite metastasis, and local metastasis. Some authors have defined satellitosis or satellite metastasis as tumor nodules within 2 cm of the primary tumor and in-transit metastasis as nodules occurring anywhere along the lymphatic drainage before the regional lymph nodes.[24] All these terms describe a similar phenomenon which has an associated poor prognosis. The 2010 AJCC staging system classifies patients with satellitosis as having regional metastatic disease. Satellitosis or in-transit metastasis are categorized as N2c disease, as these patients have outcomes similar to those with regional nodal metastases.[25] There has been considerable work done on treating in transit and satellitosis in limb melanoma. Patients with more than three nodules are considered for isolated limb perfusion therapy. Those with three or fewer nodules are treated with wide local excision.[26,27] For melanoma of the head and neck, the treatment is surgical excision. If there is any question about the histology of nodules that appear following local excision of a melanoma, either an excisional biopsy or fine needle aspiration can be performed to confirm the diagnosis. Evaluation for regional or distant metastasis should also be performed. Satellite lesions should be excised with a wide margin of 1 to 2 cm, as previously discussed.

Management of Local Recurrence

Local failure in head and neck melanoma arises from a few situations. Some recurrences are actually regrowth of residual disease following inadequate initial local treatment that leaves residual tumor. There are also true local scar recurrences following appropriate local treatment that is thought to be due to undetected microscopic disease that was present beyond the initial margin of resection. Patients also can recur locally by developing satellitosis after excision of the primary tumor. Although such satellitosis is classed as a local recurrence, the prognostic implication of this type of recurrence is similar to regional metastasis. In a series of 873 patients treated at a single center, patients who failed initial therapy were more likely to fail regionally or distantly: 10.9% recurred within 3 cm of the primary tumor, 9.9% as in-transit metastasis between the tumor and regional lymph nodes, 34.4% in regional lymph nodes, and 44.9% with distant disease.[28]

Local recurrences should be treated with surgical resection. Patients with inadequate initial treatment who recur locally should be treated as they would have been initially: with wide local resection and consideration for regional sentinel lymph node biopsy or therapeutic node dissection, as indicated. Patients with true local recurrence also should undergo wide local excision with clear margins. Satellitosis also should be excised with clear margins.

Patients who recur locally often can be salvaged with re-excision, but are at significant risk for regional and distant failure. Despite the high risk of disease recurrence elsewhere, local control should be aggressively sought, as some patients may be completely salvaged. Because local failure can result in considerable morbidity, achieving local control, even in patients who go on to fail elsewhere, can significantly improve quality of life. Patients who have a local recurrence coincident with failure at another site should still be considered for treatment of the local disease if the treatment morbidity is reasonable, given the burden and progression of disease elsewhere, and if symptomatic from the local disease.

Radiation Therapy in Localized Melanoma

Adjuvant Radiation

Adjuvant radiation therapy may improve local control in patients at high risk for local recurrence after surgery alone, although there are no randomized controlled studies that support the efficacy of radiation in this setting. One early retrospective series of 234 patients compared patients treated with excision with wide margins, excision with narrow margins, and excision with narrow margins and adjuvant radiation. Overall survival was similar in patients treated with wide local excision and those who underwent resection with narrow margins and adjuvant radiation therapy.[29] Despite this study and other small series that have demonstrated that radiation may improve local control, there are no randomized trials evaluating adjuvant radiation; therefore its use and indications remain controversial.

Patients at high risk for local failure include those with thick or deeply invasive tumors, plus those with satellitosis. In these patients, some clinicians have advocated using adjuvant radiation in an effort to improve local control. Close or positive margins also place a patient at high risk for local recurrence, and these patients should undergo re-resection when possible. If there is a contraindication to re-resection or if the patient refuses for cosmetic or functional reasons, these patients should be considered for adjuvant radiation treatment. Similarly, desmoplastic melanomas have a high rate of local recurrence and some centers consider these patients for adjuvant radiation on a routine basis following wide excision of the tumors.

Tumors that invade a named sensory or motor nerve are at high risk for local failure and should be considered for treatment along the course of the involved nerve to the skull base. Locally recurrent tumors are at increased risk of failing again after re-excision, although the greater risk is regional and distant metastasis. Some centers consider treating these patients with adjuvant radiation to both the local and regional sites. The width of the area to be targeted depends on the proximity of critical, radiosensitive structures such as the eye. Typically, 2- to 4-cm margins are treated around the target site. Because of the lack of prospective data or consensus about indications for adjuvant radiation treatment, patients with tumors that are at increased risk for local failure for any of these reasons are best evaluated on an individual basis in a multidisciplinary setting.

Primary Radiation Therapy

Radiation therapy is rarely the primary treatment for melanoma. One uncommon situation where radiation may be considered is patients with extensive lentigo malignant melanoma in a location such as the face where excision would result in severe disfigurement with poor reconstructive options. There are two trials reporting the use of radiation therapy as a primary treatment for extensive lentigo malignant melanoma of the face, either alone or following excision of the nodular portion of the tumor. Local control was obtained in 86% to 96% of the patients treated and all local failures were successfully surgically salvaged.[30,31]

Conclusions

Local treatment is a critical part of the multidisciplinary management of head and neck melanoma. Appropriate assessment including a full thickness biopsy and imaging in special circumstances is critical to successful subsequent management. Wide local excision employing adequate margins is the bedrock of local treatment. Reconstruction of the resulting defect, as discussed in subsequent chapters is critical for optimal patient outcomes. The use of adjuvant radiation or, in rare circumstances, primary radiation also may play an important role in local treatment. Surgery and adjuvant radiation comprise the primary contemporary treatments for locally recurrent melanoma.

References

1. Krown SE, Chapman PB. Defining adequate surgery for primary melanoma. *N Engl J Med.* 2004;350:823l.
2. Martin RCG, Scoggins CR, Ross MI, et al. Is incisional biopsy of melanoma harmful? *Am J Surg.* 2005;190: 927–932.
3. Austin JR, Byers RM, Brown WD, et al. Influence of biopsy on the prognosis of cutaneous melanoma of the head and neck. *Head Neck.* 1996;18(2):107–117.
4. Stell VH, Norton HJ, Smith KS, et al. Method of biopsy and incidence of positive margins in primary melanoma. *Ann Surg Oncol.* 2006;14(2):893–898.
5. Choi EA, Gershenwald JE. Imaging studies in patients with melanoma. *Surg Oncol Clin North Am.* 2007;16(2):403–430.
6. Kim JH, Kim JY, Chun KA, et al. MR imaging manifestations of skin tumors. *Eur Radiol.* 2008;18(11):2652–2661.
7. Tsao H, Atkins MB, Sober AJ. Management of cutaneous melanoma. *N Engl J Med.* 2004;351:998–1012.
8. Testori A, Rutkowski P, Marsden J, et al. Surgery and radiotherapy in the treatment of cutaneous melanoma. *Ann Oncol.* 2009;20 (suppl 6):vi, 22–29.
9. C.J. O'Brien, A.S. Coates, K. Petersen-Schaefer, et al., Experience with 998 cutaneous melanomas of the head and neck over 30 years. *Am J Surg.* 1991;162:310–314.
10. Urist MM, Balch CM, Soong S, et al., The influence of surgical margins and prognostic factors predicting the risk of local recurrence in 3445 patients with primary cutaneous melanoma. *Cancer.* 1985;55:1398–1402.
11. Balch CM, Soong SJ, Smith T, et al. Long-term results of a prospective surgical trial comparing 2 cm vs. 4 cm excision margins for 740 patients with 1–4 mm melanomas. *Ann Surg Oncol.* 2001;8(2):101–108.
12. Veronesi U, Cascinelli N, Adamus J, et al. Thin stage I primary cutaneous malignant melanoma. Comparison of excision with margins of 1 or 3 cm. *N Engl J Med.* 1988; 318: 1159–1162.
13. Khayat D, Rixe O, Martin G, et al. Surgical margins in cutaneous melanoma (2 cm versus 5 cm for lesions measuring less than 2.1 mm thick). *Cancer.* 2003;97:1941–1946.
14. Cohn-Cedermark G, Rutqvist LE, Andersson R, et al. Long term results of a randomized study by the Swedish Melanoma Study Group on 2 cm versus 5 cm resection margins for patients with cutaneous melanoma with a tumor thickness of 0.8–2.0 mm. *Cancer.* 2000; 89:1495–1501.
15. US intergroup Balch CM, Urist MM, Karakousis CP, et al. Efficacy of 2 cm surgical margins for intermediate-thickness melanomas (1 to 4 mm). Results of a multi-institutional randomized surgical trial. *Ann Surg.* 1993;218: 262–267.
16. Thomas JM, Newton-Bishop J, A'Hern R et al. Excision margins in high-risk malignant melanoma. *N Engl J Med.* 2004;350:757–766.
17. Ringborg U, Brahme EM, Drewiecki K. *Randomized trial of a resection margin of 2 cm versus 4 cm for cutaneous malignant melanoma with a tumor thickness of more than 2 mm.* Presentation at the World Congress on Melanoma, September 6–10, 2005; Vancouver, British Columbia.
18. Thompson JF, Scolyer RA, Kefford RF. Cutaneous melanoma. *Lancet.* 2005;365(9460):687–701.
19. Clark GS, Pappas-Politis EC, Cherpelis BS, Messina JL, Möller MG, Cruse CW, Glass LF. Surgical management of melanoma in situ on chronically sun-damaged skin. *Cancer Control.* 2008;15(3):216–224.
20. Lens MB, Newton-Bishop JA, Boon AP. Desmoplastic malignant melanoma: a systematic review. *Br J Dermatol.* 2005;152:673–678.
21. Beenken S, Byers R, Smith JL, et al., Desmoplastic melanoma. *Arch Otolaryngol Head Neck Surg.* 1989;115: 374–379.
22. Quinn MJ, Crotty KA, Thompson JF, et al. Desmoplastic and desmoplastic neutropenic melanoma: experience with 280 patients. *Cancer.* 1998;83:1128–1135.
23. Newlin HE, Morris CG, Amdur RJ et al. Neurotropic melanoma of the head and neck with clinical perineural invasion. *Am J Clin Oncol.* 2005;28(4):399–402.
24. Leiter U, Meier F, Schittek B, Garbe C. The natural course of cutaneous melanoma. *J Surg Oncol.* 2004;86(4):172–178.
25. Balch CM, Soong SJ, Atkins MB, et al. An evidence-based staging system for cutaneous melanoma. *CA Cancer J Clin.* 2004;54(3):131–149.
26. Fraker DL. Management of in-transit melanoma of the extremity with isolated limb perfusion. *Curr Treat Options Oncol.* 2004;5(3):173–184.
27. Hoekstra HJ. The European approach to in-transit melanoma lesions. *Int J Hyperthermia.* 2008;24(3):227–237.
28. Francken AB, Accortt NA, Shaw HM, et al. Prognosis and determinants of outcome following locoregional or distant recurrence in patients with cutaneous melanoma. *Ann Surg Oncol.* 2008;15(5):1476–1484.
29. Dickson RJ. Malignant melanoma: a combined surgical and radiotherapeutic approach. *Am J Roentgenol.* 1958;79: 1063–1070.
30. Harwood AR. Conventional fractionated radiotherapy for 51 patients with lentigo maligna and lentigo maligna melanoma. *Int J Radiat Oncol Biol Phys.* 1983;9:1019–1021.
31. Schmid-Wendtner MH, Brunner B, Konz B, et al. Fractionated radiotherapy of lentigo maligna and lentigo maligna melanoma in 64 patients. *J Am Acad Dermatol.* 2000;43:477–482.
32. Urist MM, Balch CM, Soong SJ, et al., Head and neck melanoma in 534 clinical Stage I patients. A prognostic factors analysis and results of surgical treatment. *Ann Surg.* 1984;200(6):769–775.
33. Fisher SR. Cutaneous malignant melanoma of the head and neck. *Laryngoscope.* 1989;99(8 pt 1):822–836.

25

REGIONAL MANAGEMENT OF MELANOMA IN THE CLINICALLY NODE-NEGATIVE NECK

JEFFREY E. GERSHENWALD
MATTHEW T. BALLO
JEFFREY N. MYERS

Overview

Regional lymph nodes represent the most common first site of melanoma metastasis. Although the majority of patients who present with invasive cutaneous melanoma have clinically negative regional lymph node basins, a subset of these patients actually harbor occult regional nodal metastases. Because regional nodal disease represents the dominant predictor of survival in such patients and because clinically evident disease not only may be difficult to treat but also potentially is associated with significant morbidity, emphasis on the identification and treatment of occult regional nodal (stage III) melanoma has become an important consideration for patients with newly diagnosed melanoma. In planning treatment for clinically node-negative patients with early-stage primary cutaneous melanoma arising in a site with potential lymphatic drainage to the neck, the clinician must determine: (1) the extent of wide excision of the primary tumor and how the resulting defect will be repaired and (2) whether the patient is a candidate for lymphatic mapping and sentinel lymph node biopsy, a surgical technique used to assess regional nodal basins at risk for occult stage III disease, based on primary tumor and host-related factors.

To address the primary tumor, a wide local excision to underlying fascia with radial margins appropriate for tumor thickness is performed. Guidelines for margins are based on primary tumor thickness; overall, these guidelines have been established by the results of several clinical trials, (reviewed in reference 1). Failure to widely excise using this paradigm after diagnostic biopsy has been associated with a local recurrence rate as high as 40%. Although these general recommendations regarding the extent of surgical resection are applicable to most areas of the body, certain anatomic sites are not amenable to rigid surgical criteria. For example, facial lesions often cannot be excised with more than a 1-cm margin because of adjacent vital structures; in these cases, the tumor diameter, tumor thickness, and tumor location are all considered when margin width is planned. Further discussion regarding management of the melanoma primary site is found in Chapter 24.

The AJCC Staging System and the Clinically Negative Neck

Based on a comprehensive international American Joint Committee on Cancer (AJCC) collaborative melanoma database analysis, minor changes in melanoma staging have been introduced into the 7th edition AJCC Cancer Staging manual (2009)[2] and officially implemented in January 2010 (Tables 25–1 and 25–2). Although a detailed discussion is beyond the scope of this book, criteria established as independent prognostic factors for regional metastasis in this analysis include:[2,3]

Table 25–1. Definition of the TNM Staging Categories for Cutaneous Melanoma Based on the 7th Edition Version of Melanoma Staging

Melanoma TNM Classification		
T classification	**Thickness**	**Ulceration Status**
Tis	not applicable	not applicable
T1	≤1.0 mm	a: w/o ulceration and mitosis $<1/mm^2$ b: with ulceration or mitosis $\geq 1/mm^2$
T2	1.01–2.0 mm	a: w/o ulceration b: with ulceration
T3	2.01–4.0 mm	a: w/o ulceration b: with ulceration
T4	>4.0 mm	a: w/o ulceration b: with ulceration
N classification	**No. of Metastatic Nodes**	**Nodal Metastatic Mass**
N1	1 node	a: micrometastasis* b: macrometastasis**
N2	2–3 nodes	a: micrometastasis* b: macrometastasis** c: in transit met(s)/satellite(s) *without* metastatic nodes
N3	4 or more metastatic nodes, or matted nodes, or in transit met(s)/ satellite(s) *with* metastatic node(s)	
M classification	**Site**	**Serum LDH**
M1a	Distant skin, subcutaneous, or nodal metastases	Normal
M1b	Lung metastases	Normal
M1c	All other visceral metastases	Normal
	Any distant metastasis	Elevated

*Micrometastases are diagnosed after sentinel or elective lymphadenectomy.

**Macrometastases are defined as clinically detectable nodal metastases confirmed by therapeutic lymphadenectomy or when nodal metastasis exhibits gross extracapsular extension.

Source: Used with the permission of the American Joint Committee on Cancer (AJCC), Chicago, Illinois. The original source for this material is the AJCC Cancer Staging Manual, Seventh Edition (2010) published by Springer Science and Business Media LLC, www.springer.com.

- Number of lymph nodes harboring metastatic disease (the most important criterion for N classification in recent analysis)
- Microscopic versus macroscopic tumor burden in regional lymph nodes
- Presence of satellite or in-transit metastases
- Presence or absence of ulceration in the primary lesion as an independent predictor of survival in patients with nodal disease.[3,4]

Other regional node-specific highlights include:

- Lymphatic mapping and sentinel lymph node biopsy are important components of

Table 25–2. Definition of the Stage Groupings for Cutaneous Melanoma Based on the 7th Edition Version of Melanoma Staging

Stage Groupings for Cutaneous Melanoma							
Clinical Staging*				Pathologic Staging+			
0	Tis	N0	M0	0	Tis	N0	M0
IA	T1a	N0	M0	IA	T1a	N0	M0
IB	T1b	N0	M0	IB	T1b	N0	M0
	T2a	N0	M0		T2a	N0	M0
IIA	T2b	N0	M0	IIA	T2b	N0	M0
	T3a	N0	M0		T3a	N0	M0
IIB	T3b	N0	M0	IIB	T3b	N0	M0
	T4a	N0	M0		T4a	N0	M0
IIC	T4b	N0	M0	IIC	T4b	N0	M0
III	Any T	N>N0	M0	IIIA	T1—4a	N1a	M0
					T1—4a	N2a	M0
				IIIB	T1—4b	N1a	M0
					T1—4b	N2a	M0
					T1—4a	N1b	M0
					T1—4a	N2b	M0
					T1—4a	N2c	M0
				IIIC	T1—4b	N1b	M0
					T1—4b	N2b	M0
					T1—4b	N2c	M0
					Any T	N3	M0
IV	Any T	Any N	M1	IV	Any T	Any N	M1

*Clinical staging includes microstaging of the primary melanoma and clinical/radiologic evaluation for metastases. By convention, it should be used after complete excision of the primary melanoma with clinical assessment for regional and distant metastases.

+Pathologic staging includes microstaging of the primary melanoma and pathologic information about the regional lymph nodes after partial or complete lymphadenectomy. Pathologic Stage 0 or Stage IA patients are the exception; they do not require pathologic evaluation of their lymph nodes.

Source: Used with the permission of the American Joint Committee on Cancer (AJCC), Chicago, Illinois. The original source for this material is the AJCC Cancer Staging Manual, Seventh Edition (2010) published by Springer Science and Business Media LLC, www.springer.com.

melanoma staging and should be used (and discussed with the patient) in defining occult stage III disease among patients who present with clinical stages Ib and II melanoma.

- The presence of nodal micrometastases can be defined by either H&E or immunohistochemical staining (previously, only H&E included).
- There is no lower threshold of tumor burden defining the presence of regional nodal metastasis. Specifically, inclusion of tumor deposits less than 0.2 mm in diameter (an empiric threshold previously used for defining nodal metastasis), reflects the consensus that even small amounts of metastatic tumor are clinically significant. Although the concept of isolated tumor cells (especially in subcapsular sinuses) may be valid, no evidence-based lower threshold of "false-positive" or clinically insignificant nodal metastases has yet been defined.
- Because of the prognostic importance of these criteria, pathologic evaluation of lymph nodes is required to determine a pathologic stage in all patients except those with T0 or T1a disease.[2,5]

One of the most salient findings in the recent AJCC analysis was the remarkable heterogeneity in survival among patients with regional nodal (stage III disease).[2,5] The 5-year survival rates for patients with stages IIIA, IIIB, and IIIC disease are 78%, 59%, and 40%, respectively.

According to recent database analyses of the American Joint Committee on Cancer Melanoma Task Force, 5-year survival rates for patients with stage III disease range from 81.5% for patients with nonulcerated melanomas and only 1 microscopically positive SLN to 29.2% for patients with ulcerated primary tumors and clinically evident nodal disease with more than 3 pathologically involved nodes (Table 25–3).[6] Interestingly, on multivariate analysis, for patients with nodal micrometastasis (ie, comprising the majority of contemporary patients with regional nodal disease at presentation), in addition to number of nodes involved, other factors, including age, primary tumor anatomic site, thickness, ulceration, and mitotic rate, also independently predicted survival. In contrast, among patients with regional nodal macrometastases, primary tumor features did not independently predict survival.[6]

Rationale for Lymphatic Mapping and Sentinel Lymph Node Biopsy for Melanoma

The treatment of clinically negative regional lymph node basins in patients with primary cutaneous melanoma has been controversial. Historically, some surgeons performed lymphadenectomy only for clinically evident nodal metastases (ie, *delayed, or therapeutic lymph node dissection* [TLND]). Other surgeons excised the clinically negative nodes in patients who are at increased risk of developing nodal metastases (ie, *immediate, prophylactic,* or *elective lymph node dissection* [ELND]). Advocates of the latter approach argued that "early" identification of histologically positive lymph nodes has the theoretical advantage of treating melanoma nodal metastases at a relatively early stage in the natural history of the melanoma and may be associated with a better chance for long-term survival than if clinically apparent metastases developed in the regional lymph nodes during follow-up.[7–11] The disadvantage of ELND is that many patients undergo surgery when they do not have nodal metastasis.

Only patients with known metastases undergo major lymphadenectomy with TLND, thus reducing the number of potentially unnecessary lymphadenectomies, possibly without reducing the chance for cure. The disadvantage of TLND is that delaying treatment until lymph node metastases are clinically evident may result in many patients having distant micrometastases at the time of lymphadenectomy.

Although four prospective randomized clinical trials have failed to show a benefit from ELND,[11–14] data from World Health Organization (WHO) Melanoma Group Trial 14 and the Intergroup Melanoma Surgical Trial suggested that certain subgroups of patients might benefit from this procedure.[15–17] Results from the WHO ELND trial in patients with truncal melanoma at least 1.5 mm thick indicate that patients with only microscopic regional nodal disease after pathologic analysis of the surgical specimen in

Table 25-3. Five-Year Survival Rates for Patients with Stage III Disease Stratified by Number of Metastatic Nodes, Primary Tumor Ulceration, and Nodal Tumor Burden

	Rates by Type and No. of Metastases*																	
	No. of Nodal Micrometastases									No. of Nodal Macrometastases								
	1			2–3			≥ 4			1			2–3			≥ 4		
Primary tumor ulceration	**No.†**	**%**	**SE**	**No.**	**%**	**SE**	**No.**	**%**	**SE**	**No.**	**%**	**SE**	**No.**	**%**	**SE**	**No.**	**%**	**SE**
Absent	777	81.5	1.9	246	73.2	3.7	46	38.0	8.5	75	51.6	7.2	67	46.6	7.9	50	45.4	9.1
Present	531	56.6	2.9	223	53.9	4.2	49	34.0	8.3	88	49.4	6.2	93	37.7	6.2	68	29.2	6.7

Note: Stage III disease indicates nodal metastases. Total no. of patients = 2,313.

Abbreviation: SE, standard error.

*Overall statistical significance, p <.00.

†Indicates the sample size for each subgroup.

the ELND treatment arm had improved overall survival compared with patients in whom dissection was delayed until palpable adenopathy developed after wide local excision of the primary melanoma alone[17] (5-year survival 48.2% vs 26.9% $p = 0.04$). In the Intergroup Melanoma Surgical Trial, patients who had 1- to 2-mm thick primary tumors, nonulcerated primary tumors, or were younger than 60 years also had a survival benefit with ELND.[18] Based on these subset analyses, dissection of clinically undetectable regional node metastases may lead to increased survival compared to nodal observation followed by TLND performed only when nodal metastases become clinically apparent.

An argument against a policy advocating ELND in such groups is that the majority of these patients (who do not harbor occult metastases) nonetheless would be exposed to a procedure associated with significant morbidity and potential disability. Although the survival advantage of ELND over observation in selected patients is an important finding, it is difficult to recommend a procedure with significant risks of morbid complications to a broad group of clinically node-negative melanoma patients when, overall, only 15% to 20% of such patients are found to have occult metastases. Collectively, these data called into question recommendations to delay lymphadenectomy until palpable nodal disease develops and support the use of alternative approaches to permit earlier identification of occult nodal disease.

Lymphatic Mapping and Sentinel Lymph Node Biopsy

Over the past two decades, the technique of lymphatic mapping and sentinel lymph node (SLN) biopsy has been developed as a minimally invasive procedure for identifying patients who harbor occult microscopic regional node disease.[19,20] In a now landmark report, Morton and colleagues[19,21] described this technique in melanoma, which subsequently led to a global paradigm shift in the identification of regional nodal metastases in this disease. This technique relies on two concepts: (1) different regions of the skin have specific patterns of lymphatic drainage to the regional nodal basins, and (2) for a given region of the skin there is a specific lymph node(s)—namely, SLN(s)—in the basin to which the afferent lymphatic vessels drain first.

Subsequent early studies confirmed that the SLN(s) represent the most likely first site of metastatic disease and demonstrated that if the SLN(s) are removed and are histologically negative, then the remainder of the regional lymph nodes are unlikely to contain disease, and a completion lymph node dissection need not be performed.[19,20,22,23] If, however, the SLN contains metastatic tumor cells, a completion lymph node dissection is recommended to complete the staging assessment to maximize regional basin control and potential cure. As this approach limits the number of lymph nodes submitted for pathologic evaluation (ie, fewer nodes compared to complete lymphadenectomy), the SLN(s) can be subjected to a more thorough pathologic analysis including serial sectioning and immunohistochemical analysis to assess for microscopic nodal disease.[24–31] Such an approach may accurately stage patients by identifying patients who harbor microscopic metastases and thus may potentially benefit from early therapeutic lymph node dissection and adjuvant therapy.

Goals and Benefits of SLN biopsy

Goals of surgical treatment of regional lymph nodes include: (1) pathologic regional lymph node staging, (2) regional disease control, (3) potential cure of stage III disease, and (4) desire to utilize a minimally invasive approach if possible.

Validation of SLN Biopsy

Over the past two decades, the SLN biopsy technique has gained increasing acceptance as it has been substantially refined and validated.[19,22,27,32–37] In the initial report by Morton et al,[19,21] SLN biopsy was performed with vital blue dye alone. SLNs were successfully identified in 194 (82%) of the 237 lymphatic basins. Of the 40 patients with histologically positive nodes, SLN biopsy successfully identified 38 patients (ie, 5% false-negative rate). Although these early data suggested that this new technique accurately identified patients with occult lymph node metastases,[19,21] significant room for improvement was also evident. Experience at several institutions[19,22,23,27,32,34,37–44] confirmed that nodal metastasis from cutaneous primary sites follows an orderly, nonrandom, progressive pattern and, by performing concomitant lymphadenectomy at the time of SLN biopsy,[22] that SLN status reflects the histology of the nodal basin.

Although it has been hypothesized that the nodal drainage patterns in the head and neck region might be too complex to make SLN biopsy feasible, the findings of Eicher and colleagues at MD Anderson Cancer Center have helped to dispel this notion.[45] In this study, SLNs were identified in 98% of patients in whom SLN biopsy was performed in the context of a regional lymphadenectomy in patients with intermediate thickness cutaneous melanomas arising within the head and neck region. No patients were found to have a positive non-SLN when the SLN was negative. Overall, studies reflect that the predictive value of a negative SLN approaches 99% and that the SLN procedure has a low false-negative rate (<4%).[42,46] Studies of SLN biopsy for patients with head and neck primary melanomas report a range of regional recurrence from 2 to 8% in patients who had negative SLN.[45,47–49]

Prognostic Significance

The prognostic significance of SLN pathologic status in patients with cutaneous melanoma has been convincingly demonstrated.[19,20,33,37,42,50–54] In 1999, Gershenwald and colleagues[37] showed that SLN status was the most significant independent clinicopathologic prognostic factor with respect to survival, even when primary tumor thickness and ulceration status were included in the analysis. In an updated analysis of 1487 patients who underwent SLN biopsy (median tumor thickness, 1.5 mm), the 5-year survival rate for patients with positive SLNs was 73.3%, compared with 96.8% for patients with negative SLNs. Several other multivariate regression analyses have confirmed that regional lymph node status is the most powerful predictor of recurrence and survival,[37,38,50–52,55–66] even among patients with thick melanomas.[58,67–73]

In a previous AJCC melanoma database study that compared patients with melanoma >1 mm who underwent lymphatic mapping and negative sentinel node biopsy to those who had either clinically uninvolved lymph nodes or a negative elective lymph node dissection, survival was better in those patients who underwent SLN biopsy, underscoring the improved staging among this latter cohort of patients.[52]

Tumor burden in the regional nodal basins is an important predictor of survival, making it an important determinant of stage in the current AJCC system.[2,4] Both the number of positive nodes[55,74] and the burden of disease in the nodes (macroscopic vs microscopic) are significant predictors.[55] Interestingly, recent data indicate that the extent of microscopic disease in SLNs also is associated with disease-specific survival.[51,56,60–65,68,75–81] Recent data suggest that isolated tumor cells in regional lymph nodes are clinically relevant in patients with melanoma; notably, the AJCC melanoma staging system no longer includes a lower threshold below which nodal disease is not considered significant. Others suggest that a lower threshold may exist below which metastatic deposits may not be clinically relevant.[53,56,60–65,82–85]

The concept of microscopic nodal tumor burden likely will be ever more important in this era of SLN biopsy as accurate microscopic staging of SLNs enables prognostic stratification on the basis of microscopic tumor burden. Clinical decisions regarding the need for and extent of further surgery or adjuvant therapy in the expanding stage III population with microscopic disease only may also be based on the extent of nodal tumor burden.[74,86]

Non-SLN Involvement Following Completion Lymphadenectomy

In patients with clinically negative nodal basins, most nodal metastases, when present, are identified by sentinel lymph node biopsy and are microscopic. Current standard clinical practice for patients with microscopic nodal metastases includes completion lymph node dissection, an approach also recommended by an international consensus panel of melanoma experts.[87] However, additional positive non-SLNs are identified in only 8% to 33% of completion lymph node dissection specimens,[34,38,51,53,54,56,61,64,65,68,76,80,85,88–102] suggesting that a subset of patients with a positive SLN biopsy may not benefit from completion lymph node dissection. Understanding which factors predict additional non-SLN disease may: (1) facilitate selection of patients who may benefit from the procedure and (2) spare SLN-positive patients at "minimal" risk for additional non-SLN nodal metastases from the morbidity of a CLND. In a recent study from MD Anderson of 343 patients who had CLND after the discovery of positive SLNs,[94] 14.5% had additional non-SLN disease in the lymphadenectomy specimen. Interestingly, by multivariable logistic regression analysis, measures of SLN microscopic tumor burden, tumor thickness >2 mm, and number of SLNs harvested also predicted additional disease; a model was also developed that stratified patients according to their risk for non-SLN involvement.[74]

It is important to note that the CLND specimen is not routinely histologically assessed in the same fashion as the SLN; additional disease, if present, may go undetected with standard histologic techniques, and may represent a potential source of subsequent recurrence if it were not removed. Because such recurrences are difficult to treat surgically and potentially contribute to significant morbidity, CLND performed because of microscopic disease provides the potential for improved regional control, lending additional support to the SLN approach. Although fewer than one-fifth of patients with a positive SLN have additional melanoma detected by routine histologic examination of non-SLNs, a CLND remains the standard of care for patients with a positive SLN. In the future, selection of patients for completion lymph node dissection may be based, at least in part, on the extent of SLN microscopic nodal tumor burden. The Multicenter Selective Lymphadenectomy Trial-II (MSLT-II) trial (PI, Donald Morton) has been initiated and will explore the role of completion lymphadenectomy in patients with a positive SLN as well as prospective determination of the prognostic significance of micrometastases identified by RT-PCR assessment of SLNs that show no evidence of tumor by conventional histopathologic techniques, including immunohistochemistry.

Although CLND remains the standard of care for patients with positive SLN, there are data that support the use of external beam radiation therapy to obtain regional control in patients with positive cervical SLN.[103,104] This option is potentially useful in the management of patients for whom additional surgery may be contraindicated or considered to be associated with too high of a risk.

Predictors of SLN Status

Identification of predictors of SLN metastasis has been the subject of intense investigation. Histologic status of the SLN is the dominant independent predictor of survival in clinically node-negative patients with melanoma.[38,105] In addition to their independent significance in predicting survival, tumor thickness and ulceration are dominant independent predictors of SLN metastasis in patients with clinically negative regional lymph nodes.[18,37,54,106,107] More recently, other factors, including high mitotic rate and younger patient age, have also been associated with increased SLN positivity rates.[108–110] Knowledge of the evolving factors associated with a positive SLN is necessary for appropriate patient counseling regarding treatment options and possible outcomes. (See also Indications for SLN Biopsy, below.)

Role of SLN Biopsy in Regional Disease Control

The role of sentinel lymph node biopsy in regional disease control also has been the subject of debate. It has been hypothesized that disruption of lymphatic pathways by the procedure itself might compromise regional disease control. As such, patients who have a SLN biopsy might have a higher risk of regional nodal recurrences. Gershenwald and colleagues[77] showed that SLN biopsy does not compromise regional nodal control in patients with melanoma and a positive SLN. Despite this potential risk, overall low rates of in-basin recurrence after positive SLN biopsy compare favorably with those observed after formal lymphadenectomy in patients with clinically evident nodal disease.

Pathologic Analysis of SLNs

Historically, histologic assessment of lymph nodes from CLND specimens has involved conventional hematoxylin and eosin (H&E) examination from each bisected or trisected lymph node. However, as an average of only 2 to 3 sentinel lymph nodes per nodal basin are submitted for pathologic review, the pathologist can perform a much more intense examination of the limited specimen. Optimal nodal staging requires not only accurate identification of the SLN but also careful examination of the SLN with special pathologic techniques to enhance identification of occult nodal disease (Fig 25–1).[25,27,30,38,42,111] In nearly all melanoma centers, SLNs currently are routinely examined using serial sectioning, immunostaining, or both,[24–26,28,30,31,63,91,111–113] although techniques do vary among institutions.[26,29,30,61,113–116] Importantly, immunohistochemically detected SLN metastases are formally considered evidence of node-positive disease in the 7th edition of the AJCC Melanoma Staging System.[2]

Role of Intraoperative Assessment

Multiple studies have shown that intraoperative pathologic assessment of SLNs in patients with melanoma has a low sensitivity, in large part because of the inferior quality of frozen sections compared with permanent sections.[117–121] [111,116,121,122] Given these and other limitations, frozen-section analysis of SLNs in patients with melanoma should not be routinely performed.

Clinical Relevance of Submicroscopic Disease

Molecular techniques such as reverse-transcriptase-polymerase chain reaction (RT-PCR) have been explored in assessing SLNs to detect submicroscopic disease that might not be detectable by conventional histologic methods.[123–131] Although early studies with limited follow-up suggested that the prognosis of patients with an SLN that is positive by RT-PCR but negative by histology or immunohistochemistry was worse than that of patients who had negative results by all techniques, when similar questions were addressed after longer follow-up in two of these studies, there was no difference in recurrence rates between patients, [132,133] and data suggest that the ultimate value of RT-PCR staging of SLNs is not yet clear.[129,134] Others have reported data to support the possibility that these approaches may be used to identify submicroscopic disease[135,136] and are addressing this hypothesis in the MSLT-II Trial. Overall, RT-PCR remains investigational and should not be used outside a clinical trial to direct further therapy at this time.[132,133]

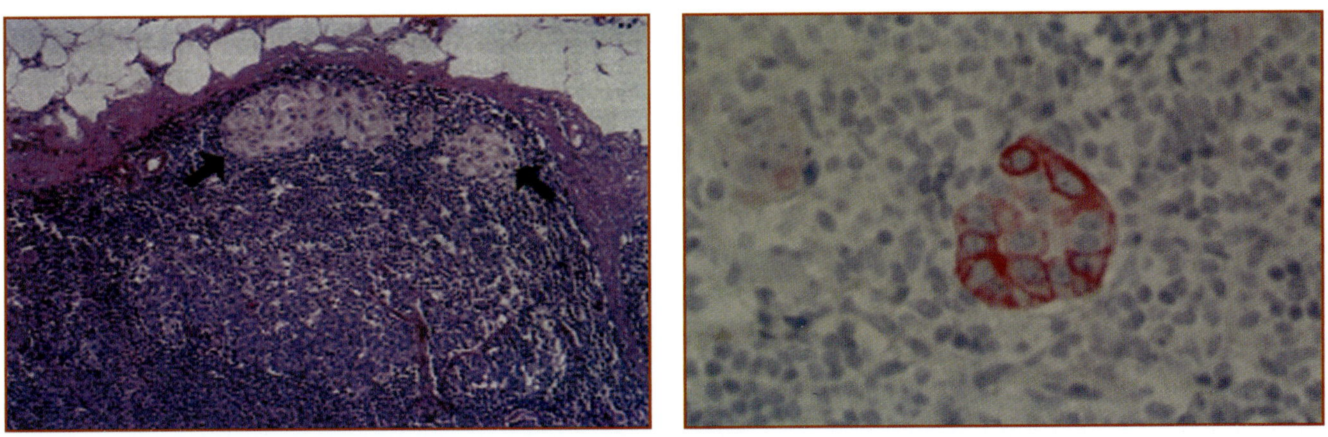

A B

Figure 25–1. Sentinel lymph node metastasis. **A.** Example of SLN metastasis (hematoxylin and eosin).[27] **B.** Sentinel node stained with HMB-45 (AEC, aminoethylcarbazol, × 40). Light hemotoxylin used as a counter stain. Note that not all melanoma cells are labeled with the antibody. (Panel B, courtesy of Victor G. Prieto, MD, PhD)

Role of SLN Biopsy in Potential Cure

The therapeutic efficacy of sentinel node biopsy is being compared with excision alone as part of a multicenter randomized phase III trial—the Multicenter Selective Lymphadenectomy Trial (MSLT-1).[105] Although interim results of this trial have not thus far demonstrated an overall survival difference after a median follow-up of 5 years,[105,137] data indicate that sentinel node biopsy followed immediately by complete dissection if the SLN contains tumor clearly prolongs disease-free survival and spares the patient the psychological trauma of anticipating possible nodal recurrence during the traditional "watch and wait" approach.[105] Interim results also demonstrate improved melanoma-specific survival in patients who underwent early TLND following a positive SLN compared to those who developed clinical recurrence after nodal observation, suggesting that failure to identify and remove occult sentinel node metastases may allow development of more extensive regional node disease.[105] The prognostic significance of sentinel node biopsy was also validated in this multicenter trial.[105,138] Further discussion of this clinical trial can be found elsewhere.[139,140] Importantly, an updated interim analysis recently reported at the 2010 Annual Meeting of the Society of Surgical Oncology confirms and strengthens these observations at median follow-up over 6 years.[137]

Patient Selection

The technique of lymphatic mapping and SLN biopsy has been shown to be highly accurate in representing the status of the regional nodal basin.[19,23,38,42,105] This approach has become a standard of care for melanoma patients,[87] providing an alternative to ELND. In nearly all melanoma centers worldwide, sentinel lymph node biopsy is routinely offered to patients with primary cutaneous melanoma whose primary tumor thickness is at least 1 mm and if the patient has no evidence of metastatic melanoma in regional lymph nodes or distant sites on physical examination and limited staging evaluation (chest radiograph and LDH levels).[38]

However, among the prevalent group of patients whose primary tumors are less than 1 mm, various clinicopathologic factors have been employed in an attempt to identify patients in this overall favorable risk group who may be at increased risk of harboring microscopic stage III disease and for whom SLN biopsy may be warranted (reviewed in reference 141). Many centers have also offered SLN biopsy to patients with a melanoma less than 1.0 mm thick, if it is at least Clark level IV or is ulcerated.[27,38,87,142] Sentinel lymph node biopsy also has been offered to patients whose thin melanomas demonstrate vertical growth phase[143–145] or have a positive deep biopsy margin.[146] Recently, several groups have offered SLN biopsy to patients whose thin primary tumors have mitotic activity (eg, ≥1 mitosis per mm^2), as this factor also has been reported to be a strong predictor of SLN positivity[108,147,148] and adverse survival among patients with T1 melanomas.[4] Although the presence of regression has been used as a criterion by which to consider individuals for SLN biopsy based on retrospective studies that identified a small number of patients with regression who subsequently developed metastases,[149] the impact of regression in primary melanoma on subsequent recurrence and overall survival is controversial;[144,149–153] recent studies have not associated regression with an increased risk of a positive SLN.[154,155] The AJCC melanoma staging system currently recommends lymphatic mapping and SLN biopsy for patients with T1b and greater melanoma.[2,4]

Patients with thick (ie, more than 4 mm) melanoma also are offered SLN biopsy.[67,69–71,73] In 2008, an international panel of expert melanoma surgeons discussed the current role of SLN biopsy in the management of patients with primary cutaneous melanoma,[87] and noted that SLN biopsy is valuable as a minimally invasive procedure to stage the regional lymph nodes with little morbidity;[105,138] it represents a standard of care, and should be discussed with all appropriate clinically node-negative melanoma patients who will undergo wide excision of a primary melanoma.[87] As noted above, most of the panelists would also discuss and offer SLN biopsy to patients whose melanomas are not thicker than 1.0 mm but have characteristics that increase the likelihood of regional node micrometastasis. Although unanimous consensus was not reached for all criteria, most panelists would consider recommending the procedure based on primary tumor ulceration, a mitotic rate ≥1 per mm^2 and/or Clark level IV/V invasion, especially if tumor thickness exceeds 0.75 mm. In fact, some of the panelists would use this tumor thickness as a sole criterion. Ulceration, mitotic rate, and Clark level would be especially relevant in patients who have no significant comorbidity, who are younger than 40 to 45 years, or whose primary tumor depth is uncertain because of tumor-positive deep margins in the biopsy specimen.[87]

Special Situations

Approach to Patients After Previous Wide Local Excision

Some patients present for consideration of lymphatic mapping and SLN biopsy following previous wide local excision of the primary melanoma. In theory, the procedure may less accurately reflect the pathologic status of the draining lymph node basins if patterns of afferent lymphatic flow from a primary tumor site were altered as a result of disruption of the lymphatic vessels from the wide local excision. Lymphatic mapping may be particularly insensitive when a melanoma was excised with particularly large margins, when a defect was covered with a rotation flap, or when the primary tumor was situated in a region of ambiguous lymphatic drainage. Our experience,[156] and that of others,[157–162] support the technical feasibility and potential utility of SLN biopsy as an accurate regional nodal staging procedure in carefully selected patients who have had a previous wide local excision without significant rotational flaps.

In contrast, the utility of SLN biopsy in patients who have undergone extensive primary excision site reconstruction remains to be defined. Overall, the data suggest that more extensive surgery may be required to accomplish accurate lymph node staging in patients who have undergone prior WLE, including the possible removal of SLNs from additional lymph node basins and as an additional surgical procedure. Therefore, to minimize morbidity and cost, concomitant WLE and SLN biopsy is strongly preferred whenever possible.[156] As melanomas with potential drainage to the neck that were widely excised prior to consideration of SLN biopsy: (1) likely arise in a region of ambiguous drainage and (2) may have been closed via extensive reconstructive techniques, the importance of proper treatment planning is further highlighted. In some centers, patients who have already had a WLE and who are considered to have a higher likelihood of a positive SLN on the basis of pathologic features of the primary tumor (eg, thicker or ulcerated lesions) or who had an excision with less than the recommended WLE criteria based on thickness alone (eg, due to functional or cosmetic concerns), are sometimes considered for adjuvant radiotherapy to the primary site and at-risk nodal basins.[103,104] Although such an approach has been reported to be associated with excellent locoregional control,[103,104] the prognostic information and risk assessment for development of distant metastatic disease that SLN biopsy provides will be lacking, and some patients may not be eligible for some clinical trials without such staging of the regional nodal basin. Therefore, patients for whom there is a particular concern about development of distant disease should be referred to a medical oncologist to discuss adjuvant treatment options.

Desmoplastic Melanoma

Desmoplastic melanoma is an uncommon histologic variant of melanoma that is characterized by an unusual spindle-cell morphology and the presence of fusiform melanocytes dispersed in a prominent collagenous stroma that most commonly present in the head and neck region.[163] From a regional melanoma standpoint, some authors have reported that desmoplastic melanoma rarely metastasizes to regional lymph nodes,[164–166] whereas others have reported lymph node metastasis rates of 8% to 15%.[167–175] Interestingly, this apparently discrepant behavior from melanoma in general may be explained by morphologic heterogeneity; specifically, some desmoplastic melanomas are characterized by a uniform desmoplasia that is prominent throughout the entire tumor (termed "pure" desmoplastic melanoma), whereas other desmoplastic melanomas appear admixed with other histologic subtypes (termed "mixed-type").[176] Distinguishing the phenotypic heterogeneity of desmoplastic melanomas has been reported to be important for stratifying patients with regard to risk of lymph node metastasis and prognosis.[176,177] Data indicate that patients with pure desmoplastic melanoma have a lower incidence of positive SLNs than do patients with mixed-type or nondesmoplastic melanoma, suggesting that SLN biopsy in patients with pure desmoplastic melanoma may not be warranted.[166,177]

Imaging Considerations

Although imaging studies historically have represented a prominent component of the initial staging workup of patients with melanoma, there is little, if any, role for routine comprehensive imaging in patients with early-stage disease[178] as numerous studies have demonstrated that they are insensitive tests to identify occult regional nodal metastases.[178] Even among patients with positive SLNs, contemporary studies indicate that the incidence of synchronous distant metastasis in asymptomatic patients with microscopic SLN metastases is low and has not been significantly impacted by recent advances in imaging. Recent studies support that most patients (except perhaps those with thick or ulcerated primaries, or with significant SLN tumor burden) can be spared formal staging evaluation before completion lymph node dissection.[178–180] A complete staging evaluation may then be pursued after completion lymph node dissection prior to consideration of adjuvant therapy or participation in adjuvant therapy trials.

Although one melanoma group has reported that preoperative ultrasound and fine-needle aspiration cytology (FNAC) may accurately identify up to 65% of SLN metastases in patients with primary cutaneous melanoma based on morphologic criteria,[181] the results of a recent study by Uren and colleagues of 716 patients suggest that preoperative ultrasound can complement but should not substitute for SLN biopsy.[182] Interestingly, the proportion of ultrasound-detected SLN metastases to the neck in this study was significantly greater than the proportion of SLN metastases detected by ultrasound in other nodal regions by univariate analysis (sensitivity: axilla, 21.1%; groin, 15.6%; neck, 45.89%; $p = 0.007$), but was associated with lower specificity when compared with SLNs in the axilla and groin.

Technical Considerations

Successful sentinel lymph node biopsy requires the integration of several disciplines, nuclear medicine, surgery, and pathology. The contemporary approach consists of three main components: (1) preoperative cutaneous lymphoscintigraphy to identify the regional nodal basins at risk and the number and location of the SLNs within the basin; (2) excisional biopsy of SLNs in all regional nodal basins at risk demonstrated by preoperative lymphoscintigraphy and intraoperative localization with vital blue dye and handheld gamma probe detection of 99Tc-labeled sulfur colloid; and (3) careful pathologic evaluation of the SLNs. Lymphatic mapping and SLN biopsy is much preferably performed at the time of wide excision of the primary tumor or biopsy site (see above). Since the introduction of lymphatic mapping and SLN biopsy, the technique has undergone several refinements that have improved detection of SLNs.

Use of a vital blue dye (isosulfan blue 1%) to help identify SLNs has been part of the lymphatic mapping and SLN biopsy procedure since its introduction. The blue dye is injected into the patient intradermally around the intact tumor or biopsy site, taken up by the lymphatic system, and carried via afferent lymphatics to the SLN. The draining nodal basin is explored, and the afferent lymphatic channels and first draining lymph nodes (the SLNs) are identified by the uptake of the blue dye. With the use of blue dye alone, an SLN is identified in approximately 85% of cases. Although this initial approach was promising, it left 15% of patients unable to benefit from SLN biopsy because no SLN was identified.

Subsequently, two additional techniques have been incorporated that have significantly improved SLN localization: (1) preoperative lymphoscintigraphy and (2) intraoperative injection of technetium-99 (^{99}Tc)-labeled sulfur colloid accompanied by intraoperative use of a handheld gamma probe. Preoperative lymphoscintigraphy using ^{99}Tc-labeled sulfur colloid (in the US) permits the identification of patients with multiple draining nodal basins and patients with lymphatic drainage to SLNs located outside standard nodal basins.[154,183–186] For the SLN biopsy technique to be accurate, all true SLNs, regardless of location, must be identified and harvested, as the histologic status of one draining basin does not predict the status of other basins in patients with melanomas that drain to multiple regional nodal basins.[187,188]

Perhaps the most important development in this technique has been the introduction of intraoperative lymphatic mapping using a handheld gamma probe. Preoperative intradermal injection of 0.5 to 1.0 mCi of ^{99}Tc-labeled sulfur colloid permits its intraoperative use with a hand-held gamma probe to transcutaneously identify SLNs to be removed. The use of both blue dye and radiocolloid increases the surgeon's ability to identify the SLN (greater than 96% to 99% accuracy) compared to the use of blue dye alone (84 to 85% accuracy).[37] Overall, radiocolloid and vital blue dye mapping techniques are complementary; to facilitate regional nodal staging, this latter technique represents the preferred approach to SLN biopsy by large academic centers and by an international consensus panel.[37,87,189]

In general, SLNs are subjected to enhanced pathologic analysis that includes both serial sectioning and immunohistochemical analysis. As noted, frozen section analysis of SLNs in patient with cutaneous melanoma is not routinely performed.[121]

When the SLNs are histologically negative, no further surgery is performed, and the remaining regional lymph nodes are left intact. When the SLNs show evidence of metastatic disease, completion lymphadenectomy of the affected nodal basin is the current standard of care. Pathologic evaluation of completion lymphadenectomy specimens often reveals no additional disease. However, it is important to recognize that completion lymphadenectomy specimens are routinely assessed with standard histologic techniques rather than the more rigorous examination reserved for SLN biopsy specimens. As a result, additional disease in the completion nodal specimen may go undetected. This disease would represent a potential source of subsequent recurrence if it were not removed. Because such recurrences are difficult to treat surgically and may contribute to significant morbidity, completion lymphadenectomy performed for microscopic disease provides the potential for improved regional control. In addition, identifying patients with minimal disease burden by using the SLN approach may help identify the group of patients who may derive an improved survival benefit from early TLND. Furthermore, knowledge of the pathologic status of the SLNs allows proper staging and facilitates decision-making regarding adjuvant treatment.

Preoperative Lymphoscintigraphy

Preoperative cutaneous lymphoscintigraphy is used to identify the regional nodal basins at risk in patients whose primary melanoma arises in a region of ambiguous nodal drainage (eg, trunk and head and neck locations), and to determine the number and location of SLNs within a given regional nodal basin. We therefore recommend that all patients with melanomas arising in an area of potentially ambiguous drainage (ie, trunk and head and neck sites) undergo lymphoscintigraphy.

At MD Anderson Cancer Center, this procedure usually is performed days before the actual operation to permit appropriate surgical planning. Following radiotracer injection, real-time images are obtained to visualize both afferent lymphatic channels and nodal basins at risk. Although images obtained in patients whose primary melanoma is remote from the regional nodal basin are often easily interpretable, it may be difficult to discern discrete lymphatic drainage patterns in patients whose melanomas are close to potential regional nodal basins, a common challenge among patients with head and neck (or truncal) primary melanomas. In these instances, multiple views often are helpful, maximizing the ability to document drainage to the regional nodal basin (Fig 25–2).

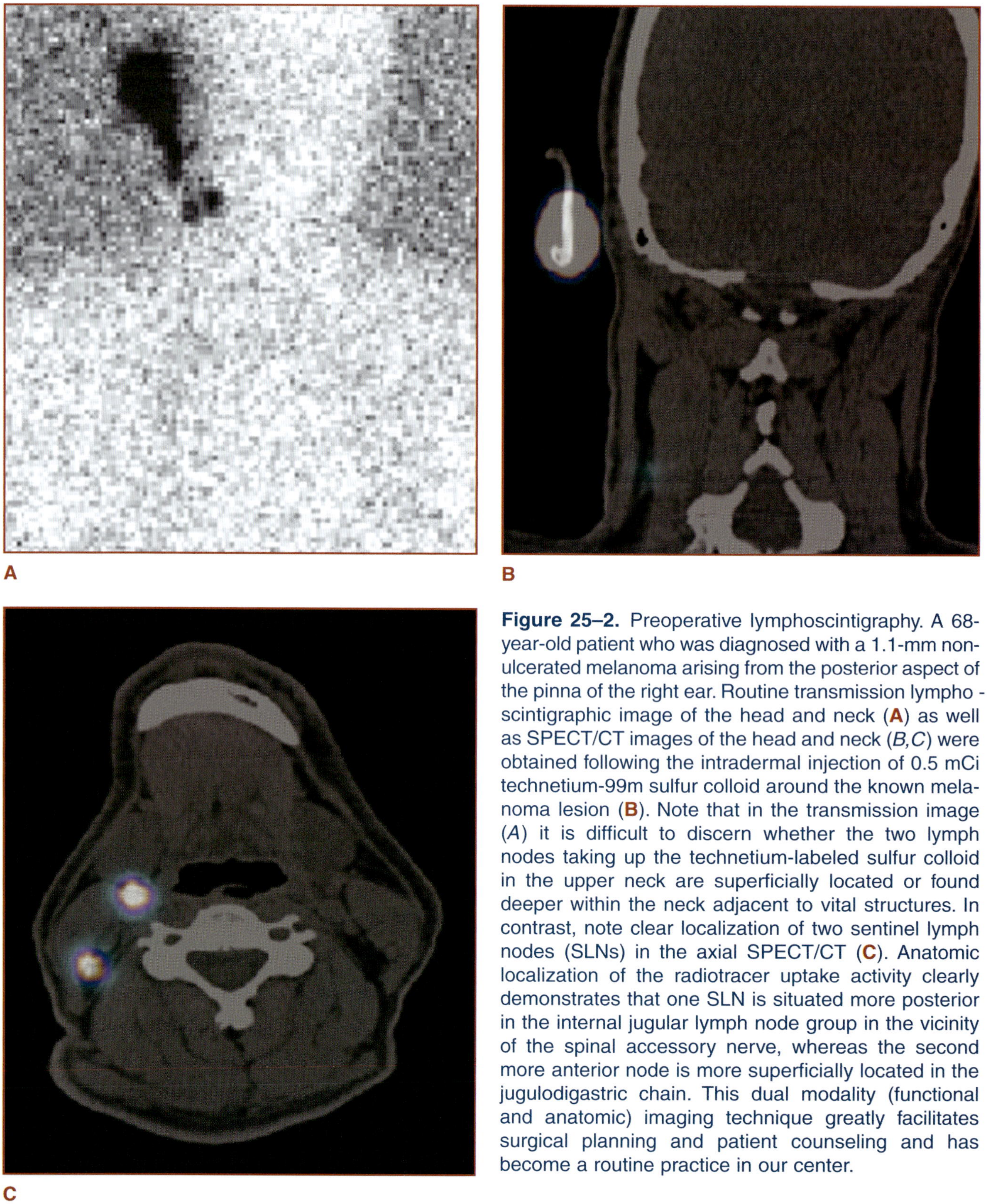

Figure 25–2. Preoperative lymphoscintigraphy. A 68-year-old patient who was diagnosed with a 1.1-mm non-ulcerated melanoma arising from the posterior aspect of the pinna of the right ear. Routine transmission lymphoscintigraphic image of the head and neck (**A**) as well as SPECT/CT images of the head and neck (*B,C*) were obtained following the intradermal injection of 0.5 mCi technetium-99m sulfur colloid around the known melanoma lesion (**B**). Note that in the transmission image (*A*) it is difficult to discern whether the two lymph nodes taking up the technetium-labeled sulfur colloid in the upper neck are superficially located or found deeper within the neck adjacent to vital structures. In contrast, note clear localization of two sentinel lymph nodes (SLNs) in the axial SPECT/CT (**C**). Anatomic localization of the radiotracer uptake activity clearly demonstrates that one SLN is situated more posterior in the internal jugular lymph node group in the vicinity of the spinal accessory nerve, whereas the second more anterior node is more superficially located in the jugulodigastric chain. This dual modality (functional and anatomic) imaging technique greatly facilitates surgical planning and patient counseling and has become a routine practice in our center.

More recently, we have used SPECT-CT imaging to enhance anatomic visualization of the SLNs, particularly in the head and neck region (Fig 25–3). This approach provides advantages over planar imaging alone, including higher sensitivity for SLN detection; detection of SLNs in new node fields; improved detection of SLNs near injection sites (where shine-through may be a significant problem; and improved SLN location by providing detailed anatomic localization (see Figs 25–2 and 25–3).[190]

It is clear that lymphatic drainage patterns from cutaneous invasive melanoma of the head and neck is highly complex, with multiple SLNs commonly draining to multiple regional nodal basins. Using this approach, Eicher and colleagues[45] found that head and neck primary sites drained to an average of 2.2 nodal basins per patient, with drainage to nonadjacent nodal basins in 42% of patients. In a subsequent effort to better understand "lessons learned" from preoperative lymphoscintigraphy performed on patients with primary melanoma of the head and neck, Reynolds et al[191] developed a three-dimensional visualization of skin lymphatic drainage patterns by employing "heat map" technology based on lymphoscintigraphy data from 929 patients with primary cutaneous melanoma on the head and neck treated at the Sydney Melanoma Unit. These data not only demonstrated inadequacies of "classical" descriptions of lymphatic drainage patterns, but also provide an important educational evidence-based tool for clinicians (Fig 25–4).

From a practical standpoint, the rare instances of failure of the radiocolloid to migrate from the injection sites may be due to subcutaneous rather than intradermal injection, especially in patients with very thin skin. Lymphoscintigraphy should be re-attempted in these patients. Preoperative lymphoscintigraphy and images also may be obtained

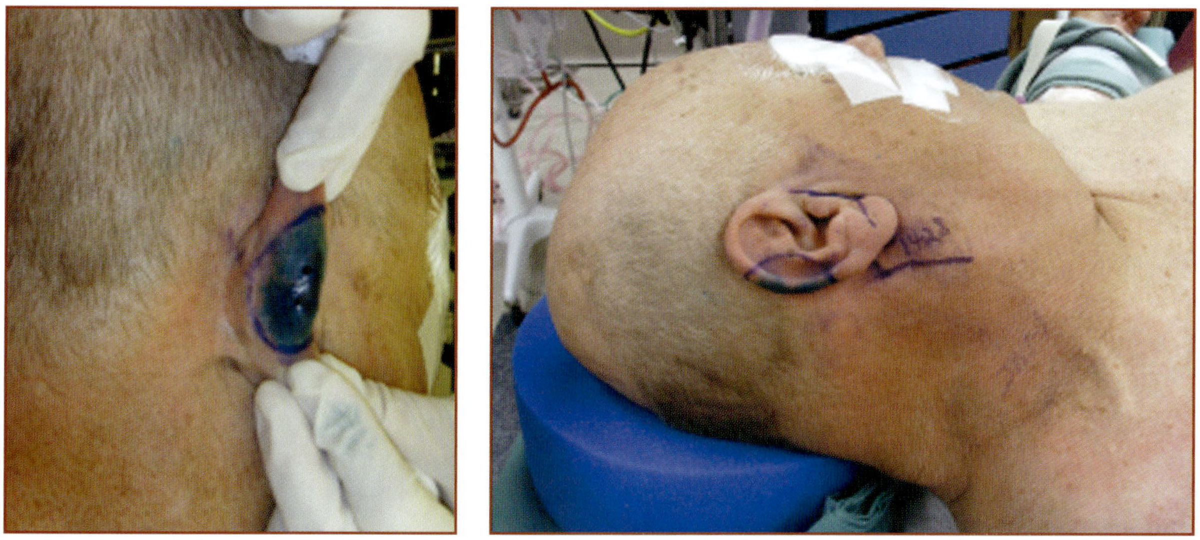

A B

Figure 25–3. Wide local excision of a right helical rim melanoma with sentinel lymph node (SLN) biopsy. The same patient with the right aurciular melanoma (Fig 25–2) returned to the nuclear medicine suite on the morning of surgery and was injected with 0.5 mCi technetium-99m sulfur colloid intradermally around the known melanoma lesion. He was then brought to the operating room where a proposed 1-cm wide local excision was outlined and an intradermal injection of 1 ml of isosulfan blue was performed (**A**). The patient was positioned and the incisions needed to harvest the SLNs from areas of increased focal radiotracer uptake activity were outlined based on hand-held gamma probe-guided SLN localization (**B**). *continues*

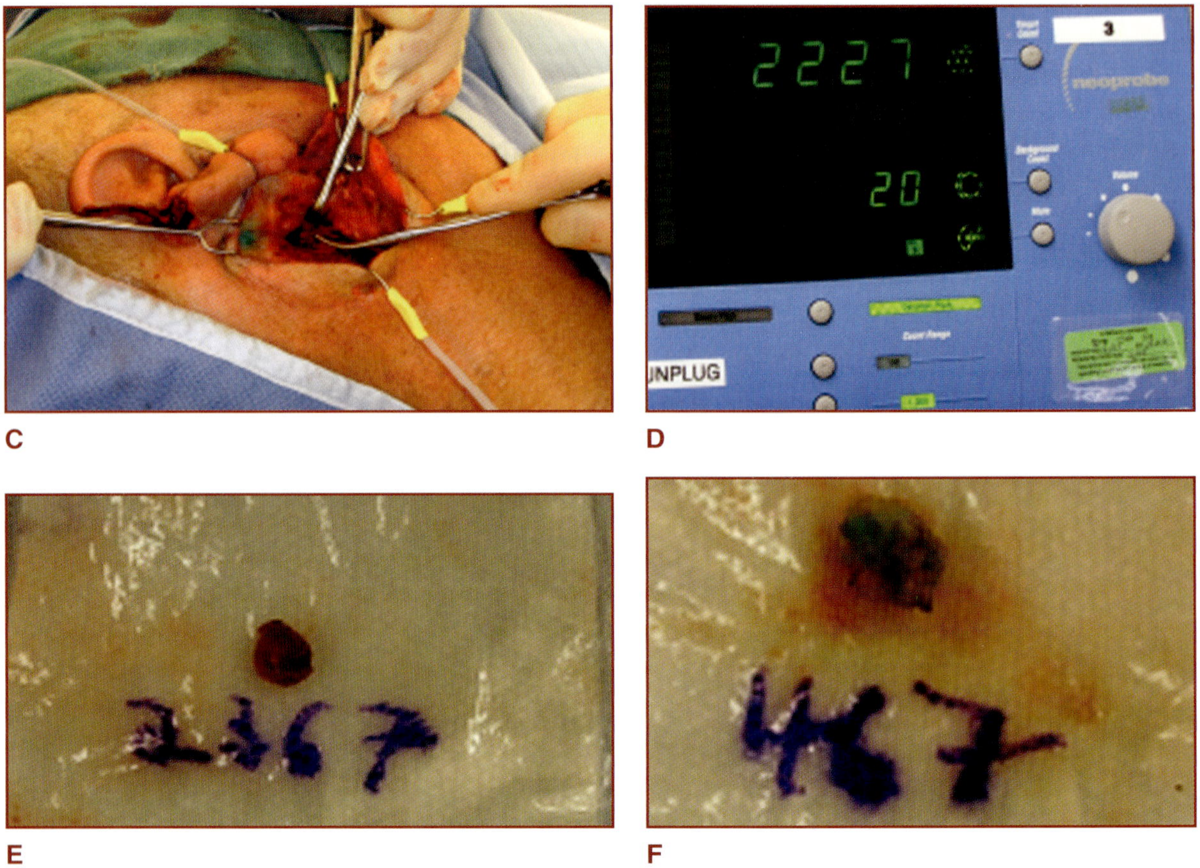

Figure 25–3. *continued* In panel **C**, a hemostat points to a SLN that had a high uptake on gamma probe evaluation (**D**) but was not stained with isosulfan blue (**E**). A second SLN had increased radiotracer uptake activty and was stained blue; it was located just anterior to a retracting double-prong skin hook (**F**). Pathologic evaluation of both SLNs by hematoxylin and eosin staining, step sectioning, and immunohistochemistry for a panel of melanoma markers failed to reveal metastatic melanoma.

immediately following technetium-labeled sulfur colloid injection on the day of surgery, an approach preferred in some institutions. Identification of all nodal basins at risk for metastatic disease is especially important with melanomas of the trunk or the head and neck (all of which may drain to the neck), where lymphatic drainage patterns cannot reliably be predicted by clinical judgment or classical anatomic guidelines and where multiple basin drainage is common.[192,193]

Intraoperative Considerations

Since 1994, lymphatic mapping and sentinel lymphadenectomy has been performed at MD Anderson using both isosulfan blue dye and technetium-labeled sulfur colloid detected using a handheld gamma probe. On the day of operation, 0.5 to 1 mCi of technetium-labeled sulfur colloid is usually injected intradermally at 4 points around the melanoma site. This procedure is scheduled to be performed approximately one hour before the scheduled start of the surgical procedure, as injection immediately before the surgical procedure may not permit enough time for the colloid to travel through afferent lymphatic channels to the SLN and an interval greater than four hours may increase the likelihood that colloid may pass through some of the SLNs to second-echelon nodes, which by definition are not the nodes most likely to contain disease.

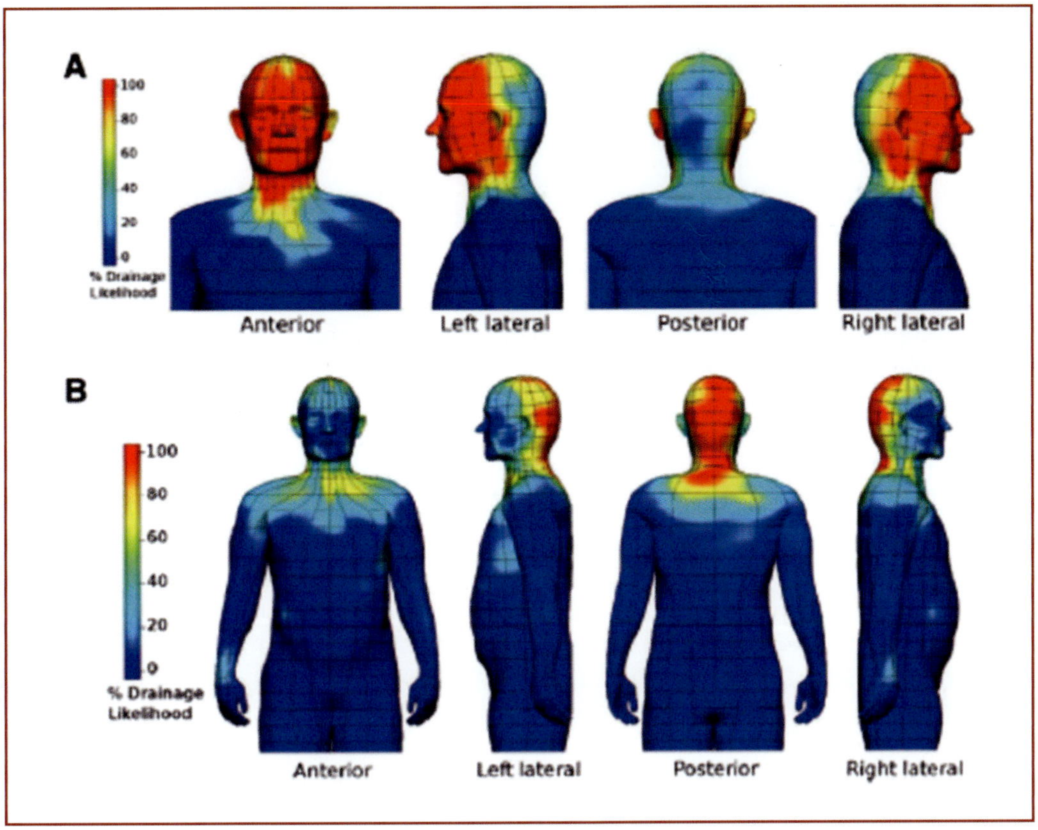

Figure 25–4. Head and neck lymphatic drainage patterns. Reynolds and colleagues from the Sydney Melanoma Unit collected lymphoscintigraphy data from 929 patients with cutaneous melanoma of the head and neck region and mapped the sentinel lymph node drainage patterns from multiple primary melanoma sites using a 3-dimensional computer model. In this example, modeling demonstrates the likelihood that a primary melanoma site will show lymphatic drainage to sentinel nodes in the (**A**) anterior node fields: preauricular, submental, cervical levels I, II, III, and IV, or (**B**) posterior node fields: postauricular, occipital, cervical level V, and supraclavicular fossa. Although posterior head and neck node fields are seen to drain the skin of the posterior head and neck region, the skin of the anterolateral neck tends to drain to nodes that are more anteriorly or laterally located. Source: Reynolds HM, et al, *Head Neck*. 2009, Wiley & Sons; 31:1316–1325.[191]

Immediately before the planned surgical procedure, it is helpful if the handheld gamma probe is used to localize areas of increased focal radiotracer activity transcutaneously in regional nodal basins. Areas of increased focal radiotracer activity are marked on the skin (see Fig 25–3B). Positioning the patient as he or she will be positioned for the actual procedure facilitates the most accurate documentation of the sites of SLNs.

Once adequate anesthesia is achieved and depending in part on the site of the primary, approximately 1 to 3 mL of isosulfan blue dye is administered intradermally, and the injection sites massaged for approximately 1 to 2 minutes to encourage uptake by the cutaneous lymphatics. Injection is usually performed using 1-mL syringes and 25- or 27-gauge needles (see Fig 25–3A).

After injection of the isosulfan blue dye, the patient is positioned and appropriately prepped and draped. Whenever possible, intraoperative lymphatic mapping and sentinel lymphadenectomy is performed before the wide local excision. If shine-through from the injected radioactivity at the primary site is a significant problem, wide local excision of the primary may be performed first. This approach often is used for head and neck primary sites given the proximity of some primary sites to draining regional nodal basins. With the patient prepped and draped, areas of increased focal radiotracer uptake in the first basin are confirmed with the handheld gamma probe.

A small incision is then made overlying the area of increased focal radiotracer activity; care is advised in making this SLN biopsy incision to ensure that it can subsequently be incorporated into a CLND incision should the SLN contain metastatic melanoma. Once identified, the blue-stained and/or highly radioactive node is secured with a suture and gently elevated (Fig 25–5). Surrounding fatty tissue is dissected with the electrocautery, and all vascular and lymphatic structures are identified and ligated to facilitate harvest of the lymph node. In certain anatomic regions within the head and neck, longer SLN biopsy incisions may be required to decrease the risk of injury to vital neurovascular structures. As shown in Figure 25–2C, the SLN at the posterior-superior aspect of level IIb of the right neck would be difficult to excise without potential significant risk of injury to the spinal accessory nerve and jugular vein without a large enough incision to expose landmarks that help the surgeon to safely identify and protect those important structures.

Although some surgeons may question need for blue dye, most surgeons believe that blue dye provides an invaluable and complementary adjunct, and remains a critical component of the lymphatic mapping technique.[37] The dye provides a visual aid that not only confirms that the lymph node is an SLN but also facilitates localization of SLNs when transcutaneous localization of colloid is unsuccessful and helps minimize dissection even when gamma probe localization is achieved. At MD Anderson, use

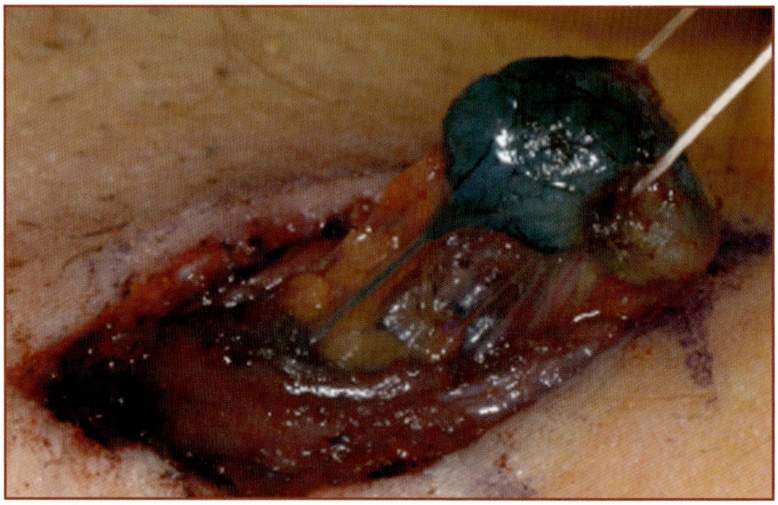

Figure 25–5. Intraoperative identification of a sentinel lymph node (SLN). Intradermal injection of a vital blue dye around the intact melanoma or biopsy site leads to uptake of the dye by the lymphatic system and transport of the dye to the draining regional nodal basins, thereby allowing for identification of SLNs. Note isosulfan blue-stained afferent lymphatic vessel leading to blue-stained SLN. (Courtesy of Jeffrey E. Gershenwald, MD. Copyright retained by the author and the University of Texas MD Anderson Cancer Center.)

of the combined-modality approach (dye and colloid) resulted in an SLN identification rate of over 99%, compared with 87% when only blue dye was used[37]; this has been cited as the preferred approach to SLN biopsy by large academic centers[37,189] and by an international consensus panel.[87]

The SLN is visually inspected for evidence of gross metastatic disease. If it has none, no frozen section analysis of the lymph node is performed. If, however, the lymph node appears grossly suspicious (eg, obvious melanin pigment and/or tumor), a frozen section examination may be performed to confirm the diagnosis if concomitant completion lymph node dissection is considered *and* has been discussed with the patient in advance. At MD Anderson and the Sydney Melanoma Unit, frozen section analysis of sentinel lymph nodes is rather uncommon, and is reserved only for highly suspicious nodes, and only if plans for possible concomitant lymph node dissection was discussed preoperatively with the patient. The "abnormal" appearance of SLNs often simply represents reaction to a previous diagnostic biopsy procedure. If frozen section analysis were performed routinely, optimal tissue for careful permanent section analysis might be lost in processing, limiting the diagnostic yield of subsequent serial section and immunohistochemistry.[121] Some investigators have employed intraoperative evaluation of sentinel lymph nodes for metastatic melanoma by imprint cytology.[194]

After removal of the SLN, the basin is rescanned using the gamma probe. If an area of increased focal radiotracer activity is again identified, the procedure is repeated in an effort to identify additional SLNs until no nodes with greater than 10% of the radiotracer uptake activity of the "hottest" SLN remain. All additional SLNs are harvested, and their uptake of blue dye and ex vivo counts are documented. The lymph nodes are numbered sequentially by order of their removal and submitted for permanent-section pathologic analysis.

Operating Room Positioning Strategies

Whereas the surgical approach to patients with melanoma arising on an extremity is relatively straightforward, the surgical approach to patients with melanoma arising in a region of potentially ambiguous lymphatic drainage (eg, trunk, head, or neck) often requires careful planning. Careful attention to patient positioning in the operating room is necessary to ensure that all components of lymphatic mapping and SLN biopsy are achievable.[195] Proper patient positioning must take into account not only the location of the primary melanoma and the regional nodal basins, but also potential in-transit or ectopic sites at risk for metastatic disease and potential donor sites for skin grafting. Careful study of the preoperative lymphoscintigram often provides most of the information necessary to develop an operative positioning strategy, incision design, and surgical plan.

Sentinel Lymph Node Biopsy and the Parotid Gland

One area of lymphatic drainage within the head and neck region worthy of additional consideration in surgical planning is the parotid gland. In one study, 44% of cutaneous lesions of the scalp, ear, face, and neck were found to drain to lymph nodes within the parotid.[45] Although several groups have shown the safety and feasibility of removing SLNs from the parotid without formal superficial parotidectomy and facial nerve dissection, there are situations in which removal of a portion of the gland may be advisable.[196,197] For example, when the SLN is deep within the substance of the gland rather than superficially located along the branches of the superficial temporal vessels, it may be worthwhile to identify the facial nerve and remove the superficial lobe of the parotid gland to avoid re-operation around the previously dissected nerve if this SLN is positive. In some centers, this approach is more readily applied if the primary tumor is thicker (>2.5 mm) and/or ulcerated.

SPECT/CT has been very helpful (compared to conventional lymphoscintigraphy) in identifying patients in whom this scenario may be likely, enabling appropriate preoperative counseling about the potential need for a more comprehensive resection of the parotid versus simple SLN removal. SPECT/CT also is particularly useful in distinguishing whether SLNs are situated within the parotid tail or in the superior external jugular lymph node chain just deep to the parotid tail.

Complications and Morbidity

Overall, SLN biopsy is associated with low morbidity.[105,138,198,199] There are substantially fewer postoperative complications after SLN biopsy than after ELND,[199,200] and the rate of lymphedema, pain, numbness, and loss of active range of motion are lower after SLN biopsy than after full anatomical dissection.[57,105,199,201,202] In addition, recent data have shown that SLN biopsy does not increase the incidence of in transit recurrence.[138,203–205]

Investigators from the Sunbelt Melanoma Trial reported overall low complication rates following SLN biopsy alone in more than 1,202 trial patients compared to the 277 patients who required a complete lymph node dissection.[199] This observation has been reiterated by others, as well as in the Multicenter Selective Lymphadenectomy Trial, whereby overall complication rates of 10% after lymphatic mapping and SLN biopsy increased to 32.7% after completion lymph node dissection.[105,138,206,207] Strategies to reduce the incidence of lymphedema, more common following formal lymphadenectomy, are also helpful.

Risk of In Transit Metastasis

Although the SLN biopsy technique has gained widespread acceptance for a number of reasons: accurate nodal staging, enhanced regional control, possible survival benefit, and limited surgical morbidity compared to formal lymphadenectomy, some authors have suggested that SLN biopsy may increase the risk of in transit metastasis (ITM), thereby reducing, eliminating, or reversing any potential survival advantage associated with the SLN biopsy technique.[208] The hypothesis that the SLN biopsy technique and subsequent completion lymph node dissection in SLN-positive patients may disturb lymph flow by mechanical disruption and lead to increased rates of ITM, if accurate, is of particular concern as SLN biopsy has been widely adopted as a standard of care. The collective experience at several large academic centers,[203,204,209] including the MSLT-1 trial,[105] provides strong support that the technique of SLN biopsy itself does not increase the risk of in transit metastasis.[105,203,204,209] Instead, the risk of in transit melanoma metastasis depends on tumor biology and not the surgical approach to regional lymph nodes.[205]

Complications Associated with Vital Blue Dye

Although allergic reactions, including anaphylactic reactions, have been reported on rare occasions following use of vital blue dye, they have occurred only rarely in large melanoma populations.[138,210] Blue dye can be retained at the primary site for more than a year. Although the color generally gradually fades with time, patients may be left with a permanent tattoo if the injected dye is not removed with WLE of the primary site. Careful attention to injection technique is particularly important in patients whose melanomas arise in cosmetically sensitive areas such as the head and neck. A small amount of residual dye may also persist for several months after WLE .

Role of Radiotherapy in the Clinical N_0 Neck

Although SLN biopsy represents a standard of care for patients with early stage melanoma at risk for regional lymph node metastasis, there are some patients with significant medical comorbidities for whom such regional nodal staging and prognostic assessment is of little relevance and for whom enrollment in a clinical trial is unlikely. For this small subset of patients otherwise at risk for occult nodal metastasis, elective cervical nodal irradiation may be superior to nodal observation with the attendant unacceptable risk of regional recurrence.[211–213]

In a retrospective analysis from MD Anderson, Bonnen and colleagues reviewed 157 patients with stage I or II cutaneous melanoma of the head and neck who received elective regional irradiation instead of lymph node dissection (in the pre-SLN biopsy era) after wide local excision of the primary site.[104] Indications for regional irradiation included primary thickness of 1.5 mm or greater or Clark level IV or V disease. There were 15 regional failures

(89% regional control at 10 years) despite an estimate that 33 to 40 patients had microscopically involved regional nodes. Six percent of patients required medical care for a clinically significant complication, with moderate hearing loss being the most common complaint ($N = 5$). Although elective nodal irradiation suffers from similar limitations as does ELND, it can effectively control nodal basins at risk for regional recurrence while avoiding significant potential surgical morbidity, as irradiation to the neck is generally well tolerated and is associated with a lower risk of lymphedema than nodal irradiation to the axilla or groin.

Among patients with regional melanoma metastases, factors associated with a high risk of subsequent regional basin recurrence after lymph node dissection include lymph nodes at least 3 cm, four or more positive lymph nodes, extracapsular extension, and recurrent disease after initial surgical resection. The role of radiation therapy for all patients with nodal disease in the adjuvant setting is somewhat controversial.[211,214] Historically, most reports consist of small retrospective comparisons of patients treated at a variety of sites, with varying doses and doses per fraction, often following surgical resections of varying extent.[211,212] Nonetheless, retrospective, and more recently phase II and phase III prospective trials support that adjuvant radiation therapy may significantly improve the locoregional control rate in these clinical settings.[211] Recently, the Trans-Tasman Radiation Oncology Group and the Australia and New Zealand Melanoma Trials group completed a randomized trial comparing nodal observation to radiation therapy after lymphadenectomy in patients with melanoma who had palpable nodal disease and one of the high-risk features.[215] Although there was no improvement in overall survival, this trial reported an acceptable acute toxicity and 2-year regional control rate of 80% with radiation therapy compared to 68% without ($p = 0.041$).[215]

Although the only randomized assessment of radiation delivery approach showed no difference in local control between conventional and hypofractionated schedules, many centers currently employ a hypofractionated regimen that is generally well tolerated and relatively convenient for patients. The impact of adjuvant radiation therapy on the incidence of distant metastasis and overall survival is, however, less clear. Although improvement in overall patient outcome will require improvements in systemic disease control, the importance of locoregional control in reducing morbidity should not be underestimated. In general, patients with multiple involved or large, matted regional nodes or with extracapsular extension of regional lymphatic metastases should be considered for adjuvant radiation therapy.[211,212,216]

Summary and Future Directions

Approximately 85% of patients diagnosed with melanoma have clinically localized disease at presentation and in general have a favorable prognosis. Nonetheless, multiple factors, both established and not yet known, lead to heterogeneity in clinical course and outcome for patients with early-stage melanoma. Over the past three decades, the approach to patients with clinically negative regional lymph nodes has significantly evolved. During this time, the technique of lymphatic mapping and SLN biopsy has emerged as the standard of care to identify patients with microscopic lymph node involvement using a minimally invasive approach that clearly has advantages over routine ELND. Overall, this technique has been shown to reliably stage the regional lymph node basins at risk and identify those patients who may benefit from completion lymph node dissection and/or adjuvant therapy, while sparing patients with negative nodes the morbidity of an additional surgical procedure. Its prognostic power and overall success is dependent on excellent communication and coordination among the surgical, nuclear medicine, radiology, and pathology teams.

Based on a comprehensive 2008 AJCC collaborative melanoma database analysis, changes in melanoma staging have been introduced in 7th edition of the AJCC Cancer Staging manual published in late 2009 and officially implemented in early 2010. Although this large analysis validated the existing staging system, among the most notable lessons learned include the importance of mitotic rate in primary melanoma and the tremendous heterogeneity of stage III disease, including the significance of tumor burden at the microscopic level.

The advent of the SLN biopsy technique has helped to usher in a new era of molecular pathologic analysis of SLNs. Rather than traditional routine histologic examination, SLNs are subjected to more extensive pathologic examination with serial sectioning, immunohistochemical staining, and, in clinical trials, evolving molecular-based strategies. Going forward, developing and maturing technologies may make possible a genomic approach to melanoma classification, potentially allowing the identification of genetic markers or expression profiles that might be important for diagnosis, determination of prognosis, and even therapy. Other frontiers in the treatment of early-stage melanoma include defining the role of SLN biopsy in patients with T1 primary tumors and determining which patients benefit the most and the least from a completion lymph node dissection following identification of a positive SLN. These represent only a few of the many questions that remain unanswered for patients with melanoma and a clinically node-negative neck.

References

1. Bedrosian I, Gershenwald JE. Surgical clinical trials in melanoma. *Surg Clin North Am.* 2003;83:385–403.
2. Balch CM. Melanoma of the Skin, in Edge SB, Byrd DR, Compton CC, et al, eds. *AJCC Cancer Staging Manual* (7th ed). New York, NY: Springer-Verlag; 2009.
3. Balch CM, Buzaid AC, Soong SJ, et al. Final version of the American Joint Committee on Cancer staging system for cutaneous melanoma. *J Clin Oncol.* 2001;19: 3635–3648.
4. Balch CM, Gershenwald JE, Soong SJ, et al. Final version of 2009 AJCC melanoma staging and classification. *J Clin Oncol.* 2009;27:6199–6206.
5. Balch CM. Melanoma of the Skin. In: Greene FL, Page DL, Fleming ID, et al, eds. *AJCC Cancer Staging Manual* (6th ed). New York, NY: Springer-Verlag; 2002
6. Balch CM, Gershenwald JE, Soong SJ, et al. Multivariate analysis of prognostic factors among 2,313 patients with stage III melanoma: comparison of nodal micro - metastases versus macrometastases. *J Clin Oncol.* In press.
7. Balch C, Soong S, Murad T, et al. A multifactorial analysis of melanoma: prognostic factors in melanoma patients with lymph node metastases (stage II). *Ann Surg.* 1981; 193:377–388.
8. Balch CM, Gershenwald JE, Soong S, et al. Melanoma staging and classification. In Balch CM, Houghton AN, Sober AJ, et al, eds. *Cutaneous Melanoma.* 5th ed. St. Louis, MO: Quality Medical Publishing, Inc; 2009:65–85.
9. McCarthy W, Shaw H, Milton G. Efficacy of elective lymph node dissection in 2,347 patients with clinical stage I malignant melanoma. *Surg Gynecol Obstet.* 1985; 161:575–580.
10. Morton DL, Wanek L, Nizze J, et al. Improved long-term survival after lymphadenectomy of melanoma. *Ann Surg.* 1991;214:491–501.
11. Reintgen D, Cox E, McCarty K, et al. Efficacy of elective lymph node dissection in patients with intermediate thickness primary melanoma. *Ann Surg.* 1983;198: 379–385.
12. Balch CM, Soong SJ, Milton GW, et al. A comparison of prognostic factors and surgical results in 1,786 patients with localized (stage I) melanoma treated in Alabama, USA, and New South Wales, Australia. *Ann Surg.* 1982; 196:677–684.
13. Sim FH, Taylor W, Pritchard D, et al. Lymphadenectomy in the management of stage I malignant melanoma: a prospective. *Mayo Clin Proc.* 1986;61:697–705.
14. Veronesi U, Adamus J, Bandiera DC, et al. Inefficacy of immediate node dissection in stage I melanoma of the limbs. *N Engl J Med.* 1977;297:627–630.
15. Balch CM, Soong S, Ross MI, et al. Long-term results of a multi-institutional randomized trial comparing prognostic factors and surgical results for intermediate thickness melanomas (1.0 to 4.0 mm). Intergroup Melanoma Surgical Trial [See comments]. *Ann Surg Oncol.* 2000;7: 87–97.
16. Balch CM, Soong SJ, Bartolucci AA, et al. Efficacy of an elective regional lymph node dissection of 1 to 4 mm thick melanomas for patients 60 years of age and younger. *Ann Surg.* 1996;224:255–263; discussion 263–266.
17. Cascinelli N, Morabito A, Santinami M, et al. Immediate or delayed dissection of regional nodes in patients with melanoma of the trunk: a randomised trial. WHO Melanoma Programme. *Lancet.* 1998;351:793–796.
18. Balch C, Soong S, Ross M, et al. Long-term results of a multi-institutional randomized trial comparing prognostic factors and surgical results for intermediate thickness melanomas (1.0 to 4.0 mm). Intergroup Melanoma Surgical Trial. *Ann Surg Oncol.* 2000;7:87–97.
19. Morton DL, Wen DR, Wong JH, et al. Technical details of intraoperative lymphatic mapping for early stage melanoma. *Arch Surg.* 1992;127:392–399.
20. Ross M, Reintgen D, Balch C. Selective lymphadenectomy: emerging role for lymphatic mapping and sentinel lymph node biopsy in the management of early stage melanoma. *Semin Surg Oncol.* 1993;9:219–223.
21. Morton DL, Wen DR, Cochran AJ. Management of early-stage melanoma by intraoperative lymphatic mapping and selective lymphadenectomy or "watch and wait." *Surg Oncol Clin North Am.* 1992;247.

22. Reintgen D, Cruse CW, Wells K, et al. The orderly progression of melanoma nodal metastases. *Ann Surg.* 1994; 220:759–767.
23. Thompson JF, McCarthy WH, Bosch CM, et al. Sentinel lymph node status as an indicator of the presence of metastatic melanoma in regional lymph nodes. *Melanoma Res.* 1995;5:255–260.
24. Abrahamsen HN, Hamilton-Dutoit SJ, Larsen J, et al. Sentinel lymph nodes in malignant melanoma: extended histopathologic evaluation improves diagnostic precision. *Cancer.* 2004;100:1683–1691.
25. Cochran AJ. The pathologist's role in sentinel lymph node evaluation. *Semin Nucl Med.* 2000;30:11–17.
26. Cook MG, Green MA, Anderson B, et al. The development of optimal pathological assessment of sentinel lymph nodes for melanoma. *J Pathol.* 2003;200:314–319.
27. Gershenwald JE, Colome MI, Lee JE, et al. Patterns of recurrence following a negative sentinel lymph node biopsy in 243 patients with stage I or II melanoma. *J Clin Oncol.* 1998;16:2253–2260.
28. Gietema HA, Vuylsteke RJ, de Jonge IA, et al. Sentinel lymph node investigation in melanoma: detailed analysis of the yield from step sectioning and immunohistochemistry. *J Clin Pathol.* 2004;57:618–620.
29. Messina JL, Glass LF, Cruse CW, et al. Pathologic examination of the sentinel lymph node in malignant melanoma. *Am J Surg Pathol.* 1999;23:686–690.
30. Prieto VG, Clark S: Processing of sentinel lymph nodes for detection of metastatic melanoma. *Ann Diagn Pathol.* 2002;6:257–264.
31. Scolyer RA, Thompson JF, McCarthy SW. Sentinel lymph nodes in malignant melanoma: extended histopathologic evaluation improves diagnostic precision. *Cancer.* 2004;101:2141–2142; author reply 2142–2143.
32. Albertini JJ, Cruse CW, Rapaport D, et al. Intraoperative radio-lympho-scintigraphy improves sentinel lymph node identification for patients with melanoma. *Ann Surg.* 1996;223:217–224.
33. Gershenwald JE, Thompson W, Mansfield PF, et al. Multi-institutional melanoma lymphatic mapping experience: the prognostic value of sentinel lymph node status in 612 stage I or II melanoma patients. *J Clin Oncol.* 1999;17:976–983.
34. Krag DN, Meijer SJ, Weaver DL, et al. Minimal-access surgery for staging of malignant melanoma. *Arch Surg.* 1995;130:654–658; discussion 659–660.
35. Reintgen D, Balch C, Kirkwood J, et al. Recent advances in the care of the patient with malignant melanoma. *Ann Surg.* 1997;225:1–14.
36. Uren RF, Howman-Giles R, Thompson JF, et al. Lymphoscintigraphy to identify sentinel lymph nodes in patients with melanoma. *Melanoma Res.* 1994;4:395–399.
37. Gershenwald JE, Tseng CH, Thompson W, et al. Improved sentinel lymph node localization in patients with primary melanoma with the use of radiolabeled colloid. *Surgery.* 1998;124:203–210.
38. Gershenwald J, Thompson W, Mansfield P, et al. Multi-institutional melanoma lymphatic mapping experience: The prognostic value of sentinel lymph node status in 612 stage I or II melanoma patients. *J Clin Oncol.* 1999; 17:976–983.
39. Godellas CV, Berman CG, Lyman G, et al. The identification and mapping of melanoma regional nodal metastases: minimally invasive surgery for the diagnosis of nodal metastases. *Am Surg.* 1995;61:97–101.
40. Gogel BM, Kuhn JA, Ferry KM, et al. Sentinel lymph node biopsy for melanoma. *Am J Surg.* 1998;176:544–547.
41. Jansen L, Nieweg OE, Peterse JL, et al. Reliability of sentinel lymph node biopsy for staging melanoma. *Br J Surg.* 2000;87:484–489.
42. Morton DL, Thompson JF, Essner R, et al. Validation of the accuracy of intraoperative lymphatic mapping and sentinel lymphadenectomy for early-stage melanoma. *Ann Surg.* 1999;230:453–465.
43. Ross MI. The case for elective lymphadenectomy. *Surg Oncol Clin North Am.* 1992;1:205.
44. Uren RF, Howman-Giles RB, Shaw HM, et al. Lymphoscintigraphy in high-risk melanoma of the trunk: predicting draining node groups, defining lymphatic channels and locating the sentinel node. *J Nucl Med.* 1993;34:1435–1440.
45. Eicher SA, Clayman GL, Myers JN, et al. A prospective study of intraoperative lymphatic mapping for head and neck cutaneous melanoma. *Arch Otolaryngol Head Neck Surg.* 2002;128:241–246.
46. Karim RZ, Scolyer RA, Li W, et al. False negative sentinel lymph node biopsies in melanoma may result from deficiencies in nuclear medicine, surgery, or pathology. *Ann Surg.* 2008;247:1003–1010.
47. Carlson GW, Page AJ, Cohen C, et al. Regional recurrence after negative sentinel lymph node biopsy for melanoma. *Ann Surg.* 2008;248:378–386.
48. Gomez-Rivera F, Santillan A, McMurphey AB, et al. Sentinel node biopsy in patients with cutaneous melanoma of the head and neck: recurrence and survival study. *Head Neck.* 2008;30:1284–1294.
49. Schmalbach CE, Nussenbaum B, Rees RS, et al. Reliability of sentinel lymph node mapping with biopsy for head and neck cutaneous melanoma. *Arch Otolaryngol Head Neck Surg.* 2003;129:61–65.
50. Clary BM, Brady MS, Lewis JJ, et al. Sentinel lymph node biopsy in the management of patients with primary cutaneous melanoma: review of a large single-institutional experience with an emphasis on recurrence. *Ann Surg.* 2001;233:250–258.
51. Cochran AJ, Wen DR, Huang RR, et al. Prediction of metastatic melanoma in nonsentinel nodes and clinical outcome based on the primary melanoma and the sentinel node. *Mod Pathol.* 2004;17:747–755.
52. Dessureault S, Soong SJ, Ross MI, et al. Improved staging of node-negative patients with intermediate to thick melanomas (>1 mm) with the use of lymphatic mapping and

sentinel lymph node biopsy. *Ann Surg Oncol.* 2001;8: 766–770.
53. Wagner JD, Davidson D, Coleman JJ 3rd, et al. Lymph node tumor volumes in patients undergoing sentinel lymph node biopsy for cutaneous melanoma. *Ann Surg Oncol.* 1999;6:398–404.
54. Wagner JD, Gordon MS, Chuang TY, et al Predicting sentinel and residual lymph node basin disease after sentinel lymph node biopsy for melanoma. *Cancer.* 2000;89:453–462.
55. Balch CM, Soong SJ, Gershenwald JE, et al. Prognostic factors analysis of 17,600 melanoma patients: validation of the American Joint Committee on Cancer melanoma staging system. *J Clin Oncol.* 2001;19:3622–3634.
56. Carlson GW, Murray DR, Lyles RH, et al. The amount of metastatic melanoma in a sentinel lymph node: does it have prognostic significance? *Ann Surg Oncol.* 2003; 10:575–581.
57. Essner R, Conforti A, Kelley MC, et al. Efficacy of lymphatic mapping, sentinel lymphadenectomy, and selective complete lymph node dissection as a therapeutic procedure for early-stage melanoma. *Ann Surg Oncol.* 1999;6:442–449.
58. Ferrone CR, Panageas KS, Busam K, et al. Multivariate prognostic model for patients with thick cutaneous melanoma: importance of sentinel lymph node status. *Ann Surg Oncol.* 2002;9:637–645.
59. McMasters KM, Sondak V, Lotze M, et al. Recent advances in melanoma staging and therapy. *Ann Surg Oncol.* 1999;6:467–475.
60. Ranieri JM, Wagner JD, Azuaje R, et al. Prognostic importance of lymph node tumor burden in melanoma patients staged by sentinel node biopsy. *Ann Surg Oncol.* 2002;9:975–981.
61. Scolyer RA, Li LX, McCarthy SW, et al. Micromorphometric features of positive sentinel lymph nodes predict involvement of nonsentinel nodes in patients with melanoma. *Am J Clin Pathol.* 2004;122:532–539.
62. Shaw HM, Scolyer RA, Thompson JF. Prognostic significance of histopathological parameters in sentinel nodes of melanoma patients. *Histopathology.* 2008;52:242; author reply 242–244.
63. Spanknebel K, Coit DG, Bieligk SC, et al. Characterization of micrometastatic disease in melanoma sentinel lymph nodes by enhanced pathology: recommendations for standardizing pathologic analysis. *Am J Surg Pathol.* 2005;29:305–317.
64. Starz H, Siedlecki K, Balda BR. Sentinel lymphonodectomy and s-classification: a successful strategy for better prediction and improvement of outcome of melanoma. *Ann Surg Oncol.* 2004;11:162S-168S.
65. Vuylsteke RJ, Borgstein PJ, van Leeuwen PA, et al. Sentinel lymph node tumor load: an independent predictor of additional lymph node involvement and survival in melanoma. *Ann Surg Oncol.* 2005;12:440–448.
66. Zettersten E, Shaikh L, Ramirez R, et al. Prognostic factors in primary cutaneous melanoma. *Surg Clin North Am.* 2003;83:61–75.
67. Cecchi R, Buralli L, Innocenti S, et al. Sentinel lymph node biopsy in patients with thick (= 4 mm) melanoma: a single-centre experience. *J Eur Acad Dermatol Venereol.* 2007;21:758–761.
68. Debarbieux S, Duru G, Dalle S, et al. Sentinel lymph node biopsy in melanoma: a micromorphometric study relating to prognosis and completion lymph node dissection. *Br J Dermatol.* 2007;157:58–67.
69. Gershenwald JE, Mansfield P, Lee J, et al. Role for lymphatic mapping and sentinel lymph node biopsy in patients with thick (> or = 4 mm) primary melanoma. *Ann Surg Oncol.* 2000;7:160–165.
70. Gutzmer R, Satzger I, Thoms KM, et al. Sentinel lymph node status is the most important prognostic factor for thick (> or = 4 mm) melanomas. *J Dtsch Dermatol Ges.* 2008;6:198–203.
71. Sassen S, Shaw HM, Colman MH, et al. The complex relationships between sentinel node positivity, patient age, and primary tumor desmoplasia: analysis of 2303 melanoma patients treated at a single center. *Ann Surg Oncol.* 2008;15:630–637.
72. Thompson J. The Sydney Melanoma Unit experience of sentinel lymphadenectomy for melanoma. *Ann Surg Oncol.* 2001;8:44S-47S.
73. Thompson JF, Shaw H. The prognosis of patients with thick primary melanomas: is regional lymph node status relevant and does removing positive regional nodes influence outcome? *Ann Surg Oncol.* 2002;9:719–722.
74. Gershenwald JE, Andtbacka RH, Prieto VG, et al. Microscopic tumor burden in sentinel lymph nodes predicts synchronous nonsentinel lymph node involvement in patients with melanoma. *J Clin Oncol.* 2008;26:4296–4303.
75. Andtbacka RH, Bedrosian I, Ross MI, et al. *AJCC nodal factors and microscopic tumor burden predict recurrence in sentinel lymph node positive stage III melanoma patients* [Abstr]. 59th Annual Cancer Symposium, Society of Surgical Oncology San Diego, CA, 2006
76. Cascinelli N, Bombardieri E, Bufalino R, et al. Sentinel and nonsentinel node status in stage IB and II melanoma patients: two-step prognostic indicators of survival. *J Clin Oncol.* 2006;24:4464–4471.
77. Gershenwald JE, Berman RS, Porter G, et al. Regional nodal basin control is not compromised by previous sentinel lymph node biopsy in patients with melanoma. *Ann Surg Oncol.* 2000;7:226–231.
78. Gershenwald JE, Prieto VG, Colome-Grimmer MI, et al. The prognostic significance of microscopic tumor burden in 925 melanoma patients undergoing sentinel lymph node biopsy, in Perry MC, ed. *Proc Am Soc Clin Oncol.* New Orleans, LA, ASCO Publications; 2000: 551a.
79. Gershenwald JE, Prieto VG, Johnson MM, et al. *Heterogeneity of microscopic stage III melanoma in the SLN era: Implications for AJCC/UICC staging and future clinical trial*

design, 6th World Congress on Melanoma. Vancouver, BC, Canada, 2005.
80. Rossi CR, De Salvo GL, Bonandini E, et al. Factors predictive of nonsentinel lymph node involvement and clinical outcome in melanoma patients with metastatic sentinel lymph node. *Ann Surg Oncol.* 2008;15:1202–1210.
81. Satzger I, Volker B, Meier A, et al. Criteria in sentinel lymph nodes of melanoma patients that predict involvement of nonsentinel lymph nodes. *Ann Surg Oncol.* 2008;15:1723–1732.
82. Satzger I, Volker B, Meier A, et al. Prognostic significance of isolated HMB45 or Melan A positive cells in Melanoma sentinel lymph nodes. *Am J Surg Pathol.* 2007;31:1175–1180.
83. Scheri RP, Essner R, Turner RR, et al. Isolated tumor cells in the sentinel node affect long-term prognosis of patients with melanoma. *Ann Surg Oncol.* 2007;14:2861–2866.
84. Scolyer RA, Murali R, Gershenwald JE, et al. Clinical relevance of melanoma micrometastases in sentinel nodes: too early to tell. *Ann Oncol.* 2007;18:806–808.
85. van Akkooi AC, de Wilt JH, Verhoef C, et al. Clinical relevance of melanoma micrometastases (<0.1 mm) in sentinel nodes: are these nodes to be considered negative? *Ann Oncol.* 2006;17:1578–1585.
86. van Akkooi AC, Nowecki ZI, Voit C, et al. Sentinel node tumor burden according to the Rotterdam criteria is the most important prognostic factor for survival in melanoma patients: a multicenter study in 388 patients with positive sentinel nodes. *Ann Surg.* 2008;248:949–955.
87. Balch CM, Morton DL, Gershenwald JE, et al. Sentinel node biopsy and standard of care for melanoma. *J Am Acad Dermatol.* 2009;60:872–875.
88. Cascinelli N, Belli F, Santinami M, et al. Sentinel lymph node biopsy in cutaneous melanoma: the WHO Melanoma Program experience. *Ann Surg Oncol.* 2000;7:469–474.
89. Reeves ME, Delgado R, Busam KJ, et al. Prediction of nonsentinel lymph node status in melanoma. *Ann Surg Oncol.* 2003;10:27–31.
90. Sabel MS, Gibbs JF, Cheney R, et al. Evolution of sentinel lymph node biopsy for melanoma at a National Cancer Institute-designated cancer center. *Surgery.* 2000;128:556–563.
91. Starz H, Balda BR, Kramer KU, et al. A micromorphometry-based concept for routine classification of sentinel lymph node metastases and its clinical relevance for patients with melanoma. *Cancer.* 2001;91:2110–2121.
92. Thompson JF, McCarthy W, Bosch C. Sentinel lymph node status as an indicator of the presence of metastatic melanoma in regional lymph nodes. *Melanoma Res.* 1995;5:255–260.
93. Shaw HM, Thompson JF. Frequency of nonsentinel lymph node metastasis in melanoma. *Ann Surg Oncol.* 2002;9:934;author reply 934–935.
94. Gershenwald JE, Andtbacka RH, Prieto VG, et al. Microscopic tumor burden in sentinel lymph nodes predicts synchronous nonsentinel lymph node involvement in patients with melanoma. *J Clin Oncol.* 2008; 26:4296–4303.
95. Dewar DJ, Newell B, Green MA, et al. The microanatomic location of metastatic melanoma in sentinel lymph nodes predicts nonsentinel lymph node involvement. *J Clin Oncol.* 2004;22:3345–3349.
96. Elias N, Tanabe KK, Sober AJ, et al. Is completion lymphadenectomy after a positive sentinel lymph node biopsy for cutaneous melanoma always necessary? *Arch Surg.* 2004;139:400–404; discussion 404–405.
97. Govindarajan A, Ghazarian DM, McCready DR, et al. Histological features of melanoma sentinel lymph node metastases associated with status of the completion lymphadenectomy and rate of subsequent relapse. *Ann Surg Oncol.* 2007;14:906–912.
98. Koskivuo I, Talve L, Vihinen P, et al. Sentinel lymph node biopsy in cutaneous melanoma: a case-control study. *Ann Surg Oncol.* 2007;14:3566–3574.
99. Lee JH, Essner R, Torisu-Itakura H, et al. Factors predictive of tumor-positive nonsentinel lymph nodes after tumor-positive sentinel lymph node dissection for melanoma. *J Clin Oncol.* 2004;22:3677–3684.
100. McMasters KM, Wong SL, Edwards MJ, et al. Frequency of nonsentinel lymph node metastasis in melanoma. *Ann Surg Oncol.* 2002;9:137–141.
101. Page AJ, Carlson GW, Delman KA, et al. Prediction of nonsentinel lymph node involvement in patients with a positive sentinel lymph node in malignant melanoma. *Am Surg.* 2007;73:674–678; discussion 678–679.
102. Sabel MS, Griffith K, Sondak VK, et al. Predictors of nonsentinel lymph node positivity in patients with a positive sentinel node for melanoma. *J Am Coll Surg.* 2005;201:37–47.
103. Ballo MT, Garden AS, Myers JN, et al. Melanoma metastatic to cervical lymph nodes: can radiotherapy replace formal dissection after local excision of nodal disease? *Head Neck.* 2005;27:718–721.
104. Bonnen MD, Ballo MT, Myers JN, et al. Elective radiotherapy provides regional control for patients with cutaneous melanoma of the head and neck. *Cancer.* 2004;100:383–389.
105. Morton DL, Thompson JF, Cochran AJ, et al. Sentinel-node biopsy or nodal observation in melanoma. *N Engl J Med.* 2006;355:1307–1317.
106. Rousseau DL, Jr., Ross MI, Johnson MM, et al. Revised American Joint Committee on Cancer staging criteria accurately predict sentinel lymph node positivity in clinically node-negative melanoma patients. *Ann Surg Oncol.* 2003;10:569–574.
107. McMasters KM, Wong SL, Edwards MJ, et al. Factors that predict the presence of sentinel lymph node metastasis in patients with melanoma. *Surgery.* 2001;130:151–156.
108. Sondak VK, Taylor JM, Sabel MS, et al. Mitotic rate and younger age are predictors of sentinel lymph node positivity: lessons learned from the generation of a probabalistic model. *Ann Surg Oncol.* 2004;11:247–258.

109. Kruper LL, Spitz FR, Czerniecki BJ, et al. Predicting sentinel node status in AJCC stage I/II primary cutaneous melanoma. *Cancer.* 2006;107:2436–2445.
110. Paek SC, Griffith KA, Johnson TM, et al. The impact of factors beyond Breslow depth on predicting sentinel lymph node positivity in melanoma. *Cancer.* 2007;109:100–108.
111. Cochran AJ, Wen D, Morton D. Occult tumor cells in the lymph nodes of patients with pathological stage I malignant melanoma: an immunohistological study. *Am J Surg Pathol.* 1988;12:612–618.
112. van Akkooi AC, de Wilt JH, Verhoef C, et al. High positive sentinel node identification rate by EORTC melanoma group protocol. Prognostic indicators of metastatic patterns after sentinel node biopsy in melanoma. *Eur J Cancer.* 2006;42:372–380.
113. Yu LL, Flotte TJ, Tanabe KK, et al. Detection of microscopic melanoma metastases in sentinel lymph nodes. *Cancer.* 1999;86:617–627.
114. Baisden BL, Askin F, Lange J, et al. HMB-45 immunohistochemical staining of sentinel lymph nodes: a specific method for enhancing detection of micrometastases in patients with melanoma. *Am J Surg Pathol.* 2000;24:1140–1146.
115. Messina JL, Glass LF. Pathologic examination of the sentinel lymph node. *J Fla Med Assoc.* 1997;84:153–156.
116. Cochran AJ, RR H, J G, et al. Current practice and future directions in pathology and laboratory evaluation of the sentinel node. *Ann Surg Oncol.* 2001;8:13–17.
117. Clary BM, Lewis J, Brady M, et al. Should frozen section analysis of the sentinel node be performed in patients with melanoma? *Eur J Nucl Med.* 1999;26:S68.
118. Gibbs JF, Huang P, Zhang P, et al. Accuracy of pathologic techniques for the diagnosis of metastatic melanoma in sentinel lymph nodes. *Ann Surg Oncol.* 1999;6:699–704.
119. Koopal SA, Tiebosch AT, Albertus Piers D, et al. Frozen section analysis of sentinel lymph nodes in melanoma patients. *Cancer.* 2000;89:1720–1725.
120. Tanis PJ, Boom RP, Koops HS, et al. Frozen section investigation of the sentinel node in malignant melanoma and breast cancer. *Ann Surg Oncol.* 2001;8:222–226.
121. Scolyer RA, Thompson JF, McCarthy SW, et al: Intraoperative frozen-section evaluation can reduce accuracy of pathologic assessment of sentinel nodes in melanoma patients. *J Am Coll Surg.* 2005;201:821–823; author reply 823–824.
122. Ariyan S, Ariyan C, Farber LR, et al. Reliability of identification of 655 sentinel lymph nodes in 263 consecutive patients with malignant melanoma. *J Am Coll Surg.* 2004;198:924–932.
123. Goydos JS, Patel KN, Shih WJ, et al. Patterns of recurrence in patients with melanoma and histologically negative but RT-PCR-positive sentinel lymph nodes. *J Am Coll Surg.* 2003;196:196–204.
124. Goydos JS, Ravikumar TS, Germino FJ, et al. Minimally invasive staging of patients with melanoma: sentinel lymphadenectomy and detection of the melanoma-specific proteins MART-1 and tyrosinase by reverse transcriptase polymerase chain reaction. *J Am Coll Surg.* 1998;187:182–188; discussion 188–190.
125. Reintgen D, Albertini J, Berman C, et al. Accurate nodal staging of malignant melanoma. *Cancer Control.* 1995;2:405–414.
126. Ribuffo D, Gradilone A, Vonella M, et al. Prognostic significance of reverse transcriptase-polymerase chain reaction-negative sentinel nodes in malignant melanoma. *Ann Surg Oncol.* 2003;10:396–402.
127. Shivers SC, Wang X, Li W, et al. Molecular staging of malignant melanoma: correlation with clinical outcome. *JAMA.* 1998;280:1410–1415.
128. Wang X, Heller R, VanVoorhis N, et al. Detection of submicroscopic lymph node metastases with polymerase chain reaction in patients with malignant melanoma. *Ann Surg.* 1994;220:768–774.
129. Chapman PB. Detection of melanoma cells in sentinel lymph nodes by PCR is not yet ready for prime time. *Pigment Cell Res.* 2007;20:343–344.
130. Mocellin S, Hoon DS, Pilati P, et al. Sentinel lymph node molecular ultrastaging in patients with melanoma: a systematic review and meta-analysis of prognosis. *J Clin Oncol.* 2007;25:1588–1595.
131. Smith B, Selby P, Southgate J, et al. Detection of melanoma cells in peripheral blood by means of reverse transcriptase and polymerase chain reaction. *Lancet.* 1991;338:1227–1229.
132. Kammula U, Ghossein R, Bhattacharya S, et al. Serial follow-up and the prognostic significance of reverse transcriptase-polymerase chain reaction-staged sentinel lymph nodes from melanoma patients. *J Clin Oncol.* 2004;22:3989–3996.
133. Scoggins CR, Ross MI, Reintgen DS, et al. Prospective multi-institutional study of reverse transcriptase polymerase chain reaction for molecular staging of melanoma. *J Clin Oncol.* 2006;24:2849–2857.
134. Tatlidil C, Parkhill WS, Giacomantonio CA, et al. Detection of tyrosinase mRNA in the sentinel lymph nodes of melanoma patients is not a predictor of short-term disease recurrence. *Mod Pathol.* 2007;20:427–434.
135. Hoon DS, Wang Y, Dale PS, et al. Detection of occult melanoma cells in blood with a multiple-marker polymerase chain reaction assay. *J Clin Oncol.* 1995;13:2109–2116.
136. Takeuchi H, Morton DL, Kuo C, et al. Prognostic significance of molecular upstaging of paraffin-embedded sentinel lymph nodes in melanoma patients. *J Clin Oncol.* 2004;22:2671–2680.
137. Morton DL, Thompson JF, Cochran AJ, et al. *Sentinel node biopsy and immediate lymphadenectomy for occult metastases versus nodal observation and delayed lymphadenectomy for nodal recurrence: Fourth Interim Analysis*

of MSLT-I. SSO 63rd Annual Cancer Symposium. St. Louis, MO, 2010.
138. Morton DL, Cochran AJ, Thompson JF, et al. Sentinel node biopsy for early-stage melanoma: accuracy and morbidity in MSLT-I, an international multicenter trial. *Ann Surg.* 2005; 242:302–311; discussion 311–313.
139. Morton DL, Cochran AJ, Thompson JF. The rationale for sentinel-node biopsy in primary melanoma. *Nat Clin Pract Oncol.* 2008;5:510–511.
140. Ross MI, Gershenwald JE. How should we view the results of the Multicenter Selective Lymphadenectomy Trial-1 (MSLT-1)? *Ann Surg Oncol.* 2008;15:670–673.
141. Andtbacka RH, Gershenwald JE. The role of sentinel lymph node biopsy in patients with thin melanoma. *JNCCN.* In press.
142. Balch CM, Morton DL, Gershenwald JE, et al. Sentinel node biopsy and standard of care for melanoma. *J Am Acad Dermatol.* In press.
143. Bedrosian I, Faries MB, Guerry DT, et al. Incidence of sentinel node metastasis in patients with thin primary melanoma (<1 mm) with vertical growth phase. *Ann Surg Oncol.* 2000;7:262–267.
144. Clark WH, Jr., Elder DE, Guerry D, et al. Model predicting survival in stage I melanoma based on tumor progression. *J Nat Cancer Inst.* 1989;81:1893–1904.
145. Karakousis GC, Gimotty PA, Czerniecki BJ, et al. Regional nodal metastatic disease is the strongest predictor of survival in patients with thin vertical growth phase melanomas: a case for SLN Staging biopsy in these patients. *Ann Surg Oncol.* 2007;14:1596–1603.
146. Gershenwald J, Sumner W, Porter G. *Role of sentinel lymph node biopsy in patients with thin (<1 mm) cutaneous melanoma.* 53rd Annual Meeting of the Society of Surgical Oncology. New Orleans, LA, 2000.
147. Azzola MF, Shaw HM, Thompson JF, et al. Tumor mitotic rate is a more powerful prognostic indicator than ulceration in patients with primary cutaneous melanoma: an analysis of 3661 patients from a single center. *Cancer.* 2003;97:1488–1498.
148. Caudle AS, Ross MI, Prieto VG, et al. *Mitotic rate predicts sentinel lymph node involvement in melanoma: Impact of the 7th edition AJCC Melanoma Staging System*, SSO 63rd Annual Cancer Symposium. St. Louis, MO; 2010.
149. Shaw HM, McCarthy SW, McCarthy WH, et al. Thin regressing malignant melanoma: significance of concurrent regional lymph node metastases. *Histopathology.* 1989;15:257–265.
150. Kelly J, Sagebiel, RW, Blois, MS. Regression in malignant melanoma: a histologic feature without independent prognostic significance. *Cancer.* 1985;56:2287–2291.
151. McGovern V, Shaw, HM, Milton, GW. Prognosis in patients with thin malignant melanoma: influence of regression. *Histopathology.* 1983;7:673–680.
152. Paladugu R, Yonemoto, RH. Biologic behavior of thin malignant melanomas with regressive changes. *Arch Surg.* 1983;118:41–44,.
153. Gershenwald JE, Thompson JF, Warneke C, et al. *(Re)Defining indications for SLN biopsy in patients with thin melanoma—preliminary results of an international thin melanoma working group* [Abstr.]. 6th Biennial International Sentinel Node Society Meeting Sydney, Australia; 2008.
154. Morris KT, Busam KJ, Bero S, et al. Primary cutaneous melanoma with regression does not require a lower threshold for sentinel lymph node biopsy. *Ann Surg Oncol.* 2008;15:316–322.
155. Manganoni AM, Farisoglio C, Farfaglia R, et al. Regression in thin melanomas does not represent a risk factor for sentinel lymph node involvement. *Eur J Dermatol.* 2007;17:95–96.
156. Gannon CJ, Rousseau DL, Jr., Ross MI, et al. Accuracy of lymphatic mapping and sentinel lymph node biopsy after previous wide local excision in patients with primary melanoma. *Cancer.* 2006;107:2647–2652.
157. Ariyan S, Ali-Salaam P, Cheng DW, et al. Reliability of lymphatic mapping after wide local excision of cutaneous melanoma. *Ann Surg Oncol.* 2007;14:2377–2383.
158. Evans HL, Krag DN, Teates CD, et al. Lymphoscintigraphy and sentinel node biopsy accurately stage melanoma in patients presenting after wide local excision. *Ann Surg Oncol.* 2003;10:416–425.
159. Kelemen PR, Essner R, Foshag LJ, et al. Lymphatic mapping and sentinel lymphadenectomy after wide local excision of primary melanoma. *J Am Coll Surg.* 1999; 189:247–252.
160. Leong SP, Thelmo MC, Kim RP, et al. Delayed harvesting of sentinel lymph nodes after previous wide local excision of extremity melanoma. *Ann Surg Oncol.* 2003; 10:196–200.
161. Leong WL, Ghazarian DM, McCready DR. Previous wide local excision of primary melanoma is not a contraindication for sentinel lymph node biopsy of the trunk and extremity. *J Surg Oncol.* 2003;82:143–146.
162. McCready DR, Ghazarian DM, Hershkop MS, et al. Sentinel lymph-node biopsy after previous wide local excision for melanoma. *Can J Surg.* 2001;44:432–434.
163. Busam KJ. Cutaneous desmoplastic melanoma. *Adv Anat Pathol.* 2005;12:92–102.
164. Jaroszewski DE, Pockaj BA, DiCaudo DJ, et al. The clinical behavior of desmoplastic melanoma. *Am J Surg.* 2001;182:590–595.
165. Thelmo MC, Sagebiel RW, Treseler PA, et al. Evaluation of sentinel lymph node status in spindle cell melanomas. *J Am Acad Dermatol.* 2001;44:451–455.
166. Pawlik TM, Ross MI, Prieto VG, et al. Assessment of the role of sentinel lymph node biopsy for primary cutaneous desmoplastic melanoma. *Cancer.* 2006;106:900–906.
167. Beenken S, Byers R, Smith JL, et al. Desmoplastic melanoma. Histologic correlation with behavior and treatment. *Arch Otolaryngol Head Neck Surg.* 1989;115:374–379.
168. Carlson JA, Dickersin GR, Sober AJ, et al. Desmoplastic neurotropic melanoma: a clinicopathologic analysis of 28 cases. *Cancer.* 1995;75:478–494.

169. Devaraj VS, Moss AL, Briggs JC. Desmoplastic melanoma: a clinico-pathological review. *Br J Plast Surg.* 1992;45:595–598.
170. Egbert B, Kempson R, Sagebiel R. Desmoplastic malignant melanoma. A clinicohistopathologic study of 25 cases. *Cancer.* 1988;62:2033–2041.
171. Payne WG, Kearney R, Wells K, et al. Desmoplastic melanoma. *Am Surg.* 2001;67:1004–1006.
172. Quinn MJ, Crotty KA, Thompson JF, et al. Desmoplastic and desmoplastic neurotropic melanoma: experience with 280 patients. *Cancer.* 1998;83:1128–1135.
173. Reed RJ, Leonard DD. Neurotropic melanoma. A variant of desmoplastic melanoma. *Am J Surg Pathol.* 1979;3: 301–311.
174. Smithers BM, McLeod GR, Little JH. Desmoplastic melanoma: patterns of recurrence. *World J Surg.* 1992; 16:186–190.
175. Su LD, Fullen DR, Lowe L, et al. Desmoplastic and neurotropic melanoma. *Cancer.* 2004;100:598–604.
176. Scolyer RA, Thompson JF. Desmoplastic melanoma: a heterogeneous entity in which subclassification as "pure" or "mixed" may have important prognostic significance. *Ann Surg Oncol.* 2005;12:197–199.
177. Hawkins WG, Busam KJ, Ben-Porat L, et al. Desmoplastic melanoma: a pathologically and clinically distinct form of cutaneous melanoma. *Ann Surg Oncol.* 2005;12:207–213.
178. Choi EA, Gershenwald JE. Imaging studies in patients with melanoma. *Surg Oncol Clin North Am.* 2007;16: 403–430.
179. Aloia TA, Gershenwald JE, Andtbacka RH, et al. Utility of computed tomography and magnetic resonance imaging staging before completion lymphadenectomy in patients with sentinel lymph node-positive melanoma. *J Clin Oncol.* 2006;24:2858–2865.
180. Gold JS, Jaques DP, Busam KJ, et al. Yield and predictors of radiologic studies for identifying distant metastases in melanoma patients with a positive sentinel lymph node biopsy. *Ann Surg Oncol.* 2007;14:2133–2140.
181. Voit C, Van Akkooi AC, Schafer-Hesterberg G, et al. Ultrasound morphology criteria predict metastatic disease of the sentinel nodes in patients with melanoma. *J Clin Oncol.* 2010;28:847–852.
182. Sanki A, Uren RF, Moncrieff M, et al. Targeted high-resolution ultrasound is not an effective substitute for sentinel lymph node biopsy in patients with primary cutaneous melanoma. *J Clin Oncol.* 2009;27:5614–5619.
183. Sumner WE, Ross MI, Mansfield PF, et al. Implications of lymphatic drainage to unusual sentinel lymph node sites in patients with primary cutaneous melanoma. *Cancer.* 2002;95:354–360.
184. Uren RF, Howman-Giles R, Thompson JF. Lymphatic drainage from the skin of the back to retroperitoneal and paravertebral lymph nodes in melanoma patients. *Ann Surg Oncol.* 1998;5:384–387.
185. Uren RF, Howman-Giles R, Thompson JF, et al. Interval nodes: the forgotten sentinel nodes in patients with melanoma. *Arch Surg.* 2000;135:1168–1172.
186. Uren RF, Howman-Giles R, Thompson JF, et al. Lymphatic drainage to triangular intermuscular space lymph nodes in melanoma on the back. *J Nuc Med.* 1996;37: 964–966.
187. Uren RF, Howman-Giles R, Thompson JF. Patterns of lymphatic drainage from the skin in patients with melanoma. *J Nuc Med.* 2003;44:570–582.
188. Uren RF, Thompson J, Howman-Giles R. Sentinel nodes, interval nodes, lymphatic lakes, and accurate sentinel node identification. *Clin Nucl Med.* 2000;25:234–236.
189. Essner R, Foshag L, Morton D. *Intraoperative radiolymphoscintigraphy: A useful adjunct to intraoperative lymphatic mapping and selective lymphadenectomy in patients with clinical stage 1 melanoma* [Abstr]. 47th Annual Cancer Symposium, Society of Surgical Oncology Houston, TX; 1994.
190. Uren RF. SPECT/CT Lymphoscintigraphy to locate the sentinel lymph node in patients with melanoma. *Ann Surg Oncol.* 2009;16:1459–1460.
191. Reynolds HM, Smith NP, Uren RF, et al. Three-dimensional visualization of skin lymphatic drainage patterns of the head and neck. *Head Neck.* 2009;31:1316–1325.
192. Norman J, Cruse CW, Espinosa C, et al. Redefinition of cutaneous lymphatic drainage with the use of lymphoscintigraphy for malignant melanoma. *Am J Surg.* 1991; 162:432–437.
193. Meyer CM, Lecklitner ML, Logic JR, et al. Technetium-99m sulfur-colloid cutaneous lymphoscintigraphy in the management of truncal melanoma. *Radiology.* 1979;131: 205–209.
194. Soo V, Shen P, Pichardo R, et al. Intraoperative evaluation of sentinel lymph nodes for metastatic melanoma by imprint cytology. *Ann Surg Oncol.* 2007;14:1612–1617.
195. Aloia TA, Gershenwald JE. Management of early-stage cutaneous melanoma. *Curr Probl Surg.* 2005;42:460–534.
196. Loree TR, Tomljanovich PI, Cheney RT, et al. Intraparotid sentinel lymph node biopsy for head and neck melanoma. *Laryngoscope.* 2006;116:1461–1464.
197. Picon AI, Coit DG, Shaha AR, et al. Sentinel lymph node biopsy for cutaneous head and neck melanoma: mapping the parotid gland. *Ann Surg Oncol.* 2006 [epub ahead of print].
198. Rayatt SS, Hettiaratchy SP, Key A, et al. Psychosocial benefits of sentinel lymph node biopsy in the management of cutaneous malignant melanoma. *Br J Plast Surg.* 2002;55:95–99.
199. Wrightson WR, Wong SL, Edwards MJ, et al:. Complications associated with sentinel lymph node biopsy for melanoma. *Ann Surg Oncol.* 2003;10:676–680.
200. Blumenthal R, Banic A, Brand C, et al. Morbidity and outcome after sentinel lymph node dissection in patients with early-stage malignant cutaneous melanoma. *Swiss Surg.* 2002;8:209–214.

201. Golshan M, Martin W, Dowlatshahi K. Sentinel lymph node biopsy lowers the rate of lymphedema when compared with standard axillary lymph node dissection. *Am Surg.* 2003;69:209–211.
202. Schijven MP, Vingerhoets AJ, Rutten HJ, et al. Comparison of morbidity between axillary lymph node dissection and sentinel node biopsy. *Eur J Surg Oncol.* 2003; 29:341–350.
203. Pawlik TM, Ross MI, Johnson MM, et al. Predictors and natural history of in-transit melanoma after sentinel lymphadenectomy. *Ann Surg Oncol.* 2005;12:587–596.
204. van Poll D, Thompson JF, Colman MH, et al. A sentinel node biopsy does not increase the incidence of in-transit metastasis in patients with primary cutaneous melanoma. *Ann Surg Oncol.* 2005;12:597–608.
205. Pawlik TM, Ross MI, Thompson JF, et al. The risk of in-transit melanoma metastasis depends on tumor biology and not the surgical approach to regional lymph nodes. *J Clin Oncol.* 2005;23:4588–4590.
206. Guggenheim MM, Hug U, Jung FJ, et al. Morbidity and recurrence after completion lymph node dissection following sentinel lymph node biopsy in cutaneous malignant melanoma. *Ann Surg.* 2008;247:687–693.
207. Kretschmer L, Thoms KM, Peeters S, et al. Postoperative morbidity of lymph node excision for cutaneous melanoma-sentinel lymphonodectomy versus complete regional lymph node dissection. *Melanoma Res.* 2008; 18:16–21.
208. Estourgie SH, Nieweg OE, Valdes Olmos RA, et al. Review and evaluation of sentinel node procedures in 250 melanoma patients with a median follow-up of 6 years. *Ann Surg Oncol.* 2003;10:681–688.
209. Kang JC, Wanek LA, Essner R, et al. Sentinel lymphadenectomy does not increase the incidence of in-transit metastases in primary melanoma. *J Clin Oncol.* 2005;23: 4764–4770.
210. Daley MD, Norman PH, Leak JA, et al. Adverse events associated with the intraoperative injection of isosulfan blue. *J Clin Anesth.* 2004;16:332–341.
211. Ballo MT, Ang KK. Radiation therapy for malignant melanoma. *Surg Clin North Am.* 2003;83:323–342.
212. Stevens G, McKay MJ. Dispelling the myths surrounding radiotherapy for treatment of cutaneous melanoma. *Lancet Oncol.* 2006;7:575–583.
213. Ang KK, Peters LJ, Weber RS, et al. Postoperative radiotherapy for cutaneous melanoma of the head and neck region. *Int J Radiat Oncol Biol Phys.* 1994;30:795–798.
214. Moncrieff MD, Martin R, O'Brien CJ, et al. Adjuvant postoperative radiotherapy to the cervical lymph nodes in cutaneous melanoma: is there any benefit for high-risk patients? *Ann Surg Oncol.* 2008;15:3022–3027.
215. Burmeister B, Henderson M, Thompson J, et al. *Adjuvant radiotherapy improves regional (lymph node field) control in melanoma patients after lymphadenectomy: Results of an intergroup randomized trial (TROG 02.01/ANZMTG 01.02).* 51st Annual Meeting of the American Society for Radiation Oncology. Chicago, IL, Elsevier, Inc; 2009:S2.
216. Mendenhall WM, Amdur RJ, Grobmyer SR, et al. Adjuvant radiotherapy for cutaneous melanoma. *Cancer.* 2008;112:1189–1196.

26

REGIONAL MANAGEMENT OF MELANOMA IN THE CLINICALLY NODE-POSITIVE NECK

JESUS E. MEDINA

Introduction

At the present time, surgery is the mainstay of treatment of patients with melanoma of the head and neck with clinically obvious lymph node metastases. The surgeon dealing with this clinical situation faces a number of questions to which the answers are still evolving. Such questions concern the extent of an appropriate diagnostic evaluation, the various prognostic implications of the presence of nodal metastases, the extent of an appropriate regional node dissection, and the role and indications for adjuvant local and systemic therapy. In this chapter, we endeavor to provide up-to-date information regarding these issues.

Diagnostic Evaluation

The rationale for a metastatic workup in patients with palpable lymph node metastases from melanoma is that the majority of them develop distant metastases in the future, suggesting that occult disease is present at the time regional disease is treated. Timely detection of distant metastatic disease could spare patients the morbidity and expense of an unnecessary lymph node dissection. The yield of computerized tomography (CT) scans in detecting unsuspected metastatic disease in patients with regional melanoma metastasis is low (7 to 15.8%); furthermore, the rate of false positive findings often equals or exceeds that of true positive findings.[1–3]

The use of PET scanning in this clinical setting has been studied by several investigators. Findings on PET scans led to a change in the planned clinical management in 15% of cases in a study by Tyler et al,[4] and in 22% in a study by Damian et al.[5] A recent prospective study by Brady et al[6] was designed to evaluate whether whole-body PET scanning in addition to standard preoperative imaging (CT scan with contrast of the chest, abdomen, and pelvis) would change management in high-risk melanoma patients. A cohort of 103 patients diagnosed with preoperative stage IIC, III, or IV disease were enrolled. Clinical or radiographic follow-up evaluation, within 4 to 6 months of the imaging studies, was used to determine the accuracy of preoperative PET and CT findings. The aim of this study was not to compare preoperative CT with PET scan, but to test the hypothesis that PET in addition to CT increases detection of occult metastatic disease. They found that PET scan in addition to standard CT was more effective than either modality alone and resulted in a change in management, most often from surgical to nonsurgical treatment, in 35% of the patients. Other studies have shown PET-CT to be superior to PET alone.[7]

PET scanning in addition to CT scanning is useful in the preoperative diagnostic evaluation of melanoma patients with clinically obvious lymph node metastases, as they are at high risk for occult systemic metastases. Obviously, a potential downside of this approach to the diagnostic evaluation is the additional cost; however, this would be easily surpassed by the cost, financial and otherwise, of futile operations.

Prognosis of the Clinically Node-Positive Neck

It is well known that patients with melanoma of the head and neck and histologically positive nodes have a worse prognosis than patients with localized disease.[8] Survival rates at 10 years are less than 30% in most series.[9–11] In these patients, there is a high correlation between the development of a recurrence in the nodal basin, distant metastasis, and survival.[12,13] Regional recurrence rates after neck dissection for positive lymph nodes are as high as 28%.[12,14] The development of a regional recurrence following therapeutic lymph node dissection portends a grave prognosis; survival rates are extremely low and distant metastases occur in almost all patients.[15–17] In a study by Fisher,[11] once a regional recurrence developed the probability of death within 2 years was 50%. Thus, the identification of risk factors for the development of regional recurrence is important in terms of prognosis for survival. It also is important to guide decisions about adjuvant therapy.

Importance of Lymph Node Tumor Burden

The metastatic tumor burden in the lymph nodes is an important determinant of prognosis. Lymph node metastases can be classified as "micrometastases," which are not detectable by clinical examination but are detected pathologically, or "macrometastases," which are evident clinically and confirmed pathologically. In the American Joint Committee on Cancer (AJCC) Database analysis, survival (calculated from the onset of primary melanoma diagnosis) was significantly higher for patients who present with micrometastases. Consequently, these patients are included in a separate staging subgroup, pathological stage IIIA (Table 26–1).

Characteristics of the primary melanoma such as tumor thickness, the presence or absence of ulceration, and increased mitotic rate are significant predictors of outcome in patients with localized disease (stages I and II) and in patients with nodal micrometastases (stage IIIA). However, they do not influence outcome in patients with macrometastases in the lymph nodes (stages IIIB and IIIC).[9,17,18]

The two most significant risk factors in patients with macrometastases from melanoma are the number of nodes harboring metastases and the presence or absence of satellites and in-transit metastases[18,19] Determination of the number of nodes involved and of the extent of the metastatic tumor in each lymph node is done more accurately through histopathologic examination of a lymphadenectomy specimen than with clinical examination or imaging studies. The Melanoma Staging Committee of the AJCC has shown that this information is essential for the identification of distinctive prognostic subgroups among patients with pathologically proven metastases (pathologic stage III).[18]

Number of Involved Nodes

The influence of the number of lymph nodes involved on the prognosis of melanoma patients has been evaluated extensively for melanomas of different sites including the head and neck.[12,17,20,21] An analysis of 17,600 patients in the AJCC Melanoma Database showed a strong correlation of 10-year survival with the number of nodes involved by metastatic tumor. From this analysis it was determined that the threshold for the N3 category should be at least 4 nodes involved.[19] Therefore, in the 2009 AJCC Staging, patients with one node involved by metastasis are categorized as N1, those with 2 to 3 nodes involved as N2 and those with 4 or more nodes involved (or matted nodes) as N3.[18]

Table 26–1. Stage III Melanoma: Clinical and Pathologic Staging

Anatomic Stage/Prognostic Groups								
Clinical Staging				**Pathologic Staging**				
III	Any T	≥N1	M0	**IIIA**	T1–4a	N1a	M0	
					T1–4a	N2a	M0	
				IIIB	T1–4b T1–4b	N1a N2a	M0 M0	1–3 **microscopic** lymph node metastases and an ulcerated primary melanoma
					T1–4a T1–4a	N1b N2b	M0 M0	1–3 **"macroscopic"** lymph node metastases and a nonulcerated primary melanoma
					T1–4a	N2c	M0	Satellites/in transit metastases without lymph node metastases
				IIIC	T1–4b T1–4b	N1b N2b	M0 M0	1–3 **"macroscopic"** lymph node metastases and an ulcerated primary melanoma
					T1–4b	N2c	M0	Satellites/in transit from ulcerated primary melanoma
					Any T	N3	M0	>4 nodes, matted nodes, satellite/in-transit with nodes

Source: Used with the permission of the American Joint Committee on Cancer (AJCC), Chicago, Ilinois. The original source for this material is the AJCC Cancer Staging Manual, Seventh Edition (2010) published by Springer Science and Business Media LLC, www.springer.com.

Satellitosis and In-Transit Metastases

Clinically obvious or microscopic satellites around a primary melanoma or in-transit metastases between the primary and the regional lymph node basin represent intralymphatic metastases and are associated with a poor prognosis.[22–25] In a study by Singletary et al,[17] in-transit metastases occurred in 12 of 287 patients after neck dissection for melanoma. Only 31% of these patients survived 2 years, and none survived 5 years. The primary melanoma was located in the face and scalp in most cases. Nine of these patients had multiple nodes involved, and seven had concomitant recurrence in cervical nodes. In the study by Calabro et al,[12] only 12% of patients with in-transit metastases after node dissection for melanoma at all body sites survived 5 years. Others have reported similar dismal survival rates for these patients.[17,19,26] The finding of satellite or in-transit metastases without metastases in the lymph nodes places the patient in stage IIIB, for which the 5-year survival ranges between 46% and 59%. On the other hand, if lymph node metastases are found in combination with satellites or in-transit metastases, the patient is categorized as stage IIIC, and the 5-year survival rate is significantly lower (26%).[22]

Staging of Regional Disease

The Melanoma Staging Committee has accounted for these prognostic factors in the 7th edition of the AJCC Staging Manual.[18] The resulting staging subgroupings for stage III melanoma are outlined in

Table 26–1. The corresponding survival rates are shown in Table 26–2. Patients with "macroscopic," palpable lymph node metastases are highlighted within pathologic stages IIIB and IIIC. As shown in detail in Table 26–2, pathologic stage IIIB is comprised of three groups of patients: those with 1 to 3 microscopic lymph node metastases and an ulcerated primary melanoma, those with 1 to 3 macroscopic metastatic nodes and a nonulcerated primary melanoma, and those with satellite or in-transit metastases, but no evidence of nodal or distant metastases. The estimated 5- and 10-year survival for stage IIIB patients in the analysis of the 2009 AJCC Melanoma Database is 59% and 43%, respectively.[18] Pathologic stage IIIC includes patients with 1 to 3 "macroscopic" lymph node metastases and an ulcerated primary melanoma, patients with satellite/in-transit metastases arising from an ulcerated primary melanoma, or any patient with N3 disease (4 or more nodes with metastases, or matted nodes, or satellite/in-transit metastases with lymph node metastases). The estimated 5- and 10-year survival rates for pathologic stage IIIC patients are significantly lower at 40% and 24%, respectively.[18]

Unknown Primary Melanoma

The site of the primary melanoma in the head and neck does not have a significant influence on the length of survival in patients with clinical stage III disease. However, in the study by Singletary et al,[17] patients with cervical lymph node metastases and an "unknown primary" site had significantly better length of survival (median 90 months) when compared with patients with primary melanomas of the scalp, face, ear and skin of the neck (median 14 to 19 months). Other investigators also have reported better outcomes for patients with "unknown primary" melanomas, with 5- and 10-year survival rates of 55% and 47%, respectively.[12,27,28]

Table 26–2. Ten-Year Survival Rates for Stage III Melanoma Substages (2008 AJCC Melanoma Staging Database)

Pathologic Stage	*N*	Survival
IIIA	1,196	68%
IIIB (including N2c)	1,391	43%
IIIB (excluding N2c)	992	38%
IIIC	720	24%

Source: Used with the permission of the American Joint Committee on Cancer (AJCC), Chicago, Ilinois. The original source for this material is the AJCC Cancer Staging Manual, Seventh Edition (2010) published by Springer Science and Business media LLC, www.springer.com.

Extent of the Regional Node Dissection

The goals of a therapeutic lymphadenectomy are to remove the lymph nodes obviously involved, as well as the lymph nodes at risk of containing metastatic tumor, and to do so with the least functional disability and cosmetic deformity. The extent of a therapeutic lymph node dissection in patients with melanomas of the head and neck is determined by the location of the primary melanoma, the location of the lymph node or nodes involved, and the extent of the tumor in the lymph nodes.

Location of the Primary Melanoma

The distribution of lymph node metastases varies with the location of the primary melanoma and can be predicted on clinical grounds in over 90% of the cases.[29] Knowledge of this distribution is helpful in determining the lymph node groups that are at risk and need to be removed, in addition to the nodes that are obviously involved by tumor. Shah et al[30] studied the distribution of lymph node metastases from cutaneous melanomas of the head and neck in 80 patients who underwent therapeutic lymphadenectomy and had histologically proven cervical metastasis. The location of the primary melanoma was listed as ear, face, anterior scalp, posterior scalp, anterior neck, and posterior neck. Lymph nodes in levels II, III, and IV were involved in melanomas of all sites, with a frequency ranging between 16% and 65%. Lymph nodes in level I, on the other hand, were involved in only 6% of the patients with melanomas of the posterior neck and scalp, and level V nodes were involved in only 12% of melanomas of the anterior scalp.

Byers[31] studied 181 patients treated with modified neck dissection for suspected or proven metastatic melanoma. Although he does not present the data, he states that the nodal groups most commonly involved in patients with melanomas of the scalp, located anterior to an imaginary line through the tragus, are the intraparotid and level II nodes; in melanomas of the scalp, posterior to the tragal line, the suboccipital and posterior cervical nodes (level V); in melanomas of the ear, the preauricular and parotid nodes; and in melanomas of the nose and anterior aspect of the face and neck, the submaxillary triangle (level I) and the jugular chain nodes (levels II–IV). Pathak et al[29] reviewed a "prospectively documented" series of 169 patients with melanomas of the head and neck and pathologically proven lymph node metastases. The aims of this study were to correlate the anatomic distribution of pathologically involved lymph nodes with the site of the primary melanoma and to compare these findings with clinically predicted patterns of metastatic spread. They found that primary tumors of the forehead metastasized to the parotid gland or neck levels I to III in 94% of the cases. Primary melanomas of the upper face also metastasized to the parotid and levels I to III in 91% of the cases. Melanomas that arose on a coronal band of the scalp equal to the width of the pinna had metastases to the parotid nodes or neck levels I to V in 85% of the cases. Patients with posterior scalp melanomas were predicted to have metastases in the suboccipital and levels II through V nodes, and this occurred in 89% of cases. Finally, 84% of patients with lower posterior neck melanomas had metastatic disease in suboccipital and levels II to V nodes. Another pertinent observation in this study was that only one lymph node was involved by tumor in 59% of the patients undergoing therapeutic lymphadenectomy, and that the lymph node group closest to the primary site was involved in 68% of the patients.

A conclusion that can be drawn from these studies is that performing a comprehensive neck dissection is the safest practice in patients with melanomas of all sites in the head and neck who undergo a therapeutic lymphadenectomy. This obviously is a sound practice, especially when there are palpable nodes in multiple levels of the neck. However, the detailed analysis presented here suggests that, for melanomas in certain locations, it may not be necessary to include all nodal levels in the dissection, especially in the presence of minimal clinical disease, namely, single palpable node. The lymph nodes in level I do not need to be removed in the majority of patients with melanomas of the posterior neck and scalp. Conversely, dissection of level V nodes may not be necessary in patients with primary melanomas of the face and anterior scalp.

In melanomas of the ear, face, and anterior scalp with palpable metastases in the neck, the risk of metastases in the parotid lymph nodes is high; therefore, an appropriate therapeutic lymphadenectomy in these cases should include a superficial parotidectomy with preservation of the facial nerve, unless the nerve was impaired preoperatively. Similarly, intra-operative findings may dictate the need to either resect the facial nerve or any of its branches, or to extend the resection to the deep lobe of the parotid if it appears involved.[30,32,33]

The Extent of the Tumor in the Lymph Nodes

Metastases from melanoma in lymph nodes are peculiar. Byers[31] has pointed out very aptly that "nodes containing metastatic melanoma rarely invade contiguous structures regardless of their size." They tend to expand in a "pushing" manner that is somewhat similar to the way in which metastases from papillary thyroid cancer grow. Consequently, it often is possible to remove these nodes adequately and preserve adjacent structures of the neck that are important for function or appearance, such as the spinal accessory nerve, the internal jugular vein, or the sternocleidomastoid muscle. This is the primary objective of the modified radical and selective neck dissections. To optimize oncologic results with these operations, it is important for the clinician to select patients properly and to perform the operation with careful attention to technical detail; it also is important to have a working understanding of the limitations of these operations and of the rationale for their combined use with adjuvant radiation therapy.

In 1986, Byers[31] reviewed retrospectively a cohort of 181 patients with melanoma of the head and neck whose actual or suspected nodal metastases were treated with a "modified neck dissection" only. All the dissections preserved the spinal accessory nerve and many preserved the internal jugular vein and the sternocleidomastoid muscle as well. In 48 patients, the dissection was therapeutic. The results in this group showed two interesting findings. First, in 42% of these patients the lymph nodes were found to be negative on pathologic examination. Second, even though these modifications of the neck dissection were performed by a group of surgeons "familiar with and expert in the surgical technique," the rate of recurrence in the neck at 5 years was 50%. Not surprisingly, the survival rate at 5 years was 37.5%. Conversely, the corresponding rates of recurrence and survival in the patients with negative lymph nodes were 5% and 70%.

Since this report was published, others have reported similar high recurrence rates in patients who were treated with radical neck dissections. Van de Vrie et al[34] reported a study comparing the results in 14 patients who underwent a therapeutic radical neck dissection (RND) with 9 patients who underwent modified radical neck dissection (MRND). The number of nodes positive pathologically, the percent of positive nodes, and the timing of the neck dissection were similar in both groups. The recurrence rate was 43% in the RND group and 44% in the MRND. The survival rate at 3 years was 35% in both groups.

Others have reported lower recurrence rates. Belli et al[35] studied 93 patients with palpable cervical lymph node metastases from melanomas of the head and neck. They underwent various types of neck dissection in a nonrandomized manner. An RND was performed in 35 patients, an MRND in 44, and a selective neck dissection (SND) in 14 patients. With an average follow-up of 7.3 years, the rates of recurrence in the neck were 11% in the RND group, 9% in the MRND, and 14% in the SND group. Subsequently, O'Brien et al[33]reported results of therapeutic neck dissections in 75 melanoma patients. The rate of recurrence in the neck at 2 years was 14% in patients who had a RND; all the patients who developed a recurrence had multiple positive nodes, and none received postoperative radiotherapy. There were no recurrences among 18 patients who underwent MRND; some of these patients received postoperative radiation therapy and some did not. All but one of these patients had only one node involved by tumor. The rate of recurrence after SND was 18%. All the patients with recurrence had only one positive node and none of them received postoperative radiation.

In 2005, Grünhagen et al[32] studied 66 consecutive patients who underwent cervical lymph node dissection for metastases from melanoma; 20 of them had a RND or an MRND and 46 had SND. The report does not specify the type of SND. It indicates, however, that the selective procedures were performed depending on the predicted or actual pattern of lymphatic drainage as established by lymphoscintigraphy. Unfortunately, the study included patients with micrometastases detected by SLNB and patients in whom the neck node metastases were not the first or only recurrent disease (3 patients had previous recurrences in the axilla or groin from melanomas in the trunk or extremities, 11 patients had previous local recurrence of the primary tumor or in-transit metastases). Furthermore, an unspecified number of patients in each group received postoperative radiation, immunotherapy, or both. Nevertheless, the results of their analysis showed that the extent of the cervical lymph node dissection, that is, RND/MRND or SND, had no influence on the overall recurrence-free survival or overall survival.

In 2009, Hamming-Vrieze et al[36] reviewed 64 cases of cutaneous melanoma with neck node metastasis. Twenty-four patients were treated with surgery only and 40 patients were treated with surgery and adjuvant postoperative radiation to the entire ipsilateral side of the neck. Surgery consisted of a modified radical neck dissection (lymph node levels I–V) or a selective neck dissection (lymph node levels I–III, II–V, or IV–V) depending on the location of the primary tumor. An MRND was performed in cases with involvement of multiple nodes. Adjuvant radiation was administered postoperatively to patients with demonstrated extracapsular extension of tumor, nodes larger than 3 cm in diameter, or 2 or more positive nodes. In the group treated with surgery alone, SND was associated with a trend toward a worse regional recurrence rate compared with the MRND, but the difference was not statistically significant in univariate analysis ($p = .08$). The type of neck dissection did not influence the regional recurrence rate in the group treated with surgery and postoperative radiation ($p = .60$).

What can be surmised from all these observations is that the extent of the tumor in the lymph nodes determines the appropriate lymphadenectomy. When involvement of multiple nodes and of nodes in multiple levels of the neck is apparent clinically, or discovered intraoperatively, a comprehensive dissection of all nodal levels involved is the most appropriate lymphadenectomy. On the other hand, a SND, sparing nodal levels at minimal risk of containing metastases, is appropriate when the metastases are limited to a single node or nodal level. In both instances, the extent of the tumor in each lymph node involved, in terms of its relationship to surrounding structures, will determine whether or not it is appropriate to preserve adjacent structures that are important for function and appearance.

The Location of the Palpable Nodes

The presence of palpable lymph node metastases in the parotid in patients with cutaneous melanomas of the head and neck creates a therapeutic dilemma: should the neck be dissected, and if so, how extensive should the neck dissection be? A study reported by O'Brien et al[37] provides useful information to guide these decisions. The aim of this study was to determine the incidence and distribution of cervical lymph node metastases in patients with clinically obvious metastases in parotid nodes, and to determine if treatment of the clinically negative neck is warranted in such patients. Among 50 patients with metastatic melanoma involving the parotid gland, 19 patients had clinically positive nodes in the neck (38%), and in all of them metastatic tumor was confirmed pathologically. The nodes in level II were involved most frequently in these patients; however, positive nodes were found in all levels of the neck. The neck nodes were deemed negative clinically in 31 patients, and 26 of them had an elective neck dissection. In 7 of these 26 patients (27%), pathologic examination demonstrated metastases in cervical lymph nodes. The nodes that were positive pathologically were confined to levels I, II, and III.

From these observations it appears that, for patients with clinically obvious metastases in the parotid, a therapeutic lymphadenectomy should consist of an appropriate parotidectomy and a comprehensive neck dissection (I–V) when there are metastases in the neck that are obvious clinically, or a selective neck dissection (I-III) when the neck is negative clinically (Fig 26–1). The extent of the parotidectomy depends on the extent of the metastatic tumor and its relationship to the facial nerve. Caldwell and Spiro[38] reported the experience of the group at Memorial Sloan Kettering with patients who underwent parotidectomy for metastases from melanoma

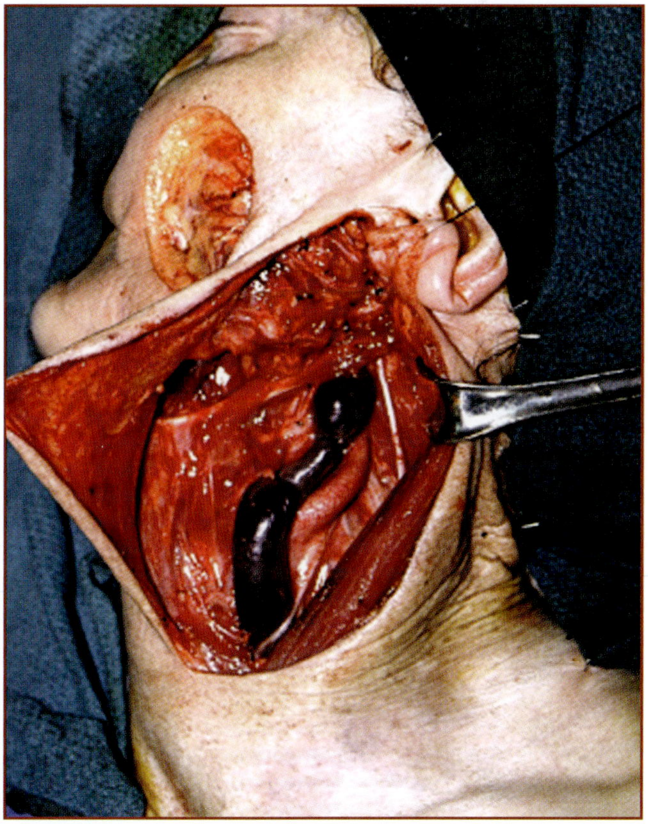

Figure 26–1. Parotidectomy and selective neck dissection of levels I–III in a patient with a melanoma of the cheek with a single palpable metastases in the parotid, without palpable metastases in the neck.

confirmed pathologically. A total parotidectomy was necessary in 14% of the patients, and a portion of the facial nerve was removed in 34% of patients. This information should be taken into consideration when counseling patients preoperatively.

Melanomas of the posterior scalp, posterior-superior aspect of the neck, and postauricular region metastasize primarily to the retroauricular and suboccipital lymph nodes, which are not included in the standard neck dissections. These nodes drain primarily into the spinal accessory nodes and secondarily into the upper jugular nodes. Therefore, a therapeutic lymphadenectomy for melanomas in these locations requires a distinct operation that has been named "posterolateral neck dissection" (Fig 26–2). This type of neck dissection was initially described by Rochlin in 1962.[39] It consists of the removal of the suboccipital and retroauricular nodes in addition to the nodes in level II–V. The main variations in surgical technique described in the literature concern the handling of the splenius capitis muscle. Some surgeons describe lymph nodes deep to the upper portion of this muscle, along the deep portion of the occipital artery, and advocate resecting it to ensure their removal.[40,41] Most surgeons, however, do not include the splenius in the resection and carry the dissection in a plane immediately superficial to this muscle.[39,42–44] Otherwise, depending on the location and extent of the nodal metastases in the neck, it often is possible to preserve the spinal accessory nerve, the internal jugular vein, and sometimes the sternocleidomastoid muscle.[44]

Adjuvant Radiation Therapy

Radiation therapy in various hypofractionated regimens has been proposed as a useful adjunct in the treatment of patients with lymph node metastases from melanomas of the head and neck. Although the effectiveness of postoperative radiation in metastatic head and neck melanoma was questioned by a large retrospective study published in 2008,[45] the results of a recent prospective, randomized trial indicate that postoperative radiation is effective in reducing the risk of regional recurrence after therapeutic lymphadenectomy.[46]

In 1990, Ang et al[47] from the MD Anderson Cancer Center reported a 2-year actuarial locoregional control rate of 85% among 48 patients with head and neck melanoma and palpable lymph node metastases, who were treated with limited neck dissection and adjuvant radiation therapy.

O'Brien et al[48] in 1997 reported, from the Sidney Melanoma Unit, a nonrandomized, prospectively documented series of 143 patients with histologically positive nodes in the neck or parotid. A total of 152 necks or parotids were dissected. Of these, 45 received postoperative irradiation and 107 were not irradiated. Radiotherapy consisted of 6 × 5.5-Gy fractions administered over 3 weeks. The regional recurrence rate was 6.5% in the irradiated group and 18.7% in the nonirradiated group (p = .055). This difference did not reach statistical significance, but the authors felt that it represented a clear beneficial trend, especially as the irradiated group had more extensive nodal involvement.

In 2003, Ballo et al[21] retrospectively reviewed the MD Anderson experience with 160 patients with cervical lymph node metastases from malignant melanoma treated with surgery and irradiation. One hundred forty-eight of these patients presented with clinically palpable nodes. Ninety of them had SND and 35 had local excision of the neck mass. Only 35 patients underwent dissection of all 5 node levels (RND or MRND). At a median follow-up of 78 months, actuarial local, regional, and locoregional control rates were 94%, 94%, and 91%, respectively. Actuarial disease-specific, disease-free, and distant metastasis-free survival rates at 10 years were 48, 42, and 43%, respectively. Complications for all patients were rare and manageable when they occurred. The authors recommended adjuvant irradiation for patients with extracapsular extension, lymph nodes 3 cm or larger in size, multiple lymph nodes, recurrent disease, or any patient having undergone a therapeutic SND.

Unfortunately, a recent, large retrospective study from the Sidney Melanoma Unit found "no evidence to support the use of adjuvant radiotherapy for "high-risk" melanoma patients."[45] This study analyzed 716 patients from a large prospective database who underwent cervical lymph node surgery between 1990 and 2004. Patients deemed high risk for regional recurrence were offered radiotherapy ($n = 129$).

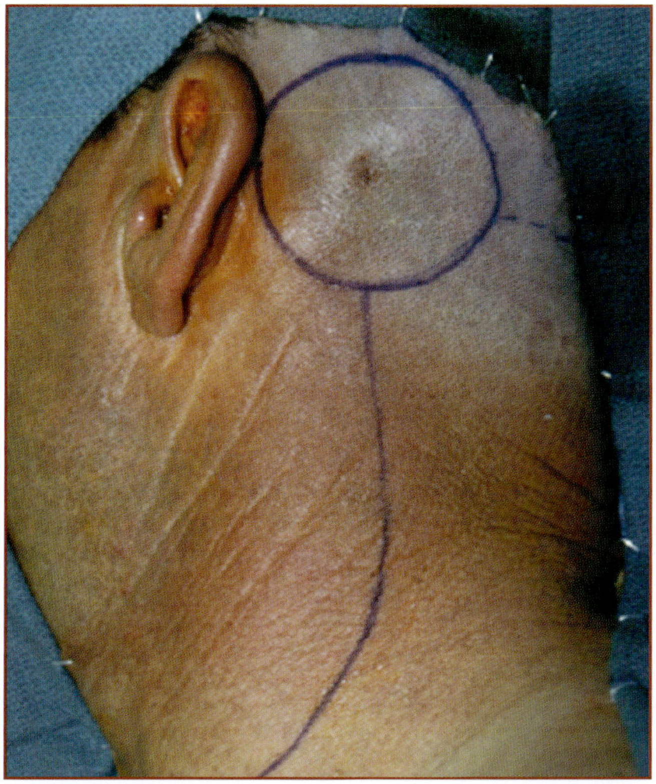

A

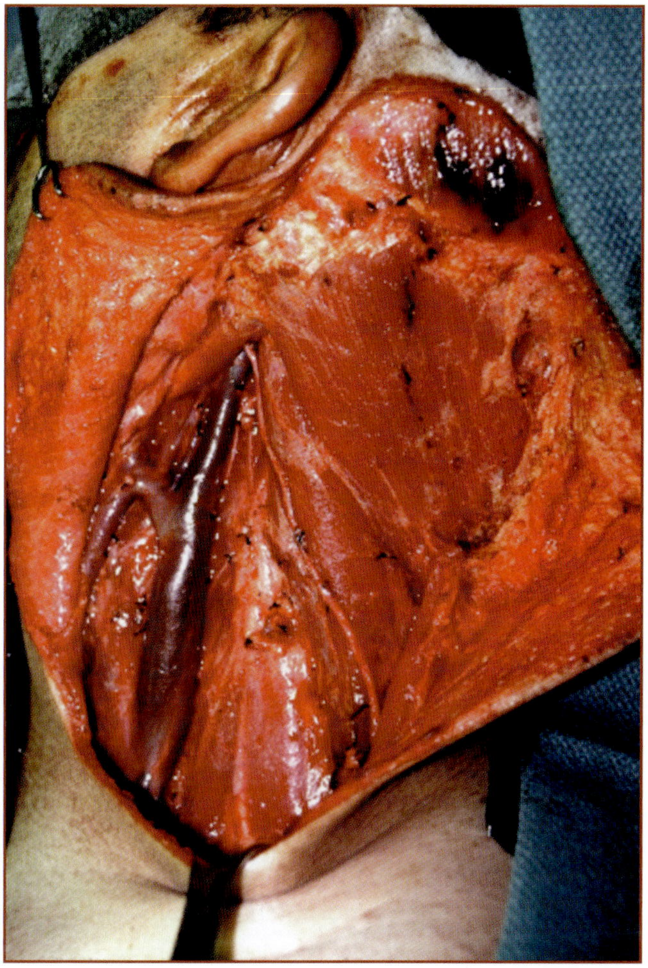

B

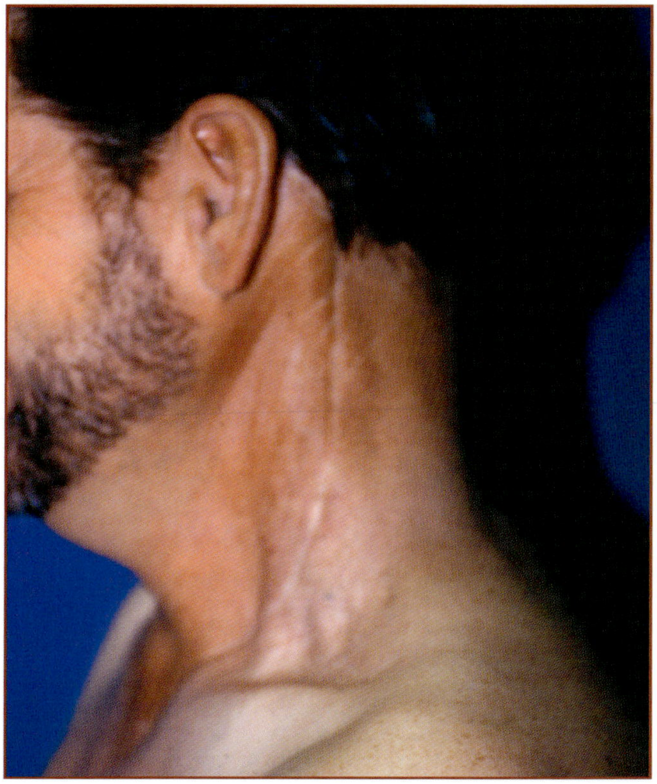

C

Figure 26–2. **A.** Melanoma in the posterior lateral aspect of the scalp. Outlined are the incision to excise the primary tumor and to perform a posterolateral neck dissection. **B.** Intraoperative photograph showing the completed posterolateral neck dissection with preservation of the spinal accessory nerve and the internal jugular vein. **C.** Patient several months after the operation.

High-risk patients exhibited extracapsular spread, parotid involvement, more than two involved nodes, or an individual node of larger than 3 cm in maximum diameter, regardless of total number of nodes involved. This group was compared with the group of patients who did not receive radiotherapy ($n = 587$) in the same period. The radiotherapy regimens varied through the years of the study, but the median radiotherapy dose administered was 33 Gy (range: 30–60 Gy), most often as a hypofractionated regimen with 5.5 Gy provided twice weekly for 3 weeks. Radiotherapy did not improve regional control in patients who had metastatic melanoma of the cervical lymph nodes ($p = 0.2$). There were 10% fewer regional recurrences in patients with extracapsular spread who received adjuvant radiotherapy, although this was not statistically significant. As would be expected, adjuvant radiotherapy conferred no overall survival benefit to patients with nodal metastases.

This controversy may be settled by the results of a prospective, randomized trial conducted in Queensland, Australia by Burmeister et al.[46] The results were presented at the annual meeting of the American Society for Radiation Oncology (ASTRO) in November of 2009. The trial included 217 patients who had complete resection of nodal metastatic melanoma and were randomized to adjuvant radiotherapy ($n = 109$) and observation ($n = 108$). The risk for recurrence in the nodal basin was considered "significant" if there were at least 1 positive parotid or 2 positive neck or axillary nodes, and 3 positive groin nodes, maximum lymph node size (30 mm or greater for parotid, neck, and axilla; 40 mm or greater for groin) and extranodal spread of tumor. The external-beam radiotherapy after lymphadenectomy consisted of 48 Gy in 20 fractions over 4 weeks. With a median follow-up of 27 months, patients treated with radiation after surgery had a statistically significant lower risk of regional recurrence than patients who did not receive radiation (19% vs 31%).

In summary, postoperative irradiation is useful in decreasing regional recurrence in melanoma patients with multiple positive nodes or extracapsular spread of tumor. Some studies suggest that it also is useful to improve results of therapeutic SNDs. However, the performance of an SND is not by itself an indication for postoperative radiation. That decision should be based on the characteristics of the tumor in the lymph nodes.

Adjuvant Chemotherapy and Immunotherapy

The high rates of distant metastasis with poor survival in stage III melanoma, compared to stages I and II, implies that the majority of patients with lymph node metastasis have subclinical distant metastasis. This observation has led to the presumption that adjuvant chemotherapy and/or immunotherapy may be of benefit by eliminating or suppressing the growth of these microscopic metastatic deposits. This has led to trials of various agents for adjuvant treatment after resection of advanced melanoma. This topic is discussed in greater detail in Chapter 27 of this text.

Biochemotherapy and Targeted Molecular Therapy

Controlled trials have produced no compelling evidence to support the value of combination chemotherapy in patients with metastatic melanoma. Similarly, the results reported to date from randomized trials using biochemotherapy do not justify its use routinely outside of a clinical trial. The intrinsic resistance of melanoma to conventional chemotherapy has led investigators to evaluate new approaches such as combinations with protein kinase inhibitors (eg, sorafenib), agents that act on cytotoxic T-lymphocyte antigen 4 (CTLA-4) or on apoptotic mechanisms (eg, oblimersen sodium, previously referred to as G3139), and antiangiogenic agents (eg, bevacizumab, SU5416, MEDI-522, PI-88). The authors of a recently published comprehensive review of the topic conclude that a discouragingly long list of targeted agents have been tested in melanoma patients and have failed.[49] New targeted therapies are urgently needed.

Interferon

Interferons are glycoproteins that have multiple biological effects including stimulation of host immune response (natural killer cells) and direct antiprolifer-

37. O'Brien CJ, McNeil EB, McMahon JD, Pathak I, Lauer CS. Incidence of cervical node involvement in metastatic cutaneous malignancy involving the parotid gland. *Head Neck.* 2001;23:744–748.
38. Caldwell CB, Spiro RH. The role of parotidectomy in the treatment of cutaneous head and neck melanoma. *Am J Surg.* 1988;156:318–322.
39. Rochlin DB. Posterolateral neck dissection for malignant neoplasms. *Surg Gynecol Obstet.* 1962;115:369–373.
40. Wander JV, Chaudhuri PK. Dissection of the posterior part of the neck. *Surg Gynecol Obstet.* 1976;143:97–100.
41. Fisher SR, Cole TB, Seigler HF. Application of posterior neck dissection in treating malignant melanoma of the posterior scalp. *Laryngoscope.* 1983;93:760–765.
42. Goepfert H, Jesse RH, Ballantyne AJ. Posterolateral neck dissection. *Arch Otolaryngol.* 1980;106:618–620.
43. de Langen ZJ, Vermey A. Posterolateral neck dissection. *Head Neck Surg.* 1988;10:252–256.
44. Medina JE. Posterolateral neck dissection. *Oper Techn Otolaryngol Head Neck Surg..* 2004;15(3):176–179.
45. Moncrief M, Martin R, O'Brien C, Shannon K, Clark J, et al. Adjuvant postoperative radiotherapy to the cervical lymph nodes in cutaneous melanoma. Is there any benefit for high risk patients? *Ann Surg Oncol.* 2008; 15(11):3022–3027.
46. Burmeister B. In nodal metastatic melanoma, radiation may be new standard of care [Abstract]. From a presentation made at the American Society for Radiation Oncology (ASTRO) Annual Meeting held on 11-3-2009. http://www.medscape.com/viewarticle/711723. Retrieved 11-3-2009. Abstract.
47. Ang KK, Byers RM, Peters LJ, et al. Regional radiotherapy as adjuvant treatment for head and neck malignant melanoma. Preliminary results. *Arch Otolaryngol Head Neck Surg.* 1990;116:169–172.
48. O'Brien CJ, Petersen-Schaefer K, Stevens GN, et al. Adjuvant radiotherapy following neck dissection and parotidectomy for metastatic malignant melanoma. *Head Neck.* 1919;(7):589–594.
49. Gogas HJ, Kirkwood JM, Sondak VK. Chemotherapy for metastatic melanoma. Time for a change? *Cancer.* 2007; 109:455–464.
50. Creagan ET, Schaid DJ, Akmann DL, Frytak S. Recombinant interferons in the management of advanced malignant melanoma. Updated review of five prospective clinical trials and long-term responders. *Am J Clin Oncol.* 1988;11:652–659.
51. Kirkwood JM, Ernstoff M. Potential applications of the interferons in oncology: lessons drawn from studies of human melanoma. *Semin Oncol.* 1986;13(suppl 2): 48–56.
52. Kirkwood JM, Ernstoff MS. Cutaneous melanoma. In: Devita VT, Hellman S, Rosenberg SA, eds. *Biologic Therapy of Cancer.* Philadelphia, PA: JB Lippincott; 1991:311.
53. Verma S, Quirt I, McCready D, Bak K, Charette M, Iscoe N. Systematic review of systemic adjuvant therapy for patients at high risk for recurrent melanoma. *Cancer.* 2006;106:1431–1442.
54. Fecher L, Flaherty K. Where are we with adjuvant therapy of stage III and IV melanoma in 2009? *J Natl Comprehens Cancer Network.* 2009;7(3):295–304.

27

ROLE OF CHEMOTHERAPY, BIOCHEMOTHERAPY, AND TARGETED SYSTEMIC THERAPIES IN THE TREATMENT OF METASTATIC MELANOMA

SAPNA P. PATEL
RICHARD W. JOSEPH
KEVIN B. KIM

Introduction

Melanoma is the most aggressive form of skin cancer. An estimated 68,720 cases of melanoma were diagnosed in the United States in 2009, and approximately 8,650 patients died of this disease.[1] Despite a high 5-year survival rate for patients with a diagnosis of malignant melanoma, patients with metastatic melanoma generally have an extremely poor prognosis, with a median survival duration of 6 to 10 months and a 5-year survival rate of less than 5%.[2,3] This poor outlook reflects the fact that the current treatment for metastatic melanoma is not effective for the majority of patients. However, a small subset of patients treated with systemic therapy have significantly prolonged survival and a long duration of disease control.

The mainstays of systemic therapy for metastatic melanoma are cytotoxic chemotherapy and immunotherapy. However, many patients so treated have a low chance of durable tumor control and/or significant side effects from the drugs. Recent advances in our understanding of the molecular pathogenesis of melanoma will likely allow us to develop better personalized therapies based on the genomic aberration of a patient's tumor. This chapter reviews current systemic therapeutic options for metastatic melanomas, including cytotoxic chemotherapeutic drugs, immunotherapeutic agents, and emerging data on targeted therapeutic drugs.

Adjuvant Systemic Therapy

Over the last few decades, researchers have made a great attempt to find an effective systemic therapy to use in an adjuvant setting for patients at high risk for melanoma recurrence. The regimens tested in a randomized clinical trial include cytotoxic drugs, immunotherapy such as Bacille Calmette-Guérin (BCG), levamisole and interferon-gamma (IFN-γ), and various types of vaccines. Unfortunately, these randomized studies all failed to show a meaningful advantage in overall survival (OS) over observation only, except in the case of high-dose interferon-alpha (IFN-α).[4,5]

The largest vaccine study to date was conducted to test the clinical efficacy of CancerVax in a randomized trial setting.[6] CancerVax is a cellular-based vaccine consisting of irradiated cells from three human melanoma cell lines, and this vaccine was administered with BCG as an immunologic adjuvant. Beginning in 1984, CancerVax was initially studied in a Phase II setting and the results suggested a superior median relapse-free survival (RFS) and median OS duration compared with matched controls who did not receive the vaccine.[7] A Phase III study examined CancerVax plus BCG adjuvant compared with placebo plus BCG in patients with completely resected stage III and IV melanoma.[6] This study was terminated early due to lack of benefit in the treatment arm but did demonstrate a high 5-year OS rate (40%) of stage IV patients, suggesting resection of metastatic disease itself could prolong survival.[6]

Granulocyte macrophage-colony stimulating factor (GM-CSF) is a growth factor with multiple known functions that affect the immune system. In vitro, GM-CSF stimulates monocytes to become cytotoxic toward human melanoma cells and is a key factor in promoting dendritic cell maturation and allowing these dendritic cells to more effectively activate T cells.[8–10] In vivo, GM-CSF has been shown to increase the functional capacity of monocytes and increases production of matrix metalloelastase by tumor-infiltrating macrophages, rendering them more capable of cellular toxicity.[11,12] Given the previous rationale, a Phase II trial tested GM-CSF in 48 patients with stage III and IV melanoma who had been rendered free of disease after surgery.[13] GM-CSF was given every 28 days until disease progression, and the median OS was 37.5 months compared with 12.2 months for matched historical controls.[13] To follow up on these results, Eastern Cooperative Oncology Group (ECOG) 4397 (a randomized Phase III trial) has been launched. Until the results of this large, randomized study re available, not enough evidence exists to recommend GM-CSF as a treatment for melanoma, and its use should therefore be reserved for clinical trials.

Interferon-alpha

IFN-α is a natural protein synthesized mainly by cells of the immune system to mount a response to infection. Melanoma has long been known to be an immunogenic tumor, and therefore the goal of many investigators has been to globally stimulate the immune system to rid the body of tumor. Although some patients with melanoma do respond to IFN-α, the response mechanism is likely mediated through manipulation of the host's immune system toward the tumor rather than by IFN-α's direct toxicity to the tumor.[14,15]

By the early 1980s, it had been established that IFN-α had a modest effect in shrinking tumors in patients with metastatic melanoma.[16] Studies were then initiated to test IFN-α in the adjuvant setting in patients with high-risk melanoma. Multiple different regimens of IFN-α doses, durations of treatment, and formulations of the drug have been studied.

In the initial randomized Phase III trial comparing the OS duration of high-dose IFN-α with observation (ECOG1684),[5] 287 patients with ≥4-mm thick primary melanoma or regional nodal metastases were randomized after the complete lymphadenectomy to receive either a high dose of IFN-α or no treatment.[5] The dosage of IFN-α was 20 million U per m^2 5 days per week via intravenous infusion for 4 weeks followed by a maintenance dose of 10 million units per m^2 subcutaneously three times weekly for 48 weeks. With a mean follow-up duration of 6.9 years, the mean RFS was 1.72 years in the IFN-α group versus 0.98 years in the observation group ($p = 0.0023$). Furthermore, there was a greater OS advantage for the IFN-α group than for the observation group (3.82 years versus 2.78 years, $p = 0.0237$). An estimated 5-year OS rate was 46% versus 37%, favoring the IFN-α group. Based on the improved RFS and OS duration observed in this study, the United States Food and Drug Administration (FDA) approved the use of IFN-α in an adjuvant setting in patients with ≥4-mm thick primary melanoma or regional nodal metastases.

However, a larger follow-up Phase III study compared the survival durations of patients in a high-dose IFN-α group, a low-dose IFN-α group, and an observation group in a similar patient population (except for the requirement of the complete lymphadenectomy in the previous study) (ECOG 1690)[17] and revealed no OS advantage of either high-dose or low-dose IFN-α over observation alone, although the RFS in the high-dose IFN-α group was superior to that in the observation group. In addition, after a longer follow-up duration of 12.9 years, the ECOG 1684 study failed to show an improvement in OS, although the improvement in RFS remained significant.[18] Furthermore, a meta-analysis of 12 randomized studies evaluating the benefit of IFN-α in the adjuvant setting showed an improvement in RFS duration but not in OS duration.[19] Despite conflicting survival data, a high-dose IFN-α regimen remains the only standard therapy in patients with a high risk for melanoma recurrence.

Recently, the Hellenic Collaborative Oncology Group tested whether the 11 months of maintenance IFN-α is necessary; the group randomly assigned 353 patients to either 1 month of a modified high-dose IFN-α regimen (15 million units per m^2 intravenous infusion 5 days a week for 4 weeks) or 1 year of IFN-α regimen (15 million units per m^2 intravenous infusion 5 days a week for 4 weeks, followed by 10 million units given in a subcutaneous injection three times a week for 48 weeks).[20] This trial demonstrated no significant difference in median PFS between the treatments (24.1 months in 1-month arm versus 27.9 months in 1-year arm, $p = 0.9$). However, this was an equivalency study with the assumption that a difference in the median RFS rates of less than 15% at 3 years is clinically equivalent. This difference of up to 15% in the median RFS rate can be clinically meaningful and moreover, this study was underpowered to detect a clinically significant difference in OS rate. A large Phase III study (ECOG 1697) is currently under way to compare the survival durations of patients receiving 4 weeks of induction IFN-α therapy at 20 million units per m^2 5 days per week via intravenous infusion with those of patients receiving no treatment and aims to answer the question of whether the 48 weeks of maintenance IFN-α is necessary.

A number of randomized studies have been conducted to compare the clinical benefit of low-dose IFN-α with the benefit of observation,[21–24] but the study results clearly indicate that the low-dose IFN-α is not useful in an adjuvant setting in patients with melanoma.

IFN-α is associated with often-severe toxicities in the majority of patients undergoing therapy. The most common toxicities include fatigue, fever, myelosuppression, nausea, vomiting, increased serum transaminases, and depression.[25] Most of the toxicities can be managed with supportive care (eg, use of acetaminophen and/or antidepressant) or an appropriate IFN-α dose reduction, and the majority of side effects are reversible with cessation of the drug. Investigators studied the effect of health-related quality of life (HRQOL) in the EORTC 18991 study and found an expected global negative effect on HRQOL in the patients receiving IFN-α.[26] To maximize the benefit of therapy and minimize unnecessary exposure of patients to IFN-α, many groups are trying to identify molecular or clinical predictors of who is most likely to benefit from adjuvant IFN-α. Until these reliable predictors are available, clinicians and patients are advised to make an individualized decision based on likelihood of disease recurrence and comorbidities of the patient.

Chemotherapeutic Treatment for Metastatic Melanoma

Cytotoxic Chemotherapy

For more than three decades, different cytotoxic chemotherapeutic drugs have been studied for use in patients with metastatic melanoma. Many clinical trials have been conducted to evaluate the clinical efficacy of a single drug or a combination of cytotoxic drugs. Although early studies with small numbers of patients with metastatic melanoma showed promising clinical response rates to chemotherapy, larger randomized studies failed to demonstrate meaningful or superior clinical benefit of one cytotoxic regimen over another.[27] To date, the only cytotoxic agent approved by the FDA is dacarbazine, and this drug has remained the standard against which other newer drugs or combination drug regimens are tested in clinical studies. Other commonly used chemotherapy drugs include alkylating agents (temozolomide), platinum analogs (cisplatin, carboplatin), vinca alkaloids (vinblastine, vincristine, vindesine), taxanes (paclitaxel, docetaxel), and nitrosoureas (lomustine, carmustine).

Alkylating Agents

Dacarbazine

In 1975, the FDA approved dacarbazine (5-[3.3-dimethyl-1-triazenyl]-imidazole-4-carboxamide; DTIC) for use in the treatment of patients with metastatic melanoma. As a single agent, dacarbazine is administered intravenously at either 850 to 1,000 mg per m^2 for 1 day or at 250 mg per m^2 for 5 days, every 3 weeks. A meta-analysis of the clinical activity of dacarbazine monotherapy from 23 randomized clinical trials found an average overall response rate of 15.3%.[28] The majority of the responses were partial responses with less than 5% complete response rates. Dacarbazine has been evaluated in several combination studies as the comparison arm with historical response rates of 12% to 20%, but OS with dacarbazine has never been compared with best supportive care in a randomized trial. The combinations of dacarbazine with additional chemotherapy, immunotherapy with interferon, or hormonal therapy with tamoxifen, however, have failed to improve survival.[27,29–31] Although dacarbazine is generally accepted as the standard therapy for patients with metastatic melanoma, many oncologists consider dacarbazine to be suboptimal therapy for this population. Unfortunately, no other therapy has been shown to have a survival advantage over dacarbazine. Common adverse events to dacarbazine are modest myelosuppression and fatigue. The availability of effective antiemetic drugs has allowed for manageable administration of dacarbazine in an outpatient regimen.

Temozolomide

Temozolomide was developed as a prodrug of dacarbazine. Temozolomide has several advantages over dacarbazine, including 100% oral bioavailability and spontaneous conversion to the active metabolite 3-methyl-[triazen-1-yl]-imidazole-4-carboxamide (MTIC) at physiologic pH. In contrast, dacarbazine requires hepatic N-demethylation for activation, which can be less than optimal in patients with hepatic dysfunction. In addition, temozolomide is able to cross the blood-brain barrier in measurable concentrations. This property of temozolomide has a potential advantage in patients with metastatic melanoma, two thirds of whom demonstrate central nervous system metastases.[32–36]

A head-to-head trial of temozolomide versus dacarbazine was published in 2000, nearly 25 years after the approval of dacarbazine for treatment of metastatic melanoma.[30] In this randomized Phase III study, 156 patients with surgically incurable or unresectable advanced melanoma were randomized to oral temozolomide (200 mg/m^2 daily for 5 days every 28 days), and 149 patients were randomized to intravenous dacarbazine (250 mg/m^2 daily for 5 days, repeating every 21 days). The primary objective of this comparison trial was the measurement of OS with the secondary objective including response rates and quality of life measures. The response rate for temozolomide, including complete responses and partial responses, was 13.5%, and the response rate for dacarbazine was 12.1%; OS was 7.7 months for temozolomide and 6.4 months for dacarbazine ($p = 0.20$). Although the difference in OS was not statistically significant, many oncologists and patients alike have interpreted this data to favor treatment with temozolomide, given its ease of administration, its favorable pharmacokinetics, and a potential antitumor activity in the central nervous system.

The oral administration of temozolomide has facilitated investigation of various dosing schedules. Continuous daily dosing has resulted in increased peripheral blood concentrations in pharmacokinetic assessments.[37] These prolonged schedules have been shown to diminish activity of peripheral blood O^6-methylguanine-DNA methyltransferase (MGMT), an enzyme that leads to tumor resistance by increasing cellular DNA repair capacity.[38] Based on this rationale, a randomized Phase III study in metastatic melanoma patients was conducted to compare temozolomide on an alternating weekly dosing schedule (150 mg/m^2 daily for 1 week, followed by 1 week of rest, repeated every 2 weeks) with dacarbazine.[39] However, in this study, no statistically significant advantage of temozolomide over dacarbazine was seen using this dosing schedule. Therefore, dacarbazine still remains the standard treatment for patients with advanced melanoma.

Platinum Analogs

Platinum analogs inhibit replication and transcription of DNA by crosslinking nucleic acids to trigger apoptosis. Cisplatin and carboplatin have been widely studied for the treatment of metastatic melanoma, mostly in combination regimens. As single agents, both cisplatin and carboplatin demonstrate only modest clinical activity. In several early trials, cisplatin exhibited response rates of 10% to 15% when used as monotherapy, including a complete response rate of 3% in doses ranging from 20 to 100 mg per m^2 every 21 to 28 days.[40,41] In Phase II studies of carboplatin at a dose of 400 mg/m^2 in patients with both untreated and previously treated advanced melanoma, response rates ranged from 11% to 19%, with complete responses reported in 2% to 7% of patients.[42–44]

Both agents have been studied further in various combinations with traditional cytotoxic chemotherapy, immunotherapy, and targeted therapy; however, the combination strategy has not been shown to be significantly superior to single-agent dacarbazine. These two platinum agents with similar mechanisms of action but differing toxicity profiles were even studied in combination in dacarbazine-refractory patients with metastatic melanoma.[45] In this small, prospective study, investigators demonstrated a 26% response rate with the combination of cisplatin and carboplatin.

Taxanes

Taxanes (cytotoxic plant hydrocarbons) are inhibitors of mitosis and specifically interfere with microtubule disassembly. The two commonly studied taxanes in melanoma are paclitaxel and docetaxel, and these taxanes have a modest antitumor activity against this refractory disease. Based on promising Phase I data[46] two Phase II studies of paclitaxel in patients with metastatic melanoma were published in the early 1990s and reported overall response rates of 12% to 14% when administered at 250 mg per m^2 as a 24-hour continuous intravenous infusion every 3 weeks.[47,48] Of 53 patients evaluable in these two studies, 3 patients had a complete response, 2 of which had durable responses lasting more than 2 years.[47,48]

Docetaxel has clinical activity similar to paclitaxel. In Phase II clinical trials of docetaxel administered at 100 mg per m^2 intravenously every 21 days, complete responses were rare and occurred in less than 3% of patients, and partial responses were reported at a rate of 2% to 17%.[49–51] Both paclitaxel and docetaxel are well tolerated at these doses; however, because clinical benefit is limited as a single agent, they are frequently combined with other cytotoxic drugs in an attempt to improve clinical responses.

Taxanes are known to induce rare hypersensitivity reactions that manifest as an urticarial rash and shortness of breath and can rapidly progress to shock. These reactions usually take place within the first half hour of infusion and primarily occur during the first or second exposure to the drug. However, reactions have been reported with later infusions, regardless of previous toxicity. Hypersensitivity is related to the solubilizers used with paclitaxel and docetaxel known as Cremophor EL and Tween 80, respectively. An albumin-bound nanoparticle form of paclitaxel (Abraxane; Abraxis BioScience, LLC, Bridgewater, NJ) utilizes "nab" technology to allow a higher concentration of paclitaxel for binding and avoid the need for Cremophor EL. In a Phase II study, this nab-paclitaxel had promising results; among 34 chemotherapy naïve patients with metastatic melanoma, the reported response rate was 27%.[52] Currently, a large Phase III randomized study comparing the clinical activities of nab-paclitaxel and dacarbazine is underway in patients with metastatic malignant melanoma.

Vinca Alkaloids

Vinca alkaloids (such as vinblastine, vincristine, and vindesine) are antimitotic or antimicrotubule agents derived from the common periwinkle plant. Vinca alkaloids inhibit cancer cell growth and induce cell death by interfering with microtubule formation, unlike taxanes, which interfere with microtubule disassembly. Vinca alkaloids exhibit antitumor activity in patients with metastatic melanoma, but the response rate is 12% to 30% and complete responses are rare.[53–57] Vinblastine also has been evaluated using differing dosing schedules, including a study evaluating protracted continuous infusion dosing, with no significant improvement in response rates but with more notable bone marrow suppression.[58] However, of the vinca alkaloids, vinorelbine appears to have the least clinical activity.[59–60] In two separate studies evaluating the clinical activity of vinorelbine in patients who have and have not received chemotherapy, no clinical response was observed.[59–60] Vinca alkaloids are mostly used in combination therapy owing to their minimal efficacy as single agents.

Nitrosoureas

Nitrosoureas are DNA alkylators and include carmustine (BCNU), lomustine (CCNU), and fotemustine. These agents exhibit clinical activity similar to dacarbazine as a single agent, with overall response rates of 13% to 18% in patients with advanced melanoma,[57,61,62] Nitrosoureas cross the blood-brain barrier and have been used alone or in combination with radiation to treat melanoma patients who have metastatic central nervous system disease, but nitrosoureas do not appear to confer meaningful clinical benefit to these patients.[63–65] In one study, radiation plus fotemustine or dacarbazine incurred a 50% response rate, four of which were complete responses.[66] These numbers have been difficult to duplicate, and patients treated with this combination rarely achieve durable remissions longer than 6 months. The most frequent adverse events associated with nitrosoureas are bone marrow suppression with neutropenia and thrombocytopenia.

Tamoxifen

Tamoxifen is an antiestrogen used primarily in hormone receptor-positive solid tumors such as breast cancer and ovarian cancer. In the 1970s, estrogen receptors were also discovered on melanoma cells.[67] This discovery prompted clinical investigation using tamoxifen to treat malignant melanoma in both adjuvant and metastatic settings. As a single agent, tamoxifen has had disappointing response rates around 10%.[68–71] Consequently, most use of tamoxifen has been in combination with cytotoxic chemotherapy and/or immunotherapy such as interleukin-2 (IL-2) or IFN-α. Among several randomized trials which compared the clinical efficacy of cytotoxic drug(s) with or without tamoxifen[72,73] all showed a lack of a survival benefit of adding tamoxifen, except one study by Cocconi and colleagues,[74] which showed a statistically significant survival benefit in dacarbazine/tamoxifen regimen over dacarbazine alone, especially in women.

The most notable of these combinations was the Dartmouth regimen, which consists of dacarbazine, cisplatin, carmustine, and tamoxifen.[62] When compared head-to-head with single-agent dacarbazine in a randomized Phase III study using patients with metastatic disease, no significant advantage in response rate (18.5% of Dartmouth regimen versus 10.5% of dacarbazine, $p = 0.09$) or median OS duration (7.7 months [95% CI, 6.3 to 8.9] of Dartmouth regimen versus 6.3 months [95% CI, 5.4 to 8.7] of dacarbazine) was seen using the Dartmouth regimen.[62] Tamoxifen has fallen out of mainstream use for melanoma patients.

Combination Chemotherapy

As discussed above, single-agent chemotherapy produces dismal response rates and rarely produces complete responses. To overcome this poor clinical efficacy, combinations of cytotoxic drugs with different mechanisms of action have been utilized in an attempt to improve response rates and ultimately prolong disease control.

Dacarbazine has been combined with cisplatin and vinblastine based on their independent clinical activity. This regimen, known as CVD, was evaluated in a prospective single-center study of metastatic melanoma patients and demonstrated a response rate that was double what had been seen with single-agent chemotherapy at 40%.[75] Additionally, the clinical responses were durable, with a 9-month median duration of response. However, in a randomized phase III study, the CVD regimen did not improve overall survival compared with dacarbazine alone.[76] As described above, the randomized phase III study of the Dartmouth regimen (a combination of dacarbazine, cisplatin, carmustine, and tamoxifen) is another example which showed no meaningful survival advantage of a combination regimen over dacarbazine alone.[62]

Despite the lack of survival benefit, these regimens have been regarded widely as palliative treatment options with a manageable toxicity for the treatment of advanced melanoma because of the superior response rate and a favorable safety profile. For patients with brain metastases or who are at high risk of developing central nervous system disease, temozolomide often has been substituted for dacarbazine to expose the meninges to effective doses of chemotherapy.

Several different combinations of cytotoxic agents have been studied in the last decade.[27] In a Phase II study, temozolomide in combination with docetaxel was shown to have a response rate of 27% with a median response duration of 9.5 months.[77] Recently, this doublet was studied with the addition of cisplatin in a Phase I study setting and demonstrated a response rate of 32% in patients who were either chemo naïve or previously treated.[78]

A number of Phase II studies have examined the clinical efficacy of the combination of carboplatin and paclitaxel in patients with metastatic melanoma.[79–81] The response rates for these studies have varied from less than 10% to 26%.[79–81] A recent randomized Phase III study that compared the efficacy of carboplatin-paclitaxel-sorafenib with that of carboplatin-paclitaxel-placebo concluded that there was no clinical benefit from the addition of sorafenib to combination carboplatin-paclitaxel, which had a response rate of 11% in a second-line treatment setting.[82] Although the response rate was only modest, the median progression-free survival (PFS) duration was nearly 18 weeks, which was longer than initially anticipated.[82] With a reasonably good tolerance, this combination of carboplatin and paclitaxel has become a popular regimen. However, these recently developed combination regimens of cytotoxic drugs have not been tested in a randomized fashion against dacarbazine.

Biochemotherapy

The use of chemotherapy with immunologic modifiers for metastatic disease became popular in the mid-1990s and has been referred to as biochemotherapy or immunochemotherapy. In 1999, a combination regimen using tamoxifen, cisplatin, and dacarbazine with IL-2 and IFN-α2b was among the first to show a trend toward improved response rates compared with tamoxifen, cisplatin and dacarbazine alone, although no improvement was seen in OS and there was, in fact, a trend toward decreased survival duration with the use of biochemotherapy.[83] A possible explanation for the inferior survival duration with biochemotherapy is that patients in the biochemotherapy arm received a less intense dose of cytotoxic drugs than did the chemotherapy arm. A more active regimen was subsequently described using the combination of cisplatin, vinblastine, dacarbazine, IL-2, and IFN-α, which had a response rate of nearly 60% in centers with much experience using this regimen.[84–88]

There have been variations in the administration and dosing schedule of the immunotherapy agents, and some investigators have modified the doses of chemotherapy. A quantitative review of biochemotherapy in metastatic melanoma verified a statistically significant advantage over chemotherapy in overall response rate.[89] In keeping with the previous studies, however, no survival advantage was seen with the use of biochemotherapy.[89] This meta-analysis of 18 trials and over 2,600 patients was careful to note that there was considerable variation in the administration of biochemotherapy in terms of doses, management of toxicities, and experience of the managing centers.[89] The effects of these confounding variables cannot be readily appreciated with statistical analyses alone but likely contribute to the conflicting data in some studies.

The unclear benefit of biochemotherapy prompted a large intergroup trial led by ECOG to compare concurrent biochemotherapy using cisplatin, vinblastine, dacarbazine, IL-2, and IFN-α-2b with chemotherapy consisting of cisplatin, vinblastine, and dacarbazine.[90] Response rates were again greater in the biochemotherapy arm along with a prolonged median PFS duration (19.5% response rate in the biochemotherapy arm versus 13.8% in the chemotherapy arm; 4.8 months of median PFS in the biochemotherapy arm versus 2.9 months in the chemotherapy arm). Unfortunately, the improved response rate did not translate into an improvement in OS and there was a significant increase in grade 3 or greater toxicities in the patients receiving biochemotherapy.[90] Of note, this multi-institutional trial involved centers with little to no experience managing the toxicities associated with biochemotherapy, a continued criticism of this study.

A different study utilizing a sequential biochemotherapy regimen in which IL-2 and IFN-α followed immediately after cisplatin, vinflastine, and dacarbazine treatment was completed within each treatment cycle, demonstrated the superiority of biochemotherapy in terms of a response rate (48% versus 25%, $p = 0.001$) and a median time to progression (4.9 months versus 2.4 months, $p = 0.008$).[88] In this study, there was a trend of an OS benefit of biochemotherapy over chemotherapy (11.9 months versus 9.5 months, $p = 0.06$).

There is a consensus among many oncologists that biochemotherapy is safe, has a manageable toxicity profile, and is effective when administered in experienced centers with a subset of patients that can have a prolonged survival duration. A large retrospective review of patients who received biochemotherapy at the University of Texas MD Anderson Cancer showed that after biochemotherapy treatment, approximately 17% and 15% of patients with advanced melanoma were alive at 5 and 10 years, respectively.[91]

Immunotherapy for Metastatic Disease

Interleukin-2

IL-2 is a naturally occurring glycoprotein produced by human T cells that stimulates the growth of T and natural killer cells through CD25.[92] Recombinant IL-2 has been shown to have potent antitumor effect in animal models, which led to the first human trials in the mid-1980s.[93] The mechanism of the antitumor effect of IL-2 occurs through a global stimulation of the acquired immune system, resulting in cellular mediated cytotoxicity. In 1993, the FDA approved high-dose bolus IL-2 as a single-agent therapy for the treatment of renal cell carcinoma, and in 1998, IL-2 was also approved for single-agent use in melanoma.

Initial studies used high-dose bolus recombinant IL-2 (600,000 to 720,000 international U/kg intravenous bolus over 15 minutes every 8 hours on days 1 to 5 and 15 to 19, with a maximum of 28 doses per course).[94] The objective response rate was 16%, with a complete response (CR) rate of 6%; 59% of patients who achieved a CR remained disease-free at 7 years.[94]

High dose IL-2 has several major toxicities that limit its use to only patients with an excellent performance status and is generally reserved for patients who have adequate pulmonary and cardiac functions. In general, the symptoms of high-dose IL-2 resemble flulike symptoms including fever, chills, nausea and vomiting, myalgias, and headache. More worrisome clinical features of high-dose IL-2 include cardiac arrhythmia, hypotension, metabolic acidosis, and renal failure, but most of these features improve with drug cessation. IL-2 is usually administered until the toxicities outweigh the safety of giving the drug.

In vitro, IFN-α upregulates tumor antigens on the cell surface, facilitating the recognition of the tumor by activated T cells.[95,96] Using this rationale, one Phase III study compared the use of the combination of high-dose IL-2 and IFN-α versus high-dose IL-2 alone.[97] The combination of IL-2 and IFN-α failed to show improvement in efficacy, with the median survival of the combination arm at 9.7 months versus 10.2 months in the IL-2–alone arm.[97]

A recent Phase III study compared the combination of high-dose IL-2 with gp-100 peptide vaccine versus high-dose IL-2 alone in patients with stage IV or unresectable stage III HLA-A2-positive metastatic melanoma.[98] The combination arm has a statistically significant increase in response rate (9.7% to 22%) and PFS (1.6 to 2.9 months) with a trend toward increased median OS (12.8 to 17.6 months). This trial was the first randomized Phase III study to demonstrate a clinical benefit for vaccines in melanoma.[98] However, because of the lack of clear OS advantage demonstrated in this study, this combination cannot be recommended on a routine basis. Research is still ongoing to improve the benefit of giving high-dose IL-2. Efforts are also being made to identify biomarkers to preselect patients who are most likely to respond to high-dose IL-2.

Anti-CTLA-4 Antibody

When T cells are stimulated through the T cell receptor, the T cell upregulates cytotoxic T-lymphocyte antigen 4 (CTLA-4) on its surface as a part of the self-regulatory process, and when bound to its ligand (CD80/86 on antigen presenting cells), CTLA-4 initiates inhibitory signals to the T cell and causes the T cell to be suppressed.[99,100] Monoclonal antibodies have been developed that prevent CTLA-4 from binding its ligand, with a net effect of stimulating the immune system by "turning off the brakes" of the T cells.[100,101] CTLA-4 antibodies have been used as antitumor agents to increase the response of a patient's immune system against a tumor. In vivo experiments demonstrated significant antitumor activity of anti-CTLA-4 in immunogenic tumors.[102]

The initial Phase I/II study of single-agent anti-CTLA-4 included 88 patients, with a total disease control rate of 39% broken down by 1 complete response, 1 partial response, and 7 stable disease.[103] Interestingly, many of the responses to the drug were late responses with at least 2 patients having consistent but small disease shrinkage 1 year after starting treatment.[103] Recently, however, a Phase III study comparing the use of tremelimumab (a fully humanized monoclonal antibody targeting CTLA-4) versus temozolomide or dacarbazine in 655 patients with unresectable stage IIIC-IV melanoma failed to show a difference in OS or response rate, and the study was terminated early because of three treatment-related deaths in the tremelimumab arm and none in the chemotherapy arm.[104] A Phase II trial comparing the combination of anti-CTLA-4 (ipilimumab) and dacarbazine versus single-agent decarbazine found an increase in disease control rate (31% vs 22%)[105] and the Phase III study with the same regimen has completed enrollment and results are pending. The moderate success of anti-CTLA-4 blockade in these early studies has also led to multiple other studies on combinations of both biologic and nonbiologic therapies, and the results of many of these studies also are pending.

The main toxicities of anti-CTLA-4 blockade are secondary to a hyperactive immune system. Development of diarrhea, skin rash, and pruritis is common from the autoimmune phenomena.[106] In addition, patients may occasionally develop hypophysitis, hepatitis, uveitis, and pancreatitis due to the CTLA-4 blockage.[106] The autoimmune symptoms can generally be managed with steroids; however, steroids should be avoided if possible so as not to blunt the theoretical antimelanoma immune effect. Pituitary disorders sometime require attention to supplement pituitary hormones to correct for primary hypothyroidism, decreased cortisol levels, and decreased sex hormones such as testosterone. In the largest study of anti-CTLA-4, 62% of subjects developed some sort of immune-related adverse event (IRAE), and interestingly, patients who developed an IRAE had a more statistically significant response to therapy.[107] As of this writing, anti-CTLA-4 is not approved for the treatment of metastatic melanoma and its use is allowed only in clinical trials.

Targeted Therapy in Melanoma

RAS/RAF/MAPK Pathway

The RAS/RAF/MAPK pathway includes a cascade of serine-threonine kinases and is initiated by activation of the RAS-family GTPases: a family of guanine-nucleotide binding proteins embedded in the inner surface of the cell membrane.[108,109] Frequently, stimulation of various membrane-bound receptor tyrosine kinases (either by ligand binding or by their mutations) activates the RAS proteins by altering its formation from a GDP-bound state to the active GTP-bound state.[110] One of the important downstream pathways resulting from the activation of RAS proteins is the mitogen-activated protein kinase (MAPK) cascade, which has been demonstrated to have an important role in regulation of cellular proliferation and survival in multiple models through the serine-threonine protein kinase RAF.[111] The activation of RAF proteins subsequently phosphorylates the MAPK/ERK kinase (MEK) protein kinases, thereby activating their serine-threonine protein kinase activity; the phosphorylated MEK further leads to the phosphorylation of the p44/42 MAPK serine/threonine protein kinases (ERK1 and ERK2), which in turn activate a number of effectors including transcription factors, cytosolic proteins, and other kinases.[111]

The RAS/RAF/MAPK pathway is constitutively active in the majority of melanomas, largely owing to functional genetic mutations of kinase proteins along this pathway.[112] Among three isoforms of RAS proteins (H-RAS, K-RAS, and N-RAS), *N-Ras* mutations are detected in approximately 15% of melanomas with *K-Ras* and *H-Ras* mutations being extremely rare.[113–115] However, the predominant mechanism of activation of the RAS/RAF/MAPK pathway in cutaneous melanomas appears to be mutation of *B-Raf*.[116,117] Davies and colleagues reported that mutations of *B-Raf* were present in 59% of the melanoma cell lines, 80% of the melanoma short-term cultures, and 67% of the melanoma clinical specimens examined. Nearly 80% of the mutations in *B-Raf* occurred at a codon 600 position on exon 15 as a single-substitution mutation (V600E), and this mutation resulted in constitutive activation of the kinase activity of B-RAF, ultimately leading to constitutive phosphorylation of downstream MEK and ERK1/2 kinases.[116] *N-Ras* and *B-Raf* mutations are mutually exclusive with rare exceptions. Interestingly, the predominance of MAPK pathway activation through *N-Ras* or *B-Raf* mutations is mostly confined to melanoma of cutaneous origin.[118,119] In noncutaneous melanoma, which accounts for less than 1% of all melanomas, these mutations occur much less frequently, and other genetic aberrations may play a more predominant role.[119]

In addition to the genetic mutations of *N-Ras* and *B-Raf*, stimulation of receptor tyrosine kinases by ligand binding in an autocrine or paracrine fashion could also activate the MAPK pathway. With all these possible mechanisms of MAPK activation, the RAS/RAF/MAPK pathway (critical to melanoma cellular proliferation and survival) is one of the most promising targets for novel molecularly targeted therapies.

Sorafenib is a small-molecule inhibitor of multiple kinases, including C-RAF, B-RAF, vascular endothelial growth factor receptor 2 (VEGFR-2), VEGFR-3, platelet-derived growth factor receptor (PDGFR), FLT-3, and C-KIT.[120] In preclinical studies, sorafenib was shown to downregulate the MAPK pathway in melanomas, which could explain its antitumor activity.[121] Although a Phase II study of sorafenib as a single agent in patients with advanced melanoma was disappointing, with none of the 34 treated patients having an objective clinical response and less than 20% of patients achieving disease stabilization,[122] sorafenib appeared to potentiate the clinical activities of cytotoxic chemotherapeutic drugs in early studies of sorafenib-containing combination regimens.[107,123] In a Phase I/II trial of the combination of paclitaxel, carboplatin, and sorafenib, 11 (31%) of 35 patients with metastatic melanoma had a partial response, and 19 (54%) had disease stabilization.[124] As predicted from preclinical data, sorafenib markedly reduced phosphorylated MEK after 3 weeks of treatment, but clinical response was not related to the status of *B-Raf* (V600E) mutation among 17 patients with available tumor samples for adequate *B-Raf* sequencing analyses.[124]

In another Phase II study, 47 patients who had not previously received temozolomide and who had not had brain metastases were treated with the combination of sorafenib and temozolomide.[123] The results were promising, with a 19% partial response rate and a 48% disease stabilization rate. In a randomized Phase II study that compared the clinical efficacy of dacarbazine alone with that of the combination of dacarbazine and sorafenib, the combination regimen was superior in terms of both response rate (24% vs 12%) and PFS rate at day 180 (41% vs 19.5%).[125] A Phase III trial randomized 270 previously treated patients with unresectable stage III or IV melanoma in a 1:1 manner to receive either the combination of carboplatin, paclitaxel, and sorafenib or the combination of carboplatin, paclitaxel, and placebo.[82] The primary endpoint of that study was to compare the PFS duration between the two groups, with the comparison of OS duration as the secondary objective; the median PFS durations were 17.4 weeks and 17.9 weeks in the sorafenib-containing combination regimen and placebo combination groups, respectively. The median OS durations were also equivalent at 42 weeks in both groups. Despite the promising results of the Phase I study, sorafenib did not show any clinical benefit in combination with carboplatin and paclitaxel in a second-line treatment setting. The same design of the Phase III randomized, placebo-controlled trial of carboplatin and paclitaxel with or without sorafenib is being investigated in chemo-naïve patients with advanced melanoma (ECOG 2603), and the final results of this study will be available shortly.

Although sorafenib initially received much attention in a field of melanoma for its inhibitory action against RAF protein, its selectivity for inhibition of mutated B-RAF is poor. A number of more potent and selective small-molecule inhibitors of mutated B-RAF protein are currently being tested. Among them are RAF265, PLX4032 (RO5185426), XL281, and GSK2118436. These drugs inhibit the kinase activity of mutated B-RAF at a nanomolar range. As of August 2009, these drugs are still being investigated in a Phase I study. A preliminary analysis of a first-in-human Phase I study of PLX4032 showed very encouraging clinical activity.[126] Among 16 patients with metastatic melanoma harboring mutated *B-Raf* who received 240 mg or higher doses of PLX4032 twice a day, 9 had partial responses and 7 had confirmed partial response by RECIST.[126] In addition, 4 other patients had minor responses, and the interim median PFS duration was at least 6 months. In comparison, all patients without such *B-Raf* mutation had early disease progression.[126] Based on the promising early clinical data, Phase II and III clinical trials are in progress to evaluate the clinical benefit of PLX4032 in patients with *B-Raf* mutation in the second-line and in the first-line treatment setting, respectively.

Several trials have evaluated the safety and clinical efficacy of inhibitors of MEK, which is the kinase activated by RAF proteins. A Phase I study of PD0325901, a potent specific MEK inhibitor, reported responses in two patients with metastatic melanoma and suggested potential for this drug.[127] Unfortunately, further clinical development of this drug is on hold because of safety concerns regarding possible ocular and cardiac events. AZD6244 is another potent selective inhibitor of MEK and has been investigated in patients with melanoma due to clinical responses observed in a Phase I study.[128] In an open-labeled Phase II study that randomized patients with metastatic melanoma in a 1:1 fashion to receive either AZD6244 or temozolomide, no differences were observed in the PFS durations (hazard ratio = 1.07) or the OS durations (hazard ratio = 1.23) between the two arms.[129] However, 5 of the 6 patients with a confirmed partial response in the AZD6244 arm had a *B-Raf* mutation, whereas only 3 of the 9 responding patients in the temozolomide arm had a *B-Raf* mutation in their tumors.[129] In addition, among patients with a *B-Raf* mutation, there was a trend for OS advantage for AZD6244 over temozolomide (Hazard ratio = 0.68). Currently, a Phase II randomized trial is underway to evaluate the clinical efficacy of the combination of AZD6244 and dacarbazine versus dacarbazine alone in selected patients with V600E *B-Raf* mutation.

PI3K/AKT/mTOR Pathway

The PI3K/AKT cascade, which is frequently activated by various growth factor receptor proteins and cell-cell contacts, is another signal transduction pathway that has been studied extensively in melanoma.[130] When extracellular signals or constitutive activation of cell surface receptor kinases activate RAS proteins, phosphoinositide 3 kinase (PI3K) phosphorylates membrane phosphatidylinositol on the 3'-hydroxyl group of the inositol ring to create polyphosphoinositides that recruit a number of pleckstrin homology (PH) domain-containing proteins to the cell membrane, including AKT (also known as protein kinase B [KB]), a serine/threonine protein kinase.[130] After AKT is recruited to the plasma membrane, AKT is phosphorylated, which leads to its activation.[130] The phosphorylated AKT further activates its downstream effectors, such as NF-κB,[131,132] TOR[133] and GSK-3β,[134] which in turn regulates cellular processes such as apoptosis, proliferation, invasion, and angiogenesis; these results suggest a role as an essential molecule in the development and progression of cancers such as melanoma. In fact, p-AKT expression was found to be correlated with melanoma progression[135]; Dai and colleagues reported that strong p-AKT expression was observed in 43% and 49% of dysplastic nevi and primary melanomas, respectively, compared with 77% of metastatic melanoma lesions.[135]

Among three members of the AKT protein kinase family (AKT1, AKT2, and AKT3), dysregulation of AKT3 appears to play the most significant role in the survival of melanoma cells and progression of disease. Stahl and colleagues[136] showed that treatment with siRNA against AKT3 downregulated p-AKT in melanoma but not with siRNA against AKT 1 or AKT2. The role of AKT3 in proliferation and survival of melanoma cells is also suggested by the discovery of a kinase activating AKT3 mutation (E17K).[136]

AKT is negatively regulated by tumor suppressor phosphatase and tensin homolog (PTEN).[138] PTEN is a dual-function lipid and protein phosphatase and dephosphorylates phosphatidylinositol 3,4,5-trisphosphate, the product of PI3K.[139,140] Aberration in PTEN function can lead to upregulation of p-AKT.[141,142] Mutations in PTEN have been identified in melanoma.[143–149] Studies have revealed PTEN mutation in 30% to 40% of melanoma cell lines and 10% of melanoma lesions[145,150] and an epigenetic PTEN silencing phenomenon is also frequently observed in melanoma.[151] These studies indicate that nonfunctional PTEN might play an important role in as many as two-thirds of sporadic melanomas.[143–151]

Despite the mounting preclinical evidence that the PI3K/AKT pathway is a promising target for antimelanoma therapy, only a small number of drugs have been investigated in the clinic so far. In a Phase II study of perifosine, a synthetic alkylphospholipid that inhibits AKT, there was no clinical response among 17 treated patients, and only 21% of patients had disease stabilization.[152,153] At this time, a number of novel small molecules are being tested in early phase clinical studies.

One of the strategies to target this pathway is inhibiting the activation of downstream mammalian target of rapamycin (mTOR), which is an important effector of AKT.[133] Temsirolimus is an ester analog of rapamycin, which has a cytostatic property by inhibiting mTOR protein in cell lines in which the PI3K pathway is activated.[154] However, in a Phase II study of temsirolimus in which 33 patients were treated with 250 mg weekly, the clinical response was observed in only 1 patient.[155] A number of small molecule inhibitors of mTOR proteins are currently being tested in clinical trial settings.

c-KIT Receptor Tyrosine Kinases

Imatinib is a small molecule that inhibits a number of protein tyrosine kinases, including the Bcr-Abl fusion protein, c-ABL, abl-related gene (ARG), PDGFR-α, PDGFR-β, and the c-KIT tyrosine kinase receptor.[156–158] Because c-KIT frequently is expressed in melanoma cells,[159] imatinib was investigated in three separate Phase II studies in patients with metastatic melanoma.[160–162] Unfortunately, only 1 patient of 62 evaluable patients in these three studies combined had a clinical response that lasted for slightly more than 1 year. In retrospect, the low clinical benefit of imatinib in patients with metastatic melanoma is not surprising because overexpression of total c-KIT protein does not necessarily indicate that it drives cell proliferation and survival.

However, it appears that c-KIT plays a significant role in melanoma survival and progression in a subset of melanoma patients, and imatinib or other c-KIT inhibiting drugs may render meaningful clinical benefit in this subset. Curtin et al[119] recently reported oncogenic mutation and/or copy number increases of c-KIT in 39%, 36%, and 28% of mucosal, acral lentiginous melanoma, and melanomas on chronically sun-damaged skin, respectively.[119] Interestingly, none of the melanomas on skin without chronic sun damage harbored the c-KIT mutation.[199] These breakthrough findings renewed the interest in c-KIT–targeting drugs in the field of melanoma, especially in this specific patient population. A number of case reports have since described the dramatic clinical response observed with imatinib treatment in patients with c-KIT mutations.[163,164] Currently, several Phase II clinical trials are testing the clinical efficacy of c-KIT–inhibiting small molecules (eg, imatinib, dasatinib, and nilotinib) in patients with c-KIT mutation or gene amplification. In a Phase II study of imatinib in melanoma patients with either c-KIT gene amplification or mutation, preliminary analyses showed that 3 of 7 treated patients had a clinical response.[165] This encouraging finding, although utilizing a very small number of patients, underscores the importance of selecting appropriate patients with a relevant target (in this case, c-KIT aberration) for targeted therapy.

Antiangiogenesis

Melanomas have been known to be highly vascular tumors, and melanoma progression is associated with induction of angiogenesis.[166–172] Among many angiogenic factors produced and secreted by melanoma cells, vascular endothelial growth factor (VEGF), basic fibroblast growth factor (bFGF), and interleukin-8 (IL-8) have appeared to play the most important role in angiogenic stimulation of melanoma progression.[138,173–179] In addition, the resistance of melanoma cells to cytotoxic drugs may be induced by these proangiogenic growth factors. Lev and colleagues demonstrated in a preclinical model that repeated treatment with dacarbazine induces chemoresistance by increasing the transcriptional upregulation of angiogenic factors such as IL-8 and VEGF in melanoma cells, leading to the selection of much more aggressive clones of melanoma cells.[180,181]

Another important class of angiogenic factors is integrins. Integrins, which are heterodimers composed of α- and β-subunit transmembrane glycoproteins, adhere to extracellular matrix proteins such as vitronectin, fibronectin, laminin, and collagen to promote endothelial cell attachment, migration, and survival.[182,183] Integrins are essential in endothelial cell proliferation and tumor angiogenesis, and integrins are widely expressed in endothelial cells in progressing melanoma lesions.[184] These findings indicate that antiangiogenic and antivascular therapies potentially can provide a clinical benefit as a treatment for patients with advanced melanoma.

However, treatments with various antiangiogenic drugs as a single agent in general have failed to show any meaningful clinical disease control. Bevacizumab is a humanized monoclonal antibody directly against VEGF and blocks the binding of VEGF to its receptors. In a randomized Phase II study of bevacizumab with or without low-dose IFN-α in patients with advanced melanoma, there were no clinical responses among 16 patients in the bevacizumab-alone arm, whereas 1 of 16 patients had a partial response in the combination arm.[185] As discussed previously, sorafenib, which inhibits VEGFRs in addition to c-RAF and b-RAF, as a single agent had minimal clinical activity with only 19% stable disease without confirmed clinical responses among 34 evaluable patients in a Phase II study.[122] Novel drugs that antagonize the action of the integrins have also been investigated for their clinical efficacies. In Phase II studies of Vitaxin (a humanized version of a monoclonal antibody against $\alpha_v\beta_3$ integrin), cilengitide (an inner salt of a cyclized pentapeptide that is a potent and selective antagonist of $\alpha_v\beta_3$ integrin), and volociximab (a high-affinity chimeric IgG_4 monoclonal antibody that specifically binds $\alpha_5\beta_1$ integrin), the clinical efficacy of these anti-integrin drugs as single agents was negligible.[186–188]

Although the clinical trials of the early antiangiogenic drugs showed discouraging results, a glimmer of optimism remains in antiangiogenic melanoma therapy. Recently, a preliminary result of a Phase II study of axitinib (an oral and selective inhibitor of VEGFR-1, -2, and -3) was reported.[189] Among 32 enrolled patients, 5 (15.6%) patients had objective clinical responses per investigators' assessment with a median PFS of 2.3 months.[189] Depending on the final analyses of this study, axitinib may be investigated further for its meaningful clinical benefit as a single agent or in combination with other drugs. Despite lower response rates of bevacizumab as a single agent, bevacizumab-containing combination regimens have been shown to improve progression-free and/or OS duration over cytotoxic chemotherapy regimens without bevacizumab in patients with advanced non-small lung cancer, colorectal cancer, or breast cancer.[190–192] We are eagerly awaiting results of a randomized clinical study that compares the PFS and OS of patients with stage IV melanoma between paclitaxel/carboplatin/placebo and paclitaxel/carboplatin/bevacizumab.

Anti-/Pro-Apoptotic Pathways

Bcl-2 (B-cell lymphoma gene-2) is implicated in the regulation of an apoptosis pathway.[193] Transfection of the *Bcl-2* gene can render neoplastic cells resistant to the induction of apoptosis by cytotoxic drugs,[194] and downregulation of Bcl-2 makes tumor cells more chemosensitive.[194–196] Oblimersen is an 18-base phosphorothioate oligonucleotide antisense to the first six codons of *bcl-2* mRNA, which causes a decrease in Bcl-2 protein translations and ultimately leads to Bcl-2 protein downregulation.[197] A randomized Phase III study of the combination of oblimersen and dacarbazine was conducted in patients with metastatic melanoma on the basis of promising preclinical and early clinical data.[198] Of 771 patients randomly assigned to receive dacarbazine either alone or in combination with oblimersen every 3 weeks, the overall response rate, complete response rate, durable response rate, and median PFS duration were all superior in the combination group over the dacarbazine-only group.[198] However, the difference in the OS durations between the two groups was not statistically different. Although the study did not meet the primary goal of improving OS duration, it was interesting that the combination group had a statistically significant OS improvement in a multivariate subset analysis of 508 patients with normal baseline serum lactate dehydrogenase (LDH) levels.[198] A randomized Phase III study comparing the same two arms in patients with normal serum LDH level was recently completed, and the outcome of the study will be available shortly.

Elesclomol is a novel anticancer drug that has proapoptotic activity through the induction of reactive oxygen species (ROS) and oxidative stress.[199] Because cancer cells have higher levels of ROS due to increased metabolic activity compared with normal cells, cancer cells have a lower threshold for apoptosis when the ROS level is further increased.[200,201] Elesclomol induces apoptosis more selectively in cancer cells by increasing ROS.[199] In a randomized Phase II study in 81 patients with stage IV metastatic melanoma, there were significant differences in the response rates and the median PFS durations between the weekly paclitaxel and elesclomol combination arm and the weekly paclitaxel and placebo combination arm, favoring the elesclomol/paclitaxel arm (overall response rate, 15.1% vs 3.6%; median PFS, 3.68 months vs 1.84 months).[202] However, a large double-blind placebo-controlled randomized Phase III study to compare the OS of the same two treatment groups in chemo-naïve patients was stopped prematurely owing to unexplained worsening of survival in the combination arm despite higher response rate and longer median PFS duration over the control arm in this study.[203] In addition, it was disappointing that the difference in the median PFS durations between the two groups was not statistically significant, although there was a trend in PFS improvement in the elesclomol/paclitaxel arm.[203]

Other Target Pathways

Currently, a number of novel targeted agents that inhibit relevant kinase proteins and pathways are being tested in clinical trials. Among these many promising targets for melanoma therapy are Poly (ADP-Ribose) Polymerase (PARP) protein, which contributes to chemoresistance by repairing DNA damages resulting from cytotoxic drugs[204]; bFGF receptors, which are involved in resistance to VEGF-targeting drugs[205]; and heat-shock protein 90 (HSP90), which contributes to cell survival through protective mechanisms as protein folding, translation between cellular compartments, and suppression of protein aggregation.[206] Drugs that inhibit these target proteins are in early clinical trial phases, and we are eager to discover the clinical usefulness of these drugs.

Future Directions for Targeted Therapy

Successful targeted therapy requires the identification of clinically relevant target proteins or genes, the selection of appropriate patient populations with these targets, and the development of potent and selective drugs against such targets. Despite disappointing results of the earlier targeted trials, we now have much enthusiasm and hope for targeted therapy in melanoma due to the discovery of clinically important targets for therapy and the promising (although preliminary) clinical activity seen in trials with selected patients with relevant targets such as *B-Raf* mutation or *c-KIT* mutations. In addition, a better understanding of complex interactions of signal pathways in melanoma likely will lead to more rational combinations of targeted drugs, and we sincerely hope that these strategies will improve survival and quality of life for patients with melanoma.

Conclusions

Despite extensive clinical investigation in a field of melanoma, cytotoxic drugs and immunotherapeutic cytokines remain the mainstay of the systemic therapy for patients with advanced melanoma. However, with a poor long-term tumor control rate of the currently available drugs, an urgent need exists for the development of novel therapeutic approaches, such as molecularly targeted therapy and/or the combination with cytotoxic agents or cytokines, and also for predictive biomarkers to maximize the clinical benefit of therapy while minimizing toxicities. Future clinical studies should incorporate correlative studies to evaluate predictive biomarkers as well as molecular effects of the treatment to define resistant mechanisms.

References

1. Jemal A et al. Cancer statistics, 2009. *CA Cancer J Clin.* 2009;59(4): 225–249.
2. Balch CM, Buzaid AC, Soong SJ, et al. Final version of the American Joint Committee on Cancer staging system for cutaneous melanoma. *J Clin Oncol.* 2001;19(16): 3635–3648.
3. Manola J, Atkins M, Ibrahim J, et al. Prognostic factors in metastatic melanoma: a pooled analysis of Eastern Cooperative Oncology Group trials. *J Clin Oncol.* 2000; 18(22):3782–3793.
4. Barth A, Morton DL. The role of adjuvant therapy in melanoma management. *Cancer* 1995;75(2 suppl):726–734.
5. Kirkwood JM, Strawderman MH, Ernstoff MS, et al. Interferon alfa-2b adjuvant therapy of high-risk resected cutaneous melanoma: the Eastern Cooperative Oncology Group Trial EST 1684. *J Clin Oncol.* 1996;14(1):7–17.
6. Morton DL et al. An international, randomized, phase III trial of bacillus Calmette-Guerin (BCG) plus allogeneic melanoma vaccine (MCV) or placebo after complete resection of melanoma metastatic to regional or distant sites [Abstract 8508]. *J Clin Oncol.* 2007;25(18 suppl).
7. Morton DL, Hsueh EC, Essner R, et al. Prolonged survival of patients receiving active immunotherapy with Canvaxin therapeutic polyvalent vaccine after complete resection of melanoma metastatic to regional lymph nodes. *Ann Surg.* 2002;236(4): 438–448; discussion 448–449.
8. Grabstein KH, Urdal DL, Tushinski RJ, et al. Induction of macrophage tumoricidal activity by granulocyte-macrophage colony-stimulating factor. *Science.* 1986; 232(4749):506–508.
9. Thomassen MJ, Barna BP, Rankin D, Wiedemann HP, Ahmad M. Differential effect of recombinant granulocyte macrophage colony-stimulating factor on human monocytes and alveolar macrophages. *Cancer Res.* 1989; 49(15):4086–4089.
10. Young JW, Szabolcs P, Moore MA. Identification of dendritic cell colony-forming units among normal human CD34+ bone marrow progenitors that are expanded by c-kit-ligand and yield pure dendritic cell colonies in the presence of granulocyte/macrophage colony-stimulating factor and tumor necrosis factor alpha. *J Exp Med.* 1995; 182(4):1111–1119.
11. Wing EJ, Magee DM, Whiteside TL. Recombinant human granulocyte/macrophage colony-stimulating factor enhances monocyte cytotoxicity and secretion of tumor necrosis factor alpha and interferon in cancer patients. *Blood.* 1989;73(3):643–646.
12. Kumar R, Dong Z, Fidler IJ. Differential regulation of metalloelastase activity in murine peritoneal macrophages by granulocyte-macrophage colony-stimulating factor and macrophage colony-stimulating factor. *J Immunol.* 1996;157(11):5104–5111.
13. Spitler LE, Grossbard ML, Ernstoff MS, et al. Adjuvant therapy of stage III and IV malignant melanoma using granulocyte-macrophage colony-stimulating factor. *J Clin Oncol.* 2000;18(8):1614–1621.
14. Lesinski GB, Anghelina M, Zimmerer J, et al. The antitumor effects of IFN-alpha are abrogated in a STAT1-deficient mouse. *J Clin Invest.* 2003;112(2):170–180.
15. Moschos SJ, Edington HD, Land SR, et al. Neoadjuvant treatment of regional stage IIIB melanoma with high-dose interferon alfa-2b induces objective tumor regression in association with modulation of tumor infiltrating host cellular immune responses. *J Clin Oncol.* 2006;24(19): 3164–3171.
16. Kirkwood JM, Ernstoff MS. Interferons in the treatment of human cancer. *J Clin Oncol.* 1984;2(4):336–352.
17. Kirkwood JM, Ibrahim JG, Sondak VK, et al. High- and low-dose interferon alfa-2b in high-risk melanoma: first analysis of intergroup trial E1690/S9111/C9190. *J Clin Oncol.* 2000;18(12):2444–2458.
18. Kirkwood JM, Manola J, Ibrahim J, et al. A pooled analysis of eastern cooperative oncology group and intergroup trials of adjuvant high-dose interferon for melanoma. *Clin Cancer Res.* 2004;10(5):1670–1677.
19. Wheatley K, Ives N, Hancock B, Gore M, Eggermont A, Suciu S. Does adjuvant interferon-alpha for high-risk melanoma provide a worthwhile benefit? A meta-analysis of the randomised trials. *Cancer Treat Rev.* 2003; 29(4):241–252.
20. Pectasides D, Dafni U, Bafaloukos D, et al. Randomized phase III study of 1 month versus 1 year of adjuvant high-dose interferon alfa-2b in patients with resected high-risk melanoma. *J Clin Oncol.* 2009;27(6):939–944.

21. Eggermont AM, Suciu S, MacKie R, et al. Post-surgery adjuvant therapy with intermediate doses of interferon alfa 2b versus observation in patients with stage IIb/III melanoma (EORTC 18952): randomised controlled trial. *Lancet.* 2005;366(9492):1189–1196.
22. Eggermont AM, Suciu S, Santinami M, et al. Adjuvant therapy with pegylated interferon alfa-2b versus observation alone in resected stage III melanoma: final results of EORTC 18991, a randomised phase III trial. *Lancet.* 2008;372(9633):117–126.
23. Cascinelli N, Belli F, MacKie RM, et al. Effect of long-term adjuvant therapy with interferon alpha-2a in patients with regional node metastases from cutaneous melanoma: a randomised trial. *Lancet.* 2001;358(9285):866–869.
24. Hancock BW, Wheatley K, Harris S, et al. Adjuvant interferon in high-risk melanoma: the AIM HIGH Study—United Kingdom Coordinating Committee on Cancer Research randomized study of adjuvant low-dose extended-duration interferon Alfa-2a in high-risk resected malignant melanoma. *J Clin Oncol.* 2004;22(1): 53–61.
25. Kirkwood JM, Bender C, Agarwala S, et al. Mechanisms and management of toxicities associated with high-dose interferon alfa-2b therapy. *J Clin Oncol.* 2002;20(17): 3703–3718.
26. Bottomley A, Coens C, Suciu S, et al. Adjuvant therapy with pegylated interferon alfa-2b versus observation in resected stage III melanoma: a phase III randomized controlled trial of health-related quality of life and symptoms by the European Organisation for Research and Treatment of Cancer Melanoma Group. *J Clin Oncol.* 2009;27(18):2916–2923.
27. Tsao H, Atkins MB, Sober AJ. Management of cutaneous melanoma. *N Engl J Med.* 2004;351(10):998–1012.
28. Lui P, Cashin R, Machado M, et al. Treatments for metastatic melanoma: synthesis of evidence from randomized trials. *Cancer Treat Rev.* 2007;33(8):665–680.
29. Falkson CI, Ibrahim J, Kirkwood JM, et al. Phase III trial of dacarbazine versus dacarbazine with interferon alpha-2b versus dacarbazine with tamoxifen versus dacarbazine with interferon alpha-2b and tamoxifen in patients with metastatic malignant melanoma: an Eastern Cooperative Oncology Group study. *J Clin Oncol.* 1998;16(5): 1743–1751.
30. Middleton MR, Grob JJ, Aaronson N, et al. Randomized phase III study of temozolomide versus dacarbazine in the treatment of patients with advanced metastatic malignant melanoma. *J Clin Oncol.* 2000;18(1):158–166.
31. Avril MF, Aamdal S, Grob JJ, et al. Fotemustine compared with dacarbazine in patients with disseminated malignant melanoma: a phase III study. *J Clin Oncol.* 2004;22(6):1118–1125.
32. Barnholtz-Sloan JS, Sloan AE, Davis FG, Vigneau FD, Lai P, Sawaya RP. Incidence proportions of brain metastases in patients diagnosed (1973 to 2001) in the Metropolitan Detroit Cancer Surveillance System. *J Clin Oncol.* 2004;22(14):2865–2872.
33. Schouten LJ, Rutten J, Huveneers HA, Twijnstra A. Incidence of brain metastases in a cohort of patients with carcinoma of the breast, colon, kidney, and lung and melanoma. *Cancer.* 2002;94(10):2698–2705.
34. Sampson JH, Carter JH Jr, Friedman AH, Seigler HF. Demographics, prognosis, and therapy in 702 patients with brain metastases from malignant melanoma. *J Neurosurg.* 1998;88(1):11–20.
35. Amer MH, Al-Sarraf M, Vaitkevicius VK. Clinical presentation, natural history and prognostic factors in advanced malignant melanoma. *Surg Gynecol Obstet.* 1979;149(5):687–692.
36. Budman DR, Camacho E, Wittes RE. The current causes of death in patients with malignant melanoma. *Eur J Cancer.* 1978;14(4):327–330.
37. Brock CS, Newlands ES, Wedge SR, et al. Phase I trial of temozolomide using an extended continuous oral schedule. *Cancer Res.* 1998;58(19):4363–4367.
38. Tolcher AW, Gerson SL, Denis L, et al. Marked inactivation of O6–alkylguanine-DNA alkyltransferase activity with protracted temozolomide schedules. *Br J Cancer.* 2003;88(7):1004–1011.
39. Patel, P.M., et al. Extended schedule, escalated dose temozolomide versus dacarbazine in stage IV malignant melanoma: final results of the randomized phase III study (EORTC 18032) [Abstract LBA8]. *Ann Oncol.* 2008;19(suppl 8):viii3.
40. Goodnight JE Jr., Moseley HS, Eilber FR, et al. Cis-dichlorodiammineplatinum(II) alone and combined with DTIC for treatment of disseminated malignant melanoma. *Cancer Treat Rep.* 1979;63(11–12):2005–2007.
41. Al-Sarraf M, Fletcher W, Oishi N, et al. Cisplatin hydration with and without mannitol diuresis in refractory disseminated malignant melanoma: a southwest oncology group study. *Cancer Treat Rep.* 1982;66(1):31–35.
42. Evans LM, Casper ES, Rosenbluth R. Phase II trial of carboplatin in advanced malignant melanoma. *Cancer Treat Rep.* 1987:71(2):171–172.
43. Casper ES. Bajorin D. Phase II trial of carboplatin in patients with advanced melanoma. *Invest New Drugs.* 1990;8(2):187–190.
44. Chang A, Hunt M, Parkinson DR, Hochster H, Smith TJ. Phase II trial of carboplatin in patients with metastatic malignant melanoma. A report from the Eastern Cooperative Oncology Group. *Am J Clin Oncol.* 1993; 16(2):152–155.
45. Guven K, Kittler H, Wolff K, Pehamberger H. Cisplatin and carboplatin combination as second-line chemotherapy in dacarbazine-resistant melanoma patients. *Melanoma Res.* 2001;11(4):411–415.
46. Wiernik PH, Schwartz EL, Einzig A, et al. Phase I trial of taxol given as a 24–hour infusion every 21 days: responses observed in metastatic melanoma. *J Clin Oncol.* 1987;5(8):1232–1239.
47. Legha SS, Ring S, Papadopoulos N, et al. A phase II trial of taxol in metastatic melanoma. *Cancer.* 1990;65(11): 2478–2481.

48. Einzig AI, Hochster H, Wiernik PH, et al. A phase II study of taxol in patients with malignant melanoma. *Invest New Drugs.* 1991;9(1):59–64.
49. Bedikian AY, Weiss GR, Legha SS, et al. Phase II trial of docetaxel in patients with advanced cutaneous malignant melanoma previously untreated with chemotherapy. *J Clin Oncol.* 1995;13(12):2895–2899.
50. Aamdal S, Wolff I, Kaplan S, et al. Docetaxel (Taxotere) in advanced malignant melanoma: a phase II study of the EORTC Early Clinical Trials Group. *Eur J Cancer.* 1994;30A(8):1061–1064.
51. Einzig AI, Schuchter LM, Recio A, et al. Phase II trial of docetaxel (Taxotere) in patients with metastatic melanoma previously untreated with cytotoxic chemotherapy. *Med Oncol.* 1996;13(2):111–117.
52. Hersh EM, O'Day SJ, Ribas A, et al. Open-label, multicenter, Phase II of ABI-007 in previously treated and previously untreated patients with metastatic malignant melanoma. *J Clin Oncol.* 2005;23(16 suppl):7558.
53. Carmichael J, Atkinson RJ, Calman KC, et al. A multicentre phase II trial of vindesine in malignant melanoma. *Eur J Cancer Clin Oncol.* 1982;18(12):1293–1295.
54. Retsas S, Newton KA, Westbury G. Vindesine as a single agent in the treatment of advanced malignant melanoma. *Cancer Chemother Pharmacol.* 1979;2(4):257–260.
55. Nelimark RA, Peterson BA, Vosika GJ, Conroy JA. Vindesine for metastatic malignant melanoma. A phase II trial. *Am J Clin Oncol.* 1983;6(5):561–564.
56. Quagliana JM, Stephens RL, Baker LH, Costanzi JJ. Vindesine in patients with metastatic malignant melanoma: a Southwest Oncology Group study. *J Clin Oncol.* 1984;2(4):316–319.
57. Anderson CM, Buzaid AC, Legha SS. Systemic treatments for advanced cutaneous melanoma. *Oncology.* (Williston Park) 1995;9(11):1149–1158; discussion 1163–1164, 1167–1168.
58. Lokich JJ, Zipoli TE, Perri J, Bothe A. Protracted vinblastine infusion. Phase I-II study in malignant melanoma and other tumors. *Am J Clin Oncol.* 1984;7(5):551–553.
59. Jimeno A, Hitt R, Quintela-Fandino M, Cortés-Funes H. Phase II trial of vinorelbine tartrate in patients with treatment-naive metastatic melanoma. *Anticancer Drugs.* 2005;16(1):53–57.
60. Whitehead RP, Moon J, McCachren SS, et al. A Phase II trial of vinorelbine tartrate in patients with disseminated malignant melanoma and one prior systemic therapy: a Southwest Oncology Group study. *Cancer.* 2004;100(8): 1699–1704.
61. Atkins MB. The role of cytotoxic chemotherapeutic agents either alone or in combination with biological response modifiers. In: Kirkwood JKE, ed. *Molecular Diagnosis, Prevention and Therapy of Melanoma.* New York, NY: Dekker; 1997:219.
62. Chapman PB, Einhorn LH, Meyers ML, et al. Phase III multicenter randomized trial of the Dartmouth regimen versus dacarbazine in patients with metastatic melanoma. *J Clin Oncol.* 1999;17(9):2745–2751.
63. Jacquillat C, Khayat D, Banzet P, et al. Chemotherapy by fotemustine in cerebral metastases of disseminated malignant melanoma. *Cancer Chemother Pharmacol.* 1990;25(4):263–266.
64. Chang J, Atkinson H, A'Hern R, Lorentzos A, Gore ME. A phase II study of the sequential administration of dacarbazine and fotemustine in the treatment of cerebral metastases from malignant melanoma. *Eur J Cancer.* 1994;30A(14):2093–2095.
65. Jacquillat C, Khayat D, Banzet P, et al. Final report of the French multicenter phase II study of the nitrosourea fotemustine in 153 evaluable patients with disseminated malignant melanoma including patients with cerebral metastases. *Cancer.* 1990;66(9):1873–1878.
66. Ulrich J, Gademann G, Gollnick H. Management of cerebral metastases from malignant melanoma: results of a combined, simultaneous treatment with fotemustine and irradiation. *J Neurooncol.* 1999;43(2):173–178.
67. Karakousis CP, Lopez RE, Bhakoo HS, et al. Estrogen and progesterone receptors and tamoxifen in malignant melanoma. *Cancer Treat Rep.* 1980;64(6–7):819–827.
68. Creagan ET, Ingle JN, Ahmann DL, Green SJ, et al. Phase II study of high-dose tamoxifen (NSC-180973) in patients with disseminated malignant melanoma. *Cancer.* 1982;49(7):1353–1354.
69. Leichman CG, Samson MK, Baker LH. Phase II trial of tamoxifen in malignant melanoma. *Cancer Treat Rep.* 1982;66(6):1447.
70. Reimer RR, Costanzi J, Fabian C. Southwest Oncology Group experience with tamoxifen in metastatic melanoma. *Cancer Treat Rep.* 1982;66(8):1680–1681.
71. Telhaug R, Klepp O, Bormer O. Phase II study of tamoxifen in patients with metastatic malignant melanoma. *Cancer Treat Rep.* 1982;66(6):1437.
72. Agarwala SS, Ferri W, Gooding W, Kirkwood JM. A phase III randomized trial of dacarbazine and carboplatin with and without tamoxifen in the treatment of patients with metastatic melanoma. *Cancer.* 1999;85(9):1979–1984.
73. Sanguino AM, et al. Long-term clinical results of the combination of cisplatin (C), vinblastine (V), DTIC (D) and interferon-alfa (I) with or without tamoxifen (T) for metastatic melanoma [Abstract 8039]. *J Clin Oncol.* 2006; 24(18S June 20 suppl).
74. Cocconi G, Bella M, Calabresi F, et al. Treatment of metastatic malignant melanoma with dacarbazine plus tamoxifen. *N Engl J Med.* 1992;327(8):516–523.
75. Legha SS, Ring S, Papadopoulos N, et al. A prospective evaluation of a triple-drug regimen containing cisplatin, vinblastine, and dacarbazine (CVD) for metastatic melanoma. *Cancer.* 1989;64(10):2024–2029.
76. Buzaid AC, Legha SS, Winn R. *Cisplatin, vinblastine, and dacarbazine versus dacarbazine alone in metastatic melanoma: preliminary results of a phase III Cancer Community Oncology Program (CCOP) trial.* Abstract in American Society of Clinical Oncology. 1993; Orlando, FL.
77. Bafaloukos D, Gogas H, Georgoulias V, et al. Temozolomide in combination with docetaxel in patients with

advanced melanoma: a phase II study of the Hellenic Cooperative Oncology Group. *J Clin Oncol.* 2002;20(2): 420–425.
78. Kim KB, Hwu WJ, Papadopoulos NE, et al. Phase I study of the combination of docetaxel, temozolomide and cisplatin in patients with metastatic melanoma. *Cancer Chemother Pharmacol.* 2009;64(1):161–167.
79. Rao RD, Holtan SG, Ingle JN, et al. Combination of paclitaxel and carboplatin as second-line therapy for patients with metastatic melanoma. *Cancer.* 2006;106(2): 375–382.
80. Zimpfer-Rechner C, Hofmann U, Figl R, et al. Randomized phase II study of weekly paclitaxel versus paclitaxel and carboplatin as second-line therapy in disseminated melanoma: a multicentre trial of the Dermatologic Co-operative Oncology Group (DeCOG). *Melanoma Res.* 2003;13(5):531–536.
81. Hodi FS, Soiffer RJ, Clark J, et al. Phase II study of paclitaxel and carboplatin for malignant melanoma. *Am J Clin Oncol.* 2002;25(3):283–286.
82. Hauschild A, Agarwala SS, Trefzer U, et al. Results of a phase III, randomized, placebo-controlled study of sorafenib in combination with carboplatin and paclitaxel as second-line treatment in patients with unresectable stage III or stage IV melanoma. *J Clin Oncol.* 2009; 27(17):2823–2830.
83. Rosenberg SA, Yang JC, Schwartzentruber DJ, et al. Prospective randomized trial of the treatment of patients with metastatic melanoma using chemotherapy with cisplatin, dacarbazine, and tamoxifen alone or in combination with interleukin-2 and interferon alfa-2b. *J Clin Oncol.* 1999;17(3):968–975.
84. Legha SS, Ring S, Bedikian A, et al. Treatment of metastatic melanoma with combined chemotherapy containing cisplatin, vinblastine and dacarbazine (CVD) and biotherapy using interleukin-2 and interferon-alpha. *Ann Oncol.* 1996;7(8):827–835.
85. Legha SS, Ring S, Eton O, et al. Development of a biochemotherapy regimen with concurrent administration of cisplatin, vinblastine, dacarbazine, interferon alfa, and interleukin-2 for patients with metastatic melanoma. *J Clin Oncol.* 1998;16(5):1752–1759.
86. McDermott DF, Mier JW, Lawrence DP, et al. A phase II pilot trial of concurrent biochemotherapy with cisplatin, vinblastine, dacarbazine, interleukin 2, and interferon alpha-2B in patients with metastatic melanoma. *Clin Cancer Res.* 2000;6(6):2201–2208.
87. Atkins MB, Gollob JA, Sosman JA, et al. A phase II pilot trial of concurrent biochemotherapy with cisplatin, vinblastine, temozolomide, interleukin 2, and IFN-alpha 2B in patients with metastatic melanoma. *Clin Cancer Res.* 2002;8(10):3075–3081.
88. Eton O, Legha SS, Bedikian AY, et al. Sequential biochemotherapy versus chemotherapy for metastatic melanoma: results from a phase III randomized trial. *J Clin Oncol.* 2002;20(8):2045–2052.
89. Ives NJ, Stowe RL, Lorigan P, Wheatley K. Chemotherapy compared with biochemotherapy for the treatment of metastatic melanoma: a meta-analysis of 18 trials involving 2,621 patients. *J Clin Oncol.* 2007;25(34): 5426–5434.
90. Atkins MB, Hsu J, Lee S, et al. Phase III trial comparing concurrent biochemotherapy with cisplatin, vinblastine, dacarbazine, interleukin-2, and interferon alfa-2b with cisplatin, vinblastine, and dacarbazine alone in patients with metastatic malignant melanoma (E3695): a trial coordinated by the Eastern Cooperative Oncology Group. *J Clin Oncol.* 2008;26(35):5748–5754.
91. Bedikian AY, Johnson MM, Warneke CL, et al. Prognostic factors that determine the long-term survival of patients with unresectable metastatic melanoma. *Cancer Invest.* 2008;26(6):624–633.
92. Lotze MT, Custer MC, Sharrow SO, et al. In vivo administration of purified human interleukin-2 to patients with cancer: development of interleukin-2 receptor positive cells and circulating soluble interleukin-2 receptors following interleukin-2 administration. *Cancer Res.* 1987;47(8):2188–2195.
93. Lotze MT, Chang AE, Seipp CA, et al. High-dose recombinant interleukin 2 in the treatment of patients with disseminated cancer. Responses, treatment-related morbidity, and histologic findings. *JAMA.* 1986;256(22): 3117–3124.
94. Atkins MB, Lotze MT, Dutcher JP, et al. High-dose recombinant interleukin 2 therapy for patients with metastatic melanoma: analysis of 270 patients treated between 1985 and 1993. *J Clin Oncol.* 1999;17(7):2105–2116.
95. Guadagni F, Schlom J, Johnston WW, et al. Selective interferon-induced enhancement of tumor-associated antigens on a spectrum of freshly isolated human adenocarcinoma cells. *J Natl Cancer Inst.* 1989;81(7):502–512.
96. Di Raimondo F, Lapushin R, Hersh EM. Synergism between alpha-interferon and interleukin-2–activated killer cells: in vitro studies. *Acta Haematol.* 1987;78 (suppl 1):77–83.
97. Sparano JA, Fisher RI, Sunderland M, et al. Randomized phase III trial of treatment with high-dose interleukin-2 either alone or in combination with interferon alfa-2a in patients with advanced melanoma. *J Clin Oncol.* 1993;11(10):1969–1977.
98. Schwartzentruber DJ, et al. A phase III multi-institutional randomized study of immunization with the gp100:209–217(210M) peptide followed by high-dose IL-2 compared with high-dose IL-2 alone in patients with metastatic melanoma [Abstract CRA9011]. *J Clin Oncol.* 2009;27(18 suppl).
99. Brunet JF, Denizot F, Luciani MF, et al. A new member of the immunoglobulin superfamily—CTLA-4. *Nature.* 1987;328(6127):267–270.
100. Leach DR, Krummel MF, Allison JP. Enhancement of antitumor immunity by CTLA-4 blockade. *Science.* 1996;271(5256):1734–1736.

101. Kwon ED, Hurwitz AA, Foster BA, et al. Manipulation of T cell costimulatory and inhibitory signals for immunotherapy of prostate cancer. *Proc Natl Acad Sci U S A.* 1997;94(15):8099–8103.
102. van Elsas A, Hurwitz AA, Allison JP. Combination immunotherapy of B16 melanoma using anti-cytotoxic T lymphocyte-associated antigen 4 (CTLA-4) and granulocyte/macrophage colony-stimulating factor (GM-CSF)-producing vaccines induces rejection of subcutaneous and metastatic tumors accompanied by autoimmune depigmentation. *J Exp Med.* 1999;190(3):355–366.
103. Weber JS, O'Day S, Urba W, et al. Phase I/II study of ipilimumab for patients with metastatic melanoma. *J Clin Oncol.* 2008;26(36):5950–5956.
104. Ribas A, et al. Phase III, open-label, randomized, comparative study of tremelimumab (CP-675,206) and chemotherapy (temozolomide [TMZ] or dacarbazine [DTIC]) in patients with advanced melanoma [Abstract LBA 9011]. *J Clin Oncol.* 2008;26(20 suppl).
105. Hersh EM, et al. Disease control and long-term survival in chemotherapy-naïve patients with advanced melanoma treated with ipilimumab (MDX-010) with or without dacarbazine [Abstract 9022]. *J Clin Oncol.* 2008; 26(May 20 suppl).
106. Weber J. Ipilimumab: controversies in its development, utility and autoimmune adverse events. *Cancer Immunol Immunother.* 2009;58(5):823–830.
107. Downey SG, Klapper JA, Smith FO, et al. Prognostic factors related to clinical response in patients with metastatic melanoma treated by CTL-associated antigen-4 blockade. *Clin Cancer Res.* 2007;13(22 pt 1):6681–6688.
108. Colicelli J. Human RAS superfamily proteins and related GTPases. *Sci STKE.* 2004;2004(250):RE13.
109. Giehl K. Oncogenic Ras in tumour progression and metastasis. *Biol Chem.* 2005;386(3):193–205.
110. Chin L, Garraway LA, Fisher DE. Malignant melanoma: genetics and therapeutics in the genomic era. *Genes Dev.* 2006;20(16):2149–2182.
111. Rubinfeld H, Seger R. The ERK cascade: a prototype of MAPK signaling. *Mol Biotechnol.* 2005;31(2):151–174.
112. Cohen C, Zavala-Pompa A, Sequeira JH, et al. Mitogen-actived protein kinase activation is an early event in melanoma progression. *Clin Cancer Res.* 2002;8(12): 3728–3733.
113. Smalley KS. A pivotal role for ERK in the oncogenic behaviour of malignant melanoma? *Int J Cancer.* 2003; 104(5):527–532.
114. Goydos JS, Mann B, Kim HJ, et al. Detection of B-RAF and N-RAS mutations in human melanoma. *J Am Coll Surg.* 2005;200(3):362–370.
115. Goel VK, Lazar AJ, Warneke CL, et al. Examination of mutations in BRAF, NRAS, and PTEN in primary cutaneous melanoma. *J Invest Dermatol.* 2006;126(1):154–160.
116. Davies H, Bignell GR, Cox C, et al. Mutations of the BRAF gene in human cancer. *Nature.* 2002;417(6892): 949–954.
117. Gray-Schopfer VC, da Rocha Dias S, Marais R. The role of B-RAF in melanoma. *Cancer Metastasis Rev.* 2005; 24(1):165–183.
118. Curtin JA, Fridlyand J, Kageshita T, et al. Distinct sets of genetic alterations in melanoma. *N Engl J Med.* 2005; 353(20):2135–2147.
119. Curtin JA, Busam K, Pinkel D, Bastian BC. Somatic activation of KIT in distinct subtypes of melanoma. *J Clin Oncol.* 2006;24(26):4340–4346.
120. Strumberg D. Preclinical and clinical development of the oral multikinase inhibitor sorafenib in cancer treatment. *Drugs Today (Barc).* 2005;41(12):773–784.
121. Panka DJ, Wang W, Atkins MB, Mier JW. The Raf inhibitor BAY 43–9006 (Sorafenib) induces caspase-independent apoptosis in melanoma cells. *Cancer Res.* 2006;66(3):1611–1619.
122. Eisen T, Ahmad T, Flaherty KT, et al. Sorafenib in advanced melanoma: a Phase II randomised discontinuation trial analysis. *Br J Cancer.* 2006;95(5):581–586.
123. Amaravadi RK, Schuchter LM, McDermott DF, et al. Phase II trial of temozolomide and sorafenib in advanced melanoma patients with or without brain metastases. *Clin Cancer Res.* 2009;15(24):7711–7718.
124. Flaherty KT, Schiller J, Schuchter LM, et al. A phase I trial of the oral, multikinase inhibitor sorafenib in combination with carboplatin and paclitaxel. *Clin Cancer Res.* 2008;14(15):4836–4842.
125. McDermott DF, Sosman JA, Gonzalez R, et al. Double-blind randomized phase II study of the combination of sorafenib and dacarbazine in patients with advanced melanoma: a report from the 11715 Study Group. *J Clin Oncol.* 2008;26(13):2178–2185.
126. Flaherty K, et al. Phase I study of PLX4032: Proof of concept for V600E BRAF mutation as a therapeutic target in human cancer [Abstract 9000]. *J Clin Oncol.* 2009; 27(15 suppl).
127. Lorusso P, et al. A phase 1–2 clinical study of a second generation oral MEK inhibitor, PD 0325901 in patients with advanced cancer. In: *Proceedings of the American Society of Clinical Oncology.* 2005. Orlando, FL.
128. Agarwal R, et al. The first-in-human study of the solid oral dosage form of AZD6244 (ARRY-142886): a phase I trial in patients (pts) with advanced cancer [Abstract 3535]. *J Clin Oncol.* 2008;26(suppl).
129. Dummer R, et al. AZD6244 (ARRY-142886) vs temozolomide (TMZ) in patients (pts) with advanced melanoma: an open-label, randomized, multicenter, phase II study [Abstract 9033]. *J Clin Oncol.* 2008. 26(suppl).
130. Downward J. PI 3–kinase, Akt and cell survival. *Semin Cell Dev Biol.* 2004;15(2):177–182.
131. Romashkova JA, Makarov SS. NF-kappaB is a target of AKT in anti-apoptotic PDGF signalling. *Nature.* 1999; 401(6748):86–90.
132. Dhawan P, Singh AB, Ellis DL, Richmond A. Constitutive activation of Akt/protein kinase B in melanoma leads

to up-regulation of nuclear factor-kappaB and tumor progression. *Cancer Res.* 2002;62(24):7335–7342.
133. Sekulic A, Hudson CC, Homme JL, et al. A direct linkage between the phosphoinositide 3–kinase-AKT signaling pathway and the mammalian target of rapamycin in mitogen-stimulated and transformed cells. *Cancer Res.* 2000;60(13):3504–3513.
134. Cross DA, Alessi DR, Cohen P, et al. Inhibition of glycogen synthase kinase-3 by insulin mediated by protein kinase B. *Nature.* 1995;378(6559):785–789.
135. Dai DL, Martinka M, Li G. Prognostic significance of activated Akt expression in melanoma: a clinicopathologic study of 292 cases. *J Clin Oncol.* 2005;23(7): 1473–1482.
136. Stahl JM, Sharma A, Cheung M, et al. Deregulated Akt3 activity promotes development of malignant melanoma. *Cancer Res.* 2004;64(19):7002–7010.
137. Davies MA, Stemke-Hale K, Tellez C, et al. A novel AKT3 mutation in melanoma tumours and cell lines. *Br J Cancer.* 2008;99(8):1265–1268.
138. Li J, Yen C, Liaw D, et al. PTEN, a putative protein tyrosine phosphatase gene mutated in human brain, breast, and prostate cancer. *Science.* 1997;275(5308):1943–1947.
139. Maehama T, Dixon JE. The tumor suppressor, PTEN/MMAC1, dephosphorylates the lipid second messenger, phosphatidylinositol 3,4,5–trisphosphate. *J Biol Chem.* 1998;273(22):13375–13378.
140. Lin H, Bondy ML, Langford LA, et al. Allelic deletion analyses of MMAC/PTEN and DMBT1 loci in gliomas: relationship to prognostic significance. *Clin Cancer Res.* 1998;4(10):2447–2454.
141. Stambolic V, Suzuki A, de la Pompa JL, et al. Negative regulation of PKB/Akt-dependent cell survival by the tumor suppressor PTEN. *Cell.* 1998;95(1):29–39.
142. Davies MA, Koul D, Dhesi H, et al. Regulation of Akt/PKB activity, cellular growth, and apoptosis in prostate carcinoma cells by MMAC/PTEN. *Cancer Res.* 1999;59(11):2551–2556.
143. Boni R, Vortmeyer AO, Burg G, Hofbauer G, Zhuang Z. The PTEN tumour suppressor gene and malignant melanoma. *Melanoma Res.* 1998;8(4):300–302.
144. Celebi JT, Shendrik I, Silvers DN, Peacocke M. Identification of PTEN mutations in metastatic melanoma specimens. *J Med Genet.* 2000;37(9):653–657.
145. Guldberg P, thor Straten P, Birck A, et al. Disruption of the MMAC1/PTEN gene by deletion or mutation is a frequent event in malignant melanoma. *Cancer Res.* 1997;57(17):3660–3663.
146. Robertson GP, Furnari FB, Miele ME, et al. In vitro loss of heterozygosity targets the PTEN/MMAC1 gene in melanoma. *Proc Natl Acad Sci U S A.* 1998;95(16):9418–9423.
147. Birck A, Ahrenkiel V, Zeuthen J, et al. Mutation and allelic loss of the PTEN/MMAC1 gene in primary and metastatic melanoma biopsies. *J Invest Dermatol.* 2000;114(2):277–280.
148. Reifenberger J, Wolter M, Boström J, et al. Allelic losses on chromosome arm 10q and mutation of the PTEN (MMAC1) tumour suppressor gene in primary and metastatic malignant melanomas. *Virchows Arch.* 2000; 436(5):487–493.
149. Poetsch M, Dittberner T, Woenckhaus C. PTEN/MMAC1 in malignant melanoma and its importance for tumor progression. *Cancer Genet Cytogenet.* 2001;125(1):21–26.
150. Tsao H, Zhang X, Benoit E, Haluska FG, et al. Identification of PTEN/MMAC1 alterations in uncultured melanomas and melanoma cell lines. *Oncogene.* 1998; 16(26):3397–3402.
151. Zhou XP, Gimm O, Hampel H, et al. Epigenetic PTEN silencing in malignant melanomas without PTEN mutation. *Am J Pathol.* 2000;157(4):1123–1128.
152. Kondapaka SB, Singh SS, Dasmahapatra GP, et al. Perifosine, a novel alkylphospholipid, inhibits protein kinase B activation. *Mol Cancer Ther.* 2003;2(11):1093–1103.
153. Ernst DS, Eisenhauer E, Wainman M, et al. Phase II study of perifosine in previously untreated patients with metastatic melanoma. *Invest New Drugs.* 2005;23(6): 569–575.
154. Investigators Brochure CCI-779, Wyeth.
155. Margolin K Longmate J, Barrata T, et al. CCI-779 in metastatic melanoma: a phase II trial of the California Cancer Consortium. *Cancer.* 2005;104(5):1045–1048.
156. Druker BJ, Lydon NB. Lessons learned from the development of an abl tyrosine kinase inhibitor for chronic myelogenous leukemia. *J Clin Invest.* 2000;105(1):3–7.
157. Okuda K, Weisberg E, Gilliland DG, Griffin JD. ARG tyrosine kinase activity is inhibited by STI571. *Blood.* 2001;97(8):2440–2448.
158. Schindler T, Bornmann W, Pellicena P, et al. Structural mechanism for STI-571 inhibition of abelson tyrosine kinase. *Science.* 2000;289(5486):1938–1942.
159. Shen SS, Zhang PS, Eton O, Prieto VG. Analysis of protein tyrosine kinase expression in melanocytic lesions by tissue array. *J Cutan Pathol.* 2003;30(9):539–547.
160. Wyman K, Atkins MB, Prieto V, et al. Multicenter Phase II trial of high-dose imatinib mesylate in metastatic melanoma: significant toxicity with no clinical efficacy. *Cancer.* 2006'106(9):2005–2011.
161. Kim KB, Eton O, Davis DW, et al. Phase II trial of imatinib mesylate in patients with metastatic melanoma. *Br J Cancer.* 2008;99(5):734–740.
162. Ugurel S, Hildenbrand R, Zimpfer A, et al. Lack of clinical efficacy of imatinib in metastatic melanoma. *Br J Cancer.* 2005;92(8):1398–405.
163. Hodi FS, Friedlander P, Corless CL, et al. Major response to imatinib mesylate in KIT-mutated melanoma. *J Clin Oncol.* 2008;26(12):2046–2051.
164. Lutzky J, Bauer J, Bastian BC. Dose-dependent, complete response to imatinib of a metastatic mucosal melanoma with a K642E KIT mutation. *Pigment Cell Melanoma Res.* 2008;21(4):492–493.
165. Carvajal RD, et al., A phase II study of imatinib mesylate (IM) for patients with advanced melanoma harboring somatic alterations of KIT [Abstract 9001]. *J Clin Oncol.* 2009;27(15 suppl).

166. Srivastava A, Laidler P, Hughes LE, et al. Neovascularization in human cutaneous melanoma: a quantitative morphological and Doppler ultrasound study. *Eur J Cancer Clin Oncol.* 1986;22(10):1205–1209.
167. Marcoval J, Moreno A, Graells J, et al. Angiogenesis and malignant melanoma. Angiogenesis is related to the development of vertical (tumorigenic) growth phase. *J Cutan Pathol.* 1997;24(4):212–218.
168. Straume O, Akslen LA. Expresson of vascular endothelial growth factor, its receptors (FLT-1, KDR) and TSP-1 related to microvessel density and patient outcome in vertical growth phase melanomas. *Am J Pathol.* 2001; 159(1):223–235.
169. Erhard H, Rietveld FJ, van Altena MC, et al. Transition of horizontal to vertical growth phase melanoma is accompanied by induction of vascular endothelial growth factor expression and angiogenesis. *Melanoma Res.* 1997;7(suppl 2):S19–S26.
170. Srivastava A, Laidler P, Davies RP, et al. The prognostic significance of tumor vascularity in intermediate-thickness (0.76–4.0 mm thick) skin melanoma. A quantitative histologic study. *Am J Pathol.* 1988;133(2):419–423.
171. Denijn M, Ruiter DJ. The possible role of angiogenesis in the metastatic potential of human melanoma. Clinicopathological aspects. *Melanoma Res.* 1993;3(1):5–14.
172. Graham CH, Rivers J, Kerbel RS, et al. Extent of vascularization as a prognostic indicator in thin (<0.76 mm) malignant melanomas. *Am J Pathol.* 1994;145(3):510–514.
173. Potgens AJ, Lubsen NH, van Altena MC, et al. Vascular permeability factor expression influences tumor angiogenesis in human melanoma lines xenografted to nude mice. *Am J Pathol.* 1995;146(1):197–209.
174. Oku T, Tjuvajev JG, Miyagawa T, et al. Tumor growth modulation by sense and antisense vascular endothelial growth factor gene expression: effects on angiogenesis, vascular permeability, blood volume, blood flow, fluorodeoxyglucose uptake, and proliferation of human melanoma intracerebral xenografts. *Cancer Res.* 1998; 58(18):4185–4192.
175. Claffey KP, Brown LF, del Aguila LF, et al. Expression of vascular permeability factor/vascular endothelial growth factor by melanoma cells increases tumor growth, angiogenesis, and experimental metastasis. *Cancer Res.* 1996; 56(1):172–181.
176. Halaban R, Kwon BS, Ghosh S, et al. bFGF as an auto - crine growth factor for human melanomas. *Oncogene Res.* 1988;3(2):177–186.
177. Becker D, Meier C, Herlyn M. Proliferation of human malignant melanomas is inhibited by antisense oligodeoxynucleotides targeted against basic fibroblast growth factor. *Embo J.* 1989;8(12):3685–3691.
178. Kunz M, Hartmann A, Flory E, et al. Anoxia-induced up-regulation of interleukin-8 in human malignant mela - noma. A potential mechanism for high tumor aggressiveness. *Am J Pathol.* 1999;155(3):753–763.
179. Zachariae CO, Thestrup-Pedersen K, Matsushima K. Expression and secretion of leukocyte chemotactic cytokines by normal human melanocytes and melanoma cells. *J Invest Dermatol.* 1991;97(3):593–599.
180. Lev DC, Onn A, Melinkova VO, et al. Exposure of melanoma cells to dacarbazine results in enhanced tumor growth and metastasis in vivo. *J Clin Oncol.* 2004;22(11): 2092–2100.
181. Lev DC, Ruiz M, Mills L, et al. Dacarbazine causes transcriptional up-regulation of interleukin 8 and vascular endothelial growth factor in melanoma cells: a possible escape mechanism from chemotherapy. *Mol Cancer Ther.* 2003;2(8):753–763.
182. Brooks PC, Montgomery AM, Rosenfeld M, et al. Integrin alpha v beta 3 antagonists promote tumor regression by inducing apoptosis of angiogenic blood vessels. *Cell.* 1994;79(7):1157–1164.
183. Varner JA, Cheresh DA. Integrins and cancer. *Curr Opin Cell Biol.* 1996;8(5):724–730.
184. Varner JA, Cheresh DA. Tumor angiogenesis and the role of vascular cell integrin alphavbeta3. *Important Adv Oncol.* 1996:69–87.
185. Varker KA, Biber JE, Kefauver C, et al. A randomized phase 2 trial of bevacizumab with or without daily low-dose interferon alfa-2b in metastatic malignant melanoma. *Ann Surg Oncol.* 2007;14(8):2367–2376.
186. Hersey P, et al. A phase II, randomized, open-label study evaluating the antitumor activity of MEDI-522, a humanized monoclonal antibody directed against the human alpha v beta 3 (avb3) integrin, ± dacarbazine (DTIC) in patients with metastatic melanoma (MM). In: *Proceedings of the American Society of Clinical Oncology.* 2005; Orlando, FL.
187. Kim KB, et al. A randomized phase II study of EMD 121974 in patients (pts) with metastatic melanoma (MM). In: *Proceedings of the American Society of Clinical Oncology.* 2007. Chicago, IL.
188. Cranmer LD, et al. Phase II study of volociximab (M200), an α5,1 anti-integrin antibody in metastatic melanoma. In: *Proceedings of the American Society of Clinical Oncology.* 2006. Atlanta, GA.
189. Fruehauf JP, et al. Axitinib (AG-013736) in patients with metastatic melanoma: a phase II study [Abstract 9006]. *J Clin Oncol.* 2008;26(suppl).
190. Sandler A, Gray R, Perry MC, et al. Paclitaxel-carboplatin alone or with bevacizumab for non-small-cell lung cancer. *N Engl J Med.* 2006;355(24):2542–2550.
191. Miller K, Wang M, Gralow J, et al., Paclitaxel plus bevacizumab versus paclitaxel alone for metastatic breast cancer. *N Engl J Med.* 2007;357(26):2666–2676.
192. Saltz LB, Clarke S, Díaz-Rubio E, et al. Bevacizumab in combination with oxaliplatin-based chemotherapy as first-line therapy in metastatic colorectal cancer: a randomized phase III study. *J Clin Oncol.* 2008;26(12): 2013–2019.
193. Vaux DL, Cory S, Adams JM. Bcl-2 gene promotes haemopoietic cell survival and cooperates with c-myc to immortalize pre-B cells. *Nature.* 1988;335(6189): 440–442.

194. Konopleva M, Zhao S, Xie Z, et al. Apoptosis. Molecules and mechanisms. *Adv Exp Med Biol.* 1999;457:217–236.
195. Maung ZT, MacLean FR, Reid MM, et al. The relationship between bcl-2 expression and response to chemotherapy in acute leukaemia. *Br J Haematol.* 1994;88(1):105–109.
196. Bedner E, Li X, Gorczyca W, et al. Analysis of apoptosis by laser scanning cytometry. *Cytometry.* 1999;35(3): 181–195.
197. Jansen B, Schlagbauer-Wadl H, Brown BD, et al. bcl-2 antisense therapy chemosensitizes human melanoma in SCID mice. *Nat Med.* 1998;4(2):232–234.
198. Bedikian AY, Millward M, Pehamberger H, et al. Bcl-2 antisense (oblimersen sodium) plus dacarbazine in patients with advanced melanoma: the Oblimersen Melanoma Study Group. *J Clin Oncol.* 2006;24(29): 4738–4745.
199. Kirshner JR, He S, Balasubramanyam V, et al. Elesclomol induces cancer cell apoptosis through oxidative stress. *Mol Cancer Ther.* 2008;7(8):2319–2327.
200. Szatrowski TP, Nathan CP. Production of large amounts of hydrogen peroxide by human tumor cells. *Cancer Res.* 1991;51(3):794–798.
201. Trachootham D, Zhou Y, Zhang H, et al. Selective killing of oncogenically transformed cells through a ROS-mediated mechanism by beta-phenylethyl isothiocyanate. *Cancer Cell.* 2006;10(3):241–252.
202. O'Day S, et al. Subgroup analysis of efficacy and safety analysis of a randomized, double-blinded controlled phase II study of STA-4783 in combination with paclitaxel in patients with metastatic melanoma [Abstract 8528]. *J Clin Oncol.* 2007;28(18 suppl).
203. Hauschild A, et al. Phase III, randomized, double-blind study of elesclomol and paclitaxel versus paclitaxel alone in stage IV metastatic melanoma (MM) [Abstract LBA9012]. *J Clin Oncol.* 2009;27(18 suppl).
204. de Murcia, G. and J. Menissier de Murcia, Poly(ADP-ribose) polymerase: a molecular nick-sensor. *Trends Biochem Sci.* 1994. 19(4):172–176.
205. Casanovas O, Hicklin DJ, Bergers G, Hanahan D. Drug resistance by evasion of antiangiogenic targeting of VEGF signaling in late-stage pancreatic islet tumors. *Cancer Cell.* 2005;8(4):299–309.
206. Whitesell L, Lindquist SL. HSP90 and the chaperoning of cancer. *Nat Rev Cancer.* 2005;5(10):761–772.

28

OCULAR MELANOMA

DAN S. GOMBOS

Introduction

As in other sites, melanomas of the eye and orbit may be primary or metastatic. In the periocular region, melanomas can arise from three distinct regions: eyelid/skin, conjunctiva, and uvea. Cutaneous melanomas can metastasize to any ocular site but most frequently involve the choroid and orbit. This chapter focuses on primary melanocytic tumors of the uvea and conjunctiva. The management of eyelid/skin melanomas is treated in a fashion similar to other cutaneous lesions with wide local excision, which is discussed in greater detail in Chapter 24.

Melanoma of the Conjunctiva

Anatomy

The conjunctiva is a thin mucosal structure that extends from the lid margin along the lid tarsus and reflects onto the globe. Pigmented lesions often are initially visualized by the patient against the white surface of the sclera. Lesions of the tarsus and fornix, however, may remain undetected unless the lids are everted and fully assessed. Any examination of this region should include a complete ophthalmic assessment with a slit lamp, eversion of the upper and lower lids, and palpation of the regional lymph nodes, including the parotid gland.

Differential Diagnosis

Pigmentation of the ocular surface in fact may represent the underlying choroid visualized due to thinning of the sclera. This can occur in the setting of rheumatologic disorders or a primary intraocular tumor such as a uveal melanoma. Nevi of the conjunctiva are not infrequent and generally are freely mobile from the underlying tissue. Lack of feeder vessels and the presence of cysts further support this diagnosis.[1,2] Sudden and rapid growth during puberty is not uncommon and does not necessarily implicate neoplastic transformation. Nonetheless, concern about such a rapid change in a young patient often compels the surgeon to consider excisional biopsy.[3]

Primary Acquired Melanosis

Unique to the conjunctiva is a condition called primary acquired melanosis, or PAM. This is a focal or diffuse pigmentation of the conjunctiva that can be diagnosed only by histopathology. PAM is further stratified to PAM with or without atypia. This distinction is important because PAM without atypia has no risk of malignant transformation. PAM with atypia is further subdivided into mild, moderate, or severe atypia.[4] Here, again, the distinction is important because recent large retrospective reviews have suggested that PAM with mild atypia has no (or very low) risk of malignant transformation.[5]

The management of PAM is complex. Small focal lesions can be completely excised. Larger diffuse regions often are assessed by map biopsy and focal resection. Thicker areas are of greatest concern because they are associated with a greater likelihood of atypia and malignant transformation. Cryotherapy and topical chemotherapy often are used in an adjuvant fashion in patients with atypia or diffuse ocular involvement where complete excision may not be possible.[6] PAM represents a recurrent risk factor for conjunctival melanoma. Such patients require lifelong ocular assessment with re-excision of suspicious lesions.

Clinical Features

Primary melanomas of the conjunctiva may arise from a region of PAM, a nevus, or de novo. The lesions are generally pigmented, raised, and demonstrate feeder vessels on the adjacent conjunctiva. The mass may be adherent to the underlying sclera. As part of their assessment, such patients should undergo neuroimaging of the head and orbits with additional assessment of the periocular lymph nodes. In our institution, this is performed with echography.

Management

The primary management of most conjunctival lesions is excisional biopsy. A "no touch" technique is employed with two sets of surgical instruments used: one set for excision of the lesion and a second set for reconstruction. Following excision, the conjunctiva can be closed in a primary fashion or left bare. Increasingly, amniotic membrane grafts are used when large portions of the conjunctiva are excised. Prior to resection, it is critical to discuss such cases with the pathologist who can anticipate the specimen.

After excision, it is best to lay the specimen flat on paper or Telfa to prevent curling of the tissue. The surgeon must ensure that the conjunctiva is oriented to the pathologist so margins are properly reported. A number of studies have correlated the thickness of the tumor with metastatic risk; therefore, the pathologist must ensure that the tissue is cut and measured in a perpendicular fashion.[7]

As with PAM, adjuvant cryotherapy or topical chemotherapy often is administered. The cryotherapy is applied to the adjacent conjunctiva and underlying sclera prior to wound reconstruction. Mitomycin-C and interferon are the two most commonly used chemotherapeutic agents used topically in this setting.[8] In cases of incomplete excision at the scleral base, adjuvant brachytherapy also can be administered in the form of a radioactive plaque. In extreme cases with diffuse disease, orbital exenteration may be indicated. A lid-sparing technique can be used in which the eyelid skin and obicularis muscle is preserved and used to cover the orbital cavity in a primary fashion.

Conjunctival melanomas spread via the lymphatics. As such, careful assessment of the periocular lymph nodes is indicated. Some institutions have advocated sentinel lymph node biopsy to identify lymphatic spread in otherwise normal appearing lymph nodes.[9] In these cases, a positive sentinel lymph node biopsy should be followed with a comprehensive neck dissection to facilitate accurate staging and optimize regional control.

Melanoma of the Uvea

The uvea is the pigmented intraocular portion of the eye that extends from the iris through the ciliary body and into the choroid. The choroid is a highly vascular region that sits between the sclera and retina. Melanomas can develop in any segment of the uveal tract, but they most commonly occur in the choroid.

Risk Factors

The majority of uveal melanomas develop de novo, but the presence of a nevus is a risk factor for tumor formation. Nevus of Ota, or oculodermal melanocytosis, and dysplastic nevus syndrome are other conditions that predispose eyes to tumor formation. Patients with such conditions should have an annual dilated funduscopic assessment.

Clinical Presentation

Most melanomas present to the ophthalmologist with painless loss of vision. Elevation of the adjacent retina may lead to an initial misdiagnosis of a rhegmatogenous retinal detachment. The accurate diagnosis is made by an experienced ocular oncologist based on clinical findings. Tissue biopsy rarely is indicated. A complete ophthalmic assessment including dilated ophthalmoscopy and slit lamp biomicroscopy is combined with noninvasive diagnostic testing such as ocular echography and fluorescein angiography to arrive at the correct diagnosis. Clinical features distinguishing uveal melanomas from nevi include larger apical dimension, presence of orange pigment, serous retinal detachment (subretinal fluid), and lack of drusen or retinal pigment epithelium (RPE) changes. Some reports also have correlated initial presence of ocular symptoms and proximity to the optic nerve with melanoma formation.[10]

Management

Management of uveal melanomas can be broadly divided into the following options: observation, local excision, primary photocoagulation or thermotherapy (laser), radiation therapy, or enucleation.[10] Many factors impact the final treatment modality selected. Most often, radiation is utilized as the primary globe-salvaging approach, whereas enucleation is reserved for larger tumors unlikely to respond well to radiation. Treatment can be administered in the form of a radioactive plaque (brachytherapy) or charged particle (teletherapy). In North America, Iodine-125 is the most common source used for treatment, and charged particle therapy is limited to a series of specialized ocular proton centers.

The Collaborative Ocular Melanoma Study (COMS) was a landmark study that had significant impact on the management of uveal melanomas. It was a large, multicenter, prospective, randomized trial sponsored by the National Eye Institute (NEI). The study had multiple arms. The medium-sized tumor trial (apical height 2.5–10.0 mm) compared melanoma-related morbidity in a cohort of patients treated with plaques versus those treated with primary enucleation. No statistically significant difference was found between the two groups, suggesting that patients treated with ocular brachytherapy or enucleation had no difference in melanoma related morbidity (ie, distant metastasis). Similarly, the large tumor trial (apical height >10.0 mm) found no benefit in pretreating large uveal melanomas with external beam radiation prior to primary enucleation.[11,12] Based on these data, most clinicians have abandoned pre-enucleation external beam radiation.

Special Considerations

Unlike conjunctival and cutaneous lesions, uveal melanomas have a unique predisposition to metastasize to the hepatic region. Once metastatic, the prognosis is poor, with few patients surviving longer than 2 years.[13] A number of factors have been associated with distant metastasis. Tumors of the cilliary body have the highest risk of metastasis; whereas iris lesions do so much less frequently. Epitheliod tumors and those with vascular arcades on histopathology correlate with higher metastatic risk. Recent data suggest that monosomy 3 and gene expression profiling correlate strongly with the likelihood of distant spread. The latter has been used to subdivide melanomas into class 1 (low risk) versus class 2 (high risk) tumors.[14,15] Although not indicated for diagnosis, a number of ocular oncologists perform fine needle aspiration biopsy for tissue prognostication. Unfortunately, even with this information, no treatment is available to halt or decrease the risk of distant spread. Once metastatic, patients are referred for systemic chemotherapy or, in select cases, hepatic chemoembolization.

Metastatic Lesions to Eye and Orbit

Metastatic cutaneous melanomas have been described in nearly every ocular structure. The orbit and choroid represent the two most common regions for periocular spread. Generally, such tumors occur in the setting of diffuse multifocal disease, although occasionally an isolated focus does occur. Orbital lesions can be treated with palliative radiation or, in select cases, excision. Choroidal lesions rarely require biopsy and management is similar to that of primary uveal melanoma. Because lesions often occur in the setting of diffuse disease with attendant poor prognosis, globe salvaging approaches (brachytherapy and laser hyperthermia) usually are preferred over enucleation.

Other Melanocytic Intraocular Tumors

Melanocytomas are benign intraocular lesions that initially are often misdiagnosed as uveal melanoma. Experienced clinicians can distinguish these lesions based on their darker appearance, echographic features, and location (generally peripapillary). Although benign, these tumors carry a small risk of malignant transformation and should be assessed annually. Similarly, congenital hypertrophy of the retinal pigment epithelium (CHRPE) occasionally is misdiagnosed as a uveal melanoma. Annual examination also is indicated due to rare transformation to adenocarcinoma.

Conclusion

The term ocular melanoma represents a broad spectrum of primary ocular tumors that may involve the eyelid/skin, uveal tract, or conjunctiva. For conjunctival lesions, excision combined with adjuvant treatment is the preferred approach. Uveal lesions can managed with globe-salvaging modalities that often carry the same risk of melanoma-related morbidity as enucleation. Although skin and conjunctival lesions can spread via the lymphatics, uveal tumors generally spread hematogenously to the liver, imparting a poor prognosis.

References

1. Folberg R, Jakobiec FA, Bernardino VB, et al. Benign conjunctival melanocytic lesions. Clinicopathologic features. *Ophthalmology.* 1989;96(4):436–461.
2. Shields CL, Fasiuddin AF, Mashayekhi A, et al. Conjunctival nevi: clinical features and natural course in 410 consecutive patients. *Arch Ophthalmol.* 2004;122(2):167–175.
3. McDonnell JM, Carpenter JD, Jacobs P, et al. Conjunctival melanocytic lesions in children. *Ophthalmology.* 1989; 96(7):986–993.
4. Jakobiec FA, Folberg R, Iwamoto T. Clinicopathologic characteristics of premalignant and malignant melanocytic lesions of the conjunctiva. *Ophthalmology.* 1989;96(2): 147–166.
5. Shields JA, Shields CL, Mashayekhi A, et al. Primary acquired melanosis of the conjunctiva: experience with 311 eyes. *Trans Am Ophthalmol Soc.* 2007;105:61–71.
6. Jakobiec FA, Rini FJ, Fraunfelder FT, et al. Cryotherapy for conjunctival primary acquired melanosis and malignant melanoma. Experience with 62 cases. *Ophthalmology.* 1988;95(8):1058–1070.
7. Esmaeli B, De Martelaere S, Ozkan Y, et al. Surgical specimen handling for conjunctival melanoma: implications for tumor thickness determination and sentinel lymph node biopsy. *Ophthal Plast Reconstr Surg.* 2006;22(3): 238–239.
8. Kurli M, Finger PT. Topical mitomycin chemotherapy for conjunctival malignant melanoma and primary acquired melanosis with atypia: 12 years' experience. *Graefes Arch Clin Exp Ophthalmol.* 2005;243(11):1108–1114.
9. Esmaeli B. Sentinel node biopsy as a tool for accurate staging of eyelid and conjunctival malignancies. *Curr Opin Ophthalmol.* 2002;13(5):317–323.
10. Damato BE. An approach to the management of patients with uveal melanoma. *Eye.* 1993;7(pt 3):388–397.
11. Diener-West M, Earle JD, Fine SL, et al. The COMS randomized trial of iodine 125 brachytherapy for choroidal melanoma, III: initial mortality findings. COMS Report No. 18. *Arch Ophthalmol.* 2001;119(7):969–982.
12. Hawkins BS. The Collaborative Ocular Melanoma Study (COMS) randomized trial of pre-enucleation radiation of large choroidal melanoma: IV. Ten-year mortality findings and prognostic factors. COMS report number 24. *Am J Ophthalmol.* 2004;138(6):936–951.
13. Woll E, Bedikian A, Legha SS. Uveal melanoma: natural history and treatment options for metastatic disease. *Melanoma Res.* 1999;9(6):575–581.
14. Singh AD, Damato B, Howard P, et al. Uveal melanoma: genetic aspects. *Ophthalmol Clin North Am.* 2005;18(1): 85–97, viii.
15. Onken MD, Worley LA, Ehlers JP, et al. Gene expression profiling in uveal melanoma reveals two molecular classes and predicts metastatic death. *Cancer Res.* 2004;64(20): 7205–7209.

29

MUCOSAL MELANOMA

SNEHAL G. PATEL
JATIN P. SHAH

Introduction

Mucosal melanomas of the head and neck (MMHN) are characterized by a generally aggressive clinical course, and in spite of advances in detection and treatment, survival outcomes remain poor. Although the first description of the tumor by Weber dates back to 1859, MMHN remained relatively obscure for several decades.[1] Moreover, the difficulty encountered in achieving an accurate histopathologic diagnosis of amelanotic melanomas, distinct from other lesions such as lymphoma and neuroendocrine tumors, also may have contributed to their relative rarity. With wider use of immunohistochemistry in diagnosis and increasing awareness, MMHN are being diagnosed more frequently, yet they remain relatively rare compared to cutaneous melanoma.

As with many rare diseases, single institutional experience in treatment of MMHN is limited and published reports suffer from small numbers and low statistical power, as well as a lack of uniformity of treatment. There is, however, little doubt that surgical resection remains the most effective treatment option. Adjuvant treatment generally consists of radiation therapy, and systemic treatment options are limited to palliation or in the context of clinical trials.

Etiology

Mucosal melanoma of the head and neck arises from melanocytes in normal mucosa; therefore, the risk of these tumors is perceived to be related to the distribution of melanocytes in the upper aerodigestive tract. The normal mucosa of the oral cavity and the nasal cavity contains approximately 1500 melanocytes per mm^3 compared to 800 per mm^3 in the abdominal skin.[2] These melanocytes are of neuroectodermal origin and migrate with the ectodermally derived mucosa. In contrast, the nonectodermally derived mucosa of the nasopharynx, larynx, esophagus, and tracheobronchial tree has a significantly lower density of melanocytes and therefore is thought to be less prone to developing MMHN.

Mucosal melanomas of the nasal cavity and paranasal sinuses are reported more frequently than those of the oral cavity, but this likely reflects detection and reporting bias rather than an actual difference.[3–7] Within the oral cavity, the hard palate and alveolus are the sites most commonly affected. The precise subsite of origin of most tumors in the sinonasal cavity is more often than not difficult to determine because of the relatively advanced nature of these tumors at detection. The nasal septum and lateral wall are the most commonly reported sites in the nasal cavity, whereas the maxillary sinus is more frequently involved compared to other paranasal sinuses.

The etiology and pathogenesis of MMHN are poorly understood. Exposure to aerosol and air pollution is thought to be contributory to the development of MMHN. The role of formaldehyde has been suggested in development of sinonasal melanoma.[8] The presence of long-term "melanosis" has been debated as a predisposing condition to MMHN without conclusive proof. Although "melanosis" of the oral cavity is quite common, the condition is not as frequently seen in the mucosa of the sinonasal tract and, in fact, has been observed to be reversible. Tobacco smoking has been suggested as an etiologic factor for laryngeal mucosal melanosis by stimulating "melanogenic metaplasia" or by increasing melanin production from mucosal melanocytes.

Epidemiology

Mucosal malignant melanoma constitutes 0.5% to 1.5% of all melanomas, and over half of all mucosal melanomas arise in the head and neck region.[9] Although there are no accurate epidemiologic data to allow direct comparison, unlike cutaneous melanoma, which is one of the fastest rising cancers in the United States, the incidence of mucosal melanomas is thought to have remained stable over the past few decades. The incidence of MMHN in the United States is estimated at 0.7 per 100,000 population.[10]

There are significant racial differences in incidence of MMHN and this appears to be inversely related to incidence of cutaneous melanoma. For instance, the incidence of MMHN is higher relative to cutaneous melanoma in Japan.[11] The incidence of mucosal melanoma of the nasal cavity has been reported to be higher in Ugandan Africans, another population where the incidence of cutaneous melanoma is low.[12]

Clinical Features and Evaluation

Physical Examination Findings

The diagnosis of MMHN is dependent in large measure on the site of the primary tumor. Lesions of the anterior oral cavity are more likely to be discovered incidentally and indeed may be noticed on routine dental evaluation or, more rarely, by the patient. Tumors of the sinonasal tract, on the other hand, typically are not diagnosed until they cause symptoms such as epistaxis and nasal obstruction, or if visual disturbances and sensory changes occur with locally advanced tumors. Cervical lymph node metastases are relatively infrequent, occurring more commonly in patients with oral cavity compared to sinonasal melanoma.

The diagnosis of MMHN generally is associated with the presence of a pigmented lesion, but not all pigmented mucosal lesions are melanomas. The typical mucosal malignant melanoma is a darkly pigmented, exophytic lesion with or without ulceration (Fig 29–1). An assortment of benign pigmented lesions is encountered at a varying frequency in the oral mucosa, and these potentially confusing lesions are listed in Table 29–1.[13] The presence of pigmentation is not essential to the diagnosis of melanoma, and the clinician should be aware that mucosal melanoma can be amelanotic, especially in the nasal cavity. The diagnosis of melanoma for these nonpigmented lesions may come as a surprise to the clinician and the patient after histopathologic examination of a biopsy or excised specimen.

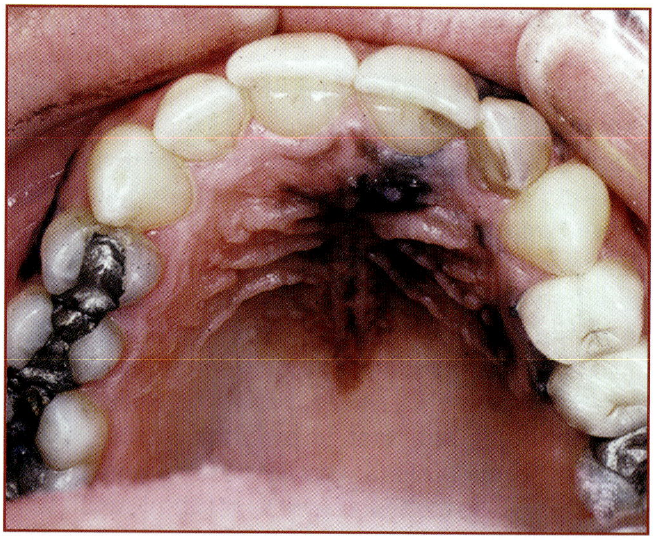

Figure 29–1. Typical clinical appearance of a mucosal malignant melanoma of the hard palate.

Table 29–1. Commonly Encountered Benign Pigmented Lesions in the Oral Cavity

Condition	Clinical Features
Diffuse pigmentation	
Melanosis	• Benign melanin-containing lesion • May represent radial phase of growth akin to lentigo maligna in skin • No prognostic importance if found with malignant melanoma
Racial pigmentation	• Reported in up to 85% of African-Americans • Benign • Requires no intervention
Smoker's melanosis	• Seen in 25 to 30% of smokers • Usually in females after the 3rd decade • Labial aspect of anterior part of lower gum • Melanin deposition in basal cell layer and lamina propria
Focal pigmentation	
Amalgam tattoo	• One of the most common causes of intraoral pigmentation • Flat, blue–black macule on gingiva or alveolus, buccal mucosa or floor of mouth • May rarely be seen on radiographs, if amalgam particles are large enough
Melanotic macule	• Most commonly seen on lower lip, gingiva, buccal mucosa, or palate • Result from increased melanin production rather than proliferation of melanocytes • Generally homogeneous light or dark brown single lesions <1 cm in diameter with well-demarcated smooth border • More common in women and young adults • Diagnosis requires biopsy and histopathologic examination
Pigmented nevi	• Brown or blue lesions • Caused by accumulation of melanocytes in basal layer of epithelium or connective tissue stroma • Location of melanocytes relative to surface epithelium determines classification into junctional, intramucosal, and compound nevi • Junctional nevi are flat dark brown lesions caused by proliferation of melanocytes at rete pegs just under the surface epithelium • Intramucosal and compound nevi have proliferating melanocytes deeper in connective tissue stroma • Proliferation of melanocytes in deep connective tissue results in blue nevus • Most common type is intramucosal nevus seen on buccal mucosa • Blue nevus seen most frequently on palate • Clinical differentiation from melanoma may require biopsy • No conclusive proof that nevi transform to melanoma but excision prudent for most significant lesions
Oral melanoacanthoma	• Benign, flat dark brown or black lesion generally seen on buccal mucosa of young black females • May grow rapidly raising concern but is not malignant • Histologically characterized by hyperkeratotic epithelium containing proliferating dendritic melanocytes • May disappear spontaneously or after incisional biopsy

Imaging

Clinical examination of accessible lesions such as those in the oral cavity and inferior nasal cavity is reliable at assessing local extent. For most other lesions, especially those arising in the paranasal sinuses, radiographic imaging is indispensable. Contrast-enhanced computed tomography (CT) scan of the sinuses is an excellent initial examination and provides superior assessment of the tumor relative to relevant bony anatomy. Unlike the more commonly encountered squamous cell carcinoma, which tends to invade and destroy bone, sinonasal melanoma generally causes regressive remodeling of bone (Fig 29–2).

Most patients with sinonasal melanoma will benefit from an MRI scan because MRI is better able to differentiate tumor from retained mucous secretions, rendering MRI excellent for delineating soft tissue extent. The tumor can be bright on T1-weighted MRI because of its melanin content and blood, but the usual appearance is isointense to muscle or dark on T2-weighted MRI (Fig 29–3). MRI and CT also complement each other in the evaluation of orbital invasion, perineural invasion, and intracranial extension. The cost effectiveness of FDG-PET imaging in initial workup remains to be elucidated, but it is generally useful for surveillance after treatment.[14]

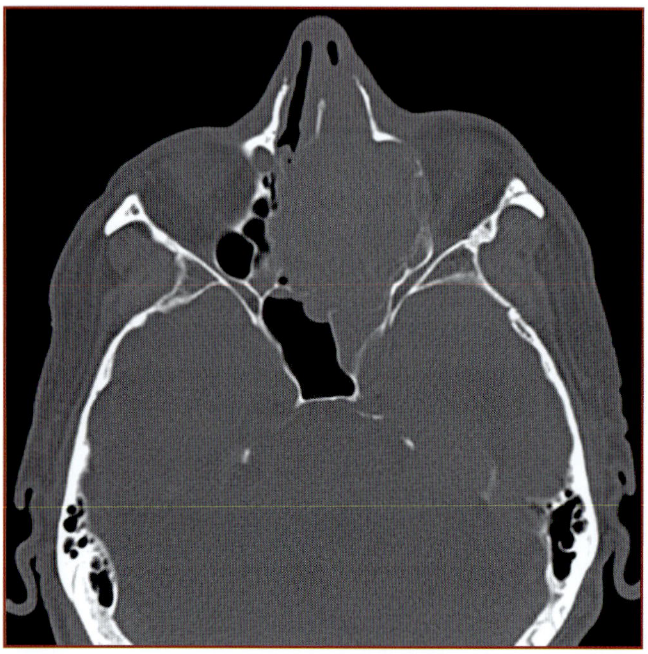

Figure 29–2. Axial CT scan (bone algorithm) shows regressive remodeling of the medial wall of the left orbit by a melanoma of the nasal cavity.

Biopsy and Histopathologic Assessment

Accurate diagnosis of a suspicious pigmented mucosal lesion requires biopsy and histopathological evaluation. Photographic documentation of the lesion prior to biopsy is recommended, as this visual information is crucial for the head and neck surgeon at the time of surgical resection. Oral cavity lesions generally are accessible for an incisional biopsy, whereas lesions in the nasal cavity generally are diagnosed after punch biopsy, endoscopic biopsy, or endoscopic excision of a "polyp." Excisional biopsy of a suspected mucosal melanoma is not recommended because adequate margins are unlikely if histopathology reveals a melanoma. Re-excision of the biopsy scar to exclude residual tumor in these situations is especially problematic because of the difficulty in identifying the precise extent of the lesion.

The histopathologic hallmark of melanoma is the demonstration of intracellular melanin.[15] Histopathologic distinction from other small round bluecell tumors can be difficult, especially if the tumor is amelanotic and located in the sinonasal tract. The differential diagnosis in these cases includes poorly differentiated carcinoma, lymphoma, small cell carcinoma, and esthesioneuroblastoma. Conventional light microscopy examination with hematoxylin and eosin, or Fontana stains can be significantly augmented by immunohistochemistry. Melanomas stain strongly for specific antibodies to S-100, HMB-45, tyrosinase, Melan-A/Mart-1, microphthalmia-associated transcription factor, and PNL2.[16] However, the pathologist generally relies on a panel of antibodies to characterize the cells and the diagnosis of melanoma is often reached by a process of excluding other tumors based on the immunohistochemical profile.

Staging

Until recently, MMHN were not assigned a TNM stage by the national or international community,

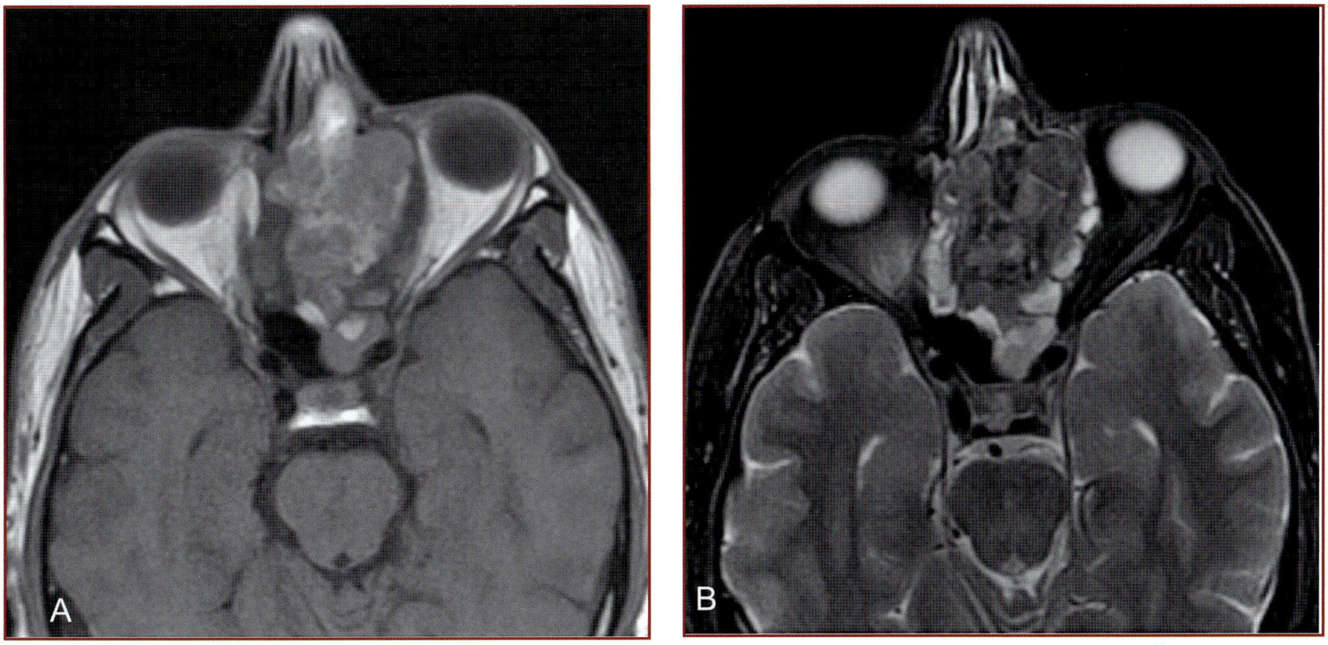

Figure 29–3. MRI scan of the patient shown in Figure 29–2. **A.** The melanoma is bright on T1-weighted sequence, whereas (**B**) the T2-weighted sequence is excellent at delineating tumor compared to postobstructive changes in the ethmoid air cells bilaterally, and in the sphenoid sinus. Note minimal protrusion of tumor into the otherwise uninvolved sphenoid sinus.

and a relatively simple staging system that stratified patients into stage I (local disease), stage II (regional nodal metastases), and stage III (distant metastases) was in use for several decades.[17] In view of the uniquely aggressive behavior of MMHN, the 7th edition of the American Joint Commission on Cancer (AJCC) staging system now categorizes these tumors distinctly from cutaneous melanoma (Tables 29–2 through 29–5).[18]

This new T-staging system designates anatomically "early" lesions restricted to the mucosa as T3, and the lowest possible stage grouping for MMHN is stage III. Further stratification for localized MMHN (without nodal or distant disease) can be achieved using a histologic system that uses the histologic architecture, tumor differen-

Table 29–2. T-Staging Criteria for Mucosal Melanoma of the Head and Neck

T3	Mucosal disease
T4a	Moderately advanced disease Tumor involving deep soft tissue, cartilage, bone, or overlying skin.
T4b	Very advanced disease Tumor involving brain, dura, skull base, lower cranial nerves (IX, X, XI, XII), masticator space, carotid artery, prevertebral space, or mediastinal structures.

Source: Used with permission of the American Joint Committee on Cancer (AJCC), Chicago, Illinois. The original source for this material is the AJCC Cancer Staging Manual, Seventh Edition (2010) published by Springer Science and Business Media LLC, www.springer.com.

Table 29–3. N-Staging Criteria for MMHN

NX	Regional lymph nodes cannot be assessed
N0	No regional lymph node metastases
N1	Regional lymph node metastases present

Source: Used with permission of the American Joint Committee on Cancer (AJCC), Chicago, Illinois. The original source for this material is the AJCC Cancer Staging Manual, Seventh Edition (2010) published by Springer Science and Business Media LLC, www.springer.com.

Table 29–4. M-Staging Criteria for MMHN

MX	Distant metastasis cannot be assessed
M0	No distant metastasis
M1	Distant metastasis present

Source: Used with permission of the American Joint Committee on Cancer (AJCC), Chicago, Illinois. The original source for this material is the AJCC Cancer Staging Manual, Seventh Edition (2010) published by Springer Science and Business Media LLC, www.springer.com.

Table 29–5. Stage Grouping for MMHN

T3, N0, M0	Stage III
T4a, N0, M0	Stage IVA
T3-T4a, N1, M0	Stage IVA
T4b, any N, M0	Stage IVB
Any T, Any N, M1	Stage IVC

Source: Used with permission of the American Joint Committee on Cancer (AJCC), Chicago, Illinois. The original source for this material is the AJCC Cancer Staging Manual, Seventh Edition (2010) published by Springer Science and Business Media LLC, www.springer.com.

tiation and the depth of invasion of the tumor.[19] However, the major limitation of this system is that it is based on histopathologic parameters that would be applicable only for patients who are treated with definitive surgical resection of the primary tumor.

Treatment and Therapeutic Outcomes

Surgery, radiation therapy, chemotherapy, and immunotherapy are the currently available options for treatment of MMHN. Surgical resection of MMHN with negative margins offers the best chance for local control and cure. Radiation therapy is used most often in the postoperative setting as adjuvant therapy. As for cutaneous melanoma, systemic options are relatively limited and currently are best used within the context of a clinical trial.

The overall outcomes for patients with MMHN are dismal, as depicted in Figure 29–4. Patients with mucosal melanoma of the ethmoid or paranasal

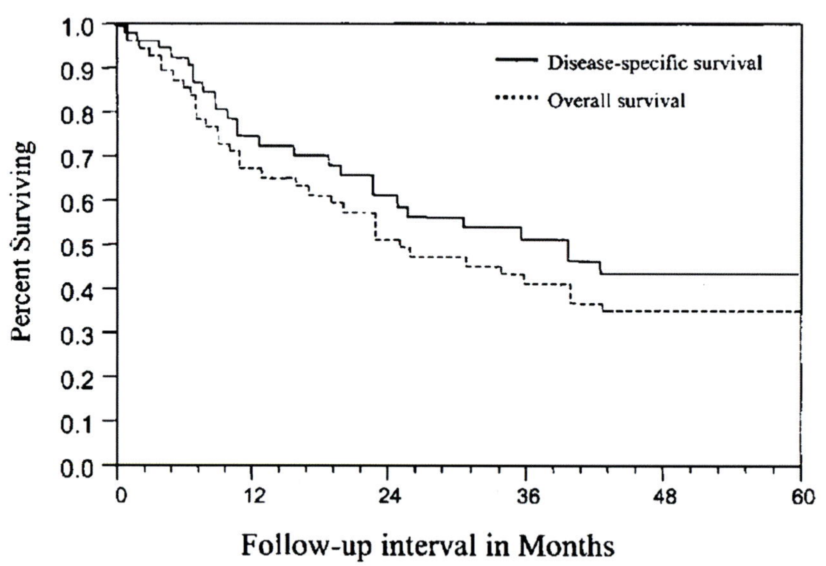

Figure 29–4. Disease-specific survival for mucosal melanoma of the head and neck. From Patel SG, Prasad ML, Escrig M, et al. Primary mucosal malignant melanoma of the head and neck. Head and Neck; 24(3): 247–257. Reprinted with permission.

sinuses approaching the skull base have a particularly poor prognosis, even after undergoing craniofacial resection (Fig 29–5). In spite of significant advances including improved pretreatment assessment, better surgical technique, and availability of more precise radiation therapy, control of disease remains difficult in the majority of patients with MMHN.

Local failure and distant metastases are relatively common, with regional neck failure in up to 25% of patients (Fig 29–6). Local failure, in particular, is a significant problem, occurring in over half of patients with MMHN.[7,20] Only a minority of patients with locally recurrent disease are amenable to successful salvage. These are generally patients with a relatively indolent clinical course who started

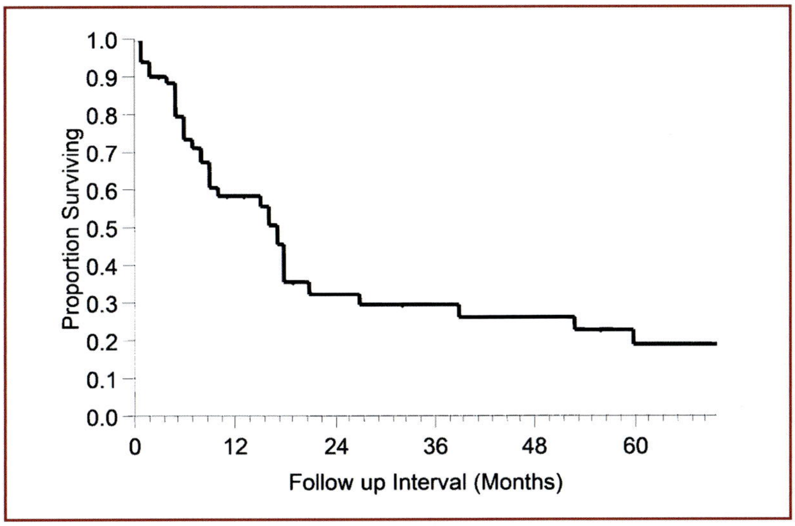

Figure 29–5. Disease-specific survival in patients requiring craniofacial resection for malignant melanoma. From Ganly I, Patel SG, Singh B, et al. Craniofacial resection for malignant melanoma of the skull base: Report of an international collaborative study. Arch Otolaryngol Head Neck Surg: 2006; 132(1): 73-78. Reprinted with permission.

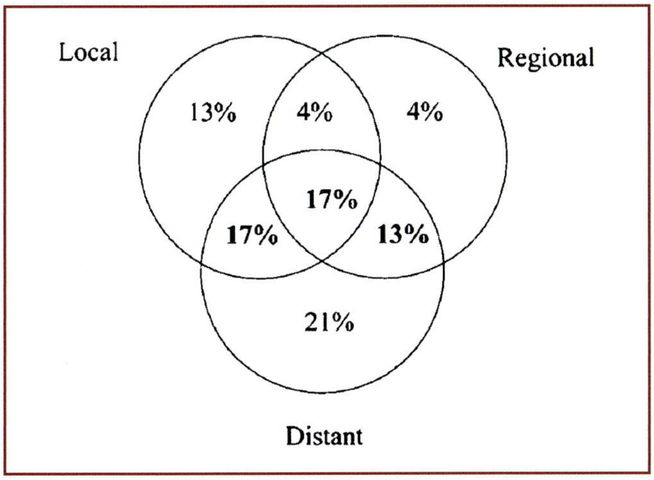

A

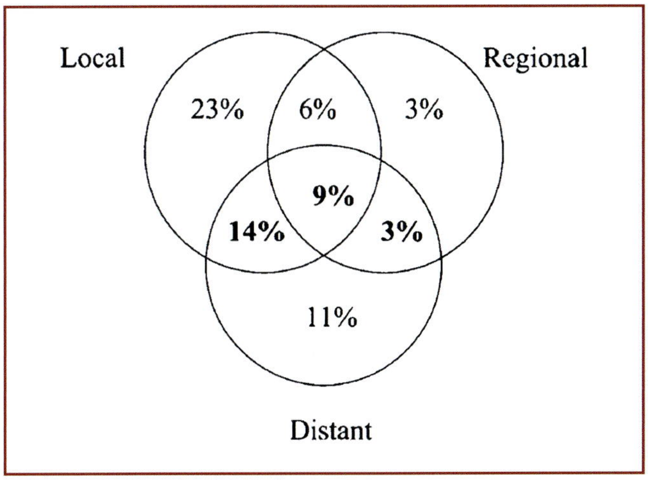

B

Figure 29–6. Patterns of recurrence in MMHN. **A.** Oral cavity. **B.** Sinonasal. From Patel SG, Prasad ML, Escrig M, et al. Primary mucosal malignant melanoma of the head and neck. Head and Neck; 24(3): 247–257. Reprinted with permission.

with limited local disease without regional or distant metastases. The high incidence of local failure has been attributed to diffuse involvement of submucosal lymphatics by tumor and to the presence of subclinical premalignant changes in the surrounding mucosa. Moreover, local failure rates likely are related to the difficulty in achieving "wide" margins of resection.

The incidence of regional nodal failure is higher for lesions of the oral cavity compared to sinonasal lesions. A particularly troublesome feature of MMHN is the relatively high incidence of distant failure. The lungs and the brain are the most common sites for distant metastases, and the median survival after diagnosis of distant metastases is only about 6 months.

It is important to realize that, although complete surgical resection affords the best chance for cure, local control does not necessarily portend improved survival. The propensity of these tumors for distant metastases has been shown to overwhelm all other prognostic features, underscoring the importance of developing effective systemic therapy.[21] The extent of surgical resection is determined largely by the location of the tumor. Transnasal endoscopic surgery has been used for treatment of various benign and malignant sinonasal tumors including melanoma.[22] It has been argued that these approaches may be especially relevant in patients with mucosal melanoma as outcomes are dismal even with more radical surgical resection. However, combined craniofacial resection represents the most effective contemporary surgical option for treatment of sinonasal melanoma approaching or involving the skull base.[23]

Managing the Orbit

Management of the orbit is another major consideration in surgical management of locally advanced sinonasal tumors, and orbital preservation is an obvious goal if possible.[24,25] The decision for orbital exenteration is relatively easy if there is intraconal extension of tumor, gross involvement of the globe, or orbital apex involvement. Orbital exenteration also may be a better option if the eye is predicted to be nonfunctional postoperatively, especially as the vast majority of patients with locally advanced tumors will require adjuvant radiation. Although loss of vision generally occurs gradually in the radiated orbit, sequelae such as radiation keratitis and panophthalmitis are of immediate concern and can be debilitating. The functional and cosmetic sequelae of treatment can therefore be drastic, and the surgeon should carefully balance quality of life issues against overall prognosis for each individual patient.

Neck Dissection

In spite of the relatively high rate of neck failure, nodal metastasis at presentation is not frequent and occurs more commonly in oral melanoma (<25%) than in sinonasal melanoma (<10%). Elective treatment of the clinically and radiographically negative neck, therefore, is not indicated for sinonasal melanoma, but patients with oral melanoma should be considered for elective neck dissection as part of their initial surgical treatment.

Radiation Therapy

The role of radiation therapy in treatment of MMHN remains controversial. Melanoma cells are believed to be relatively resistant to conventional fractionated radiation therapy because of their ability to repair cellular damage.[26] Therefore, hypofractionated schedules have been advocated for cutaneous melanoma, based largely on laboratory evidence and some clinical data.[27] The radiation dose of 2400 cGy is delivered in three fractions of 800 cGy each on days 0, 7, and 21 or four fractions of 600 cGy.

Initially, it was believed that these hypofractionated schedules would result in higher local toxicity related to the optic structures. However, recently published data suggest that hypofractionated intensity-modulated radiation therapy (IMRT) appears to be well tolerated.[28] However, another retrospective study reported a higher rate of locoregional failure with hypofractionated radiation compared to conventional fractionation, raising the possibility that poorer outcomes with the hypofractionation schedule were related to the lower total dose administered.[21] The use of hyperfractionated radiation therapy with combined chemotherapy also has been reported in a small series of patients.[29]

Adjuvant Radiation Therapy

External beam radiation therapy is routinely used in the postoperative adjuvant setting for sinonasal melanoma. The most obvious indication for adding postoperative radiation therapy (PORT) in sinonasal melanoma is the presence of close or positive margins. A majority of patients with locally advanced sinonasal melanoma will be eligible for PORT by default, because the regional anatomy often precludes wide margins in the conventional sense. There are no randomized data assessing the efficacy of PORT in MMHN. Some retrospective studies report enhanced local control with an unclear benefit on survival, but improvement in local control or survival rates was observed in patients treated with PORT in a cohort of MMHN patients treated at Memorial Hospital.[7,30–32] This could be the result of selection bias in that higher risk patients with adverse tumor factors would be selected for PORT, which can be assumed to have improved their outcome to a level comparable to that of lower risk patients in whom PORT was not deemed indicated. Recently, a multi-institutional analysis of patients requiring craniofacial resection for sinonasal melanoma demonstrated improved local control and survival with the addition of PORT.[23]

Primary Radiation Therapy

Primary radiation therapy for treatment of MMHN with conventional photons has been reported with varying efficacy.[33–35] Although some studies report complete response rates of up to 80% with long-term control over 50%, radiation therapy generally is not accepted as primary treatment of MMHN. This is especially true for melanomas of the oral cavity, which are more amenable to surgical resection than sinonasal melanomas.

Conversely, primary radiation therapy may provide effective palliation by relieving compressive symptoms in patients with surgically unresectable or inoperable disease.[36] Neutron beam therapy has been used in the past with impressive response and local control rates but one in five patients develop significant treatment-related sequelae.[37] The efficacy of radiation therapy in treating MMHN can be expected to improve with evolving technology such as proton beam therapy and carbon ion radiation therapy.[38,39]

Systemic Therapy

Systemic therapy options for MMHN include chemotherapy and immunotherapy. Chemotherapy is largely used with palliative intent in management of recurrent, metastatic, or unresectable disease.[40,41] There has been an enormous amount of research in the basic developmental pathways of melanoma with the aim of identifying molecular targets of clinical relevance. Approximately 25% of patients with melanoma have been shown to have KIT mutations or amplifications.[42] The efficacy of targeted therapy using imatinib (Gleevec®) in patients who have tumors exhibiting c-kit alterations is currently being investigated in two Phase II trials, one at Memorial Sloan-Kettering Cancer Center (Protocol IDs: MSKCC-07014, 7754, 07-014, NCT00470470) and the other at the Dana Farber Cancer Institute (Protocol IDs: 06-056, NCT00424515). Other small molecules being studied include nilotinib (Protocol IDs: 08-244, DUS11T, NCT00788775) and dasatinib (Protocol IDs: ECOG-E2607, E2607, NCT00700882).

Immunotherapy with biologic response modifiers such as Bacillus Calmette-Guérin (BCG), interferon α-2b, and interleukin-2 has been studied extensively, but the only immunotherapy currently approved for standard clinical use by the FDA is interferon α-2B.[43–45] Vaccine-based immunotherapy of melanoma also has been studied extensively, initially with vaccines derived from autologous or allogeneic melanoma cells, or using molecules such as proteins, peptides, or gangliosides.[46] Another approach is to use cell-mediated immunity including dendritic-cell vaccines.[47] These approaches were shown to be of limited efficacy, and strategies using DNA-based vaccines are currently thought to offer more promise.[48]

Conclusion

Treatment outcomes of MMHN have improved only marginally over the past several decades, despite advances in diagnosis, surgical treatment, and radiation therapy. Systemic treatment approaches have been disappointing, and currently there are no available options that are effective. Considerable research is ongoing with the goal that effective biological therapeutic options will become available in the future. Until improved systemic therapy is devised, the overall nature of MMHN should be kept in mind when designing treatment programs so that quality of life and function are preserved as best as possible in this unique group of patients whose fate is decided more by the biology of their disease than by any available treatment.

References

1. Weber CO. *Chirurgische Erfahrungen und Untersuchungen: nebst zahlreichen Beobachtungen aus der chirurgischen Klinik und dem evangelischen Krankenhause zu Bonn.* Berlin, Germany: Reimer; 1859.
2. Szabo G. The number of melanocytes in human epidermis. *Br Med J.* 1954;1(4869):1016–1017.
3. Shah JP, Huvos AG, Strong EW. Mucosal melanomas of the head and neck. *Am J Surg.* 1977;134(4):531–535.
4. Stern SJ, Guillamondegui OM. Mucosal melanoma of the head and neck. *Head Neck.* 1991;13(1):22–27.
5. Andersen LJ, Berthelsen A, Hansen HS. Malignant melanoma of the upper respiratory tract and the oral cavity. *J Otolaryngol.* 1992;21(3):180–185.
6. Nandapalan V, Roland NJ, Helliwell TR, et al. Mucosal melanoma of the head and neck. *Clin Otolaryngol Allied Sci.* 1998;23(2):107–116.
7. Patel SG, Prasad ML, Escrig M, et al. Primary mucosal malignant melanoma of the head and neck. *Head Neck.* 2002;24(3):247–257.
8. Holmstrom M, Lund VJ. Malignant melanomas of the nasal cavity after occupational exposure to formaldehyde. *Br J Ind Med.* 1991;48(1):9–11.
9. Chang AE, Karnell LH, Menck HR. The National Cancer Data Base report on cutaneous and noncutaneous melanoma: a summary of 84,836 cases from the past decade. The American College of Surgeons Commission on Cancer and the American Cancer Society. *Cancer.* 1998; 83(8):1664–1678.
10. McLaughlin CC, Wu XC, Jemal A, et al. Incidence of noncutaneous melanomas in the U.S. *Cancer.* 2005;103(5): 1000–1007.
11. Takagi M, Ishikawa G, Mori W. Primary malignant melanoma of the oral cavity in Japan. With special reference to mucosal melanosis. *Cancer.* 1974;34(2):358–370.
12. Lewis MG, Martin JA. Malignant melanoma of the nasal cavity in Ugandan Africans. Relationship of ectopic pigmentation. *Cancer.* 1967;20(10):1699–1705.
13. Kauzman A, Pavone M, Blanas N, Bradley G. Pigmented lesions of the oral cavity: review, differential diagnosis, and case presentations. *J Can Dent Assoc.* 2004;70(10): 682–683.
14. Goerres GW, Stoeckli SJ, von Schulthess GK, Steinert HC. FDG PET for mucosal malignant melanoma of the head and neck. *Laryngoscope.* 2002;112(2):381–385.
15. Batsakis JG, Regezi JA, Solomon AR, Rice DH. The pathology of head and neck tumors: mucosal melanomas, part 13. *Head Neck Surg.* 1982;4(5):404–418.
16. Busam KJ. The use and application of special techniques in assessing melanocytic tumours. *Pathology.* 2004;36(5): 462–469.
17. Ballantyne AJ. Malignant melanoma of the skin of the head and neck. An analysis of 405 cases. *Am J Surg.* 1970; 120(4):425–431.
18. Edge SB BD, Compton CC, Fritz AG, Greene FL, Trotti A, eds *AJCC Cancer Staging Manual.* 7th ed. New York, NY: Springer; 2010.
19. Prasad ML, Patel SG, Huvos AG, Shah JP, Busam KJ. Primary mucosal melanoma of the head and neck: a proposal for microstaging localized, Stage I (lymph node-negative) tumors. *Cancer.* 2004;100(8):1657–1664.
20. Manolidis S, Donald PJ. Malignant mucosal melanoma of the head and neck: review of the literature and report of 14 patients. *Cancer.* 1997;80(8):1373–1386.
21. Moreno MA, Roberts DB, Kupferman ME, et al. Mucosal melanoma of the nose and paranasal sinuses, a contemporary experience from the M. D. Anderson Cancer Center. *Cancer.* 2010;116(9):2215–2223.
22. Hanna E, DeMonte F, Ibrahim S, et al. Endoscopic resection of sinonasal cancers with and without craniotomy: oncologic results. *Arch Otolaryngol Head Neck Surg.* 2009; 135(12):1219–1224.
23. Ganly I, Patel SG, Singh B, et al. Craniofacial resection for malignant melanoma of the skull base: report of an international collaborative study. *Arch Otolaryngol Head Neck Surg.* 2006;132(1):73–78.
24. Andersen PE, Kraus DH, Arbit E, Shah JP. Management of the orbit during anterior fossa craniofacial resection. *Arch Otolaryngol Head Neck Surg.* 1996;122(12):1305–1307.
25. Imola MJ, Schramm VL Jr. Orbital preservation in surgical management of sinonasal malignancy. *Laryngoscope.* 2002;112(8 pt 1):1357–1365.
26. Bentzen SM, Overgaard J, Thames HD, et al. Clinical radiobiology of malignant melanoma. *Radiother Oncol.* 1989;16(3):169–182.
27. Ang KK, Peters LJ, Weber RS, et al. Postoperative radiotherapy for cutaneous melanoma of the head and neck region. *Int J Radiat Oncol Biol Phys.* 1994;30(4):795–798.
28. Wu AJ, Gomez J, Zhung JE, et al. Radiotherapy after surgical resection for head and neck mucosal melanoma. *Am J Clin Oncol.* 2010;33(3):281–285.
29. Albertsson M, Tennvall J, Andersson T, et al. Malignant melanoma of the nasal cavity and nasopharynx treated with cisplatin and accelerated hyperfractionated radiation. *Melanoma Res.* 1992;2(2):101–104.

30. Owens JM, Roberts DB, Myers JN. The role of postoperative adjuvant radiation therapy in the treatment of mucosal melanomas of the head and neck region. *Arch Otolaryngol Head Neck Surg.* 2003;129(8):864–868.
31. Temam S, Mamelle G, Marandas P, et al. Postoperative radiotherapy for primary mucosal melanoma of the head and neck. *Cancer.* 2005;103(2):313–319.
32. Kingdom TT, Kaplan MJ. Mucosal melanoma of the nasal cavity and paranasal sinuses. *Head Neck.* 1995; 17(3):184–189.
33. Harwood AR, Cummings BJ. Radiotherapy for mucosal melanomas. *Int J Radiat Oncol Biol Phys.* 1982;8(7): 1121–1126.
34. Gilligan D, Slevin NJ. Radical radiotherapy for 28 cases of mucosal melanoma in the nasal cavity and sinuses. *Br J Radiol.* 1991;64(768):1147–1150.
35. Trotti A, Peters LJ. Role of radiotherapy in the primary management of mucosal melanoma of the head and neck. *Semin Surg Oncol.* 1993;9(3):246–250.
36. Wada H, Nemoto K, Ogawa Y, et al. A multi-institutional retrospective analysis of external radiotherapy for mucosal melanoma of the head and neck in northern Japan. *Int J Radiat Oncol Biol Phys.* 2004;59(2):495–500.
37. Blake PR, Catterall M, Errington RD. Treatment of malignant melanoma by fast neutrons. *Br J Surg.* 1985;72(7): 517–519.
38. Chan AW, Liebsch NJ. Proton radiation therapy for head and neck cancer. *J Surg Oncol.* 2008;97(8):697–700.
39. Yanagi T, Mizoe JE, Hasegawa A, et al. Mucosal malignant melanoma of the head and neck treated by carbon ion radiotherapy. *Int J Radiat Oncol Biol Phys.* 2009;74(1): 15–20.
40. Guzzo M, Grandi C, Licitra L, Podrecca S, Cascinelli N, Molinari R. Mucosal malignant melanoma of head and neck: forty-eight cases treated at Istituto Nazionale Tumori of Milan. *Eur J Surg Oncol.* 1993;19(4):316–319.
41. Jacquillat C, Khayat D, Banzet P, et al. Final report of the French multicenter phase II study of the nitrosourea fotemustine in 153 evaluable patients with disseminated malignant melanoma including patients with cerebral metastases. *Cancer.* 1990;66(9):1873–1878.
42. Garrido MC, Bastian BC. KIT as a therapeutic target in melanoma. *J Invest Dermatol.* 2010;130(1):20–27.
43. Kirkwood JM, Strawderman MH, Ernstoff MS, Smith TJ, Borden EC, Blum RH. Interferon alfa-2b adjuvant therapy of high-risk resected cutaneous melanoma: the Eastern Cooperative Oncology Group Trial EST 1684. *J Clin Oncol.* 1996;14(1):7–17.
44. Kirkwood JM, Ibrahim JG, Sondak VK, et al. High- and low-dose interferon alfa-2b in high-risk melanoma: first analysis of intergroup trial E1690/S9111/C9190. *J Clin Oncol.* 2000;18(12):2444–2458.
45. Legha SS, Ring S, Eton O, et al. Development of a biochemotherapy regimen with concurrent administration of cisplatin, vinblastine, dacarbazine, interferon alfa, and interleukin-2 for patients with metastatic melanoma. *J Clin Oncol.* 1998;16(5):1752–1759.
46. Chapman PB. Melanoma vaccines. *Semin Oncol.* 2007; 34(6):516–523.
47. Engell-Noerregaard L, Hansen TH, Andersen MH, et al. Review of clinical studies on dendritic cell-based vaccination of patients with malignant melanoma: assessment of correlation between clinical response and vaccine parameters. *Cancer Immunol Immunother.* 2009;58(1):1–14.
48. Yuan J, Ku GY, Gallardo HF, et al. Safety and immunogenicity of a human and mouse gp100 DNA vaccine in a phase I trial of patients with melanoma. *Cancer Immun.* 2009;9:5.

30

MICROSCOPICALLY ORIENTED HISTOGRAPHIC SURGERY (MOHS): INDICATIONS, PRINCIPLES, AND TECHNIQUE

MICHAEL R. MIGDEN

Introduction

Mohs micrographic surgery has evolved as a widely accepted technique for the management of cutaneous malignancy, particularly in the head and neck. Its nomenclature credits the surgeon who devised the technique. For cutaneous malignancies of the head and neck, Mohs micrographic surgery constitutes an excellent primary or adjunctive modality, and it is a cornerstone of the multidisciplinary management of these tumors.

History and Evolution

In 1933, Dr. Frederic Mohs (Fig 30–1) began his pioneering work in microscopic chemosurgery as a research assistant at the University of Wisconsin in the department of zoology.[1] He assessed the effects of injecting platinum and other chemicals into cancers implanted in rats. The effects of the various chemicals were evaluated by shaving a specimen from the injected implanted tumors parallel to the skin surface and examining them in the horizontal excision plane. When zinc chloride was injected, excellent histologic structural features were unexpectedly preserved. This led to the concept of "micrographic" observation of tumor surgical margins that were "fixed" in vivo by applying zinc chloride paste

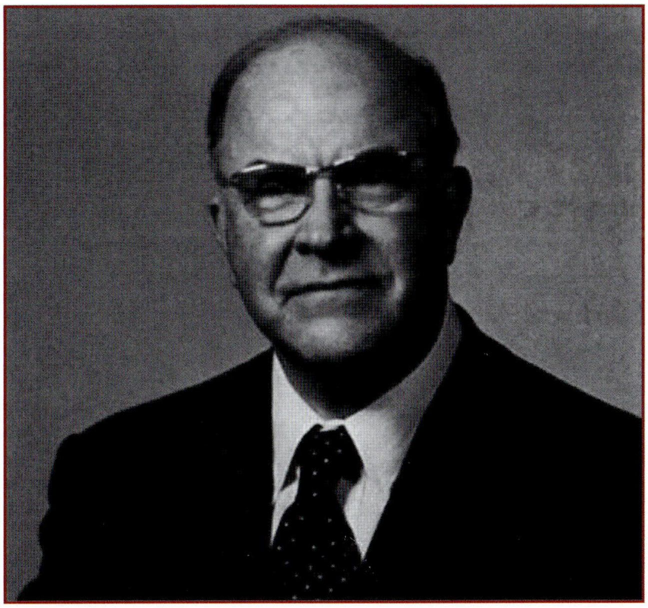

Figure 30–1. Frederic Mohs, father of Mohs micrographic surgery.

to the lesion, thereby allowing confirmation of complete tumor removal. The term micrographic recognizes both components of microscopic examination and mapping of the surgical resection plane.

In 1936, when Dr. Mohs began using his micrographic chemosurgery method to treat patients, the method was considered controversial. In vivo chemosurgical tissue fixation led to pain and tissue morbidity, and although later debunked, there was a common belief at the time that cutting through malignancy would trigger local spread or metastasis. To minimize objections, early applications of the technique were restricted to patients with extremely advanced cancers who were considered to be incurable.[1] In 1941, Dr. Mohs reported high cure rates treating these advanced tumors.

Evolution of the technique to incorporate fresh frozen sections began out of necessity. While making an instructional film demonstrating the Mohs technique, Dr. Mohs needed to complete a multistage excision of an eyelid basal cell carcinoma within a single day to accommodate the camera crew and equipment. Replacing the in vivo fixation with frozen sections prepared from fresh tissue allowed the filming to be completed on schedule.

The decreased inflammation noted on microscopic evaluation using this modification led Dr. Mohs to use the fresh tissue technique for removal of eyelid cancers from that date forward. The rationale for adopting the micrographic fresh frozen section approach over traditional chemosurgery was based on the obvious benefits of changing the procedure from a multiday process to a single day procedure, producing less tissue inflammation, and eliminating in vivo tissue fixation pain.[1] With increasing experience, Mohs micrographic surgery has evolved to be a widely accepted modality in the armamentarium against cutaneous malignancy of the head and neck.

Margin Control—Methods and Considerations

In cutaneous cancer surgery, the goal of treatment is complete removal of the tumor while sparing as much normal tissue as possible to optimize function, structural integrity, and cosmesis (Table 30–1). Achieving this goal depends on cancer screening and early detection of the smallest possible primary lesion, before it becomes locally destructive, exhibits greater subclinical extension, or develops in-transit or distant metastasis. Complete excision of a naïve primary tumor affords the best protection against developing a larger, more locally destructive, recurrent tumor or metastasis. Simply put, the best opportunity for total cure is early entire tumor extirpation.

Intuitively, one may reason that more aggressive tumors demand larger margins of excision in order to decrease the likelihood of incomplete removal, local extension, or metastasis. Commonly accepted wide local excision margins are based on tumor type, subtype, grade, and stage as well as other features such as depth of invasion, ulceration, and perineural involvement. Margin size dictates the amount of additional tissue beyond the clinical tumor that should be taken to include, and thereby contain, the irregular subclinical extension of tumors which often occur. However, in the absence of known local metastasis, substantially increasing margins beyond what will completely clear the primary tumor has not been demonstrated to provide benefit in decreasing recurrence rate or increasing long-term survival.

Wide Local Excision

Most wide local excision specimens are evaluated by transverse sectioning of tissue in "bread loaf" orientation, providing a survey of excision margins. These parallel cross sections are performed in series from one end of the specimen to the other. Although each section from a "bread-loafed" specimen contains a component of the peripheral margin, the

Table 30–1. Core Treatment Goals for Cutaneous Malignancy

- Eliminate tumor while preserving normal tissue
- Preserve function whenever possible
- Restore structural form and cosmesis

sum of all the peripheral margins from these sections may encompass less than 1% to 2% of the complete peripheral margin available in the excision specimen (Fig 30–2).

Standard "bread loaf" sectioning is appropriate for tumors with less potential subclinical extension and regular edges. For tumors with a high degree of irregular subclinical extension, a root or vein of the malignancy may fall between transverse sections (see Fig 30–2), allowing a negative margin to be erroneously reported. Adherence to the recommended margins appropriate for tumor type and subtype often compensates for some of this subclinical irregular extension, but attempts to narrow standard margins may result in incomplete excision. Timely and more detailed scrutiny of selected areas may be achieved through intraoperative en face frozen sections, which may be combined with tumor mapping of the regions evaluated. The challenge with standard intraoperative frozen sections is to predict which portion of the total margin should receive en face evaluation during the procedure.

Wide local excision constitutes the primary treatment modality for cutaneous malignancies that are not appropriate for Mohs surgery. Such lesions include noncontiguous tumors and deeply invasive lesions that involve bone or are beyond the reach of Mohs surgery, as performed under local anesthesia. These lesions may appear fixed to deeper structures on preoperative exam, or there may be radiographic evidence of substantially deeper extension. Standard wide local excision also may be indicated in patients who are not willing to undergo a longer procedure under local anesthesia.

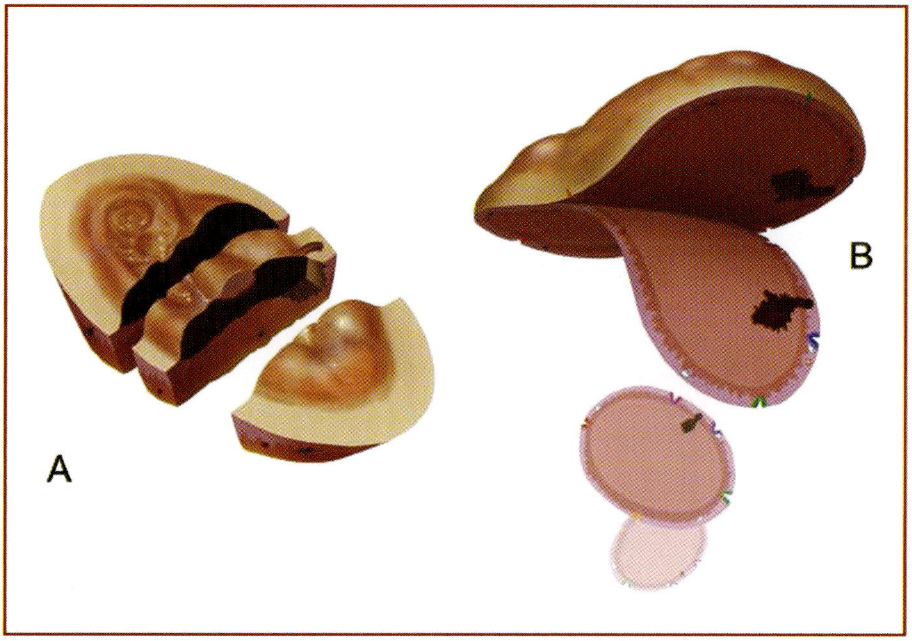

Figure 30–2. Standard "bread-loaf" (*A*) versus Mohs micrographic (*B*) sectioning of a cutaneous specimen. **A.** Transverse sectioning of tissue in "bread loaf" orientation consists of parallel cross-sections in series from one end of the specimen to the other. Less than 1% to 2% of the total margin is evaluated in this manner, with the potential for a false negative margin, if a root or vein of malignancy falls between sections. **B.** Mohs micrographic surgery (MMS) specimens are processed to examine 100% of the contact area between the Mohs specimen and the wound bed.

Mohs Surgery

In contrast to standard excision, Mohs micrographic surgery (MMS) specimens are not cross-sectioned. They are processed to examine 100% of the contact area between the Mohs specimen and the wound bed. This "complete view" is similar to compiling a mosaic of all possible adjacent contiguous en face sections, with each face parallel to a specific portion of the total contact area (see Fig 30–2). If the Mohs excision specimen were thought of as a freshly baked pie and the wound bed as a pie pan, the Mohs frozen sections would examine all of the pie crust where it contacts the pie pan, including the sides as well as the bottom. By evaluating 100% of the margin of excision, the chance of missing a root or vein of malignancy is substantially decreased.

Proponents argue that one primary advantage of Mohs surgery is that a single physician exerts continuity across all aspects of the Mohs process. One Mohs surgeon performs all steps of the resection process including resection of Mohs layer specimens while maintaining strict anatomical orientation, meticulous specimen mapping, interpretation of frozen section slides, and precise identification of residual disease on the Mohs map to guide further resection. This continuity and approach to margin assessment, in turn, provides complete margin control.

Precisely mapped, comprehensive margin evaluation with Mohs frozen sections provides the surgeon with the information necessary to continue surgical excision by tracking irregular, subclinical extension of the tumor. Although complex cases may be quite time consuming, MMS is performed while the wound bed is "fresh," and complete resection occurs prior to the development of extensive inflammation and granulation tissue, which can complicate histologic interpretation. Staged excisions with paraffin sections also are subject to postsurgical wound distortion and contraction that can alter the surgical site's contour and render accurate orientation more difficult.

With its advantages of precise orientation and comprehensive margin assessment, Mohs micrographic surgery has become the primary technique in the treatment of many skin cancers including basal cell carcinoma (BCC) and squamous cell carcinoma (SCC).[2,3] The success with which MMS has been applied to BCC and SCC is evidenced by its superior cure rates for most skin cancers.[2,3] Maintaining the delicate balance between comprehensive tumor extirpation and tissue preservation ultimately lowers the risk of functional loss and postoperative morbidity. When the tumor composition allows clearance with a resultant smaller surgical defect, less extensive reconstruction is required, improving the opportunity for optimal functional and aesthetic restoration.[1]

Mohs Surgery Training

To appreciate the basis for Mohs surgeons reading their own frozen section histology, it may be helpful to look at the scope of pathology training during dermatology residency and its practice within the specialty.

Dermatology is the only specialty other than pathology where diagnostic histopathology training in relevant diseases, dermatopathology, comprises a substantial portion of the overall training during residency. In order to become board-certified in dermatology, the candidate must demonstrate competency in diagnosing skin diseases by reading glass slide specimens during the dermatology board examination. Dermatologists are qualified to read and generate reports on the skin biopsies they perform. It also is the only medical specialty other than pathology where, upon completing residency, diplomates can apply for subspecialty dermatopathology fellowship training that is certified by the American Board of Pathology.

Accreditation Council for Graduate Medical Education (ACGME)-approved fellowship training after residency prepares the Mohs practitioner for the multiple roles of cutaneous oncologic surgeon, Mohs frozen section dermatopathologist, and cutaneous restorative surgeon.

Mohs Surgery Fundamentals

Patient Evaluation and Selection

Safe and effective Mohs resection begins with a thorough preoperative patient evaluation. A comprehensive medical history including comorbidities, relevant cancer history, medications, and allergies is reviewed. Specifically, the patient should be queried about symptoms suggestive of aggressive disease such as formication, numbness, paresthesias, and neck swelling or masses. Prior skin malignancies or lesions, as well as previous radiation therapy or exposure, should be elicited. Risk factors for aggressive cutaneous malignancy are reviewed elsewhere in this text.

Physical examination should focus on surface features such as ulceration, fixation to underlying tissues, and proximity to vital structures. Palpation of the "Z" axis, or thickness, is carried out to assess for apparent depth of invasion and whether the tumor is freely mobile. The Mohs surgeon must evaluate the tumor to determine if it meets the criteria for Mohs surgery in the outpatient setting under local anesthesia. Factors that may prompt additional evaluation such as scouting biopsies and imaging (computed tomography (CT) or magnetic resonance imaging (MRI)) include: suspicion of in-transit metastasis, perineural disease, lymph node involvement, and deep structural invasion of bone or muscle.

Patients having extraordinarily large lesions, clinical or radiographic perineural tumor invasion, an unusual number of local recurrences, or regional metastases benefit from multidisciplinary evaluation. A cutaneous oncology team that includes Mohs surgeons, head and neck surgeons, medical oncologists, and radiation therapists among others may provide valuable perspectives to optimize patient care. Certain extensive, more complex tumors may be amenable to combined resection of the tumor, using both Mohs micrographic and standard, en bloc, techniques.[4] MMS may be used to obtain clear peripheral margin under local anesthesia, followed by en bloc extirpation of the disease and involved structures, including cranial nerves in the setting of clinical or gross perineural invasion and lymph node involvement (Fig 30–3).

If the Mohs surgeon anticipates the defect to be too extensive or the patient is deemed inappropriate for reconstruction in the outpatient setting under local anesthesia, preoperative consultation with a plastic surgeon should be accomplished. Mohs surgical resection is readily performed in combination with delayed facial plastic surgery reconstruction.

Minimum selection criteria for Mohs micrographic surgery are depicted in Table 30–2.

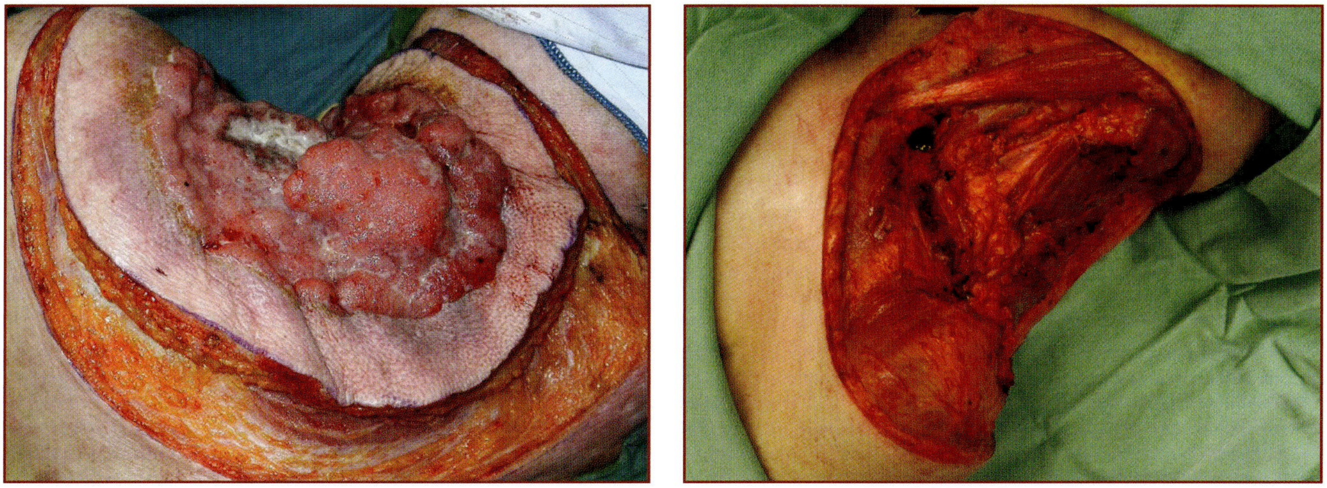

A B

Figure 30–3. Neglected basal cell carcinoma on the left posterolateral neck of a 63-year-old female. The peripheral margins were cleared by Mohs micrographic surgery (**A**), and then the patient underwent en bloc resection of the lesion, including platysma and modified radical neck dissection the following morning (**B**).

Table 30–2. Prerequisites for Mohs Micrographic Surgery

1. Contiguous tumor
2. Tumor type that is identifiable on frozen section histology
3. Extent of tumor does not preclude obtaining clear margins in the outpatient surgical setting under local anesthesia
4. Patient preference and comorbidities do not preclude a prolonged, awake procedure

MMS Technique

Correct identification of the biopsy site is accomplished with the patient using preoperative biopsy site photos if available. The patient is asked to verify this site as correct while viewing it in a mirror as part of the surgical "time-out." The clinical lesion is assessed for precise tumor marking under optimal lighting conditions, with or without wood's lamp, polarized magnification, or surgical loupes. The outer edge is then marked with a surgical marker or gentian violet liquid, and a 1- to 5-mm uninvolved margin is also precisely marked outside of the clinical tumor, depending on histology, grade, status as a primary or recurrent lesion, and other known features from the biopsy such as perineural invasion.

The Mohs surgeon may choose a round, oval, or an angulated outer margin based on the size and shape of the tumor. Choice of an appropriate size, shape, and thickness of a tissue layer that can be prepared in the Mohs frozen section histology lab can be complex, and it depends on the size, tumor grade, anatomic location, perceived depth of tumor, and tissue involved (Fig 30–4). Preoperative markings frequently include short "hash marks" that traverse the marked Mohs margin. After infiltrating local anesthetic, the patient is prepped and draped in the standard surgical fashion.

The first stage of resection is performed with a beveled edge that ranges from 30° to 90°, depending on the preference of the surgeon and the tissue involved. When the incision is perpendicular to the skin, it is termed a "no bevel" Mohs layer. The outer margin "hash marks" may be scored with short superficial transverse nicks placed lightly for accurate and secure specimen orientation. Prior to resection of the first stage, the central component of the lesion may be surgically debulked, curetted, or managed with intraoperative relaxing incisions. These techniques facilitate tissue processing by allowing the peripheral skin edge to more freely rotate down to the level of the deep tissue plane to promote contiguous 100% evaluation of both the deep and peripheral margins. Properly performed, these center specimen maneuvers do not violate any of the outer margins of the specimen, which constitutes the key portion of the Mohs layer (Fig 30–5).

Tissue Processing and Assessment

The first Mohs stage is placed on the transfer medium with appropriate annotation of precise specimen orientation. The transfer medium may include a photograph or drawing of the surgical site that matches the same design on the Mohs map, and the specimen is taken to the lab for processing. Depending on the specimen, it may be submitted as a single piece of tissue or divided into smaller sections, the sum of which will be analyzed to evaluate the complete margin. Processing is performed to allow visualization of the entire bottom as well as all of the sides of the specimen.

Processing may be simple or very complex, depending on the technique of the Mohs surgeon and the individual case. The advanced techniques required to process more difficult specimens are an essential part of Mohs surgery fellowship training. Improper processing of the specimen can lead to frozen sections that are impossible to evaluate or that contain substantial artifact that limits assessment. The specimen is precisely marked with colored tissue stain to accurately maintain orientation.

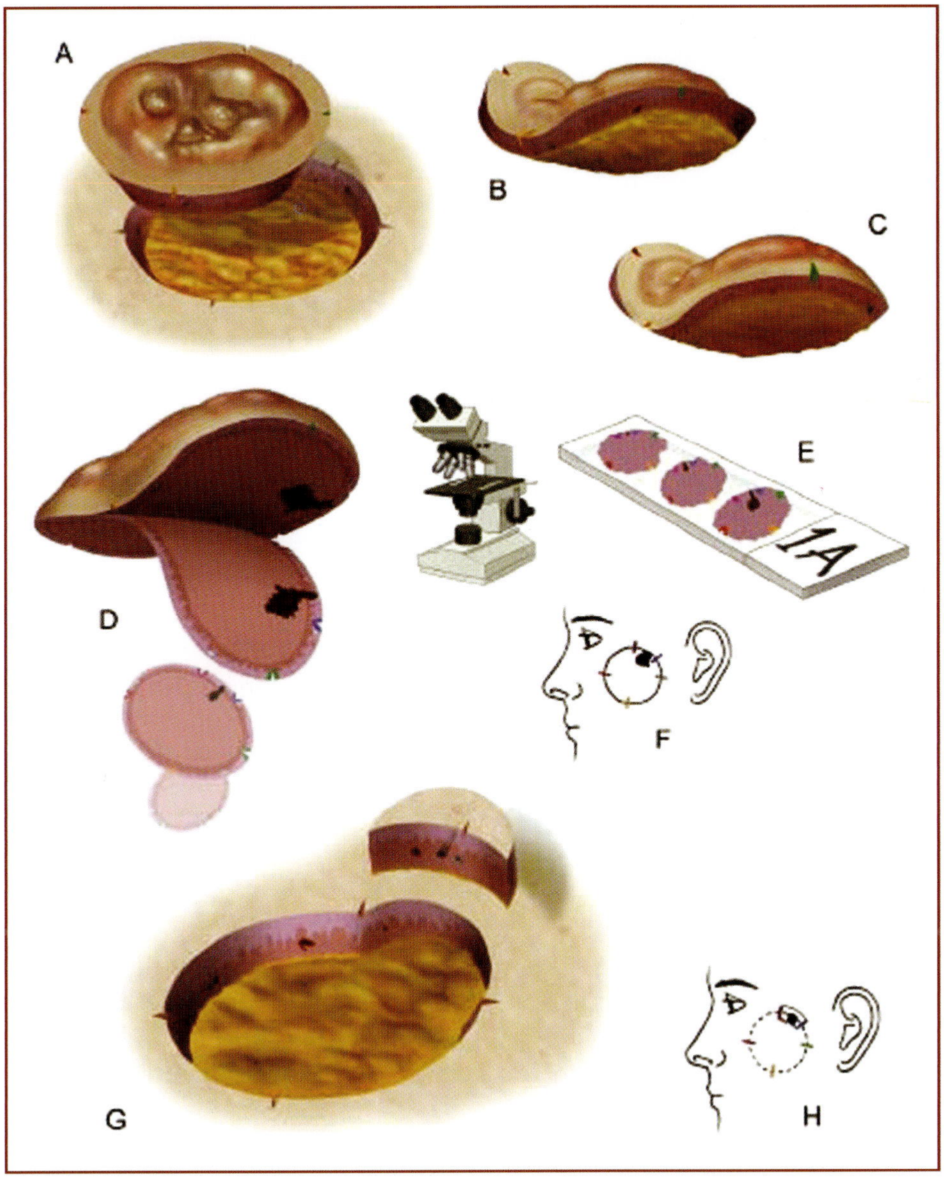

Figure 30–4. Process of Mohs micrographic surgery. **A.** Preoperative markings frequently include short "hash marks" that traverse the marked Mohs margin. **B.** The first stage of resection is performed with a beveled edge that ranges from 30° to 90°. **C.** Through a variety of maneuvers, the peripheral skin edge is rotated down to the level of the deep margin, thereby allowing simultaneous evaluation of 100% of the margin. **D.** The tissue is processed to visualize the entire bottom and sides of the lesion. **E.** The specimen is precisely marked with colored tissue stain to accurately maintain orientation. **F.** A precise representation of the Mohs layer is drawn on the Mohs map with the same color markings used on the specimen. **G.** If residual tumor is identified, it is precisely marked on the Mohs map to guide the next Mohs resection layer. **H.** The process is repeated until the margins are clear. Visual Art: © 2010 The University of Texas M.D. Anderson Cancer Center.

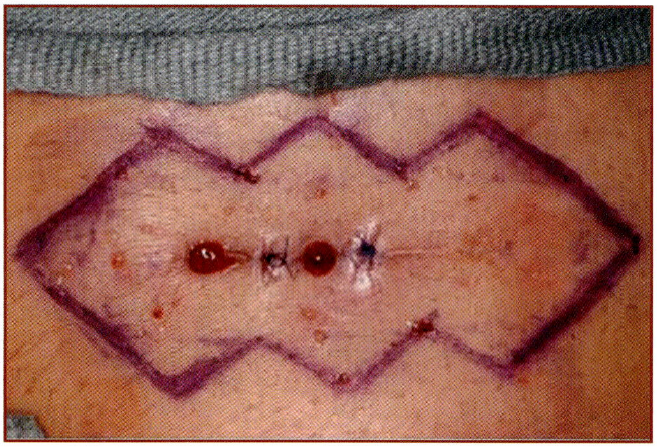

A

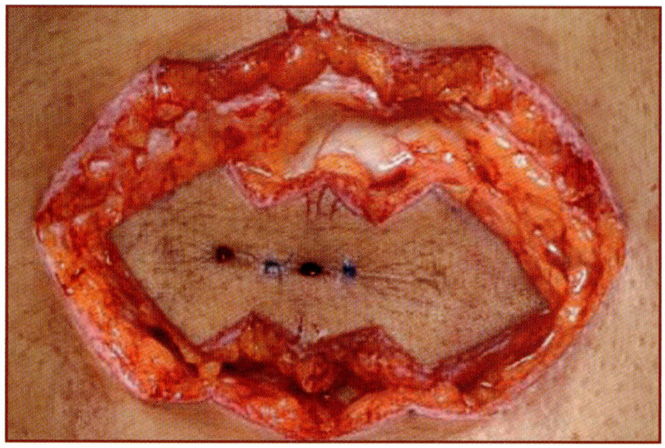

B

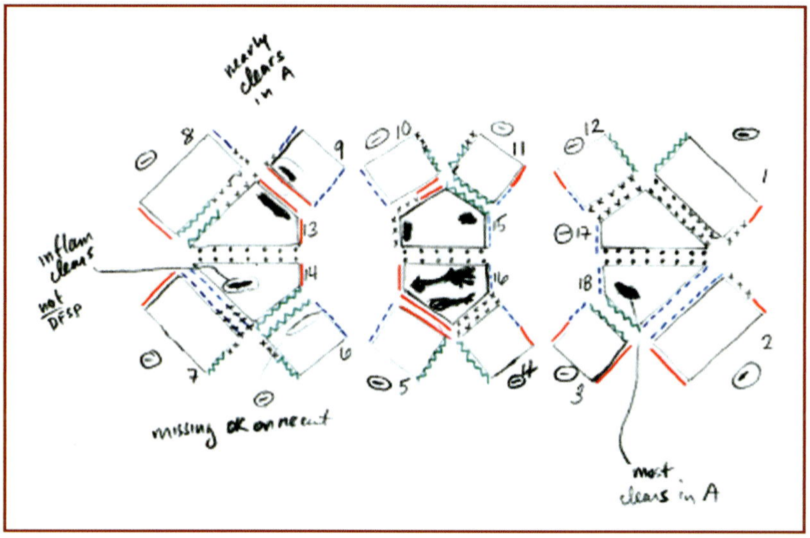

C

Figure 30–5. A. Preoperative markings for a dermatofibrosarcoma protuberans of the cheek. **B.** Angulated Mohs resection in situ. **C.** Comprehensive Mohs map of this complex specimen.

Furthermore, a precise representation of the Mohs layer is drawn on the Mohs map with the same color markings used on the specimen (Fig 30–6).

The specimen is embedded in optimal cutting temperature compound (OCT), and frozen sections are prepared. Glass slides are then stained in hematoxylin and eosin or toluidine blue. Once cover slipped, the frozen section slides are ready for evaluation by the Mohs surgeon. Immunohistochemical frozen section staining also can be performed to provide additional information in select cases and specific tumor types.

Tumor Clearance and Reconstruction

The corresponding Mohs map for the slides evaluated is placed adjacent to the microscope. If tumor is identified, it is precisely marked and annotated for subtype and tissue depth. Positive margins demand another focused resection stage, and this process is repeated until the margins are clear. Following tumor clearance, the majority of Mohs defects are reconstructed by the Mohs surgeon under local anesthesia. The benefits of this approach are many and include clinical-pathologic correlation, continuity of care,

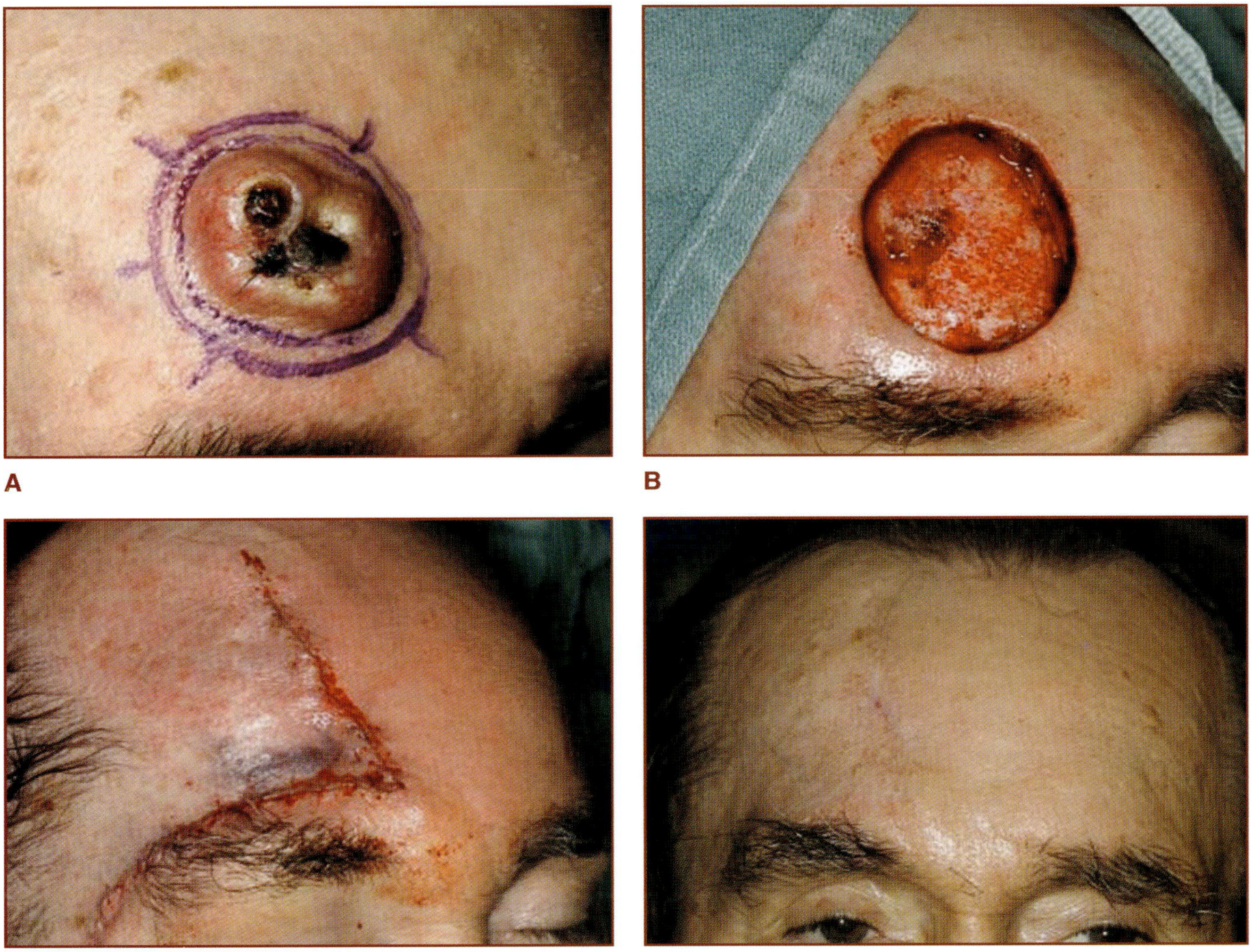

A B C D

Figure 30–6. **A.** Recurrent basal cell carcinoma of the forehead in a 74-year-old male with preoperative Mohs markings. **B.** Comprehensive tumor clearance was achieved, including resection of the periosteum. **C.** The defect was reconstructed with a local advancement-rotation flap. **D.** Postoperative result.

patient convenience, efficiency, and cost-effectiveness. Clinical-pathologic correlation refers to the awareness of surrounding precancerous changes both histologically and clinically. This often is identified by the Mohs surgeon during Mohs frozen sections and can be factored into the reconstructive plan. Under some circumstances, however, a reconstructive referral should be scheduled based on patient preference, nature of defect, or anesthesia requirements.

Indications for Mohs Surgery

Although Mohs surgery has been shown to be very effective in treating a wide range of skin cancers, there is no multidisciplinary consensus that requires its use to treat these malignancies. It is an extremely valuable technique in the multidisciplinary management of cutaneous malignancy. A detailed review of indications for MMS has been published by the Guidelines/Outcomes Committee of the American Academy of Dermatology.[5] These indications have been accepted across specialty lines, reflecting the widespread acceptance of this technique.[6] MMS often constitutes the ideal treatment for a given cutaneous neoplasm, based on its clinical features, histology, and patient considerations.

Clinical Features

Contiguous Tumor

Most skin cancers grow contiguously and therefore are appropriate to treat with Mohs surgery. Careful physical examination is essential to identify significantly multifocal lesions or in transit metastases that would render a tumor inappropriate for MMS.

Location

Mohs surgery is appropriate for most skin tumors of the head and neck. This encompasses the higher risk "H"-zone or mask area of the face, including the periorbital, perioral, periauricular, nasal, and glabellar units, as well as the functional areas of the ears, lips (cutaneous and mucosal), eyelids, and distal intranasal vestibule. Recurrence rates for treating SCC of the lip have been reported to be lower with Mohs surgery than with non-Mohs treatments.[3,7] The central face has extensive contour variation and is often composed of thin skin or mucosa overlying muscle, cartilage, and glands, in addition to blood vessels, sensory organs, and nerves. Skin cancers frequently invade these structures, potentially leading to substantial destruction. In these areas, contour variation and proximity to vital structures can make resection of recommended standard excision margins much more difficult, while avoiding anatomic distortion and functional compromise.

Although MMS is useful in reducing distortion and functional change, en bloc resection is commonly performed when bone, periocular tissue within the orbital septum, substantial oral cavity tissue beyond the lips, or intranasal tissue other than the distal vestibule are involved. Other locations where Mohs surgery is indicated include the hands, feet, digits, anogenital region, and pretibial lower extremity skin. These areas share a common theme of a limited tissue reservoir available for reconstruction and major structures located very superficially below the skin.

Size

In addition to clinical features such as location and for recurrent lesions, larger tumors may be amenable to Mohs surgery because they are higher risk neoplasms. Increasing tumor size correlates with an increased risk for wider subclinical extension and recurrence. Based on size alone, BCC and SCC lesions greater than 2 cm in any location are appropriate to consider for treatment with Mohs surgery.[2,3,6]

Clinical Presentation

Tumors that are recurrent, ill-defined, rapidly growing, ulcerated, or associated with significant pain or formication may be appropriate to treat with Mohs surgery.[6] Marjolin's ulcer, a particularly aggressive SCC that arises in an area of trauma, chronic inflammation, scar, or burn injury may be suitable for MMS if the size and degree of local extension are clinically appropriate. When very large or deeply invasive, Marjolin tumors should be managed with a multidisciplinary approach and en bloc resection.[6]

Histologic Considerations

Basal Cell Carcinoma

High risk basal cell carcinoma subtypes include infiltrative, morpheaform (also known as sclerosing), basosquamous, and micronodular. These subtypes are appropriate for treatment with Mohs surgery independent of their size and location. Perineural BCC may be a harbinger of aggressive behavior that is well suited for treatment with MMS. Gross perineural involvement may require adjunctive therapy using a multidisciplinary approach. Tumor extension of the infraorbital nerve, for example, is effectively tracked by Mohs surgery up to the infraorbital foramen. Continued extension beyond the foramen, however, requires bony resection under general anesthesia and postoperative radiation therapy. Ill-defined, multifocal, superficial basal cell carcinoma may be appropriate for treatment with MMS if treatment with a medical modality or curettage is not effective.[2,5,6]

Smaller, less aggressive subtypes of basal cell carcinoma outside of the central face and other functionally limiting locations can be treated effectively with a wide variety of non-Mohs modalities such as simple excision, electrodessication and curettage, cryotherapy, topical chemotherapy with imiquimod or 5-fluorouracil, intralesional interferon injection, or photodynamic therapy. Small, well-defined superficial and nodular subtype basal cell carcinoma are examples that may be appropriate for these non-Mohs excisional and destructive treatments.

Squamous Cell Carcinoma

SCC is a higher risk cutaneous malignancy than BCC for recurrence, metastasis, and, rarely, even death.[7] When there are clinical features that increase the risk for metastasis such as very deeply invasive lesions (substantially beyond the subcutaneous tissues), very large lesions involving the lips, orbits, or ears, signs or symptoms of perineural invasion, or lymphovascular invasion, multidisciplinary evaluation is essential.[8,9] Although the primary lesion may be managed with MMS, regional lymphadenectomy or adjuvant therapy may be necessary. In such cases, this author also recommends preoperative consultation with a head and neck surgeon for contingency scheduling in the event of extraordinary subclinical extension is found beyond what is reasonable to resect under local anesthesia. If imaging identifies an appropriate tumor, potential planned surgical collaboration may be considered.

Other features of SCC that increase risk for metastasis include moderately/poorly differentiated tumor, acantholytic subtype, desmoplastic tumor, and tumor with spindle cell features.

Squamous cell carcinoma in situ (SSCIS), also known as Bowen disease, may be treated with superficial destruction or topical therapy. MMS may be useful in larger lesions, or when the skin adnexa are involved. Verrucous carcinoma is also amenable to MMS, particularly in larger lesions with the potential for greater disruption of adjacent tissues. Similarly, keratoacanthoma, a rapidly growing neoplasm that may histologically resemble well-differentiated SCC and be locally destructive is appropriate for treatment with MMS.[1,5,6,8]

Other Nonmelanoma Skin Cancers

Although Mohs surgery is most frequently used for basal cell carcinoma and squamous cell carcinoma, the most common skin cancers, MMS has also been demonstrated to be effective in a variety of other cutaneous malignancies.

Microcystic Adnexal Carcinoma. Microcystic adnexal carcinoma (MAC), also called sclerosing sweat duct carcinoma, is an uncommon, very invasive, facial malignancy that clinically is often poorly defined and may be difficult to diagnose. The subclinical extent of the tumor is frequently found to extend far beyond the initial impression, potentially accounting for a high rate of recurrence with wide local excision. One study found that MAC is misdiagnosed in 30% of cases and MMS techniques tracking tumor extension resulted in a mean defect 4 times the size of the initial lesion.[10] This locally aggressive, but usually slow growing, tumor has a predilection for perioral, periocular, perinasal, or scalp tissue. Perineural invasion is often encountered, but metastases are rare. Local excision has an approximately 50% recurrence rate; whereas Mohs surgery has been reported to have an approximately 5% to 10% recurrence rate.[10,11] Due to the poorly defined nature of this disease, mapped scouting biopsies prior to treatment may provide a better starting point for the first stage of Mohs surgery.

Dermatofibrosarcoma Protuberans. Although dermatofibrosarcoma protuberans (DFSP) most frequently occurs on the trunk and upper limbs, the head and neck is also commonly involved. Although slow growing and rarely metastatic, DFSP may be locally destructive with a growth pattern of irregular tentacle-like strands of tumor that invade deeply and widely. Again, the clinically apparent tumor usually is much smaller than the subclinical spread, which may explain higher rates of local recurrence. Recurrence rates after WLE for DFSP of the head and neck treated with have been reported in the range of 50% to 75%.[12–14]

Due to the lack of randomized, controlled studies and few comparative studies, controversy over the ideal treatment method continues. A large 2008 comparative study using available treatment data pooled from the literature reported a recurrence rate 25 times lower with MMS than with WLE for head and neck tumors: 1.9% with MMS versus 51.8% with WLE.[15] Recurrence rates for standard margins have been reported to be as high as 39.7% for 2-cm and 15.5% for 3-cm margins.[16] Because larger excision margins can be difficult in the cosmetically and functionally sensitive head and neck, Mohs surgery may provide precise tumor mapping and excision of tumor tentacles while maximally sparing normal tissue. When using MMS to treat DFSP, the first stage margin should be increased to 5 to 10 mm from the periphery of the lesion, with subsequent stage margins 3 to 5 mm from the previous. The addition of CD34 immunohistochemistry staining of the Mohs frozen sections may differentiate DFSP from normal fibroblasts, which is particularly useful at the margins as tumor trails off into less cellular tissue.[16,17]

Atypical Fibroxanthoma. Atypical fibroxanthoma (AFX) commonly presents as an ulcerated nodule on sun damaged areas of the head and neck. It can be identified easily on frozen section as haphazardly arranged, pleomorphic, spindle cells that are frequently associated with multinucleated giant cells. Although AFX usually is found within the dermis, it may extend into deeper tissues and be locally destructive. It is considered a tumor with low metastatic potential, and most recurrences are believed to be due to incomplete excision. Reported recurrence rates range from 0% to 6.9% with MMS, and 9% to 16% with non-Mohs surgical treatment.[18–20]

Sebaceous Carcinoma. Sebaceous carcinoma (SC) is a relatively rare tumor found most commonly on the upper eyelids of patients over 60, although other areas of the head and neck can be involved. It can present as a painless yellowish-to-pink papule or nodule that may be mistaken for chalazion, blepharitis, or conjunctivitis. Muir-Torre syndrome should be considered in patients with SC, and the lesions may have basaloid or squamous features, potentially leading to misdiagnosis as BCC or SCC.[21] Regional lymph node metastases are estimated to occur in 17% to 30% of cases, with a 5-year survival rate of 50%.[21–23] Distant metastasis to muscle, liver, spleen, viscera, and the brain are uncommon, but portend a dismal 5-year survival rate.

Accurate early diagnosis with complete surgical extirpation within the first 6 months of presentation correlates with a much more favorable prognosis. Sebaceous carcinoma exhibits the potential for multifocal organization in up to 6% of cases, making any method of surgical resection challenging.[21] Even with this limitation, MMS has been reported to offer a reduced recurrence rate and better tissue sparing of vital eyelid and ocular structures when compared with WLE.[24] Potential adjunctive measures to MMS that are designed to maximize local control in SC include combining conjunctival map biopsies with Mohs surgery to track pagetoid conjunctival spread, resecting an additional Mohs layer of tissue beyond the stage appearing to clear the tumor, and submitting tissue for paraffin sections to confirm negative frozen margins.[25–28] Recurrence rates with MMS have been reported to be approximately 11% to 12%, compared to approximately 32% with WLE.[24,29]

Close collaboration with oculoplastic and head and neck surgeons is integral to the multidisciplinary approach to treatment of SC. Adjuvant, controlled cryotherapy to treat conjunctival extension, radiotherapy, chemotherapy, and lymph node dissection have been used in conjunction with both MMS and WLE, but radiotherapy alone may be ineffective.[26] Chemotherapy and elective lymph node dissection following local surgery have not been shown to improve disease-free survival.[21] Topical mitomycin-C treatment of conjunctival disease is controversial, but it may play a role in high-risk tumors.[30–32] Meticulous and frequent postoperative follow-up is essential to identify recurrences in this aggressive neoplasm.

Horizons of MMS in NMSC

Merkel cell carcinoma (MC) and cutaneous angiosarcoma (AS) represent aggressive cutaneous malignancies that commonly arise on the head and neck. These tumors frequently recur and metastasize, leading to generally poor survival rates in both conditions. Although wide excision is the traditional standard for local control in these malignancies, recent reports document the successful application of MMS in MC and AS. Contemporary recommendations for the management of these neoplasms are discussed elsewhere in this text. Applications of MMS to other rare cutaneous malignancies of the head and neck are continually evolving.

Merkel Cell Carcinoma. Merkel cell carcinoma forms in sun-exposed areas, and head and neck lesions are associated with high rates of local recurrence. A review of 86 patients with MC by O'Connor documented a marginal persistent rate in 12 patients who underwent MMS to be 8.3%, versus 31.7% in 41 patients who underwent WLE.[33] Regional lymph node metastases also were noted to occur less frequently in patients undergoing MMS compared to standard excision, although the follow-up is limited in the MMS patients.[33] Management of MC is best accomplished with a multidisciplinary approach, as sentinel lymph node biopsy with aggressive treatment of draining lymphatics by radiation or surgery may improve disease control.[34,35] Radiation therapy constitutes a critical consideration in the management of the primary site as well, regardless of surgical margin size or technique.[36]

Cutaneous Angiosarcoma. Cutaneous AS may present as an ill-defined, dusky red-to-violaceous patch that trails off into adjacent normal skin, often on the sun-exposed skin on the head and neck. It is very aggressive with an exceedingly low 5-year survival rate. There are only limited reports of MMS being used to treat AS, and the recurrence rate in these small groups is similar to that of WLE.[37,38] MMS also may play a role as an alternative to multiple scouting biopsies in delineating the tumor borders prior to radiation or electron-beam therapy.[39]

Melanoma In Situ and Invasive Malignant Melanoma

Although the topic remains controversial, treatment of invasive malignant melanoma (MM) and melanoma in situ (MIS) with Mohs surgery has been reported to be effective in multiple published case series. A pivotal 15-year study by Zitelli compared treatment of 553 primary stage I melanomas, including 369 invasive tumors, with MMS to historical data of 15,798 melanomas treated by WLE.[40] The first stage of MMS was taken with a 6-mm margin. Treatment with MMS demonstrated a 0.5% overall local recurrence rate and a 1.2% local recurrence rate on the head, neck, hands and feet. After stratification by Breslow depth into 5 groups, the metastasis and 5-year survival rates of the MMS groups were either equivalent to, or better than, those in the WLE group. The majority of melanomas were completely excised using 6-mm margins (83%), and 95% of lesions were cleared with margins less than 1 cm, regardless of Breslow thickness. However, most of the lesions requiring greater than 1 cm margins for clearance were found on the head, neck, hands, and feet.[40]

The authors acknowledge that their results are dependent on the Mohs surgeon's experience, as well as ensuring the highest standards of tissue processing in the Mohs histology laboratory.[40] This study was followed by a 2006 case series of 202 melanomas treated with MMS, including 69 invasive tumors, that employed a 5-mm initial margin for stage 1 of resection with excellent local control over a mean follow-up of 29.8 years.[41]

Similarly, lentigo maligna (LM) type of MIS, which is notorious for frequently having ill-defined clinical margins and higher local recurrence rates, may be well suited for treatment with MMS, particularly in anatomically sensitive locations.[41–43] Some authors recommend that MMS be combined with paraffin section confirmation of margins when treating LM.[43,44] Still others prefer the "square technique" of staged excision with en face permanent section evaluation of the margins prior to delayed resection of the central portion of the lesion over both MMS and standard WLE for treating LM.[45–47]

However, there is no current consensus recommending MMS for treatment of MM and LM. There is debate within the dermatopathology community about the ability to accurately identify melanoma on frozen section and whether en face sectioning without assessment of cross-sectional architecture is adequate to provide a diagnosis of clear margins.[48] The data supporting MMS in melanocytic lesions is evolving, and these additional studies may further support the technique.

More recent advances in the use of immunohistochemistry for frozen section assessment may pave the way for more widespread applications of MMS in melanoma and LM. Use of immunostains such as MART-1 will likely augment the accurate, high-quality, thin Mohs section technique used in other malignancies to render MMS increasingly accepted within the surgical oncology community.[49,50] Although the American Academy of Dermatology and the National Institutes of Health have acknowledged the benefits of Mohs micrographic surgery in treating melanoma, additional studies, particularly randomized, prospective trials, may help resolve this controversy.[51,52]

Regardless of the technique employed, invasive malignant melanoma of the head and neck is best treated using a multidisciplinary approach, based on accurate clinical and pathologic staging, to identify patients who need sentinel lymph node biopsy and adjuvant therapy.

Patient Considerations

There are many patient-specific variables that are valid when considering treatment with Mohs surgery. MMS is appropriate in individuals with multiple skin cancers from any cause, or in patients whose tumors display aggressive features, placing them at increased risk for substantial tissue destruction and functional loss. Patients with extreme environmental exposure manifest with overwhelming sun damage, and they frequently develop multiple skin cancers. By undergoing MMS, these patients can maximally spare their cutaneous "real estate" as a tissue reservoir that will be available during treatment of future lesions. Chronically immunosuppressed patients such as solid organ transplant recipients, those with chronic lymphocytic leukemia or other leukemia/lymphoma, and HIV/AIDS patients also are reasonable candidates for MMS. Patients with certain genetic conditions, like basal cell nevus syndrome, albinism, and xeroderma pigmentosum, that lead to a large number of skin cancers also may benefit from MMS.

Elderly patients are more likely to have significant medical comorbidities that may make place them at "high risk" for complications from general anesthesia, but they may be ideally suited for treatment with Mohs surgery under local anesthesia. When substantial comorbidities are identified, patients should be evaluated preoperatively to make sure that they are stable enough even for Mohs surgery performed in an outpatient setting. MMS also is appropriate in young patients with skin cancer from early substantial ultraviolet exposure as they are at risk for not only more aggressive lesions, but also an increased number of cutaneous malignancies over their lifetimes.

Treatment Alternatives to Mohs Surgery

MMS is a detailed, time-consuming process that is indicated for appropriate higher risk cutaneous malignancies. Several contraindications to MMS are summarized in Table 30–3. When review of tumor

Table 30–3. Relative Contraindications to Mohs Surgery

1. Tumor that is not contiguous
2. Tumor not readily identifiable in Mohs frozen sections
3. Anatomic access is limited
   a. External auditory canal
   b. Nasal vestibule
4. Location with substantial risk for tissue fragmentation
   a. Lacrimal crest
5. Structure is not amenable to resection in the outpatient environment
   a. Bone
   b. External auditory canal
   c. Muscle
   d. Salivary glands
   e. Intraconal ocular structures
   f. Major neurovascular trunks
6. Limitations of local anesthesia
   a. Extensive tumor in low threshold pain sensitive patient
   b. Anticipated prolonged procedure
7. Patient has a strong psychological aversion to procedure performed under local anesthesia
8. Advanced age or extreme comorbidities that may be associated with increased patient fatigue

type, size, anatomic location, and patient considerations are unfavorable for MMS, other treatment modalities should be pursued. En bloc resection with wide margins remains the mainstay in significantly higher risk, very deeply invasive disease and for other very extensive tumors not appropriate for resection under local anesthesia. On the other end of the spectrum, in less aesthetically concerning anatomic locations, wide local excision or one of the various methods of local destruction can treat lower risk skin cancers safely and cost-effectively with acceptable cure rates.

References

1. Brodland DG, Amonette R, Hanke CW, Robins P. The history and evolution of Mohs micrographic surgery. *Dermatol Surg*. 2000;26(4):303–307.
2. Rowe DE, Carroll RJ, Day CL, Jr. Long-term recurrence rates in previously untreated (primary) basal cell carcinoma: implications for patient follow-up. *J Dermatol Surg Oncol*. 1989;15(3):315–328.
3. Rowe DE, Carroll RJ, Day CL Jr. Prognostic factors for local recurrence, metastasis, and survival rates in squamous cell carcinoma of the skin, ear, and lip. Implications for treatment modality selection. *J Am Acad Dermatol*. 1992;26(6):976–990.
4. Ducic Y, Marra DE, Kennard C. Initial Mohs surgery followed by planned surgical resection of massive cutaneous carcinomas of the head and neck. *Laryngoscope*. 2009;119(4):774–777.
5. Drake LA, Dinehart SM, Goltz RW, et al. Guidelines of care for Mohs micrographic surgery. American Academy of Dermatology. *J Am Acad Dermatol*. 1995;33(2 pt 1): 271–278.
6. Minton TJ. Contemporary Mohs surgery applications. *Curr Opin Otolaryngol Head Neck Surg*. 2008;16(4):376–380.
7. Clayman GL, Lee JJ, Holsinger FC, et al. Mortality risk from squamous cell skin cancer. *J Clin Oncol*. 2005;23(4): 759–765.
8. Holmkvist KA, Roenigk RK. Squamous cell carcinoma of the lip treated with Mohs micrographic surgery: outcome at 5 years. *J Am Acad Dermatol*. 1998;38(6 pt 1): 960–966.
9. Moore BA, Weber RS, Priete V, et al. Lymph node metastasis from cutaneous squamous cell carcinoma of the head and neck. *Laryngoscope*. 2005;115(9):1561–1567.
10. Chiller K, Passaro D, Scheuller M, Singer M, McCalmont T, Grekin RC. Microcystic adnexal carcinoma: forty-eight cases, their treatment, and their outcome. *Arch Dermatol*. 2000;136(11):1355–1359.
11. Snow S, Madjar DD, Hardy S, et al. Microcystic adnexal carcinoma: report of 13 cases and review of the literature. *Dermatol Surg*. 2001;27(4):401–408.
12. Barnes L, Coleman JA, Jr., Johnson JT. Dermatofibrosarcoma protuberans of the head and neck. *Arch Otolaryngol*. 1984;110(6):398–404.
13. Snow SN, Gordon EM, Larson PO, Bagheri MM, Bentz ML, Sable DB. Dermatofibrosarcoma protuberans: a report on 29 patients treated by Mohs micrographic surgery with long-term follow-up and review of the literature. *Cancer*. 2004;101(1):28–38.
14. Sondak VK, Cimmino VM, Lowe LM, Dubay DA, Johnson TM. Dermatofibrosarcoma protuberans: what is the best surgical approach? *Surg Oncol*. 1999;8(4):183–189.
15. Paradisi A, Abeni D, Rusciani A, et al. Dermatofibrosarcoma protuberans: wide local excision vs. Mohs micrographic surgery. *Cancer Treat Rev*. 2008;34(8):728–736.
16. Ratner D, Thomas CO, Johnson TM, et al. Mohs micrographic surgery for the treatment of dermatofibrosarcoma protuberans. Results of a multiinstitutional series with an analysis of the extent of microscopic spread. *J Am Acad Dermatol*. 1997;37(4):600–613.
17. Huether MJ, Zitelli JA, Brodland DG. Mohs micrographic surgery for the treatment of spindle cell tumors of the skin. *J Am Acad Dermatol*. 2001;44(4):656–659.
18. Zalla MJ, Randle HW, Brodland DG, Davis JL, Roenigk RK. Mohs surgery vs wide excision for atypical fibroxanthoma: follow-up. *Dermatol Surg*. 1997;23(12):1223–1224.
19. Davis JL, Randle HW, Zalla MJ, Roenigk RK, Brodland DG. A comparison of Mohs micrographic surgery and wide excision for the treatment of atypical fibroxanthoma. *Dermatol Surg*. 1997;23(2):105–110.
20. Fretzin DF, Helwig EB. Atypical fibroxanthoma of the skin. A clinicopathologic study of 140 cases. *Cancer*. 1973; 31(6):1541–1552.
21. Cook BE, Jr, Bartley GB. Treatment options and future prospects for the management of eyelid malignancies: an evidence-based update. *Ophthalmology*. 2001;108(11): 2088–2098; quiz 2099–2100, 2121.
22. Ratz JL, Luu-Duong S, Kulwin DR. Sebaceous carcinoma of the eyelid treated with Mohs' surgery. *J Am Acad Dermatol*. 1986;14(4):668–673.
23. O'Neal ML, Brunson A, Spadafora J. Ocular sebaceous carcinoma: case report and review of the literature. *Compr Ther*. 2001;27(2):144–147.
24. Snow SN, Larson PO, Lucarelli MJ, Lemke BN, Madjar DD. Sebaceous carcinoma of the eyelids treated by mohs micrographic surgery: report of nine cases with review of the literature. *Dermatol Surg*. 2002;28(7):623–631.
25. Arora A, Barlow RJ, Williamson JM, Olver JM. Eyelid sebaceous gland carcinoma (SGC) treated with "slow" Mohs micrographic surgery. *Eye (Lond)*. 2004;18(8):854–855.
26. Cook BE, Jr., Bartley GB. Treatment options and future prospects for the management of eyelid malignancies: an evidence-based update. *Ophthalmology*. 2001;108(11): 2088–2098; quiz 2099–2100, 2121.

27. Yount AB, Bylund D, Pratt SG, Greenway HT. Mohs micrographic excision of sebaceous carcinoma of the eyelids. *J Dermatol Surg Oncol.* 1994;20(8):523–529.
28. Dzubow LM. Sebaceous carcinoma of the eyelid: treatment with Mohs surgery. *J Dermatol Surg Oncol.* 1985; 11(1):40–44.
29. Spencer JM, Nossa R, Tse DT, Sequeira M. Sebaceous carcinoma of the eyelid treated with Mohs micrographic surgery. *J Am Acad Dermatol.* 2001;44(6):1004–1009.
30. Rudkin AK, Muecke JS. Mitomycin-C as adjuvant therapy in the treatment of sebaceous gland carcinoma in high-risk locations. *Clin Experiment Ophthalmol.* 2009; 37(4):352–356.
31. Tumuluri K, Kourt G, Martin P. Mitomycin C in sebaceous gland carcinoma with pagetoid spread. *Br J Ophthalmol.* 2004;88(5):718–719.
32. Shields CL, Naseripour M, Shields JA, Eagle RC, Jr. Topical mitomycin-C for pagetoid invasion of the conjunctiva by eyelid sebaceous gland carcinoma. *Ophthalmology.* 2002;109(11):2129–2133.
33. O'Connor WJ, Roenigk RK, Brodland DG. Merkel cell carcinoma. Comparison of Mohs micrographic surgery and wide excision in 86 patients. *Dermatol Surg.* 1997; 23(10):929–933.
34. Schmalbach CE, Lowe L, Teknos TN, Johnson TM, Bradford CR. Reliability of sentinel lymph node biopsy for regional staging of head and neck Merkel cell carcinoma. *Arch Otolaryngol Head Neck Surg.* 2005;131(7):610–614.
35. Lawenda BD, Arnold MG, Tokarz VA, et al. Analysis of radiation therapy for the control of Merkel cell carcinoma of the head and neck based on 36 cases and a literature review. *Ear Nose Throat J.* 2008;87(11):634–643.
36. Gillenwater AM, Hessel AH, Morrison WH, et al. Merkel cell carcinoma of the head and neck—effect of surgical excision and radiation on recurrence and survival. *Arch Otolaryngol Head Neck Surg.* 2001;127(2):149–154.
37. Muscarella VA. Angiosarcoma treated by Mohs micrographic surgery. *J Dermatol Surg Oncol.* 1993;19(12): 1132–1133.
38. Goldberg DJ, Kim YA. Angiosarcoma of the scalp treated with Mohs micrographic surgery. *J Dermatol Surg Oncol.* 1993;19(2):156–158.
39. Bullen R, Larson PO, Landeck AE, et al. Angiosarcoma of the head and neck managed by a combination of multiple biopsies to determine tumor margin and radiation therapy. Report of three cases and review of the literature. *Dermatol Surg.* 1998;24(10):1105–1110.
40. Zitelli JA, Brown C, Hanusa BH. Mohs micrographic surgery for the treatment of primary cutaneous melanoma. *J Am Acad Dermatol.* 1997;37(2 pt 1):236–245.
41. Temple CL, Arlette JP. Mohs micrographic surgery in the treatment of lentigo maligna and melanoma. *J Surg Oncol.* 2006;94(4):287–292.
42. Cohen LM, McCall MW, Zax RH. Mohs micrographic surgery for lentigo maligna and lentigo maligna melanoma. A follow-up study. *Dermatol Surg.* 1998;24(6): 673–677.
43. Cohen LM, McCall MW, Hodge SJ, Freedman JD, Callen JP, Zax RH. Successful treatment of lentigo maligna and lentigo maligna melanoma with Mohs micrographic surgery aided by rush permanent sections. *Cancer.* 1994; 73(12):2964–2970.
44. Zitelli JA. Mohs surgery for lentigo maligna. *Arch Dermatol.* 1991;127(11):1729–1730.
45. Zalla MJ, Lim KK, Dicaudo DJ, Gagnot MM. Mohs micrographic excision of melanoma using immunostains. *Dermatol Surg.* 2000;26(8):771–784.
46. Johnson TM, Headington JT, Baker SR, Lowe L. Usefulness of the staged excision for lentigo maligna and lentigo maligna melanoma: the "square" procedure. *J Am Acad Dermatol.* 1997;37(5 pt 1):758–764.
47. Huilgol SC, Selva D, Chen C, et al. Surgical margins for lentigo maligna and lentigo maligna melanoma: the technique of mapped serial excision. *Arch Dermatol.* 2004;140(9):1087–1092.
48. Smith-Zagone MJ, Schwartz MR. Frozen section of skin specimens. *Arch Pathol Lab Med.* 2005;129(12):1536–1543.
49. El Tal AK, Abrou AE, Stiff MA, Mehregan DA. Immunostaining in Mohs micrographic surgery: a review. *Dermatol Surg.* 2010;36(3):275–290.
50. Whalen J, Leone D. Mohs micrographic surgery for the treatment of malignant melanoma. *Clin Dermatol.* 2009; 27(6):597–602.
51. Guidelines of care for malignant melanoma. Committee on Guidelines of Care. Task Force on Malignant Melanoma. *J Am Acad Dermatol.* 1993;28(4):638–641.
52. NIH Consensus Conference. Diagnosis and treatment of early melanoma. *JAMA.* 1992;268(10):1314–1319.

31

MOHS SURGERY: ADJUNCTIVE TREATMENT OF SKIN CANCER

VALENCIA D. THOMAS
KIMBERLY THOMAS

Introduction

The nonsurgical management of premalignant and malignant tumors of the skin has evolved over the past century. Although surgery remains the cornerstone of treatment for aggressive or recurrent nonmelanoma skin cancer (NMSC), medical treatments and superficial destructive measures serve as alternative primary or adjunctive measures. Treatment with topical medications, intralesional medications, and superficial destructive methods constitute the vast majority of the nonsurgical management of cutaneous premalignant and malignant conditions. The recent development of topical immunomodulators has further expanded the breadth of topical treatment to potentially include melanoma in-situ and extramammary Paget's disease (EMPD). The decision to pursue nonsurgical treatment modalities either as primary or adjuvant therapy is based on tumor type, clinical context, patient compliance, and overall treatment expectations. Table 31–1 summarizes presently available nonsurgical therapies.

Premalignant and Malignant Tumors of Epidermal Origin Amenable to Nonsurgical Modalities

Actinic Keratoses (AK)

Actinic keratoses are precancerous lesions displaying partial-thickness epidermal atypia; they represent the earliest and least aggressive tumor on the keratinocytic spectrum of malignancies. These lesions arise from excess ultraviolet light exposure and it has been estimated that more than 60% of individuals over the age of 40 are affected.[1] In cases of severe sun damage, confluent AKs may be identified on sun-exposed areas. In one study, the rate of transformation from AK to SCC in the first year was reported to be 0.6%.[2,3]

Basal cell carcinomas may also arise from AK precursor lesions. Variants of AK include hypertrophic (thick), hyperkeratotic (scaly), and acantholytic

Table 31–1. Dosing and Treatment Guidelines in the Management of AK and NMSC

Agent	Tumor	Recommended Dosing	FDA-Approved
5-Fluorouracil cream or solution	AK	• 2 or 5% solution or cream topically twice daily for 2–6 weeks • 0.5% microsphere formulation once daily for up to 4 weeks	Yes
	SCCIS	• Dosing and timing not yet determined • SBCC: 5% cream or solution twice daily for 3–12 weeks	No
	SCC	• 0.8 to 3 ml intralesionally of 50 mg/ml solution every 1–3 weeks for 8 weeks or until clinically resolved	No
Imiquimod cream	AK	• Apply nightly for at least 8 hours twice weekly for 6 weeks	Yes
	SBCC	• Apply nightly for 8 hours 5 days per week for 6 weeks • Tumors ranging from 0.5 to 1 cm require a 10 mg (4-mm diameter of cream); 1 to 1.5-cm tumors require 25-mg (5-mm droplet); and tumors 1.5 to 2 cm require 40 mg of cream (7 mm of cream)	Yes
Interferon alpha 2B	SCC, BCC	• 1.5×10^6 IU intralesionally 3 times a week for 3 weeks or • 1.0 to 2.5×10^6 IU intralesionally 3 times a week for 3 weeks	No
Bleomycin	SCCIS	• Bleomycin in 1% lignocaine intralesionally every 3–6 week intervals to a cumulative total of 6.35 U	No
Diclofenac	SCCIS	• 3% diclofenac in 2.5% hyaluronic acid gel topically twice a day for 90 days	Yes

AK: actinic keratosis; BCC Basal cell carcinoma; SBCC Superficial basal cell carcinoma; SCCIS squamous cell carcinoma in situ; SCC squamous cell carcinoma.

(weepy or erosive due to loss of adhesion between keratinocytes) types. Follicular or proliferative AKs represent lesions that involve hair follicles or adnexal structures. Although the follicular variant is still considered to be a premalignant lesion, involvement of adnexal structures may be more difficult to treat because the lesion may have a reservoir in the adnexal epithelium.

Squamous Cell Carcinoma in Situ (SCCIS, Bowen's Disease) and Squamous Cell Carcinoma (SCC)

Squamous cell carcinomas (SCC) represent about 200,000 to 300,000 of the more than 1 million non-melanoma skin cancers identified annually in the

United States, with approximately 75% of these tumors arising on the head and neck.[4,5] Cutaneous SCCs are a malignancy of the epidermal keratinocytes, which usually arise in response to prolonged ultraviolet radiation. Other risk factors for the development of SCCs include older age, male sex, chemical exposure (arsenic), chronic ulcers, fair skin, blond or red hair, blue eyes, and chronic scarring conditions.[6] Solid organ transplant recipients have a risk of developing skin cancer that is up to 250-fold greater than that of the general population.[7–9]

Most cutaneous SCCs do not metastasize, with an overall metastatic rate between 3% to 5%.[10] Metastatic disease usually involves regional lymph nodes, particularly in the parotid gland, but a small proportion of tumors spread to distant sites. Although the case-fatality rate for cutaneous SCC is only approximately 1%, more people die from SCC than from melanoma.[6,11,12] Among organ transplant recipients, the mortality rate reaches 8%.[9] Squamous cell carcinoma in situ (SCCIS) represents the intraepidermal form of SCC that displays full-thickness epidermal atypia. These lesions are notable for their hyperkeratosis with the formation of occasional cutaneous horns. Unlike AK, most SCCIS tend to involve terminal hair follicles and often arise in association with warts. The association between oncogenic human papilloma virus (HPV) and squamous cell carcinoma is well known, although the vast majority of lesions arise from excess sun exposure. If the malignant proliferation extends through the basement membrane, then the lesion is termed invasive squamous cell carcinoma (SCC). Commonly, AK and SCCIS can be found at the margins of SCC excisions. Myriad nonsurgical treatments are available for SCCIS, including topical 5-fluorouracil, imiquimod, and topical tretinoin. Complete surgical extirpation is the mainstay of treatment for uncomplicated, invasive SCC. High reported cure rates are achieved with Mohs micrographic surgery (MMS), with rates reaching 95% to 98%. Intralesional therapy has been used in the past as a viable alternative for patients with nonaggressive SCC who are not good surgical candidates or for those who decline surgery. Intralesional medications including 5-fluorouracil, bleomycin, or interferon alpha-2a may be effective in the treatment of nonaggressive SCC. There have been reports of excisions with positive margins being treated with adjunctive intralesional therapy.[13] Recurrent tumors after nonsurgical therapy merit complete surgical tumor extirpation. Following complete excision, recurrent SCCs may represent a category of high-risk SCCs that may benefit from adjuvant chemotherapy or radiotherapy.

Nonsurgical therapies for aggressive SCC is strongly discouraged. High-risk cutaneous SCC typically is defined as a lesion with a greater than 5% chance of subclinical metastases; aggressive clinical behavior (as evidenced by prior recurrence, involvement of deep tissues, depth greater than 4 mm, occurrence in prior scars, or tumor size greater than 2 cm); aggressive histologic features (poorly differentiated tumor histology, lymphovascular invasion, or perineural invasion), location in high-risk areas such as the temporoparietal region or midface; and host immunosuppression from solid-organ transplantation, hematologic malignancy, or HIV infection, among other causes.[14–17] The metastatic rate of tumors larger than 2 cm may be triple that of lesions less than 2 cm, with lesions exceeding 4 cm significantly correlating with disease-specific mortality.[5,6,17] Dermal invasion of the tumor greater than 4 mm and beyond the subcutis also independently correlates with an increased risk of subclinical metastases.[16] Such atypical, aggressive lesions may require postoperative radiation therapy to decrease the risk of recurrence or metastasis.

Superficial Basal Cell Carcinoma (SBCC) and Basal Cell Carcinoma (BCC)

Basal cell carcinoma (BCC) is the most common cancer in humans and is overwhelmingly associated with prolonged sun exposure. Of the more than 1 million nonmelanoma skin cancers diagnosed in the US every year, 800,000 to 900,000 will be BCC. A malignancy of basal layer keratinocytes, the disease exhibits many histologic subtypes.

Superficial basal cell carcinoma (SBCC) is a variant of BCC that projects directly from the epidermis and is most commonly found on the trunk. Superficial and nodular BCC represent the vast majority of BCC, and they are highly responsive to most interventions. Treatment options include routine topical, destructive, or surgical methods such as imiquimod, 5-fluorouracil, interferon-alpha 2b, photodynamic therapy, electrodessication and curettage, cryotherapy, or laser ablation. Intralesional therapy may be used in the management of nodular BCC alone or after incomplete excision.

Recurrent lesions or more aggressive subtypes such as infiltrative/morpheaform, micronodular, and basosquamous lesions, although less common, require surgical excision with clear surgical margins or Mohs-assisted excision to achieve local disease control.[18–22] Up to 3% of infiltrative, or morpheaform, and basosquamous subtypes of BCC are estimated to have perineural invasion (PNI).[22] Aggressive basal cell carcinomas are most commonly located on the head and neck. As with squamous cell carcinoma, BCCs displaying PNI are associated with an aggressive growth pattern, recurrence, larger tumor size, and significant subclinical extension.[23] Unlike SCC, basal cell carcinomas tend to invade via direct tumor extension, rarely metastasizing to regional lymph nodes, but occasionally demonstrating hematogenous spread to the viscera and bone.[24,25]

As with SCC, high-risk tumors with the above aggressive features are not suitable for conservative management with topical or superficial destructive methods—they may even require aggressive adjunctive therapy to increase the likelihood of cure. The main adjunctive therapies for aggressive BCC include radiation therapy for local disease and chemotherapy for metastatic disease. Platinum-based chemotherapy regimens constitute the most effective therapy for metastatic disease, with overall response rates up to 77%.[26,27] Other agents, including 5-fluorouracil, doxorubicin, vincristine, docetaxel, prednisone, and interferon have been used, although currently there is not a systemic agent appropriate for control of local disease.[22]

Medical Adjunctive Treatments for AK and NMSC

5-Fluorouracil (5-FU)

5-Fluorouracil is a pyrimidine antimetabolite that inhibits DNA and RNA synthesis during the S phase of the cell cycle. This DNA and RNA inhibition preferentially affects rapidly dividing cells, resulting in abnormal growth and cell death.[28] Topical 5-FU cream and solution have been widely used for the treatment of AK, SCCIS, and SBCC.[29]

The successful treatment of AK can be achieved with twice-daily application of 2% or 5% cream or solution for 2 to 6 weeks (Fig 31–1). Total clearance of AK after 4 weeks of therapy has been reported to be 43% at a follow-up of 4 weeks.[30] Topical application of 5-FU cream or solution 5% twice daily for 3 to 6 weeks up to a total of 10 to 12 weeks has also been approved by the Food and Drug Association (FDA) for the treatment of superficial BCC.[28]

Although effective, this cream causes local erythema, crusting, scaling with occasional itching, ulceration, photosensitivity, and pain at the treatment site. In an attempt to overcome these side effects, a 0.5% microsphere formulation has been formulated that reportedly causes fewer cutaneous reactions. Dosing for AK is daily for up to 4 weeks with the 0.5% microsphere formulation.

Although successful treatment of SCCIS, erythroplasia of queryat, and condyloma acuminatum has been described, the exact dosing regimen for these conditions has not been determined. The recurrence rate of 5-FU for the treatment of SCCIS has been reported as 14% within 5 years.[31] Use of this antimetabolite is contraindicated in patients with dihydropyrimidine dehydrogenase enzyme

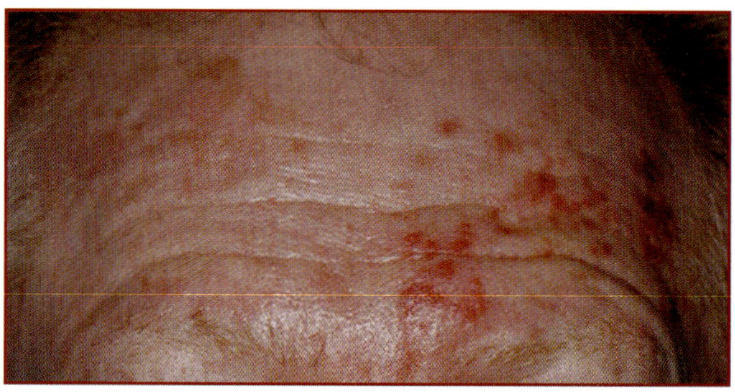

Figure 31–1. Actinic keratoses treated with 5-fluorouracil cream. The right side of the forehead is one-month status-post 3 weeks of 5-fluorouracil cream applied twice a day. The left side of the forehead is currently undergoing treatment with 5-fluorouracil cream.

deficiency and in patients with a hypersensitivity to fluorouracil or capecitabine. 5-FU is pregnancy category X and the World Health Organization (WHO) recommends avoiding breastfeeding if using this drug. Following topical treatment with 5-FU, supportive care with moisturizers or topical steroids may be indicated to control inflammation and to promote healing.[28]

Intralesional administration of fluorouracil solution, 50 mg/ml, has been described to successfully treat invasive squamous cell carcinoma, but the FDA has not approved this indication. Reported treatment regimens of intralesional 5-FU for SCC range from 0.8 to 3 ml every 1 to 3 weeks for 8 weeks, or until full clinical resolution is achieved.[32,33] Intravenous 5-FU is reserved for the treatment of metastatic squamous cell carcinoma.

Imiquimod

Imiquimod is an immune modulator whose efficacy derives from the local upregulation of tumor necrosis factor alpha (TNF-α). Although it does not have explicit antiviral properties, this topical medication was initially approved for the treatment of external condyloma acuminatum. The upregulation of TNF-α was later found to be efficacious in the treatment of nonhyperkeratotic, nonhypertrophic AKs on the face and neck, as well as SBCC of the trunk, neck, or extremities. The recommended dose of imiquimod for AK requires local application for 8 hours at bedtime twice weekly for 16 weeks. Total clearance of AK using this regimen is reported to be 45%.[34] Use of the cream nightly for 8 hours 5 days per week for 6 weeks is recommended for the treatment of SBCC.

The amount of imiquimod recommended varies according to tumor size. Tumors ranging from 0.5 to 1 cm require a 10 mg (4-mm diameter of cream); 1 to 1.5-cm tumors require 25 mg (5-mm droplet); and tumors 1.5 to 2 cm require 40 mg of cream (7 mm of cream).[35] Imiquimod has been used off-label for the treatment of SCCIS, melanoma in situ, and EMPD, but dosing recommendations have not been standardized.[36–41]

Continued follow-up is critical to the successful use of this immune modulator, regardless of the tumor treated and the dosing regimen used. As with all nonsurgical methods, the lack of histologic confirmation of clear surgical margins mandates close continued clinical follow-up. Side effects during therapy include local site reactions (erythema, itching, pain, discomfort) and rare reports of flulike symptoms. Imiquimod is pregnancy category C and the effects of the cream during breastfeeding are not known.[35]

Interferon Alpha-2B (IFNα-2B)

Since their discovery in 1957, the family of glycoproteins known as interferons has been extensively investigated and found to be an important part of the immune response. Secreted in response to viral infections, these agents have been found to have immunomodulatory and antiproliferative effects.[42] IFNα-2b is secreted primarily by white blood cells and is FDA-approved for the treatment of AIDS-related Kaposi's sarcoma, hairy cell leukemia, follicular lymphoma, chronic hepatitis C, malignant melanoma, and condyloma acuminatum.[43]

Treatment of SCC and BCC with IFNα-2b is off-label. In the initial pilot tudy by Greenway in 1986, intralesional injections of 1.5×10^6 IU IFNα-2b were administered 3 times a week for 3 weeks.[44] The efficacy of this treatment modality has subsequently been widely established, with successful doses ranging from 1.0 to 2.5×10^6 IU and clinical resolution noted at approximately 8 weeks.[42,44,45] The overall cure rate is estimated to range between 75% to 81%, although only one placebo-controlled study exists.[45,46] Treatment efficacy should be assessed at 16 weeks.[46]

IFNα-2b is not a first-line therapy for the treatment of SCC and BCC because surgical excision and other treatment modalities offer a better cure rate, so this treatment is not FDA-approved.[46] If this modality is pursued, it is likely that the patient is a poor surgical candidate or that surgery would result in excessive morbidity or disfigurement. When successful, this modality may produce excellent cosmetic results. Side effects of intralesional IFNα-2b include flulike symptoms, fatigue, hair-loss, diarrhea, or neurologic or psychiatric issues. IFNα-2b is contraindicated in patients with autoimmune hepatitis, decompensated liver disease, or hypersensitivity to interferons.[43]

Bleomycin

Bleomycin is a cytotoxic antibiotic that is widely used as a systemic chemotherapeutic agent in the treatment of squamous cell carcinomas arising from mucosal epithelium, including squamous cell carcinoma of the head and neck, cervix, penis, and vulva. Off-label applications of this drug have been widely reported in the treatment of verruca vulgaris and SCCIS. Verruca vulgaris may be treated with 1 unit per mL administered in multiple punctures.

The use of intralesional bleomycin for cutaneous malignancies is not a common practice. A case of SCCIS treated with bleomycin in 1% lignocaine was injected at 3- to 6-week intervals to a cumulative total of 6.35 U resulted in clinical clearance with without recurrence at 18 months.[47] Electrochemo - therapy, the administration of local chemotherapy followed by electric pulses, using bleomycin has been reported to be successful, although no standard protocol exists.[48] This cytotoxic agent may result in pulmonary fibrosis at doses greater than 400 units and is pregnancy category D.[47]

Retinoids

Retinoids can play a critical role in the chemoprevention, rather than the treatment, of nonmelanoma skin cancers. Topical and systemic retinoids are powerful agents that are structurally similar to vitamin A and act via a family of steroid nuclear receptors with direct effects on DNA and RNA synthesis. Although the exact mechanism of action of these agents is not known, these drugs display antiproliferative, antineoplastic, and keratolytic effects. Retinoids are thought to prevent genomic damage, epigenetic damage, and the progression of damage sustained by cells undergoing malignant transformation.[49] Retinoids are FDA-approved for the treatment of acne and acute promyelocytic leukemia in the oral form, and topical retinoids are approved for the treatment of fine lines and wrinkles, tactile roughness, and hyperpigmentation of the skin.[50]

Although studies have shown efficacy of topical retinoids in promoting regression of AKs, their variable efficacy supports their role as an adjunctive measure when used in combination with other therapies.[50] Otley et al[51] delineated the general and specific indications for the use in NMSC. In general, patients with more than five skin cancers per year with or without actinic keratoses, those with eruptive keratoacanthomas, or those with aggressive NMSC may benefit from prophylactic therapy with acitretin or tretinoin. Specifically, solid-organ transplant, immunosuppressed, or tumor syndrome patients (basal cell nevus, Bazex, or Rombo syndrome) who are at significantly higher risk of NMSC may benefit from oral retinoid therapy. Recommended dosing regimens for acitretin begins at 10 mg orally every other day for 2 weeks followed by 10 mg daily for 2 weeks, and finally 20 mg orally daily as tolerated. The recommended tretinoin dose is 0.25 mg per kg every other day for one month, 0.25 mg per kg daily for one month, and 0.5 mg per kg thereafter, titrated to tolerance.[51]

Side effects of oral retinoid therapy include hypertriglyceridemia, hyperlipidemia, elevated liver function tests, eye dryness, and xerosis (dry skin).[51] Routine blood tests to check lipid levels and liver function are recommended monthly for every 3 months following dose changes. The use of retinoids is contraindicated in those with hypersensitivity to retinoids, chronically elevated liver enzymes, patients on methotrexate or tetracyclines, and in pregnant patients or those who desire pregnancy in the 3 years following therapy.[49] Topical retinoids are pregnancy category D with topical tazarotene being pregnancy category X. Oral retinoids are pregnancy category X.[49]

Diclofenac

Diclofenac is a nonsteroidal antiinflammatory agent with antitumor activity. Although the exact mechanism of action is unclear, this drug specifically blocks cyclo-oxygenase-2 and thus disrupts prostaglandin synthesis.[52] Other proposed mechanisms of action include the induction of apoptosis, disruption of angiogenesis, and actions via nuclear hormone receptors.[53–55] The FDA-recommended method for the treatment of AK is to apply the 3% diclofenac in 2.5% hyaluronic acid gel twice a day for 90 days. This results in a total clearance of 50% of lesions at 30 days.[56]

Adverse cutaneous effects include application site reactions such as erythema and irritation. Diclofenac carries a "black box" warning from the FDA due to an increased risk of serious and potentially fatal cardiovascular thrombotic events, myocardial infarction, and stroke observed with the use of NSAIDS. Additionally, gastrointestinal events, including bleeding and ulceration, are noted. This drug is contraindicated in individuals with a history of hypersensitivity or allergic reactions to aspirin and NSAIDS, as well as in patients with preoperative pain in the setting of coronary artery bypass graft. This medication is pregnancy category C in the first 2 trimesters and D in the third trimester. Risks of this medication during lactation cannot be ruled out.[57]

Procedure-Based Adjunctive Treatments for AK and NMSC

Photodynamic Therapy

The destruction of premalignant or malignant lesions can be achieved by administering a photosensitizing drug that is selectively absorbed by the abnormal cells, followed by exposure to a light source. This is the fundamental principle of photodynamic therapy (PDT). Although the treatment has been around since the early 1900s, short-acting photosensitizers that could be applied topically to the skin with a short duration of action (24 to 48 hours) were not developed until the late 20th century.[58,59]

The primary photosensitizer used in dermatology is 5-aminolevulinic acid (5-ALA), which is converted to protoprophyrin IX by the mitochondria of skin cells. This photosensitizing porphyrin results in intracellular free-radical formation, singlet oxygen species, and cell damage. An alternative cutaneous photosensitizer is methyl aminolevulinic acid (MAL), and it has demonstrated more selective accumulation in premalignant and malignant tissues.[60–64] The light source used to activate 5-ALA or MAL PDT must produce wavelengths within the absorption spectrum of protoporphyrin IX: 400 to 700 nm (visible light). Incandescent bulbs, intense pulse light sources, and lasers all have been used successfully in this capacity.

The original FDA recommendation for the treatment of actinic keratoses included application of the 5-ALA solution for 14 to 18 hours followed by illumination with blue light for 16 minutes. Shorter incubation times of 1 to 3 hours with ALA and MAL have been reported to result in clearance of 90% of AKs with less pain.[65,66] Off-label applications of 5-ALA and MAL PDT for the treatment of SBCC result in clearance rates ranging from 76% to 97%, and 64% to 92% for nodular BCC.[59] Preprocedure reduction of the tumor burden with curettage or debulking may also increase treatment efficacy. SCCIS has also been successfully treated with 5-ALA PDT. Clearance of SCCIS ranges from 54% to 100% initially, and from to 31% to 100% at 12 to 36 months.[58,59] Treatment protocols incorporate various 5-ALA incubation periods, ranging from 3 to 20 hours and including the use of various light sources. The most effective light sources are red light or the pulsed dye laser (585–595 nm).[58,59]

Side effects of PDT include pain, itching, burning, stinging, and redness. This treatment modality is contraindicated in patients with porphyria, with hypersensitivity reactions to any component of 5-ALA, and patients with photosensitivity within the wavelengths of visible light. This treatment is pregnancy category C and risk during breastfeeding cannot be ruled out.[59]

Chemical Peel/Laser Resurfacing

Both chemical peels and resurfacing laser therapy for actinically damaged skin involve the controlled, superficial destruction of the skin with the goal of epidermal regeneration. The depth of tissue destruction is determined by the type of peel or laser chosen. Superficial peels damage the epidermis; medium-depth peels cause damage to the epidermis and the superficial papillary dermis; and deep peels damage the epidermis, penetrating beyond the papillary dermis. Increasing the depth of tissue injury into the dermis increases the risk of postprocedural scarring.

After either a chemical peel or a resurfacing laser treatment, the epidermis is reconstituted from epidermal stem cells thought to be located within the hair follicle at the insertion of the arrector pilli muscle, a location termed "the bulge." Chemical peels and laser ablation that cause damage superficial to the bulge can effectively destroy abnormal epidermal tissue and allow for epidermal regeneration. However, damage of sufficient depth to destroy the bulge will destroy the epidermal stem cells, resulting in scarring.[67] Unfortunately, many of the reports about treating premalignant skin conditions with chemical peels and resurfacing lasers are subjective, making quantification of successful disease clearance difficult.[68,69]

Medium-depth chemical peels may provide the ideal balance between epidermal tissue destruction and regeneration without scarring. Trichloroacetic acid (TCA), ranging in concentration from 35% to 50%, and Jessner's solution, in combination with TCA less than 35%, result in medium-depth peels. To perform a chemical peel, the skin is first degreased with acetone or alcohol, eye protection is provided, and the appropriate solution is applied to the skin. Both TCA and Jessner's solution are self-neutralizing, so the key to successful treatment is selection of the appropriate peel concentration. Tissue rehydration and sun protection are very important after the procedure to optimize the healing environment. The side effects of medium-depth peels include desquamation, pain, scarring, erythema, and pigmentary alteration.[69]

Both ablative and nonablative resurfacing lasers also can be effective in the removal of abnormal superficial epidermal tissue.[70] A laser's depth of penetration is contingent on its wavelength and the target chromophore. Resurfacing lasers usually have wavelengths in the infrared, near infrared, or far-infrared spectrum, and they utilize water in the skin as their chromophore.[71] Nonablative lasers also can be used to address superficial premalignant and malignant lesions of the skin if used in conjunction with a photosensitizer that can amplify the effects of the device, as previously discussed with PDT. The risks of these resurfacing procedures include pain, erythema, scabbing, desquamation, ulceration, burns, scarring, pigmentary alteration, and edema. Preoperative treatment with acyclovir may be indicated in individuals with a history of herpes simplex virus infection (HSV), to minimize periprocedural outbreaks and subsequent scarring.[72]

Electrodessication and Curettage (ED&C)

Electrodessication and curettage (ED&C) is a cost-effective treatment modality that has been used for years in the management of cutaneous malignancies. Superficial BCC, SCCIS, BCC, and SCC have all been reported to have 5-year clearance rates ranging from 92% to 96% for tumors less than 1 cm in maximum dimension that are located in low-risk areas.[73,74] This treatment consists of gentle curettage of the lesion followed by electrodessication or electrofulguration of the lesion base. One cycle may be sufficient for superficial tumors, whereas 2 to 3 cycles may be required for invasive tumors. ED&C is not indicated for aggressive lesions greater than 2 cm, recurrent lesions, lesions occurring in the setting of immunosuppression, or lesions occurring in high-risk areas such as the central face, ear, and chin.[74,75] Scarring and pigmentary alteration are the primary risks of the procedure.[75]

Cryosurgery

Cryosurgery utilizes the inflammation triggered by cold to destroy superficial or minimally invasive cutaneous lesions, depending on the amount of tissue cooling. One freeze-thaw cycle of 5 to 7 seconds with liquid nitrogen is sufficient to cause the rapid production of intracellular ice crystals, leading to regression of AKs (Fig 31–2). Thicker tumors, such as SCCIS and SBCC, may require debulking or multiple freeze-thaw cycles to increase efficacy.[76] Unfortunately, the recurrence rate after cryosurgery for SCCIS has been reported as 34% within 5 years.[31]

Cryosurgery used for the treatment of invasive BCC and SCC requires a greater duration of cooling, and thus creates a greater depth of tissue destruction. When used for the treatment of BCC and SCC, cryosurgery has reported cure rates of upwards of 97% after two, 40- to 90-second freeze-thaw cycles under local anesthesia. However, reported recurrence rates range from 3% to 17%.[78] Although the treatment is easily administered, pain, scarring, and pigmentary alteration limit the use of cryosurgery. Wound healing may be protracted in cases of SCC and BCC treatment due to the depth of ulceration and tissue injury.

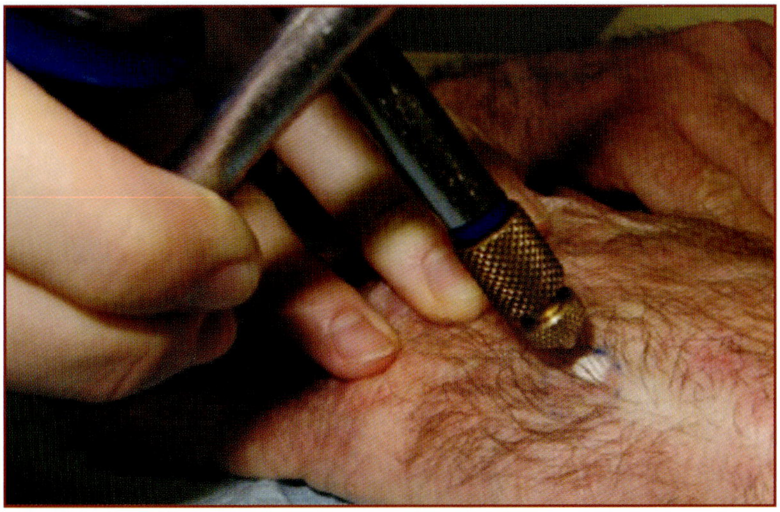

Figure 31–2. Treatment of an actinic keratosis with cryotherapy. The patient is undergoing cryosurgery for the treatment of an actinic keratosis. Note the area of superficial ice crystals on the skin.

Neither aggressive nor ill-defined lesions should be treated with cryosurgery. Furthermore, this treatment modality should not be used for invasive lesions located in critical areas such as the central face and ears that carry a significant risk of morbidity if tumor is incompletely treated.[79]

Radiation Therapy

Radiation therapy (RT) may be used as a primary or adjunctive treatment for the treatment of nonmelanoma skin cancers. In general, young patients and solid organ transplant patients who are at risk for developing cutaneous malignancies in the future should be discouraged from pursuing RT for uncomplicated primary cutaneous malignancies amenable to other treatments.[79,80] Conversely, the most common adjunctive therapy for high-risk, invasive SCC and BCC after excision is RT. Radiation therapy may be delivered in the form of orthovoltage RT, electron beam RT, proton beam RT, high-energy photons, and interstitial brachytherapy.

Orthovoltage RT offers the ability to concentrate the maximum dose at the skin surface without significant penetration of eye shields, but higher exit doses and higher tissue differentials for cartilage and bone with respect to that of electrons limit the use of this form in some cases.[81] RT is delivered in fractionated doses to allow for tissue recovery between treatments, and typical courses of RT range from 50 to 70 Gy in 25 to 35 daily fractions.[80,83] Common early side effects include erythema and desquamation, followed by sclerosis, atrophy, hypopigmentation, and telangiectasias after therapy. Exposure to ionizing radiation is an independent risk for cutaneous malignancy, and the risk of developing skin cancer after radiation therapy is 1 per 1000, underscoring the need for judicious application of this technology as primary treatment.[82]

Indications for adjuvant RT in the treatment of SCC include positive surgical margins, multiple recurrences, clinical or asymptomatic perineural invasion, and deep invasion of cartilage or bone, unless adequate clear surgical margins are achieved.[84] RT is contraindicated in patients with Gorlin's syndrome (basal cell nevus syndrome) and xeroderma pigmentosum because of the risk of inducing additional skin malignancies.[80] Currently, systemic chemotherapeutic agents are not indicated for localized disease.

As with squamous cell carcinomas, high-risk BCC displaying aggressive features may require adjunctive radiation therapy to increase the likelihood of cure. BCCs, however, are less radioresponsive than SCC, so there is no clear consensus on the role of radiation therapy in the management of BCC.[85] Adjuvant RT for BCC with perineural involvement is determined on a case-by-case basis, weighing patient age, the risks of the tumor, and the risks of the RT into the decision.[84]

Patients with SCC and incidental PNI have a local control rate of 80% to 90% with RT, with about 50% to 55% for those with clinical PNI.[84] Microscopic residual disease in certain locations, such as the medial canthus, may greatly benefit from the additional of RT, where local control is usually upwards of 90% at 10 years with orthovoltage RT.[85] Tumors displaying PNI with extension toward the skull base may benefit from the addition of RT in the form of megavoltage photons or proton beam.[85] In a review of 12 patients treated with MMS and adjunctive radiotherapy for the treatment of BCCs displaying PNI, no recurrences were noted after 3 to 32 months of follow-up.[23] Similarly, the optimal treatment for patients with clinically positive nodes is surgery and postoperative RT.[86,87]

Summary

Although surgery remains one of the preferred treatments for aggressive cutaneous tumors, nonsurgical treatment modalities remain an essential part of the arsenal for the treatment of premalignant and early malignant cutaneous tumors. These interventions expand the treatment options for cutaneous tumors, and they can be used in combination with surgical interventions or with each other. Integration of these new and developing treatments into our current treatment plans will allow physicians to offer a variety of treatment options and provide the best opportunity for cure.

References

1. Drake LA, Ceilley RI, Cornelison RL, et al. Guidelines of care for AKs. *J Am Acad Dermatol.* 1995;32(1):95–98.
2. Criscione VD, Weinstock MA, Naylor MF, Luque C, Eide MJ, Bingham SF; Department of Veteran Affairs Topical Tretinoin Chemoprevention Trial Group. Actinic keratoses: natural history and risk of malignant transformation in the Veterans Affairs Topical Tretinoin Chemoprevention Trial. *Cancer.* 2009;115(11):2523–2530.
3. Quaedvlieg PJ, Tirsi E, Thissen MR, Krekels GA. Actinic keratosis: how to differentiate the good from the bad ones? *Eur J Dermatol.* 2006;16:335–339.
4. American Cancer Society. Overview: Skin cancer—basal and squamous cell: How many people get basal and squamous cell skin cancers? ACS Web site. http://www.cancer.org/docroot/CRI/content/CRI_2_2_1X_How_many_people_get_nonmelanoma_skin_cancer_51.asp?sitearea=.
5. Clayman GL, Lee JJ, Holsinger FC, et al. Mortality risk from squamous cell skin cancer. *J Clin Oncol.* 2005;23(4):759–765.
6. Bivens MM, Bhosle M, Balkrishnan R, et al. Nonmelanoma skin cancer: is the incidence really increasing among patients younger than 40? A re-examination using 25 years of U.S. outpatient data. *Dermatol Surg.* 2006;32(12):1473–1479.
7. Kim NN, Boone SL, Ortiz S, et al. Squamous cell carcinoma in solid organ transplant recipients: influences on perception of risk and optimal time to provide education. *Arch Dermatol.* 2009;145(10):1196–1197.
8. Hartevelt MM, Bavinck JN, Kootte AM, et al. Incidence of skin cancer after renal transplantation in the Netherlands. *Transplantation.* 1990;49(3):506–509.
9. Stockfleth E, Ulrich C, Meyer T, Christophers E. Epithelial malignancies in organ transplant patients: clinical presentation and new methods of treatment. *Recent Results Cancer Res.* 2002;160:251–258.
10. Martinez JC, Otley CC, Okuno SH, et al. Chemotherapy in the management of advanced cutaneous squamous cell carcinoma in organ transplant recipients: theoretical and practical considerations. *Dermatol Surg.* 2004;30(4 pt 2):679–686.
11. Nolan RC, Chan MTL, Heenan PJ. A clinicopathologic review of lethal nonmelanoma skin cancers in Western Australia. *J. Am. Acad. Dermatol.* 2005;52(1):101–108.
12. Pickle LW, Mason TJ, Howard N, et al. *Atlas of U.S. Cancer Mortality Among Nonwhites: 1950–1980.* Bethesda, MD, NIH Publication 90-1582, 1990.
13. De Silva SP, Dellon AL. Recurrence rate of positive margin basal cell carcinoma: results of a five-year prospective study. *J Surg Oncol.* 1985;28(1):72–74.
14. Veness MJ. Defining patients with high-risk cutaneous squamous cell carcinoma. *Australas J Dermatol.* 2006;47(1):28–33.
15. Cherpelis BS, Marcusen C, Lang PG. Prognostic factors for metastasis in squamous cell carcinoma of the skin. *Dermatol Surg.* 2002;28(3):268–273.
16. Johnson TM, Rowe DE, Nelson BR, Swanson NA. Squamous cell carcinoma of the skin (excluding lip and oral mucosa). *J Am Acad Dermatol.* 1992;26(3 pt 2):467–484.
17. Lang PG. Management of squamous cell carcinomas and lymph node evaluation. In: Wheeland RG, ed. *Cutaneous Surgery.* Philadelphia, PA: WB Saunders; 1994:752–787.

18. Mosterd K, Krekels GA, Nieman FH, et al. Surgical excision versus Mohs' micrographic surgery for primary and recurrent basal-cell carcinoma of the face: a prospective randomised controlled trial with 5-years' follow-up. *Lancet Oncol.* 2008;9(12):1149–1156.
19. Feasel AM, Brown TJ, Bogle MA, et al. Perineural invasion of cutaneous malignancies. *Dermatol Surg.* 2001;27(6): 531–542.
20. Ratner D, Lowe L, Johnson TM, Fader DJ. Perineural spread of basal cell carcinomas treated with Mohs micrographic surgery. *Cancer.* 2000;88(7):1605–1613.
21. Mendenhall WM, Amdur RJ, Williams LS, et al. Carcinoma of the skin of the head and neck with perineural invasion. *Head Neck.* 2002;24(1):78–83.
22. Walling HW, Fosko SW, Geraminejad PA, et al. Aggressive basal cell carcinoma: presentation, pathogenesis, and management. *Cancer Metastasis Rev.* 2004;23(3–4):389–402.
23. Leibovitch I, Huilgol SC, Selva D, et al. Basal cell carcinoma treated with Mohs surgery in Australia III. Perineural invasion. *J Am Acad Dermatol.* 2005;53(3):458–463.
24. Snow SN, Sahl W, Lo JS et al. Metastatic basal cell carcinoma. Report of five cases. *Cancer.* 1994;73(2):328–335.
25. Elghissassi I, Mikou A, Inrhaoun H, et al. Metastatic basal cell carcinoma to the bone and bone marrow. *Int J Dermatol.* 2009;48(5):481–483.
26. Schwartz RA, De Jager RL, Janniger CK, et al. Giant basal cell carcinoma with metastases and myelophthisic anemia. *J Surg Oncol.* 1986;33(4): 223–226.
27. Jefford M, Kiffer JD, Somers G, et al. Metastatic basal cell carcinoma: rapid symptomatic response to cisplatin and paclitaxel. *ANZ J Surg.* 2004;74(8):704–705.
28. Thomson Micromedex. Fluorouracil. M.D. Anderson Online Web site, 2010. Retrieved February 2, 2010 from https://mdajun.mdanderson.org/hcs/librarian/ND_T/HCS/ND_PR/Main/CS/217F26/DUPLICATIONSHIELDSYNC/B6B8E0/ND_PG/PRIH/ND_B/HCS/SBK/1/ND_P/Main/PFActionId/hcs.common.RetrieveDocumentCommon/DocId/236390/ContentSetId/100/SearchTerm/5/SearchOption/,DanaInfo=www.thomsonhc.com+BeginWith#secN108E0.
29. Gross K, Kircik L, Kricorian G. 5% 5-Fluorouracil cream for the treatment of small superficial basal cell carcinoma: efficacy, tolerability, cosmetic outcome, and patient satisfaction. *Dermatol Surg.* 2007;33(4):433–439.
30. Loven K, Stein L, Furst K, et al. Evaluation of the efficacy and tolerability of 0.5% fluorouracil cream and 5% fluorouracil cream applied to each side of the face in patients with actinic keratosis. *Clin Ther.* 2002;24(6): 990–1000.
31. Thestrup-Pedersen K, Ravnborg L, Reymann F. Morbus Bowen: a description of the disease in 617 patients. *Acta Derm Venereol.* 1988;68(3):236–239.
32. Hadley JC, Tristani-Firouzi P, Florell SF, et al. Case series of multiple recurrent reactive keratoacanthomas developing at surgical margins. *Dermatol Surg.* 2009;35(12):2019–2024.
33. Morse LG, Kendrick C, Hooper D, Ward H, Parry E. Treatment of squamous cell carcinoma with intralesional 5-fluorouracil. *Dermatol Surg.* 2003;29(11):1150–1153.
34. Lebwohl M, Dinehart S, Whiting D, et al. Imiquimod 5% cream for the treatment of actinic keratosis: results from two Phase III, randomized, double-blind, parallel group, vehicle-controlled trials. *J Am Acad Dermatol.* 2004;50(5): 714–721.
35. Thomson Micromedex. Imiquimod. M.D. Anderson Online Website, 2010. Retrieved February 1, 2010 from https://mdajun.mdanderson.org/hcs/librarian/ND_T/HCS/ND_PR/Main/CS/899EFE/DUPLICATIONSHIELDSYNC/987852/ND_PG/PRIH/ND_B/HCS/SBK/1/ND_P/Main/PFActionId/hcs.common.RetrieveDocumentCommon/DocId/924239/ContentSetId/100/SearchTerm/imiquimod/SearchOption/,DanaInfo=www.thomsonhc.com+BeginWith .
36. Love WE, Bernhard JD, Bordeaux JS. Topical imiquimod or fluorouracil therapy for basal and squamous cell carcinoma: a systematic review. *Arch Dermatol.* 2009;145(12): 1431–1438.
37. Rosen T, Harting M, Gibson M. Treatment of Bowen's disease with topical 5% imiquimod cream: retrospective study. *Dermatol Surg.* 2007;33(4):427–431.
38. Missall TA, Fosko SW. The use of imiquimod to minimize the surgical defect when excising invasive malignant melanoma surrounded by extensive melanoma in situ, lentiginous type. *Dermatol Surg.* 2009;35(5):868–874.
39. Powell AM, Robson AM, Russell-Jones R, Barlow RJ. Imiquimod and lentigo maligna: a search for prognostic features in a clinicopathological study with long-term follow-up. *Br J Dermatol.* 2009;160(5):994–998.
40. Wang LC, Blanchard A, Judge DE, et al. Successful treatment of recurrent extramammary Paget's disease of the vulva with topical imiquimod 5% cream. *J Am Acad Dermatol.* 2003;49(4):769–772.
41. Zampogna JC, Flowers FP, Roth WI, Hassenein AM. Treatment of primary limited cutaneous extramammary Paget's disease with topical imiquimod monotherapy: two case reports. *J Am Acad Dermatol.* 2002;47(4 suppl): S229–S235.
42. Kim KH, Yavel RM, Gross VL, Brody N. Intralesional interferon alpha-2b in the treatment of basal cell carcinoma and squamous cell carcinoma: revisited. *Dermatol Surg.* 2004;30(1):116–120.
43. Thomson Micromedex. Interferon Alpha-2B. M.D. Anderson Online Web site, 2010. Retrieved February 1, 2010 from https://mdajun.mdanderson.org/hcs/librarian/ND_T/HCS/ND_PR/Main/CS/35DBF8/DUPLICATIONSHIELDSYNC/7739B7/ND_PG/PRIH/ND_B/HCS/SBK/1/ND_P/Main/PFActionId/hcs.common.RetrieveDocumentCommon/DocId/301640/ContentSetId/100/SearchTerm/interferon/SearchOption/,DanaInfo=www.thomsonhc.com+BeginWith .
44. Greenway HT, Cornell RC, Tanner DJ, et al. Treatment of basal cell carcinoma with intralesional interferon. *J Am Acad Dermatol.* 1986;15(3):437–443.
45. Edwards L, Berman B, Rapini RP, et al. Treatment of cutaneous squamous cell carcinomas by intralesional interferon alfa-2b therapy. *Arch Dermatol.* 1992;128(11):1486–1489.

46. Cornell RC, Greenway HT, Tucker SB, et al. Intralesional interferon therapy for basal cell carcinoma. *J Am Acad Dermatol.* 1990;23(4 pt 1):694–700.
47. Dyall-Smith D. Intralesional bleomycin. *Australas J Dermatol.* 1998;39(2):123–124.
48. Heller R, Jaroszeski MJ, Reintgen DS, et al. Treatment of cutaneous and subcutaneous tumors with electrochemotherapy using intralesional bleomycin. *Cancer.* 1998;83(1):148–157.
49. Dragnev KH, Rigas JR, Dmitrovsky E. The retinoids and cancer prevention mechanisms. *Oncologist.* 2000;5(5):361–368.
50. Peck GL. Topical tretinoin in actinic keratosis and basal cell carcinoma. *J Am Acad Dermatol.* 1986;15(4 pt 2):829–835.
51. Otley CC, Stasko T, Tope WD, Lebwohl M. Chemoprevention of nonmelanoma skin cancer with systemic retinoids: practical dosing and management of adverse effects. *Dermatol Surg.* 2006;32(4):562–568.
52. Fecker LF, Stockfleth E, Nindl I, et al. The role of apoptosis in therapy and prophylaxis of epithelial tumours by nonsteroidal anti-inflammatory drugs (NSAIDs). *Br J Dermatol.* 2007;156(suppl 3):25–33.
53. Adamson DJ, Frew D, Tatoud R, et al. Diclofenac antagonizes peroxisome proliferator-activated receptor-gamma signaling. *Mol Pharmacol.* 2002;61(1):7–12.
54. Lu X, Xie W, Reed D, et al. Nonsteroidal antiinflammatory drugs cause apoptosis and induce cyclooxygenases in chicken embryo fibroblasts. *Proc Natl Acad Sci U S A.* 1995;92(17):7961–7965.
55. Merk HF. Topical diclofenac in the treatment of actinic keratoses. *Int J Dermatol.* 2007;46(1):12–18.
56. Wolf Jr JE, Taylor JR, Tschen E, et al. Topical 3.0% diclofenac in 2.5% hyaluronan gel in the treatment of actinic keratoses. *Int J Dermatol.* 2001;40(11):709–713.
57. Thomson Micromedex. Diclofenac. M.D. Anderson Online Web site, 2010. Retrieved February 2, 2010 from https://mdajun.mdanderson.org/hcs/librarian/ND_T/HCS/ND_PR/Main/CS/0A738D/DUPLICATIONSHIELDSYNC/99E103/ND_PG/PRIH/ND_B/HCS/SBK/2/ND_P/Main/PFActionId/hcs.common.RetrieveDocumentCommon/DocId/178000/ContentSetId/100/SearchTerm/diclofenac%20/SearchOption/,DanaInfo=www.thomsonhc.com+BeginWith .
58. Dougherty TJ, Kaufman JE, Goldfarb A, et al. Photoradiation therapy for the treatment of malignant tumors. *Cancer Res.* 1978;38(8):2628–2635.
59. Tierney E, Barker A, Ahdout J, Hanke CW, Moy RL, Kouba DJ. Photodynamic therapy for the treatment of cutaneous neoplasia, inflammatory disorders, and photoaging. *Dermatol Surg.* 2009;35(5):725–746.
60. Kennedy JC, Pottier RH, Pross DC Photodynamic therapy with endogenous protoporphyrin IX: basic principles and present clinical experience. *J Photochem Photobiol B.* 1990;6(1–2):143–148.
61. Lehmann P. Methyl aminolaevulinate-photodynamic therapy: a review of clinical trials in the treatment of actinic keratoses and nonmelanoma skin cancer. *Br J Dermatol.* 2007;156(5):793–801.
62. Morton CA. Methyl aminolevulinate: actinic keratoses and Bowen's disease. *Dermatol Clin.* 2007;25(1):81–87.
63. Szeimies RM. Methyl aminolevulinate-photodynamic therapy for basal cell carcinoma. *Dermatol Clin.* 2007;25(1):89–94.
64. Calzavara-Pinton PG, Venturini M, Sala R. Photodynamic therapy: update 2006. Part 1: photochemistry and photobiology. *J Eur Acad Dermatol Venereol.* 2007;21(3):293–302.
65. Alexiades-Armenakas MR, Geronemus RG. Laser-mediated photodynamic therapy of actinic keratoses. *Arch Dermatol.* 2003;139(10):1313–1320.
66. Gold MH. The evolving role of aminolevulinic acid hydrochloride with photodynamic therapy in photoaging. *Cutis.* 2002;69(6 suppl):8–13.
67. Nelson BR, Fader DJ, Gillard M, et al. Pilot histologic and ultrastructural study of the effects of medium-depth chemical facial peels on dermal collagen in patients with actinically damaged skin. *J Am Acad Dermatol.* 1995;32(3):472–478.
68. Witheiler DD, Lawrence N, Cox SE, Cruz C, Cockerell CJ, Freemen RG. Long-term efficacy and safety of Jessner's solution and 35% trichloroacetic acid vs 5% fluorouracil in the treatment of widespread facial actinic keratoses. *Dermatol Surg.* 1997;23(3):191–196.
69. Fulton JE, Porumb S. Chemical peels: their place within the range of resurfacing techniques. *Am J Clin Dermatol.* 2004;5(3):179–187.
70. Ostertag JU, Quaedvlieg PJ, Neumann MH, Krekels GA. Recurrence rates and long-term follow-up after laser resurfacing as a treatment for widespread actinic keratoses on the face and scalp. *Dermatol Surg.* 2006;32(2):261–267.
71. Hruza GJ. Laser treatment of epidermal and dermal lesions. *Dermatol Clin.* 2002;20(1):147–164.
72. Fischer TC, Perosino E, Poli F, et al. Chemical peels in aesthetic dermatology: an update 2009. *J Eur Acad Dermatol Venereol.* 2009 Sep 8. (epub ahead of print).
73. Werlinger KD, Upton G, Moore AY. Recurrence rates of primary nonmelanoma skin cancers treated by surgical excision compared to electrodesiccation-curettage in a private dermatological practice. *Dermatol Surg.* 2002;28(12):1138–1142.
74. Sheridan AT, Dawber RP. Curettage, electrosurgery and skin cancer. *Austral J Dermatol.* 2000;41(1):19–30.
75. An KP, Ratner D. Surgical management of cutaneous malignancies. *Clin Dermatol.* 2001;19(3):305–320.
76. Tull S, Nunley K, Sengelmann R. Nonsurgical treatment modalities for primary cutaneous malignancies. *Dermatol Surg.* 2008;34(7):859–872.
77. Thissen MR, Neumann MH, Schouten LJ. A systematic review of treatment modalities for primary basal cell carcinomas. *Arch Dermatol.* 1999;135(10):1177–1183.
78. Veness M, Richards S. Role of modern radiotherapy in treating skin cancer. *Aust J Dermatol.* 2003;44(3):159–166.

79. Tavin E, Persky M. Metastatic cutaneous squamous cell carcinoma of the head and neck region. *Laryngoscope.* 1996;106(2 pt 1):156–158.
80. Neville JA, Welch E, Leffell DJ. Management of nonmelanoma skin cancer in 2007. *Nat Clin Pract Oncol.* 2007; 4(8):462–469.
81. Veness MJ. Treatment recommendations in patients diagnosed with high-risk cutaneous squamous cell carcinoma. *Aust Radiol.* 2005;49(5):365–376.
82. Geist DE, Garcia-Moliner M, Fitzek MM, Cho H, Rogers GS. Perineural invasion of cutaneous squamous cell carcinoma and basal cell carcinoma: raising awareness and optimizing management. *Dermatol Surg.* 2008;34(12): 1642–1651.
83. Mendenhall WM, Amdur RJ, Hinerman RW, Cognetta AB, Mendenhall NP. Radiotherapy for cutaneous squamous and basal cell carcinomas of the head and neck. *Laryngoscope.* 2009;119(10):1994–1999.
84. Cernea CR, Ferraz AR, de Castro IV, et al. Perineural invasion in aggressive skin carcinomas of the head and neck. *ORL J Otorhinolaryngol Relat Spec.* 2009;71(1):21–26.
85. Swanson EL, Amdur RJ, Mendenhall WM, Morris CG, Kirwan JM, Flowers F. Radiotherapy for basal cell carcinoma of the medial canthus region. *Laryngoscope.* 2009; 119(12):2366–2368.
86. Ceilley RI, Del Rosso JQ. Current modalities and new advances in the treatment of basal cell carcinoma. *Intl Dermatol.* 2006;45(5):489–498.
87. Gluck I, Ibrahim M, Popvtzer A, et al. Skin cancer of the head and neck with perineural invasion: defining the clinical target volumes based on the pattern of failure. *Intl J Radiat Oncol Biol Phys.* 2009;74(1):38–46.

32

PRINCIPLES OF HEAD AND NECK CUTANEOUS RECONSTRUCTION

ROXANNA BARATELLI
BRIAN A. MOORE
MATTHEW M. HANASONO

Introduction

Defects of the head and neck arising from cutaneous malignancy can have devastating effects on a patient's appearance and function, potentially resulting in significant disability and social isolation. The desire to alleviate these problems led to the development of reconstructive surgery as early as 3000 BC. The Edwin Smith Surgical Papyrus, from ancient Egypt, described the first surgical management of facial trauma, including the treatment of mandibular and nasal fractures.[1] Nasal reconstruction by adjacent tissue transfer from the forehead and the cheek was described in northern India by Sushruta in the 6th century, BC.[2] Later advances in surgical technique, the introduction of general anesthesia, the advent of antibiotics and blood transfusions, and improved survival and cure rates have emboldened head and neck tumor excision, subsequently driving the evolution of reconstructive surgery. Despite these advances, the ideal reconstruction of cutaneous defects remains a challenge due to the precise demands of form and function in the head and neck.

The contemporary reconstructive surgeon possesses a vast armamentarium to combat defects arising from cutaneous malignancy of the head and neck. These tools have evolved to incorporate all components of the reconstructive ladder—from primary closure and secondary healing to microvascular free tissue transfer and advanced prostheses. The fundamental principle in oncologic cutaneous reconstruction is to replace "like" tissue with "like" tissue in terms of appearance and function, whenever possible, while minimizing donor site morbidity. Cutaneous reconstruction is predicated on thoughtful defect analysis, the availability and appropriateness of flap and graft donor tissues, patient and oncologic factors, and the skill and experience of the reconstructive surgeon. Each defect within each anatomic subsite presents unique demands; there is no panacea in head and neck cutaneous reconstruction.

Goals of Reconstruction

Treatment of cutaneous malignancy of the head and neck requires a multidisciplinary approach, particularly in advanced disease. The extirpative plan should evolve in concert with the reconstructive plan through close communication. When appropriate, incisions should be designed to promote the maximum availability of reconstructive options. However, the primary intent of surgery for cutaneous malignancy of the head and neck is eradication of disease, and the oncologic sanctity of an operation, in terms of margins, incisions, and dissection, should never be compromised to simplify reconstruction. Although patient positioning, operating room preparation, and incision placement can be performed in such a way as to facilitate the reconstruction as much as possible, the true challenge in oncologic reconstruction is to accommodate the requirements of the resection while making every effort to optimize the resultant outcome.

For aesthetic restoration of the skin of the head and neck, consideration must be given not only to the best color match, but also to the texture and thickness of the reconstructed tissues. Functional considerations include minimizing ocular distortion, protecting the globe, maintaining a patent oral and nasal airway, preserving oral competence, and covering vital anatomic structures such as the craniofacial skeleton, dura, and great vessels. In addition to restoring form and function, the reconstruction must also promote quick (or at least timely) recovery and withstand adjuvant therapy, if necessary.

Reconstruction Planning

Patient Factors

Patients with cutaneous malignancy of the head and neck frequently have a history of prior similar lesions, particularly when they present with advanced disease.[3] As such, they may have undergone multiple prior surgeries or previous radiation therapy, which would limit the reconstructive options. The reconstructive team should complete a thorough history and physical, with particular focus on any history of skin lesions, biopsies, or procedures, as well as any evidence of healed incisions or scars. Previous radiation therapy leads to fibrosis and relative tissue hypoxia; therefore, well-vascularized tissue must be brought into the wound in previously irradiated patients for reliable healing, which may necessitate regional or free flaps in wounds that might otherwise heal using less complicated techniques.[4]

Patients with advanced or recurrent disease usually require adjuvant therapy, adding yet another dimension to surgical planning. As with patients with prior adjuvant therapy, particularly radiation, reconstruction with well-vascularized tissue is requisite. If postoperative radiation therapy is planned, single-staged reconstruction also should be employed when possible, as multistaged procedures may delay the initiation of adjuvant therapy, with a potential impact on disease control and survival.[5] In cases where a multistaged procedure is indicated, delayed reconstruction may be the best compromise in terms of achieving optimal functional and aesthetic results. Another issue in patients with advanced or recurrent disease is that the prognosis for long-term cure or survival may be poor or guarded. In such cases, the simplest reconstruction that minimizes the risk for complications may be the best choice.

Medications such as steroids or immunosuppressive drugs, underlying comorbidities like cardiovascular disease and diabetes, and smoking also can compromise tissue viability and wound healing.[6] Patients with significant medical comorbidities may not tolerate a prolonged reconstructive procedure, so a more expeditious modality should be considered. In some cases, such as when the indication for reconstruction is completely aesthetic, reconstruction may not be performed or delayed until the patient can better tolerate extensive surgery. In patients who are poor surgical candidates, prosthetic rehabilitation may have significant advantages over autologous tissue reconstruction and should discussed with patients as part of their multidisciplinary plan of care.

Defect Analysis

Historically, there are three general categories of head and neck defects: defects that require mandatory coverage (exposed dura, eye, great vessels, etc), those that yield a significant functional deficit, and those with significant aesthetic consequences.[7] The wounds created by the extirpation of cutaneous malignancy in the head and neck often fit all three categories. As mentioned, in some circumstances, a rapid, although less cosmetically ideal, modality such as skin grafting may be chosen to facilitate margin control or adjuvant therapy, with a plan to revise the wound at a later time.

Each defect must be analyzed for size, depth, tissues involved, critical structures placed at risk, and the appearance and mobility of adjacent tissue.

In patients with widespread actinic damage, adjacent skin that could be used for reconstruction may exhibit cancerous or precancerous lesions as well. The potential impact of various reconstructive options on nearby critical features, such as the lip, ala, and eyelid, should be evaluated. The effect of cicatricial contracture must also be anticipated (eg, lower lid ectropion after excision and reconstruction of cheek lesions) and a plan to prevent undesirable results must be made.

The face is unique in that it has been divided into aesthetic regions and subunits, with implications for both resection and reconstruction (Fig 32–1). Many of the facial regions have been further divided into subunits, based on differences in contour that affect the way light and shadow interact. For example, the nose is usually divided into subunits for the purposes of reconstruction, and many surgeons advocate resecting the remainder of a subunit, when reasonable, to optimize the cosmetic result (see Chapter 33).[8] Each unit or subunit may merit an individualized approach, and definitive reconstruction may incorporate multiple techniques.[9,10] Additionally, the face and neck demonstrate lines of relaxed skin tension that run perpendicular to the mimetic musculature, which provide reliable areas to camouflage incisions and orient scars (Fig 32–2).[11,12]

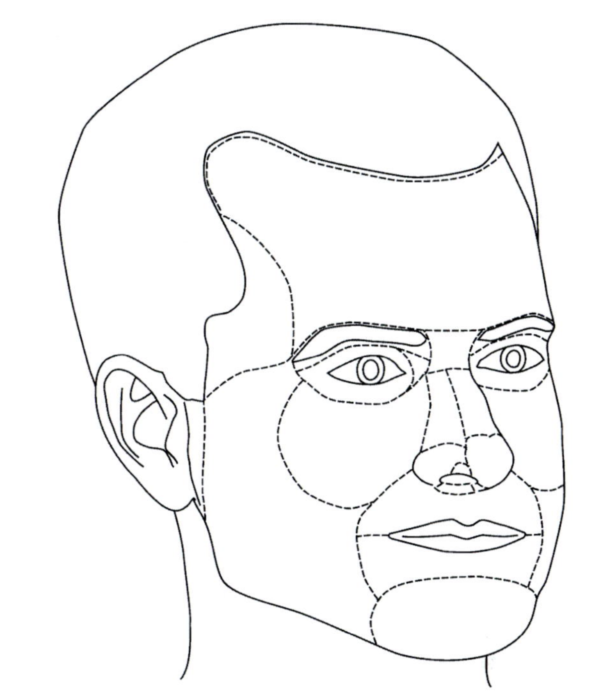

Figure 32–1. Facial aesthetic units. Adapted, in part, from Burget GC, Menick FJ. Subunit principle in nasal reconstruction. *Plast Reconstr Surg.* 1985;76:239–247, with permission.

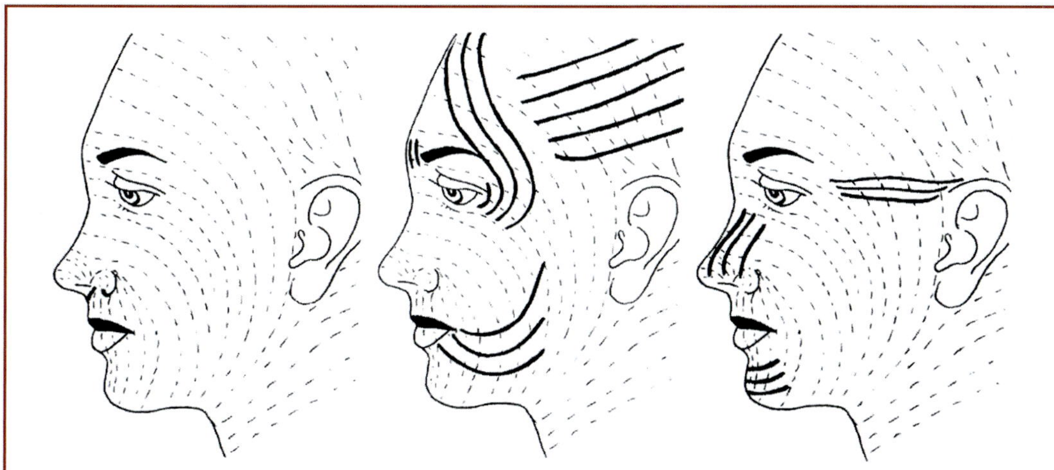

Figure 32–2. Relaxed skin tension lines and potential incisions, as depicted by Borges (*left*), Langer (*center*), and Kraissl (*right*). Incisions for elective facial procedures placed in Borges' lines led to better cosmetic outcomes. From Wilhelmi BJ, Blackwell SJ, Phillips LG. Langer's lines: To use or not to use. *Plast Reconstr Surg.* 1999;104(1):208–214, with permission.

The depth of the wound, more specifically, the layers involved, is a particularly important concept in head and neck reconstruction. Facial wounds may involve the covering skin; subcutaneous structures such as supporting cartilages, mimetic muscles, and facial bones; mucosal lining (in the cases of nasal, eyelid, cheek, or lip wounds); or critical underlying tissues and organs, like the dura or eye. Therefore, a three-dimensional appreciation of the defect is paramount in preoperative planning, and the reconstructive surgeon should anticipate potentially involved structures. Skin edges may be freshened if delayed reconstruction is pursued, and the beveled edges that often result from Moh micrographic excision should be straightened. Flap and recipient bed edges also can be thinned to ensure a smooth transition across the reconstructed tissues.[13] The unique demands of each anatomic site in the head and neck and their preferred reconstructive options are addressed in the focused chapters that follow. An overview of the reconstructive options available for each anatomic site is provided in Table 32–1.

The Reconstructive Armamentarium

Reconstruction traditionally follows the concept of the reconstructive ladder, beginning with the simplest solution and progressing to more elaborate reconstructions only if needed. No single reconstructive method is optimal for every defect, and an individualized defect-oriented approach defines our philosophy in head and neck cutaneous reconstruction. Following a thorough defect analysis, the appropriate technique(s) may be selected, and some anatomic sites are more amenable to simple techniques than others, demanding the full range of skill from the reconstructive surgeon.[14]

Secondary Healing

Secondary intention healing is an alternative to primary reconstruction wherein the entire thickness of the wound is closed by means of contraction and reepithelialization. A variety of dressings, including negative pressure therapy, may be chosen to facilitate healing by secondary intention. In general, reepithelialization may be accelerated by maintaining a moist environment with an agent as elementary as antibacterial ointment.[15,16] This approach requires meticulous wound care, and a discussion of the techniques, products, and medications currently available is beyond the scope of this chapter.

Small (<1 cm), superficial wounds located on concave surfaces such as the medial cheek, dorsal nose, medial canthus, auricular fossae, and temple heal satisfactorily by this method.[15,17] Secondary intention healing also can be considered for larger defects in critically ill patients who have not been previously irradiated, as well as in the setting of a failed or partially failed local flap prior to later revision, if necessary. The skin laxity and pigmentation changes that define the skin of the elderly render secondary intention healing ideal in older patients.[18] The disadvantages of this approach include longer healing time and an increased risk of hypertrophic scarring and scar contracture. Secondary healing is contraindicated in defects involving the free edge of the lips, nasal ala, or eyelids, as it can result in notching or retraction, with the potential for oral incompetence, nasal obstruction, or exposure keratitis.[15]

Primary Closure

For many cutaneous defects, primary closure is preferred, but not always possible. Incisions should be placed within or parallel to the relaxed skin tension lines as a means of camouflage, wide undermining should be accomplished to facilitate a tension-free wound closure.[11] Primary closure with or without undermining usually is reserved for smaller defects anywhere in the head and neck that allow tension-free closure without distortion of surrounding structures, significant standing cone deformities, or associated loss of function.[19] Typical locations for primary closure include lax regions of the cheek, forehead, temple, nasal dorsum, and neck. During the immediate postablation evaluation of the defect, the impact of primary closure on adjacent critical structures should be assessed, and this modality abandoned if distortion appears likely.

Table 32–1. Options for Reconstruction of Head and Neck Cutaneous Defects

Location	Challenges and Special Considerations	Reconstructive Choices

Lip	Focal point of appearance
	Oral competence
	Projection of emotion
	Access to oral cavity for food and dental appliances
	Meticulous approximation of vermilion border
		Wedge excision with primary closure
		Local advancement flaps
		  V-Y advancement
		  Stairstep advancement
		  A-T closure
		Lip/Cheek advancement
		  Webster-Bernard flap
		  Karapandzic flap
		  Gilles fan flap
		  Melolabial flap
		Lip switch procedures
		  Abbe flap
		  Estlander flap
		Free tissue transfer

Nose	Three layers: cover, support, mucosa
	Remember nasal subunits
	Multiple procedures are common
		Mucosal coverage
		  Skin grafts on flap undersurface
		  Turnover cutaneous flaps
		  Hinge flaps from septum/turbinate
		  Free flaps
		Support
		  Cartilage grafts from septum, auricle, rib
		  Full-thickness auricle grafts
		Cover
		  Secondary intention
		  Primary closure
		  Small defects (<1.5 cm)
		    Banner (note) flap
		    Dorsal nasal flap
		    Bilobed flap
		    Full-thickness grafts from auricle
		  Larger defects
		    Paramedian forehead flap
		    Melolabial flap
		    Free tissue transfer
		    Prosthetics

continues

Table 32–1. *continued*

Location	Challenges and Special Considerations	Reconstructive Choices
Orbital/Periorbital	Thin skin Risk of ectropion, exposure keratopathy Remember concepts of anterior and posterior lamella Ensure meticulous alignment of the tarsus	Small wounds Secondary intention Primary closure (<50% marginal defect) Full thickness grafts from upper lid Larger wounds Single or bipedicled transposition flaps Cross-lid techniques Hughes tarsoconjunctival flap Cutler-Beard composite flap Cervicofacial flaps Lateral defects Primary closure V-Y advancement flap Rhomboid flap Posterior lamella Free cartilage grafts Free mucosal grafts
Auricle	Anatomic detail requires planning Multiple procedures are common Size of reconstructed ear may be sacrificed for normal appearance Prosthetics are an option	Small rim defects Primary closure Star excision Large rim defects Antia-Buch advancement flaps Conchal bowl defects Secondary intention Full/split-thickness skin grafts Postauricular flaps Extensive defects of temporal bone Temporalis flap Pedicled trapezius or latissimus flap Free tissue transfer
Cheek	Primary goal is optimal color and texture match Orient in concert with relaxed skin tension lines Complex wounds must address mucosal lining and external cover	Small wounds Secondary intention Primary closure Local flaps Banner (note) flaps Rhomboid flaps Bilobed flaps Larger wounds Cervicofacial flap Free tissue transfer

Table 32–1. *continued*

Location	Challenges and Special Considerations	Reconstructive Choices
Scalp	Tissue has limited flexibility Tissue expansion may be an option Must preserve perichondrium for skin-graft survival Beware of skin grafts in a radiated field	Small wounds Secondary intention Primary closure Full/split-thickness skin grafts Larger wounds Scalp flaps Local transposition flaps Extensive defects Free tissue transfer

Source: From "Skin cancer of the head and neck" by B.A. Moore and R.S. Weber in Practical Head and Neck Oncology (pp. 162–163) by G.J. Petruzzelli: (Ed.).

Skin Grafts

Skin grafts constitute a rapid and reliable method of head and neck cutaneous reconstruction with a broad range of applications. Skin grafts are the preferred reconstructive technique in critically ill patients who demand minimal operative time, when initial margin status in unclear, or rapid adjuvant therapy is required, or if the patient prefers such a minimalist approach, when primary closure is not feasible. Patients should be extensively counseled prior to skin grafting, as the final cosmetic result often evolves over time, and revision procedures may be required.[20]

Skin grafts consist of the entire epidermis and a dermal component of variable thickness (Fig 32–3). If less than the entire thickness of the dermis is included, this graft is referred to as a split-thickness skin graft (STSG). STSGs are categorized further as thin (0.005 to 0.012 inch), intermediate (0.012 to 0.018 inch), or thick (0.018 to 0.030 inch), based on the thickness of the harvested graft.[21] Full-thickness skin grafts (FTSG) include the epidermis and dermis, as well as a variable amount of subdermal fat that should be thinned prior to placement. The choice between full- and split-thickness grafting depends on wound condition, location, thickness, size, and aesthetic concerns.[20–24] Other grafts employed in head and neck cutaneous reconstruction include cartilage grafts, bone grafts, and composite grafts, such as those consisting of skin and cartilage harvested from the auricle.[20]

Skin grafts are transferred from the donor site to the defect without an independent blood supply. Graft survival within the first 24 to 48 hours is predicated on plasmatic imbibition, in which the graft basically is ischemic and derives its nutrients from the extracellular fluid of the recipient bed. During the next phase, termed inosculation, blood vessels and capillaries penetrate into the graft until the final phase of revascularization ensues, with anastomoses and subsequent flow between vessels in the graft and recipient bed over the next 48 to 72 hours. Adherence to a well-vascularized recipient bed is critical for skin graft survival, making placement in a previously irradiated area fraught with difficulty.[20]

STSGs tend to demonstrate more reliable take than FTSGs, although they result in more wound contracture, and, often, a less desirable cosmetic outcome due to color, texture, and thickness mismatches. Specifically, STSGs, often hypo- or hyperpigment, are depressed compared to the surrounding facial skin, and exhibit a shiny appearance that renders the reconstruction obvious to the eye in a potentially unpleasing way.[23,24] STSG are most commonly used to resurface large wounds, line cavities or mucosal defects, close flap donor sites, and cover muscle flaps; they often are used in concert with another reconstructive technique such as a latissimus dorsi muscle free flap in scalp reconstruction (Fig 32–4). Their reliability and rapid harvest makes STSGs a reasonable choice for wound coverage in critically ill patients who cannot tolerate prolonged

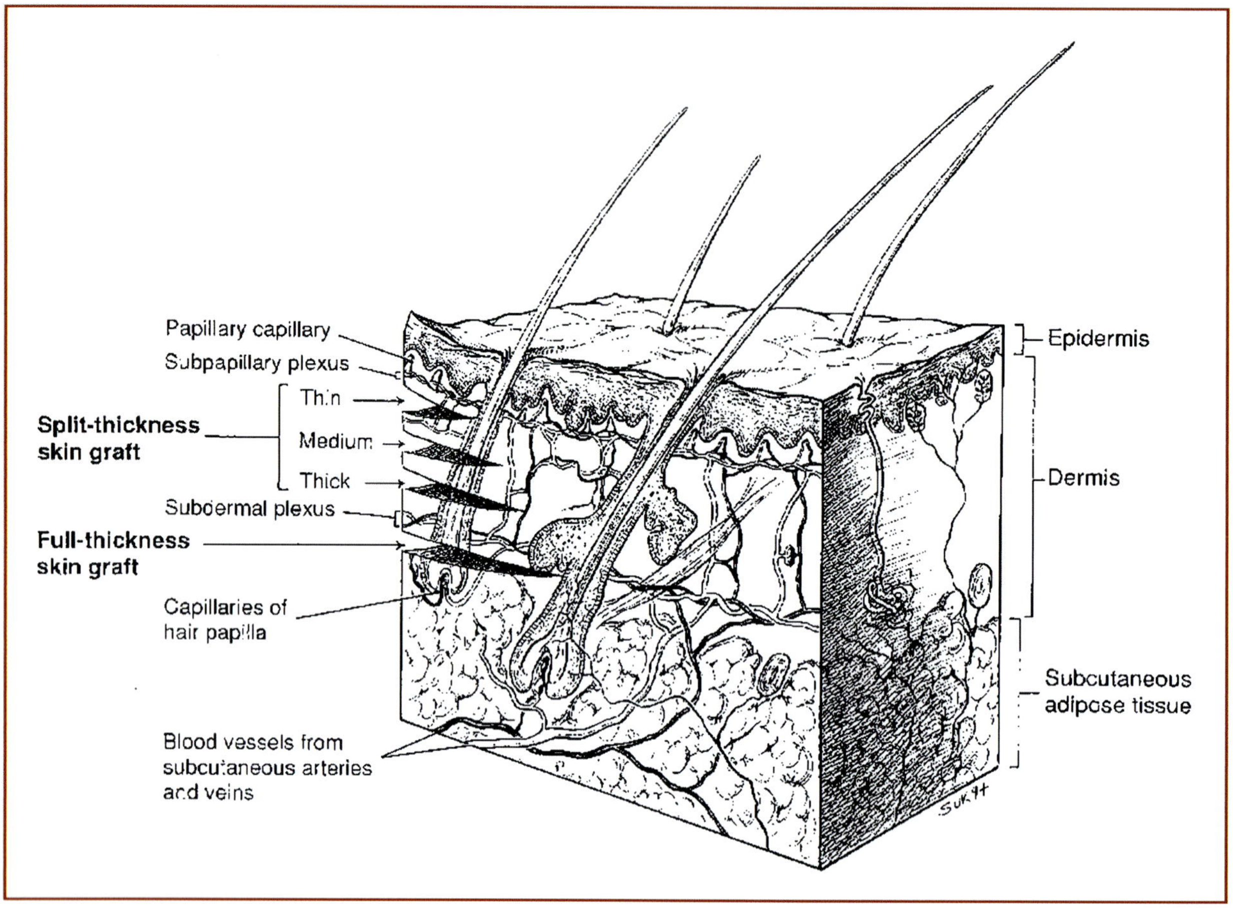

Figure 32–3. Graphic depiction of skin anatomy pertinent to the thickness of skin graft harvest. From Reece GP, Kroll SS. Skin grafts. In: Weber RS, Miller MJ, Goepfert H, eds. *Basal and Squamous Cell Skin Cancers of the Head and Neck*. Baltimore, MD: Williams and Wilkins; 1996;225–242, with permission.

procedures, or when coverage is needed to facilitate definitive margin control or easy monitoring for recurrence.[20] However, they are quite fragile and may not withstand subsequent radiation therapy. STSGs may be harvested by hand, often from the supraclavicular fossa or pre- or postauricular region, or with a dermatome from the upper thigh or buttock, and the resultant donor defect may be closed primarily or allowed to heal by secondary intention (Fig 32–5).[20]

FTSGs frequently are preferred over STSGs for head and neck cutaneous reconstruction because they demonstrate improved texture, thickness, and color match to native tissues, and they are subject to less contracture. These grafts have wide applicability in the head and neck, constituting the modality of choice in certain defects such as small wounds of the scalp or auricle, or a reasonable secondary choice in total nasal resurfacing (see Table 32–1). A FTSG may be harvested from the supraclavicular region, an incision modeled around a cervical or facial crease, the upper eyelid, the pre- or postauricular tissues, or the inguinal region. The donor site typically can be closed primarily. However, FTSGs have higher metabolic needs and require optimal conditions for survival, resulting in higher failure rates.[22,24]

Cartilage grafts consisting of cartilage and perichondrium are particularly important in nasal reconstruction, reconstituting the support structures, and they often are performed coincident with other

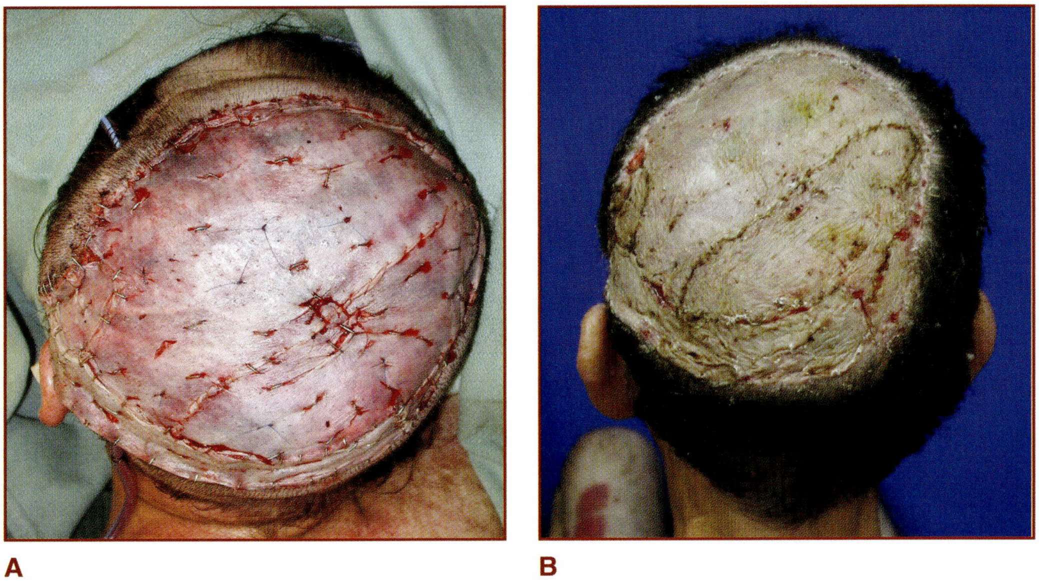

Figure 32–4. Reconstruction of a massive scalp wound following resection of a multiply recurrent basal cell carcinoma of the scalp, including craniectomy and dural resection with a latissimus dorsi muscle free flap covered with split-thickness skin grafts. The intraoperative (**A**) and early postoperative (**B**) views demonstrate complete graft take and gradual atrophy of the muscle resulting in excellent contour.

techniques to provide cover and lining. Common donor sites for cartilage grafts include the nasal septum, conchal bowl, helix, antihelix, and rib, with the choice dependent on the volume of support needed and the patient's prior surgical history.[20] Composite grafts of two types of tissue, most often skin and cartilage, are ideal for small (<1 cm) defects of the nasal ala, and auricular helix, and they frequently are harvested from the helix, antihelix, or conchal bowl. Similar to FTSGs, composite grafts must not exceed 1 cm in maximum dimension because their survival may be compromised.[20]

Flaps

Flap reconstruction of the head and neck is a nonspecific term that indicates the reconstructed tissue carries its own blood supply, either randomly or via a named local, regional, or distant vessel. Because of their superior vascularity, flaps contract less than skin grafts and often produce more durable coverage and superior cosmetic results. Postoperatively, flaps maintain their original color, thickness, and texture, and they may manifest sensation and hair growth similar to the donor site. As a generic term, flaps range from simple skin advancement or transposition of tissue to composite flaps containing many different tissues such as skin, muscle, bone, fat, and fascia. Flaps are classified based on their blood supply (random and axial pattern), donor site location, type of tissue transferred, or the method of transfer. Tissue may be transferred from an area adjacent to the defect (local flaps) or from a noncontiguous anatomic site (regional or distant flap). Distant flaps may be either pedicled, indicating that they remain attached to their original blood supply, or free, which requires a microvascular anastomosis at the recipient site.[25]

Local Random Flaps

A random pattern flap derives its blood supply from the communication of vessels in the dermal-subdermal plexus. Design of these flaps usually follows a 4 to 1 ratio of flap length to width due to this

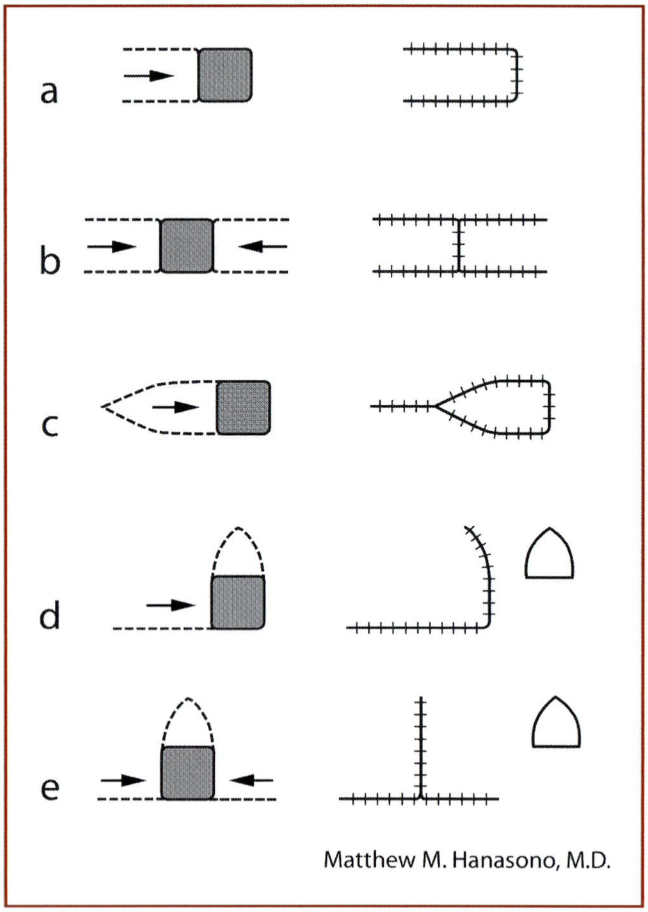

Figure 32–5. Types of local advancement flaps: simple advancement flap (*a*), bilateral advancement flap (*b*), V to Y flap (*c*), wedge (Burow's) advancement flap (*d*), and A to T flap (*e*).

blood supply pattern. The majority of cutaneous flaps in the face are random pattern flaps. Local random flaps are ideal for repairing defects resulting from excision of small skin cancers of the nose, cheek, and periauricular area. Local random flaps from adjacent tissues generally provide excellent color, texture, and thickness match to the defect. Common variants of local random flaps include advancement, rotation, and transposition flaps, which are described in more detail below.[26,27]

Local random flaps are heavily influenced by design, technique, and patient factors such as prior radiotherapy, and smoking. Random local flaps may not be ideal for larger defects or in patients who smoke or who have been previously radiated due to limited vascular supply to these flaps.[25,26] Other complications of local flaps include partial or total flap loss, standing cone deformities, "pin cushioning," or the "trap-door" effect, from concentric scarring, distortion of critical structures like the eyelid, lip, and nasal alae, and potentially undesirable redistribution of hair.[27] Another risk of local random flaps is the potential to transfer diseased or damaged tissue into the extirpative defect.

Advancement Flaps. Advancement flaps are among the most versatile techniques in head and neck cutaneous reconstruction. Through broad undermining of adjacent mobile skin in a subdermal plane to include some fat with the flap, advancement flaps may be employed to close both small and large defects in multiple aesthetic regions. In general, a minimum 3 to 1 length to width ratio should be designed to minimize the risk of distal flap necrosis. Variations of advancement flaps include single and double advancement flaps, V to Y flaps, Burow's triangle or wedge flaps, and A to T flaps (see Fig 32–5). A to T flaps, which are essentially bilateral wedge flaps that leave a "T"-shaped scar, are valuable at the hairline, lip, and chin, when one edge of a defect tolerates minimal to no distortion. The V to Y flap, which is an island pedicled advancement flap that results in a "Y"-shaped scar, has wide applicability in the head and neck.[28–30]

Rotation Flaps. Similar to advancement flaps, rotation flaps comprise a straightforward method of cutaneous reconstruction, utilizing closely matched, adjacent tissue to redistribute tension and potentially camouflage incisions within RSTLs.[31] Common indications include the nasal dorsum and cheek. For example, the cervicofacial rotation flap provides excellent coverage of cheek and lower eyelid lesions, and it can be modified as needed to cover more extensive defects (Fig 32–6).[32,33] Larger wounds of the cheek may merit extension of a cervicofacial flap onto the chest, and these flaps should be elevated as composite flaps, incorporating the platysma or superficial musculoaponeurotic system (SMAS), to maximize the vascularity (Fig 32–7).[27,33,34]

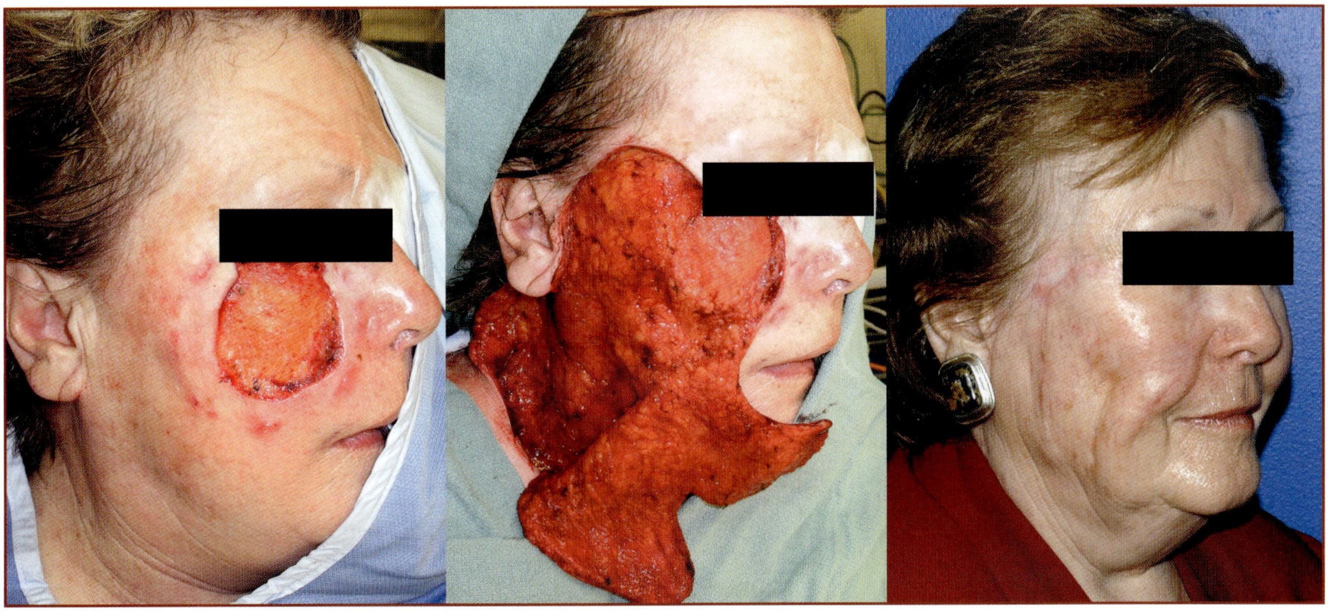

A B C

Figure 32–6. Intraoperative (**A**) and postoperative (**B** and **C**) views of a cervicofacial flap used to reconstruct a defect resulting from excision of a malignant melanoma.

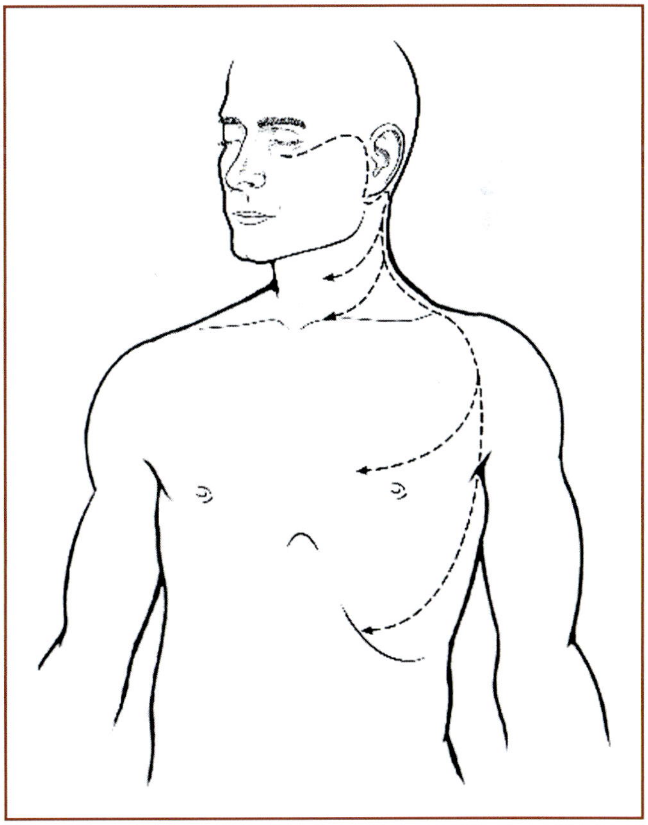

Figure 32–7. Incision options for large cervicofacial or cervicothoracic rotation flaps. From Moore BA, Wine T, Netterville JL. Cervicofacial and cervicothoracic rotation flaps in head and neck reconstruction. *Head Neck.* 2005;27(12):1092-1101, with permission.

Disadvantages of rotation flaps include the potential need for extensive undermining of adjacent tissues. Standing cone deformities, or "dog-ears," also are common. As with advancement flaps, prior incisions or radiotherapy may limit the extension or arc of rotation as well as the viability of the distal portions of the flap, and, therefore, the applicability of rotation flaps in the head and neck.[27]

Transposition Flaps. Transposition flaps demonstrate wide applicability to cutaneous defects of the head and neck, and are predicated on meticulous planning and defect analysis. They range from the simple note or banner flap utilized in cheek or nasal reconstruction to rhombic flaps and bilobed flaps, which are ideal for a variety of nasal defects.[35,36] In general, transposition flaps are frequently utilized on the nose, particularly the dorsum and side walls, due to tissue laxity in these areas. The bilobed flap, a unique variant of transposition flap that requires a double movement of tissue, has gained widespread acceptance for use in nasal wounds up to 1.5 cm in maximum dimension, as demonstrated in Figure 32–8.[27,37]

Rhombic flaps demonstrate great utility for both cheek and nasal wounds, but demand careful design. In the classic description, or Limberg flap, a rhomboid defect with angles of 60 and 120 degrees is defined and then the flap is oriented in one of four directions off the short axis, in order to hide it in an RSTL and minimize tension or distortion of adjacent structures.[27,38] The initial version has been modified over time to accommodate circular wounds, improve redistribution of tension, and limit the scar length and potential standing cone deformity.[39,40] Rhombic flaps are useful in areas of tissue laxity such as the cheek and temple (Fig 32–9).

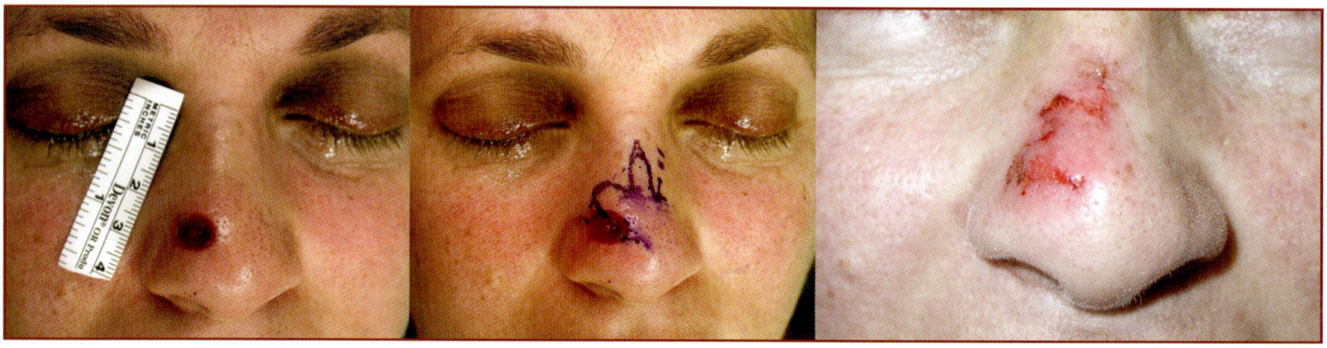

A B C

Figure 32–8. Intraoperative (**A, B**) and early postoperative (**C**) views of a 1.2-cm dorsal nasal defect resulting from Mohs micrographic surgery that was reconstructed with a bilobed flap.

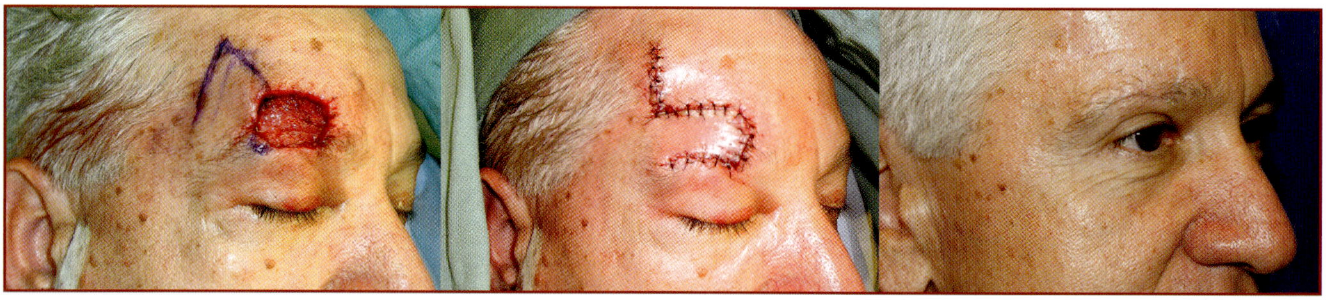

A B C

Figure 32–9. Intraoperative (**A, B**) and postoperative (**C**) view of a rhombic flap used to reconstruct a right temporal defect resulting from Mohs micrographic surgery to remove a basal cell carcinoma.

Axial Pattern Flaps

Axial pattern flaps are defined by an anatomically recognized arteriovenous circulation derived from a named artery that follows the long axis of the flap and branches to the dermal-subdermal plexus. Unlike random pattern flaps, the vascularity of axial flaps is determined by the length of the specific axial vessel within the flap, rather than width-to-length ratio. The length is not entirely limited by the length of the named vessel: additional tissue at the distal tip with random blood supply from the subdermal plexus may provide additional length. When dissecting an axial pattern flap, the plane of dissection extends deeply to include the fascia containing the relevant named artery.[25]

The pre-eminent axial pattern flap in head and neck cutaneous reconstruction is the interpolated paramedian forehead flap. It is called an interpolated flap because the base of the flap is not contiguous with the defect, differentiating it from a transposition flap.[41] The interpolated paramedian forehead flap is based on the supratrochlear artery, whereas another interpolated flap commonly used in the head and neck, the melolabial flap, is based on branches of the facial artery. Although reliable, these flaps often require multiple stages, with division of the main flap pedicle and definitive inset occurring several weeks after initial elevation once neovascularization occurs into the flap from tissues adjacent to the recipient bed.[13]

The interpolated paramedian forehead flap constitutes the primary modality for resurfacing large (>1.5 cm) defects of the distal nasal dorsum, tip, and ala, as well as select wounds in the medial upper cheek and lower eyelid. It is based on the supratrochlear artery, and can be modified as necessary to increase flap length, typically by extending the superior limit into the hairline or dropping the incisions at the base below the orbital rim. The pedicle may be designed as narrow as 1.2 cm, and bilateral flaps are possible. The donor defect typically is closed primarily across the forehead, and the superior extent may be left to heal by secondary intention. A hearty flap, the distal skin may be thinned primarily or at a later stage. The pedicle is frequently divided at a second stage 3 to 6 weeks later, once distal neovascularization occurs.[13]

Similarly, the nasolabial or melolabial flap is another versatile interpolated flap in facial reconstruction. Based on branches of the facial artery, this flap may be pedicled proximally or distally and used to resurface defects of the nasal ala or sidewall, lip, or even intraoral wounds. It is a hybrid flap, in the sense that it also may be elevated as an island subcutaneous flap or advanced in one stage.[41]

Other Pedicled Flaps. An array of regional pedicled flaps are also available for use in head and neck cutaneous reconstruction: the submental island flap, the temporalis flap, the superficial temporoparietal fascia flap, the supraclavicular flap, and various permutations of the scalping flap.[42–44] Unfortunately, donor site morbidity is a limiting factor with many of these flaps, as the secondary defect often is as significant as, if not worse than, the primary wound. Many of these modalities are of historic significance only, but they may retain utility in austere settings or as salvage procedures. When a larger volume of tissue is required, distal pedicled flaps such as the pectoralis major, latissimus dorsi, and trapezius system flaps can provide necessary bulk, although applications may be limited by arc of rotation and the distance from the defect.[45–47]

Free Tissue Transfer

The advent of free tissue transfer in head and neck oncologic reconstruction has made single-stage resection and reconstruction of composite facial defects possible. Simply put, free tissue transfer requires the vascular detachment of an isolated and specific region of the body followed by transfer of that tissue to another region of the body with reattachment of the divided artery and vein to the recipient site artery and vein. Tissues transferred by this method include skin, fat, fascia, muscle, and bone, as well as composites of these tissues. Many local and regional pedicled flaps also can be used as free flaps, such as the rectus abdominis muscle or myocutaneous flap. Free flaps commonly used in head and neck cutaneous reconstruction include the anterolateral thigh, rectus abdominis muscle/myocutaneous, latissimus dorsi muscle/myocutaneous, fibula osseous/osteocutaneous, and radial forearm fasciocutaneous/osteocutaneous flaps.[48]

The ability to reconstruct complex three-dimensional defects with composite tissue is one of the primary advantages of free tissue transfer, potentially improving cosmetic and functional outcomes. It liberates ablative surgeons to accomplish comprehensive tumor extirpation without sacrificing margins due to limitations of local or regional reconstructive options. Similarly, it allows reconstructive surgeons to incorporate well-vascularized tissue into challenging wounds in previously irradiated areas that would not be amenable to conventional local or regional pedicled flap reconstruction (Fig 32–10). Free flaps are very reliable, with success rates exceeding 95% in most recent series, and they facilitate single-stage reconstruction of difficult wounds.[48–51]

However, there is a learning curve of success in head and neck microvascular surgery, and the operations tend to occupy more operating room time. Special training, experience, and equipment are required both intraoperatively and perioperatively. Because the donor sites often do not have similar color, texture, and thickness to the recipient tissues, free flaps often result in an obvious tissue mismatch. Unfortunately, as with any large flap reconstruction, tumor recurrences can be obscured by the added bulk.[48]

Prosthetic Rehabilitation

Prosthetic rehabilitation, rather than reconstruction with living tissue, may produce the best aesthetic result in certain instances, such as in re-creating the aesthetics of the globe after orbitectomy or orbital exenteration. In others, it may produce at least an equal result, but in significantly fewer stages, such as in nasal and auricular reconstructions for substantial or total defects. In these cases, prosthetic rehabilitation may be preferred to extensive and multiply staged surgeries, in patients with multiple medical comorbidities making them poor surgical candidates. Prosthetic rehabilitation also may be favored when there are limited options in donor tissues for flap and graft reconstructions. Downsides of prostheses include problems with fit and fixation, cost, availability, need for periodic replacement, and

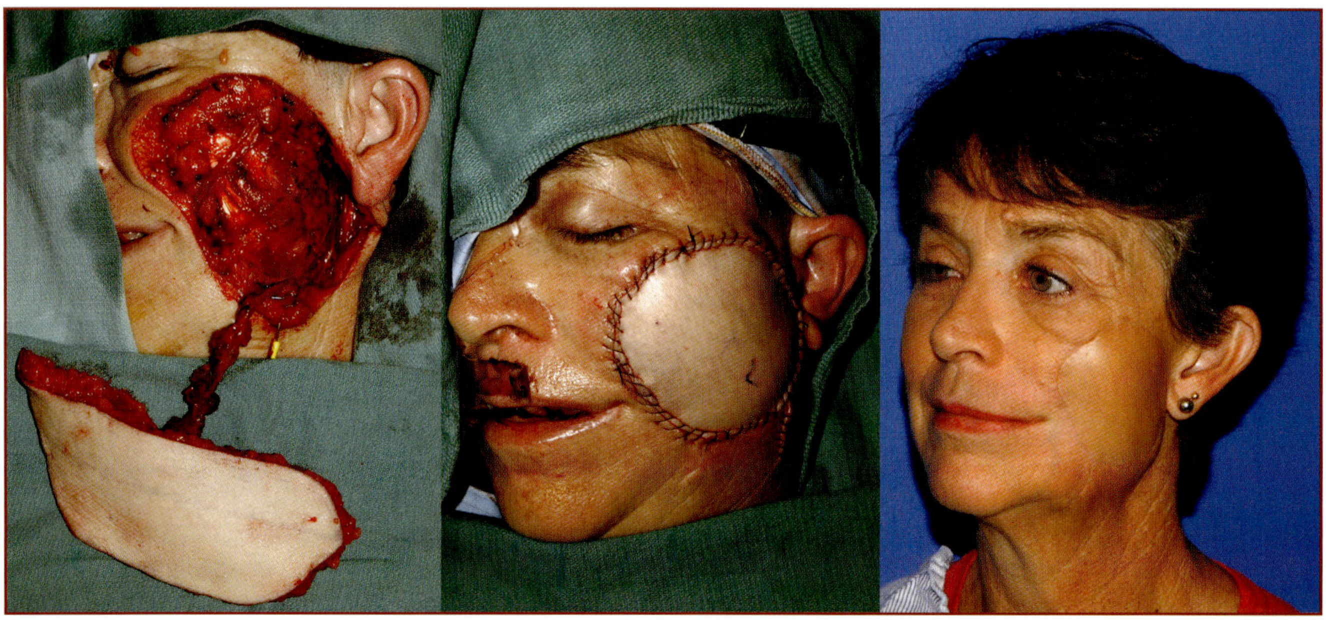

A B C

Figure 32–10. Intraoperative (**A, B**) and postoperative (**C**) views of a left cheek defect resulting from excision of a previously irradiated, recurrent malignant melanoma reconstructed with an anterolateral thigh free flap.

the sense that they are not "natural" part of one's body. Details of prosthetic rehabilitation are discussed in Chapter 39.

Conclusions

The management of cutaneous malignancy of the head and neck requires a multidisciplinary approach, and reconstructive surgeons are integral to this process to optimize the functional and aesthetic outcome. Although reconstructive considerations should not impact the oncologic sanctity of an operation, proper preoperative planning incorporates the reconstructive team to accommodate multiple options.

Head and neck cutaneous reconstruction begins with a thoughtful analysis of the defect, with particular attention paid to the size, components, and surrounding structures. Optimal outcomes are achieved with local or regional tissue that demonstrates excellent color, texture, and thickness match to the adjacent tissues, and this can be accomplished with a multitude of techniques that encompass the entire reconstructive ladder. Free tissue transfer has expanded the possibilities for functional and aesthetic reconstruction of larger defects with multiple tissue components, particularly for lesions occurring in compromised settings of prior surgery or radiation where reliable local and regional options are few. Each anatomic site in the head and neck presents unique challenges, so there is no ideal modality or flap. We advocate a defect-oriented approach, which is discussed in great detail in the chapters that follow.

References

1. Stiefel M, Shaner A, Schaefer SD. The Edwin Smith Papyrus: the birth of analytical thinking in medicine and otolaryngology. *Laryngoscope.* 2006;116(2):182–188.
2. Whitaker IS, Karoo RO, Spyrou G, Fenton OM. The birth of plastic surgery: the story of nasal reconstruction from the Edwin Smith Papyrus to the twenty-first century. *Plast Reconstr Surg.* 2007;120(1):327–336.
3. Clayman CL, Lee JJ, Holsinger FC, et al. Mortality risk from squamous cell skin cancer. *J Clin Oncol.* 2005;23(4):759–765.
4. Olascoaga A, Vilar-Compte D, Poitevin-Chacon A, Contreras-Ruiz J. Wound healing in radiated skin: pathophysiology and treatment options. *Int Wound J.* 2008;5(2):246–257.
5. Rosenthal DI, Liu L, Lee JH, et al. Importance of treatment package time in surgery and postoperative radiation therapy for squamous cell carcinoma of the head and neck. *Head Neck.* 2002;24(2):115–126.
6. Kinsella JB, Rassekh CH, Wasmuth TD, et al. Smoking increases facial skin flap complications. *Ann Otol Rhinol Laryngol.* 1999;108:139–142.
7. Hanna DC. Present and future trends in reconstructive surgery for head and neck cancer patients. *Laryngoscope.* 1978;88(1 pt2 suppl 8):96–100.
8. Burget G, Menick FJ. The subunit principle in nasal reconstruction. *Plast Reconstr Surg.* 1985;76:239–247.
9. Robinson JK. Segmental reconstruction of the face. *Dermatol Surg.* 2004;30(1):67–74.
10. Levasseur JG, Mellette JR, Jr. Techniques for reconstruction of perialar and perialar-nasal ala combined defects. *Dermatol Surg.* 2000;26(11):1019–1023.
11. Borges AF. Relaxed skin tension lines (RSTL) versus other skin lines. *Plast Reconstr Surg.* 1984;73(1):144–150.
12. Wilhelmi BJ, Blackwell SJ, Phillips LG. Langer's lines: to use or not to use. *Plast Reconstr Surg.* 1999;104(1):208–214.
13. Jewett BS. Interpolated forehead and melolabial flaps. *Facial Plast Surg Clin North Am.* 2009;17:361–377.
14. Hurvitz KA, Kobayashi M, Evans GR. Current options in head and neck reconstruction. *Plast Reconstr Surg.* 2006;118(5):122e–133e.
15. Van der Eerden PA, Lohuis PJ, Hart AA, Mulder WC, Vuyk H. Secondary intention healing after excision of nonmelanoma skin cancer of the head and neck: statistical evaluation of prognostic values of wound characteristics and final cosmetic results. *Plast Reconstr Surg.* 2008;122(6):1747–1755.
16. Svensjo T, Pomahac B, Yao F, et al. Accelerated healing of full-thickness wounds in a wet environment. *Plast Reconstr Surg.* 2000;106(3):602–612.
17. Zitelli JA. Secondary intention healing: an alternative to surgical repair. *Clin Dermatol.* 1984;2(3):92–106.
18. Goldwyn RM, Rueckert F. The value of healing by secondary intention for sizeable defects of the face. *Arch Surg.* 1977;112(3):285–292.
19. Weber SM, Baker SR. Management of cutaneous nasal defects. *Facial Plast Surg Clin North Am.* 2009;17(3):395–417.
20. Ratner D. Skin grafting. *Sem Cut Med Surg.* 2003;22(4):295–305.
21. Petruzzelli GJ, Johnson JT. Skin grafts. *Otolaryngol Clin North Am.* 1994;27(1):25–37.
22. Rudolph R. The effect of skin graft preparation on wound contraction. *Surg Gynecol Obstet.* 1976;142(1):49–56.

23. Ratner D. Skin grafting: from here to there. *Dermatol Clin.* 1998;16(1):75–90.
24. White N, Hettiaratchy S, Papini RP. The choice of split-thickness skin graft donor site: patients' and surgeons' preferences. *Plast Reconstr Surg.* 2003;112(3):933–934.
25. Mathes SJ, Hansen SL. Flap classification and applications. In: Mathes SJ. *Plastic Surgery. Vol. I: General Principles.* 2nd ed. Philadelphia, PA: Saunders; 2005:365–482.
26. Tschoi M, Hoy EA, Granick MS. Skin flaps. *Clin Plast Surg.* 2005;32(2):261–273
27. Chu EA, Byrne PJ. Local flaps I: bilobed, rhombic, and cervicofacial. *Facial Plast Surg Clin N Am.* 2009;17:349–360.
28. Krishnan R, Garman M, Nunez-Gussman J, Orengo I. Advancement flaps: a basic theme with many variations. *Dermatol Surg.* 2008;31(8 pt 2):986–994.
29. Pribaz JJ, Chester CH, Barrall DT. The extended V-Y flap. *Plast Reconstr Surg.* 1992;90(2):275–280.
30. Tomich JM, Wentzell JM, Grande DJ. Subcutaneous island pedicle flaps. *Arch Dermatol.* 1987;123(4):514–518.
31. Jackson IT. Local flap reconstruction after excision of nonmelanoma skin cancer. *Clin Plast Surg.* 1997;24(4): 747–767.
32. Mustarde JC. The use of flaps in the orbital region. *Plast Reconstr Surg.* 1970;45(2):146–150.
33. Moore BA, Wine T, Netterville JL. Cervicofacial and cervicothoracic flaps in head and neck reconstruction. *Head Neck.* 2005;27(12):1092–1101.
34. Kroll SS, Reece GP, Robb G, Black J. Deep-plane cervicofacial rotation-advancement flap for reconstruction of large cheek defects. *Plast Reconstr Surg.* 1994;94(1):88–93.
35. Zitelli JA. The bilobed flap for nasal reconstruction. *Arch Dermatol.* 1989;125(7):957–959.
36. Field LM. The glabellar transposition "banner" flap. *J Dermatol Surg Oncol.* 1988;14(4):376–379.
37. Zitelli JA, Fazio MS. Reconstruction of the nose with local flaps. *J Dermatol Surg Oncol.* 1991;17(2):184–189.
38. Limberg AA. *Mathematical Principles of Local Plastics Procedures on the Surface of the Human Body.* Leningrad, Russia: Medgis; 1946.
39. Quaba AA, Sommerlad BC. A square peg into a round hole: a modified rhomboid flap and its clinical application. *Br J Plast Surg.* 1987;40(2):163–170.
40. Fee WE Jr., Gunter JP, Carder HM. Rhomboid flap principles and common variations. *Laryngoscope.* 1976;86(11): 1706–1711.
41. Baker SR. Flap classification and design. In: Baker SR, ed. *Local Flaps in Facial Reconstruction.* 2nd ed. Philadelphia, PA: Mosby; 2007:71–106.
42. Chow TL, Chan TT-F, Chow T-K, et al. Reconstruction with submental flap for aggressive orofacial cancer. *Plast Reconstr Surg.* 2007;120(2):431–436.
43. Chiu ES, Liu PH, Friedlander PL Supraclavicular artery island flap for head and neck oncologic reconstruction: indications, complications, and outcomes. *Plast Reconstr Surg.* 2009;124(1):115–123.
44. Papadopoulos O, Karypidis D, Moustaki M, et al. Double scalping flap: a versatile technique in scalp reconstruction. *J Craniofac Surg.* 2009;20(5):1484–1491.
45. Ariyan S. The pectoralis major myocutaneous flap. *Plast Reconstr Surg.* 1979;63(1):73–81.
46. Hayden RE, Kirby SD, Deschler DG. Technical modifications of the latissimus dorsi pedicled flap to increase versatility and viability. *Laryngoscope.* 2000;110(3):352–357.
47. Netterville JL, Panje WR, Maves MD. The trapezius myocutaneous flap. *Arch Otolaryngol Head Neck Surg.* 1987; 113(3):271–281.
48. Wax M. Free Tissue transfer in the reconstruction of massive skin cancer. *Facial Plast Surg Clin North Am.* 2009; 17(2):279–286
49. Beasley NJ, Gilbert RW, Gullane PJ et al. Scalp and forehead reconstruction using free revascularized tissue transfer. *Arch Facial Plast Surg.* 2004;6(1):16–20.
50. Funk GF, Laurenzo JF, Valentino J et al. Free tissue transfer reconstruction of midfacial and cranio-orbito-facial defects. *Arch Otolaryngol Head Neck Surg.* 1995;121(3):293–303.
51. Lipa JE, Butler CE. Enhancing the outcome of free latissimus dorsi muscle flap reconstruction of scalp defects. *Head Neck.* 2004;26(1):46–53.

33

NASAL RECONSTRUCTION

MATTHEW M. HANASONO
ROBERT L. WALTON
ELISABETH K. BEAHM

Introduction

The function of the nose is to act as a conduit for respired air, warming and humidifying it while directing it past the olfactory sensors. Aesthetically, the nose dominates the central face and, when it is absent or deformed, has a profound effect on facial appearance and self-image. The ideal reconstruction is performed with autologous tissues and produces a result that is as close as possible to the color, texture, and contour of the original nose. However, the goal of creating a stable, refined, and three-dimensionally accurate nasal reconstruction remains one of the most challenging to achieve in reconstructive surgery. Although an entire text could be devoted to the various techniques used for nasal reconstruction, this chapter will attempt to provide broad principles and useful technical pearls for basic nasal reconstruction that can be applied to the majority of nasal defects encountered following skin cancer resection.

Nasal Anatomy

It is most convenient to conceptualize nasal defects based on an evaluation of what tissue components are missing, including the covering skin, bony or cartilaginous skeletal support, and epithelial or mucosal lining. These components, the "cover," "support," and "lining," vary in thickness, texture, pliability, and, in the case of the external skin, color between different regions of the nose. To functionally and aesthetically restore the nose, all resected components must be replaced as part of the reconstruction.

The external nose can be further divided into visual "subunits" based on concavities or convexities that are perceived as regions of light or shadow (Fig 33–1). These subunits, defined and later refined by Burget and Menick, can be used as a guide to plan the most aesthetic placement of scars as transition lines between subunits are hidden by natural shadows and, therefore, are less noticeable.[1–3] Although a subject of debate, it also has been suggested that, when reasonable, the entire subunit should be replaced if more than 50% of that subunit has been resected for cancer, excising viable, noncancerous skin if need be, so that visible scarring and "patchiness" due to color mismatches are minimized.

Skin characteristics of the various subunits of the nose differ substantially. The skin of the dorsum and sidewalls is thin, smooth, pliable, and mobile, making this area a good donor site for local flaps. The skin of the columella and alar rims is thin but densely adherent. The skin of the soft triangles, which are the small regions of skin spanning the angle formed by the columella and alae, is also thin and not pliable. The skin of the tip is thick and stiff, and has a high density of sebaceous glands.

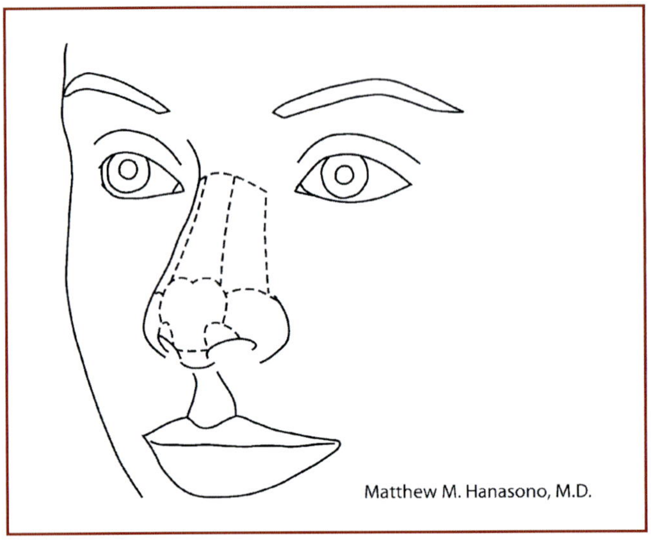

Figure 33–1. External nasal subunits. Adapted from: Burget GC, Menick FJ. Subunit principle in nasal reconstruction. *Plast Reconstr Surg.* 1985;76:239–247 with permission.

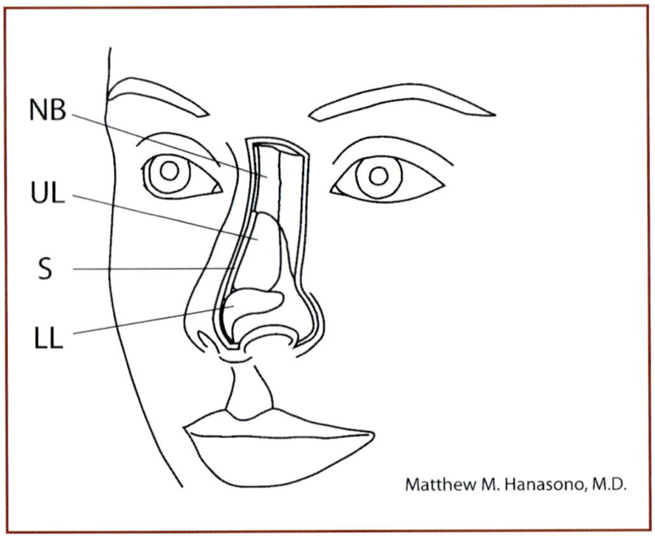

Figure 33–2. The bony and cartilaginous skeletal support of the nose, including the paired nasal bones (NB), upper lateral cartilages (UL), septum (S), and lower lateral cartilages (LL).

The underlying skeletal structure divides the nose into thirds (Fig 33–2). The paired nasal bones support the upper third of the nose. Paired upper and lower lateral cartilages support the middle and lower thirds of the nose, respectively. The medial crura of the lower lateral cartilages are in apposition to each other and support the nasal tip, while the genu and lateral crura give shape to the tip. The alae do not have cartilaginous or bony support and maintain their shape solely due to the density of the fibrofatty tissue within them. Additionally, the nasal septum provides dorsal support to the nose and lies between the medial borders of the paired upper lateral cartilages.

The nasal lining is composed of stratified squamous epithelium in the region of the vestibule and membranous septum. Deep to these areas, the nasal lining is composed of mucosa, which produces mucus and contains cilia that propel the mucus posteriorly toward the nasopharynx. The nasal mucosa is highly vascular due to the rich anastomotic network of feeding blood vessels, which include branches of the facial artery, anterior and posterior ethmoid arteries, sphenopalatine artery, and internal maxillary artery.

Reconstructive Approach

The length to which one goes to restore the nose as closely as possible to its original form is dictated by the desires of the patient and his or her suitability for one or multiple surgeries. Only very small defects in areas of mobile skin can be closed primarily without distorting the nasal shape. However, in some patients, the simplicity of primary closure, even with a moderate amount of disfigurement may be the best choice. Defects of the skin can also be allowed to heal by secondary intention with the understanding that distortion of the nasal shape may occur due to tissue contraction in wounds larger than about 5 mm in diameter.[4]

During delayed reconstruction or revision of a prior, unsatisfactory reconstruction, it is common to underestimate the size of the defect. An initial step during the reconstructive process is to release or excise all scar tissues and relocate the remaining nasal elements to their original positions. Once this is done, the size of the defect can be considerably larger than originally suspected. Creating a template from suture packet foil is often a very useful technique for measuring the true size and extent of the defect, particularly when the defect is large or irregularly shaped.

As mentioned above, when 50% or more of an external skin subunit has been resected, consideration should be given to removing the remainder of the subunit and replacing the entire subunit as long as there are adequate local and/or regional tissues to reconstruct that subunit. Skin defects can be divided into smaller defects, which can be closed with local tissues, and larger defects, which need regional flaps for reconstruction. As a general rule, most local flaps are restricted to about 1.5 to 2 cm in diameter. Cheek and other facial defects generally should be addressed separately from nasal defects, as attempting to reconstruct both with a single reconstructive flap generally will result in a poorly defined nose and a compromised final aesthetic outcome.

For patients who are suboptimal candidates for surgery, based on medical, surgical, or psychosocial conditions, a prosthesis may be the best reconstructive option. Another indication for a prosthesis is when the risk of recurrence is high. In such cases, a prosthesis can be a good temporary solution while allowing reasonable time to pass to rule out an early recurrence in histologically aggressive or recurrent cancers, or while adjuvant therapy is being given. Timely administration of adjuvant therapy may not be possible before completing multistaged reconstructions or it may be preferable to perform reconstructions with tissues not affected by radiation, thus avoiding radiation-associated tissue fibrosis and contracture, which can compromise the final reconstructive result. For large or composite tissue defects, a high quality prosthetic may provide excellent aesthetic results. Prosthetic rehabilitation of nasal and other facial defects is addressed in Chapter 39.

External Skin Replacement

Skin Grafts and Composite Grafts

Skin grafts may be an acceptable reconstructive option for defects of the nasal skin if the wound bed is adequate. Graft take is not reliable over cartilage or bone devoid of perichondrium or periosteum, respectively. Skin grafts should be full-thickness to minimize contracture, and donor sites that are close in texture and color, such as the preauricular, postauricular, or supraclavicular neck skin, are preferred. Even still, some color mismatch is usually anticipated. The graft itself will tend to atrophy and may look shiny in comparison to the surrounding skin once healed. Grafts usually look better on the upper two-thirds of the nose where the skin is thin and smooth, and appear more patch-like and depressed in the lower nose.

Composite chondrocutaneous grafts from the external ear can be used to reconstruct small defects (less than 1.0 to 1.5 cm) of the alar rim and columella.[5–7] Such grafts are harvested from the rim or the root of the auricular helix (Fig 33–3). Although attractive in that external skin, cartilaginous support, and internal lining may be replaced simultaneously, composite auricular grafts often shrink and result in a poor color match to the surrounding tissues. Because composite grafts revascularize from the edges, grafts should be no larger than 1.5 cm in diameter so that the center is never more than 5 to 8 mm away from the blood supply, as a general guideline. Cooling the graft has been suggested as a way to lower the metabolic rate while waiting for revascularization to take place.[8] These grafts theoretically do better if one of the surfaces, internal or external, is denuded of skin and placed on a well-vascularized wound bed, either of the native tissue in partial thickness defects or against a flap. Incomplete graft take is not uncommon and compromised wound vascularity, such as after radiation, are contraindications for using this technique.

Local Flaps

Local flaps do not add skin to the nose. Instead, they rearrange the remaining skin and redistribute it. Local flaps should, therefore, be designed so that they are harvested from areas of relative skin laxity, such as the dorsum of the nose, so that the wound tension after flap inset is not so great as to distort the shape of the nose. Local flaps tend to "pincushion" so the depth of the defect should at least match the thickness of the flap. Often, secondary thinning procedures or corticosteroid injections are beneficial.

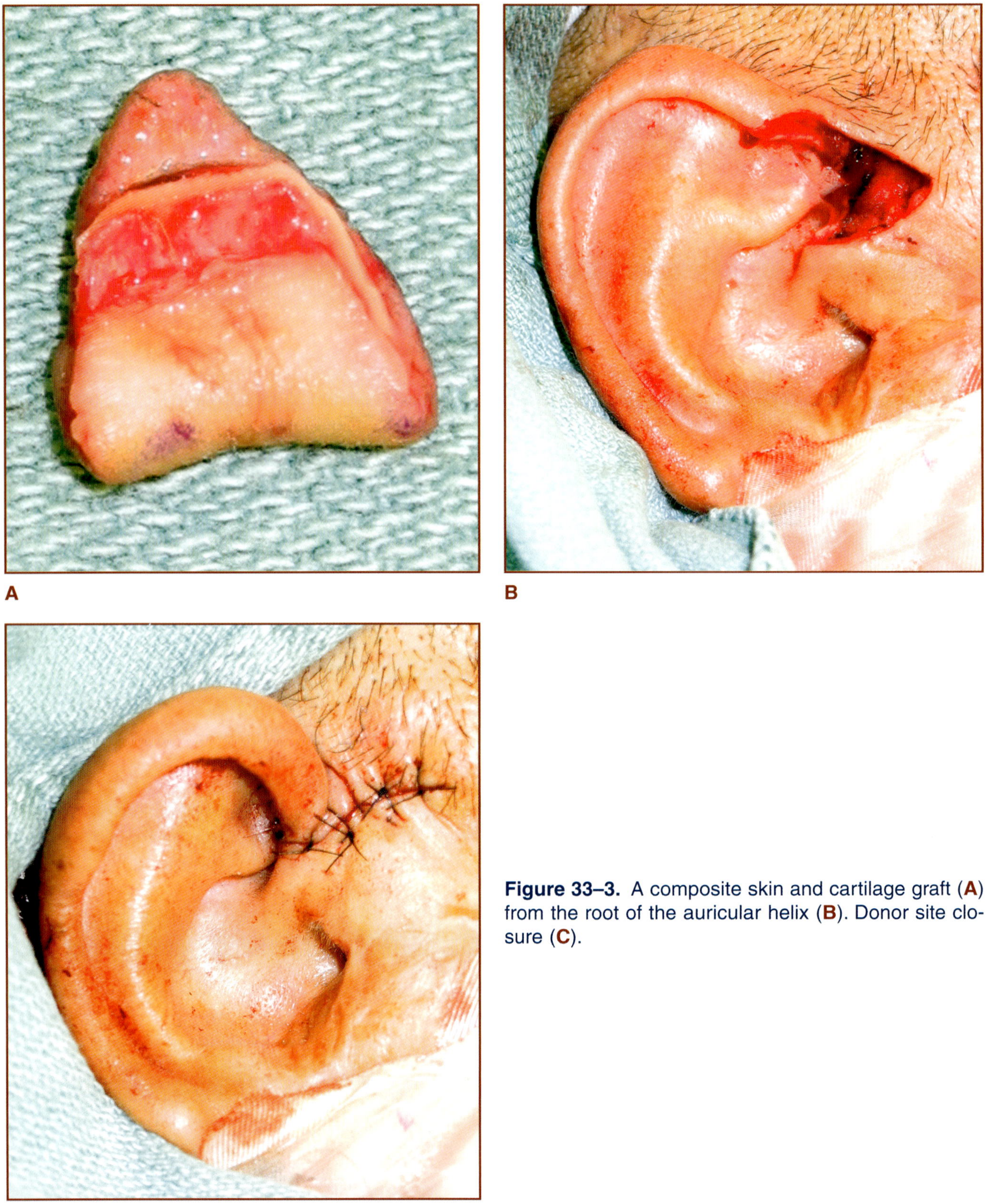

A

B

C

Figure 33–3. A composite skin and cartilage graft (**A**) from the root of the auricular helix (**B**). Donor site closure (**C**).

Single-lobe transposition flaps, also known as banner flaps, are used for small defects, generally under 1.5 cm in greatest diameter.[9] Commonly, banner flaps are harvested from and used to reconstruct external skin defects of the mobile skin of the upper third of the nose as a better matching alternative to skin grafts. Banner flaps and other local flaps should be elevated in a submuscular fashion, within the loose areolar plane above the perichondrium, to preserve vascularity. One criticism of the banner flap is its tendency to distort surrounding nasal landmarks due to tension on the donor site, resulting in elevation of the alar margin.

Bilobed flaps are used for defects of up to 1.5 cm in the thick-skinned areas of the tip and ala.[10,11] They are based on the concept of distributing tension from lax areas of the nose to tight, adherent areas of the nose in a graded fashion by placing a small secondary flap ("lobe") from an area of laxity (i.e., the upper two-thirds of the nose) into the donor defect of the primary flap ("lobe"), which is used to close the original defect (Fig 33–4). The second lobe donor defect takes advantage of the tissue laxity at its donor site and is closed primarily. Because tension is distributed over two transposition flaps, many surgeons favor the bilobed over the banner flap. Each lobe should be transposed about 45 degrees. The diameter of the first lobe should equal the diameter of the defect, and the diameter of the second lobe should be smaller to facilitate primary closure of its donor site defect. A Burow's triangle of skin is excised between the defect and the flap pivot point. Wide undermining above the perichondrial plane is advised to allow transposition and closure without excessive tension and redraping of the nasal skin so that the shape of the nose is not distorted.

The dorsal nasal flap is used to resurface defects of the dorsum and tip by rotating and advancing the majority of the remaining dorsal skin (Fig 33–5).[12] The defect size limitation is between 1.5 and 2.0 cm in diameter, somewhat larger than can be reconstructed with a banner or bilobed flap. The flap itself is richly vascularized, based laterally on the angular vessels. The dorsal nasal flap should not be used for defects that extend past the ala or to the columella in order to prevent alar distortion or elevation of the tip cephalad, respectively. A Burow's triangle excision in the glabellar region may be performed to facilitate donor site closure, if needed.

Regional Flaps

Forehead Flap

The forehead flap is considered by many to be the workhorse of nasal reconstruction due to its excellent color and texture match, reliability, and ability to resurface the entire nose if needed. The forehead is richly vascular and numerous variations of the forehead flap have been described based on both random and axial blood supplies. Most commonly, the forehead flap is designed along a vertical paramedian axis, based on a single supratrochlear artery (Fig 33–6).[13–16] The location of this vessel can be confirmed with a hand-held Doppler ultrasound. For proximal defects, this flap is usually designed to extend from the brow to the hairline. The reach of the flap can be increased significantly by lowering the pivot point into the brow and extending the distal tip into the hair-bearing scalp.

As with other flaps used in nasal reconstruction, the size of the flap should precisely match the size of the skin defect. In heminasal reconstructions, the ipsilateral paramedian forehead provides the maximum arc of rotation. A left-sided flap is rotated clockwise and a right-sided flap is rotated counterclockwise to obtain the shortest distance between the flap pivot point and the nasal defect. The base of the forehead flap should be approximately 1.2 to 1.5 cm in width. Wider based flaps actually risk flap perfusion due to kinking of the pedicle after rotation.

When the location of the defect requires extension of the flap into the hair-bearing scalp, the possibility of hair growth on the reconstructive flap needs to be discussed with the patient preoperatively to avoid undue distress on their part. In nonsmoking patients, hair can be depilated primarily at the time of flap harvest by thinning the distal 1 to 1.5 cm of the flap, removing the hair follicles. However, if there is any doubt regarding the blood supply to the flap, it is best to defer depilation to a later stage. Attempts to avoid hair on the distal flap by designing the flap obliquely so that it avoids the hair-bearing scalp usually result in poor viability of the distal flap and also may compromise the final appearance of the donor site. Angling the distal flap toward the contralateral forehead also may preclude the use of a second flap if needed later.

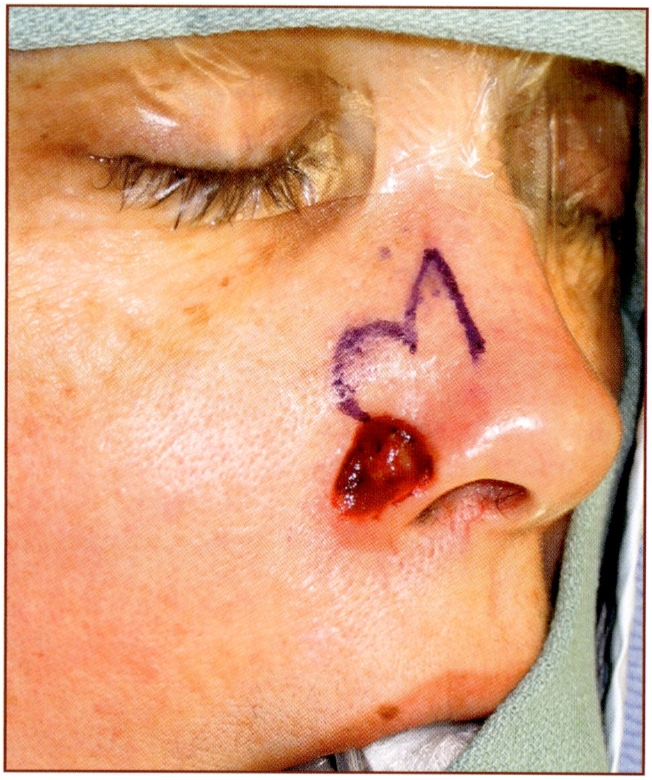

A

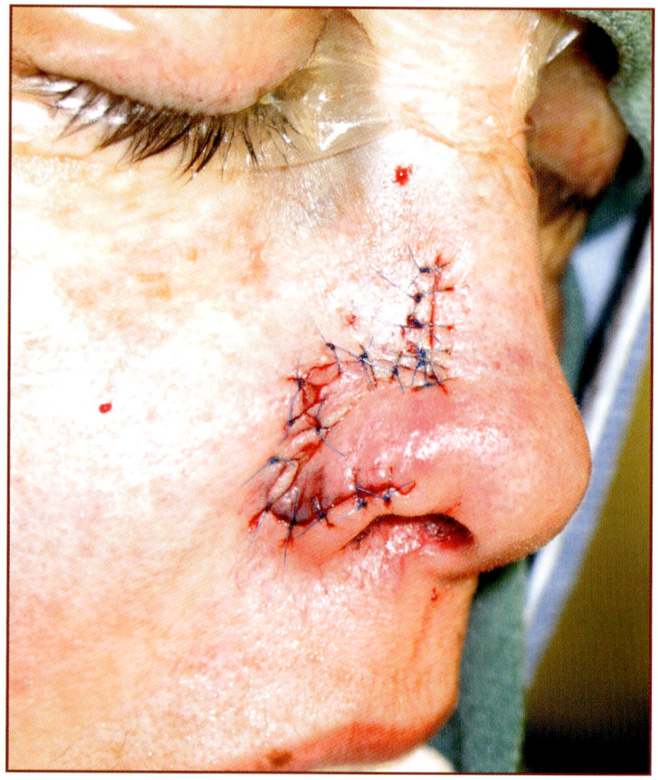

B

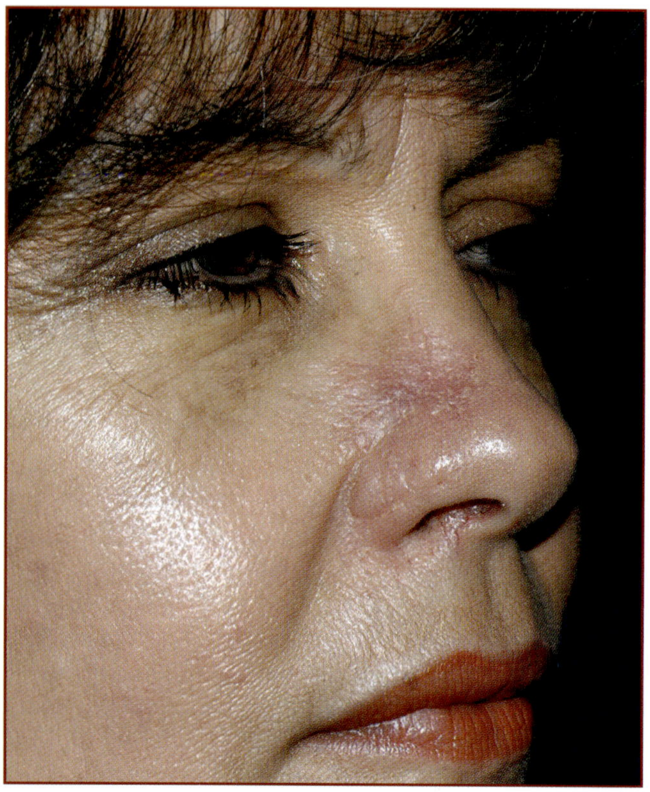

C

Figure 33–4. Example of a defect reconstructed with a bilobed flap (**A**), rotation of the first lobe into the oncologic defect and the second lobe into the donor defect of the first lobe (**B**). The donor defect of the second lobe is closed primarily. Postoperative result (**C**).

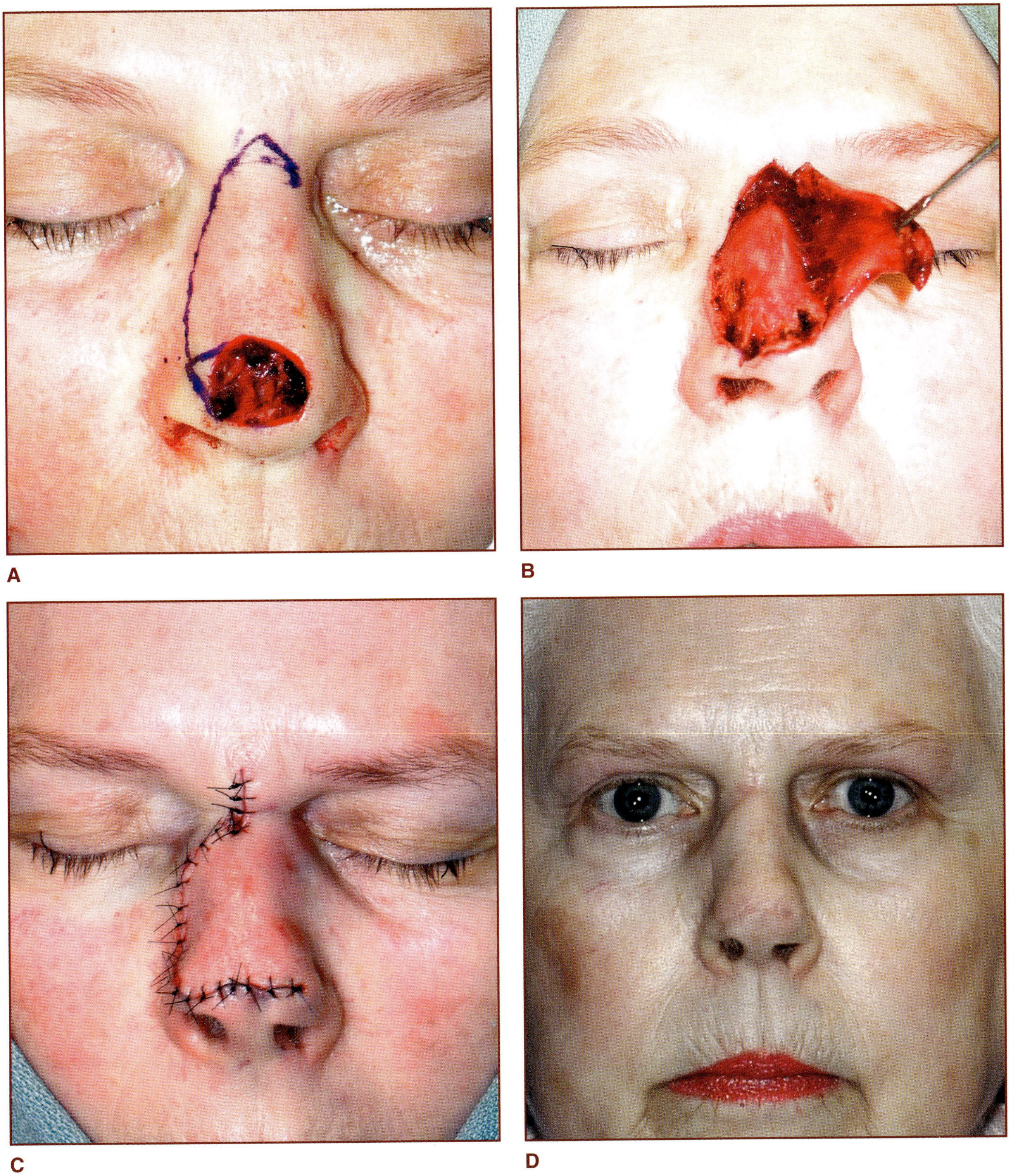

Figure 33–5. Dorsal nasal flap based laterally on the angular branch of the facial artery. Planned incision (**A**), flap elevation (**B**), and closure (**C**). A glabellar "dog-ear" is removed, but this is often not necessary. Postoperative result (**D**).

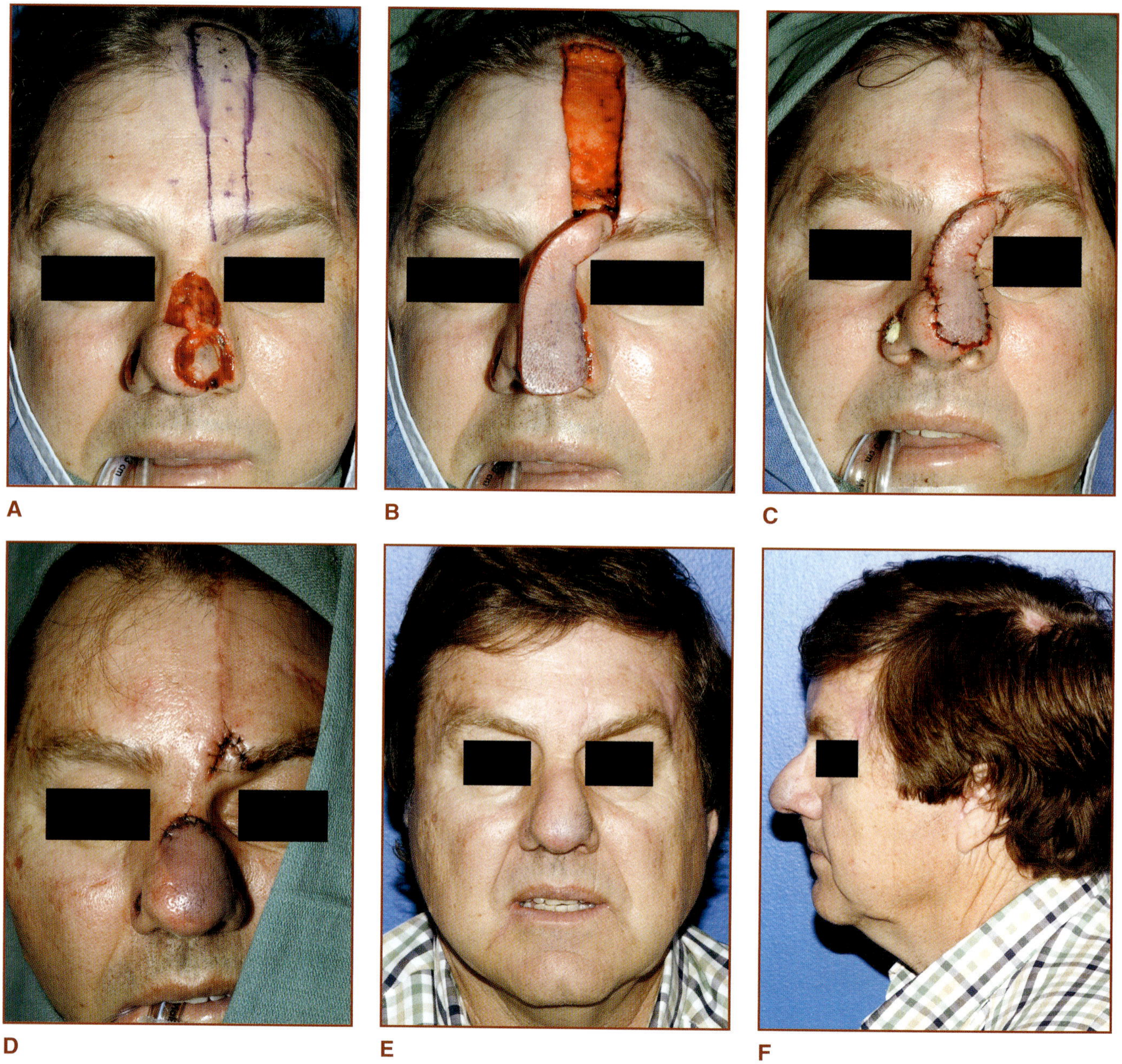

Figure 33–6. A left paramedian flap is designed for a central and lateral nasal cutaneous defect (**A**). It is rotated counterclockwise for maximum reach (**B**). The flap is divided and inset approximately 3 weeks later (**C** and **D**). Postoperative result after a third surgery for thinning of the distal flap (**E** and **F**).

The flap is elevated from distal to proximal in the loose areolar plane above the periosteum for most of its course. The distal flap can be thinned by excising the frontalis muscle and some of the subcutaneous fat if it appears well perfused once elevated and rotated, and there are no underlying risk factors for compromised circulation, such as smoking. The frontalis muscle must be included in the proximal portion of the flap, as the blood vessels that supply the flap course through this layer.

Once rotated, the flap is inset from distal to proximal. An overly tight inset can compromise the vascularity of the distal forehead flap or distort other elements of the nasal reconstruction in cases of composite defects. The flap is carefully evaluated for perfusion. Signs of compromise may necessitate removal of one or more sutures to release tension on the flap, or, if the compromise is significant, return the flap to its donor site and delay transfer. Once the flap is inset, the underside of the pedicle may be dressed with petroleum-impregnated gauze and left to heal by secondary intention or, as the authors prefer, covered with a skin graft to avoid crusting and drainage.

The donor site should be closed without undue tension. Wide undermining of the forehead and scalp above the periosteum facilitates closure. Care is taken to align the hairline accurately. It is preferable to leave a portion of the donor site open to heal by secondary intent and contraction than to perform an overly tight closure that will lead to an unfavorable scar. Provided the periosteum has been left intact over the frontal bone, the wound should heal within 6 to 8 weeks leaving behind a favorable appearing scar. Any open donor site areas should be meticulously cared for by dressing with antibiotic ointment and packing with petroleum-impregnated gauze to prevent desiccation of the periosteum and nonhealing of the wound. Tissue expansion prior to forehead flap elevation has been recommended by some to allow primary closure of the donor site defect when a wide flap is needed.[14,16] However, skin expansion delays the repair, results in a thick flap due to capsule formation, and may be associated with "rebound" contraction of the flap, which can distort the nasal reconstruction.

Traditionally, the forehead flap is transferred in two stages. Approximately 2 to 3 weeks after elevation and distal insetting, the pedicle is divided, the proximal flap is debulked and the inset completed. In smokers or for large defects, a three-stage approach is recommended.[13] In this approach, the flap is initially transposed without thinning. Three weeks after the first operation, the distal flap is elevated at a superficial level, retaining 2 to 3 mm of fat on the skin. The wound bed is debrided of frontalis muscle and fat, and underlying grafts used for support are revised as necessary, if present. The pedicle is then divided at a third stage 3 weeks later unless other revisions are needed. The pedicle base is inset in an inverted "V" shape. Later revisions may be necessary to achieve optimal results. Such revisions usually are carried out after allowing the flap to mature and the edema to resolve.

Nasolabial Flap

The nasolabial flap, also known as the melolabial flap, is primarily useful for reconstruction of alar defects, although it is occasionally used for defects of the nasal sill (anterior floor), columella, and lining (Fig 33–7).[17–19] When greater than 50% of the alar subunit is missing, it is best to discard the residual normal skin. For alar reconstruction, the flap is superiorly based and rotated medially into the defect. Using a reversed suture foil template made from the ala of the contralateral side, the entire subunit is replaced. The medial border of the flap is positioned within or just a millimeter or two lateral to the nasolabial crease.

The flap is elevated distal to proximal. The most distal portion can be thinned to retain only a few millimeters of subcutaneous fat. The proximal portion should be elevated in a plane just above the facial musculature to retain robust circulation from a perforating branch of the angular artery, which arises in the vicinity of the levator labia muscle. The nasolabial flap is commonly harvested as a traditional pedicled flap, leaving an intact skin bridge between the pivot point of the flap and the nasal defect that is divided and inset 2 to 3 weeks later. Alternatively, the flap may be harvested as an island flap, doing away with the skin bridge and keeping the distal flap perfused by an axial blood supply existing within the subcutaneous fat. This adipose pedicle is tunneled into the defect, potentially eliminating a secondary procedure to divide the pedicle. This modification should not be used in cases of questionable flap vascularity. In practice, undermining the skin between the donor site and the defect and the bulk of the pedicle produces a result that may be suboptimal or require a revision regardless.

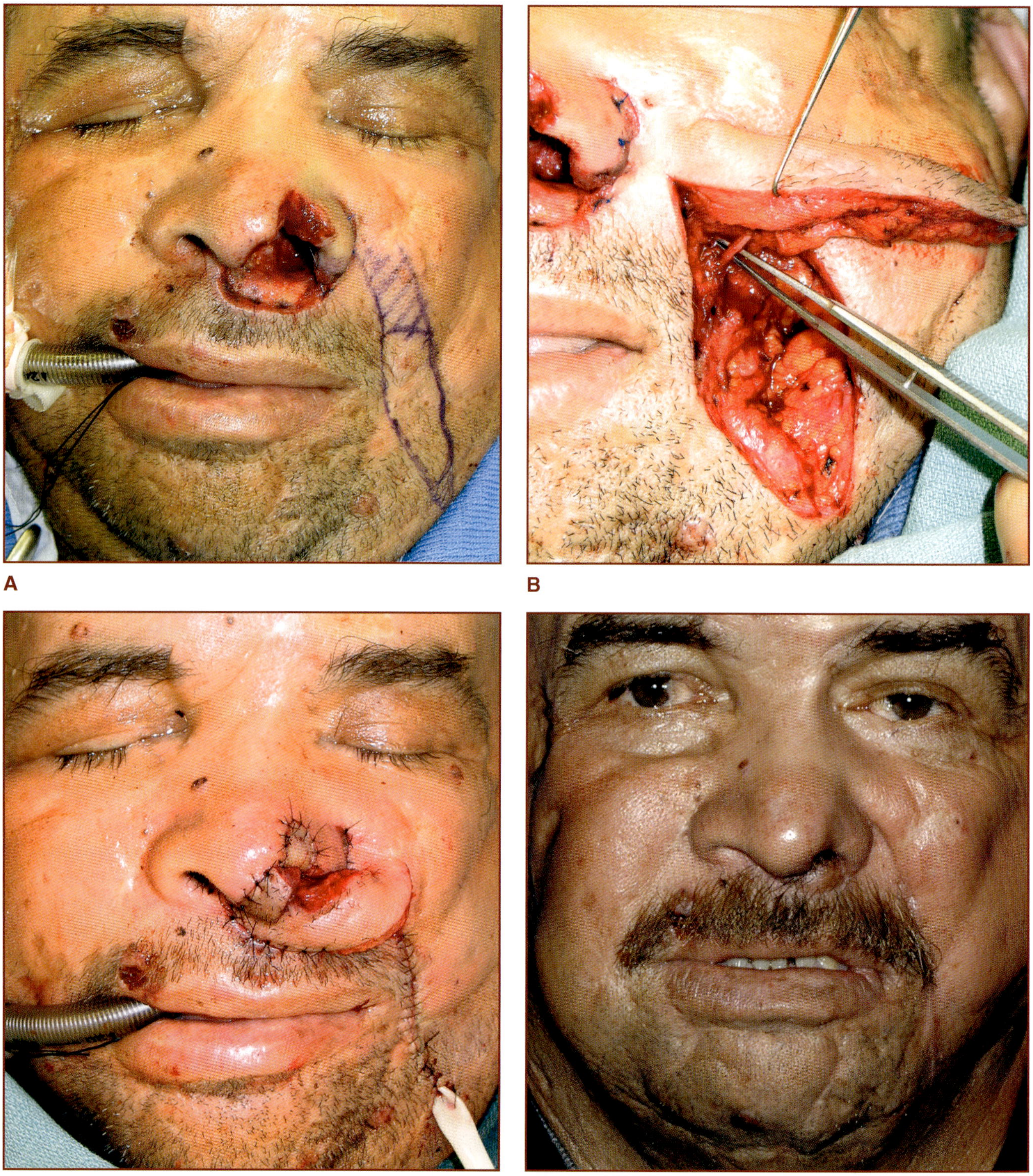

A B C D

Figure 33–7. A superiorly based nasolabial flap is planned for a defect of the nasal floor and columella (**A**). A close-up view shows that this flap derives its blood flow from a branch of the facial artery (**B**). The flap inset (**C**). Note that a composite auricular graft was used to reconstruct the alar rim. Postoperative result (**D**).

Its length and arc of rotation limit the nasolabial flap's use in tip, dorsum, or sidewall defects. The width of the flap also is limited by the ability to close the donor site, which is dependent on skin laxity. For large defects, such as those that extend to the tip or nasal sidewall, the forehead flap is a better choice. In young patients, the nasolabial donor site scar may be prominent and unattractive on an otherwise smooth face. Conversely, in older patients, there may be flattening of a previously deep nasolabial fold after flap harvest. The flap itself may be unreliable in patients who are smokers or have undergone radiation treatment. In all patients, the nasolabial flap does not reliably cross the midline.

Cheek Advancement Flaps

Advancement flaps from the cheek are limited to nasal sidewall defects. In individuals with lax skin, they can close lateral nasal defects up to 2.5 cm. The axis of this flap should follow the nasolabial crease to minimize visible donor site scarring. The flap is most reliably elevated above the SMAS layer, taking care not to injure the facial nerve while dissecting superficial to the zygomaticus major and minor muscles. The flap should be widely undermined for a tension-free inset to avoid distorting the lower eyelid and mouth. A Burow's triangle may need to be excised from the alar base and nasolabial area. Secondary procedures may be required to define the alar crease or nasal-lip-cheek interface. The flap may blunt the nose-cheek junction somewhat when used to reconstruct the nasal sidewall, and should never be used to reconstruct the ala for this reason.

Nasal Support

When resected, the supporting framework for the nose must be replaced to maintain nasal shape. Composite septal flaps can be used to provide both lining and support (see the section on "Nasal Lining," below). Otherwise, autologous cartilaginous or bony grafts are used to restore nasal support. Septal and auricular cartilage grafts, as well as rib costal cartilage grafts, are most commonly used. Septal cartilage is rigid and useful for structural support, and, when not involved in the resection, provides a large quantity of graft material, even when dorsal and anterior septal struts are left intact, as they should be. Auricular cartilage is thin and curved, and useful primarily for restoring the curved lower lateral cartilages and nasal tip. Rib cartilage can provide ample material when harvested from the "floating" 12th rib or, when a larger amount of graft material is needed, confluence of the 6th and 7th ribs, which lies beneath the rectus abdominis muscle. One caveat is that rib cartilage may be brittle and calcified in the elderly, rendering it unusable. Bone grafts, used primarily in total nasal reconstructions for reconstructing the nasal dorsum, usually are harvested from the iliac crest or the outer table of the calvarium.

Occasionally, cadaver cartilage allografts may be used. Irradiated cartilage preserved in saline seems to be less prone to softening and resorption than lyophilized irradiated cartilage, based on our experience. Alloplasts are also available but have a higher propensity for infection and extrusion. In cases of repeated infection or repeated wound breakdown, vascularized bone or cartilage microsurgical flaps have been described.[20,21]

The structural requirements to reestablish the shape of the nose with supporting grafts differs from the cartilaginous and bony skeleton of the native nose.[22–24] Once bony and cartilaginous structures are resected, the nose has greater requirement for support, requiring both anatomic and nonanatomic element to resist the forces of scar contracture. Supportive grafts may include a dorsal buttress, a sidewall brace, tip and columellar grafts, and alar margin (batten) grafts, although no cartilage exists in the native ala, which derives adequate support from fibrofatty tissues (Fig 33–8).

Structural grafts are fixed in place with fine permanent suture using tapered needles. Dorsal and columellar elements are replaced first, establishing the appropriate nasal height, length, and projection. The columellar strut is anchored to the nasal spine through an intraoral, gingivolabial sulcus incision. The dorsal graft is anchored to the nasal bone, occasionally requiring screw fixation. Nasal sidewall grafts are then placed, shaped based on foil templates. Thin, curved alar rim grafts are then placed. Although nonanatomic, alar grafts are needed to maintain the curved shape of the ala and to prevent

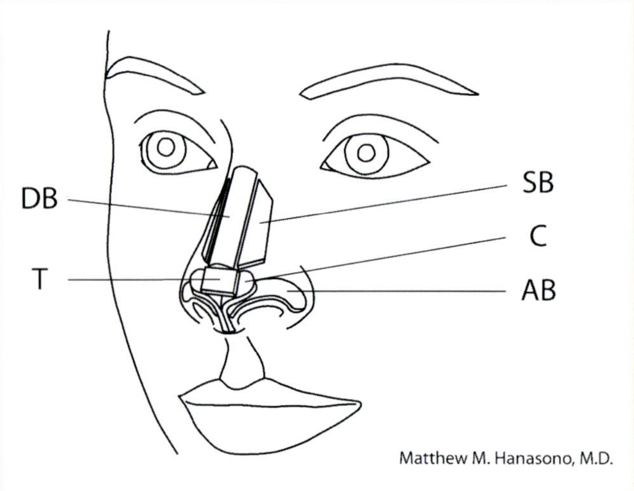

Figure 33–8. Schematic diagram of various grafts used for nasal support, including: dorsal buttress (DB), sidewall brace (SB), columellar (C), alar batten (AB), and tip (T) grafts. Adapted from: Burget GC, Menick FJ. Nasal support and lining: the marriage of beauty and blood supply. *Plast Reconstr Surg*. 1989;84:189 with permission.

their collapse during inspiration. A tip graft, which, like alar rim grafts, is also nonanatomic, is placed between the crura of the alar rim grafts.

In extensive resections, the septum may also be absent. The lower septum, separating the left and right nasal cavities does not necessarily need to be replaced. However, some form of midline dorsal support must be re-established or the dorsum and tip will inevitably collapse. One option is a rib cartilage or bone graft cantilevered off the nasal bones and extending to the nasal tip. This cantilevered reconstruction, however, is prone to fracturing or buckling over time due to lack of columellar support at the nasal tip. A more stable option is an "L"-shaped bone or cartilage graft fixed to the maxilla, although it will tend to produce a wide columella.

Nasal Lining

Nasal lining, although not a visible part of the reconstruction once it is complete, is a critical component for reconstruction of full-thickness defects. Unlined flaps used for external reconstruction contract, resulting in distortion of the nasal shape and obstruction of the nasal airway. Numerous techniques for restoring the nasal lining have been described, including grafts, nasal mucosal flaps, local and regional flaps, and free flaps. As usual, the size and location of the defect as well as the availability of donor tissue dictates the choice of technique. The ideal lining is thin, supple, and well vascularized. Making a template of suture package foil can be invaluable in planning reconstruction of the lining, just as it is in planning reconstruction of external skin defects.

Small vestibular defects can be reconstructed with full-thickness skin grafts provided they are not used to resurface immediately placed cartilage grafts.[25] They can, however, be used to resurface the underside of an external skin cover flap, such as a forehead flap. In such cases, a cartilage graft can be placed secondarily, ideally within about 3 weeks, between the forehead skin and the frontalis muscle to provide structural support if needed to preserve nasal shape. Attempts at prelamination, in which composite grafts from the ear or septum or separate cartilage and skin grafts are placed under the distal end of a forehead flap at a preliminary operation prior to flap rotation should be reserved only for very small defects as the results for anything more extensive can be unpredictable and are usually suboptimal.

Septal and Vestibular Flaps

Local flap options for reconstructing the nasal lining with mucosal tissues include septal flaps and vestibular flaps. These flaps are thin and can support the primary placement of cartilage grafts due to their rich vascularity. Placement of mucosal flaps near the alar rim may result in a persistent discharge of mucus from the nostril, which can be troublesome to the patient, although often difficult to avoid. Prior to elevation, local anesthetic with epinephrine is infiltrated submucosally (subperichondrially in septal flaps) to minimize bleeding.

The septal flap can be mucosal or a composite of mucosa and cartilage. Design of a composite septal flap should leave adequate septal structural support for the nasal dorsum and tip. Practically speaking, this means leaving 1 to 1.5 cm of dorsal septal cartilage intact, in addition to leaving the same amount of anterior septal cartilage for tip support. Septal flaps can be based superiorly (dorsally) on the anterior ethmoid artery, or based inferiorly (anteriorly) on the superior labial artery. The septal flap should have a base width of about 1.3 cm to maintain vascularity.

Alternately, a composite septal transposition flap can be used to restore lining and support for small- to medium-sized defects of the lateral nasal sidewall. The ipsilateral septal mucosa is incised and undermined and a "trapdoor" flap of septal cartilage and contralateral septal mucosa is swung or transposed into the lateral dorsal defect. Problems with this technique including limited reach and flap size, as well as postoperative contracture of the septum toward the harvest side, leading to curvature of the septum toward the contralateral nose and a reduced nasal airway on that side.

Small alar lining defects can be reconstructed using residual vestibular mucosal flaps above the defect. Vestibular flaps are often designed as bipedicled flaps for enhanced blood supply and are used to resurface alar rim lining defects up to 6 to 10 mm in width (Fig 33–9). The bipedicled vestibular flap reconstructs the alar lining and the septal flap reconstructs the donor site of the vestibular flap. For larger defects, the vestibular flap can be combined with a septal mucosal or composite flap. Cartilage grafts for nasal support can be placed primarily over vestibular and septal lining flaps.

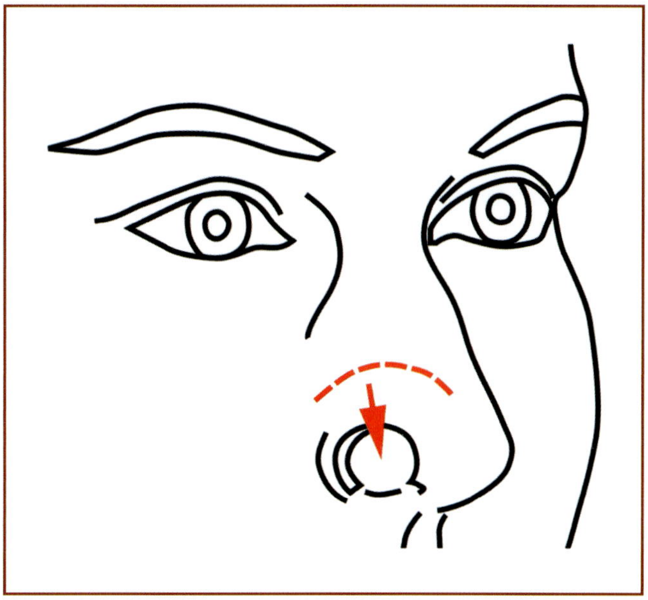

Figure 33–9. Schematic diagram of a bipedicled vestibular nasal flap for defects of the alar rim lining. Adapted from: Burget GC, Menick FJ. Nasal support and lining: the marriage of beauty and blood supply. *Plast Reconstr Surg.* 1989;84:189 with permission.

Facial Artery Musculomucosal (FAMM) Flap

The facial artery musculomucosal (FAMM) flap can also be used for nasal lining. This flap is a flap of buccal mucosa vascularized by retrograde flow from the angular branch of the facial artery, which is divided in the distal (inferior) end of the flap.[26] The flap is generally limited to a size of 2 cm wide by 4 cm long. It can be used to provide lining to the nasal floor or lateral nasal cavity. The flap is designed over the facial artery located intraoral by hand-held Doppler ultrasound, taking care not to include or disturb Stensen's duct. Dissection proceeds from inferior to superior, including the facial artery as its axial blood supply in a plane just deep to the facial vessels, including as little buccinator muscle and buccal fat as possible. The flap is transposed through a hole in the oral cavity within the gingivobuccal sulcus and the donor site is closed primarily in layers. The FAMM flap may be bulky and require later thinning. Additionally, the mucosa of the FAMM flap may tend to dry and fissure. Finally, there is risk to injuring the distal facial nerve branches, the levator anguli oris muscle, and the orbicularis oris muscle during dissection.

Skin Flaps for Nasal Lining

For delayed reconstructions, small defects of the nasal lining can be repaired using local nasal flaps abutting the defect margins that are "turned-in" to the defect. For immediate reconstruction or for larger defects, facial skin flaps, separate from those used for external coverage, can be used for lining, such as the nasolabial flap. This flap is usually based superiorly and both transposed and twisted into the defect. The pedicle base usually is excised or revised in a secondary procedure several weeks later. Alternately, a single stage procedure using an island flap variant of the nasolabial flap can be performed, as described above for external cover reconstructions. The nasolabial flap usually is used to line the alar vestibule, floor, or middle nasal vault. It is usually excessively thick and necessitates a secondary thinning procedures.

The distal forehead flap can be folded over on itself to supply lining and external cover for alar defects simultaneously.[13] This technique results in a very bulky reconstruction that precludes primary placement of cartilage graft support. The resulting alar rim is thick, shapeless, and unsupported. However, early (within 3 weeks) elevation of the external skin along its superior margin and thinning with placement of a cartilage graft to support the ala can then be performed.

Major lining defects may require a second forehead flap or free tissue transfer, which can supply a nearly limitless quantity of tissue. Uses and limitations of microvascular free flaps, such as the radial forearm flap, are described in the following section.

Total Nasal Reconstruction

The principles outlined above, which utilize local and regional flaps and grafts to restore nasal lining, support, and cover in a way that takes into account nasal subunits, are the current gold standard for reconstruction of partial nasal defects. For near-total and total defects, however, local and regional tissues often are inadequate to restore the entire surface and volume of the nose. Moreover, attempts to reconstruct the nose with local and regional tissues usually result in compromised nasal airways.

For near-total and total nasal defects prosthetic rehabilitation may be the best option, particularly in patients who are not candidates for or are unwilling to go through extended and multistaged procedures. A prosthesis can produce excellent aesthetic result in a single, nonsurgical procedure. Disadvantages associated with prosthetic rehabilitation revolve around the need for periodic replacement, problems with securing the prosthesis, which may sometimes be remedied by osseointegrated implant fixation when there is adequate bone stock, inconvenience of removal and attachment, and the sense that the prosthetic nose is not a "natural" part of one's body.

In patients with an acceptable medical, surgical, and psychosocial functional status, who desire autologous reconstruction, microvascular free flaps provide an abundant source of tissue for reconstruction. In general, free flaps are best used for nasal lining while still deriving external skin coverage from the forehead, if available.[27–30] The color and texture match of free flaps harvested from distant sites to facial tissues is poor. Only when the forehead is not available as a flap donor site, such as after truly massive resections, is free tissue transfer considered.

Several free flaps have been used for replacement of nasal lining in near-total and total nasal defects. The radial forearm free flap is currently the preferred flap based on its pliability, thinness, versatility, and reliable vascular supply. Suprafascial harvest can help to further thin the flap without reducing its viability. Even still, flap thickness, resulting in a narrow nasal airway, remains a problem. Efforts have been made to prelaminate free flaps with skeletal support elements, such as bone and cartilage grafts, in order to minimize the period of time that the patient must endure with a partial reconstruction on his or her face.[31] In any case, near-total and total nasal reconstructions require a multistaged approach.

Conclusions

Nasal reconstruction remains one of the most challenging surgeries. Smaller cutaneous defects can be managed with local flaps and occasionally with grafts. Larger cutaneous defects usually require regional flaps, such as the forehead flap and nasolabial flap. The most challenging defects require composite reconstruction. Strict adherence to reconstructing each of the three nasal layers, the cover, support, and lining, are critical for long-term success.

References

1. Burget GC, Menick FJ. Subunit principle in nasal reconstruction. *Plast Reconstr Surg.* 1985;76:239–247.
2. Burget GC. Aesthetic restoration of the nose. *Clin Plast Surg.* 1985;12:463–480.
3. Burget GC, Menick FJ. Nasal reconstruction: seeking a fourth dimension. *Plast Reconstr Surg.* 1986;78:145–157.
4. Becker CD, Adams LA, Levin BC. Nonsurgical repair of perinasal skin defects. *Plast Reconstr Surg.* 1991;88: 768–776.
5. Brown JB, Cannon B. Composite free grafts of skin and cartilage from the ear. *Ann Surg.* 1946;124:1101–1107.
6. Clairmont AA, Conley JJ. Uses and limitations of auricular composite grafts. *J Otolaryngol.* 1978;7:249–255.
7. Avelar JM, Psillakis JM, Viterbo . Use of large composite grafts in the reconstruction of deformities of the nose and ear. *Br J Plast Surg.* 1984;37:55–60.
8. Conley JJ, Von Fraenkel PH. The principle of cooling as applied to the composite graft in the nose. *Plast Reconstr Surg.* 1956;17:444–451
9. Masson JK, Mendelson BC. The banner flap. *Am J Surg.* 1977;13:419–423.
10. Zitelli JA. The bilobed flap for nasal reconstruction. *Arch Dermatol.* 1989;125:957–959.
11. McGregor JC, Soutar DS. A critical assessment of the bilobed flap. *Br J Plast Surg.* 1981;34:197–205.
12. Reiger RA. A local flap for repair of the nasal tip. *Plast Reconstr Surg.* 1967;40:147–149.
13. Menick FJ. Ten-year experience in nasal reconstruction with the three-stage forehead flap. *Plast Reconstr Surg.* 2002;109:1839–1855.
14. Adamson JE. Nasal reconstruction with the expanded forehead flap. *Plast Reconstr Surg.* 1988;81:12–20.
15. Kroll SS, Rosenfield L. Delayed pedicle separation in forehead flap nasal reconstruction. *Ann Plast Surg.* 1989;23:327–334.
16. Bolton LL, Chandaseker B, Gottlieb ME. Forehead expansion and total nasal reconstruction. *Ann Plast Surg.* 1988; 21:210–216.
17. Herbert DC, Harrison RG. Nasolabial subcutaneous pedicle flaps. *Br J Plast Surg.* 1975;28:85–89.
18. Heller N. Subcutaneous pedicle flaps in facial repair. *Ann Plast Surg.* 1991;27:421–428.
19. Cameron RR, Latham WD, Dowling JA. Reconstruction of the nose and upper lip with nasolabial flaps. *Plast Reconstr Surg.* 1973;52:145–150.
20. Walton RL, Burget GC, Beahm EK. Microsurgical reconstruction of the nasal lining. *Plast Reconstr Surg.* 2005;115: 1813–1829.
21. Burget GC, Walton RL. Optimal use of microvascular free flaps, cartilage grafts, and a paramedical forehead flap for aesthetic reconstruction of the nose and adjacent facial units. *Plast Reconstr Surg.* 2007;120:1171–1207.
22. Millard DR Jr. Reconstructive rhinoplasty for the lower half of a nose. *Plast Reconstr Surg.* 1974;53(2):133–139.
23. Millard DR Jr. Reconstructive rhinoplasty for the lower two-thirds of the nose. *Plast Reconstr Surg.* 1976;57(6): 722–728.
24. Burget GC, Menick FJ. Nasal support and lining: the marriage of beauty and blood supply. *Plast Reconstr Surg.* 1989;84:189.
25. Menick FJ. The use of skin grafts for nasal lining. *Clin Plast Surg.* 2001;28:311–321.
26. Pribaz J, Stephens W, Crespo L, Gifford G. A new intraoral flap: facial artery musculomucosal (FAMM) flap. *Plast Reconstr Surg.* 1992;90:421–429.
27. Walton RL, Burget GC, Beahm EK. Microsurgical reconstruction of the nasal lining. *Plast Reconstr Surg.* 2005; 115(7):1813–1829.
28. Upton J, Ferraro N, Healy G, et al. The use of prefabricated fascial flaps for lining of the oral and nasal cavities. *Plast Reconstr Surg.* 1994;94(5):573–579.
29. Marshall DM, Amjad I, Wolf SA. Use of the radial forearm flap for deep, central midfacial defects. *Plast Reconstr Surg.* 2003;111(1):56–64.
30. Winslow CP, Cook TA, Burke A, Wax MK. Total nasal reconstruction: utility of the free radial forearm fascial flap. *Arch Facial Plast Surg.* 2003;5:159–163.
31. Pribaz JJ and Fine NA. Prelamination: defining the prefabricated flap–a case report and review. *Microsurgery.* 1994;15:618–623.

34

LIP RECONSTRUCTION

HOWARD N. LANGSTEIN
HANI SBITANY

Introduction

Lip defects have a large impact on both form and function. Cosmetically, they are readily visible, owing to the lip's position in the center of the face. In addition, these defects can negatively affect the many functions for which the lip is an integral part, namely speech, eating, and facial expression. Appearance of the reconstruction is always important, and any procedure should attempt to re-create a normal appearing lip mound. However, function should take precedence over form, as failure to restore oral competence may result in potentially debilitating problems such as constant drooling or difficulty eating. Most surgeons strive to achieve a result that restores the ability to perform these normal activities, and, if necessary, will tolerate a suboptimal appearance to produce a functional reconstruction.[1]

The majority of lip defects requiring reconstruction can be broadly categorized as congenital or acquired. Congenital conditions, such as cleft lip, the most prevalent one, often are addressed in infancy and are not covered in this chapter. Acquired defects of the lip are seen at all ages. Common mechanisms for these acquired defects include chronic exposure to sunlight, tobacco smoke, and alcohol consumption, leading to skin cancer and subsequent tumor extirpation. In addition, traumatic injuries and inflammatory conditions often result in lip defects requiring reconstruction. Although defects caused by these differing mechanisms may warrant varying definitive treatment plans, reconstructive principles for the defects remain largely similar, as they are usually dependent on defect size and location of the defect on the lip mound.[2]

The task of the reconstructive surgeon repairing defects of the lip is aided by the presence of a rich vascular network, as well as the existence of redundant lip tissue in the majority of patients. As is true with most surgical repairs of the facial region, lip reconstructive scars usually heal well, providing a result that can remain inconspicuous, if performed properly.[3] This chapter highlights the knowledge, treatment algorithms, and procedures necessary to produce the goal of a normally functioning oral sphincter with restoration of a natural appearance.

Pertinent Anatomy

The outermost cutaneous layer of the upper and lower lip complexes is the vermilion layer. The vermilion can be divided into dry and wet regions. The dry vermilion is completely surrounded by facial skin, also termed the *white lip*. The border between the dry vermilion and the *white lip* is a prominent junction known as the *white roll* or vermilion border. The vermilion border is of great significance in surgical repair.[4] Misalignment of as little as 1 mm in the vermilion border is noticeable at a conversational distance. The contractile force of the underlying orbicularis oris muscle sphincter gives the vermilion its characteristic vertical creases.

The philtrum is the midline portion of the upper lip, between the paired philtral columns. The midline portion of the upper mucocutaneous line, at the base of the philtrum, is known as *Cupid's bow*. Topographically, the tubercle of the upper lip is the area of dry vermilion lying below Cupid's bow. Laterally, the upper and lower lips come together on each side at the lateral commissures.

The upper and lower lips are primarily muscular structures. The orbicularis oris muscle, lying immediately beneath the vermilion, is the circular muscle that gives the lip its shape and allows it to function as a sphincter. Its upper and lower divisions on each side interdigitate at the modiolus, which lies just beneath the lip commissure.

Unlike the orbicularis, the other muscles controlling lip movement are rarely individually manipulated during lip reconstruction. Elevators of the upper lip include the levator labii superioris, the zygomaticus major and minor, and the levator anguli oris. Lower lip depression is controlled by the depressor anguli oris and the depressor labii inferioris, and to a variable degree by the platysma. The mentalis muscle, in the midline, allows the lower lip to advance superiorly.

The orbicularis oris receives its motor innervation from the buccal branch of cranial nerve VII. Sensory innervation to the upper lip is supplied by the infraorbital nerve (V_2), whereas sensory innervation to the lower lip is supplied by the mental nerve (V_3).

The lip receives a paired blood supply from the superior and inferior labial arteries, both branches of the ascending facial artery. Venous drainage is through the paired venae comitantes.[5,6] These vessels usually are found in a plane superficial to the orbicularis muscle, in the subcutaneous tissue deep to the vermilion lip.

Lymphatic drainage of the lip is through both the submandibular nodes (upper and lateral lower lip) and the submental nodes (central lower lip).

Reconstructive Strategy

The reconstructive surgeon should categorize lip defects by the amount of the upper and/or lower lip absent, as well as the thickness of the defect (full vs partial). In addition, the degree of involvement of the adjacent white lip or cheek must be considered.

When analyzing the total lip subunit for reconstructive assessment, calculations can be made by estimating the lip as a circular unit.[7] The average circumference of this circle in adults is 16 cm. Taking into account that circumference = $\pi \times$ diameter, then average diameter is approximately 5 cm, representing the intercommissural distance. It also is important to keep in mind that in adults, the upper hemi-lip is longer than the lower by an average of 1 cm. In some patients, the average intercommissural distance is actually closer to 6 cm, because the sphincter is more oval than circular.

The utility of this exercise is that it allows the surgeon to calculate the reduced size of the reconstructed lip preoperatively, assuming the operation will not add any additional tissue. Thus, the extent of postoperative microstomia may be estimated. For example, if a patient presents with 12 cm of remaining lip, then a reconstruction will create a lip subunit with an intercommissural distance of approximately 3.8 cm. This is above the lower limit of acceptable microstomia (~3 cm), does not significantly impair eating or oral competence, and is thus an acceptable outcome.

Lip defects also are classified by the thickness of the defect (lip tissues involved). Partial thickness defects of the lip are those that do not traverse through all layers of the lip in an anterior-posterior dimension (skin, mucosa, and muscle on both sides). Thus, they do not form a direct communication between the outer skin and the intraoral mucosa. Conversely, a full-thickness defect is one in which all layers of the lip have been violated and require reconstruction. The choice of reconstructive technique will depend on the thickness of the defect.

Reconstructive Options

Partial-Thickness Defects

The reconstructive ladder for partial-thickness defects of the lip involves three general strategies:

skin grafting, local flap reconstruction, and conversion to full-thickness defect with subsequent local flap reconstruction.

Skin Grafting

If skin grafting is used, full-thickness grafts are preferable to spilt-thickness grafts for definitive reconstruction because of improved cosmesis and lower degree of secondary contracture. Both the preauricular and supraclavicular areas are acceptable donor sites for these grafts. Split-thickness skin grafts are best used as a temporary closure until definitive reconstruction can be achieved.

Local Flap Reconstruction

The strategy of defect resurfacing with local tissue flaps is especially useful in female patients, given the reconstruction of non-hair-bearing areas with similarly non-hair-bearing tissue. The V to Y advancement of nasolabial or adjacent tissue in such a manner can be used to reconstruct defects of both the red and white lip. Similarly, in men, hair-bearing upper lip skin can be reconstructed using V to Y advancement flaps taken from local hair-bearing areas.[9,10] If necessary, as dictated by the defect, such flaps may incorporate orbicularis oris muscle in addition to mucosa.

For isolated vermilion defects, a common reconstructive choice is an advancement flap utilizing adjacent, intact vermilion.[11] When designing these advancement flaps, incisions are made longitudinally along the vermilion-white lip border. Additionally, care is taken to incise across the vermilion border at a 90-degree angle, so as to traverse this area in the direction of least tension. If the area of the vermilion defect exceeds the area able to be covered by local vermilion advancement, local oral mucosa can aid in reconstruction. This mucosal advancement can be preformed in a bipedicle fashion, to improve vascularity of the flap.

For partial thickness defects less than one-third of the lip area, with muscle and vermilion loss, a myomucosal flap may be utilized.[12,13] This flap can be designed as either an advancement from the same lip, or as a cross-lip unipedicle flap. In either case, this is an axial pattern flap, based on the labial artery. In cases where this flap is rotated from the opposite lip, it is done as a two-stage procedure; thus, it is reserved for use in patients in which there are no issues involving airway management, as well as those who are able to conform to oral restrictions and soft diet for 2 to 3 weeks.[14]

In addition to these local flaps, there are other, less commonly utilized options. Labial-buccal advancement flaps can be performed for larger defects, as can axial flaps such as the facial artery myomucosal (FAMM) flap.[15] In addition, tongue mucosal flaps can be used in a pedicled, two-stage procedure to reconstruct large defects.[16] However, such reconstruction has fallen out of favor, given poor cosmesis and severe oral restrictions experienced by the patient between the two operative stages. Finally, for superficial vermilion loss, full-thickness free vermilion grafts can be harvested from the opposite lip.

Conversion to Full-Thickness Defect, Followed by Local Flap Reconstruction

The strategy of converting a partial-thickness defect to a full-thickness defect, followed by primary closure, is especially useful in upper lip defects in men involving less than one-third of the lip and not crossing the philtral column.[17] In this strategy, a hair-bearing defect is reconstructed with hair-bearing tissue. Because the upper lip serves more of a static function in the oral sphincter relative to the lower lip, shortening it in this way is more acceptable. Furthermore, male patients are better able to, and often do, hide the incisions from this procedure by allowing their facial hair to grow. With lateral upper lip defects, the incision is often carried high enough to create peri-nasal alar crescents on the ipsilateral side (Fig 34–1). This technique greatly facilitates flap advancement.[18] Prior to infiltrating and distorting the lip with local anesthetic, dye should be used to mark both the red and white lip in the area adjacent to the defect, as this will facilitate proper alignment of the vermilion border at closure. As previously stated, the incision across the vermilion border should be made in a perpendicular direction. Wound closure should be achieved in multiple layers, including muscle and mucosa.

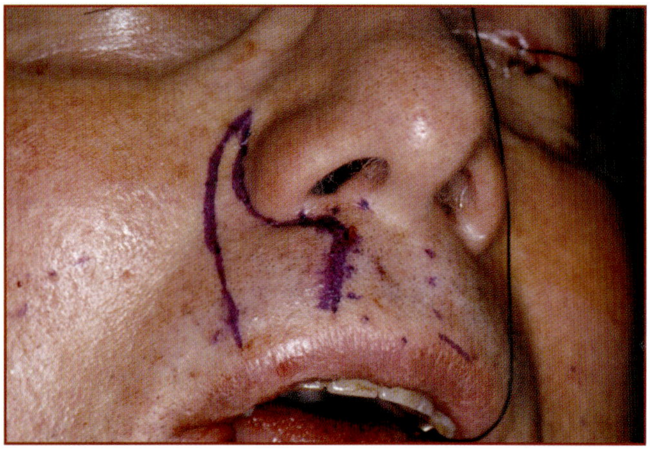

Figure 34–1. Upper lip marked for full-thickness excision followed by primary closure. Note the planned creation of pernasal alar crescents, to eliminate excess tissue.

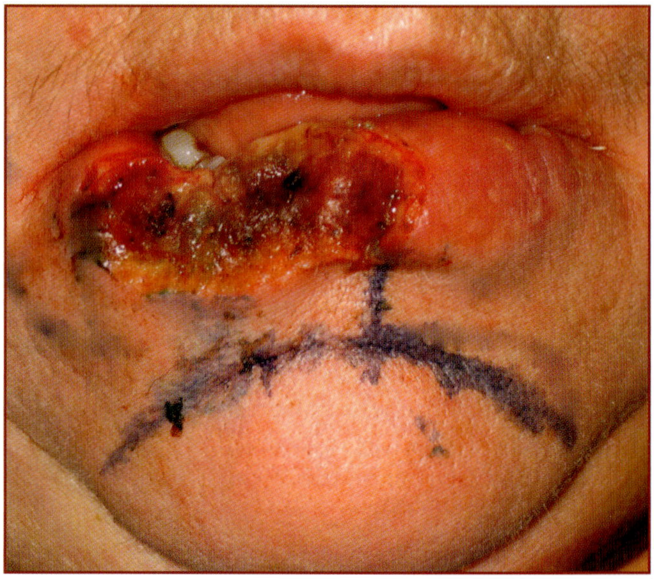

Figure 34–2. Preoperative view of planned lower lip resection. Note the markings for incision along the extent of the labiomental groove just above the chin, to allow for improved mobility of the lower white lip on advancement.

Full-Thickness Defects

When analyzing full-thickness defects of the lip for reconstruction, an algorithmic approach to defining the defect should be utilized, taking into account the lip involved, as well as size of the defect.

Defect Involving up to One-Third of the Lip

For either lip, a defect involving up to one-third of the lip in most cases may be closed primarily. This leaves the patient with an acceptable degree of microstomia and a fully functional oral sphincter. As with the closure of advancement flaps on any area of the body, primary closure of lip defects results in a certain degree of excess tissue, or "dog-ear," on the side not being advanced. In order to achieve acceptable cosmesis, this redundant tissue must be accounted for when planning a primary closure. In the upper lip, redundant tissue may be minimized by planning a peri-alar crescent into the excision plan prior to closure.[19] This removes a wedge of tissue around the ipsilateral alar base of the nose, including the nasolabial fold, in the shape of a half-moon. In the lower lip, a good result may be achieved by planning excision of a rim of tissue from the ipsilateral labiomental groove at the inferior rim of the advancement flap (Fig 34–2). For central defects of the lower lip, it may be necessary to excise tissue from the labiomental grooves bilaterally and advance each side to the midline.

Defects Involving One-Third to Two-Thirds of the Lip

For defects between one-third and two-thirds of either lip, and no involvement of the lip commissure, the initial choice considered for lip reconstruction is the Abbé flap. This is a lip sharing procedure, in which a portion of the opposite lip is harvested on a maintained vascular pedicle and inset into the defect. Sufficient time for the flap to incorporate into its new location and for vascular inosculation to occur is 2 to 3 weeks in most cases. Following this, a second procedure is performed to divide the pedicle and complete inset of the flap.[20]

When designing the Abbé flap, certain principles must be kept in mind. First, the primary defect must be prepared for reconstruction. If possible, an attempt should be made to shorten this defect.

If this is to be done, relaxing incisions should be placed in the aesthetic regions (perialar crescent for the upper lip, labiomental groove for the lower lip) (Fig 34–3). Second, the reconstructive segment from the opposite lip must be designed. The reconstructive segment does not need to be equal in lip width to the defect because stretching will occur following flap inset. The ratio of flap size to defect size, in terms of the amount of red lip included, is dictated by the amount of defect narrowing that has been achieved. In general, if the defect has been narrowed, then the ratio should be 3 to 4. If no narrowing of the defect has been achieved, then the ratio is 1 to 2. Third, one must decide on the amount of white lip to incorporate into the flap. The labial artery pedicle supplying vascularity to the flap is capable of perfusing a large amount of tissue. In lower lip flaps, this pedicle can supply flaps extending beyond the extent of the white lip, and onto the chin. There have also been descriptions of incorporating underlying mandibular bone into lower lip Abbé flaps. Such composite flaps may be beneficial in the reconstruction of complex midface defects involving the columella or other aesthetic units of the nose.[21]

As previously stated, every attempt must be made to facilitate closure and aesthetic outcome by planning incisions such that the relaxing incisions are placed in certain areas. For flaps based on the lower lip, incisions should extend along the labiomental groove. Flaps based in the upper lip should be designed to include a perialar crescent. In all cases, undermining should be carried out just superficial to the orbicularis oris muscle, at the base of the subcutaneous tissue, to maintain vascular supply of the labial artery. When possible, every attempt should be made to avoid inclusion of the philtrum into a flap based on the upper lip, although total elimination of this landmark can still lead to an acceptable result.

As mentioned, the Abbé flap is a two-stage procedure to achieve lip reconstruction. Thus, when selecting this flap for reconstruction of a lip defect, the surgeon must be confident in the patient's ability to temporarily eat and carry on daily activities with a transoral pedicle for a few weeks. A result of this pedicled design is that the patient will have two oral stomas during this time, both of reduced size (see Fig 34–3C). The relative sizes of the stomas will depend on whether the flap is based on the ipsilateral or contralateral labial artery, each of which is an acceptable approach.

When based on the ipsilateral labial artery, the result is one oral stoma that is significantly larger than the other. This larger, contralateral stoma is more functional, and allows the patient greater facility in performing activities such as suctioning through a straw. The ipsilateral, smaller stoma can be functionally closed without difficulty. When the Abbé flap is based on the contralateral labial artery, the result is two smaller stomas, which more readily approximate each other in size. Each of these stomas is less functionally adaptive during the temporary period than the one larger opening created by the ipsilateral-based flap. Thus, the ipsilateral approach is the preferred, although both are acceptable.

Regardless of the pedicle laterality chosen, inset of the flap is similar. Once the flap has been inset, closure is achieved in a systematic approach, from deep to superficial (ie, intraoral mucosa, orbicularis, and finally, skin). As with primary lip repairs, alignment of the vermilion border is of utmost importance when insetting the Abbé flap. In order to achieve appropriate approximation on both sides, the incision on the flap adjacent to the pedicle must be carried up into the superficial vermilion. This provides an arc of rotation amenable to vermilion approximation. Care must be taken, however, to avoid constricting the pedicle because this will compromise perfusion to the flap.[22]

The amount of time that is required for vascularization of the transferred flap is dependent on the size of the flap and the amount contact between the soft tissue of the inset flap and the defect. Prior to pedicle division, it is wise to assess new vascular supply to the transferred segment by manually occluding the pedicle and then check the capillary refill of the flap. If sufficient angiogenesis has occurred, as indicated by brisk capillary refill, then pedicle division may proceed. This is achieved in as little as 2 weeks, and perhaps earlier.

The pedicle is best divided at its midpoint, thus leaving sufficient vermilion for closure of both the donor and recipient areas. The vermilion can be folded over, aligned at the borders, and any excess tissue trimmed as necessary (see Fig 34–3D). Following pedicle division, a certain degree of clinically apparent venous congestion should be expected.

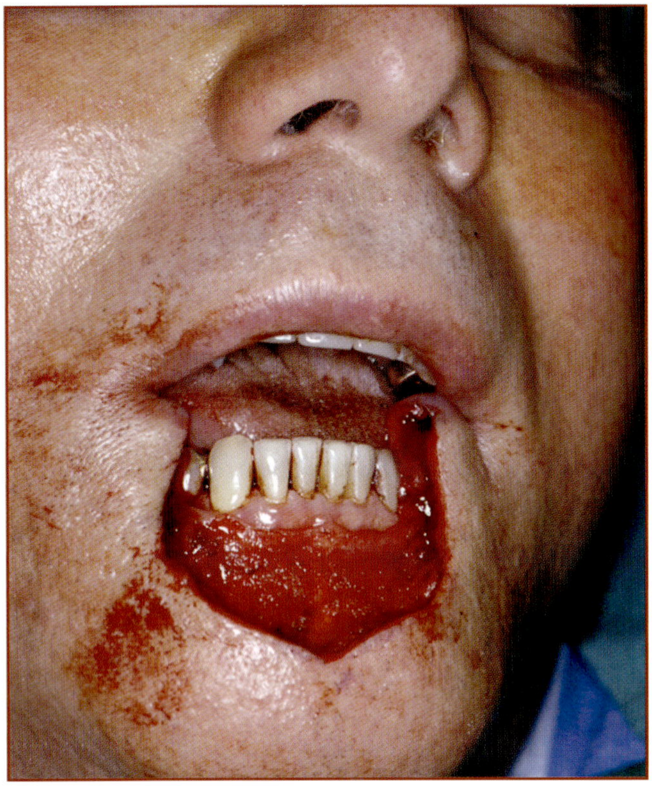

A

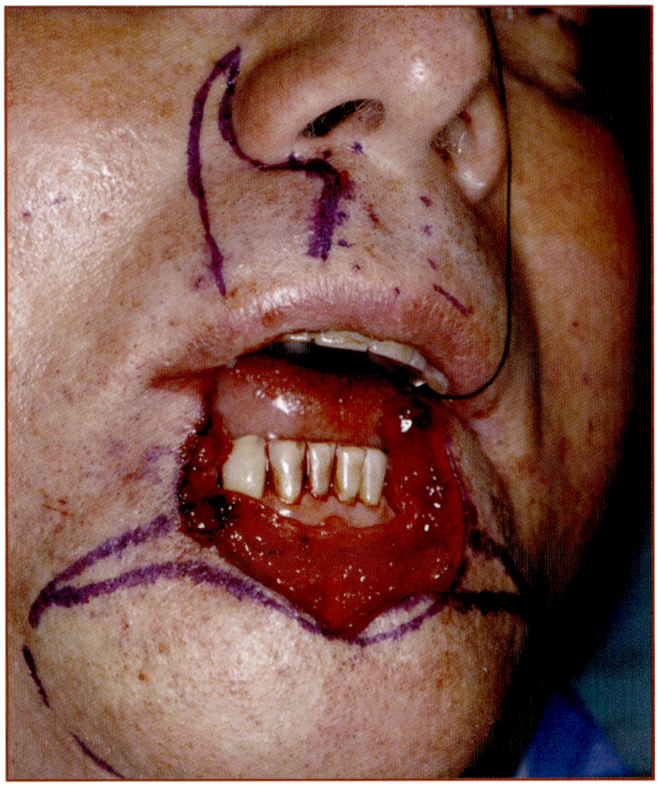

B

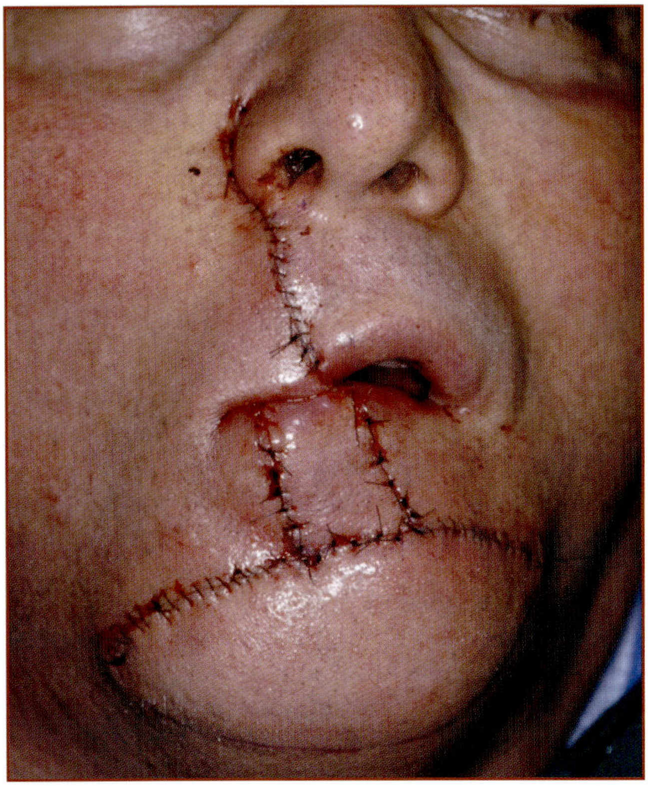

C

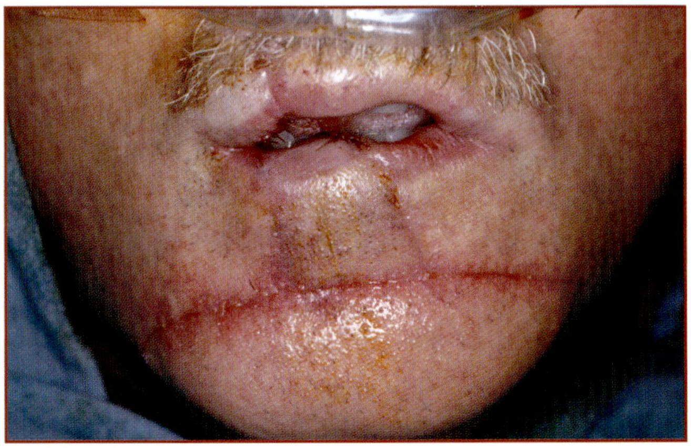

D

Figure 34–3. **A.** Lower lip defect to be reconstructed with Abbé flap from the right upper lip. **B.** Abbé flap designed with extension into nasal peri-alar area to eliminate excess skin; also, primary defect shortened with planned labiomental groove excisions and tissue advancement towards the midline. **C.** Postoperative view of patient following rotation of Abbé flap, demonstrating existence of two oral stomas. **D.** Patient following division of Abbé flap pedicle, 3 weeks after initial flap rotation.

It is common for this to remain up to a few hours, and invariably resolves spontaneously following this period. Flap edema also is very common. In many cases, this postoperative swelling is extremely pronounced and can be worrisome to the physician. In most instances, the edema resolves gradually over a few months. Finally, it is important to remember that it will take approximately 1 year for resumption of motor activity of the orbicularis muscle incorporated in the flap.

When performed in this way, the Abbé flap is the method of choice for reconstruction of central or lateral defects not involving the commissure, in which there is sufficient remaining lip stock for reconstruction. However, when such defects involve the commissure, the treatment plan changes. For such extreme lateral defects, the flap of choice for reconstruction is the Estlander flap.

The Estlander flap is similar to the Abbé flap in that it is a lip switch procedure, with a full-thickness flap transferred on a pedicle. However, the Estlander flap is a one-stage procedure. The flap is designed from the lateral-most portion of the donor lip, with the pedicle based on the contralateral labial artery. In this way, following rotation of the flap into the defect, the pedicle is hidden in the new commissure, and no further division is necessary (Figs 34–4A and 34–4B).

The general principles for designing the Estlander flap are similar to those for the Abbé flap. Flap width ranges from one-half that of the original

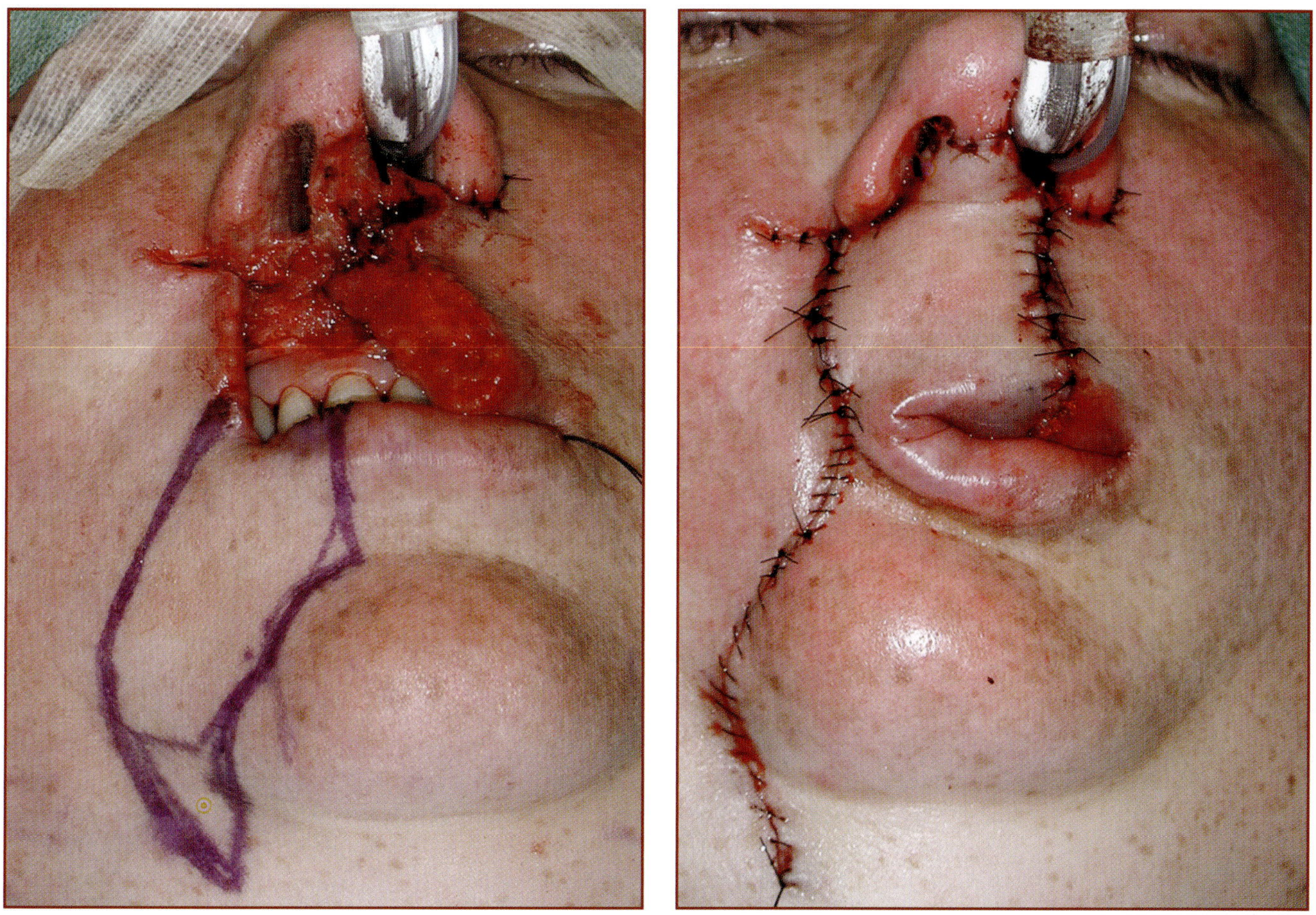

A B

Figure 34–4. **A.** Preoperative view of patient with large right upper lip defect involving right oral commissure. **B.** Postoperative view of patient following defect reconstruction with single-stage Estlander flap rotation.

defect if it has not been narrowed, to three-fourths of the narrowed defect, to account for stretching. For improved cosmesis, every attempt should be made to place the incision in the melolabial sulcus. When the width is accurately judged for this flap, the result is that the lips generally remain of even size.[23]

Patients must be counseled preoperatively that, after this operation, the commissure will be rounded. Although this may normalize spontaneously, it may necessitate a secondary commissure-plasty in the future. Furthermore, this procedure carries a higher rate of insensate lip, which may result in subsequent drooling.

Another procedure deserving mention, useful for reconstruction of central or commissural defects of either lip with sufficient lip tissue remaining, is the Karapandzic flap. Although this flap can be used for a multitude of defects, it is most commonly employed to reconstruct defects of the lower lip. This flap is favored because it transfers lateral lip segments to a medial position while maintaining their innervation. Thus, this flap restores a competent, circular oral sphincter, at the expense of some degree of microstomia.[1,2,22] Although this procedure can be performed as a unilateral flap, it is more often performed as bilateral flaps, to restore optimal form and function.[24–27]

When designing the Karapandzic flap, the height of the defect is measured in a cephalocaudad direction. This distance is then used as the radius for the two semicircular limbs. These semicircles begin at the lowermost border of the defect, and move laterally, traveling superiorly for defects of the lower lip, and inferiorly for defects of the upper lip (Fig 34–5A). One

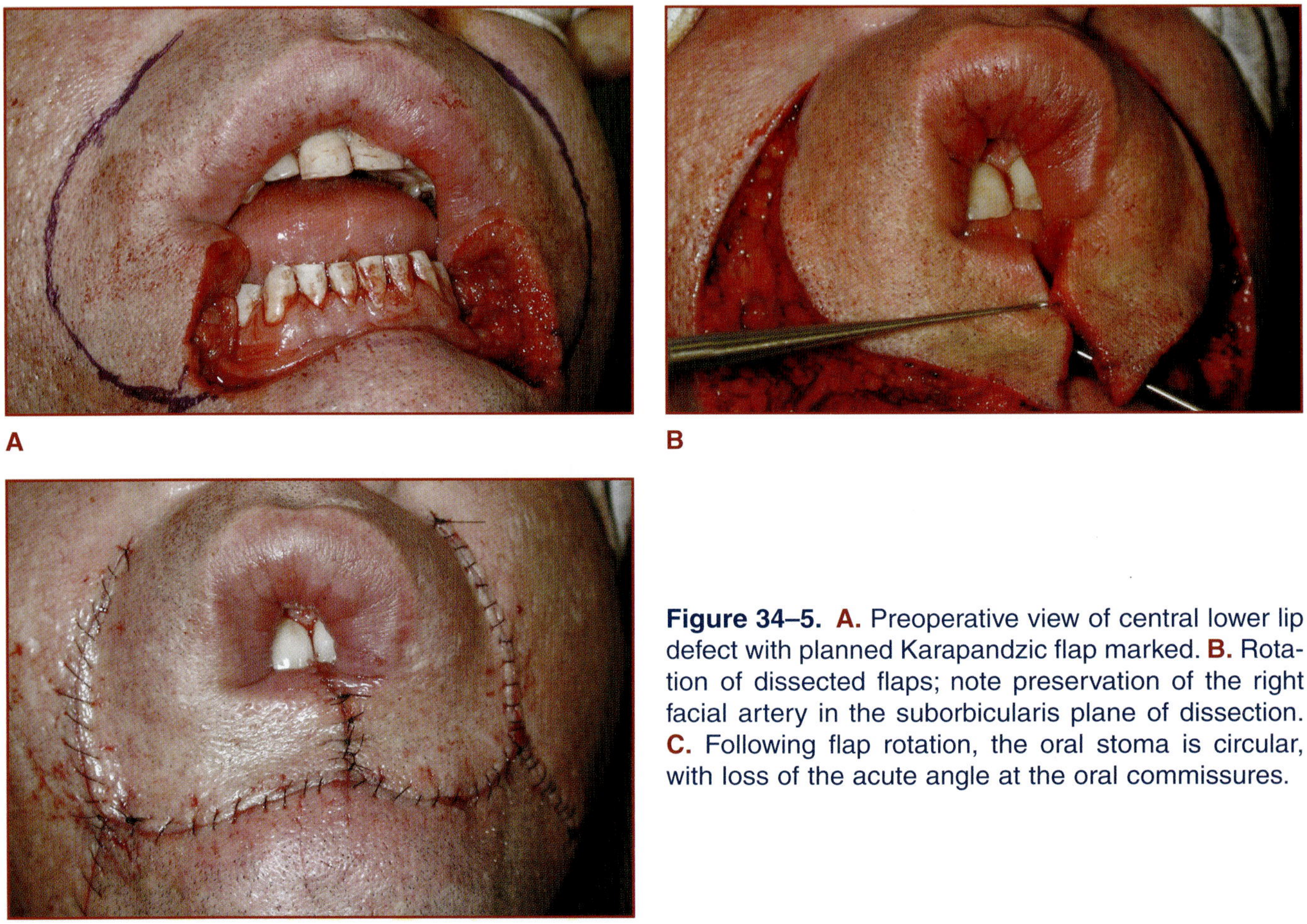

A

B

C

Figure 34–5. A. Preoperative view of central lower lip defect with planned Karapandzic flap marked. **B.** Rotation of dissected flaps; note preservation of the right facial artery in the suborbicularis plane of dissection. **C.** Following flap rotation, the oral stoma is circular, with loss of the acute angle at the oral commissures.

can also use the nasolabial grooves for incision placement, but the semicircular incisions heal quite well.

When creating the semicircular limbs, the correct plane of dissection is sub-orbicularis and premucosal (Fig 34–5B). Karapandzic's original description of this technique involved a methodical lysis of facial suspensory muscles, but in fact, all one needs to do is to dissect and spare both the labial artery and the motor nerve branches to the orbicularis (buccal and marginal mandibular branches of CN VII). With careful technique, the labial artery and vein are easily identified with spreading techniques, and preserved. If necessary, a nerve stimulator may be used to identify the branches of the facial nerve, which are immediately under the vessels.

Following full dissection, any tissues preventing rotation of the flaps toward the defect must be divided. Additional muscles are lysed only to provide mobility of the flap segments; mucosa is generally preserved. This generally involves myotomy of the superficial muscles attached to the flap. However, great care must be taken to leave the modiolus and all inserting muscles intact and undivided. Transection of the modiolus may compromise the functionality of the reconstructed oral sphincter.

The lead portion of each advancement flap is a full-thickness flap, encompassing skin, subcutaneous tissue, muscle, and mucosa. However, it is not necessary to incise mucosa over the full extent of the semicircular flaps. It is released just enough to allow for advancement and mucosal approximation between the two flaps. The remainder of the mucosa will stretch as the flap is advanced.

Once the flaps have been fully released, and the lead points approximated, a three-layer closure is performed. The immediate result is a spherical mouth, with loss of its sharp angles (34–5C). If the modiolus and its attaching muscles are spared on each side, the lip retains its function, and the commissures may re-form over time. A secondary commissureplasty may be contemplated, but is rarely needed.

Of note, advancement of the Karapandzic flaps may result in excess tissue in the cheek, along the line of advancement. If this occurs, a triangular excision of skin and subcutaneous tissue may be performed, generally in the area of the commissure, to eliminate the dog-ear.

The previous methods of lip reconstruction discussed all utilize existing lip tissue to reconstruct defects, that is, using lip for lip in a zero sum game. However, in cases where there remains a paucity of existing lip tissue to aid in reconstruction, these flaps are less desirable. This is seen in certain defects measuring one-third to two-thirds of lip length, and all defects involving greater than two-thirds of the lip surface area.

In such cases, if sufficient lax cheek tissue exists, as in elderly patients, it may be used to reconstruct either lip. This is the case in the Webster-Bernard advancement. In this procedure, lateral cheek skin, subcutaneous tissue, and mucosa is released on each side, and advanced in a horizontal fashion to the midline to form a new oral sphincter.[1,22,28–31] Because this procedure does not depend on the limited lip stock available for reconstruction, it minimizes the incidence of microstomia.

In order to facilitate advancement of the cheek segment, relaxing incisions are made bilaterally in both the labiomental groove and the nasolabial fold area (Fig 34–6A). In the labiomental groove, a triangular wedge of tissue is excised. This excision involves skin and subcutaneous tissue, while leaving the mucosa intact. If necessary to facilitate advancement without too much stretch, small incisions can be made in the mucosa. The upper excision is an upright triangle, with its medial border along the nasolabial fold, and its lateral limb placed to allow the necessary amount of advancement towards the midline. This upper triangular excision is partial thickness, removing skin and subcutaneous tissue. An incision is then extended from the medial base of this upper triangle to the lip commissure. This incision is full-thickness through the skin, subcutaneous tissue, and muscle; mucosa is also incised, along a line intraorally, 6 to 7 mm above the external incision (Fig 34–6B). This step-cut allows the mucosa to roll out and reconstruct new vermilion.

Following advancement to the midline, the cheek flaps are sutured to each other in three layers, excess mucosa is advanced extra-orally and sutured to the superior edge of the advancement flaps, thus reconstructing vermilion (Figs 34–6C and 34–6D).

As with the Karapandzic flap, sufficient medial advancement of the cheek flaps during a Webster-Bernard may require selective myotomy of facial

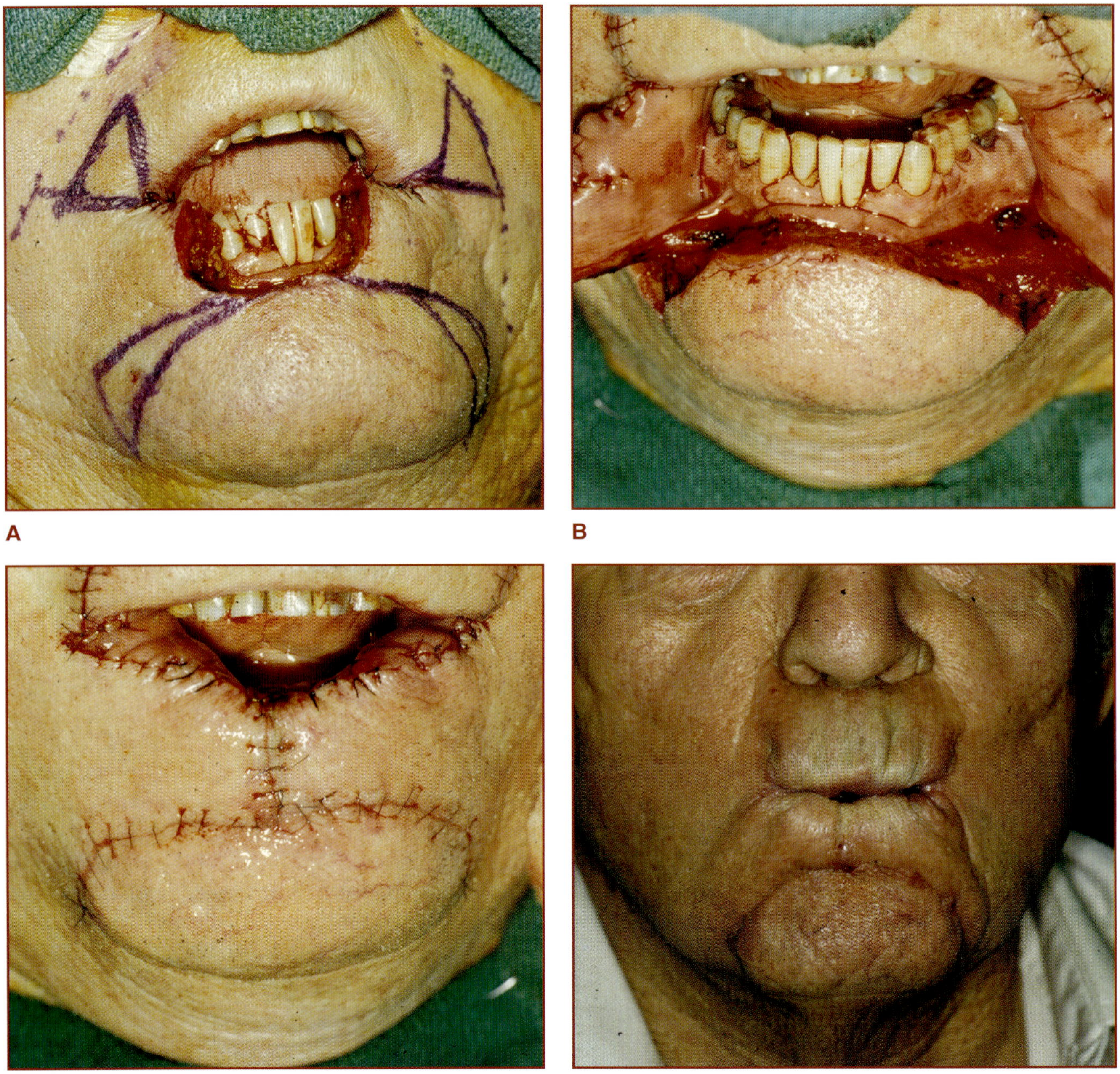

A B C D

Figure 34–6. **A.** Preoperative markings for planned Webster-Bernard flap reconstruction of large lower lip defect. **B.** Mobilization of full-thickness cheek flaps. **C.** Closure is achieved in three layers at all levels. **D.** Postoperative view of patient, demonstrating competent oral stoma.

musculature. Experience has shown that the lower facial muscles often limit the advancement, and are the ones that necessitate considerable lysis.

Finally, it has been noted that, on occasion, the vertical fusion line between the two advancement flaps in the midline may lead to contracture, and a subsequent reduction in the cephalocaudal length of the reconstructed lip. This may be alleviated by incorporating a z-plasty into this incision at the conclusion of the reconstruction, or by planning a zigzag incision. This can alleviate the issue of vertical height reduction.

Defects Greater Than Two-Thirds Lip Stock

For the majority of defects greater than two-thirds, and certainly greater than 80%, distant tissue is often needed for reconstruction. As such, defects of this size are less amenable to local tissue rearrangement using either lip tissue (Karapandzic flap) or cheek (Webster-Bernard flap).

For the upper lip, there is less demand on transfer of functional, mobile tissue, as the role of the upper lip in the oral sphincter mechanism is less important. For this reason, the most common method of large upper lip defect reconstruction is free tissue transfer. The preferred flaps for the upper lip are the free radial forearm flap, and more recently, the free anterolateral thigh flap. Each provides a flap of adequate thickness, and a pedicle of sufficient length. Due to its thinner nature and long vascular pedicle, the free radial forearm flap remains the more popular choice.[1,22] Paramount to this procedure is meticulous trimming and inset of the flap, to approximate the upper lip. The most common donor vessels for such flaps remain the facial vessels, and vein grafts are rarely needed.

For near-total defects of the lower lip, restoration of function is of utmost importance, because the sphincter function of the lower lip maintains oral competence, and prevents chronic drooling. Reconstruction of these defects is also carried out most commonly with microvascular free tissue transfer, also most commonly using the free radial forearm flap.[1,22,32–35] As for the upper lip, this flap is generally harvested with intact palmaris longus tendon. The cephalic vein also is preferentially harvested for venous drainage, as the vena comitantes of the radial artery can be of smaller caliber. The nondominant hand is preferred for flap harvest, and Allen's test is performed to ensure that the radial artery may be safely harvested. It is useful to design the flap to approximate the defect as closely as possible, using a template.

Following vascular anastomosis, which is commonly performed to the facial artery and vein, the palmaris tendon can be attached as a support for the flap. This is done by either anchoring the tendon to the maxilla or tunneling it through to the upper lip and suturing it there. The latter option allows for greater control over restoration of a circular oral sphincter (Figs 34–7A, 34–7B, and 34–7C).

With free radial forearm flap reconstruction of the lower lip, some surgeons have advocated neurotizing the reconstruction for sensory restoration. This is done by maintaining the lateral antebrachial cutaneous sensory nerve on the flap and performing a neurrorhaphy repair to the mental nerve. Although this has shown good results in returning sensibility to the reconstructed lower lip, many flaps regain some amount of sensation without such neurotization, so it may not be necessary.

Such free tissue reconstructions of the lower lip generally result in good satisfaction. The key is to place them under the appropriate amount of tension, such that they function well as a physical barrier to leakage from the mouth. When the flap is anchored to the upper lip through the palmaris tendon, the upper lip further augments the lower lip sling through compensatory mechanisms, because the flap is adynamic.

Some surgeons advocate the use of a neurotized free muscle transfer for resumption of sphincter motor activity of the lower lip.[36] This has been carried out with a neurotized gracilis flap, anastomosing the obturator nerve to a branch of the facial nerve. This option has great theoretical benefit; however, the main hurdle to this procedure is the bulk provided by the gracilis flap. The flap is larger than desired for lower lip reconstruction, and trimming is difficult if the motor function of the flap is to be preserved. Other potential neurotized muscle flap donors include the pectoralis minor and slips of the serratus anterior muscle.

Although the presence of a near-total lip defect poses a distinct reconstructive dilemma, the composite defect involving both cheek and lip tissue poses an even greater reconstructive challenge. Similar to

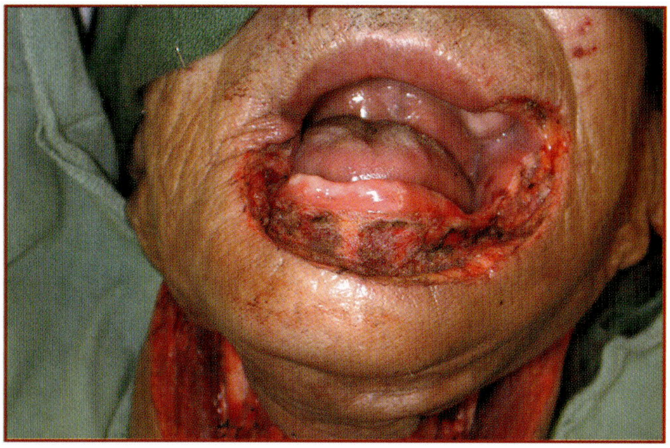

A

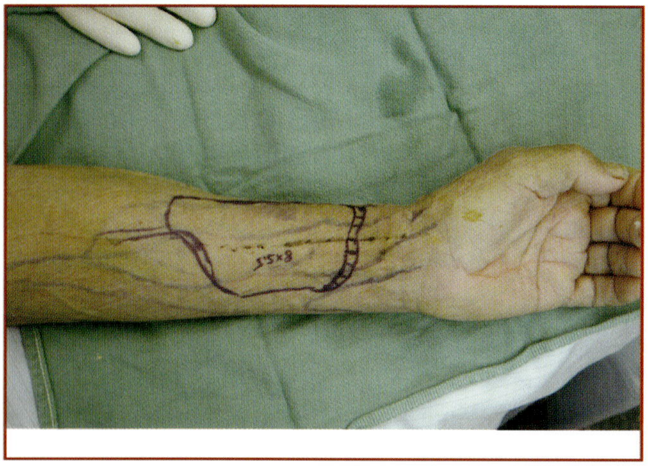

B

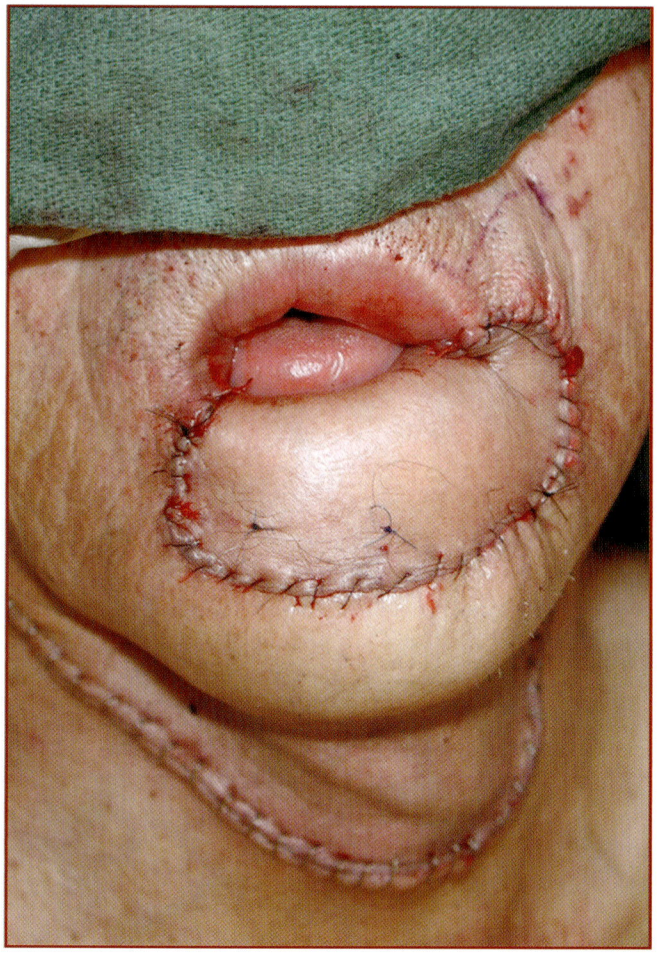

C

Figure 34–7. A. Large defect consisting of total lower lip, partial upper lip, and chin. **B.** Marking for planned reconstruction with radial forearm free flap. **C.** Radial forearm free flap following inset.

reconstruction of other regions of the body, it is probably not preferable to reconstruct anatomically and functionally separate regions with a single flap, but rather best to separate the task into multiple defects. In the case of the lip and cheek, such a reconstruction requires a flap of greater soft tissue bulk, such as a rectus abdominus myocutaneous flap (Fig 34–8).[37] This flap should be performed for such defects to restore soft tissue to both external and intra-oral lining of the lip and cheek, with every effort to inset and fold the flap in such a way as to demarcate the lip and cheek.[1,22,38–40] Furthermore, this is to be done with the understanding that later revision of the flap will likely be necessary, with some combination of debulking and lip rebalancing.

This rebalancing often is performed with previously discussed techniques, such as Abbé or Estlander flaps. Through the combined use of free tissue transfer and lip switch procedures, reconstruction of the composite defect can both restore static soft tissue bulk and recreate the oral sphincter with mobile tissue. Thus, composite defects are best addressed with combined procedures.

Regional tissue transfers also are a viable option for reconstruction of the lip and cheek. Flaps such as the deltopectoral flap or cervicofacial flap serve a similar purpose of delivering large amounts of

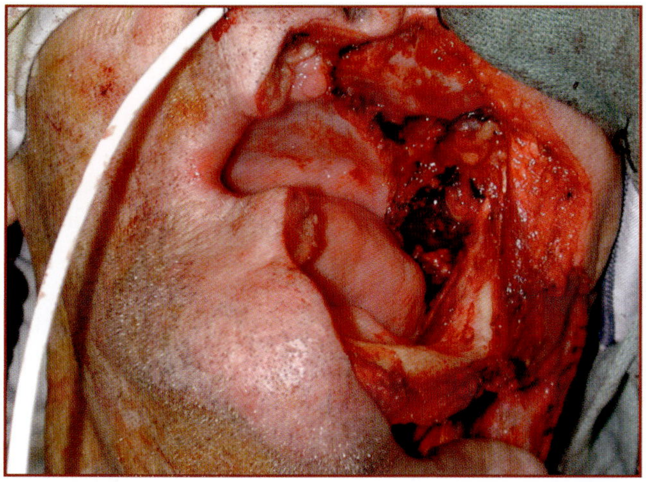

A

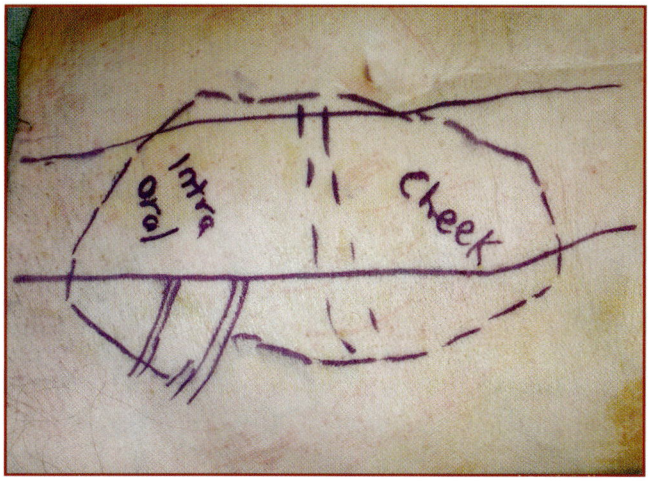

B

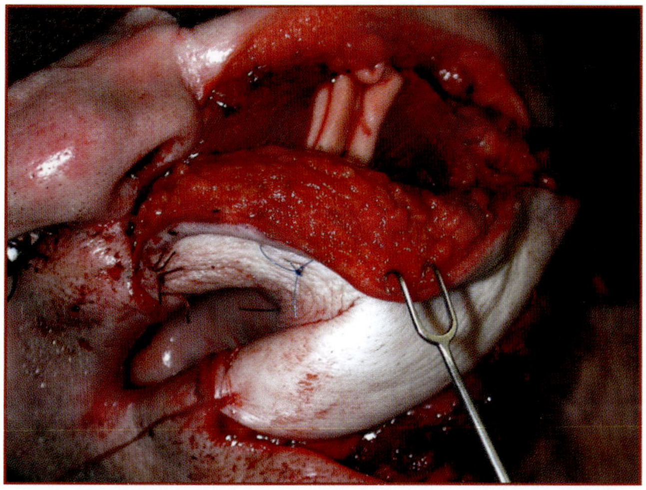

C

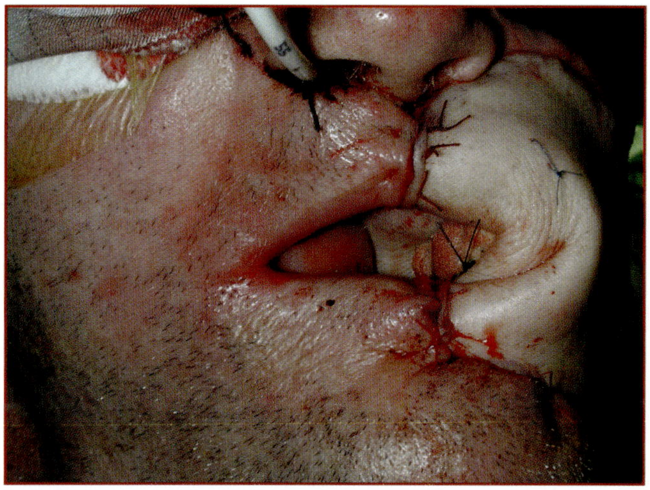

D

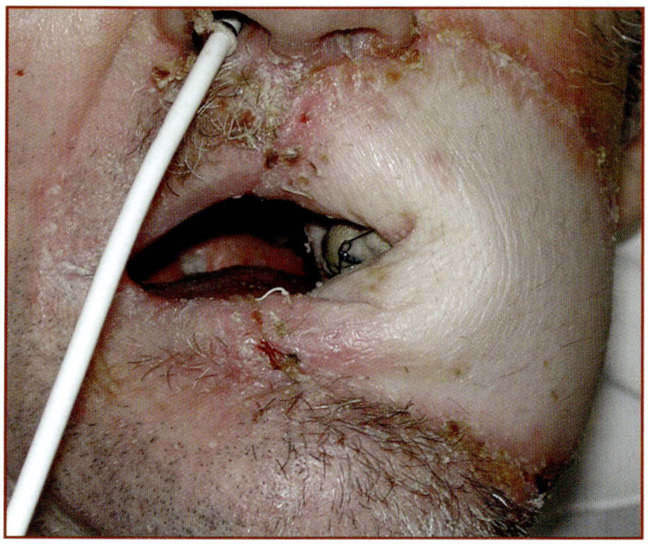

E

Figure 34–8. **A.** Large near-hemifacial defect in need of extensive soft tissue coverage. **B.** Markings for rectus abdominis myocutaneous flap; note preoperative diagramming of separate intraoral and cheek skin paddles. **C.** Rectus abdominis myocutaneous flap following inset; note acellular dermis sling used to anchor static upper lip and prevent collapse and newly created lip commissure. **D.** Final position of myocutaneous flap, illustrating both intraoral and cheek skin paddles. **E.** One-month postoperative view.

soft tissue bulk for reconstruction. However, with advances in microsurgical techniques, and improved success rates, regional tissue transfer is regarded as a secondary or salvage option for composite defect lip reconstructions.

When such large composite defects involve loss of mandible as well as soft tissue, microsurgical reconstruction remains the best reconstructive option. The free fibular osteocutaneous flap will restore mandibular osseous domain as well as intraoral lining. Following this, the lip soft tissue must be reconstructed, with either a second free flap or the remaining lip.[41] There are no viable options for reconstructing such defects without the use of microvascular techniques.

These large lip defect reconstructions continue to be hindered by significant microstomia when remaining lip stock is used to replace missing lip tissue. Although lip stretching through therapy and secondary lip rebalancing through lip switch procedures alleviate this problem somewhat, the microstomia remains distressing to many patients.

To overcome some of these limitations, one can use an "extended" variant of the Karapandzic for restoration of lip domain in very large defects (Figs 34–9A and 34–9B). Although designed with the same semicircular flaps, the distal flap portions are extended, to recruit additional "cantilevered" vascularized tissue from the lower medial cheeks. The main difference is seen in the distal portion of each flap, where the borders are no longer in continuity with the defect. Instead, the incision lines are dropped down from the defect edges, to the lowest extent of the oral cavity, while still maintaining a width equal to the defect height (Fig 34–9C).

In this way, additional tissue is recruited from the labiomental groove and chin region, and microstomia is minimized. The remainder of the flap, as it is designed superiorly, continues as that of the standard Karapandzic flap (Figs 34–9D and 34–9E). Thus, the height of the defect equals the radius of the semicircle. Closure of the buccal portion of the flap incisions invariably requires excision of triangular wedges, to avoid bunching of tissue. Although the distal-most portion of these advancement flaps may not be completely innervated, patients have been observed to exhibit good immediate postoperative function.

Postoperative Care

At the completion of surgery, the incisions are dressed with a topical antibiotic ointment. On the second postoperative day, the patient is encouraged to begin gently cleansing the lip with saline or water. Simultaneously, intraoral care with saline irrigations may begin.

Removal of external permanent sutures occurs on postoperative days 5 to 7, to avoid leaving permanent suture marks in the skin of the red and white reconstructed lip.

Patients undergoing two-stage procedures with pedicled flaps that obstruct the oral stoma (eg, Abbé flap reconstruction) may require assistance to maintain adequate hydration and nutrition between the stages of the operation. For some, eating and drinking may be difficult with the reduced size of the temporary oral stoma. Nasogastric feeding tubes may be needed to replace or supplement oral dietary intake.

For patients undergoing free flap lip reconstruction, routine flap monitoring is carried out for 5 days. This consists of careful flap monitoring every 1 to 2 hours.

Complications

The complications encountered with lip reconstruction are similar to those encountered in other types of lip procedures. Scarring remains a primary cosmetic concern, but is unavoidable in the majority of patients, especially with incisions carried into the perialar crescent areas and the labiomental or melolabial creases. This is especially true in larger lower lip reconstructions, when the lip flap is inset under some tension, to retain lower lip functionality.

Similar to any lip procedure, extreme care must be taken to realign the vermilion borders during closure. Failure to do so will result in a noticeable mismatch of this landmark following healing. Scar contracture, especially in the vertical midline scar of Karapandzic flap reconstruction, may produce a noticeable notch in the lower lip; thus, it is advisable to model this closure in a stair-step fashion or perform a Z-plasty upon completion.

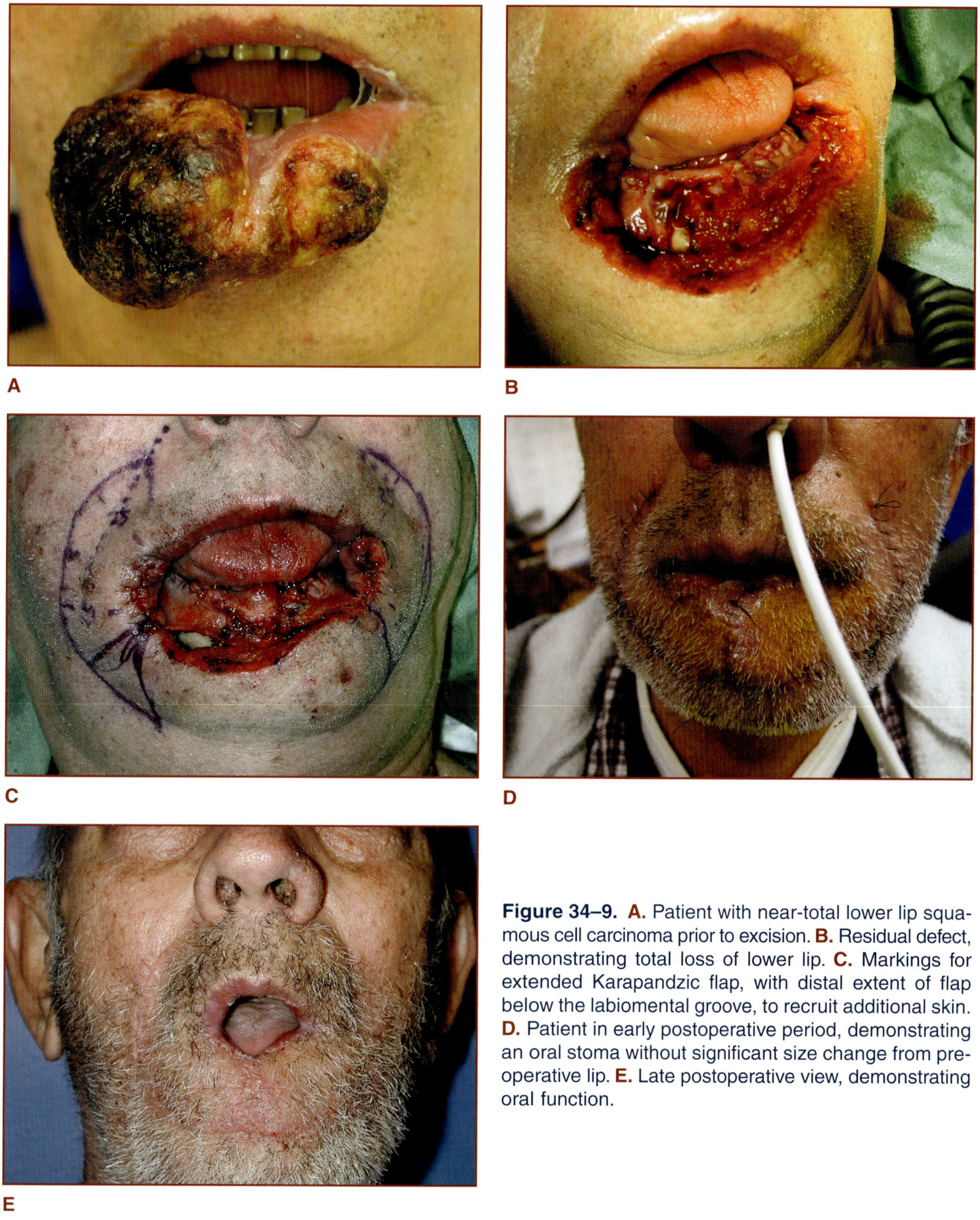

Figure 34–9. **A.** Patient with near-total lower lip squamous cell carcinoma prior to excision. **B.** Residual defect, demonstrating total loss of lower lip. **C.** Markings for extended Karapandzic flap, with distal extent of flap below the labiomental groove, to recruit additional skin. **D.** Patient in early postoperative period, demonstrating an oral stoma without significant size change from preoperative lip. **E.** Late postoperative view, demonstrating oral function.

Finally, microstomia should always be considered when designing the reconstruction of a large defect with available lip stock. As mentioned earlier, it is important to remember that function always precedes form in lip reconstruction. If microstomia inhibits functioning of the oral sphincter, then lip rebalancing procedures should be performed. However, if it is a question of form, it is important to remember that the reconstructed lip will invariably stretch with time.

Conclusions

The modern reconstructive surgeon has a variety of local and regional flap options for repair of lip defects. The choice can often be approached in an algorithmic manner and is dictated by the lip involved, the size of the defect, commissural involvement, the presence or absence of adequate remaining lip stock, and involvement of surrounding cheek or bone in the defect.

The reconstructive surgeon should categorize lip defects by the amount of hemilip absent, as well as the thickness of the defect (full vs partial); the degree of involvement of the adjacent white lip or cheek must also be noted. Partial thickness defects can be treated by either local tissue rearrangement or by conversion to a full-thickness defect followed by closure. Full-thickness defects up to 40% can be closed primarily. For those defects up to two-thirds of either lip and not involving either commissure, the Abbé flap is an excellent choice for reconstructing the defect with opposite lip stock. Commissural defects of a similar size may be reconstructed with an Estlander flap, another variant of the lip switch procedure.

With larger defects and no commissural involvement, the Karapandzic flap is an excellent choice for reconstruction with innervated lip stock. If such larger reconstructions are limited by the creation of function-limiting microstomia, then it may be necessary to borrow adjacent lip tissue for the reconstruction. The Webster-Bernard flap advances lateral cheek tissue toward the midline, and uses this tissue to reproduce the white lip; following this, intraoral mucosa may be rolled out to reconstruct the red lip. For defects too large to be reconstructed with such local tissue transfers, or for composite defects involving lip and cheek, a microvascular free flap reconstruction is necessary.

Regardless of the option utilized, the key is to allow function to take precedence over form. An excellent lip reconstruction may restore the maximal amount of oral sphincter function possible at the expense of cosmesis. Restoration of a dynamic sphincter, without debilitating microstomia, invariably will define excellent reconstructions, and produce extremely satisfied patients. The ultimate goal, however, is to restore both function and form.

References

1. Langstein HN. Reconstructive lip surgery. In: Guyuron B, Eriksson E, Persing JA, eds. *Plastic Surgery Indications and Practice*. Philadelphia, PA: Saunders Elsevier; 2009: 807–816.
2. Anvar BA, Evans BC, Evans GR. Lip reconstruction. *Plast Reconstr Surg*. 2007;120(4):57e–64e.
3. Nabili V, Knott PD. Advanced lip reconstruction: functional and aesthetic considerations. *Facial Plast Surg*. 2008;24(1):92–104.
4. Langstein HN, Robb GL. Lip and perioral reconstruction. *Clin Plast Surg*. 2005;32(3):431–445.
5. Edizer M, Mağden O, Tayfur V, et al. Arterial anatomy of the lower lip: a cadaveric study. *Plast Reconstr Surg*. 2003;111(7):2176–2181.
6. Mağden O, Edizer M, Atabey A, Tayfur V, Ergür I. Cadaveric study of the arterial anatomy of the upper lip. *Plast Reconstr Surg*. 2004;114(2):355–359.
7. Langstein, HN. Lip reconstruction. In: Butler CE, Evans GR, eds. *Head and Neck Reconstruction; Procedures in Reconstructive Surgery*. Vol 1. Philadelphia, PA: Saunders Elsevier; 2009;127–138.
8. Walton RL, Beahm EK, Brown RE, et al. Microsurgical replantation of the lip: a multi-institutional experience. *Plast Reconstr Surg* 1998;102(2):358–368.
9. Carvalho LM, Ramos RR, Santos ID, et al. V-Y Advancement flap for the reconstruction of partial and full-thickness defects of the upper lip. *Scand J Plast Reconstr Surg Hand Surg*. 2002;36(1):28–33.
10. Bocchi A, Baccarani A, Bianco G, et al. Double V-Y advancement flap in the management of lower lip reconstruction. *Ann Plast Surg*. 2003;51(2):205–209.
11. Okazaki M, Hisatomi T, Sarukawa S. Aesthetic upper lip reconstruction with vermilion submucosal-pedicle cross-lip flap. *J Craniofac Surg*. 2006;17(6):1259–1262.

12. Lane JE, Kent DE. Repair of vermilion Mohs defect with unilateral axial myocutaneous advancement flap. *Dermatol Surg.* 2007;33(12):1502–1504.
13. Pribaz, JJ, Meara JG, Wright S, et al. Lip and vermilion reconstruction with the facial artery musculomucosal flap. *Plast Reconstr Surg.* 2000;105(3):864–872.
14. Zide MF, Fuselier C. The partial-thickness cross-lip flap for correction of postoncologic surgical defects. *J Oral Maxillofac Surg.* 2001;59(10):1147–1153.
15. Demirseren ME, Afandiyev K, Ceran C. Reconstruction of the perioral and perinasal defects with facial artery perforator flaps. *J Plast Reconstr Aesthet Surg.* 2009;62(12): 1616–1620.
16. Tezel E, Guerrerosantos J, Trabanino C. Reconstruction of the lower lip with a tongue flap. *Plast Reconstr Surg.* 2002;110(6):1603–1604.
17. Godek CP, Weinzweig J, Bartlett SP. Lip reconstruction following Mohs' surgery: the role for composite resection and primary closure. *Plast Reconstr Surg.* 2000;106(4): 798–804.
18. Wang SQ, Behroozan DS, Goldberg LH. Perialar crescentic advancement flap for upper cutaneous lip defects. *Dermatol Surg.* 2005;31(11 pt 1):1445–1447.
19. Kouba DJ, Fincher EF, Moy RL. Crescentic complex closure of perialar upper lip defects. *Dermatol Surg.* 2008; 34(4):561–566.
20. Culliford A 4th, Zide B. Technical tips in reconstruction of the upper lip with the Abbé flap. *Plast Reconstr Surg.* 2008;122(1):240–243.
21. Naficy S, Baker SR. The extended Abbé flap in the reconstruction of complex midfacial defects. *Arch Facial Plast Surg.* 2000;2(2):141–144.
22. Langstein HN, Robb GL. Reconstruction for extensive defects of the lip. *Oper Tech Otolaryngol.* 2005;16(1):2–9.
23. Roldán JC, Teschke M, Fritzer E. Reconstruction of the lower lip: rationale to preserve the aesthetic units of the face. *Plast Reconstr Surg.* 2007;120(5):1231–1239.
24. Ethunandan M, Macpherson DW, Santhanam V. Karapandzic flap for reconstruction of lip defects. *J Oral Maxillofac Surg.* 2007;65(12):2512–2517.
25. Karapandzic M. Reconstruction of lip defects by local arterial flaps. *Br J Plast Surg.* 1974;27(1):93–97.
26. Rashid M, Hanif MS, Illahi I, et al. Reconstruction of lip defects with the Karapandzic technique. *J Coll Physicians Surg Pak.* 2003;13(4):219–222.
27. Ong WC, Lim J, Lim TC. A modification of the bilobed and Karapandzic flap used for reconstruction of the lower lip. *Plast Reconstr Surg.* 2005;115(7): 2154–2155.
28. Orsi VV, Pinto Oliveria AC. Lower lip reconstruction: Rudkin technique and Bernard-Webster technique. *Plast Reconstr Surg.* 2004;113(4):1296.
29. Williams EF 3rd, Setzen G, Mulvaney MJ. Modified Bernard-Burow cheek advancement and cross-lip flap for total lip reconstruction. *Arch Otolaryngol Head Neck Surg.* 1996;122(11):1253–1258.
30. Westreich R, Meisner J, Reino A, Lawson W. The use of combined Bernard-Webster and Karapandzic flaps for subtotal lower lip reconstruction. *Plast Reconstr Surg.* 2008;121(5):340e–341e.
31. Wechselberger G, Gurunluoglu R, Bauer T, et al. Functional lower lip reconstruction with bilateral cheek advancement flaps: revisitation of Webster method with a minor modification in the technique. *Aesthetic Plast Surg.* 2002; 26(6):423–428.
32. Cinar C, Arslan H, Ogur S. Reconstruction of massive lower lip defect with the composite radial forearm-palmaris longus free flap: empowered static and partial dynamic reconstruction. *J Craniofac Surg.* 2007;18(1):237–241.
33. Jeng SF, Kuo YR, Wei FC, Su CY, Chien CY. Total lower lip reconstruction with a composite radial forearm-palmaris longus tendon flap: a clinical series. *Plast Reconstr Surg.* 2004;113(1):19–23.
34. Gurlek A, Aslan A, Celik M, et al. A total lower lip reconstruction with a composite radial forearm-palmaris longus tendon flap: a clinical series. *Plast Reconstr Surg.* 2005;115(3):949.
35. Carroll CM, Pathak I, Irish J, Neligan PC, Gullane PJ. Reconstruction of total lower lip and chin defects using the composite radial forearm-palmaris longus tendon free flap. *Arch Facial Plast Surg.* 2000;2(1):53–56.
36. Ninkovic M, Spanio di Spilimbergo S, Ninkovic M. Lower lip reconstruction: introduction of a new procedure using a functioning gracilis muscle free flap. *Plast Reconstr Surg.* 2007;119(5):1472–1480.
37. Jallali N, Malata CM. Reconstruction of concomitant total loss of the upper and lower lips with a free vertical rectus abdominis flap. *Microsurgery.* 2005;25(2):118–120.
38. Corderiro PG, Santamaria E. Primary reconstruction of complex midfacial defects with combined lip-switch procedures and free flaps. *Plast Reconstr Surg.* 1999;103(7): 1850–1856.
39. Kuo YR, Jeng SF, Wei FC, et al. Functional reconstruction of complex lip and cheek defect with free composite anterolateral thigh flap and vascularized fascia. *Head Neck.* 2008;30(8):1001–1006.
40. Jeng SF, Kuo YR, Wei FC, et al. Reconstruction of concomitant lip and cheek through-and-through defects with combined free flap and an advancement flap from the remaining lip. *Plast Reconstr Surg.* 2004;113(2):491–498.
41. Kuzon WM Jr. Jejurikar S, Wilkins EG, et al. Double free-flap reconstruction of massive defects involving the lip, chin, and mandible. *Microsurgery.* 1998;18(6):372–378.

35

PERIORBITAL RECONSTRUCTION

STEPHEN R. KLAPPER
CHARLES N.S. SOPARKAR
JAMES R. PATRINELY

Introduction

An understanding of the basic principles and approaches of periorbital and eyelid wound repair is essential for dermatologic, oculofacial, and plastic reconstructive surgeons managing cutaneous malignancies involving the ocular adnexa. The standard of care for the surgical management of common nonmelanoma facial skin cancers is complete tumor excision often with microscopic tissue margin control guided by Mohs micrographic resection, intraoperative frozen sections, and/or postoperative permanent histopathologic analysis.[1–5] Mohs micrographic surgery permits maximal preservation of normal tissue and may be the preferred resection technique for malignant epithelial lesions involving the canthal and pericanalicular areas, and for aggressive, extensive, poorly defined, or recurrent eyelid lesions.[6–10] Even following tissue-sparing Mohs micrographic surgical techniques, postresection defects typically are 4 to 6 times the original clinical tumor dimensions.[7,11] Similarly, melanomatous lesions require wide, often staged, surgical excision extending typically 5 to 10 mm beyond the clinical tumor margin. Therefore, oculofacial reconstructive surgeons will often need to repair large soft tissue defects for even relatively small cutaneous lesions.

In determining the most appropriate surgical approach to repair a periorbital defect, the surgeon must consider how to optimally achieve the functional goals of eyelid reconstruction which primarily include: restoration of a stable eyelid margin, normalization of eyelid position and excursion, approximation of the lacrimal apparatus to the tear lake, protective eyelid closure, and development of a smooth, epithelialized posterior surface. Furthermore, the purpose and goals of periorbital reconstructive surgery must be clearly outlined for the patient, and expectations must be aligned with the surgeon's abilities and realistic outcomes. Surgeons should remind patients that, even with optimal results, a reconstructed eyelid often will not match the unoperated contralateral eyelid or be the same as it was prior to surgical intervention. Continued reassurance by the surgeon often is critical while both the functional and cosmetic results improve for up to a year or more after surgery, as wound maturation results in scar softening and natural tissue coloration.

Periorbital Defect Assessment

Successful periorbital reconstruction requires an understanding of eyelid anatomy and the relationship of the eyelids to the adjacent structures of the mid-face. Evaluation of an eyelid defect should include assessment of the anterior (skin and orbicularis oculi muscle) and posterior (tarsus and conjunctiva) lamellae. The orbital septum, levator aponeurosis and muscle, and Müller's muscle are sometimes referred to as the middle lamella. The levator and Müller's muscles elevate and stabilize the upper eyelid, whereas the capsulopalpebral fascia and inferior tarsal muscle are analogous structures in the lower eyelid. Significant disruption of these structures may require primary or secondary repair. The orbital septum is a critical anatomic landmark but is not utilized in most conventional eyelid repair techniques. The presence of orbital fat should alert the surgeon to postseptal wound extension.

In determining which techniques to use in eyelid reconstruction, the presence of eyelid margin loss, canthal tendon involvement, and/or lacrimal structure injury should be considered. The surgical goals of eyelid reconstruction should be to attempt to restore a thin, elastic cutaneous surface, a semirigid internal supporting structure, and an internal nonkeratinized mucous membrane lining while recreating a functioning eyelid structure in near-normal anatomic position. Adequate blood flow to the donor tissues must be maintained, typically by utilizing adjacent vascularized flaps.

Periorbital Defects Not Involving the Eyelid Margin

Selected superficial wounds may heal well by second intention. Unlike most other areas of the head and neck, laissez-faire wound healing in certain areas of the ocular adnexa is occasionally a useful and cosmetically acceptable alternative to surgical repair. Small, nonmarginal, partial-thickness eyelid defects can be repaired by direct closure. Undermining of the adjacent skin and subcutaneous tissues may assist in reapproximation of the wound edges. If distortion of the eyelid margin results or eyelid function is significantly altered, then full-thickness skin grafting, local flap advancement, or transposition may be indicated. Skin grafts are straightforward to perform; however local tissue flaps often provide a better aesthetic result and, when designed appropriately, may help avoid postoperative eyelid malposition.

Second-Intention Wound Healing

Healing by primary intention involves reapproximation of full-thickness wound edges. Sutures provide wound apposition during the first week of healing until collagen deposition begins and wound tensile strength increases. Re-epithelialization and wound contraction have a minor role in primary wound healing, whereas these are important components of healing in wounds left to heal by second intention.

During the lag phase in the first week of wound healing, an open full-thickness wound demonstrates minimal change in size. Healing then proceeds at a constant rate and is dependent on various factors including depth of injury, available blood supply, and geometric shape. Superficial wounds heal more quickly than deeper wounds, or when cartilage or bone is exposed. Linear or fusiform-shaped wounds contract more efficiently than circular defects with the same area since healing time is dependent on the diameter of the largest circle contained within the wound margins. Most wounds will re-epithelialize over the course of 2 to 6 weeks.

The ideal location of a wound permitted to heal by second intention would be a superficial defect surrounded by lax skin that lies within a concavity where contraction will minimize the depression.[12] The concave surfaces of the nose (alar and nasolabial folds), medial canthus, and lower eyelid are the most amenable areas of the mid-face to heal well by second intention.[13–19] Medial canthal wounds evenly distributed above and below the medial canthal tendon are exceptionally well suited for spontaneous granulation.[13–16,20] If a canthal defect extends into the upper or lower eyelids, guiding sutures placed across the wound perpendicularly to that of the contraction vector to be prevented may be helpful to prevent eyelid distortion caused by wound contraction.[21] Small, anterior lamellar defects along the eyelid margin often heal well without surgical closure.[16] Second-intention wound healing typically is less noticeable in light-colored skin than in darkly pigmented or telangiectatic skin.

Laissez-faire wound healing is often the simplest, most appropriate strategy in elderly or debilitated patients. If the risk of recurrence or residual tumor in the wound bed is significant, then second-intention wound healing may reduce the risk of masking residual tumor by allowing for close visual surveillance of the surgical site.[22–24] Unfortunately, in some cases, thick granulation tissue may be difficult to distinguish from recurrent tumor. Recurrent or large cutaneous malignancies that occur in the medial and lateral canthal regions are at greatest risk of incomplete tumor removal and require more vigilant postoperative surveillance.[25–28]

Wound care initially is directed by ensuring hemostasis and maintaining a clean, granulating tissue base. Avoidance of dessication and crust formation accelerates re-epithelialization.[29–30] Antibiotic ointment and a temporary, nonadherent absorptive dressing should be applied for the first 24 to 48 hours. Gauze or an eye pad can be placed over the nonadherent, fluid-permeable dressing. After removal of this dressing, antibiotic ointment should be reapplied at least three to four times per day until the wound is epithelialized. Some patients will develop a toxoallergic dermatitis to prolonged use of some topical antibiotic ointments (eg, bacitracin, neomycin, tobramycin) so these should be administered with caution after the first week. Mupirocin 2% is an antibiotic that is useful in slowly healing open wounds. SilverMed™ (MPM Medical Inc, Irving, TX) is a nonprescription alternative. Dilute baby shampoo washes twice daily followed by the application of shortening oil, such as Crisco™ (Orrville, Ohio) is an inexpensive treatment that can be used successfully for prolonged wound care. For patients unable to tolerate available topical antibiotic ointments, applying honey to the wound postoperatively may help keep wounds moist and perhaps aid in healing. Hydrogen peroxide should be avoided near the eyes and may lead to devitalization of the wound and delayed wound healing. Occlusive or semiocclusive dressings are rarely necessary in the periocular area. After the second postoperative day, wounds generally can be left uncovered or a light, nonadherent dressing can be used for patient convenience and cosmesis.

Full-Thickness Skin Grafting

Nonmarginal, partial-thickness eyelid defects not amenable to direct closure may require augmentation or replacement of the anterior lamella of the eyelid (Fig 35–1). Although local tissue flaps generally are preferred because of their superior color match and inherent blood supply, it is not always possible to design an adequate flap from the adjacent myocutaneous tissues. In these circumstances, full-thickness skin grafting should be considered. Partial-thickness skin grafts rarely are indicated and typically avoided, as aesthetic and functional results are frequently suboptimal. Contralateral upper eyelid skin is the best donor site for full-thickness skin grafts if adequate dermatochalasis is present. Ipsilateral upper eyelid skin also may be used in lower eyelid reconstruction. In larger defects or when limited upper eyelid skin is present, skin from both upper eyelids may be combined. Retroauricular or preauricular skin can be used if the upper eyelid skin is inadequate or when larger defects involve the thicker skin of the lower eyelid-cheek junction.[31,32] The non-hair-bearing areas of the supraclavicular fossa or inner arm are nontraditional alternatives when large skin grafts are necessary, or when prior facelift surgery scarring precludes the use of periauricular skin.[33] Thinning the thicker dermis and removal of the associated adnexal structures will improve graft match from these areas. As with healing by second intention, full-thickness skin grafts have a greater risk of developing unacceptable scars when used to repair cutaneous defects of the convex areas of the cheek, nasal, temporal, or forehead areas (see Fig 35–1).

Graft failure is the most common early postoperative host site complication following full-thickness skin grafting.[34] Trauma and shearing forces may lead to disruption of graft vascularization. Hematoma or seroma formation beneath the graft and wound infection are less common early complications but may also contribute to graft failure. Two to three days of gentle postoperative graft compression is probably helpful in promoting graft adhesion and revascularization. This can be achieved with an antibiotic ointment, nonstick dressing, and standard overlying bolsters. In the periocular area, an eye pad can be securely placed to provide the necessary graft compression. Following careful removal of the dressing around the third postoperative day, a successfully placed skin graft typically

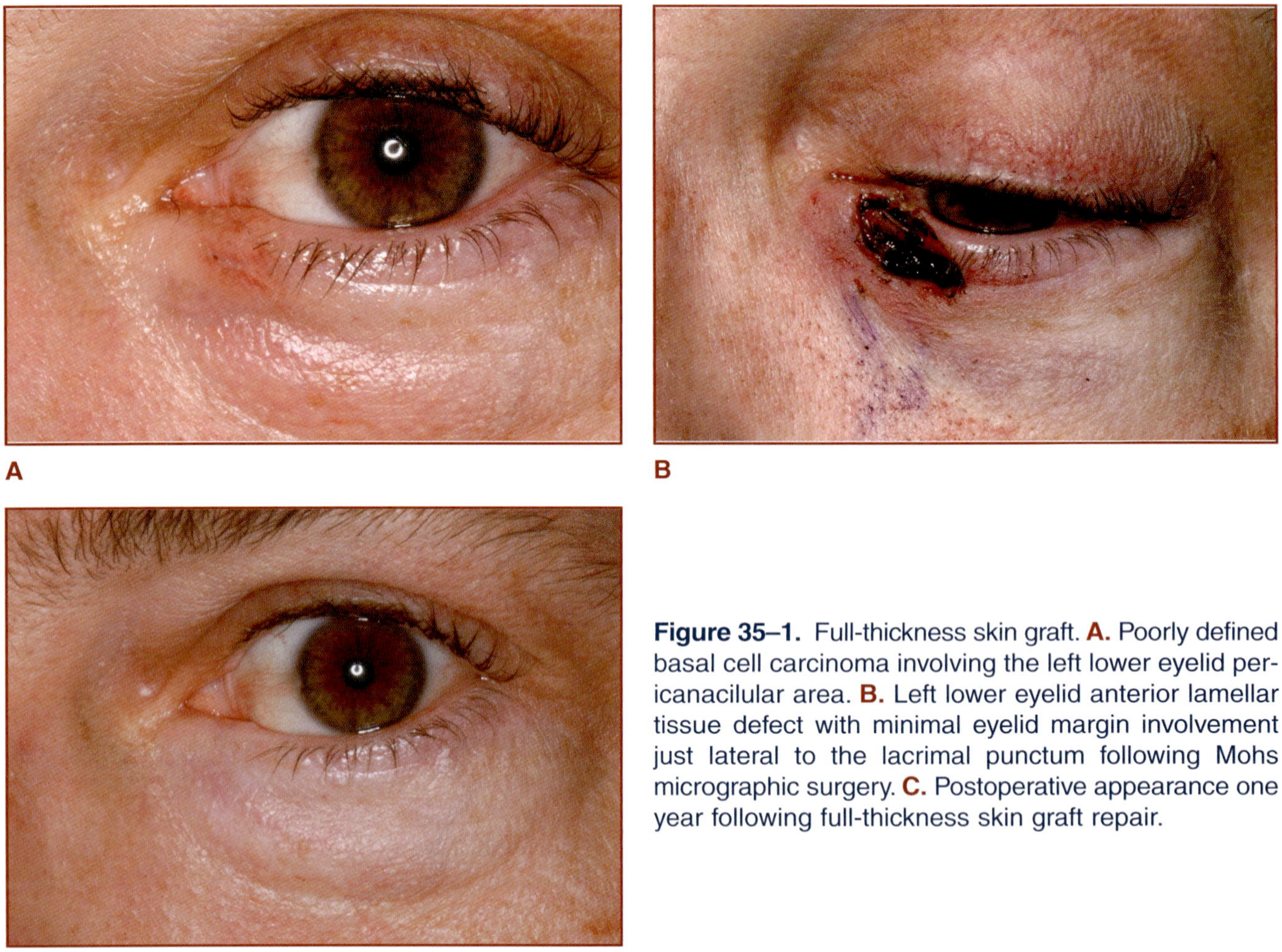

Figure 35–1. Full-thickness skin graft. **A.** Poorly defined basal cell carcinoma involving the left lower eyelid pericanacilular area. **B.** Left lower eyelid anterior lamellar tissue defect with minimal eyelid margin involvement just lateral to the lacrimal punctum following Mohs micrographic surgery. **C.** Postoperative appearance one year following full-thickness skin graft repair.

will appear light pink in color but occasionally will be darker red or purple. A black graft is evidence of necrosis and partial or total failure. A nonviable skin graft is generally left in situ as a biologic dressing, and epithelialization often proceeds beneath the necrosed graft, providing an acceptable outcome despite graft failure. A plastic or metallic eye shield may be worn to protect periorbital skin grafts from inadvertent trauma. Soft cloth ("pirate patch") occlusion may lead to adherence of the graft to the patch and should be avoided.

The most common late postoperative complications are graft hypertrophy, contraction, and/or hyper- or hypopigmentation.[34,35] Contracture of grafts in the periocular area can result in eyelid malposition and web formation. Graft contraction results from centripetal movement of the unapposed elastic fibers causing variable amounts of shrinkage.[34] Contracture can result in loss of up to one-third of a graft's initial size.[36] Therefore, it is important to oversize full-thickness skin grafts to account for anticipated graft shrinkage. Eyelid traction sutures may keep a graft on stretch during the first few weeks following surgery and potentially minimize graft contracture. Large defects in the medial canthal area may be at greater risk for hypertrophy and contracture, since a single skin graft may overlap the confluence of multiple aesthetic subunits.[37] For this reason, using separate grafts that come to a confluence at the base of the medial canthal concavity may provide a better result than a large skin graft over the entire medial canthal defect.

Periorbital Skin Flaps

Local skin and skin-muscle flap repair of partial thickness eyelid and periorbital defects is generally preferred over full-thickness skin grafting. In contrast to skin grafts, flaps provide superior color and texture matches and bring a rich blood supply. Flaps also can be combined with free posterior lamellar grafts when full-thickness eyelid reconstruction is necessary. It is important for the oculofacial reconstructive surgeon encountering nonmarginal eyelid, periorbital, and facial defects secondary to cutaneous tumor resection to understand the physiological and biomechanical principles of skin flap survival and orientation.

Successful cutaneous flap design begins with placement of surgical incisions that will result in minimally conspicuous scar formation and limited traction on the eyelids and periorbital tissues. It is preferable to place incisions within or parallel to the various facial "lines" that develop from the specific orientation of collagen and elastin fibers and are modified by the effects of gravity and facial muscle contraction. Relaxed skin tension lines (RSTL) correspond to the directional pull that is present in relaxed skin and generally correspond to the lines of facial expression.[38] Wrinkle lines typically are perpendicular to the long axis of subjacent muscles. Contraction of the orbicularis oculi sphincteric muscle raises the lower eyelid and closes the upper eyelid. Wrinkle lines in the eyelid, therefore, are perpendicular to the action of the muscle but parallel to the muscle fibers. In the periorbital region, RSTL run horizontally across the eyelids, lateral canthal area, forehead, and glabella, and parallel to the nasolabial fold. The dermis has a differential extensibility due to the topographic arrangement of collagen and elastic fibers allowing greater laxity in one direction than another.[39] These lines of maximum extensibility (LME) are perpendicular to the RSTL. Conversely, the RSTL are oriented in the direction of minimum extensibility.

Preoperative surgical planning should include consideration of all possible sites and orientations of flap design.[40] Although defect shape and location influence skin flap selection, the wound may be altered to increase surgical options for closure. Flaps should be slightly oversized to account for minor contracture, to include redundancy at the base of the flap, and to minimize tension on closure of the recipient wound. Extensive subcutaneous undermining and attention to the LME are both helpful in minimizing tension on recipient and donor site wound closure. Proper reconstructive planning should avoid distortion of important anatomic landmarks (eyebrow, medial and lateral canthus) and free margins (eyelid margin, nasal alae, and lips). Dog-ear formation (ie, "tissue bunching") should be addressed to prevent cone development and disfigurement.[52]

Sliding Cutaneous Flaps

Simple Ellipse. The most common configuration for skin lesion excision and closure is the simple ellipse. The elliptical facial incision should be oriented with its long axis parallel to a wrinkle line, contour line, line of dependency, or a RSTL. If closure is oriented about a RSTL, then the resultant tension on wound closure is in the direction of the LME. The simple ellipse sacrifices normal skin up to 1.5× the original lesion area. The long axis should be about four times the short axis creating an ellipse angle of around 30°. If the long axis is shorter, then bunching at the wound ends is more prominent. Minimizing tension on closure reduces scar formation and prevents secondary deformation of tissues.

Modified Ellipses. A variety of modifications of the simple ellipse may be utilized to diminish uninvolved tissue removal, a particularly critical goal in periorbital soft tissue repair. The "double-S" ellipse sacrifices half the normal tissue of a simple ellipse. A simple ellipse is designed but only alternate halves of the ellipse are excised. The resulting suture line has a mild S-shape.[41]

A double rotation advancement flap (O-to-Z plasty) may be used to close circular defects. Wound tension can be redirected along the long axis of the ellipse (with the RSTL).[42] An O-to-Z plasty is useful in lower eyelid defects where tension can be directed parallel to the eyelid margin minimizing the risk of ectropion and retraction. Beginning near points 180° from one another on that part of the circular defect furthest from the RSTL bisecting the lesion or defect, curved incisions are made centrifugally to end approximately where they meet lines parallel to the RSTL running tangentially to the defect. Each flap will be about twice the diameter of the circular defect and the flap tips typically require trimming to round the distal ends.

The M-plasty is a modified ellipse used to reduce the amount of normal skin removed and to produce a shorter scar (Fig 35–2).[43] A standard ellipse is outlined around a circular defect. The midpoint of each arm of the ellipse is connected to the midpoint of the side of defect near where the RSTL bisects the defect. Angles of about 30° are created at the base of each "M." The M-tips are closed with a half-buried horizontal mattress suture and the remainder of the ellipse is closed in standard fashion.

If uninvolved skin cannot be sacrificed to lengthen the incision in a standard ellipse or modified ellipse closure technique, then a subcutaneous–pedicle triangular skin flap is another option.[44,45] One or two triangles of skin are outlined with the bases of the triangles on the perimeter of the circular defect and the long axis of the flap placed near the RSTL or what would be a suitable line for a standard ellipse. The triangles are then cut taking care to preserve the flap's subcutaneous blood supply. Undermining and/or gentle spreading is only

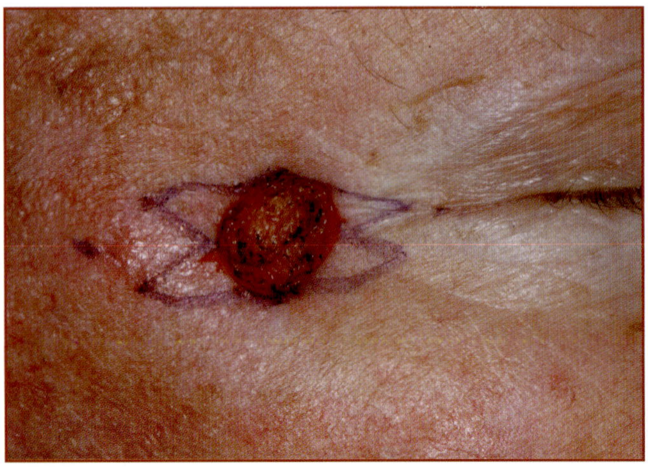

A

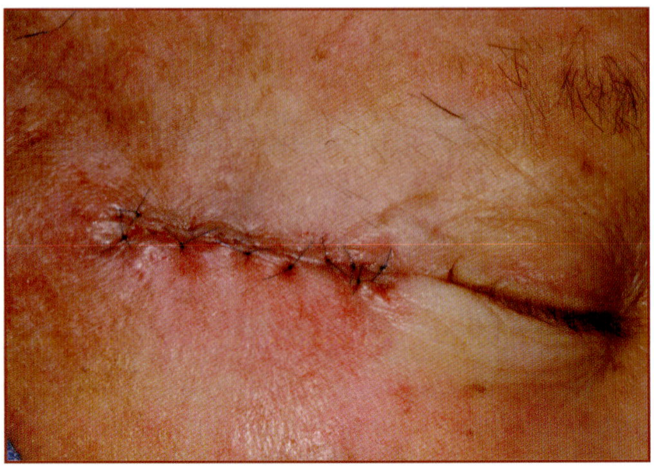

B

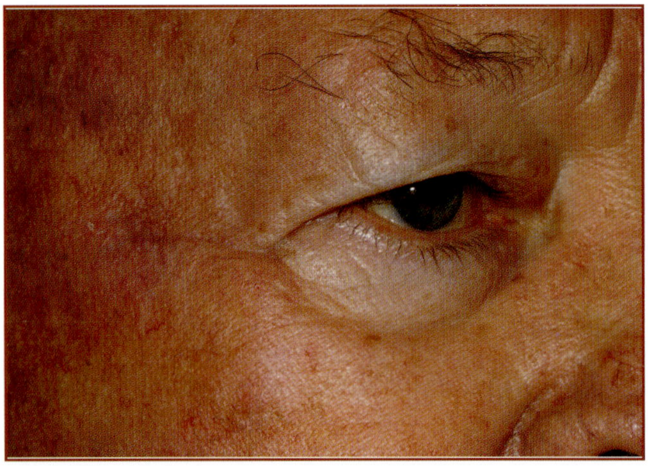

C

Figure 35–2. M-plasty. **A.** Right lateral canthal area Mohs surgical defect. M-plasty design minimizes normal tissue removal. **B.** Layered closure of wound within crow's feet or natural folds of lateral canthal region. **C.** Short, well-concealed scar 4 months following repair.

performed lateral to the flap(s) so as not to disturb the underlying muscular pedicle. The angles at the bases of the flap are trimmed and the advanced flap(s) sutured to the perimeter of the circle or to the opposing flap for a standard V-to-Y closure. A similar method of closure using a V-to-Y skin flap on a muscular pedicle (kite flap) has been described for the repair of lower eyelid defects where the base of the Y is positioned laterally outside of the eyelid to avoid eyelid distortion and to place the scar within existing crow's feet.[46]

Advancement Flaps

Skin or myocutaneous rectangular advancement flaps are useful in pretarsal and preseptal defects, particularly in the eyebrow and medial eyelids. Although the LME are oriented vertically in the eyelids, excess tension in a periocular skin-muscle flap should be directed parallel to the eyelid margin along the RSTL to reduce the risk of cicatricial ectropion and/or retraction.[40]

A circular defect involving the anterior lamella of the upper or lower eyelid can be converted into a square defect. A single or double rectangular flap constructed as wide as the defect then can be advanced horizontally in the eyelid.[47] The flap's base may be designed wider than its distal portion to maximize blood supply. Careful undermining in the preseptal plane permits adequate mobilization of skin and orbicularis muscle and recruits skin from the more lax soft tissues of the lateral periorbital area. Excision of each Burow's[48] triangle (lateral to the flap's base) aids in aligning the flap and adjacent wound margins prior to layered wound closure. A superiorly hinged blepharoplasty skin advancement flap may also be used to recruit redundant skin from the lateral periorbital area for repair of medial upper eyelid defects.[49]

A V-Y advancement flap is used to lengthen structures or to close a donor site.[40] This also is a useful method to transfer glabellar skin into medial canthal defects less than 2.5 cm. After a V-shaped incision is made, the skin on each side of the V is advanced with the defect closed as a Y. A Y-V flap is the opposite of the V-to-Y flap and can be used to lessen the distance between the medial canthi in epicanthus or in serial fashion to release skin contracture.[40]

Rotation Flaps

A rotation flap is a semicircular flap of skin and subcutaneous tissue that rotates about a pivot point into a defect. The donor site typically is repaired with wide undermining and direct, layered closure. The vector of greatest tension is directed from the pivot point outward to the defect's farthest radial point. Tension can be released by making a short back cut from the pivot point along the base of the flap or by making a small incision in the middle of the flap perpendicular to the line of tension.[40] Undermining of the tissue apposing the radial aspect of the flap also helps diminish the tension on wound closure. The Tenzel semicircular flap[50] and some cheek flaps are examples of rotational flaps used in the periorbital region.

Glabellar Flap. A traditional glabellar flap is a rotational flap that shifts skin from the glabellar region into the medial canthus. Glabellar flaps are useful for deep defects that extend down to periosteum or bone (Fig 35–3). These thick flaps provide a good blood supply from both the subdermal plexus and, with appropriate design, the supratrochlear vessels. An incision is made from the superior aspect of the defect toward the middle of the glabella. The incision is then turned down toward the opposite medial canthus to create an inverted "V" with an angle of about 60°. Each arm of the "V" should extend below the eyebrow. The flap is rotated into the defect and anchored to the medial canthal tendon and associated deep tissues to maintain the normal canthal concavity and to prevent webbing. The donor site is closed primarily. In some cases, secondary debulking of the thick, rotated glabellar flaps may be required; however, this can usually be prevented by trimming the flap intraoperatively to the desired thickness.[51] For larger medial canthal defects with eyelid involvement, glabellar flaps can be thinned and divided to cover medial upper and lower eyelid wounds, as well as used concomitantly with laterally based horizontal orbicularis oculi myocutaneous advancement flaps.[52]

In order to prevent drawing the eyebrows together, the redundant triangular tip of the flap can be excised and placed as a graft between the eyebrows.[53] Others have described a modification

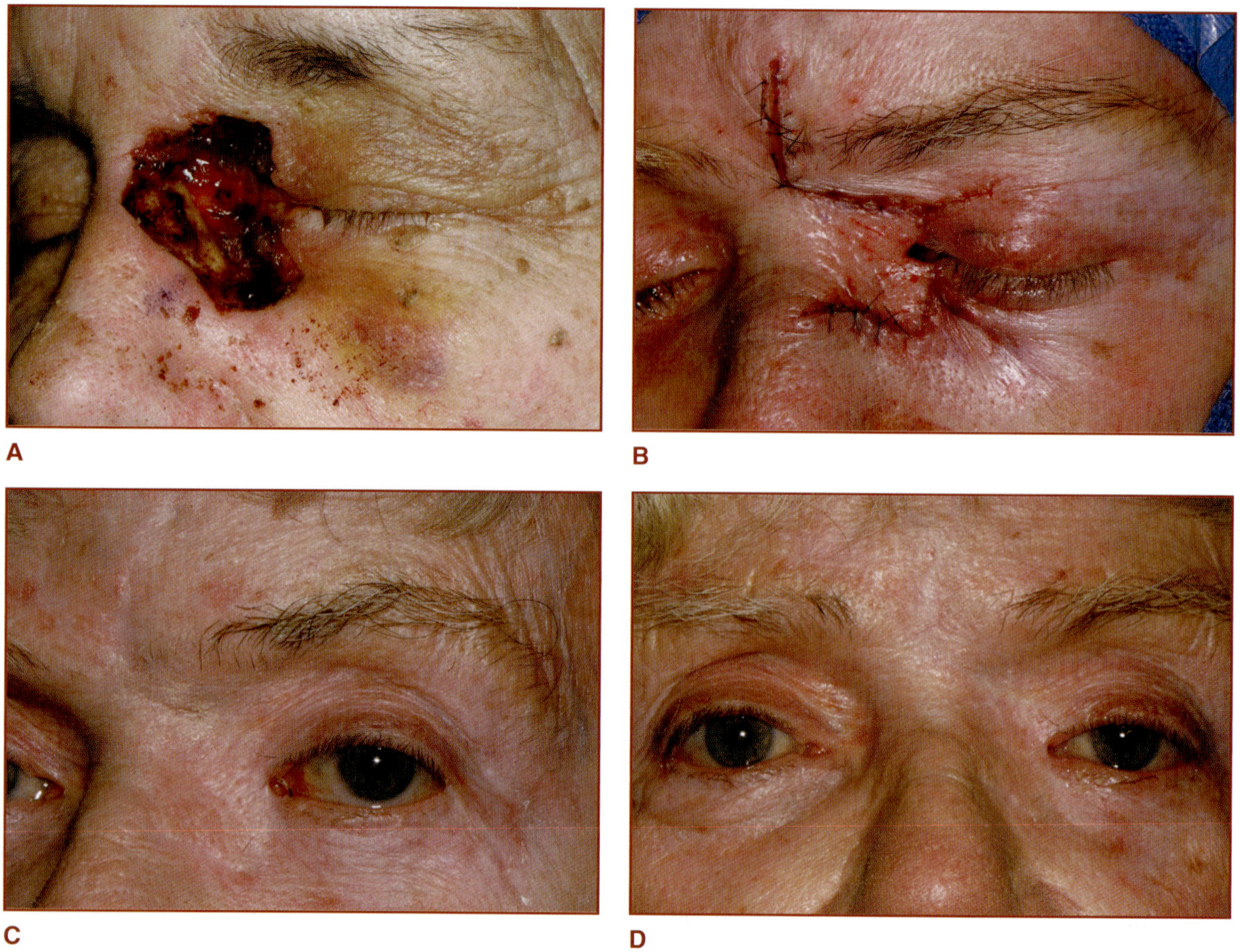

Figure 35–3. Glabellar flap. **A.** Defect following removal of a squamous cell carcinoma of the left medial canthus, involving both superior and inferior puncta and canaliculi. **B.** Glabellar flap with tip bifurcation to cover upper and lower eyelid wounds and re-establish medial canthal angle. **C.** Nine months following reconstruction. Annular lacrimal stent in place. **D.** One year after glabellar flap repair.

referred to as a "flap in flap" technique where a traditional V-shaped flap is rotated into a medial canthal or nasal dorsum defect and an adjacent second V-shaped flap extending superiorly into the glabella region is closed in V-Y fashion to relieve tension on the primary glabellar flap wound closure and minimize disruption of eyebrow spacing.[54]

Another modification of glabellar flap repair of the medial canthus utilizes a rectangular skin flap from the superior nasal dorsum and inferior glabella that is rotated on a caudal subcutaneous vascular pedicle into the adjacent defect.[55] A Rintala flap is then advanced inferiorly to fill the donor site. The advancement flap is secured to the underlying periosteum and Burow's triangles are resected near the head of each eyebrow.

Transposition Flaps

In a transposition procedure, a flap of skin or skin-muscle is transposed on a vascularized pedicle to fill a non adjacent defect. A cutaneous flap with a single pedicle based in the medial or lateral canthal areas may be raised using standard blepharoplasty techniques and transposed into canthal or lower eyelid defects. This unipedicle flap with its superiorly oriented traction vector is particularly useful when attempting to correct or prevent ectropion.[56] A single pedicled myocutaneous transposition from the upper eyelid to the lower eyelid is referred to as a modified Tripier flap based on the first reported description in of an innervated musculocutaneous flap by Tripier in 1889.[57] We have also found a bipedicled myocutaneous flap from the upper eyelid to the lower eyelid useful to reconstruct the anterior lamella in large full-thickness lower eyelid defects requiring posterior lamellar free tarsal grafts and an overlying vascularized flap. Blunting of the canthal angles and pincushioning may result with these eyelid transposition flaps necessitating subsequent cosmetic revisions. Bipedicled myocutaneous flaps from the subbrow region may be transposed into the inferior aspect of the upper eyelid in the reconstruction of large anterior lamellar defects.

Defects involving the lateral upper and lower eyelids may be closed with lateral transposition skin flaps. Our preferred flap design utilizes a vertical skin flap, up to 1.5 cm wide, that begins from the lateral edge of the defect and ends lateral to and above the eyebrow as needed. The skin flap is undermined including only subcutaneous tissue and avoiding deep dissection (below the superficial fascia) to prevent injury to branches of the facial nerve. The skin flap is transposed into the defect and bifurcated, if necessary, to fill the upper and lower eyelid anterior lamellar defects. The donor area is closed in layers. Temporal lower and upper eyelid full-thickness defects often require a periosteal flap hinged at the lateral orbital rim to provide posterior support (see Lateral Semicircular Rotational Flap and Lateral Periosteal Flap).[58,59] The transposed skin flaps can be secured to the underlying periosteal grafts with 6-0 plain gut suture, taking care to recess the skin flaps 1 to 2 mm from the reconstructed eyelid margin.

Cone formation "dog-ears" and the challenges of closing large donor sites make transposition flaps less attractive than other reconstructive surgical options available to repair large periorbital defects. As with traditional glabellar flaps, many periorbital transposition flaps create scars oriented perpendicular to RSTL. The midline forehead flap, which is a vertically oriented flap based in the glabellar area, can be rotated to reconstruct the medial canthi, eyebrows, and nasal defects.[60] These usually are designed as an interpolation flap with the pedicle bridging intact intervening skin and the base excised as a secondary procedure. Medially based upper eyelid myocutaneous flaps also can be designed as interpolation flaps with skin and muscle from a traditional upper blepharoplasty dissection transposed on a medial orbicularis oculi pedicle through a subcutaneous tunnel into the medial canthal region.[61,62] This versatile flap may be a good alternative to avoid utilizing the thicker skin of the glabella or forehead, such as when repairing defects involving the lateral nasal area or the bony nasal dorsum.

Bilobed Transposition Flaps. Single and bilobed transposition flaps can be used to close round defects.[63] The double transposition flap is a random-pattern cutaneous flap that consists of two lobes separated by an angle and sharing a pedicle with the smaller, second flap filling the donor defect and the larger lobe filling the primary defect. The bilobed flap enables recruitment of skin from a distant area of laxity to a defect where the adjacent tissue lacks adequate distensibility. Each rounded flap is undersized to share the tension of wound closure with the first lobe approximately 75% of the defect size and the second lobe about 75% of the size of the first lobe and usually one-half its width. The secondary flap can be 45° to 90° from the primary flap to ideally place it in the direction of the LME with the resulting scar parallel to the RSTL. After undermining and transposition of each of the flaps, the wound is closed in layers with deep absorbable sutures used to anchor the first lobe to the deep fibrous tissue, periosteum, or medial canthal tendon in order to minimize wound tension and web deformities.

The bilobed flap takes advantage of the sum of laxity along two different axes and is particularly useful in reconstruction of nasojugal and nasal sidewall defects where there is generally minimal tissue laxity.[64] In the periorbital region, these double transposition flaps are most useful in reconstruction of the medial canthal aesthetic subunit where tissue can be recruited from the nasofacial sulcus, nasal dorsum, or glabella.[65–67] In the medial canthus, the bilobed flap may help minimize distortion and webbing that can occur with larger transposition or advancement flaps. Defects that involve multiple medial canthal aesthetic subunits require a combination of flap techniques to achieve the best cosmesis.[37]

Reconstruction of large lateral canthal with lateral eyelid anterior lamellar defects utilizing bilobed flaps also have been described.[68]

Rhombic Flaps. The rhomboid (oblique-angled parallelogram with unequal adjacent sides) flap and its rhombic (form of a rhombus which has four equal sides) variants are the most useful and versatile transposition flaps for the primary repair of medial canthal and lateral periorbital quadrangular or circular defects.[69–71,72] These flaps also can be used to repair cheek and forehead defects using a combination of skin rotation and advancement. The main advantage of this technique is that transfer of the flap redistributes and redirects wound closure tension and helps with closure of the donor area. These flaps may leave less extensive scar lines than glabellar flaps when used in medial canthal wound repair.[70–73]

Classically, a round defect (often following Mohs micrographic surgery) is converted into a 60°/120° rhomboid shape (a parallelogram) by drawing lines tangential to the defect. Ideally, these lines should be parallel to the lines of maximum extensibility. However, it is more important to orient the rhombic flap to place the tension of the donor site closure parallel to the eyelid margin or to otherwise minimize deformation of the free eyelid margin, canthi, or eyebrow. A line is marked from the center of the 120-degree angles equal in length to the sides of the defect and bisecting the angle. Designing the flap off the short axis of the defect minimizes the size of the secondary defect. Another line is drawn in both directions parallel to the rhombic–shaped defect and equal in length to any side.

Of the four potential three-sided flaps based off the short axis of the defect, only two have diagonals (lines of closure) in line with the LME for lateral defects or parallel to the eyelid margin for central defects. Because all sides are intended to appose each other after transfer, they must all be identical in length. Proper orientation conceals the dipper-shaped scar, places the donor site's tension of closure parallel to the eyelid margin, and minimizes trap-door lymphedema.[71–74] The flap is transposed into the defect, and the donor site is closed after wide undermining. The disadvantages of the classic rhombic flap design include the loss of normal tissue when converting a round defect to rhombic shaped wound and the significant tension placed at the closure point of the secondary defect.

Alternatively, uninvolved tissue adjacent to a round or ovoid defect can be preserved and a smaller, quasi-triangular flap can be developed.[75,76] An infinite number of flap orientations is possible and the smaller donor site may be easier to close. As closure of the donor site results in a tension vector parallel to the unincised flap base, the base of the flap is oriented parallel to the eyelid margins. The initial incision bisects the circular defect, extends out radially, and is slightly shorter than the diameter of the circular wound. The second incision is equal in length to the first incision and is drawn back toward the defect at a 60° angle from the endpoint of the radial incision. The flap should be raised at a depth based on the depth of the defect, and extensive undermining is critical to permit adequate flap transposition. A Burow's triangle may be excised from the base of the flap to minimize cone formation, and squaring off of the defect opposite the flap base will facilitate closure of the distal aspect of the transposed flap. The primary and secondary wounds should be closed in layers.

Flap Repair of Large Nonmarginal Periocular Defects

The surgical management of periocular cutaneous malignancies often extends beyond the eyelids to other areas of the upper and middle face. Functional and aesthetic eyelid concerns must be considered when addressing defects in these contiguous areas. Small and medium-sized nonmarginal defects may be repaired by direct approximation, full-thickness skin grafting, advancement flaps, or rotational flaps as described elsewhere in this chapter. Large facial defects resulting from Mohs micrographic surgery or wide excision of a cutaneous melanoma require a combination of reconstructive options to minimize the aesthetic costs resulting from the use of large free skin grafts and extensive rotational flaps. Harris and colleagues have expertly outlined many of the important principles that guide our approach to these challenging oculofacial cases.[77,78] These include wide undermining of the tissues adjacent to the facial defect, direct wound approximation where possible, and the utilization of advancement and rotational flaps with deep, anchored fixation. Wound everting skin closure with vertical mattress suture techniques should be performed in the thicker skin of the midface and forehead.

Eyebrow, Glabella, and Forehead Advancement Flaps

The tissues of the glabella, forehead, and temple comprise a highly visible, major aesthetic unit of the upper face. Forehead reconstruction is reviewed in greater detail in Chapter 37. Reconstruction of eyebrow defects should include extensive undermining below the level of the hair follicles followed by direct closure with 3-0 or 4-0 polyglactin or polyglycolic acid sutures passed in buried, interrupted fashion to achieve secure subdermal support. Direct alignment of upper and lower rows of brow hairs followed by excision of superior and/or inferior tissue redundancy (Burow's triangles) preserves eyebrow continuity and an acceptable aesthetic result despite creation of a scar that is oblique to the RSTL of the brow area. The skin is closed with 6-0 nylon or polypropylene sutures in vertical mattress fashion to achieve good wound eversion. The excised Burow's triangles can be used as small full-thickness skin grafts if the entire defect cannot be closed with direct wound approximation (Fig 35–4). Similar techniques can be used for midline glabellar defects. Removal of medial brow hairs may be necessary as the heads of each brow are advanced medially.

Cheek and Lower Eyelid Rotation-Advancement Flaps

Mohs micrographic surgical resection of cutaneous malignancies involving the ocular adnexa often extends beyond the lower eyelid to the cheek. The repair of large cheek defects is also covered in Chapter 38. Repair of large mid-face defects must account for the differences in wound depth, skin thickness,

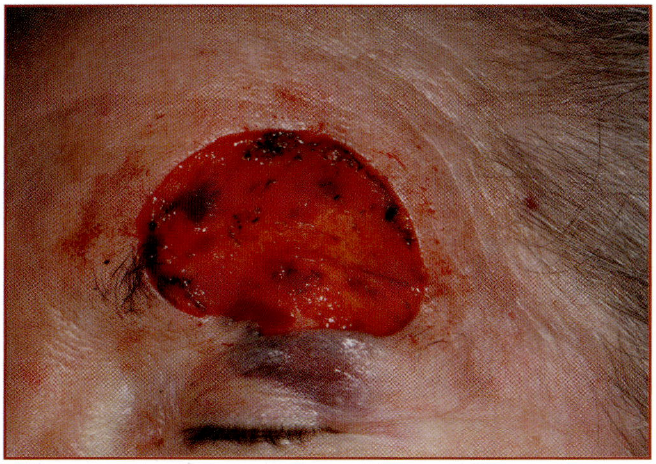

A

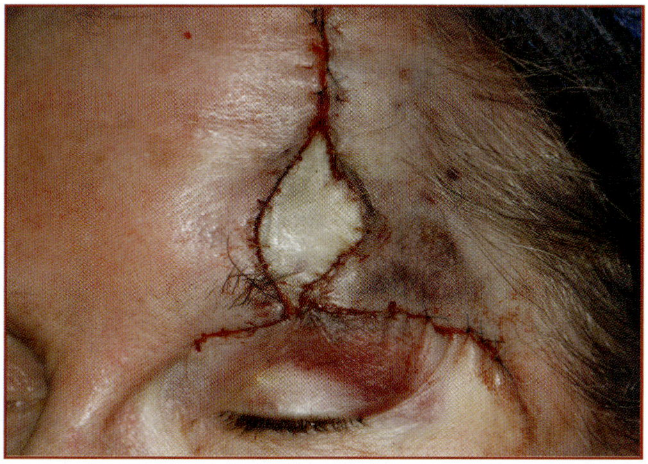

B

Figure 35–4. Eyebrow reconstruction. **A.** Left eyebrow and forehead defect after Mohs micrographic surgery for a morpheaform basal cell carcinoma. **B.** Wide cutaneous undermining permits sliding advancement closure of most of the eyebrow and forehead defect. Excised Burow triangle is used as a full-thickness skin graft to complete repair. *continues*

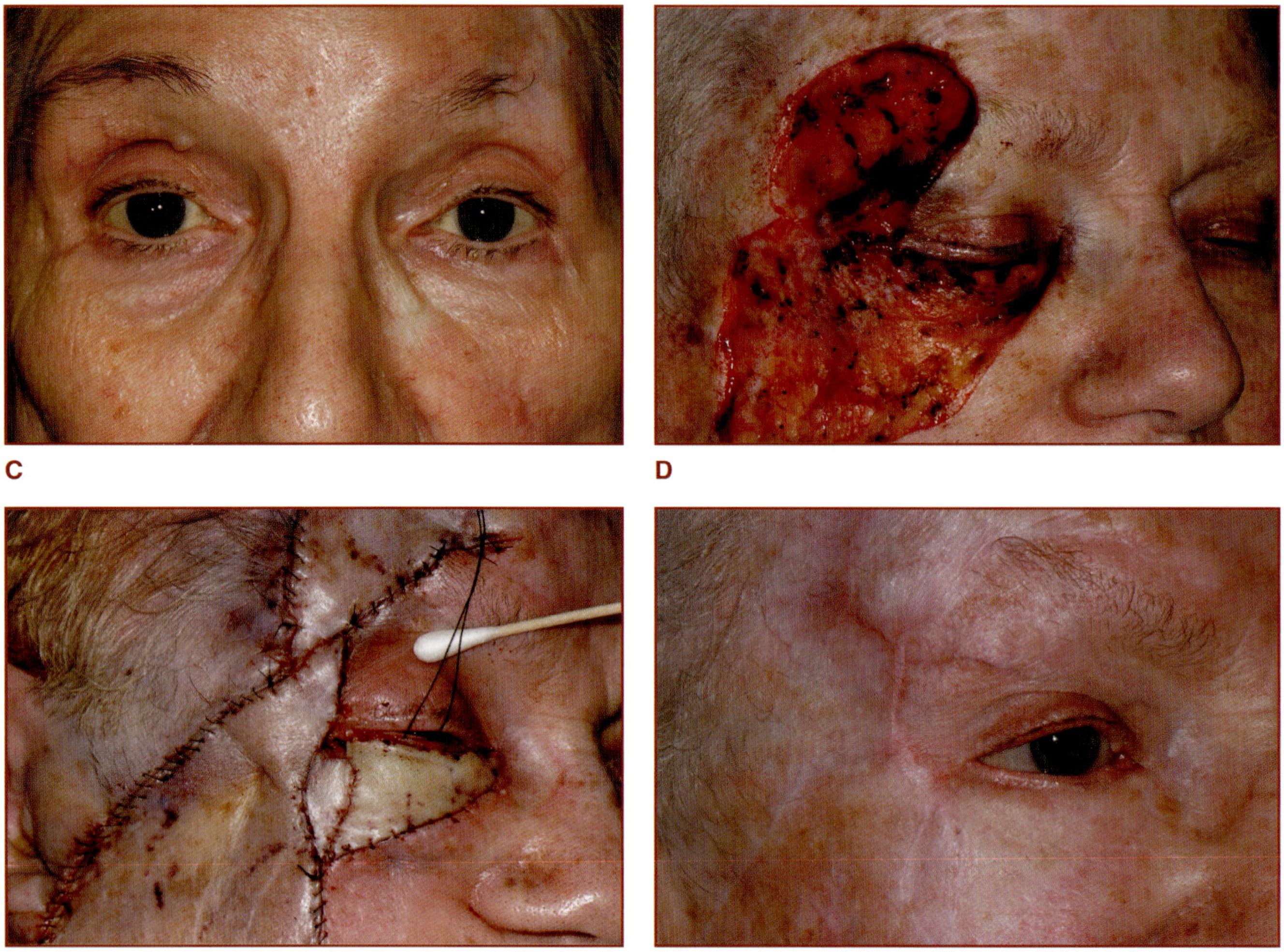

C D E F

Figure 35–4. *continued* **C.** One year following eyebrow and forehead defect reconstruction. **D.** Wide excision resulting in extensive defect of right eyebrow, lower eyelid, and cheek areas. *continues* **E.** Combination of cheek and forehead rotational and advancement flaps permits closure of most of the surgical defect. The excised Burow triangle and the redundant skin from the tip of the advanced forehead flap are used as full-thickness skin grafts to complete repair of the right lower eyelid anterior lamellar wound. **F.** One year following cutaneous flap and graft reconstruction.

and subjacent fat pads. Reconstructive techniques near or involving the lower eyelid must contend with the free margin of the lower eyelid that is susceptible to both gravitational and cicatricial forces. Flap repair of midface defects provides the ideal skin color match and can resurface wounds of varying depth with the necessary tissue thickness. Incisions within the horizontally oriented RSTL of the lower eyelid and midface allow angle rotation flaps to create favorable traction vectors that help counteract postoperative downward forces on the lower eyelid.[79]

Construction of a cheek flap begins with an incision at the superior aspect of the defect extending laterally within a RSTL toward the preauricular area. For defects in the lateral aspect of the eyelid-cheek complex, a medial based advancement flap permits additional tissue recruitment. Nasal and temporal incision length and the amount of flap dissection are determined by the surgeon following an intraoperative assessment of defect size and tissue elasticity. Skin flap mobilization is carried out by dissection above the orbicularis muscle in the lower eyelid and within the subcutaneous fat of the midface.

When wound proximity and lower eyelid laxity increase the risk of postoperative lower eyelid malposition, a lateral tarsal strip eyelid tightening procedure is also performed.[80] Large advancement flaps should be anchored to deep, stable tissue to help prevent flap distortion of the lower eyelid and canthi. Anchor points include the medial canthal tendon, maxillary periosteum inferior to the tendon, and the periosteum overlying the inferior or lateral orbital rim or malar eminence. A 4-0 polyglactin suture passed in buried fashion through the subcutaneous tissue of the flap and appropriate anchor point usually is adequate. A larger caliber suture may be required in some flaps with minimal inherent tissue laxity and significant tension with flap advancement. Subdermal, buried 4-0 or 5-0 polyglactin sutures can then be used to approximate the subcutaneous wound edges under minimal tension. Skin closure is completed with 6-0 nylon or polypropylene sutures in interrupted, vertical mattress, or running fashion as indicated. Tissue redundancy at the inferior aspect of the defect is typically excised, and the skin is not discarded in case full-thickness skin grafting is necessary for cutaneous defects remaining after flap advancement.

The Mustardé semirotational cheek advancement flap is another classic technique used to repair large lower eyelid defects.[81,82] Most large, full thickness lower eyelid defects do not require an extended facial incision and can be repaired with a more limited temporal eyelid rotational or advancement flap or a brow transposition flap.

Eyelid Defects Involving the Eyelid Margin

If eyelid margin involvement is evident, then the size of the defect should be assessed by carefully grasping the wound edges with an appropriately sized forceps with teeth and gently pulling the wound together to determine local tissue laxity and full-thickness wound size. Similar techniques may be used for small to medium full-thickness defects of the upper and lower eyelids, whereas different techniques are often indicated for large and total defects of the eyelids. Although vascularized flaps generally are superior to skin grafts in the eyelids for the same reasons as they are in other areas of head and neck reconstruction, full-thickness skin grafting also has a role in the reconstruction of full-thickness eyelid defects. As previously mentioned, reconstruction of full-thickness eyelid defects generally requires preservation of blood flow to the anterior or posterior lamella of the eyelid.

Direct Closure

Closure of lower eyelid defects that are less than one-fourth to one-third of the horizontal length of the eyelid often may be accomplished by direct wound approximation. In older patients with greater canthal tendon laxity, defects involving up to one-third to one-half of the horizontal dimension of the eyelid may be reapproximated with direct closure. A lateral canthotomy and lysis of the inferior crus of the lateral canthal tendon may gain an additional 5 to 10 mm in the horizontal dimension and permit closure with minimal tension for larger eyelid defects. With adequate pre-existing eyelid laxity, transconjunctival lysis of the inferior or superior crura of the lateral canthal tendon may be performed and a lateral canthotomy avoided in central eyelid defects.[83] If rounding of the lateral canthus or horizontal phimosis results due to inadequate eyelid laxity, then a lateral canthotomy should be performed with the canthal tendon lysis.

A full-thickness, vertical, pentagon-shaped defect with the point near the conjunctival fornix is created to minimize tarsal buckling and eyelid margin notching. The cut tarsal edges are reapproximated with two or three 5-0 or 6-0 polyglactin sutures on a spatula needle passed in interrupted fashion through partial thickness tarsus to avoid suture exposure on the conjunctival side of the wound. Inadequate tarsal reapproximation frequently will result in eyelid margin entropion. Minimizing tension on closure of the tarsus and performing buried orbicularis muscle closure when anterior lamellar wound tension is present help reduce the risk of wound dehiscence and unintended scar formation. A subciliary incision with horizontal myocutaneous wound advancement also has been suggested to minimize vertical scar formation.[84]

Meticulous reapproximation of the eyelid margin strut and realignment of the eyelid margin landmarks with wound eversion are critical steps to minimize the risk of postoperative trichiasis or eyelid margin notching. Classically, the meibomian gland orifices and anterior and posterior eyelash line are then meticulously realigned with three 6-0 silk vertical mattress sutures.[85] The skin is closed without tension using 6-0 plain gut suture incorporating the long ends of the marginal sutures to prevent corneal irritation. Alternatively, a single absorbable 7-0 poly - glactin vertical mattress suture passed through the Meibomian gland orifices eliminates the need for suture removal and may diminish the risk of wound margin dehiscence.[86] To help prevent suture knot-induced conjunctival and corneal contact, a "buried" vertical mattress 7-0 polyglactin suture pass is begun and completed about 3 to 4 mm away from the eyelid margin deep within the tarsal wound.[87] This is our preferred technique. Similarly, 6-0 and 7-0 chromic gut sutures have also been advocated for eyelid margin re-approximation[88,89] (Fig 35–5).

Lateral Semicircular Rotational Flap and Lateral Periosteal Flap

If tarsal or eyelid margin reapproximation cannot be achieved with release of the canthal attachments, then mobilization of the lateral canthal and temporal tissues may permit reconstruction of defects involving up to one-half of the central and lateral eyelid.[50,58,90] Although the risk of wound dehiscence and notch formation is increased with increasing wound tension, acceptable aesthetic results can be achieved even when large full-thickness wounds are closed with moderate to considerable wound tension.[91] Canthal tendon laxity, inherent eyelid elasticity, straightening of the normal eyelid curvature by globe displacement, and mechanical tissue creep are proposed mechanisms that contribute to postoperative eyelid relaxation.

After a pentagon-shaped defect is created, a rounded myocutaneous flap then can be recruited from the lateral canthal area to augment the anterior lamellar tissues of the eyelid and provide a helpful superolateral vector of support. For lower eyelid defects, a semicircular incision is directed from the lateral canthal angle superiorly toward the tail of the brow before curving laterally. The lateral aspect of the incision typically is flattened and does not complete the semicircle. In upper eyelid defects, the semicircular flap initially arches inferotemporally, ending below the lateral extent of the eyebrow. A lateral canthotomy and inferior (lower eyelid repair) or superior (upper eyelid repair) cantholysis is performed to mobilize any remaining lateral eyelid tissue. The musculocutaneous flap is undermined, rotated nasally, and attached to the medial edge of the eyelid defect. Separate posterior lamellar grafts are often not necessary as the conjunctiva will mucosalize the underside of the advanced flap. Donor site closure may be facilitated by performing a temporal Z-plasty with the horizontal rotational flap.[92] This combined flap technique transfers available vertical laxity in the temple area to the horizontal deficiency resulting from rotation of the semicircular flap into the eyelid defect (see Fig 35–5).

For larger full-thickness defects requiring additional structural support, a hinged periosteal flap from the superolateral orbital rim may provide a stable posterior platform for anterior lamellar reconstruction. The periosteum of the lateral rim is exposed and two parallel cuts are made 1.5 to 2.0 cm apart, beginning at the inner aspect of the lateral orbital rim and continuing through the periosteum into the temporalis fascia. Less frequently, the periosteal flap may be constructed from the periorbita of the lateral orbital wall within the orbital cavity. If the defect involves the lateral aspects of both the upper and lower eyelids, then the periosteal flap is bisected horizontally and inferior flap is crossed with the superior flap to recreate the lateral canthal angle.[93] The periosteal flap is secured to the cut edge of the tarsal wound with 5-0 or 6-0 polyglactin sutures passed in partial-thickness fashion through the intact tarsal plate. The underside of the musculocutaneous flap is fixated to the lateral orbital rim periosteum at the desired canthal angle also using absorbable sutures such as 4-0 or 5-0 polyglactin to curve the eyelid inward along the contour of the globe. Addi-

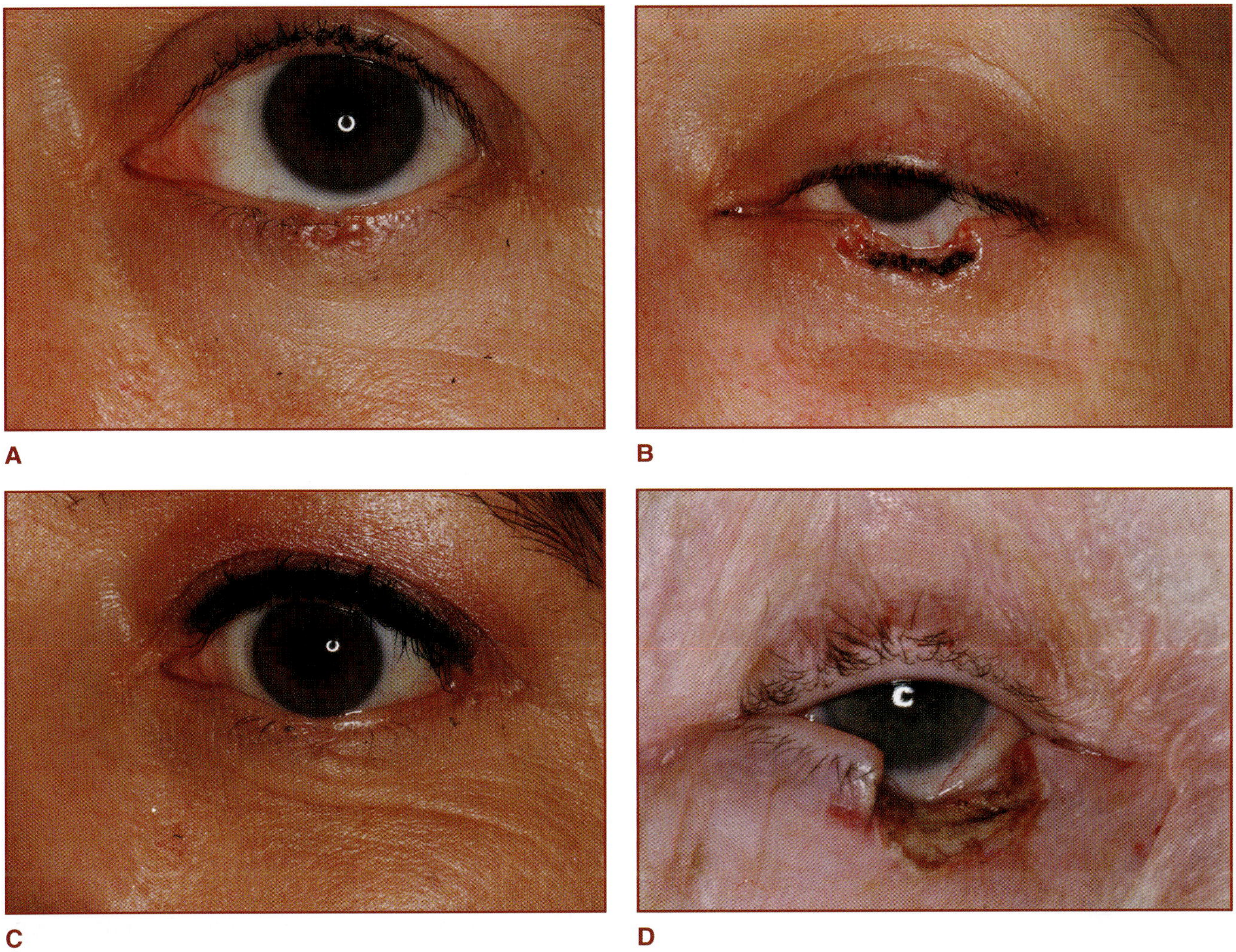

Figure 35–5. Small-medium full-thickness eyelid repair. **A.** Left lower eyelid margin basal cell carcinoma. Note ulcerated appearance. **B.** Small-medium full-thickness pentagonal wound of left lower eyelid. **C.** Ten weeks following direct closure of lower eyelid wound. **D.** Medium-sized right lower eyelid defect after basal cell carcinoma resection. *continues*

tional sutures fixated deeply to the lateral orbital rim periosteum may be needed to minimize tension on flap wound closure. The skin muscle flap can be sutured to the underlying periosteal flap to ensure an acceptable eyelid margin contour.

An alternative technique for the repair of large lateral canthal wounds with full-thickness defects of the upper and lower eyelids uses temporalis fascia grafts for posterior lamellar reconstruction and a trilobed, transposition skin flap with each of the elliptical lobes developed at 45-degree angles to one other in the premalar region, cheek, and preauricular area for anterior lamellar repair.[94] The superior lobe is used to close the upper eyelid defect, the middle lobe is used for the lower eyelid repair, and the third lobe is transposed into the donor site. Disadvantages of this technique include multiple, midface incisions that are not as easily concealed as with a temporal transposition flap and exposure of the deep temporalis fascia requiring a second operative site unlike anchored periosteal strip flaps that help maintain appropriate eyelid position and tone.

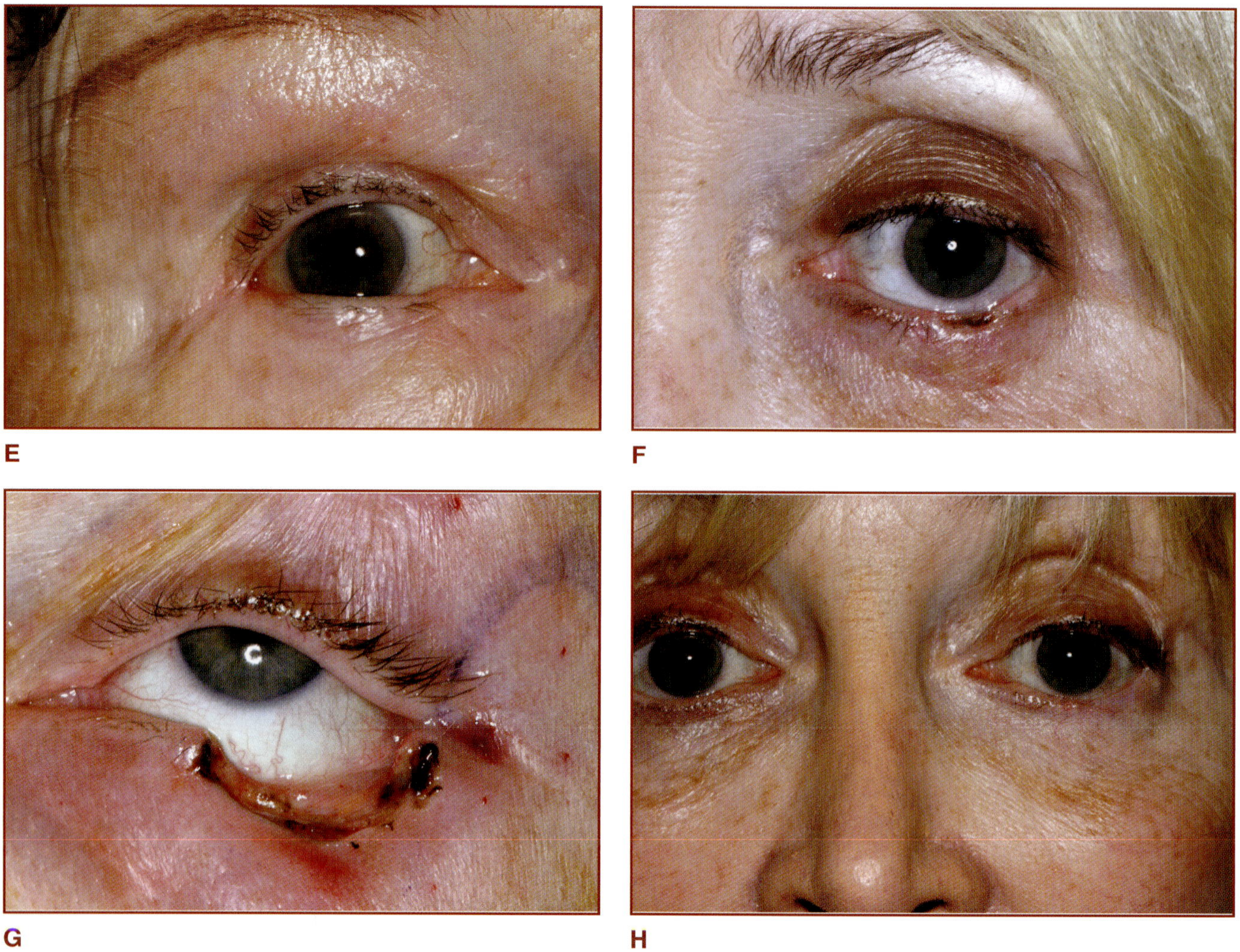

Figure 35–5. *continued* **E.** Three months following reconstruction with semicircular rotational flap and direct wound closure. **F.** Left lower eyelid margin basal cell carcinoma **G.** Medium-large pentagonal wedge defect. Note marking of superiorly directed semicircular flap. **H.** Four months following semicircular rotational flap wound repair.

Sliding Tarsoconjunctival Flap

One of techniques that we find useful in the repair of medium-sized (approximately one-third to two-thirds of the horizontal dimension of the eyelid) upper and lower posterior eyelid defects is the fornix-based, sliding tarsoconjunctival flap. A 4-0 silk traction suture is placed through the eyelid margin, and the eyelid is everted over a Desmarres retractor. Relaxing incisions are made in the tarsus to create a flap just slightly smaller than the width of the defect. At least 2 mm of the lower eyelid margin tarsus and 3 to 4 mm of upper eyelid margin tarsus is left intact at the donor area to maintain eyelid shape and stability. The superior relaxing incision should extend beyond the tarsoconjunctival border. The flap is elevated with careful dissection and transposed horizontally into the posterior lamellar defect. Slight vertical overcorrection is desirable in anticipation of conjunctival contracture which can create an eyelid margin depression. The free edge of the tarsal flap is secured to the edge of the defect in a similar fashion as described for direct eyelid margin closure.[95] For lesions near the lateral canthus, it may be necessary to secure the flap to the remnant of the lateral canthal tendon, to the periosteum, or to a hinged periosteal flap. The anterior lamella is reconstructed with a full-thickness skin graft, rotational flap or advanced myocutaneous flap (see Periorbital Defects Not Involving the Eyelid Margin, above). The anterior lamellar tissue is recessed 1 mm from the reconstructed eyelid margin and closed with an absorbable suture.

When Mohs micrographic surgical resection of a marginal malignancy results in a shallow, full-thickness lower eyelid defect, then the residual tarsal strip may be utilized as a modified "sliding tarsal flap" to reconstruct the posterior lamella.[96] After the orbital septal attachments to the intact tarsal strip are released, an oblique incision is made inferiorly from one margin of the defect through the inferior tarsal remnant. The transected tarsal segments are then advanced obliquely to overlap and recreate an intact tarsal layer of near normal height. Anterior lamellar repair is then carried out with either a full-thickness skin graft or local flap.

Sharing Tarsoconjunctival Bridge Flap: Modified Hughes Procedure

One of the first descriptions of an upper eyelid tarsoconjunctival flap for reconstructing lower eyelid defects was by Kollner in 1911.[97] Wendell Hughes' classic initial report was in 1937 and reviewed again almost 40 years later.[98–100] Traditionally, the Hughes tarsoconjunctival flap is a useful lid-sharing technique for shallow wounds involving up to two-thirds of the horizontal length of the lower eyelid. For more extensive defects of the lower eyelid, often following Mohs micrographic tumor, a lateral periosteal flap provides additional posterior lamellar support.[58–59] Some authors also have found medial periosteal flaps useful in the repair of large lower eyelid defects.[101,102] The primary advantages of the Hughes procedure are its simplicity, blood supply, and its postoperative vertical traction, which helps prevent lower eyelid ectropion and eyelid retraction. Temporary obstruction of the visual axis is the main disadvantage of this eyelid-sharing technique. Careful patient selection and preoperative counseling are essential for patients to accept the impact of 2 to 6 weeks of restricted vision.

The upper eyelid is everted over a malleable or Desmarres retractor using a 4-0 silk suture through the eyelid margin for traction. A full-thickness tarsal incision, approximately 10 to 25% smaller than the horizontal length of the recipient defect, is made parallel to the upper eyelid margin leaving 3 mm of intact tarsus along the eyelid margin. Vertical cuts in the tarsus are then made extending beyond the upper border of the tarsal plate. The levator aponeurosis and pretarsal tissue attachments are meticulously dissected from the tarsal plate, and the dissection is carried superiorly and posteriorly into the superior fornix. Müller's sympathetic muscle is recessed as failure to adequately release the upper eyelid retractor muscles may contribute to postoperative upper eyelid retraction. The mobilized tarsoconjunctival flap is advanced inferiorly into the lower eyelid defect. The leading margin of the flap is secured to the recipient conjunctiva and lower eyelid retractors with interrupted or running 6-0 absorbable sutures with the suture knots oriented away from the globe. The medial and lateral edges of the advanced tarsus are attached to the intact tarsus of the lower eyelid with 5-0 or 6-0 polyglactin sutures on a spatulated needle to ensure partial thickness tarsal suture placement. The superior tarsal border of the upper eyelid flap will become the reconstructed lower eyelid margin. The anterior lamellar defect is repaired with either a full-thickness skin graft from the ipsilateral eyelid superior to the advanced flap, the contralateral upper eyelid, or from a pre- or postauricular site. A local eyelid or cheek advancement flap is also an option for anterior lamellar repair (Fig 35–6).

Second stage flap takedown traditionally is performed around 4 weeks postoperatively. Division of the tarsoconjunctival pedicle may be performed as early as 7 to 14 days following the primary operation.[103,104] The palpebral fissure is opened by dividing the tarsoconjunctival flap just slightly above the desired new lower eyelid margin position. This second stage procedure is performed in an office setting under topical and infiltrative anesthesia using a straight, blunt-tipped scissors (Steven's tenotomy)

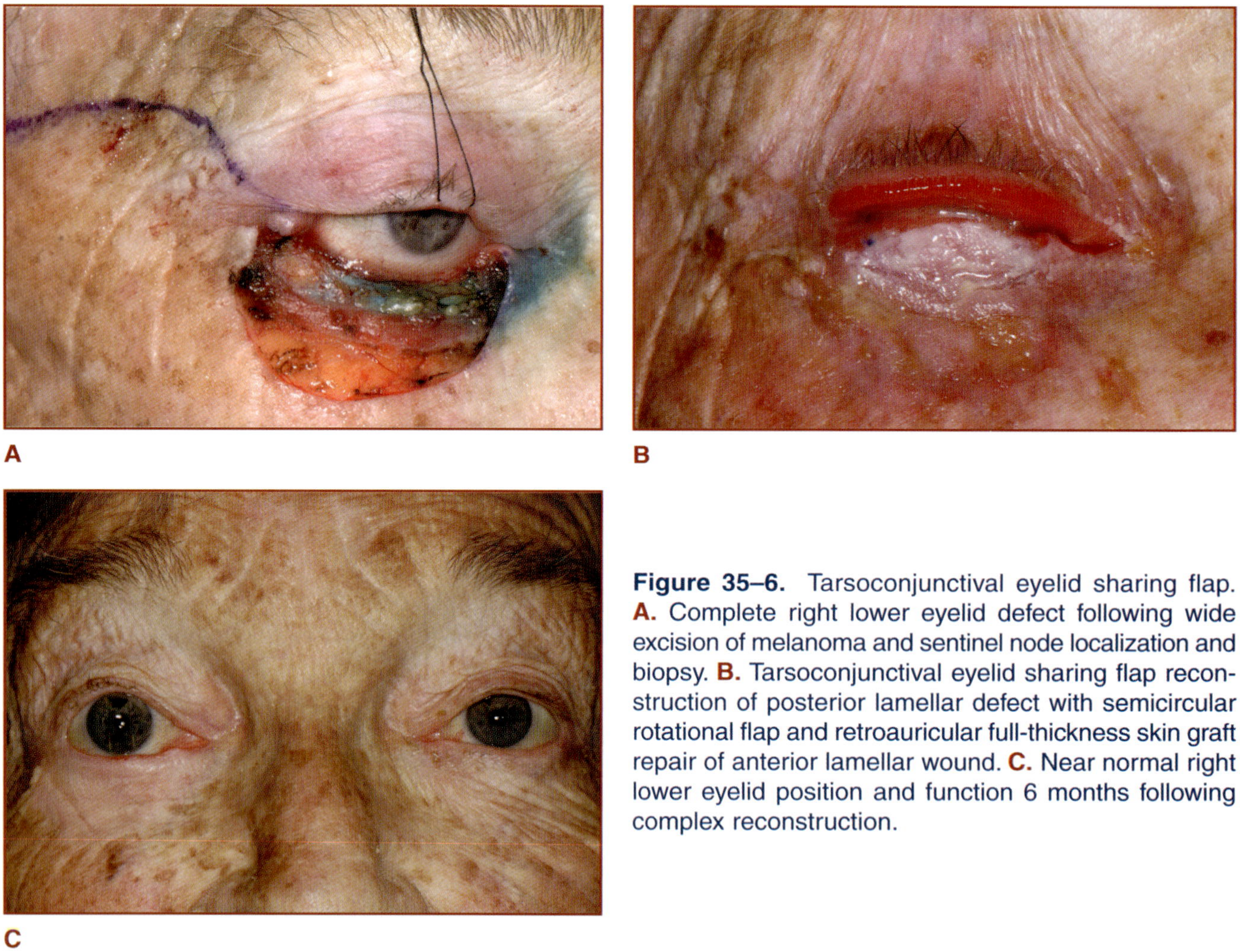

Figure 35–6. Tarsoconjunctival eyelid sharing flap. **A.** Complete right lower eyelid defect following wide excision of melanoma and sentinel node localization and biopsy. **B.** Tarsoconjunctival eyelid sharing flap reconstruction of posterior lamellar defect with semicircular rotational flap and retroauricular full-thickness skin graft repair of anterior lamellar wound. **C.** Near normal right lower eyelid position and function 6 months following complex reconstruction.

to divide the flap while the eyelids are distracted away from the cornea. The upper eyelid is everted over a Desmarres retractor and the residual donor pedicle is dissected between Müller's muscle and the levator aponeurosis to the superior fornix and excised to help prevent postoperative upper eyelid retraction. Light cautery may be indicated for hemostasis of the transected vascular pedicle. Allowing the mucocutaneous line to form spontaneously minimizes the postoperative thickness and redness of the eyelid margin.[105] Contouring of the eyelid margin can be performed, as needed, after the eyelid is allowed to heal for a few months. Artificial eyelashes and eyeliner are recommended for cosmesis if desired by the patient.

If a tarsoconjunctival lid-sharing flap is not a viable option because there is insufficient tarsus in the ipsilateral upper eyelid from prior reconstruction, or because eye occlusion must be avoided, a free tarsoconjunctival graft harvested from the ipsilateral or contralateral upper eyelid can be used for posterior lamellar lower eyelid reconstruction. A vertically advanced myocutaneous flap from the lower eyelid or a laterally based myocutaneous transposition flap from the upper eyelid can provide for a vascularized repair of the lower eyelid anterior lamella.[106] If adequate lower eyelid conjunctiva remains following tumor resection, then superior conjunctival advancement combined with an overlying V-Y myocutaneous flap is a recently presented alternative technique for one-stage reconstruction of lower eyelid defects.[107]

Free Mucosa-Lined Grafting (Autogenous Tarsus, Hard Palate Mucosa)

Reconstruction of large upper eyelid defects presents unique challenges not encountered in lower eyelid repair. The upper eyelid has greater contact with the cornea during normal eyelid blinking and closure. Irregularities tolerated in the posterior eyelid surface of the lower eyelid may cause significant corneal irritation if present in the upper eyelid. Additionally, greater eyelid excursion must be maintained in the eyelid to permit facile opening and closing.

In order to utilize host tarsoconjunctival tissues for posterior lamellar reconstruction, subtotal and total upper eyelid defects traditionally have been repaired with lower eyelid switch flaps and lower eyelid bridge flaps.[108–110] If a remnant of superior tarsus greater than 3 mm remains following tumor resection, it may be advanced inferiorly to reconstruct the upper eyelid margin and posterior lamella in a single-stage procedure.[111] Some surgeons have advocated nasal chondromucosal flaps based on the dorsal nasal artery.[112] Others have proposed using acellular dermal graft material as an alternative tarsal substitute in the repair of large upper eyelid full-thickness defects.[113–114]

For years, attempts have been made to develop one-stage, autogenous surgical repair of the posterior lamella in total upper eyelid reconstruction. Moschella and Cordova[115] described their use of mucosa from inside the lower lip to replace absent superior tarsoconjunctival tissue. Unfortunately, this abundant tissue does not provide adequate rigid support and is prone to substantial contraction. Venous wall grafts from the propulsive veins of the distal forearm or leg have been suggested as autogenous posterior lamellar replacements in upper and lower eyelid reconstruction.[116]

Hard palate mucosal grafts (HPMGs) are mucosally lined, flexible tissues traditionally used in lower eyelid posterior lamellar reconstruction.[117] Although hard palate graft use in the lower eyelid is a well accepted reconstructive technique, these grafts are associated with numerous potential complications including graft contraction with eyelid retraction, donor site morbidity (hemorrhage, oronasal fistula, candida infection), and mucus production from minor salivary glands located within the graft.[118] Limited success with HPMG in the upper eyelid has been described.[119] However, as with lower reconstruction, placement of HPMGs in the upper eyelid has been reported to result in a substantial incidence of ocular irritation, keratopathy, and overlying skin flap necrosis.[120] Hard palate mucosal grafts may not differentiate to nonkeratinized epithelium following transplantation.[121] Postoperative keratinization of HPMGs can cause ocular irritation and disruption of the corneal epithelium. A bandage soft contact lens may be helpful to minimize corneal trauma when HPMGs are used in upper eyelid repair.

For full-thickness large or total upper eyelid defects, we have found that a free tarsoconjunctival graft (FTG), periosteal strip flap, and overlying ipsilateral, bipedicle myocutaneous flap is an effective one-stage technique that is aesthetically and functionally superior to the Cutler-Beard flap.[122] Alternatively, the FTG may be covered by a bipedicled orbicularis muscle flap with an overlying full-thickness skin graft. This one-stage technique permits immediate visual rehabilitation, provides functional orbicularis muscle to help preserve eyelid blinking and closure, and gives an acceptable aesthetic result. We have not experienced significant donor site morbidity and typically can harvest adequate tarsal tissue from the unaffected, contralateral upper eyelid. A similar technique also can be used for subtotal and total lower eyelid reconstruction if the previously described rotational flaps or lid-sharing procedures are inadequate or contraindicated.[123]

To harvest a FTG the upper eyelid is everted over a malleable or Desmarres retractor using a 4-0 silk suture through the eyelid margin for traction.[124] A full-thickness tarsal incision, equal to the length of the recipient defect, is made parallel to the upper eyelid margin leaving 2 to 3 mm of intact tarsus along the eyelid margin. Vertical cuts in the tarsus are then made to the superior border of the tarsal plate. The pretarsal tissues (levator aponeurosis and orbicularis muscle) are dissected away from the tarsus, the superior conjunctival attachments incised, and the graft is delivered. The donor site is left to heal by second intention. The mucosalized tarsal graft is placed in the recipient defect with the conjunctival side against the globe and is sutured to the forniceal conjunctiva with a running 6-0 mild gut suture with the suture knots buried subconjunctivally. The medial and lateral edges of the tarsal graft are sutured to the host tarsus with 5-0 or 6-0 polyglactin sutures passed in partial-thickness fashion to avoid suture contact with the ocular surface. If there are no tarsal edges or tendon remnants, a hinged periosteal flap from just inside the lateral orbital rim may be reflected into the defect for additional posterior lamellar support. In many cases, the levator superioris muscle will transmit contractile forces through conjunctival attachments and not require advancement. For large upper eyelid defects, reattachment of the levator aponeurosis to the donor tarsus may be indicated. Complications from FTG use in upper eyelid reconstruction are generally limited to avoidable donor site problems such as eyelid contour abnormalities.[120]

The anterior lamella must be reconstructed with a vascularized tissue flap such as a vertically advanced or transpositional myocutaneous flap. A bipedicle skin-muscle flap from the superior margin of the eyelid defect is an excellent option for large marginal defects with intact subbrow upper eyelid tissue (Fig 35–7).[122] The myocutaneous flap should be

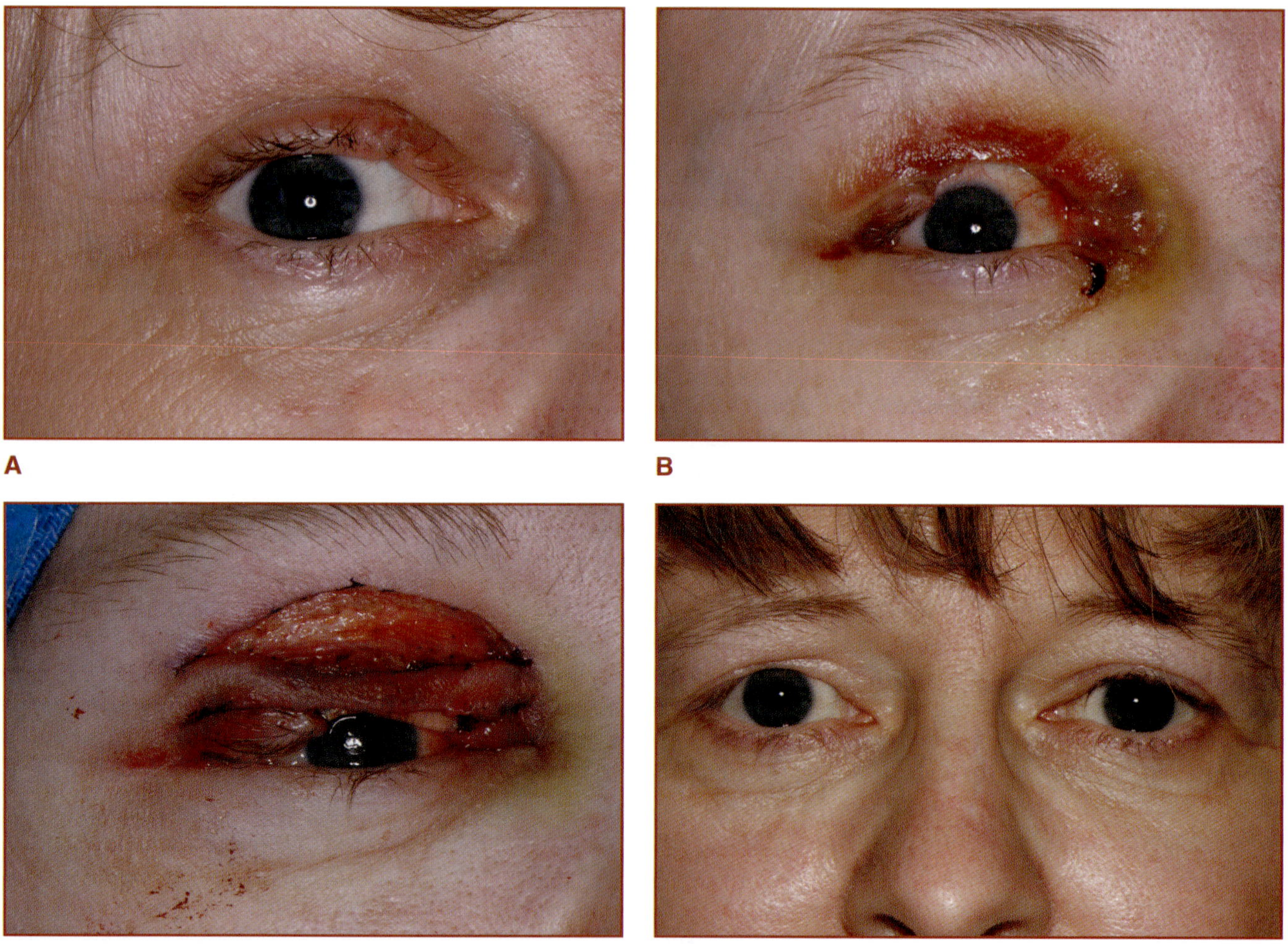

A B C D

Figure 35–7. Free tarsoconjunctival graft **A.** Right upper eyelid sebaceous cell carcinoma. **B.** Large right upper eyelid defect following wide excision of sebaceous cell carcinoma. **C.** Free tarsoconjunctival graft in place covered by bipedicle myocutaneous flap. **D.** One year following repair of large right upper eyelid full-thickness defect.

recessed 1 mm from the tarsal graft margin and secured to the donor tarsus with a running 6-0 mild chromic suture. In some cases, sufficient residual skin is available adjacent to the donor site permitting primary closure. More commonly, the flap donor site is closed with a full-thickness skin graft from the contralateral upper eyelid or retroauricular area. A less aesthetically desirable option for donor site closure is to utilize a supra-eyebrow cutaneous unipedicle transposition flap.[119] Ophthalmic antibiotic ointment, a nonstick dressing, and a light pressure patch are placed over the operated area for two to three days.

Medial Canthal Reconstruction

Reconstruction of the medial canthus can be a surgical challenge even for the experienced oculofacial reconstructive surgeon. The deep concavity of the medial canthus represents the convergence of multiple aesthetic subunits that differ in skin quality, thickness, and contour.[37] Mohs micrographic surgical resection of cutaneous malignancies is a common indication for reconstruction in this anatomically complex periocular region. Second-intention healing, full-thickness skin grafting, and local flap repair are reconstructive options that have been individually reviewed in this chapter. A combination of these techniques may be indicated to achieve an optimal aesthetic result. Skin grafting and flap closure can diminish the size of a large defect allowing the remaining wound to heal by second-intention.

Some complex defects may not respect the aesthetic subunits of the periorbital region and medial canthus, requiring a combination of local flaps to repair a large medial canthal defect.[37,125] Component flaps that have been reviewed in this chapter include: an inverted V-Y flap (glabellar region), rhombic flap, bilobed transposition flap (nasal sidewall), upper and lower eyelid rectangular advancement flaps, cheek advancement and semirotational flaps, and direct closure of brow defects. These flaps are each anchored to the anterior limb of the medial canthal tendon or adjacent deep fibrous tissue using buried 4-0 or 5-0 polyglactin sutures. By individually fixating the component flaps, traction forces are appropriately directed and web deformities are minimized. Periosteal fixation of the advanced lower eyelid and cheek flaps will help recreate the natural canthal concavity and diminish the risk of postoperative wound dehiscence as well as punctal and eyelid malposition. The skin is closed with interrupted and vertical mattress 6-0 plain gut and/or 6-0 nylon sutures.

Closure of full-thickness medial canthal defects may be also be initiated by developing tarsoconjunctival flaps in both the upper and lower eyelids and advancing these flaps medially. The tarsal attachments are then secured in the area of the desired medial canthal tendon near the superior aspect of the posterior lacrimal crest. Posterior fixation is critical to prevent medial distraction of the eyelid from the globe and may be achieved with a slowly absorbing or permanent suture (on a small semicircular needle) passed through the periosteum or by using a Y-shaped titanium microplate with the arms secured to the frontal process of the maxilla and the single leg bent down and back into the orbit allowing for fixation of the medial canthal remnant or tarsal attachments to a hole in the plate.[126] Alternatively, a resorbable poly-L-lactic acid-polyglycolic acid screw has been advocated to provide medial canthal bone fixation.[127] More complex transnasal wiring techniques are rarely necessary.

Canalicular Repair

Mohs micrographic surgical resection of medial canthal or paracanalicular cutaneous malignancies often results in damage to the canalicular system. Primary canalicular repair should be considered in all patients undergoing reconstruction of the medial eyelids where canalicular injury has occurred.[128,129] The critical aspects of canalicular repair include temporary, atraumatic placement of a well-tolerated endocanalicular stent, meticulous anastomosis of pericanalicular tissues, and anatomic closure of the eyelid margin and medial canthal wounds.

Reifler[130] has provided an excellent review of the different methods of locating the medial lacerated canaliculus. Over the past 35 years, silicone tubing has become the most widely accepted stent material.[130,131] Silicone stents are designed from a soft, malleable, and inert material with little risk of tissue erosion or globe irritation. We have found bicanalicular intubation utilizing loupe magnification, in most cases, to be the simplest and most effective method of repairing monocanalicular or bicanalicular lacerations. Silicone tubing can be passed into the nose or in an annular configuration. Initial reports using the pigtail probe for annular stent placement were associated with unacceptable complication rates.[132,133] These problems were later identified as resulting from defective instrumentation design, poorly tolerated stent materials, and inadequate canalicular anastomosis.[129] Avoidance of Worst's barbed-tip spiral instrument and careful use of the round-tipped, eyed pigtail probe has greatly minimized iatrogenic injury to the canalicular system.[129,134–136]

The technique described by Jordan et al,[129] is simple, quick, and facilitates location of the medial cut end of the canaliculus. Additionally, manipulation of the lacrimal sac and nasolacrimal duct is avoided, the risk of stent prolapse is virtually eliminated, and the silicone stent provides an effective anchor for eyelid reconstruction by realigning the traumatized tissues and facilitating medial canthal repair and pericanalicular tissue anastomosis. Pericanalicular tissue alignment over a canalicular stent is sufficient to restore a patent canaliculus.[137] The silicone tubing typically is removed in the office 3 to 6 months following placement.

If a pigtail probe is not available or the absence of a common canaliculus makes use of the probe difficult, then conventional bicanalicular intubation into the nose using a Crawford stent system may be necessary. A variety of monocanalicular intubation techniques have been described.[138,139] Newly designed silicone stents swaged to round tip steel probes (Collarette Monoka, FCI Ophthalmics, Marshfield Hills, MA) may prove to be effective when bicanalicular intubation is not feasible and may be more practical for the office surgical setting.

Conclusion

The reconstructive surgeon confronted with periorbital and eyelid defects must have a firm understanding of the standard techniques utilized in the repair of soft tissue defects in other areas of the face. Second-intention wound healing, full-thickness skin grafting, and myocutaneous flaps are all common methods of managing oculofacial wounds. The use of these techniques in the ocular adnexa must account for some of the unique anatomic features of the eyelids and periorbital tissues. To formulate a surgical plan the surgeon must be able to conceptualize different options for periorbital reconstruction and consider the advantages and disadvantages of standard eyelid reconstructive techniques.

This chapter highlights a variety of periorbital reconstructive techniques that can be utilized to achieve the functional goals of maintaining a stable eyelid margin, normal eyelid position and excursion, adequate eyelid closure, and lacrimal drainage. Repair of full thickness eyelid defects should result in the development of a smooth, epithelialized posterior surface with semirigid posterior lamellar support, as well as an aesthetically acceptable anterior lamellar substitute.

References

1. Older JJ, Quickert MH, Beard C. Surgical removal of basal cell carcinoma of the eyelids utilizing frozen section control. *Trans Am Acad Ophthalmol Otolaryngol.* 1975;79:658–663.
2. Chalfin J, Putterman AM. Frozen section control in the surgery of basal cell carcinoma of the eyelid. *Am J Ophthalmol.* 1979;87:802–809.
3. Mohs FE. Micrographic surgery for the microscopically controlled excision of eyelid cancers. *Arch Ophthalmol.* 1986;104:901–909.
4. Rapini RP. Comparison of methods for checking surgical margins. *J Am Acad Dermatol.* 1990;23:288–294.
5. Otley CC, Salasche SJ. Mohs surgery: efficient and effective. *Br J Ophthalmol.* 2004;88:1228.
6. Pieh S, Kuchar A, Novak P, et al. Long term results after surgical basal cell carcinoma excision in the eyelid region. *Br J Ophthalmol.* 1999;83:85–88.
7. Carter KD, Nerad JA, Whitaker DC. Clinical factors influencing periocular surgical defects after Mohs micrographic surgery. *Ophthalmic Plast Reconstr Surg.* 1999;15:83–91.
8. Lindgren G, Lindblom B, Larkö O. Mohs micrographic surgery for basal cell carcinomas on the eyelids and medial canthal area. *Acta Ophthalmol Scand.* 2000;78:430–436.

9 Nemet AY, Deckel Y, Martin PA, et al. Management of periocular basal and squamous cell carcinoma: a series of 485 cases. *Am J Ophthalmol.* 2006;142:293–297.
10. Anderson RL, Ceilley RI. A multispecialty approach to the excision and reconstruction of eyelid tumors. *Ophthalmology.* 1978;85:1150–1163.
11. Nerad JA, Whitaker DC. Periocular basal cell carcinoma in adults 35 years of age and younger. *Am J Ophthalmol.* 1988;106:723–729.
12. Thomas JR, Frost TW. Immediate versus delayed repair of skin defects following resection of carcinoma. *Otolaryngol Clin North Am.* 1993;23:203–213.
13. Fier RH, Older JJ. Spontaneous repair of the medial canthus after removal of basal cell carcinoma. *Ophthalmic Surg.* 1982;13:737–740.
14. Harrington JN. Reconstruction of the medial canthus by spontaneous granulation (laissez-faire): a review. *Ann Ophthalmol.* 1982;14:956–970.
15. Moscona R, Pnini A, Hirshowitz B. In favor of healing by secondary intention after excision of medial canthal basal cell carcinoma. *Plast Reconstr Surg.* 1983;71:189–195.
16. Mehta HK. Simultaneous spontaneous and primary surgical repair of eyelids. *Br J Ophthalmol.* 1989;73:488–493.
17. Becker GD, Adams LA, Levin BC. Nonsurgical repair of perinasal skin defects. *Plast Reconstr Surg.* 1991;88:768.
18. Lowry JC, Bartley GB, Garrity JA. The role of second-intention healing in periocular reconstruction. *Ophthal - mic Plast Reconstr Surg.* 1997;13:174–188.
19. DaCosta J, Oworu O, Jones CA. Laissez-faire: how far can you go? *Orbit.* 2009;28:12–15.
20. Fox SA, Beard C. Spontaneous lid repair. *Am J Ophthalmol.* 1964;58:947–952.
21. Albright III SD. Placement of "guiding sutures" to counteract undesirable retraction of tissues in and around functionally and cosmetically important structures. *J Dermatol Surg Oncol.* 1981;7:446–449.
22. Albom MJ. The management of recurrent basal-cell carcinomas: please, no grafts or flaps at once. *J Dermatol Surg Oncol.* 1977;3:382–384.
23. Koplin L, Zarem HA. Recurrent basal cell carcinoma: a review concerning the incidence, behavior, and management of recurrent basal cell carcinoma, with emphasis on the incompletely excised lesion. *Plast Reconstr Surg.* 1980;65:656–664.
24. Mordick TG, Hamilton R, Dzubow LM. Delayed reconstruction following Mohs' chemosurgery for skin cancers of the head and neck. *Am J Surg.* 1990;160:447–449.
25. Taylor GA, Barisoni D. Ten years' experience in the surgical treatment of basal-cell carcinoma: a study of factors associated with recurrence. *Br J Surg.* 1973;60:522–525.
26. Levine HL, Bailin PL. Basal cell carcinoma of the head and neck: identification of the high risk patient. *Laryngoscope.* 1980;90:955–961.
27. Dzubow LM. Chemosurgical report: recurrence (persistence) of tumor following excision by Mohs surgery. *J Dermatol Surg Oncol.* 1987;13:27–30.
28. Dzubow LM. False-negative tumor-free margins following Mohs surgery. *J Dermatol Surg Oncol.* 1988;14:600–602.
29. Svensjo T, Pomahac B, Yao F, et al. Accelerated healing of full-thickness skin wounds in a wet environment. *Plast Reconstr Surg.* 2000;106:602–612.
30. Brown CD, Zitelli JA. Choice of wound dressings and ointments. *Otolaryngol Clin North Am.* 1995;28:1081–1091.
31. Breach NM. Pre-auricular full-thickness skin grafts. *Br J Plast Surg.* 1978;31:124–126.
32. Dryden RM, Wulc AE. The preauricular skin graft in eyelid reconstruction. *Arch Ophthalmol.* 1985;103:1579–1581.
33. Custer PL, Harvey H. The arm as a skin graft donor site in eyelid reconstruction. *Ophthalmic Plast Reconstr Surg.* 2001;17:427–430.
34. Leibovitch I, Huilgol SC, Hsuan JD, Selva D. Incidence of host site complications in periocular full thickness skin grafts. *Br J Ophthalmol.* 2005;89:219–222.
35. Valencia IC, Falabella AF, Eaglstein WH. Skin grafting. *Dermatol Clin.* 2000;18:521–532.
36. Stephenson AJ, Griffiths RW, La Hausse-Brown TP. Patterns of contraction in human full thickness skin grafts. *Br J Ophthalmol.* 2000;53:397–402.
37. Harris GJ, Logani SC. Multiple aesthetic unit flaps for medial canthal reconstruction. *Ophthalmic Plast Reconstr Surg.* 1998;14:352–359.
38. Borges AF. Relaxed skin tension lines (RSTL) versus other skin lines. *Plast Reconstr Surg.* 1984;73:144–150.
39. Gibson T, Kenedi RM. Biomechanical properties of skin. *Surg Clin North Am.* 1967;47:279–294.
40. Patrinely JR, Marines HM, Anderson RL. Skin flaps in periorbital reconstruction. *Surv Ophthalmol.* 1987;31:249–261.
41. Alvarado A. Reciprocal incisions for closure of circular skin defects. *Plast Reconstr Surg.* 1981;67:482–490.
42. Webster RJ, Benjamin BJ, Smith RC. Closure of circular defects. *Laryngoscope.* 1978;88:534–538.
43. Webster RC, Davidson TM, Smith RC. M-plasty techniques. *J Dermatol Surg Oncol.* 1976;2:393–396.
44. Emmett AJJ. The closure of defects by using adjacent triangular flaps with subcutaneous pedicles. *Plast Reconstr Surg.* 1977;59:52.
45. Saunders DH, Shannon GM. Subcutaneous-based triangular skin flaps. *Ophthalmic Surg.* 1980;11:437–439.
46. Marchac D, Lange A, Bine-bine H. A horizontal V-Y advancement lower eyelid flap. *Plast Reconstr Surg.* 2009;124:1133–1141.
47. Demir Z, Yuce S, Karamursel S, Celebioglu S. Orbicularis oculi myocutaneous advancement flap for upper eyelid reconstruction. *Plast Reconstr Surg.* 2008;121:443–450.
48. Burow A. Zur blepharoplastik. *Monatsschr Med Augenh Chir.* 1838;1:57.
49. Then SY, Malhotra R. Superiorly hinged blepharoplasty flap for reconstruction of medial upper eyelid defects

following excision of xanthelasma palpebrum. *Clin Experiment Ophthalmol.* 2008;36:410–414.
50. Tenzel RR. Reconstruction of the central one half of an eyelid. *Arch Ophthalmol.* 1975;93:125–126.
51. Emsen IM, Benlier E. The use of the superthinned inferior pedicled glabellar flap in reconstruction of small-to-large medial canthal defect. *J Craniofac Surg.* 2008;19:500–504.
52. Chao Y, Xin X, Jiangping C. Medial canthal reconstruction with combined glabellar and orbicularis oculi myocutaneous advancement flaps. *J Plast Recon Aesthet Surg.* 2009;1–5.
53. Meadows AER, Manners RM. A simple modification of the glabellar flap in medial canthal reconstruction. *Ophthalmic Plast Reconstr Surg.* 2003;19:313–315.
54. Turgut G, Ozcan A, Yesiloglu N, Bas L. A new glabellar flap modification for the reconstruction of medial canthal and nasal dorsal defects: "flap in flap" technique. *J Craniofac Surg.* 2009;20:198–200.
55. Onishi K, Maruyama Y, Okada E, Ogino A. Medial canthal reconstruction with glabellar combined Rintala flaps. *Plast Reconstr Surg.* 2007;119:537–541.
56. Anderson RL, Hatt MU, Dixon R. Medial ectropion: a new technique. *Arch Ophthalmol.* 1979;97:521–524.
57. Labbe D, Benateau H, Rigot-Joliver M. Homage to Leon Tripier. Description of the first musculocutaneous flap and current indications. *Ann Chir Plast Esthet.* 2000;45: 17–23.
58. Tenzel RR, Stewart WB. Eyelid reconstruction by the semicircle flap technique. *Ophthalmology.* 1978;85: 1164–1169.
59. Weinstein GS, Anderson RL, Tse DT, Kersten RC. The use of a periosteal strip for eyelid reconstruction. *Arch Ophthalmol.* 1985;103:357–359.
60. Dortzbach RK, Hawes MJ. Midline forehead flap in reconstructive procedures of the eyelids and exenterated socket. *Ophthalmic Surg.* 1981;12:257–268.
61. Jelks GW, Glat PM, Jelks EB, Longaker MT. Medial canthal reconstruction using a medially based upper eyelid myocutaneous flap. *Plast Reconstr Surg.* 2002;110: 1636–1643.
62. Tezel E, Sonmez A, Numanoglu A. Medial pedicled orbicularis oculi flap. *Ann Plast Surg.* 2002;49:599–603.
63. Zimany A. The bi-lobed flap. *Plast Reconstr Surg.* 1953; 11:424–434.
64. Morgan BL, Samhan MZ. Advantages of the bilobed flap for closure of small defects of the face. *Plast Reconstr Surg.* 1973;52:35–37.
65. Sullivan TJ, Bray LC. The bilobed flap in medial canthal reconstruction. *Aust N Z J Ophthalmol.* 1995;23:42–48.
66. Meadows AER, Rhatigan M, Manners RM. Bilobed flap in ophthalmic plastic surgery: simple principles for flap construction. *Ophthalmic Plast Reconstr Surg.* 2005; 21:441–444.
67. Perry JD, Taban M. Superiorly based bilobed flap for inferior medial canthal and nasojugal fold defect reconstruction. *Ophthal Plast Reconstr Surg.* 2009;25:276–279.
68. Emsen IM. Additional and different application of the bilobed flap: bilobed in bilobed flap for reconstruction of the lower-upper lid and lateral canthal defects. *Aesthetic Plast Surg.* 2008;32:542–545.
69. Limberg AA. *Mathematical Principles of Local Plastic Procedures on the Surface of the Human Body.* Leningrad, Russia: Medgiz; 1946.
70. Bullock JD, Koss N, Flagg SV. Rhomboid flap in ophthalmic plastic surgery. *Arch Ophthalmol.* 1973;90:203–205.
71. Becker FF. Rhomboid flap in facial reconstruction: new concept of tension lines. *Arch Otolaryngol.* 1979;105: 569–573.
72. Borges AF. The rhombic flap. *Plast Reconstr Surg.* 1981; 67:458–466.
73. Ng SGJ, Inkster CF, Leatherbarrow B. The rhomboid flap in medial canthal reconstruction. *Br J Ophthalmol.* 2001;85:556–559.
74. Shotton FT. Optimal closure of medial canthal surgical defects with rhomboid flaps: "rules of thumb" for flap and rhomboid defect orientations. *Ophthalmic Surg.* 1983;14:46–52.
75. Quaba AA, Sommerlad BC. "A square peg into a round hole": a modified rhomboid flap and its clinical application. *Br J Plast Surg.* 1987;40:163–170.
76. Teske SAH, Kersten RC, Devoto MH, Kulwin DR. The modified rhomboid transposition flap in periocular reconstruction. *Ophthalmic Plast Reconstr Surg.* 1998;14: 360–366.
77. Harris GJ, Garcia GH. Advancement flaps for large defects of the eyebrow, glabella, forehead, and temple. *Ophthalmic Plast Reconstr Surg.* 2002;18:138–145.
78. Harris GJ, Perez N. Anchored flaps in post-Mohs reconstruction of the lower eyelid, cheek, and lateral canthus: avoiding eyelid distortion. *Ophthal Plast Reconstr Surg.* 2003;19:5–13.
79. Boutros S, Zide B. Cheek and eyelid reconstruction: the resurrection of the angle rotation flap. *Plast Reconstr Surg.* 2005;116:1425–1430.
80. Anderson RL, Gordy DD. The tarsal strip procedure. *Arch Ophthalmol.* 1979;97:2192–2196.
81. Mustarde JC. *Repair and Reconstruction in the Orbital Region.* Edinburgh, UK: Churchill Livingstone; 1971.
82. Callahan MA, Callahan A. Mustarde flap lower lid reconstruction after malignancy. *Ophthalmology.* 1980; 87:279–286.
83. Lewis CD, Perry JD. Transconjunctival lateral cantholysis for closure of full-thickness eyelid defects. *Ophthal Plast Reconstr Surg.* 2009;25:469–471.
84. Rosser P, McCormick A. Horizontal skin wound closure in full thickness eyelid excision. *Clin Experiment Ophthalmol.* 2008;36:709–711.
85. Divine RD, Anderson RL. Techniques in eyelid wound closure. *Ophthalmic Surg.* 1982;13:283–287.
86. Devoto MH, Kersten RC, Teske SA, Kulwin DR. Simplified technique for eyelid margin repair. *Arch Ophthalmol.* 1997;115:566–567.

87. Burroughs JR, Soparkar CNS, Patrinely JR. The buried vertical mattress: a simplified technique for eyelid margin repair. *Ophthalmic Plast Reconstr Surg.* 2003;19:323–335.
88. Perry JD, Aguilar CL, Kuchtey R. Modified vertical mattress technique for eyelid margin repair. *Dermatol Surg.* 2004;30:1580–1582.
89. Custer PL, Vick V. Repair of marginal eyelid defects with 7-0 chromic sutures. *Ophthal Plast Reconstr Surg.* 2006; 22:256–258.
90. Boynton JR. Semicircle flap reconstruction "plus." *Ophthalmic Surg.* 1993;24:826–830.
91. Thaller VT, Then KY, Luhishi E. Spontaneous eyelid expansion after full thickness eyelid resection and direct closure. *Br J Ophthalmol.* 2001;85:1450–1454.
92. Khan JA, Garden VS. Combined flap repair of moderate lower eyelid defects. *Ophthalmic Plast Reconstr Surg.* 2002;18:202–204.
93. Leone Jr CR. Lateral canthal reconstruction. *Ophthalmology.* 1987;94:238–241.
94. Copcu E, Sivrioglu N, Koc B, Er S. Reconstruction of the lateral canthus with trilobed skin flap and temporalis fascia graft. *Plast Reconstr Surg.* 2006;117:2514–2516.
95. Klapper SR, Patrinely JR, Soparkar CNS. Eyelid reconstruction. In: Evans GRD, ed. *Operative Plastic Surgery.* New York, NY: McGraw-Hill, 2000:241–254.
96. deSousa JL, Malhotra R, Davis G. Sliding tarsal flap for reconstruction of large, shallow lower eyelid tarsal defects. *Ophthal Plast Reconstr Surg.* 2007;23:46–48.
97. Köllner H. Verfahren für den plastischen Ersatz des Unterlides. *Munch Med Wochenschr.* 1911;41:2166–2168.
98. Hughes WL. A new method for rebuilding a lower lid: report of a case. *Arch Ophthalmol.* 1937;17:1008–1017.
99. Hughes WL. Reconstruction of the lids. *Am J Ophthalmol.* 1945;28:1203–1211.
100. Hughes WL. Total lower lid reconstruction: technical details. *Trans Am Ophthalmol Soc.* 1976;74:321–329.
101. Glatt HJ. Tarsoconjunctival flap supplementation: an approach to reconstruction of large lower eyelid defects. *Ophthalmic Plast Reconstr Surg.* 1997;13:90–97.
102. Leibsohn JM, Hahn F. Medial canthal tendon reconstruction with nasal periosteum. *Ophthalmic Plast Reconstr Surg.* 1992;8:35–40.
103. McNab AA, Martin P, Benger R, et al. A prospective randomized study comparing division of the pedicle of modified Hughes flaps at two or four weeks. *Ophthalmic Plast Reconstr Surg.* 2001;17:317–319.
104. Bartley GB, Messenger MM. The dehiscent Hughes flap: outcomes and implications. *Trans Am Ophthalmol Soc.* 2002;100:61–66.
105. Bartley GB, Putterman AM. A minor modification of the Hughes' operation for lower eyelid reconstruction. *Am J Ophthalmol.* 1995;119:96–110.
106. Zinkernagel MS, Catalano E, Ammann-Rauch D. Free tarsal graft combined with skin transposition flap for full-thickness lower eyelid reconstruction. *Ophthal Plast Reconstr Surg.* 2007;23:228–231.
107. Garces JR, Guedes A, Alegre M, Alomar A. Double mucosal and myocutaneous island flap: a one-stage reconstruction for full-thickness lower eyelid defect. *Dermatol Surg.* 2009;35:779–785.
108. Cutler NL, Beard C. A method for partial and total upper lid reconstruction. *Am J Ophthalmol.* 1955;39:1–7.
109. Mustardé JC. Major reconstruction of the eyelids: functional and aesthetic considerations. *Clin Plast Surg.* 1981;8:227–231.
110. Mauriello Jr JA, Antonacci R. Single tarsoconjunctival flap (lower eyelid) for upper eyelid reconstruction ("reverse" modified Hughes procedure). *Ophthalmic Surg.* 1994;25:374–378.
111. Jordan DR, Anderson RL, Nowinski TS. Tarsoconjunctival flap for upper eyelid reconstruction. *Arch Ophthalmol.* 1989;107:599–603.
112. Scuderi N, Ribuffo D, Chiummariello S. Total and subtotal upper eyelid reconstruction with the nasal chondromucosal flap: a 10-year experience. *Plast Reconstr Surg.* 2005;115:1259–1265.
113. Pushpoth S, Tambe K, Sandramouli S. The use of AlloDerm in the reconstruction of full-thickness eyelid defects. *Orbit.* 2008;27:337–340.
114. Hayek B, Hatef E, Nguyen M, et al. Acellular dermal graft (Alloderm) for upper eyelid reconstruction after cancer removal. *Ophthal Plast Reconstr Surg.* 2009;25: 426–429.
115. Moschella F, Cordova A. Upper eyelid reconstruction with mucosa-lined bipedicled myocutaneous flaps. *Br J Plast Surg.* 1995;48:294–299.
116. Barbera C, Manzoni R, Dodaro L, et al. Reconstruction of the tarsus-conjunctival layer using a venous wall graft. *Ophthal Plast Reconstr Surg.* 2008;24:352–356.
117. Bartley GB, Kay PP. Posterior lamellar eyelid reconstruction with hard palate mucosa grafting. *Am J Ophthalmol.* 1989;107:609–612.
118. Kim JW, Kikkawa DO, Lemke BN. Donor site complications of hard palate mucosal grafting. *Ophthal Plast Reconstr Surg.* 1997;13:36–39.
119. Fujiwara M. Upper eyelid reconstruction with a hard palate mucosa-lined bipedicled myocutaneous flap. *J Craniofac Surg.* 2006;17:1011–1015.
120. Leibovitch I, Malhotra R, Selva D. Hard palate and free tarsal grafts as posterior lamella substitutes in upper lid surgery. *Ophthalmology.* 2006;113:489–496.
121. Weinberg DA, Tham V, Hardin N, et al. Eyelid mucous membrane grafts: a histologic study of hard palate, nasal turbinate, and buccal mucosal grafts. *Ophthal Plast Reconstr Surg.* 2007;23:211–216.
122. Patrinely JR, O'Neal KD, Kersten RC, Soparkar CNS. Total upper eyelid reconstruction with mucosalized tarsal graft and overlying bipedicle flap. *Arch Ophthalmol.* 1999;117:1655–1661.
123. Leone Jr CR, Van Gemert JV. Lower lid reconstruction using tarsoconjunctival grafts and bipedicle skin-muscle flap. *Arch Ophthalmol.* 1989;107:758–760.

124. Stephenson CM, Brown BZ. The use of tarsus as a free autogenous graft in eyelid surgery. *Ophthalmic Plast Reconstr Surg*. 1985;1:43–50.
125. Motomura H, Taniguchi T, Harada T, Muraoka M. A combined flap reconstruction for full-thickness defects of the medial canthal region. *J Plast Reconstr Aesthet Surg*. 2006;59:747–751.
126. Howard GR, Nerad JA, Kersten RC. Medial canthoplasty with microplate fixation. *Arch Ophthalmol*. 1992; 110:1793–1797.
127. Sharma V, Nemet A, Ghabrial R, et al. A technique for medial canthal fixation using resorbable poly-L-lactic acid-polyglycolic acid fixation kit. *Arch Ophthalmol*. 2006;124:1171–1174.
128. Hawes MJ, Segrest DR. Effectiveness of bicanalicular silicone intubation in the repair of canalicular lacerations. *Ophthalmic Plast Reconstr Surg*. 1985;1:185–190.
129. Jordan DR, Nerad JA, Tse DT. The pigtail probe, revisited. *Ophthalmology*. 1990;97:512–519.
130. Reifler DM. Management of canalicular laceration. *Surv Ophthalmol*. 1991;36:113–132.
131. Baylis HI, Axelrod R. Repair of the lacerated canaliculus. *Ophthalmology*. 1978;85:1271–1276.
132. Saunders DH, Shannon GM, Flanagan JC. The effectiveness of the pigtail probe method of repairing canalicular lacerations. *Ophthalmic Surg*. 1978;9:33–40.
133. Kennedy RH, May J, Dailey J, Flanagan JC. Canalicular laceration. An 11-year epidemiologic and clinical study. *Ophthalmic Plast Reconstr Surg*. 1990;6:46–53.
134. Worst JG. Method for reconstructing torn lacrimal canaliculus. *Am J Ophthalmol*. 1962;53:520–522.
135. Walter WL. The use of the pigtail probe for silicone intubation of the injured canaliculus. *Ophthalmic Surg*. 1982;13:488–492.
136. Jordan DR, Gilberg S, Mawn LA. The round-tipped, eyed pigtail probe for canalicular intubation: a review of 228 patients. *Ophthal Plast Reconstr Surg*. 2008;24:176–180.
137. Kersten RC, Kulwin DR. "One-stitch" canalicular repair. A simplified approach for repair of canalicular laceration. *Ophthalmology*. 1996;103:785–789.
138. Dibble RF, Friedel SD. A simplified method of monocanalicular silicone intubation. *Ophthalmic Surg*. 1990; 21:134–135.
139. Jordan DR, Anderson RL, Patrinely JR. Unicanalicular stent for nasolacrimal duct obstruction. *Can J Ophthalmol*. 1989;24:251–253.

36

AURICULAR RECONSTRUCTION

LOK HUEI YAP
SEAN G. BOUTROS
CHARLES E. BUTLER

The Part always has a tendency to reunite with its Whole in order to escape from Imperfection.

—Leonardo da Vinci[1]

History

According to Converse's[2] detailed description of the history and evolution of ear reconstruction, the Indian surgeon Sushruta was recorded as having reconstructed ear lobules using local cheek flaps in approximately 600 BC.[3] In 1597, Tagliacozzi[4] described using a pedicled flap from the arm to reconstruct the ear. The use of a buried rib cartilage graft in ear reconstruction was described by Gillies[5] in the 1920s; in the 1930s Pierce[6] modified Gillies' approach by using a skin graft to recreate the postauricular sulcus and augmenting the helix with tubed skin. In the 1950s, Tanzer[7] ushered in the modern era of ear reconstruction through his use of a fabricated cartilage frame. These techniques were further refined by Converse[8] and by contemporary surgeons such as Brent[9] and Nagata.[10]

Anatomy

The external ear, or pinna, is a complex, trilaminar structure consisting of anterior skin, auricular cartilage, and posterior skin.

Proportions and Orientation of the Ear

As shown in Figure 36–1, the ear's outer segment, the helix, is supported by a girderlike, curved cartilaginous strut known as the antihelix. The antihelix

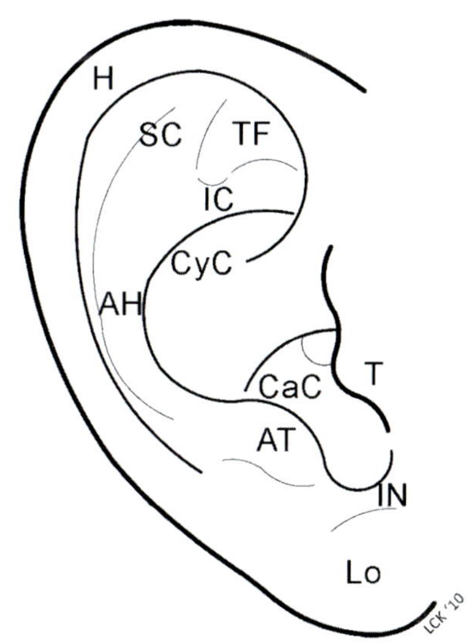

Figure 36–1. Standard nomenclature for components of the pinna. The components of the pinna are as follows: helix (*H*), antihelix (*AH*), superior crus (*SC*), inferior crus (*IF*), triangular fossa or scaphoid fossa (*TF*), cymba concha (*CyC*), cavitas concha (*CaC*), tragus (*T*), antitragus (*AT*), intertragic notch (*IN*), and lobule (*Lo*).

divides into the superior and inferior crura, which between them subtend a concave space known as the scaphoid fossa, or triangular fossa. Below the inferior crus is the cymba concha, which rests just superior to the root of the helix. Farther below, posterior to the external auditory meatus, is the concavity of the cavitas concha. The tragus is a quadrangular elevation of cartilage that shields the acoustic meatus anteriorly, and diagonally opposite the tragus is the antitragus, which is connected to the lower crescent of the antihelix. Between the tragus and antitragus lies the intertragic notch, or the incisura intertragica.

It is essential for the reconstructive surgeon to have a precise and intimate understanding of the normal aspects of the ear. Anatomical canons have been in use for centuries[11] and were highlighted during the Renaissance through the work of artists such as Leonardo da Vinci.[12] Just as the face is easily divided by the planes of the anterior hair line, glabella, alar base, and mentum, so the pinna is divided into equal halves by the Frankfort horizontal plane (a horizontal plane connecting the inferior orbital foramen and the upper edge of the external auditory meatus). The line of the inferior crus is located about one-third of the way down from the top of the pinna (as measured from the superior helical margin).

Tolleth[13] described the ideal orientation of the ear and its components (Fig 36–2). The longitudinal

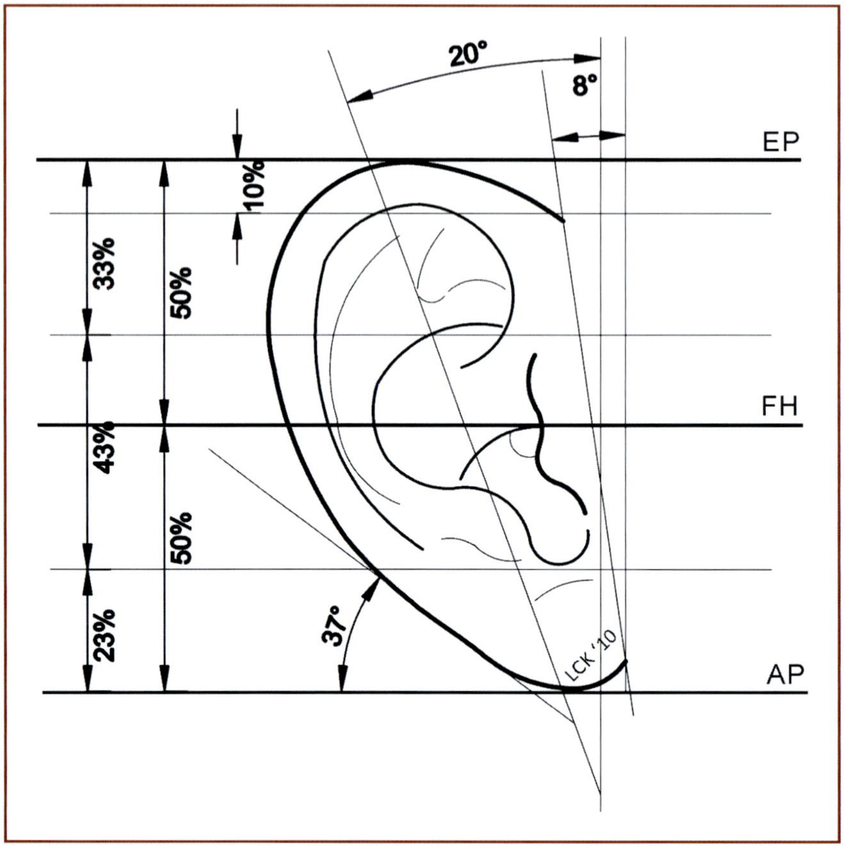

Figure 36–2. Anatomic location and ratios of the pinna. The pinna is located anatomically between the planes of the lateral edge of the eyebrow (*EP*) and the alar base (*AP*). The pinna is centered on the Frankfort horizontal plane (*FH*), which passes just above the auditory canal. The longitudinal axis of the ear is offset from the vertical plane by approximately 20°.

axis of the pinna is offset 20° from vertical, whereas the root of the helix is located at a point that is offset 8° from vertical. Vertically, the pinna extends from the horizontal plane of the lateral edge of the eyebrow to the horizontal plane of the alar base; horizontally, the pinna begins one ear length posterior to the vertical plane of the lateral edge of the eyebrow.

Despite variations among patients, these anatomical locators help the surgeon in correctly sizing and placing the reconstructed pinna. These locators play an especially important role when bilateral deformities are present. Congenital deformities, such as craniofacial microsomia, may involve translocation of the auditory meatus, and their impact on facial skeletal growth may distort normal anatomical markers. Nevertheless, the opposite ear (if present) should be the primary reference for planning the reconstructed pinna. The final position and size of the ear should represent a synthesis of ideal anatomical position, measured against the patient's own ears, with consideration of the availability of both soft and cartilaginous tissues for reconstruction, as described below.

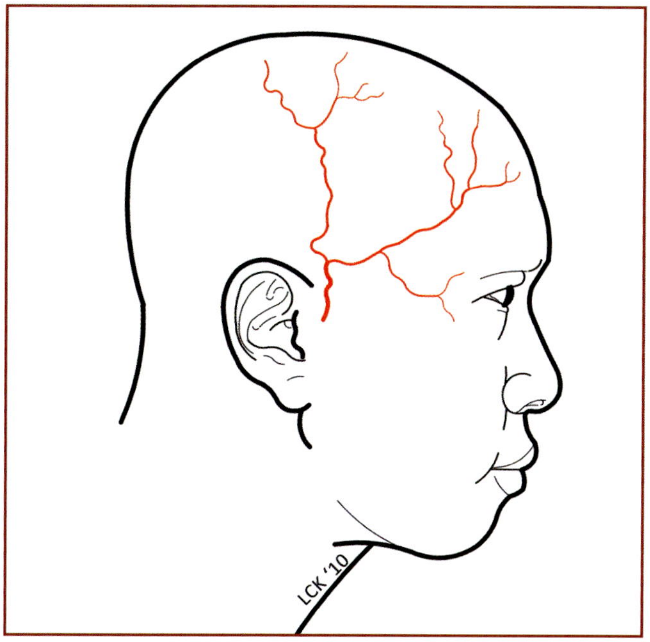

Figure 36–3. Superficial temporal artery and branches.

Blood Supply

The superficial temporal and posterior auricular arteries supply blood to the ear.[14] The venous system of the ear drains to the superficial temporal, retromandibular, and external jugular veins. The lymphatic drainage goes to the parotid, superior cervical, mastoid, and infraclavicular nodes.

The superficial temporal artery,[15] one of the terminal divisions of the external carotid artery (Fig 36–3), measures approximately 2 mm in diameter at its origin within the parotid gland. From this position behind the condylar neck of the mandible, the superficial temporal artery passes through the deep fascia of the face 5 mm anterior to the tragus. As the superficial temporal artery crosses the zygomatic process of the temporal bone, it lies anterior to the auriculotemporal nerve and the superficial temporal vein. Approximately 3 cm above the zygomatic arch, the superficial temporal artery divides into two terminal branches. The anterior, or frontal, branch supplies all layers of the scalp, running anteriorly and superiorly to anastomose with its opposite number as well as with the supratrochlear and supraorbital arteries on the same side. The posterior, or parietal, branch passes almost vertically upward and backward, accompanying the main branch of the superficial temporal vein.

The posterior auricular artery comes off the posterior border of the external carotid artery above the posterior belly of the digastric muscle, adjacent to the stylohyoid muscle, and runs in the sulcus between the cartilaginous pinna and the mastoid process (Fig 36–4). The posterior auricular artery divides into the auricular branch and the occipital branch. The auricular branch ascends vertically, deep to the auricularis posterior muscle, to supply the skin and posterior aspect of the pinna. Two fairly constant perforating branches from this vessel penetrate the cartilage of the pinna to reach the anterior auricular surface; one is near the inferior crus, and the other is just above the intertragic notch. The auricular branch also branches to supply the upper pole of the pinna, and these branches anastomose with branches from the posterior branch of the superficial temporal artery. The occipital branch of the posterior auricular artery runs horizontally backward from the sternomastoid to supply the

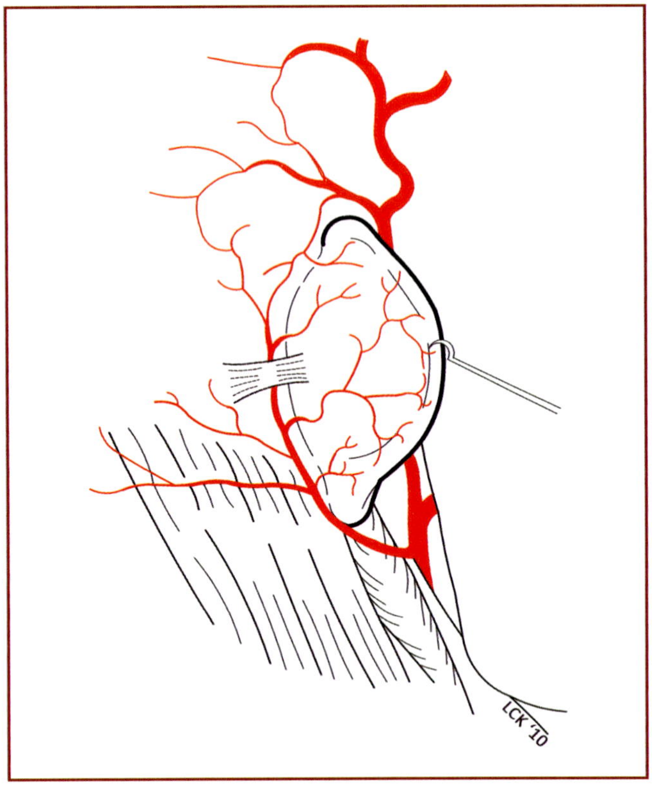

Figure 36–4. Posterior auricular artery and branches.

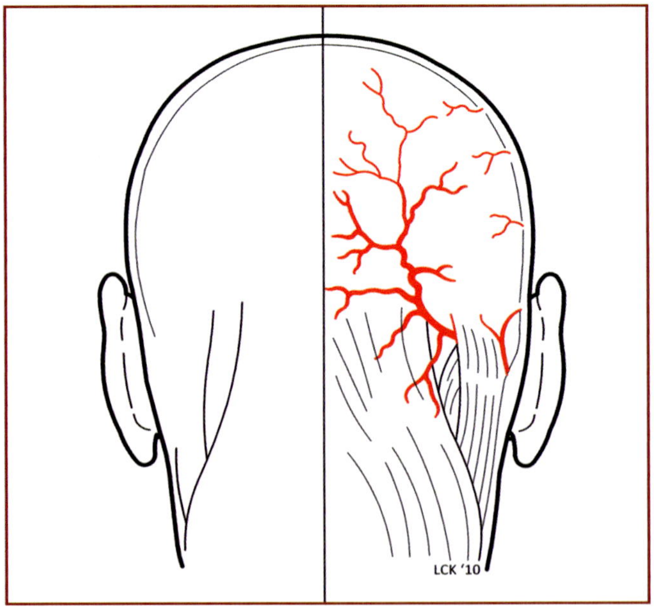

Figure 36–5. Occipital artery and branches.

posterior scalp and to anastomose with branches from the occipital artery.

Another important regional artery is the occipital artery, which arises from the posterior border of the external carotid artery opposite the origin of the facial artery (Fig 36–5). The occipital artery runs backward below the posterior belly of the digastric muscle, crosses the internal jugular vein, and lies medial to the mastoid process underneath the splenius capitis and sternomastoid muscles. The occipital artery gives off the following branches: sternomastoid branches, which supply the upper end of the sternomastoid muscle and its overlying skin; an auricular branch, which continues up to meet the posterior branches of the posterior auricular artery; a trapezius branch; occipital branches, which run up to the apex of the cranium and anastomose with the posterior auricular and superficial temporal artery branches of the same side; and descending branches, which supply the skin and muscle over the posterior cervical region.

The vessels listed above are critical in providing vascularized regional tissue for ear reconstruction. In patients with large ear defects, the available blood vessels are the basis for choosing the type of reconstruction to be performed.

Sensory Nerve Supply

Sensation to the ear is derived from the following nerves: the auriculotemporal nerve (from cranial nerve V), which innervates the anterior surface of the ear, the tragus, and the anterior half of the exterior auditory canal; the lesser occipital nerve (from cranial nerve IX), which innervates the superior and mastoid regions; the great auricular nerve (from the second and third cervical nerves), which innervates the ear lobe and posterior auricular region; and the facial nerve (cranial nerve VII), which innervates the conchal skin at the external meatus; Arnold's nerve, the auditory branch of the vagus nerve (cranial nerve X), which innervates the posterior half of the external auditory canal and Jacobson's nerve, the auricular branch of the glossopharyngeal nerve (cranial nerve IX), which innervates the medial aspect of the tympanic membrane (the lateral surface of the tympanic membrane is innervated by the auriculotemporal nerve and Jacobson's nerve). Thus, the ear receives sensory innervation from four cranial nerves as well as from branches of the cervical plexus, a fact to bear in mind when considering local anesthetic blocks to the pinna and skin of the external meatus.

Types of Defects

Its anatomic location on the side of the head leaves the ear exposed to solar radiation and vulnerable to various types of trauma.

Oncologic Resection

Skin cancers caused by actinic exposure are common in the head and neck region. A recent review reported that 57% of basal cell carcinomas occurred on the head or neck, with 10% of these situated on the ear.[16] Malignancies of the ear are frequently treated by Mohs micrographic surgery to minimize the sacrifice of uninvolved tissues. The recurrence rate for squamous cell carcinomas of the ear treated with Mohs surgery has been reported to be 5.3%, compared to 18.7% for those treated with conventional surgical techniques,[17] and patients in the latter group are more likely to require ear reconstructions.

Principles of Reconstruction

Multidisciplinary Management

Ideally, all ear reconstruction patients should be managed in a multidisciplinary team environment comprising specialties such as otolaryngology, plastic surgery, prosthodontics, radiation oncology, medical oncology, audiology, speech and language therapy, and clinical psychology. In such an environment, patients would receive a comprehensive treatment plan, designed by the best available experts in each field, including adjuvant therapy for cancer and treatment of concurrent conditions, such as clinical hearing loss.

Defining the Goals of Reconstruction

In planning ear reconstruction, the multidisciplinary team should first define the goals of the procedure and assess the expectations of the patient. As in other areas of reconstructive plastic surgery, patients' expectations of the surgical outcome may differ widely according to their sex, age, level of education, understanding of the procedure, disease process, and social background.

Patients with skin cancer may focus primarily on their oncologic treatment and be less concerned about reconstruction of the ear. Even in contemporary practice, many patients remain satisfied with unrepaired postresection defects of the pinna, such as straight-line scars. When they do choose reconstruction, some such patients may be prepared to accept a surgical technique that is simple but offers less anatomical accuracy, such as a wedge excision and closure; however, some patients in this situation may have higher aesthetic requirements and request a more complex, anatomically accurate reconstruction.

The primary goal of reconstruction is usually to create as normal and natural a replacement as possible for the entire ear or for those parts of the ear that have been damaged or removed. This aim is moderated, however, by a measured consideration of whether complete accuracy in reconstruction is achievable, which is determined through an assessment of the size and nature of the defect; the local and regional tissues available for reconstruction; the patient's desires in terms of healing time, hospital stay, cost, and discomfort; requirements for wound care and dressings; and the option of using an implant-based prosthetic reconstruction.

Clinical Assessment and Preoperative Workup

Significant Medical History

The medical history should note physiologically significant cardiovascular conditions, pulmonary disease, diabetes, hypertension, and autoimmune disease. Concurrent use of medications such as anticancer agents, aspirin, steroids, and hormones should be noted, as well as the patient's use of tobacco products or recreational drugs. A full preoperative workup, including lab work and an anaesthetic risk assessment, should be undertaken.

Extent of the Auricular Defect

Scaled clinical photographs, including standard facial views and close-ups, should be taken of both ears. The defect should be measured and its location on the pinna recorded. The height of the normal ear should be recorded as a guide to the required height of the reconstructed ear.

At this point, the reconstructive surgeon should consider the defect in the context of the trilaminar structure of the pinna to determine which layer or layers, anterior skin, auricular cartilage, or posterior skin, need reconstruction. The surrounding skin of the ear in the supra-, post-, and infra-auricular regions should be inspected to assess the amount of healthy, vascularized, and relatively elastic skin available for reconstruction. Associated scarring, both new and chronic, should be noted, and the severity of local and regional scars can be used to assess the patient's potential for hypertrophic or keloid scarring.

Local and Regional Blood Supply

The local vasculature, particularly that of the superficial temporal artery, should be assessed clinically and by Doppler ultrasonography. If there has been significant regional trauma, angiography of the external carotid artery may be used to assess regional vascular flow, particularly in situations requiring subtotal or total ear reconstruction and/or a source of reliable vascularized tissue.

Source of Cartilage

The patient should be asked about previous surgery or trauma to the potential sites of cartilage harvest, the contralateral concha and the costal margin. These sites should be inspected for adequate cartilage volume and, if the patient has undergone a prior harvest, for tissue healing and scarring. A chest radiograph may be helpful if the patient has a history of chest trauma. If a decision is made to harvest costal cartilage, the surgeon and patient must discuss from which side of the chest the cartilage will be harvested. Some surgeons may prefer to take costal cartilage from the side whose convex curvature is closer to the shape of the frame to be constructed.

Assessment by Prosthetics Team

It is helpful, in the multidisciplinary assessment process, for the prosthetics team to determine the patient's suitability for prosthetic rehabilitation, including adhesive-based prostheses and clinical camouflage. As part of the process of choosing the type of reconstruction to be done, the patient ideally will have the opportunity to examine prepared prostheses, discuss the maintenance protocol for osseointegrated prosthetic devices, and consider the full range of prosthetic options. For delayed reconstructions, molds can be taken of both the defect and the normal ear for planning purposes, and three-dimensional models can be produced to guide surgical reconstruction.

Fabrication of Templates

Surgeons vary in the type of template they use to size the reconstruction. Many surgeons use radiographic film to trace an outline of the opposite, normal ear to obtain normative data for the patient. If both ears are absent, some surgeons will obtain a tracing from an age-matched control as a reference. This tracing, which carries information about ear height and width, can be superimposed over the auricular defect. The defect then can be traced onto the template, giving the surgeon an outline of the amount of tissue required to reconstruct the ear.

Nagata published details of an anthropometric, idealized framework for ear reconstruction based on anatomical landmarks and an analysis of the height-width ratios of each pinna.[10] This is analogous to constructs and considerations for nasal framework reconstruction. Idealized templates can be created and printed for ears of different sizes. If a patient has a unilateral defect, the template is matched to the measured height of the contralateral ear; if the patient has bilateral defects, the template is matched to the anatomic landmarks of the lateral eyebrow margin, the Frankfort horizontal plane, and the alar base plane, obviating the use of age-matched controls. The template can be sterilized and used intraoperatively as a guide for framework and soft tissue fabrication.

It is possible to generate a three-dimensional, silicone template based on an impression taken from the normal ear, which is mirrored to produce a life-size sculpture. A model created in this way can be sterilized for intraoperative use, providing the surgeon with an instant three-dimensional reference against which the reconstructed ear can be compared. The projection and angulation of the pinna can also be preserved in the model by extending the impression to include the mastoid region. This is helpful to assess the "set" of the reconstructed ear and saves the surgeon having to turn the patient's head frequently during the operation to compare the ears. Figure 36–6 shows idealized and three-dimensional templates being used together.

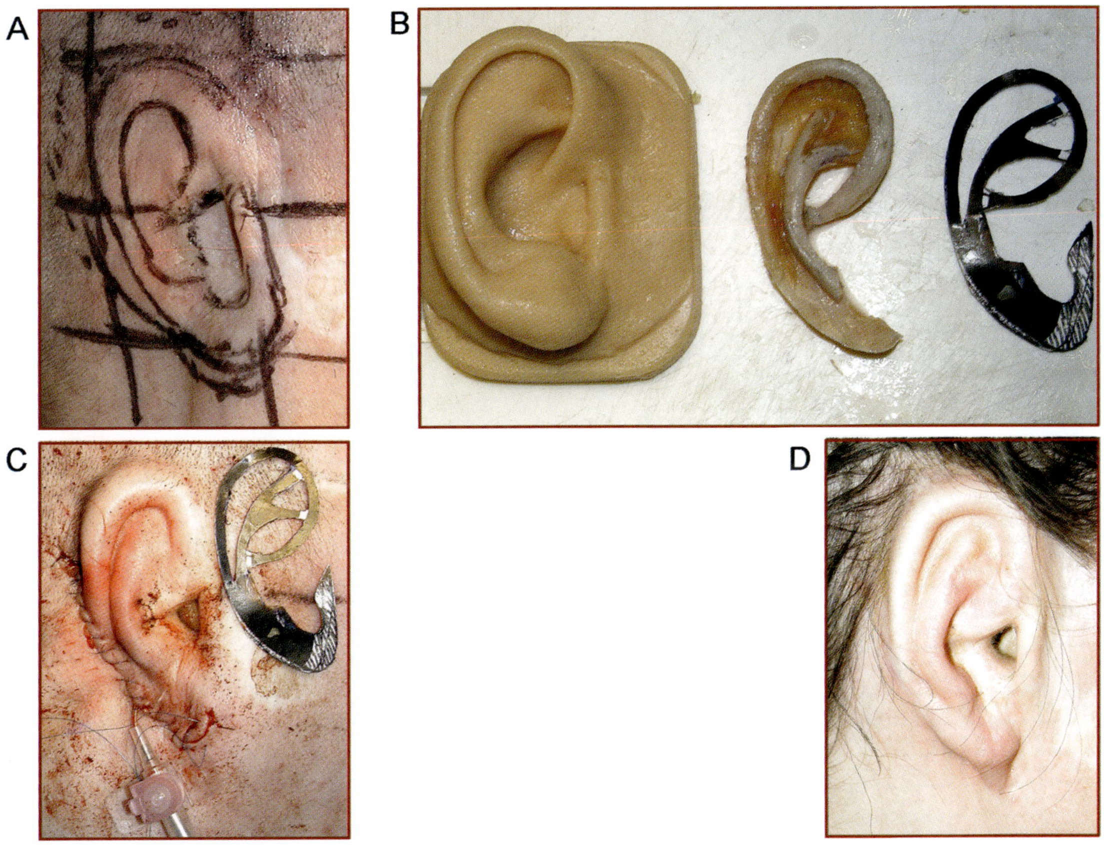

Figure 36–6. Full auricular frame reconstruction. A 28-year-old patient was ejected from a moving car and sustained a severe shearing injury to the side of the head, which resulted in complete traumatic amputation of the ear. **A.** Preoperative markings helped the surgeon position the proposed ear construct. The reconstruction was planned for two stages. **B.** An idealized template based on measurements suggested by Nagata and Tolleth was digitized and printed on acetate film (*right*), and a three-dimensional, silicone template (*left*) of the proposed ear was based on the normal contralateral ear. The actual cartilage frame (*middle*) was fabricated using the method of Nagata, with dimensions that incorporated details from both templates. **C.** The patient is shown immediately after the first stage of reconstruction. **D.** The patient is shown 6 months after the first stage of reconstruction.

Choice of Reconstruction Technique

The primary considerations for choosing an ear reconstruction technique are the degree of complexity of the reconstructive surgery and the patient's desired level of anatomical accuracy in reconstruction. Generally, the more accurate the reconstruction, the more surgical effort is required. In reconstructions following cancer resection, oncological clearance and the possibility of recurrence are additional factors to be weighed. Therefore, a detailed preoperative cost-benefit analysis should be carried out for each patient.

The source material on which the surgeon is basing the reconstruction also should be assessed. The first decision should be whether the reconstruction will comprise autologous or alloplastic tissue. As discussed above, this is based on the patient's fitness for surgery, the patient's preference, the availability of source materials, and the likelihood of success. Where possible, native ear tissue should be preserved and utilized, unless the tissue has been devitalized or comprises areas of scarring, which may interfere with vascular supply to the reconstruction.

Cartilage

Defects of up to 15% of the total ear may be reconstructed using local tissues only, as discussed below, provided there is adequate support remaining. Defects of the concha are less likely to require complex reconstructions than are defects involving the antihelix because the cartilage of the antihelix provides vertical and anterior-posterior strut support to maintain the height and shape of the pinna.

The soft tissues of the ear have a tendency to fibrose and tighten after reconstruction; therefore, the framework used in reconstruction must be strong enough to resist the deformational constrictive forces of secondary scarring. Costal cartilage is uniquely suited for this purpose because it is stronger than auricular cartilage, integrates well with local tissues, and has a low risk of infection when integrated. Because of the thickness and height of the costal cartilages, as well as the dimensional requirements of the frame, several cartilage segments may have to be assembled together to create an adequate frame.

Cartilage frames are also required to repair larger defects. In general, a cartilage frame will be essential if a defect includes more than 20% of the original area of the ear. However, smaller defects also can benefit from the insertion of a small, custom-designed piece of carved cartilage, as the definition achieved with a correctly carved cartilage segment is superior to that achieved using soft tissue alone. If a cartilage frame is used, it can be created slightly larger than the defect for which it is intended and then be trimmed to fit, with a small overlap to allow accurate dovetailing into the remaining ear frame.

Skin

The skin required to repair a segmental defect is more than double the area of the defect visible on a lateral view of the ear; the additional skin is required to provide anterior and posterior skin and also to replicate the convex and concave undulations of the pinna. Thus, there may not be sufficient local tissue to complete the "wrap-around" in a single setting, and the reconstruction may have to be staged, with the replacement of the frame and anterior skin in the first stage, followed by the elevation of the frame and the re-creation of the posterior skin in the second stage.

For example, if a frame is constructed with a single base-plate piece with a rudimentary helical rim, the surface area of skin required to cover the frame will be less than that required to cover a fully detailed frame of the correct projection and contours, which may involve full reconstruction of the crura and antihelix. Staging the procedure and delaying the posterior surface reconstruction allows the surgeon to utilize more skin and create a more lifelike frame, but this is done at the cost of an additional procedure.

A good vascular supply to the soft tissues is a prerequisite for safe reconstruction of the ear. If significant scarring has occurred around the ear, the use of regional tissues supplied by the superficial temporal artery and/or the occipital artery branches should be considered instead rather than tissue with a random blood supply.

Timing of Reconstruction

Ideally, reconstructive surgery should be carried out immediately after the resection of a lesion. Whether or not immediate reconstruction can be carried out depends on the multidisciplinary team's confidence that oncologically clear surgical margins were achieved and on the availability of suitable soft tissue and tissue beds for reconstructive surgery.

For larger, more complex defects, reconstructive surgery may be too complex to be carried out along with the initial resection. For some patients, the best course of action is a staged, delayed reconstruction using an initial simple closure. A delay of 3 to 4 months will aid reconstruction by allowing some softening of induration and scarring. An extended period of 12 to 24 months before proceeding to the second stage of a complex reconstruction may clarify the risk of local or regional cancer recurrence. On the other hand, early prosthetic reconstruction can be used for larger defects to provide a reasonable quality of life in patients with advanced tumors.

One further consideration is the timing of reconstruction in relation to postoperative irradiation, if such treatment is required. If possible, radiotherapy should be deferred for 4 weeks after complex autologous reconstructive procedures to allow for complete healing and secondary vascularization of the tissues and to avoid wound breakdown and loss of skin.

Reconstructive Techniques

Reconstruction for Small Defects

According to the basic principles of reconstructive surgery, if possible, small defects should be closed primarily. The possibility of primary closure depends not only on the size of the defect but also on the location (upper pole, lower pole) and on the involved structures (skin only, skin and cartilage, or lobe only).

Skin-Only Defects

Skin overlying the cartilage of the anterior pinna is held down relatively firmly to the underlying perichondrium by fibrous extensions. The skin here has relatively little subcutaneous fat and is well supplied by perforating branches of the posterior auricular artery as well as branches of the superficial temporal artery. The skin of the posterior pinna is slightly less well tethered than that of the anterior pinna and consequently has slightly more mobility. The posterior pinna skin has a marginally thicker subcutaneous fat layer.

The underlying cartilage of the auricular frame can be a help but also a hindrance to primary closure. In skin-only defects over the anterior auricular frame, the adherence of skin to the surrounding cartilage limits mobility and therefore limits the maximum size of defects that can potentially be closed by direct apposition. Thus, defects with widths as small as 3 mm to 4 mm may not be closeable primarily. In such cases, a skin graft may be the surgical technique of choice, provided there is a sufficiently vascular underlying tissue bed, such as a vascularized perichondrial layer, available to graft onto. Skin grafts are discussed in more detail below.

If the defect includes the anterior perichondrial layer, then use of a skin graft becomes difficult. In this situation, it may be necessary to convert the defect into a skin and cartilage defect by removing the cartilage layer while retaining the opposing layer of skin on the anterior or posterior surface. This procedure provides an additional anatomical layer of excision in cases of skin cancer resection and also presents a new vascular surface for the application of a graft. This technique is useful when excision of the cartilage will not compromise the integrity or shape of the cartilage frame. Cartilage sections up to 1-cm wide can be removed in the conchal bowl. However, additional care must be taken in the upper pole or helical rim area to avoid creating a secondary flop-down deformity as a result of the cartilage excision.

The perichondrium is important in reconstruction because its fibrous outer layer provides support for the auricular framework's vascular network while its cellular inner layer comprises chondrocytes and chondroblasts that merge with the underlying cartilage matrix.

Skin and Cartilage Defects

For small skin and cartilage defects close to the helical rim, primary closure is usually possible. In potentially infected cases, it may be necessary to debride the wound and loosely suture the wound edges to allow primary healing before considering a secondary, formal reconstruction or revision.

For small defects of the helical rim, the standard reconstructive technique would be direct closure in the form of a wedge excision with the closing angle of the wedge toward the central area of the pinna.

A wedge-type excision and closure will typically result in a small redundancy of cartilage near the apex of the angle, and this can be managed by a keyhole-type, or "bilateral-closing-triangles-type," subcutaneous excision of cartilage (Figs 36–7 and 36–8).[18] Figure 36–9 shows other wedge-type excisions.

The cartilage edges should be approximated as accurately as possible by using atraumatic needles to avoid fracturing the cartilage at the suture points and by using monofilament sutures to reduce the risk of secondary infection.

Central skin and cartilage defects can be closed by direct grafting to the remaining skin surface as described above.

Lobule-Only Defects

Defects of the lobule are closed more easily than are defects on the upper two-thirds of the pinna because of the lobule's relative lack of cartilage and the abundance and elasticity of the lobule's skin (Fig 36–10).

The simplest types of resection/reconstruction for skin cancers on the lobule are amputation-type resections. These can be carried out along a curved line to approximate the curvature of the lower border of the lobule. Most of the procedures will result in some loss of volume or height of the lobule; however, a number of local flap procedures utilizing postauricular and neck skin can restore some of the tissue in this region if desired (Fig 36–11).[19,20]

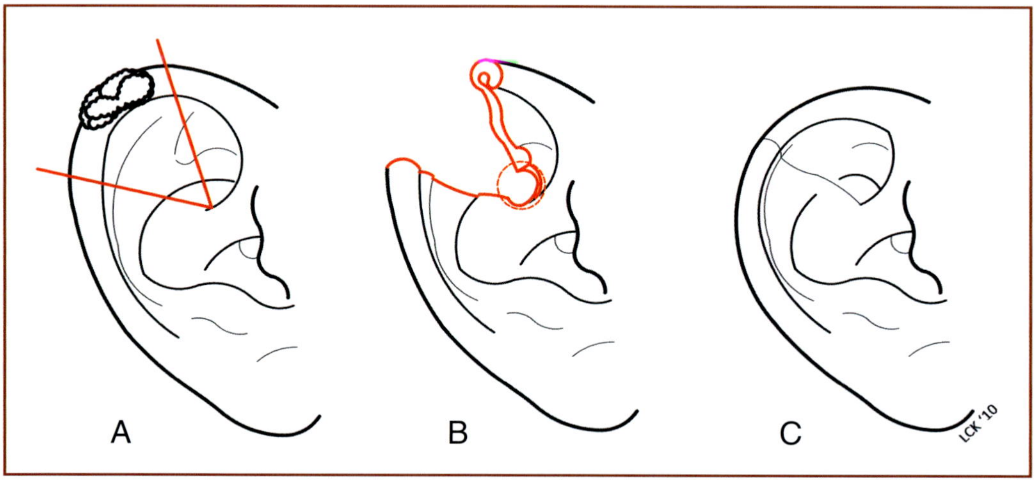

Figure 36–7. Wedge excision. **A.** The excision is marked out as a wedge, subtending the tumor to include adequate margins. **B.** Excising a larger, circular amount of cartilage subcutaneously in a keyhole-type cut can facilitate closure of the wedge without creating a central buckle of cartilage. **C.** The disadvantage of a wedge closure is that it can reduce the height or width of the normal ear; however, the technique may still allow a reasonable approximation of a normal pinna shape.

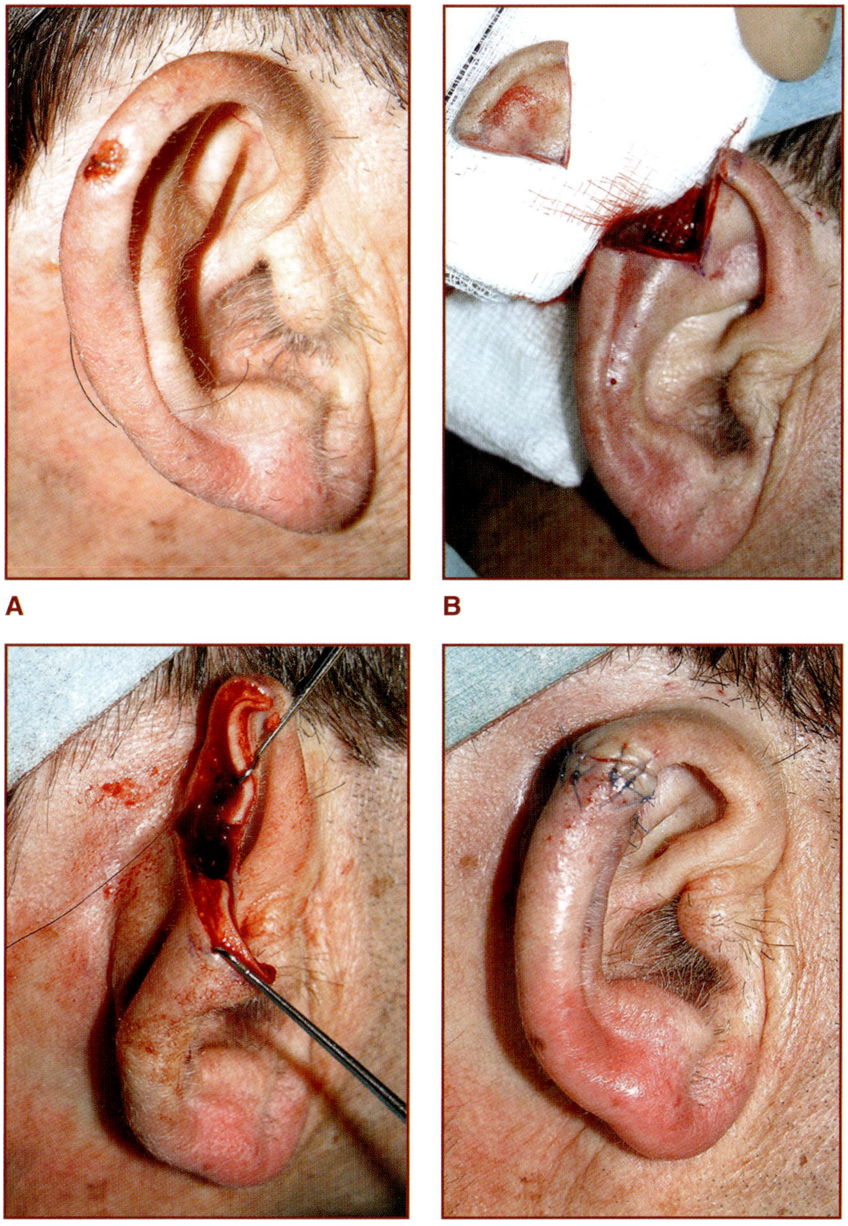

A B C D

Figure 36–8. Wedge excision. **A.** A patient with skin cancer on the helical rim. **B.** A wedge excision is planned and executed. **C.** A small keyhole cut is made in the apex of the wedge to facilitate closure. **D.** The wedge excision is closed, maintaining continuity of the rim.

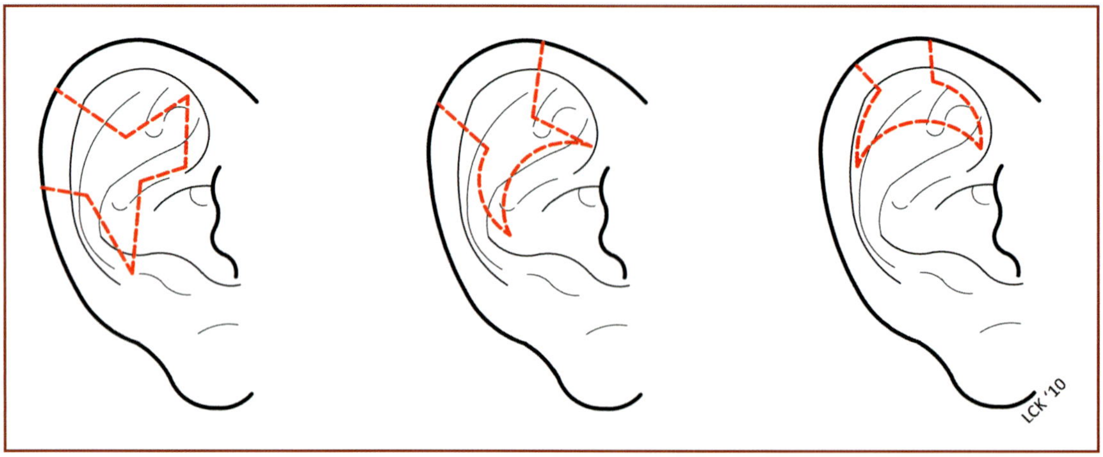

Figure 36–9. Alternative types of wedge excision. **A.** Excisions may be marked out with linear closing angles. It is possible to design variations of wedge excisions based on more than one closing angle. **B.** The central incisions can be based around a curve along the lower edge of the anti-helix. **C.** The central incision may also be based around a curve along the upper edge of the antihelix.

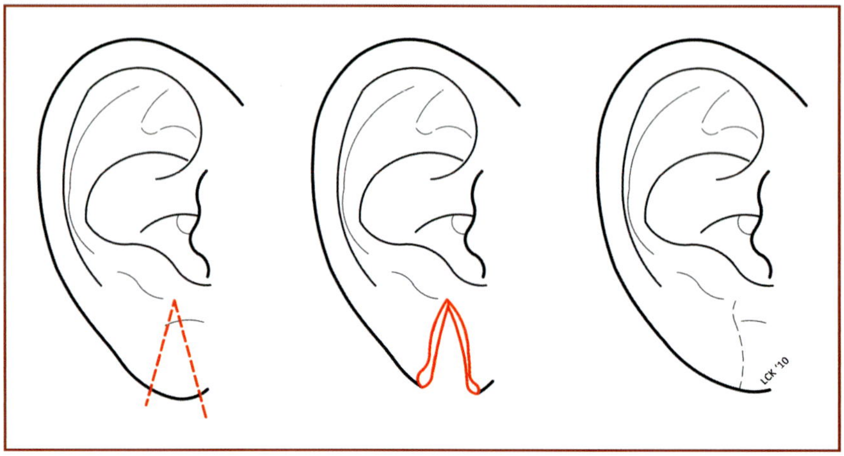

Figure 36–10. Lobule lesion excision with direct closure.

Skin Grafts

A full-thickness skin defect of the ear can often be repaired using a skin graft (Figure 36–12). The use of a graft requires that a suitable vascular bed is available. Thus, if the skin defect overlies auricular cartilage, then a graft necessitates the preservation of a vascularized layer, usually perichondrium. If this is not available, then other tissue such as local vascularized fascia should be transposed or advanced to cover the defect before a graft is applied. Alternatively, the surgeon may elect to transpose or advance skin and/or cartilage into the defect.

Skin grafts can be either split-thickness or full-thickness. Split-thickness grafts, being thinner, generally have a higher primary take rate than do full-thickness grafts, but split-thickness grafts also have a greater tendency to contract after transfer.

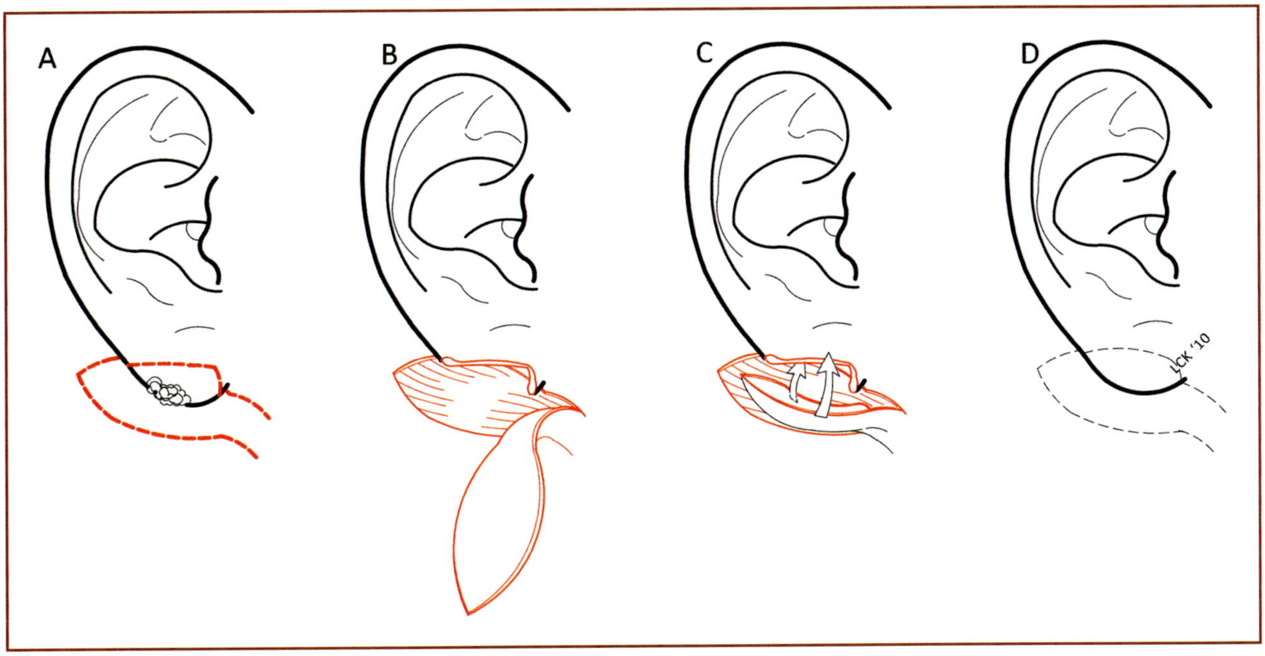

Figure 36–11. Lobule lesion excision with local flap closure. **A.** The lesion is excised. **B.** A skin flap from the region based on the posterior auricular artery is used for reconstruction. **C.** The flap is folded along its long axis to approximate the superior and inferior edges of the lobule. **D.** The flap is inset to re-create the lobule's inferior curvature.

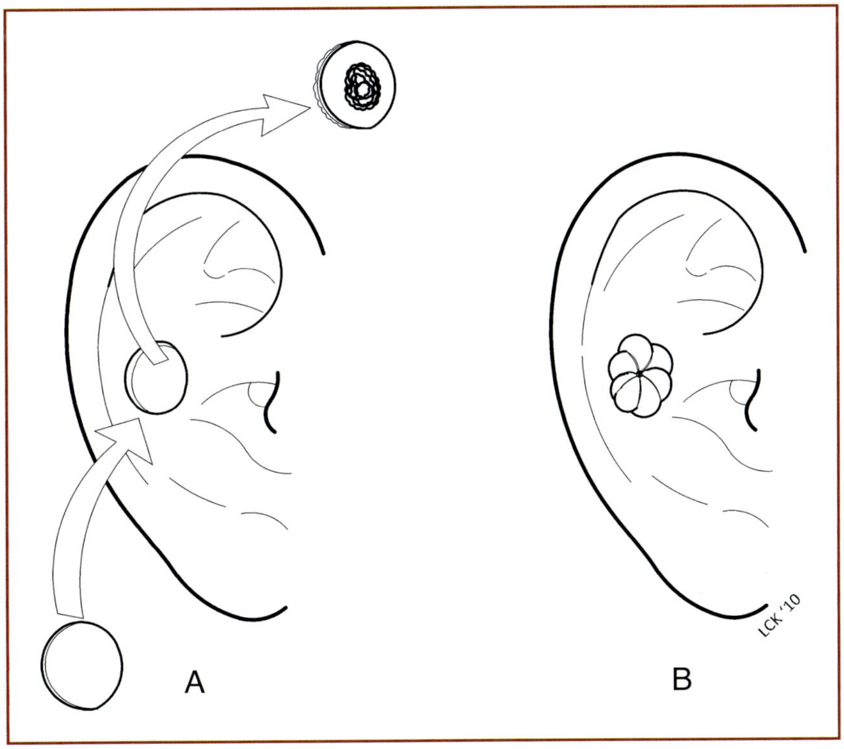

Figure 36–12. Excision of lesion and skin graft. **A.** For small skin cancers, excision as a disc or an ellipse may be an option. **B.** The defect can then be repaired with a similarly sized skin graft that is secured with a standard tie-over bolster dressing.

A split-thickness skin graft from the scalp will provide a good color match for the ear. When this donor area is not available, split-thickness skin grafts can be obtained from the thigh or other sites. Full-thickness skin grafts can be harvested from the opposite postauricular sulcus, the neck, or the lower abdomen. Care should be taken not to inadvertently transfer lower abdominal or groin hair follicles with the skin.

Local Flaps

Local flaps available in the periauricular region both random-pattern flaps and axial-pattern flaps. Most of the flaps used to repair skin-only auricular defects will have a random pattern of blood supply from branches of either the postauricular artery or the superficial temporal artery. Examples of local flaps used in auricular reconstruction are described below.

Posterior Auricular Flap

Posterior auricular flaps used in ear reconstruction can be based superiorly, inferiorly, or in the middle portion of the ear (Figs 36–13 and 36–14). A superiorly based, vertical flap can be used to re-create tissue of the upper pole or helical rim. An inferiorly based, caudally located flap can be used to refashion the lobule. Skin-only defects of the middle part of the posterior auricular surface can be resurfaced with transposition or advancement flaps based on branches of the posterior auricular artery.[21]

Antia-Buch flap

For helical rim defects, especially in the upper pole, the semicircular shape of the rim can be used to create a local rotation-advancement flap that advances into the rim defect. The Antia-Buch flap[22] is the archetypal helical rim advancement flap (Fig 36–15). This flap is useful for the repair of defects of the upper and middle third of the helix. An incision in the helical sulcus is made through the anterior skin, continuing through the auricular cartilage. With undermining of the posteromedial skin, the helix can be mobilized and advanced as a chondrocutaneous pedicled flap based on the blood supply of posterior auricular skin.

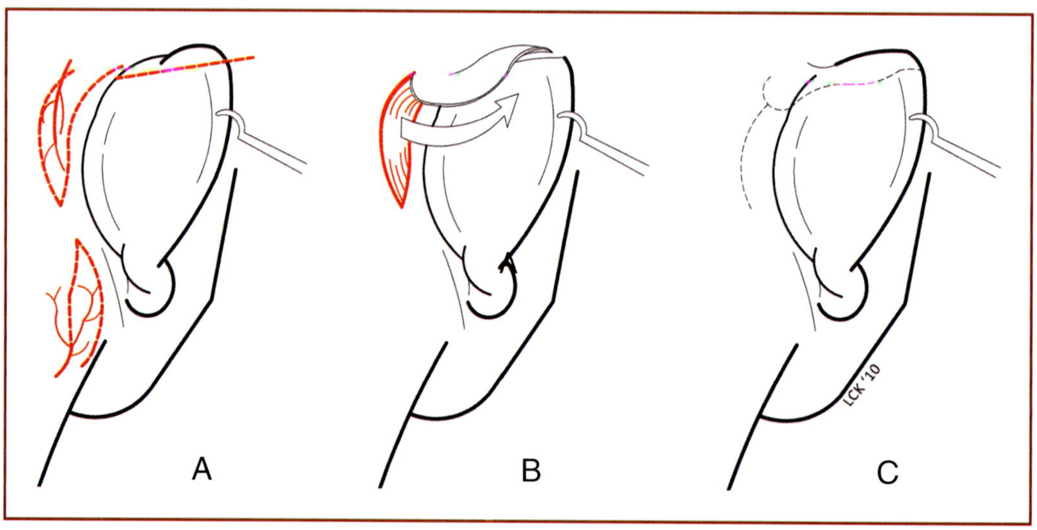

Figure 36–13. Posterior auricular flap. **A.** The posterior auricular artery can be used to vascularize superiorly based or inferiorly based flaps. **B.** This flap can be used for marginal reconstructions. **C.** Reconstruction of the upper part of the pinna is shown. After excision of the upper helical portion, a flap is designed with a superiorly based pedicle, along the line of the auricular sulcus. This is pivoted and inset into the upper part of the helix. The donor site is then closed directly.

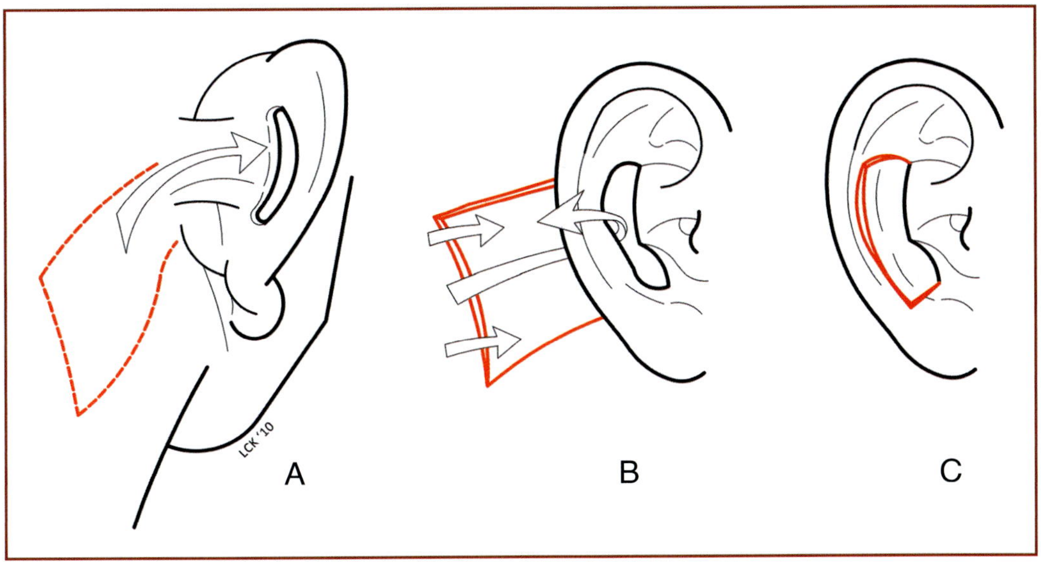

Figure 36–14. Posterior auricular trapdoor flap. **A.** The pedicle is based on ascending and descending branches of the posterior auricular artery. **B.** The flap is tunneled through the posterior aspect of a conchal defect. **C.** The flap is inset in the fashion of a trapdoor.

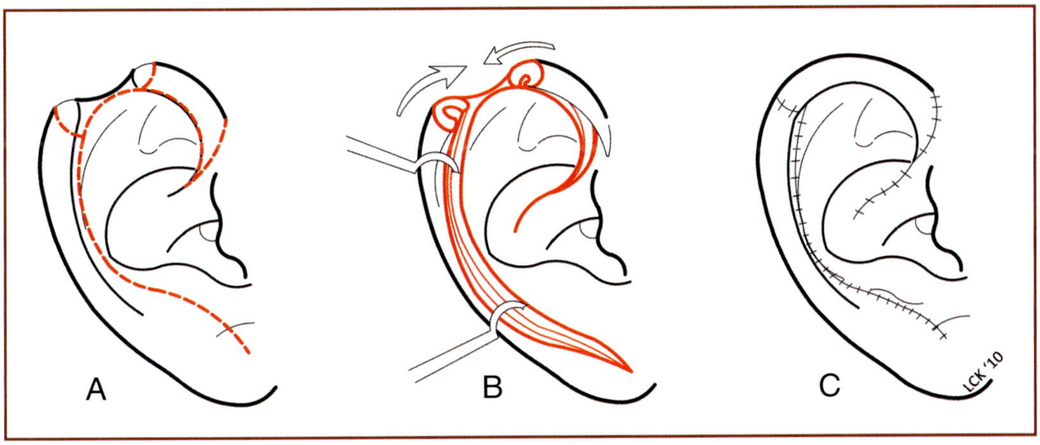

Figure 36–15. The Antia-Buch chondrocutaneous flap. **A.** The Antia-Buch flap utilizes a posteriorly based chondrocutaneous segment. **B.** This segment can be advanced around the helical rim. **C.** The procedure may reduce the pinna height, but preservation of the auricular curve may be possible.

If the defect is small, advancement of only the inferior (lateral) segment of the helix may be sufficient for closure. If the defect is larger, both the superior (medial) and inferior segments may have to be mobilized to achieve sufficient advancement for closure. The superior segment can be mobilized based on the anterior auricular skin and advanced as a V-Y flap to meet the inferior segment. Modifications of this technique have greatly expanded its application, allowing the repair of defects that extend into the scaphal hollow[23] and of those involving the middle and/or lower third of the ear.[24] If the helical rim defect is larger, the rim's height can be reduced by including crescentic chondrocutaneous excisions (as described above for wedge excisions), and closure of the rim can be effected with a modified Antia-Buch flap.

The Antia-Buch procedure has the disadvantage of slightly reducing the height of the pinna; the opposite ear can be similarly reduced to improve symmetry,[22] although this approach generally is not recommended.

Dieffenbach Flap

The Dieffenbach flap is a staged, posteriorly based flap used mainly for defects of the middle third of the pinna.[25,26] In the first stage, a posteriorly based flap is elevated and advanced anteriorly in a horizontal configuration. This is used to recreate the anterior pinna skin, as illustrated in Figure 36–16. The flap can be laid over a cartilage graft if required, although the original description specified a skin flap only. At a second stage (6 to 8 weeks later, after secondary revascularization), the posterior aspect of the flap is divided. The ear can then be elevated and the flap inset posteriorly to complete the reconstruction. Larger defects can be repaired using a novel modification involving an extended retroauricular advancement flap.[27]

Vascularized Island Flap

A random-pattern or axial-pattern flap can be created using skin from either the mastoid region or the postauricular region. The flap of skin can be elevated on a thinned vascular pedicle, or "islanded"; the flap can then be transferred from to replace anterior tissue replacement (Fig 36–17).[28,29] Care should be taken to avoid kinking of the vascular pedicle or excessive pressure on it. This flap's reach is in fact limited by the dimensions of its vascular pedicle.

Reconstruction of the Frame

Alloplastic Materials for Frame Reconstruction

In lieu of cartilage frames, prefabricated or molded frames of different materials have been used in ear reconstruction.

Silicone has been used in ear reconstructions because of its relative success as an implant elsewhere in the body.[30] However, liquid forms of silicone used as injectable implants can cause granulomas and severe tissue reactions in the ear, and formed implants made of solid silicone have been shown to have high rates of complications such as tissue reaction and framework extrusion when used in ear reconstruction.[31] Rates of framework extrusion and/

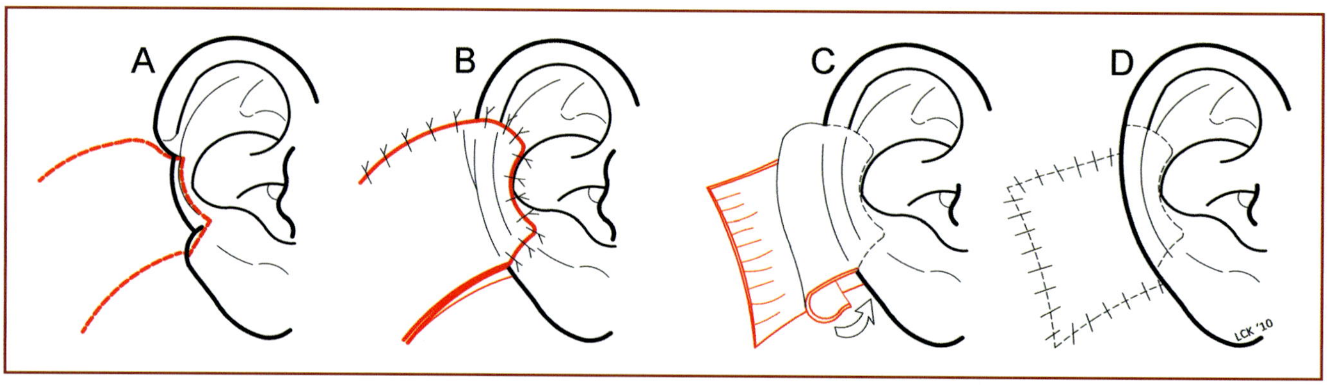

Figure 36–16. The Dieffenbach flap. **A.** In the first stage, a horizontal skin flap is raised from the mastoid area. **B.** The skin flap is used to reconstruct the anterior lamina of the middle ear while retaining its pedicle attachment. **C.** After secondary vascularization is satisfactory, with blood flow across the helical attachment, the posterior end of the flap is divided. **D.** The flap is advanced to reconstruct the posterior lamina of the auricular skin.

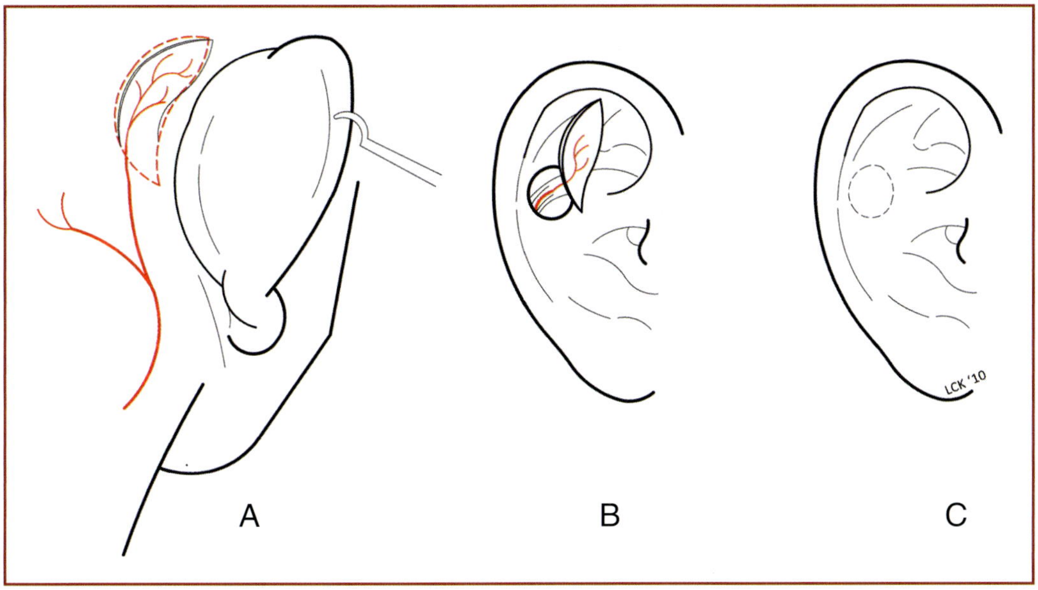

Figure 36–17. Vascularized island flap. To reconstruct defects of the anterior lamina, an islanded flap based on the branches of the postauricular artery may be used. **A.** The harvest site can be placed superior to the anterior defect to increase the reach of the vascular pedicle. **B.** The flap can be isolated on a pedicle and tunneled subcutaneously to reach the defect anteriorly. **C.** The flap can then be inset in the usual fashion.

or exposure ranging from 27%[32] to 81%[33] have been reported. Silicone therefore is not recommended in ear reconstruction.

Polytetrafluoroethylene also has been used to construct formed implants for ear reconstruction. Like silicone, polytetrafluoroethylene is an inert substance but does not incorporate well into auricular tissues. To improve tissue integration, expanded polytetrafluoroethylene implants with a foamlike structure, with microscopic channels for vessel and tissue ingrowth, have been designed. Originally, these were intended to be inserted directly underneath auricular skin, but the implants showed a higher incidence of local tissue complications[34] compared to autologous cartilage. Now, it is suggested that vascularized tissue, such as a superficial temporal artery (temporoparietal) fascial flap, be used as an envelope for this type of frame, and there are some isolated reports of success with this method.[35,43] However, should there be complications, the removal of this type of implant can be difficult because of tissue ingrowth into the foam channels.

Suture Materials in Frame Reconstruction

Because of its lack of primary vascularity, cartilage heals differently than skin or bone, and apposed cartilage pieces do not form firm bonds but instead undergo a modified type of fibrous union. For larger frames, it therefore is important to have stable joints between elements of the framework. In the context of ear reconstruction, the suture materials used to join these elements can be considered nonvascularized grafts. Many different permanent suture materials have been used for assembling cartilage pieces for ear reconstruction, including monofilament materials such as polypropylene and nylon.

One material that is now frequently used in ear reconstruction is fine stainless steel wire.[36] This well-known material provides a nonreactive, long-lasting suture anchor. There has been concern about the possible extrusion of wire sutures,[37] but the risk of this occurrence can be reduced by burying the wire ends in the reconstructed cartilage frame.[38] Stainless steel has a higher tensile strength than polymeric monofilament sutures and helps provide a strong and stable structure for cartilage frames.

Autologous Cartilage for Frame Reconstruction

The cartilage of choice for auricular frame reconstruction is costal cartilage because it is strong and its rigidity resists secondary deformation.[26] Costal cartilage has better structural strength than auricular cartilage—an important consideration as strong scar contractures can occur in auricular skin after surgery and can cause considerable distortion of the reconstructed auricular frame.

Although autologous cartilage itself is nonvascularized, when used as the framework for ear reconstruction, it can obtain a secondary blood supply from surrounding tissue. This blood supply helps keep the chondrocytes within the frame nourished and helps the frame itself resist infection. Recent reviews show extrusion or complication rates of 1% to 2% in pinnae reconstructed with autologous cartilage.[39,40] In contrast, extrusion/exposure rates of approximately 7% have occurred in ears reconstructed using polytetrafluoroethylene frameworks, even when covered with superficial temporal and/or galeal vascularized fascia.[41] Another series reported an exposure rate at 5.7%, with an overall complication rate of 17%, when extra-auricular implants were included in the analysis.[42]

Reconstruction for Larger Defects with Adequate Local Skin

For simple defects that are limited to 25% of the pinna, cartilage from the contralateral ear can be used to provide structural support and contour restoration. For larger, more complex defects, the surgeon can use autologous costal cartilage in the reconstructive framework to create a detailed yet natural appearance. There is a constant need to balance detail in the frame with the amount of available tissue for repair. This influences the decision about immediate versus delayed reconstruction of the posterior ear surface, as discussed above.

As noted previously, the template for the reconstructed ear can take the form of an idealized acetate template, a tracing from the contralateral ear, a tracing from an age-matched control, or a sculpted model that mirrors the contralateral ear. The template is used to estimate the amount of cartilage to be harvested. A subperichondrial harvest allows the surgeon to maintain the outline of the costal margin, minimizing the donor site morbidity[43] by making possible the return of unused cartilage for partial regeneration (Fig 36–18).[44]

The framework is carved using a combination of appropriately sized sculpture knives, or gouges, for shaping the required segments and surgical blades for sharp dissection. The segments are then assembled as a framework of the appropriate dimensions (Fig 36–19).

When using a template, one factor to bear in mind is the thickness of the skin covering the pinna, typically 2 mm. This means that the cartilaginous frame should be fabricated smaller than the corre-

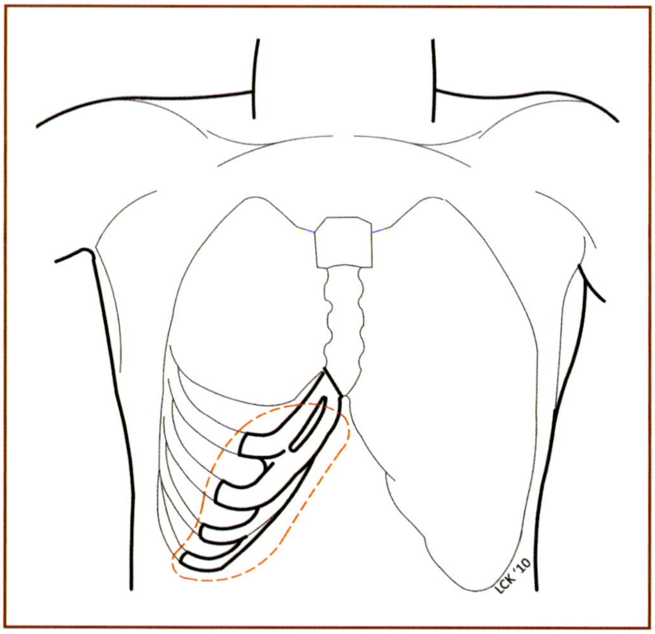

Figure 36–18. Region for costal cartilage harvest. Costal cartilage can be harvested from the anteromedial aspect of the costal margin through an oblique or transverse incision. Cartilage from ribs 6, 7, 8, or 9 can be used. A subperichondrial dissection helps reduce the risk of pneumothorax and may be useful in aiding reconstitution of the costal margin by return of unused cartilage blocks.

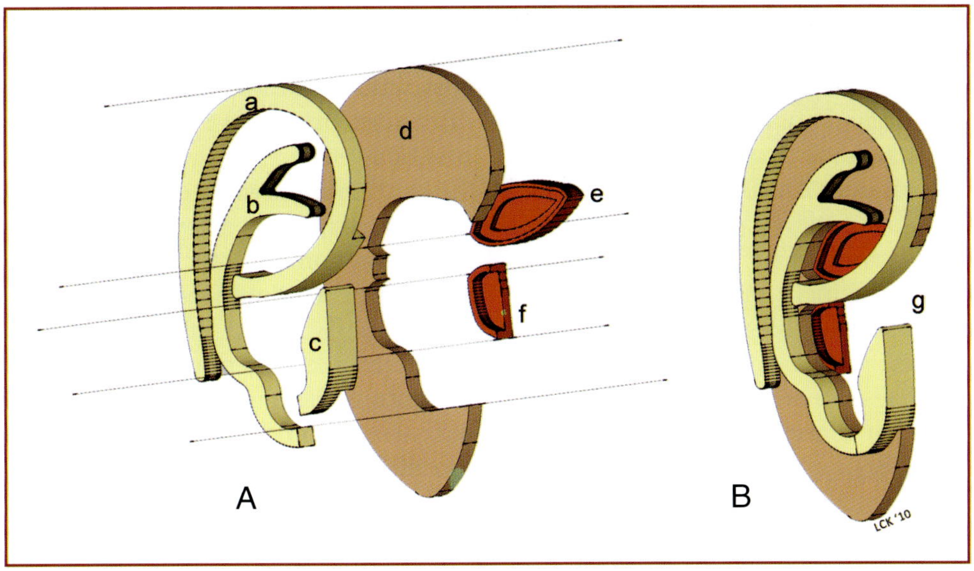

Figure 36–19. Full cartilage frame assembly. This diagram illustrates a typical full cartilage frame assembly in the style of Nagata. **A.** The components include the helix (*a*), antihelix (*b*), tragus (*c*), base plate (*d*), cymba concha (*e*), and cavitas concha (*f*) segments. These can be coapted using stainless steel wire sutures to form the complete auricular frame (*g*). The frame can be modified or formed in part to address smaller or subtotal defects if required. **B.** This figure illustrates the fit of the segments. In vivo, the cartilage frames are fabricated with smooth edges and as few right-angle edges as possible.

sponding molded template; in a total ear reconstruction, the frame height should be 4 mm shorter than the measured full normal ear.

For segmental defects, it is helpful to create a thin flange above the margin of the defect for use as a dovetail segment. Care should be taken to thin the flange so that it is not visible after reconstruction; however, if made too thin, the flange may fracture easily, resulting in loss of retention. The cartilage frame can be attached to the margins of the defect using thin monofilament sutures or stainless steel wire sutures, with the knots set in a position not likely to extrude through the skin.

The pocket for the cartilage frame must be adequately dissected, especially for larger or staged reconstructions, to reduce tension at the projection points of the frame and hence the risk of skin necrosis. Wide elevation of the skin for 1 cm to 2 cm around the frame is recommended to allow easier redraping of the skin envelope over the cartilage frame and also to create a gentle transition from the scalp surface to the frame contour. A gentle and meticulous technique is crucial in avoiding unnecessary tissue injury and excessive bleeding. Hemostasis is important but should be carried out judiciously to avoid full-thickness burns to the skin envelope.

Numerous methods can be used to close the incision sites around a cartilage frame. Avoidance of hematoma, and therefore delayed fibrous organization and scarring, is important for maintaining the definition and accuracy of the reconstruction. Coaptation of skin to the underlying framework helps by promoting healing, reducing swelling, and improving adhesion of the skin to the underlying cartilage. Some surgeons recommend negative pressure application through the use of suction drains,[39] whereas others use bolster sutures to avoid skin necrosis.[10] Skin glues have been used to prevent leakage at the closure site.[45]

If a staged reconstruction is planned, the elevation of the framework can be carried out 4 to 6 months after the first stage. This wait allows neovascularization to occur between the anterior skin and the cartilage. Soft tissue cover for the postauricular and mastoid surfaces can be provided by elevating local soft tissue with the reconstructed frame and placing a skin graft[26] or by using a turndown vascularized flap combined with a skin graft.[46] These techniques are described below.

Reconstruction for Larger Defects Without Adequate Local Skin

Tissue Expansion

One method for obtaining tissue cover in patients who have larger defects without adequate local skin is serial expansion of the skin using a tissue expander.[47,48] The tissue expander is inserted into the subcutaneous tissues in the periauricular region. Serial injections of saline solution over several weeks increase the volume of the tissue expander and thus the amount of skin covering it by gradual stretching and new tissue growth. The surgeon thus can increase the recruitment and availability of the tissue surrounding the defect, allowing advancement of these tissues over the defect to cover an auricular frame.

This method has several limitations. First, there is a tendency for the expanded skin to contract after reconstruction. This is of particular concern in auricular skin because operated skin in the pinna has a tendency to constrict postoperatively, with strong secondary scar contractures. Second, the local soft tissues may not always be suitable for tissue expansion, particularly if there has been previous surgery or scarring. Finally, tissue expansion has been associated with significant rates of infection and extrusion of the expander, particularly with rapid expansion.[49]

Vascularized Tissue

In patients with larger defects who do not have adequate skin coverage, the use of vascularized tissue should be considered.

The surface area of skin required to repair larger defects often is greater than may be initially apparent. The amount of skin to be reconstituted is often underestimated because the auricular skin covers three surfaces: the anterior auricular surface, the postauricular surface, and the mastoid.

As discussed previously, for defects whose reconstruction requires a detailed or complex frame, most of the available local skin may be used to form an anteriorly based Dieffenbach flap to cover the primary reconstruction. In such cases, the posterior skin reconstruction is staged. At the second stage, neovascularization of the tissues underneath the frame should have been completed so that when the frame is elevated, a skin graft can be applied to re-create the postauricular and mastoid skin.[9] However, it has been suggested that patients with Fitzpatrick type III or type IV skin may have a higher incidence of graft and scar contracture in the postauricular region, causing loss of projection, possible collapse of the cartilage framework, and an unsatisfactory result. In these patients, vascularized flaps such as a superficial temporal artery turndown fascial flap for posterior auricular skin reconstruction can deliver a better blood supply to the posterior tissues and reduce the risk of contracture.[10] The vessels that are useful for vascularizing larger flaps of tissue in the periauricular region are the superficial temporal artery, the posterior auricular artery, and the occipital artery.

In general, the superficial temporal artery flap is considered the workhorse regional flap for vascularized reconstruction (Fig 36–20).[10,50] The superficial temporal artery supplies the superficial temporal fascia, which overlies the temporalis muscle and is just beneath the subcutaneous adipose layer of the temporal skin. The fascia extends superiorly to join the galea at the temporal crest line and is contiguous with the superficial musculoaponeurotic system anteriorly and inferiorly.

It is possible to harvest a fascial flap 6 cm to 8 cm wide that extends to within 2 cm of the vertex and is based (usually) on the posterior branch of the superficial temporal artery. This flap can be carried on a fascial pedicle approximately 2-cm to 3-cm wide, including the superficial temporal artery pedicle. A flap with these dimensions would be sufficient to cover the anterior surface of a normal pinna.

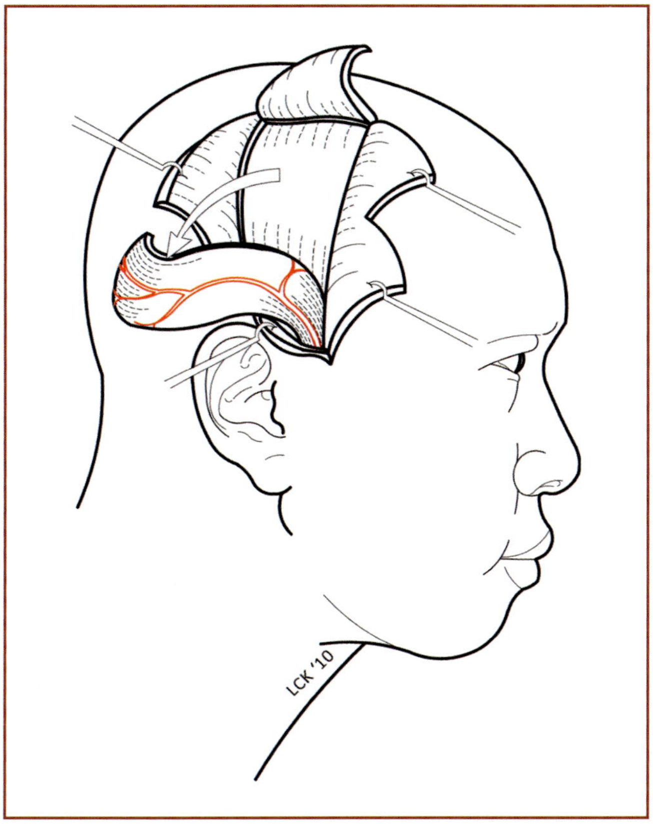

Figure 36–20. Superficial temporal artery flap. The flap can be elevated on either the anterior or posterior branches of the superficial temporal artery. Access incisions can be planned according to the arc of the flap's rotation relative to the site of the defect. Care must be taken in harvesting this flap because the superficial temporal artery lies immediately superficial to the superficial temporal fascia.

The transfer of tissue for the reconstruction of soft tissue cover can include fascia only or fascia with overlying skin. Harvesting both the fascia and skin layers for transfer usually is not feasible with a superficial temporal artery flap because of the hair-bearing nature of the skin of the parietal and temporal regions; a full-thickness harvest would lead to significant donor-site alopecia and unacceptable cosmetic sequelae. Harvesting both skin and fascia is possible for smaller defects with the use of a posterior auricular artery flap because the donor site is not hair-bearing and the wound at the donor site can be closed directly or with a skin graft.

If the harvested tissue comprises fascia only, a further skin graft must be added to the reconstruction to complete the resurfacing. As discussed previously, split-thickness skin from the scalp provides an excellent color match for this purpose.

Auricular Prosthetics

Alloplastic prosthetic devices may be considered in patients in whom autologous-tissue reconstruction has failed, in patients who have severe soft tissue or skeletal hypoplasia or acquired total or subtotal traumatic or ablative auricular defects, in patients who are poor anesthesia risks, or in patients who may benefit from the shorter operating times in implant-based reconstructions.[51,52] Implant-retained ear prostheses have the advantages of better color match and camouflage, consistent cosmetic results, a shorter time for rehabilitation, and reduced donor site morbidity compared to autologous-tissue techniques (Figs 36–21 and 36–22).[53] There also is the possible advantage of earlier detection of tumor recurrence in oncologic cases.

A prosthesis can be either bone anchored or not, and it can be partial or total. The prosthesis usually is constructed from a combination of silicone polymers and plastics and is tailored to fit an existing defect (partial) or an entire ear (total). Partial prostheses are applied to the ear or ear skin using a skin adhesive and matched, using makeup, to the surrounding skin. They are not easy to apply, and many patients find retention of the prosthesis difficult.

Total prostheses are secured by an implant attached to the bony base of the reconstruction site. The surface of the implants can be plain, textured or treated (eg, sandblasted, etched, sprayed), or coated (eg, with hydroxyapatite).

The implant has external threading to anchor it securely in the bone. Extraoral implants anchored in the mastoid bone for ear reconstruction typically are 3 mm to 4 mm long to allow for the thinner bone. Intraoral implants are longer, 7 mm to 20 mm, and may have better retention rates owing to their longer implant-bone interfaces.

Within the implant are internal threads to which a skin-penetrating abutment can be connected. The abutment can be used to support prosthetic

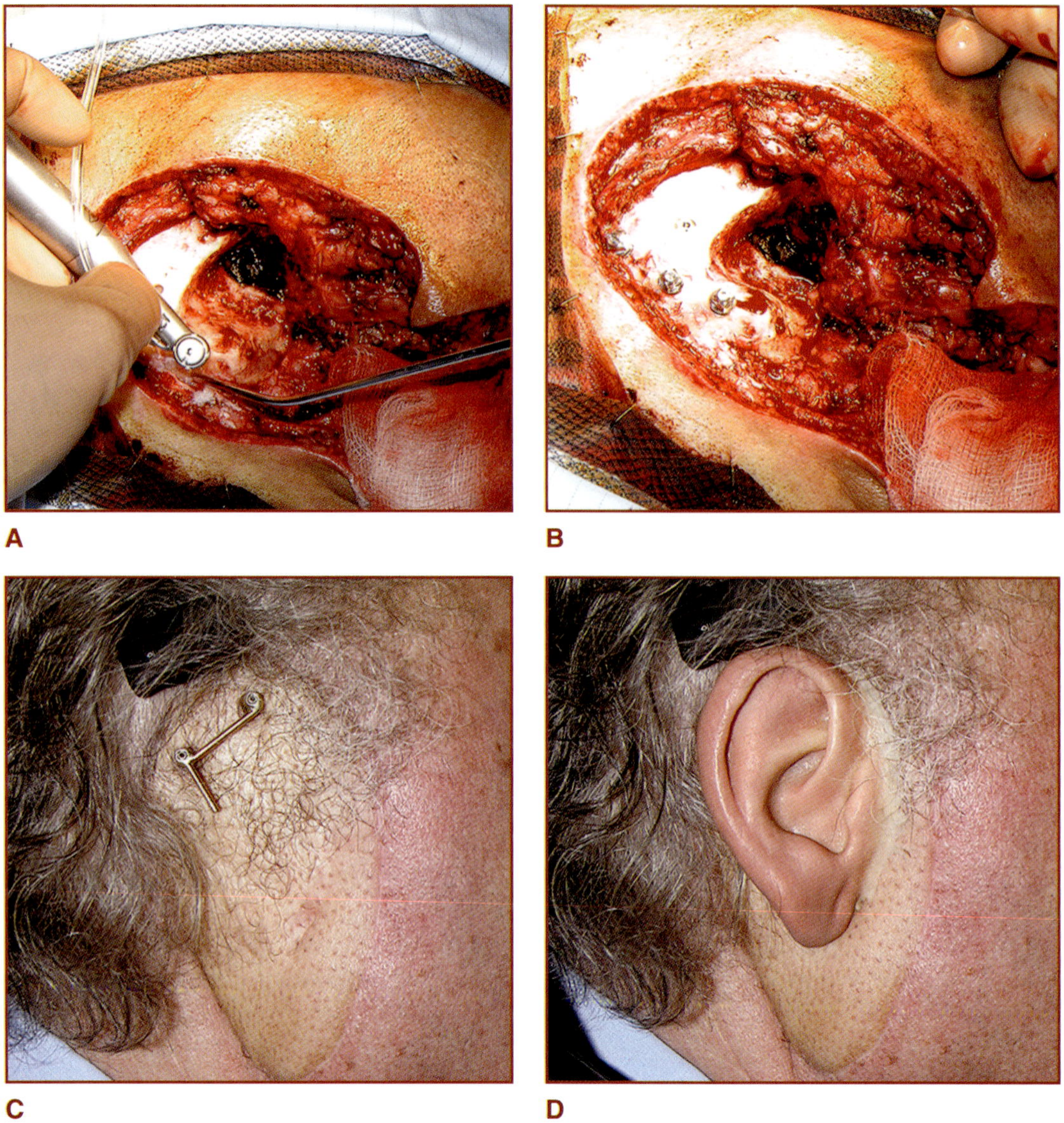

Figure 36–21. Osseointegrated prosthesis reconstruction. A 67-year-old patient presented with a rapidly growing, large, invasive squamous cell carcinoma extending into the ear canal. This required wide excision in the form of total pinnectomy with temporal bone resection for clearance. **A, B.** The patient underwent immediate placement of titanium screws for implant rehabilitation. **C.** Soft tissue cover was achieved using a free anterolateral thigh microsurgical flap, hearing was improved using a bone-anchored hearing aid, and a mounting bracket for the prosthesis was implanted. **D.** The patient is shown with the prosthesis in place.

components to which a retentive framework can be attached. Prosthetic retention can be achieved by clips or by magnets placed within the auricular frame. Implant osseointegration is usually a two-stage operation. With bone-anchored osseointegrated prostheses, a period of 6 weeks is allowed for osseointegration before the healing plates are uncovered and the prosthesis attached.

One advantage of prosthetic reconstructions over autologous-tissue ear reconstruction is that any

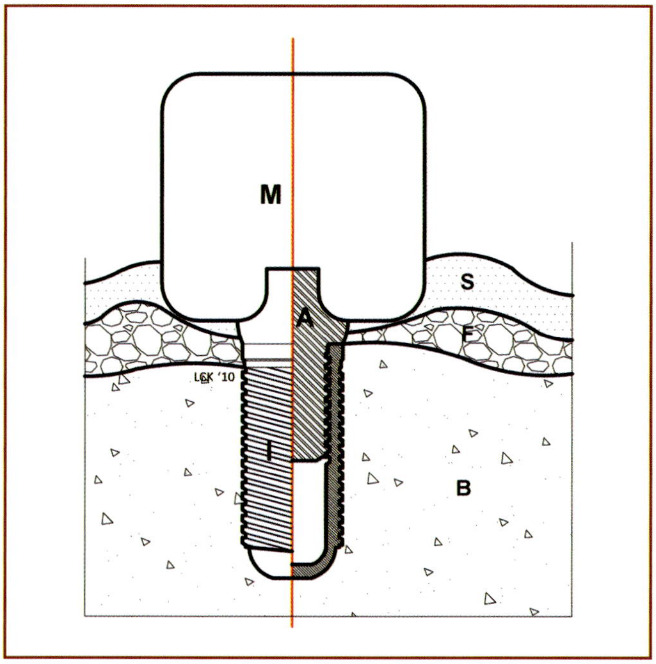

Figure 36–22. Typical osseointegrated prosthesis. An osseointegrated prosthesis includes an osseointegrated implant (*I*), which has outer threads allowing anchorage to the bone (*B*); and a skin-penetrating abutment (*A*), which is secured to the implant through an internal thread. The abutment can be used to carry prosthetic components to which a retentive framework (*M*) can be attached. The abutment passes through skin (*S*) and fat (*F*), and meticulous skin hygiene is required to minimize the risk of infection.

errors in shape and size can be corrected with revisions to the prosthesis. The color of the prosthesis can also be revised over time, as needed. However, unlike the patient's normal skin, the color is fixed and therefore some patients have a summer ear as well as a winter one.

A disadvantage of prosthetic reconstruction is that the patient must adhere to a lifelong regimen of follow-up and care; prosthetic abutments require daily, careful cleaning, and patients occasionally experience granulation, tissue overgrowth at the prosthesis-skin interface, or (less commonly) infection.[54] An infection of the bony anchor can result in osteomyelitis and, ultimately, failure of the prosthetic implant. In addition, although the surgical techniques required in a prosthetic rehabilitation are less demanding than those needed for autologous-tissue reconstruction, construction of the prosthesis is time-consuming and requires considerable expertise.[51,52] Furthermore, the polymer substance and color of the prosthesis do not last indefinitely, and many patients must return to the laboratory for maintenance or replacement of the prosthesis every 2 to 3 years, on average. Fabrication of a prosthetic pinna also is expensive, and over the lifetime of a patient, this may represent an unacceptable cost to both patient and insurance provider.

Some patients find the use of a prosthesis simple and rewarding. Others, however, find that the use of an artificial implement unappealing and are unwilling to consider a prosthesis. Further details involving prosthetic rehabilitation are discussed in Chapter 39.

Conclusions

Reconstruction of the pinna is challenging. The surgeon should have a thorough understanding of the blood supply and soft tissue characteristics of the ear and periauricular regions as well as an appreciation for the normal anatomical projection, position, and dimensional ratios of the ear.[55] A multidisciplinary approach is helpful during the planning of reconstruction. Although reconstruction of this complex structure is affected by multiple variables related to causative and patient factors, with the correct attention to detail, satisfactory outcomes can be achieved.[56,57]

References

1. Leonardo da Vinci, XIX: Philosophical maxims, morals, polemics and speculations. In: Richter JP, *The Literary Works of Leonardo Da Vinci.* Vol 2. London, England: S. Low, Marston, Searle & Rivington; 1883: Phrase 1142.
2. Converse JM. Reconstruction of the auricle—part I. *Plast Reconstr Surg.* 1958;22(2):150–163.
3. Bhishagratna KKL. *An English Translation of the Sushruta Samhita.* Calcutta, India: Wilkins Press; 1907:chap XVI.
4. Tagliacozzi G. *De Curtorum Chirurgia per Institionem.* Venice, Italy: Gaspare Bindonus; 1597.

5. Gillies H. *Plastic Surgery of the Face.* London, England: H. Frowde, Hodder & Stoughton; 1920.
6. Pierce GW. Reconstruction of the external ear. *Surg Gynecol Obstet.* 1930;50:601.
7. Tanzer RC. Total reconstruction of the external ear. *Plast Reconstr Surg.* 1959;23(1):1–15.
8. Converse JM. Reconstruction of the auricle—Part II. *Plast Reconstr Surg.* 1958;22(2):230–249.
9. Brent B. The correction of microtia with autogenous cartilage grafts: I. The classic deformity. *Plast Reconstr Surg.* 1980;66(1):1–12.
10. Nagata S. A new method of total reconstruction of the auricle for microtia. *Plast Reconstr Surg.* 1993;92(2):187–201.
11. Vitruvius. On symmetry: in temples and in the human body. In: Morgan MH, trans. *The Ten Books of Architecture.* Book III. London, England: Humphrey Milford, Oxford University Press; 1914:chaps 1–3.
12. Leonardo da Vinci. VII: On the proportions and on the movements of the human figure. In: Richter JP; *The Literary Works of Leonardo Da Vinci.* Vol 1. London, England: S. Low, Marston, Searle & Rivington; 1883:310, plate VII.
13. Tolleth H. Artistic anatomy, dimensions, and proportions of the external ear. *Clin Plast Surg.* 1978;5(3):337–345.
14. Park C, Lineaweaver WC, Rumly TO, Buncke HJ. Arterial supply of the anterior ear. *Plast Reconstr Surg.* 1992;90(1): 38–44.
15. Nakajima H, Imanishi N, Minabe T. The arterial anatomy of the temporal region and the vascular basis of various temporal flaps. *Br J Plast Surg.* 1995;48(7):439–450.
16. Richmond-Sinclair NM, Pandeya N, Ware RS, et al. Incidence of basal cell carcinoma multiplicity and detailed anatomic distribution: longitudinal study of an Australian population. *J Invest Dermatol.* 2009;129,323–328.
17. Rowe DE, Carroll RJ, Day C Jr. Prognostic factors for local recurrence, metastasis, and survival rates in squamous cell carcinoma of the skin, ear, and lip: implications for treatment modality selection. *J Am Acad Dermatol.* 1992; 26(6):976–990.
18. Tanzer RC. Congenital deformities (of the auricle). In: Converse JM, ed. *Reconstructive Plastic Surgery.* Vol 3. 2nd ed. Philadelphia, PA: WB Saunders; 1977:1671–1719.
19. Yotsuyanagi T, Yamashita K, Sawada Y. Reconstruction of congenital and acquired earlobe deformity. *Clin Plast Surg.* 2002;29(2):249–255, vii.
20. Singh A, Singh G. Earlobe reconstruction using a Limberg flap in six ears. *Br J Plast Surg.* 2003;56(1):33–36.
21. Van Geertruyden JP. Earlobe reconstruction with a reverse-flow chondrocutaneous flap. *Br J Plast Surg.* 2002;55(3):253–255.
22. Talmi YP, Horowitz Z, Bedrin L, Kronenberg J. Auricular reconstruction with a postauricular myocutaneous island flap: flip-flop flap. *Plast Reconstr Surg.* 1996;98(7): 1191–1199.
23. Antia NH, Buch VI. Chondrocutaneous advancement flap for the marginal defect of the ear. *Plast Reconstr Surg.* 1967;39(5):472–477.
24. Butler CE. Reconstruction of marginal ear defects with modified chondrocutaneous helical rim advancement flaps. *Plast Reconstr Surg.* 2003;111(6):2009–2013.
25. Butler CE. Single-stage reconstruction of middle-and lower-third helical rim defects using chondrocutaneous helical rim and lobular advancement flaps and a scaphal reduction cartilage graft. *Plast Reconstr Surg.* 2008;122(2): 403–467.
26. Dieffenbach, JF. *Die Operative Chirurgie.* Leipzig, Germany: FA Brockhaus; 1845.
27. Brent B. Reconstruction of the Auricle. In: McCarthy, JG, ed. *Reconstructive Plastic Surgery.* Vol 3. 1st ed. Philadelphia, PA: WB Saunders; 1990:2094–2152.
28. Butler CE. Extended retroauricular advancement flap reconstruction of a full-thickness auricular defect including posteromedial and retroauricular skin. *Ann Plast Surg.* 2002;49(3); 317–321.
29. Turan A, Turkaslan T, Kul Z, Isler C, Ozsoy Z. Reconstruction of the anterior surface of the ear using a postauricular pull-through neurovascular island flap. *Ann Plast Surg.* 2006;56(6):609–613.
30. Dessy LA, Figus A, Fioramonti P, Mazzocchi M, Scuderi N. Reconstruction of anterior auricular conchal defect after malignancy excision: revolving-door flap versus full-thickness skin graft. *J Plast Reconstr Aesthet Surg.* 2010;63(5):746–752.
31. Cronin TD, Greenberg RL, Brauer RO. Follow-up study of Silastic frame for reconstruction of external ear. *Plast Reconstr Surg.* 1968;42(6):522–529.
32. Spitalny HH, Lemperle G. Long-term experience with silicone implants in the face. *Handchir Mikrochir Plast Chir.* 1982;14(1):29–35.
33. Lynch JB, Pousti JE, et al. Our experiences with silastic ear implants. *Plast Reconstr Surg.* 1972;49(3):283–285.
34. Wray RC, Hoopes JE. Silastic frameworks in total reconstruction of the auricle. *Br J Plast Surg.* 1973;26(3):296–297.
35. Wellisz T. Clinical experience with the Medpor porous polyethylene implant. *Aesthetic Plast Surg.* 1993;17(4): 339–344.
36. Yang SL, Zheng JH, Ding Z, et al. Combined fascial flap and expanded skin flap for enveloping Medpor framework in microtia reconstruction. *Aesthetic Plast Surg.* 2009;33(4):518–522.
37. Edlich RF, Drake DB, Rodeheaver GT, et al. Syneture stainless STEEL suture. A collective review of its performance in surgical wound closure. *J Long Term Eff Med Implants.* 2006;16(1):101–110.
38. Brent B. Microtia repair with rib cartilage grafts: a review of personal experience with 1000 cases. *Clin Plast Surg.* 2002;29(2):257–271, vii.
39. Nagata S. Total auricular reconstruction with a three-dimensional costal cartilage framework. *Ann Chir Plast Esthet.* 1995;40(4):371–399; discussion 400–403.
40. Brent B. Auricular repair with autogenous rib cartilage grafts: two decades of experience with 600 cases. *Plast Reconstr Surg.* 1992; 90(3): 355–374.

41. Chen J, Yang Q, Wang X, et al. Fabrication of a three-dimensional autogenous costal cartilage framework in auricular reconstruction: experience with 250 cases of Asian lobule-type microtia. *J Otolaryngol Head Neck Surg.* 2008;37(6):901–908.
42. Reinisch JF, Lewin S. Ear reconstruction using a porous polyethylene framework and temporoparietal fascia flap. *Facial Plast Surg.* 2009;25(3):181–189.
43. Sevin K, Askar I, Saray A, Yormuk E. Exposure of high-density porous polyethylene (Medpor) used for contour restoration and treatment. *Br J Oral Maxillofac Surg.* 2000; 38(1):44–49.
44. Kawanabe Y, Nagata S. A new method of costal cartilage harvest for total auricular reconstruction: part I. Avoidance and prevention of intraoperative and postoperative complications and problems. *Plast Reconstr Surg.* 2006; 117(6):2011–2018.
45. Kawanabe Y, Nagata S. A new method of costal cartilage harvest for total auricular reconstruction: part II. Evaluation and analysis of the regenerated costal cartilage. *Plast Reconstr Surg.* 2007;119(1):308–315.
46. Hallock GG. Expanded applications for octyl-2-cyanoacrylate as a tissue adhesive. *Ann Plast Surg.* 2001;46(2): 185–189.
47. Nagata S. Modification of the stages in total reconstruction of the auricle: Part IV. Ear elevation for the constructed auricle. *Plast Reconstr Surg.* 1994;93(2):254–266;discussion 267–268.
48. Bauer BS. The role of tissue expansion in reconstruction of the ear. *Clin Plast Surg.* 1990;17(2):319–325.
49. Sasaki GH. Tissue expansion in reconstruction of acquired auricular defects. *Clin Plast Surg.* 1990;17(2):327–338.
50. Jing C, Hong-Xing Z. Partial necrosis of expanding postauricular flaps during auricle reconstruction: risk factors and effective management. *Plast Reconstr Surg.* 2007;119(6):1759–1766.
51. Park C, Lew DH, Yoo WM. An analysis of 123 temporoparietal fascial flaps: anatomic and clinical considerations in total auricular reconstruction. *Plast Reconstr Surg.* 1999;104(5):1295–1306.
52. Thorne CH, Brecht LE, Bradley JP, et al. Auricular reconstruction: indications for autogenous and prosthetic techniques. *Plast Reconstr Surg.* 2001;107(5):1241–1252.
53. Wilkes GH, Wolfaardt JF. Osseointegrated alloplastic versus autogenous ear reconstruction: criteria for treatment selection. *Plast Reconstr Surg.* 1994; 93(5):967–979.
54. Federspil PA. Ear epistheses as an alternative to autogenous reconstruction. *Facial Plast Surg.* 2009;25(3): 190–203.
55. Hamming KK, Lund TW, Lander TA, Sidman JD. Complications and satisfaction with pediatric osseointegrated external ear prostheses. *Laryngoscope.* 2009;119(7): 1270–1273.
56. Suutarla S, Rautio J, Klockars T. The learning curve in microtia surgery. *Facial Plast Surg.* 2009;25(3):164–168.
57. Horlock N, Vögelin E, Bradbury ET, Grobbelaar AO, Gault DT. Psychosocial outcome of patients after ear reconstruction: a retrospective study of 62 patients. *Ann Plast Surg.* 2005;54(5):517–524.
58. Steffen A, Klaiber S, Katzbach R, et al. The psychosocial consequences of reconstruction of severe ear defects or third-degree microtia with rib cartilage. *Aesthet Surg J.* 2008;28(4):404–411.

37

SCALP RECONSTRUCTION

MELISSA A. CROSBY

Introduction

Scalp defects following oncologic resection present a reconstructive challenge requiring precise planning. The lack of redundant tissue on the scalp and presence of thick, nonpliable connective tissue complicates ease of closure. In addition, many cancer patients have had prior scalp surgery and have undergone or will undergo radiation therapy. Some patients also may present with infected or exposed devascularized bone or alloplastic material after craniotomy, complicating the reconstruction further. As with all forms of reconstruction, the reconstructive technique chosen must provide durable and reliable coverage with minimal donor site morbidity. In addition, aesthetic issues, including minimizing alopecia, distortion of the hairline or brow, and symmetric contour, should be considered.

Anatomy

The scalp is made up of five layers often remembered by the mnemonic SCALP: skin, subcutaneous tissue, aponeurosis, muscle and loose areolar tissue, and pericranium[1] (Fig 37–1). The skin and subcutaneous tissue are often treated as one layer owing to the lack of cleavage plane between these two layers. Within these layers lie the hair follicles, sweat glands, and fat cells. The scalp skin is unique in that it is the thickest in the body, measuring 3 to 8 mm, actually making it a good donor site for split-thickness skin graft harvest.[2] Beneath the subcutaneous layer lies the musculoaponeurotic layer, also known as the galea aponeurotica. The galea aponeurotica consists of fibrous tissue continuous with the frontalis muscle anteriorly, occipitalis muscle posteriorly, and the temporoparietal (superficial temporal) fascia laterally. This layer provides the strength layer to the scalp and extends anteriorly into the face as the superficial musculoaponeurotic system described by Mitz and Peyronie[3] and later modified by Jost.[4] Beneath the galea lies the loose areolar layer, also known as the subgaleal or innominate fascia or subaponeurotic plane. This dissection within the plane of this layer allows for scalp mobility when creating rotation or advancement flaps for reconstruction. The greatest mobility of the scalp occurs in the parietal regions in the areolar plane between the temporoparietal fascia and the deep temporal fascia. The deepest layer of the scalp is the pericranium, which is the periosteum to the calvaria. This layer is vascular and serves a reliable recipient site for skin grafting. In addition, this layer is often raised to provide pericranial flaps for dural reconstruction.

The scalp has a vast and rich vascular plexus with extensive collateralization between four vascular territories supplied primarily by branches off the internal and external carotid arteries (Fig 37–2). The anterior territory is supplied by the supraorbital

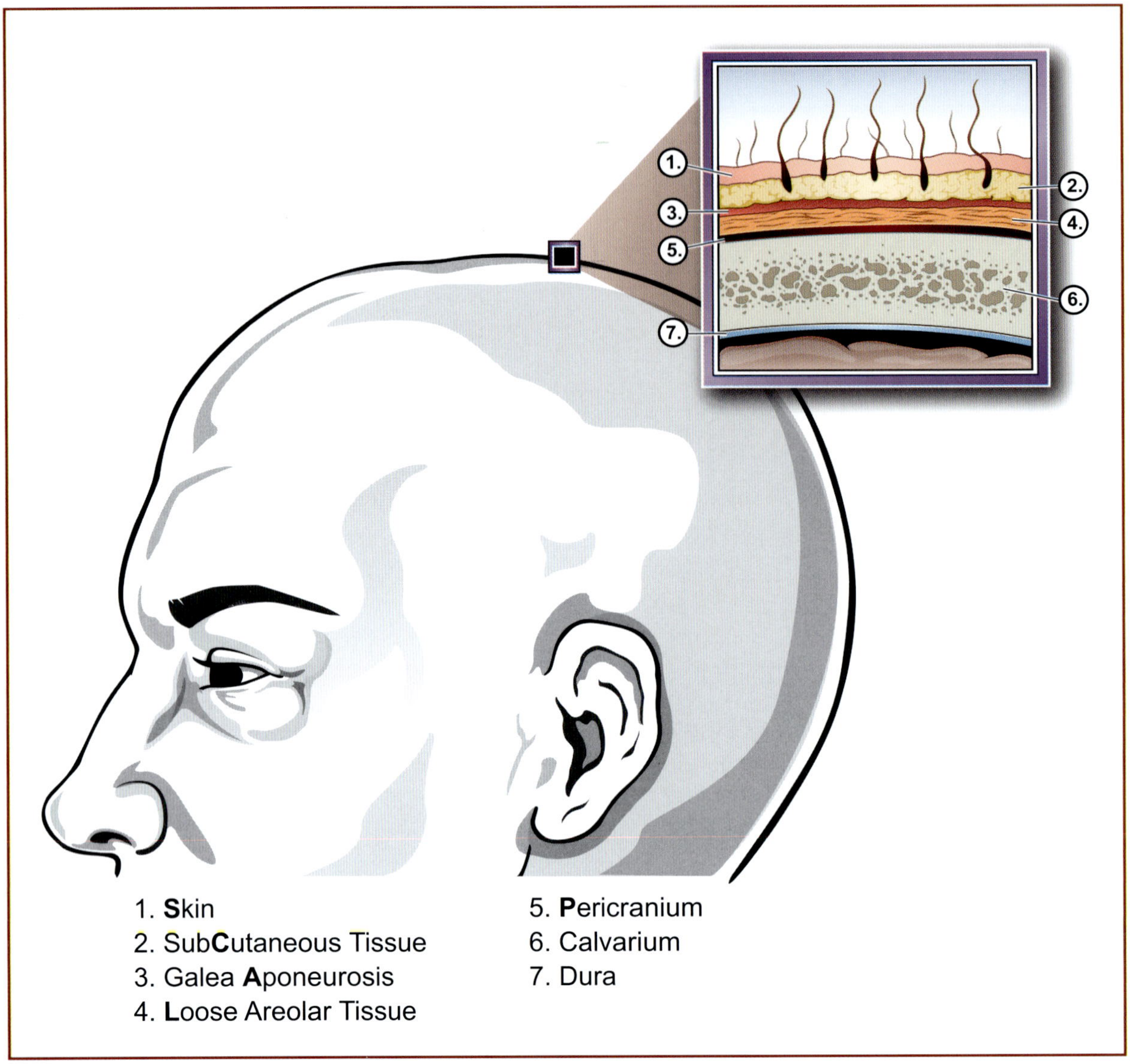

Figure 37–1. Layers of the scalp.

and supratrochlear arteries arising from the ophthalmic artery, which is a branch of the internal carotid artery. The lateral and largest vascular territory is supplied by the superficial temporal artery, a terminal branch off the external carotid artery, which bifurcates at the superior helix into frontal and parietal branches. The occipital arteries supply the posterior scalp cephalad to the nuchal line. Caudal to the nuchal line, perforating branches of the trapezius and splenius capitus muscles supply the posterior scalp. The posterior auricular artery also supplies the posterolateral scalp territory as a terminal branch of the external carotid artery system. The venous system parallels the arterial system. Because of the vast overlap between vascular territories, scalp replantation based on a single arterial anastomosis (although usually accompanied by several venous anastomoses) and large axial flaps designed

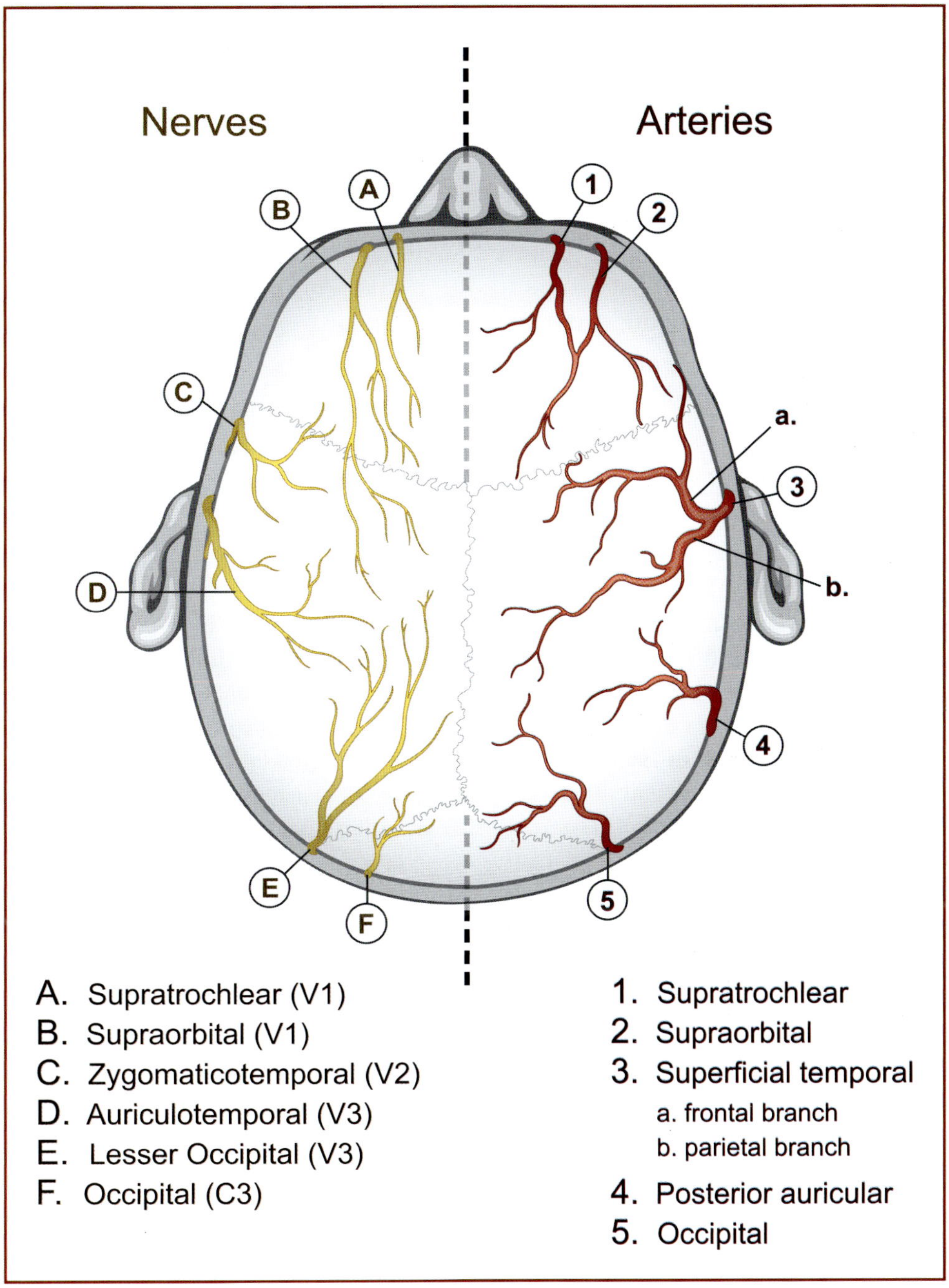

Figure 37–2. Blood supply and sensation of the scalp.

around one vascular territory are possible with minimal to no vascular compromise.

Innervation to the scalp involves both motor and sensory nerves. Motor nerves to the scalp and forehead include the temporal branches of the facial nerve. These nerves are found on the deep surface of the temporoparietal fascia within the loose areolar plane along an imaginary line connecting the ear lobe and a point 1.5 cm above the lateral brow (Pitanguy's line). The temporal branch crosses the middle third of the zygoma, and therefore, dissection is performed in a plane deep to the superficial layer of the deep temporal fascia to prevent nerve injury. The occipitalis muscle is supplied by the posterior auricular branch originating from the facial nerve as it exits the stylomastoid foramen. The temporalis muscle is supplied by the posterior and anterior deep temporal nerves arising from the trigeminal nerve.

Sensory innervation comes from branches of the trigeminal nerve, including the supratrochlear (V1); supraorbital (V1); zygomaticotemporal (V2); auriculotemporal (V3) nerves; and branches of the cervical plexus, including the lesser occipital (C2, C3) and greater occipital nerves (C2) (see Fig 37–2). The supratrochlear and supraorbital nerves provide sensation to the forehead and anterior scalp, the zygomaticotemporal nerve to the temporal region, the auriculotemporal nerve anterior to the ear, and the occipital nerve to the posterior scalp.

The scalp itself does not contain lymph nodes. Lymphatic vessels travel within the subcutaneous plane draining into nodes located within the parotid gland, preauricular region, upper neck, and occipital region. Skin neoplasms of the scalp tend to spread via local extension rather than through lymphatic or vascular channels.[5]

Reconstruction

Surgical treatment of cutaneous malignancies may range from resections involving only superficial layers of the scalp to more complex resections involving calvarium and dura, depending on the invasiveness of the malignancy. Methods of reconstruction include healing by secondary intention, primary closure, skin grafting, tissue expansion, local flaps, and free tissue transfer. The choice of reconstructive technique is often dependent on many variables, including the size, depth, and location of the defect; recipient bed vascularity; mobility of the surrounding tissue; flap donor site availability; prior treatments or surgeries; and the need for adjuvant radiation. Whenever possible, Millard's principle of replacing like tissue with like should be followed.[6] Extensive preoperative planning and intraoperative attention to detail such as maintaining meticulous hemostasis, placing incisions parallel to hair follicles, and avoiding excessive tension on wound closure can provide for improved aesthetic results and reduced complications.[7] In addition, meticulous postoperative wound care, including head elevation to minimize edema, and positioning to reduce compression on the reconstruction, which might compromise vascularity of the transferred tissue, are vital to reconstructive success.

Healing by Secondary Intention

Healing by secondary intention may be indicated in patients who may not be able to undergo a surgical intervention due to extensive comorbidities. The optimal wound to heal by secondary intention is one in which the defect is partial thickness or the pericranium is intact providing a vascularized bed for healing. In situations in which the pericranium has been removed and the calvarium is exposed, awaiting closure by secondary intention may result in calvarial desiccation and subsequent infection unless a strict moist wound care regimen is maintained.

Options in this situation may include transferring a pericranial flap or a temporoparietal fascia flap from beneath adjacent intact scalp to provide a vascularized base for healing. Some authors advocate the removal of the outer cortical layer of the calvarium, exposing the vascular diploic space.[8] Dressing changes or a vacuum-assisted closure device then could be applied, allowing for granulation tissue formation. However, Becker and colleagues[9] have reported good results without superficial decortication of exposed bone in 38 patients undergoing Mohs treatment with a mean area of exposed bone reported to be 1074 mm^2. The mean time for the exposed bone to re-epithelialize was reported to be 13 weeks. As demonstrated by this study, the downside to closure by secondary intention is the time and care necessary to heal a wound. In addition, the resulting scar is often atrophic and hairless, resulting in a less aesthetic result than might be accomplished with other methods of closure. This method of closure is probably unlikely to succeed in patients who have received prior radiation therapy owing to the compromised vascularity of the scalp tissue and calvarial bone.

Primary Closure

Primary closure of a scalp defect often is possible when the defect is less than 3 cm in diameter and extensive subgaleal undermining is performed.[10] The use of primary closure has the advantage of maintaining hair-bearing areas of the scalp with minimal scarring. Careful planning can reduce tension on closure by recruiting the laxity of the scalp to close the defect and by planning resections along a sagittal plane/orientation where lines of minimal tension run. Areas of greater laxity occur in the frontal, parietal, and occipital regions. Scoring the galea often assists in the recruitment of tissue and also assists in utilization of intrinsic viscoelastic properties, including stress relaxation and creep, to close defects.[11] These relaxing incisions should be placed approximately 1 cm apart and perpendicular to the direction of the scalp advancement. Raposio et al[12] have shown that these incisions provide 1.67 mm of additional scalp advancement per relaxing incision and can reduce the closing tension by 40%.

When performing galeotomies, one must be careful not to injure the underlying blood vessels superficial to the galea, because this may result in decreased vascularity and hematomas. Reduced tension on closure also results in lessening the alopecia that can result along surgical scars. Rapid intraoperative tissue expansion also has been described as an adjunct to primary closure.[13–16] The process usually involves cyclic expansion and deflation of a balloon device under the tissue surrounding the defect. Although controversial, reportedly 1 to 3 cm of additional flap length can be obtained with this technique because of fragmentation of elastin and collagen fiber realignment (creep) and reduction of interstitial fluid intraoperatively.[14,15]

Skin Grafting

Split- and full-thickness skin grafting can be used if a sufficiently vascularized recipient bed is available. For partial-thickness defects and when periosteum is left intact, a skin graft can be applied with good results. Burring of the outer table to expose the diploe and application of a skin graft also is an option if periosteum is absent. Graft take may be increased by allowing an interval of granulation tissue to form with dressing changes followed by delayed placement of a split-thickness skin graft.[17,18] The primary advantage of skin grafting is that it is technically simple. The downside is the cosmetically inferior appearance of the skin graft compared with other forms of reconstruction that provide hair-bearing tissue. Also, the long-term stability of this type of reconstruction on full-thickness wounds (particularly on bare bone) can be a problem due to its susceptibility to trauma; hence, in patients who are to receive or have received radiation therapy as an adjunct to their cancer treatment, skin grafting is not recommended if another form of reconstruction is available. Most often, skin grafting is used as part of a staged reconstruction, such as with tissue expansion to provide temporary wound coverage or as an adjunct to local flaps providing coverage of the donor site when primary closure is not possible (Fig 37–3).

Tissue Expansion

Tissue expansion often is reserved for secondary revisions rather than in primary reconstruction in scalp defects resulting after oncologic resection. Intraoperative expansion has been reported as described above, but usually only as an adjunct to primary closure of small defects. Tissue expansion is used most commonly for removal of giant congenital nevi or of other lesions of low or no malignant potential, or for secondary revisions to remove skin grafts and replace non–hair-bearing scars with hair-bearing, sensate, adjacent tissue through the use of rotation, transposition, or advancement flaps.

From 30% to 75% of the scalp can be reconstructed with the use of tissue expansion but requires staged operations with a lengthy interval period.[19,20] Many sizes of tissue expanders exist, and the shape of the tissue expander base affects the amount of tissue gain. Rappard et al[21] determined that expanders with a round base, a crescentic base, and a rectangular base give tissue gains of 25%, 32%, and 38%,

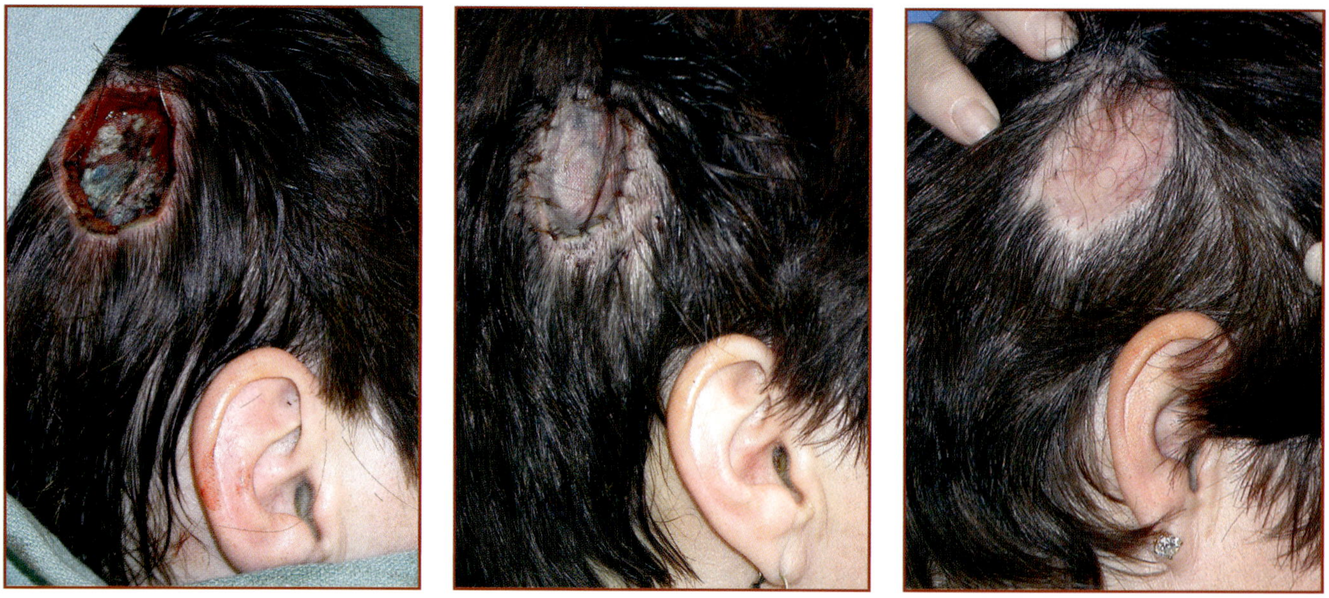

A B C

Figure 37–3. A scalp defect after excision of a malignant melanoma (**A**) reconstructed with a split-thickness skin graft (**B**). **C.** Postoperative result.

respectively. The tissue expander is placed in the subgaleal plane through an incision that can be incorporated into the final scalp reconstruction if at all possible.[22] Expansion usually begins 2 weeks after placement and continues weekly until the expander is filled "to provide an area" 2 to 2.5 times the size of the defect to account for innate tissue recoil. To calculate the expanded flap size, the length of the base of the expander is subtracted from the length over the top of the expander.[23] Advancement flaps generally are preferred in tissue expander reconstruction so that the orientation of hair follicles is not disrupted. Scoring the nondistensible capsule is preferable to capsulectomy to achieve increased length when necessary.

Expanded tissue has been shown to have an enhanced blood supply, allowing longer flaps to be harvested that are reported to be more resistant to infection.[24] Despite this, complication rates with expansion of the scalp range from 3.1% to 17%.[19,25,26] In addition, expanders should not be used in patients with irradiated skin and adjacent infected wounds because of potential increased complication rates. Decreased hair density because of the increased surface area of the scalp that results from expansion also may be noticeable postoperatively, especially for large expansions or when hair is sparse preoperatively. Tissue expanders generally are considered contraindicated in children under the age of 3 years owing to the presence of open cranial sutures.[23] Anecdotally, however, the bony changes that do occur in young children have been observed to reverse over time.[27] Despite the potential advantages of tissue expansion reconstruction of the scalp, the process places a physical and emotional burden on patients and their families; therefore, support and education are vital when considering the use of this technique in scalp reconstruction.

Local Flaps

A variety of local tissue rearrangements can be employed in scalp reconstruction, including transposition, advancement, and rotation flaps either alone or in combination when primary closure is not possible (Fig 37–4). The advantage of these flaps is that they can provide large areas of hair-bearing tissue,

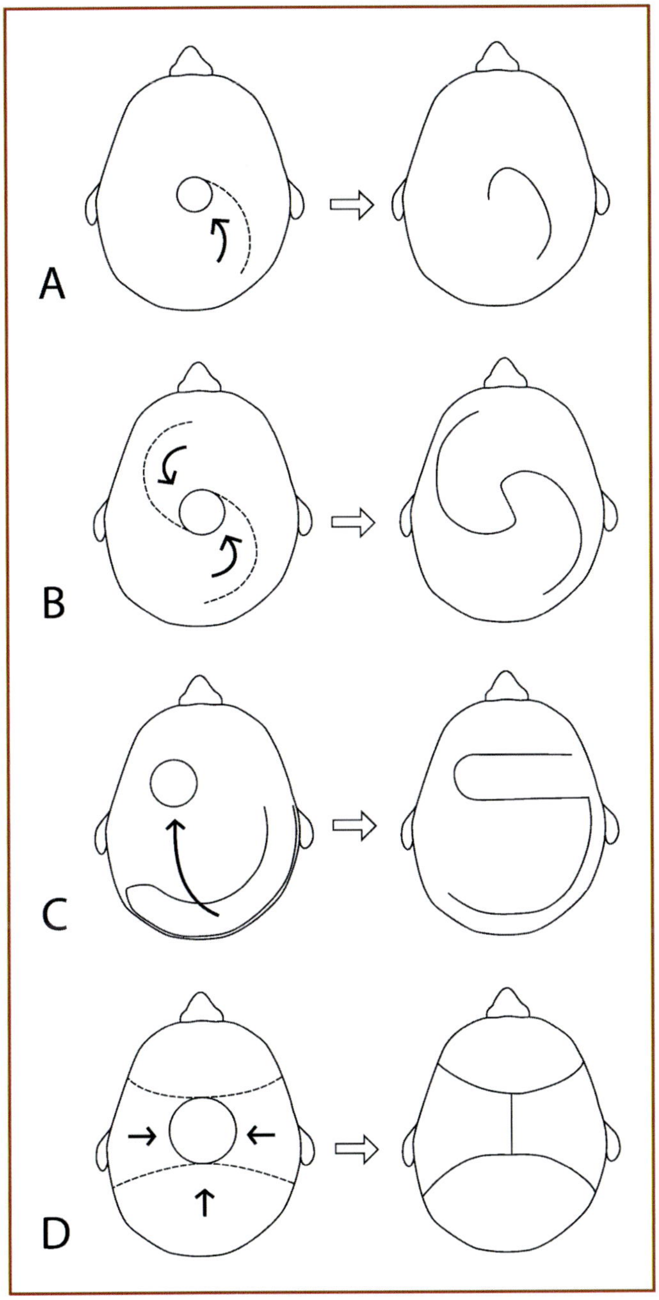

Figure 37–4. Examples of local flaps used in scalp reconstruction. **A.** Rotation flap, **B.** Double opposing rotation flaps (yin-yang flaps), **C.** Juri flap, **D.** Orticochea tripartite flaps.

unlike many other forms of scalp reconstruction.[28] We find that double opposing flaps (the so-called "yin-yang" flap) are most useful for smaller defects up to about 5 to 6 cm in diameter (Fig 37–5).[29] Larger flaps with a broad base that include a named vessel or vascular territory allow for improved survival of the transferred tissue but may require skin grafting of the donor site. For defects of the central scalp, multiple flaps often are necessary.

Orticochea described a four-flap reconstructive technique and later a three-flap technique based on known vascular territories of the scalp to reconstruct defects as large as 30% of the scalp.[30–32] Orticochea's tripartite flap is designed with two smaller advancement flaps on either side of the defect, with each of these advancement flaps having a width at least 50% the width of the defect, and the third flap drawn posterior to the defect to close the donor site created by the other two flaps. The temporoparietal-occipital flaps, as described by Juri, are useful flaps in reconstructing the anterior hairline of the scalp.[33–36] These long flaps are transposed after a delay, and the donor site is closed primarily in the temporal, occipital, and parietal regions. Local flaps should be raised in the subgaleal plane, and careful galeal scoring parallel to the subaponeurotic blood supply and perpendicular to the line of maximal tension may be necessary for gaining increased length and reducing wound tension. Leaving the pericranium intact allows the surgeon to skin graft flap donor site defects when larger flap coverage is necessary (Fig 37–6).[23,37,38] In addition, approximating galea to galea reduces tension on the skin and consequently reduces the amount of alopecia and wound complications that may occur along the incision.

When using a rotation flap, a redundant area of tissue (ie, dog-ear) is often formed at the point of rotation. It is important to resist the temptation to excise this dog-ear during the inset of the rotation flap because this may narrow the base of the flap and ultimately compromise the blood supply, leading to necrosis at the tip of the flap where tissue is most needed. Dog-ears on the scalp often flatten over time and can be excised as necessary in a delayed fashion.[28,39,40] In patients who have had prior radiation therapy, the adjacent scalp tissue may be fibrotic, limiting the use of local flaps.[41,42] Newman et al[38] reported low major complication rates of 3.4% with the use of local flaps for moderate-sized defects (average, 52 $cm^2 \pm 37\ cm^2$) but found an increased overall complication rate (17.1% vs 37.5%)

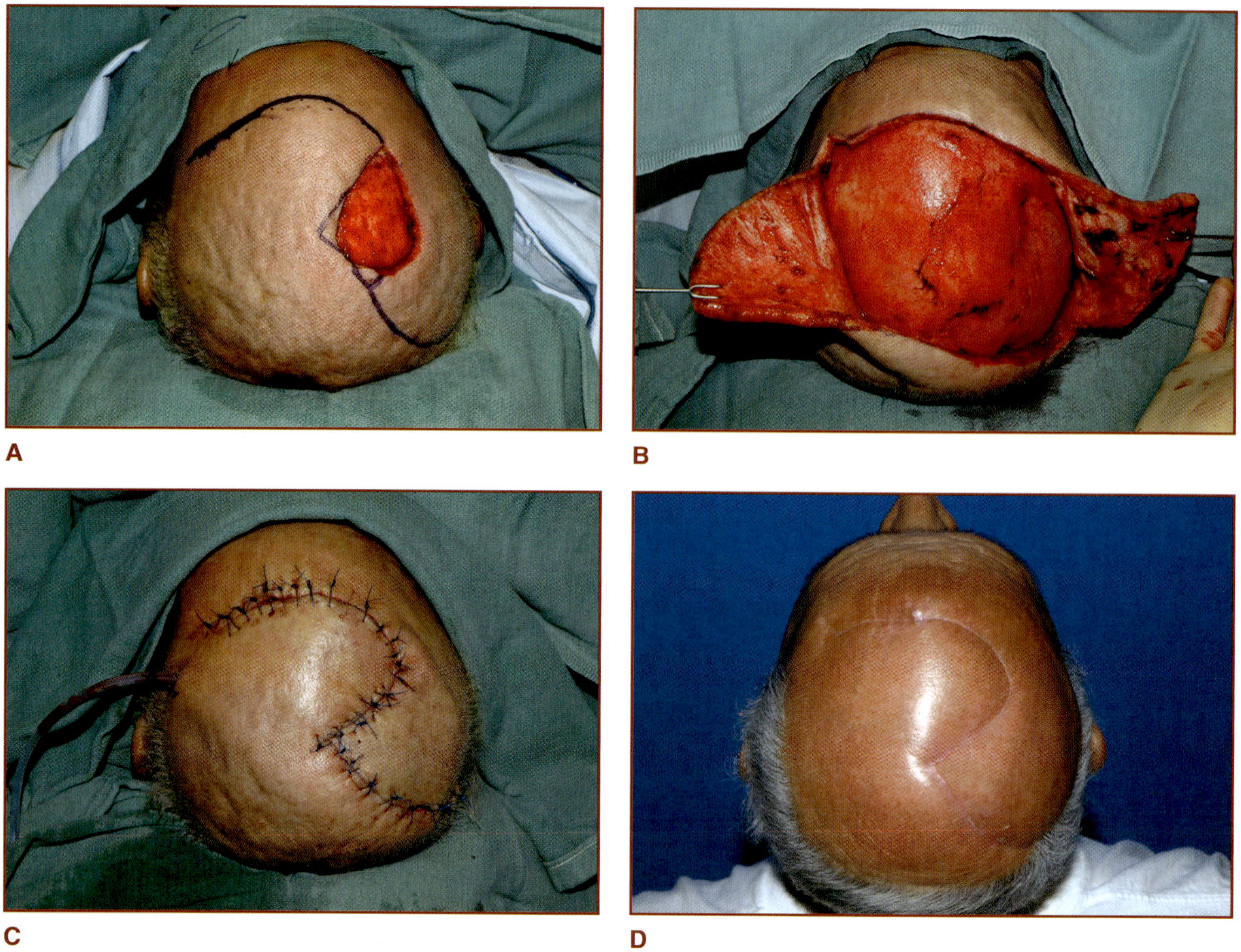

Figure 37–5. A scalp defect after excision of a malignant melanoma (**A**) reconstructed with a "yin-yang" flap (**B** and **C**). **D.** Postoperative result. Matthew M. Hanasono, MD.

in patients who had received prior radiation therapy. In patients receiving postoperative radiation therapy or who need coverage of calvarial reconstructions, the use of local flaps may be limited, and more durable coverage such as free tissue transfer may be required.

Regional Flaps

The application of regional flaps often is limited in scalp reconstruction owing to restrictions in the length and arc of rotation of the available flaps and their vascular pedicles. Regional flaps for coverage of the temporal region include the temporoparietal fascia flap and temporalis muscle flap. Harvesting of the temporalis muscle results in a contour depression at the donor site, unless the flap is split and the anterior third of the muscle is left in situ. The pectoralis major myocutaneous flap, despite being a workhorse in head and neck reconstruction, is limited to the mastoid and temporal regions of the scalp and often requires extensive mobilization including transection of the clavicle and inclusion of

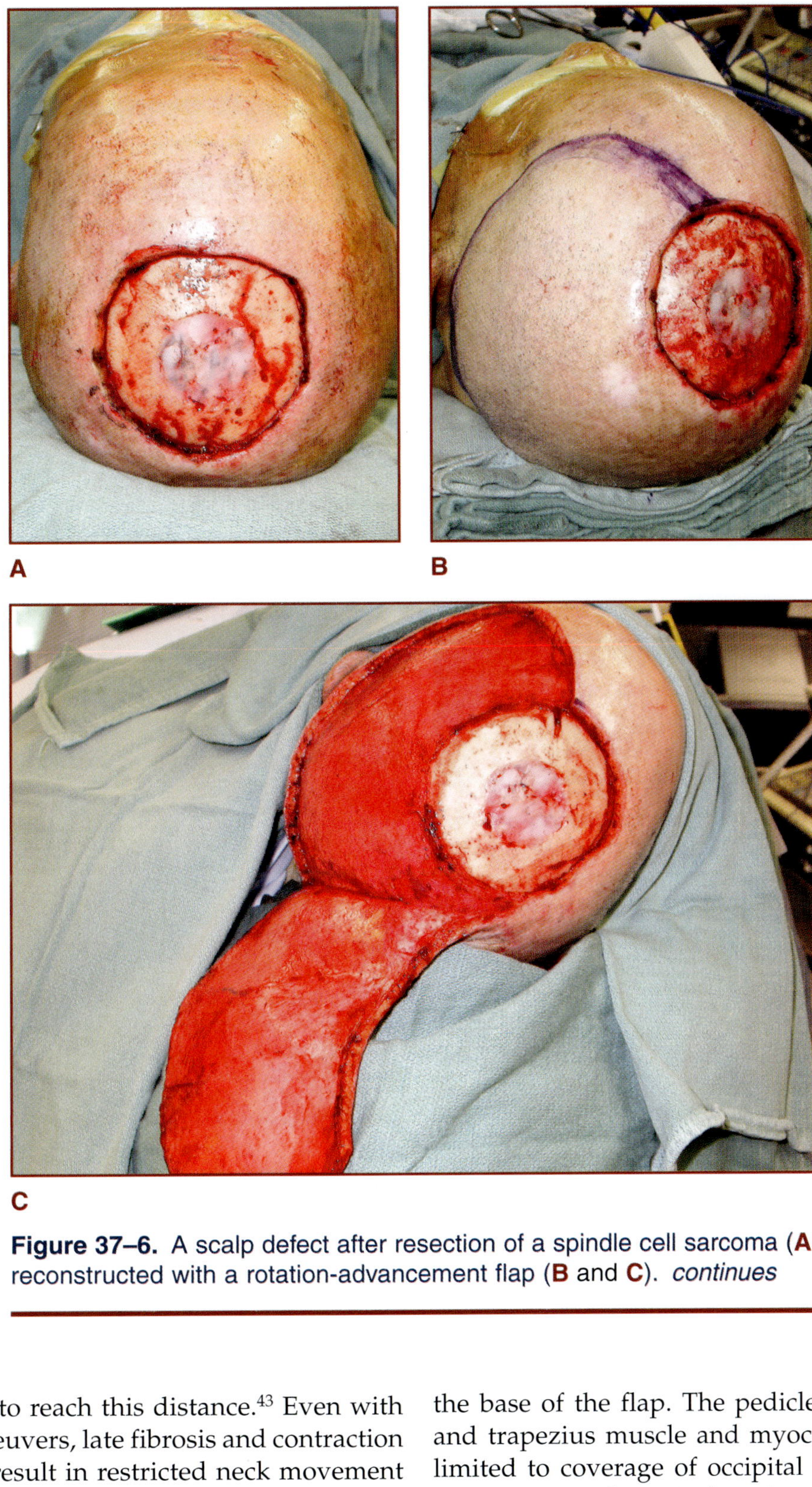

Figure 37–6. A scalp defect after resection of a spindle cell sarcoma (**A**) reconstructed with a rotation-advancement flap (**B** and **C**). *continues*

the rectus fascia to reach this distance.[43] Even with use of these maneuvers, late fibrosis and contraction of the flap may result in restricted neck movement and an unattractive bulge in the lower neck near the base of the flap. The pedicled latissimus dorsi and trapezius muscle and myocutaneous flaps are limited to coverage of occipital scalp defects only. Transverse and vertical variants of the trapezius

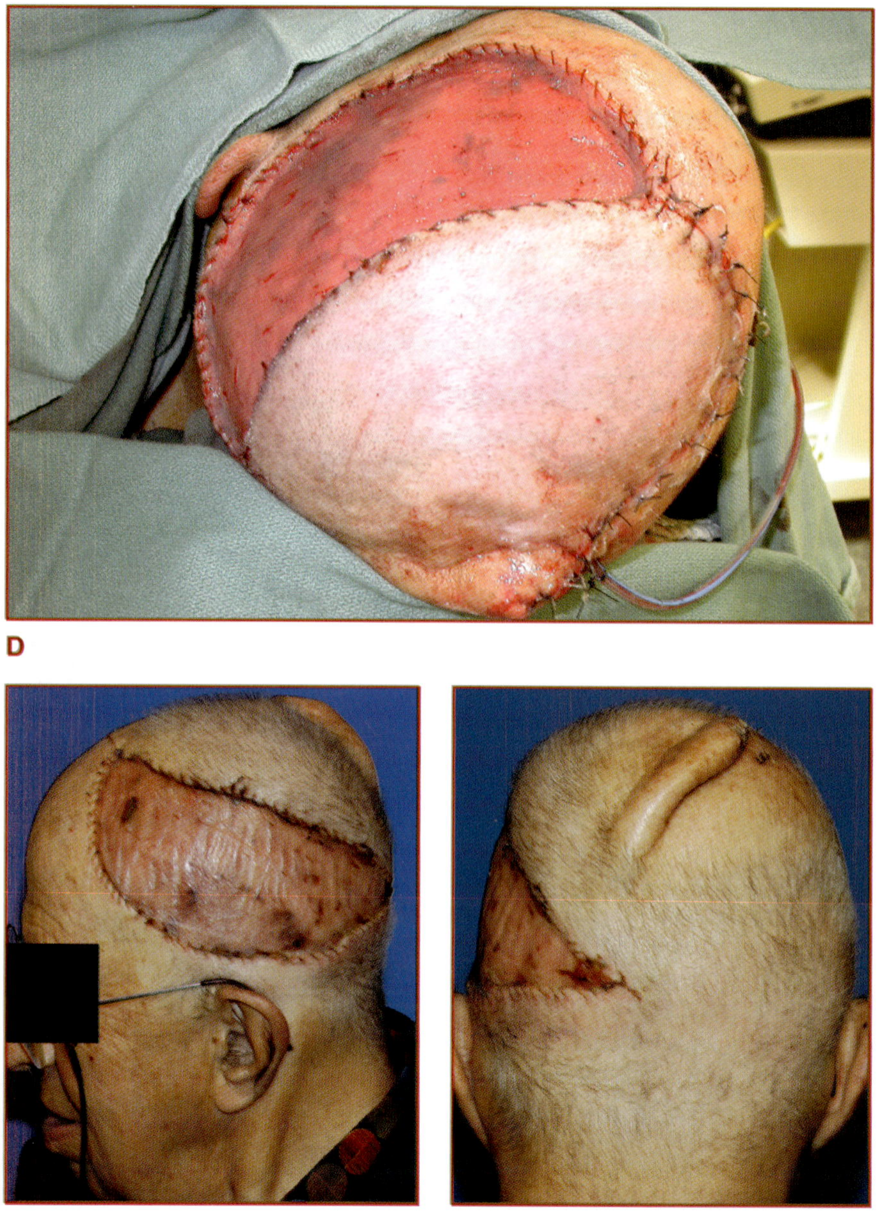

Figure 37–6. *continued* **D.** The donor site defect was reconstructed with a split-thickness skin graft. **E** and **F.** Postoperative result with 100% skin graft take and demonstration of a "dog-ear" at the base of the flap, which can be excised at a later time.

myocutaneous flap have been described. The vertical flap provides posterior coverage of the scalp without the risk of injury to the spinal accessory nerve resulting in shoulder drop, which can occur with harvest of the transverse flap.[44–47]

Microvascular Free Flaps

Microvascular composite free tissue transfer is most often used in large defects when neighboring tissue is unavailable or is compromised from prior radiation therapy, infection, or injury.[48] These flaps also are an excellent option for complex composite wounds with exposed dura and for wound beds with alloplastic plating. Many flaps have been described for scalp reconstruction, the most common being the latissimus dorsi, serratus anterior, scapular and parascapular, radial forearm, omental, rectus abdominis, and, more recently, the anterolateral thigh flap. Studies demonstrating successful reconstruction with free tissue transfer of complex scalp defects are numerous.[49–53] The greater omentum was the first free flap to be described for extensive scalp coverage. The flap requires a skin graft for coverage and provides a pedicle length of up to 12 to 20 cm, which allows for anastomosis to the neck vessels when necessary. Because of the need for a laparotomy to harvest the flap and the risk of postoperative intestinal adhesions, the omental flap has fallen out of favor as a first-line flap.[54,55]

The latissimus dorsi muscle covered with a split-thickness skin graft is the most commonly used flap for extensive scalp defects because it provides relatively thin, broad (maximum muscle dimensions, 40 × 20 cm), and well-vascularized coverage (Fig 37–7).[56,57] The muscle is supplied by the thoracodorsal artery and vein, which arise from the subscapular vessels and can provide up to a 10-cm pedicle length. The muscle atrophies over time, allowing for excellent contour match to the native scalp. In most patients, the donor site morbidity of harvesting this flap is minimal. The latissimus dorsi flap can be harvested with the serratus anterior muscle as a chimeric flap for additional coverage as needed. The serratus anterior muscle can be harvested alone for smaller defect coverage (about 10 × 10 cm), providing muscle coverage and a long pedicle length of approximately 16 cm if the subscapular vessels are included within the pedicle. In addition, the sixth or seventh rib can be harvested with the serratus anterior muscle flap to provide a vascularized segment of bone if there is a calvarial defect.

The rectus abdominis muscle flap with or without a skin paddle is a frequently used flap in scalp reconstruction for mid-sized defects. The flap may be harvested at the same time as the scalp resection and provides coverage for scalp defects smaller (average muscle size, 30 cm long × 6 cm wide) than those covered by the latissimus dorsi muscle flap. The pedicle also is slightly shorter (8 to 10 cm), and the donor site is at some risk of hernias and bulges due to fascial dehiscence and weakening. The flap can be harvested either through a vertical or paramedian incision or, for a more aesthetic donor site scar, thru a low horizontal abdominoplasty-like incision. With any of these incisions, muscle only flaps or flaps including a skin paddle may be harvested, depending on the orientation of the coverage necessary.[58] A muscle-only flap covered with a split-thickness skin graft usually has better aesthetic results due to the amount of subcutaneous adipose tissue in the myocutaneous flap that leads to a bulky reconstruction which does not atrophy with time.

Fasciocutaneous flaps also may be a good option in scalp coverage because of the thin and pliable skin and tissue coverage they provide.[59] The radial forearm fasciocutaneous flap is useful for smaller defects, particularly, those involving the forehead subunit. The flap provides a long pedicle up to 20 cm, which can reach the neck vessels for anastomosis. The donor site often requires a thick split-thickness or full-thickness skin graft for functional and aesthetic coverage. Prior to harvest, a preoperative Allen's test must be performed to confirm that sacrifice of the radial artery will not result in vascular compromise of the hand.[60,61] The parascapular and scapular flaps also have been advocated for scalp coverage and large composite defects involving the face and forehead due to the color match and large skin island that they can provide.[62,63]

The anterolateral thigh flap can be harvested as a fasciocutaneous flap or with a portion of the vastus lateralis muscle for reliable and versatile coverage of extensive or composite scalp defects (Fig 37–8).[64–66] The donor site can be closed either primarily (flaps up to 8 to 10 cm width) or with a skin graft, depending on the dimensions of the flap harvested, with minimal to no functional morbidity. The leg fascia can be harvested with the flap to cover dura mater when calvarial reconstruction is not performed, and the vastus lateralis muscle also can be included to fill dead space when deeper defects exist.[66] Disadvantages of this flap include the fact that not all patients have thin thighs available for harvesting a thin and pliable flap, and anatomic variations of the vascular pedicle exist, sometimes requiring tedious perforator dissection.[67–69] Thinning of the

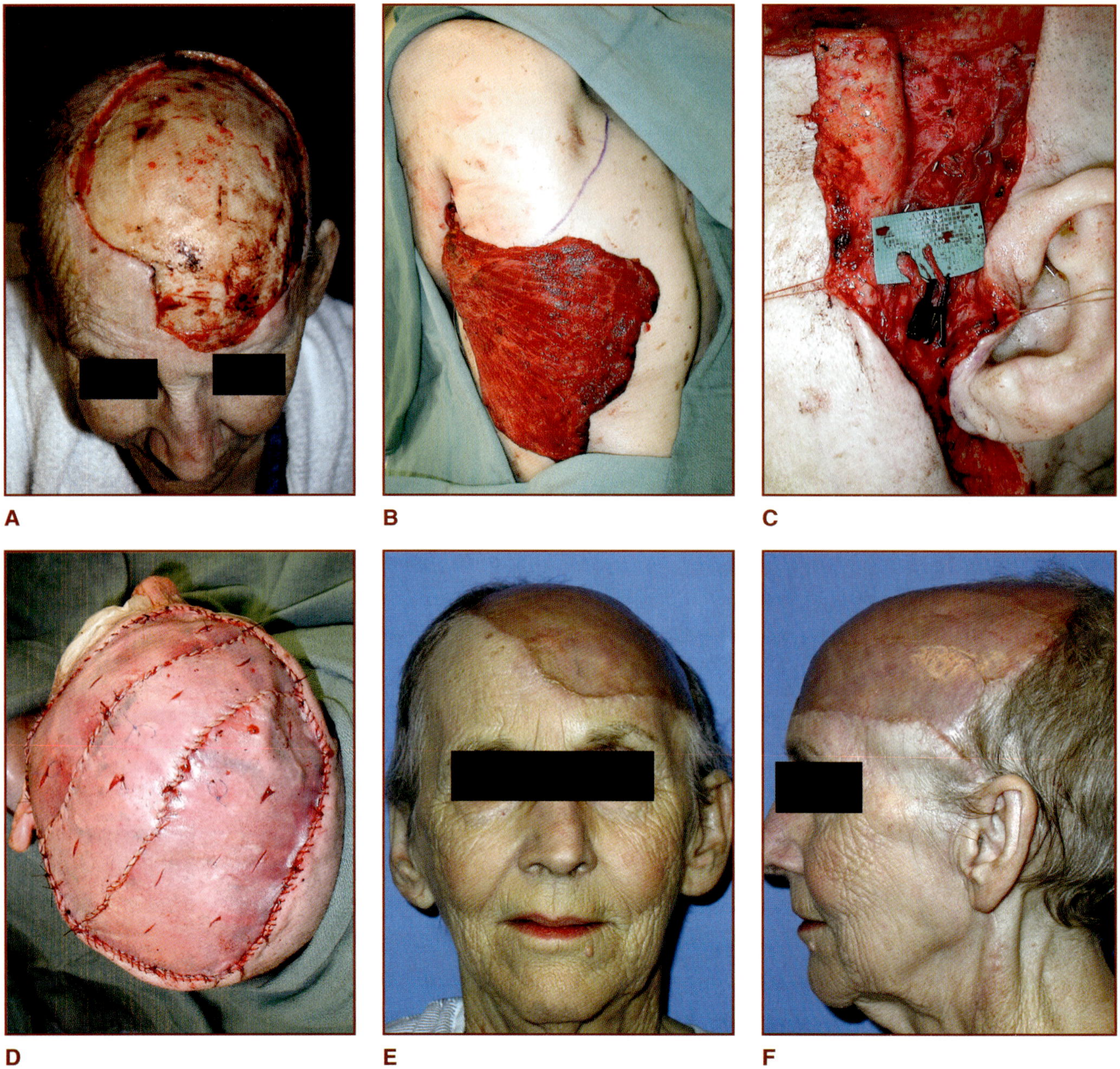

Figure 37–7. A scalp defect after multiple resections for a desmoplastic melanoma (**A**) reconstructed with a free latissimus dorsi muscle flap (**B**) anastomosed to the left superficial temporal vessels (**C**) and covered with a split-thickness skin graft (**D**). **E** and **F.** Postoperative result.

flap intraoperatively has been described, but requires care in order to not injure the perforators within the flap. Preservation of at least 0.5 cm of subcutaneous tissue is recommended to preserve subdermal plexus viability.[67]

Recipient vessels for free tissue transfer to the scalp include the superficial temporal artery and vein as well as multiple branches of the external carotid vascular network. The choice of recipient vessel depends on the defect location, pedicle length

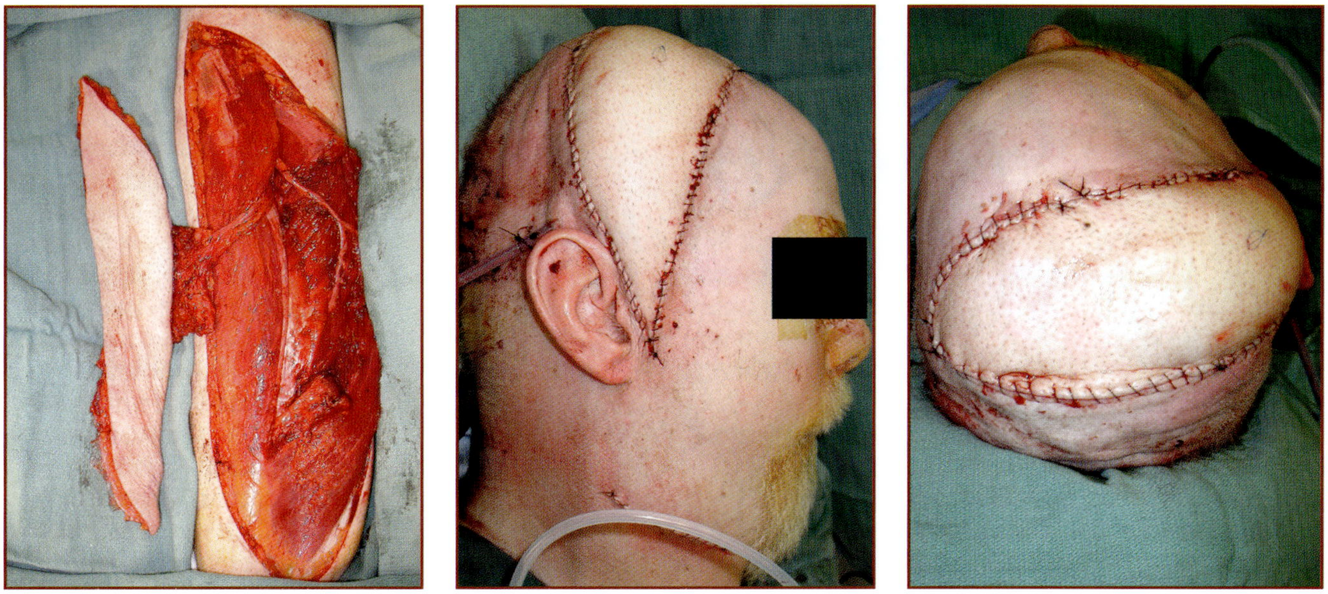

A B C

Figure 37–8. An open scalp wound after tumor resection and radiation therapy, reconstructed with an anterolateral thigh free flap. Right thigh showing flap harvest (**A**) and flap inset to scalp wound (**B** and **C**).

of the harvested flap, and the availability and size of the recipient vessels. The superficial temporal vessels are located anterior to the root of the helix and bifurcate at the level of the superior helix into the frontal and parietal branches.[70] These vessels often are smaller in caliber and require delicate dissection because of the fragile nature of their thin walls. Anastomoses performed as proximal as possible will allow for increased vessel caliber and decreased risk of postoperative vasospasm that often can lead to flap compromise.

If the superficial temporal vasculature is unavailable for anastomosis, branches of the external carotid system can be utilized, but this often requires a long pedicle length or vein grafting to provide the adequate length to reach these recipient vessels. Posteriorly, the occipital artery and vein can be used but are frequently limited by small caliber size. Anteriorly, the facial artery and vein provide good recipient vessels but often require tunneling along the facial skin for pedicle placement.[37] Care must be taken to provide a large enough tunnel to prevent pedicle kinking or compression, which may compromise blood flow to the flap.

Calvarial Reconstruction

Calvarial reconstruction may be necessary if the tumor invades the bony cortex requiring full-thickness excision. Reconstruction using alloplastic materials such as titanium mesh, methyl methacrylate, or prefabricated polymers such as polyetheretherketone (PEEK) is convenient and avoids the need for an autologous donor site.[71] Involvement of a neurosurgeon is important for preventing and monitoring for cerebrospinal fluid leaks, which may compromise reconstructive efforts. Autologous bone grafts such as calvarial grafts or split rib grafts can be used for calvarial reconstruction, but the availability of donor tissue limits this technique to relatively smaller defects. Because of the increased risk of infections associated with nonvascularized bone and alloplastic materials, it is critical that healthy vascularized coverage is available over the calvarial reconstruction. Free flap coverage often is indicated in the setting of prior surgery, infection, or radiation (Fig 37–9).

Some free flaps, such as rib with the serratus anterior muscle as described above, can restore both

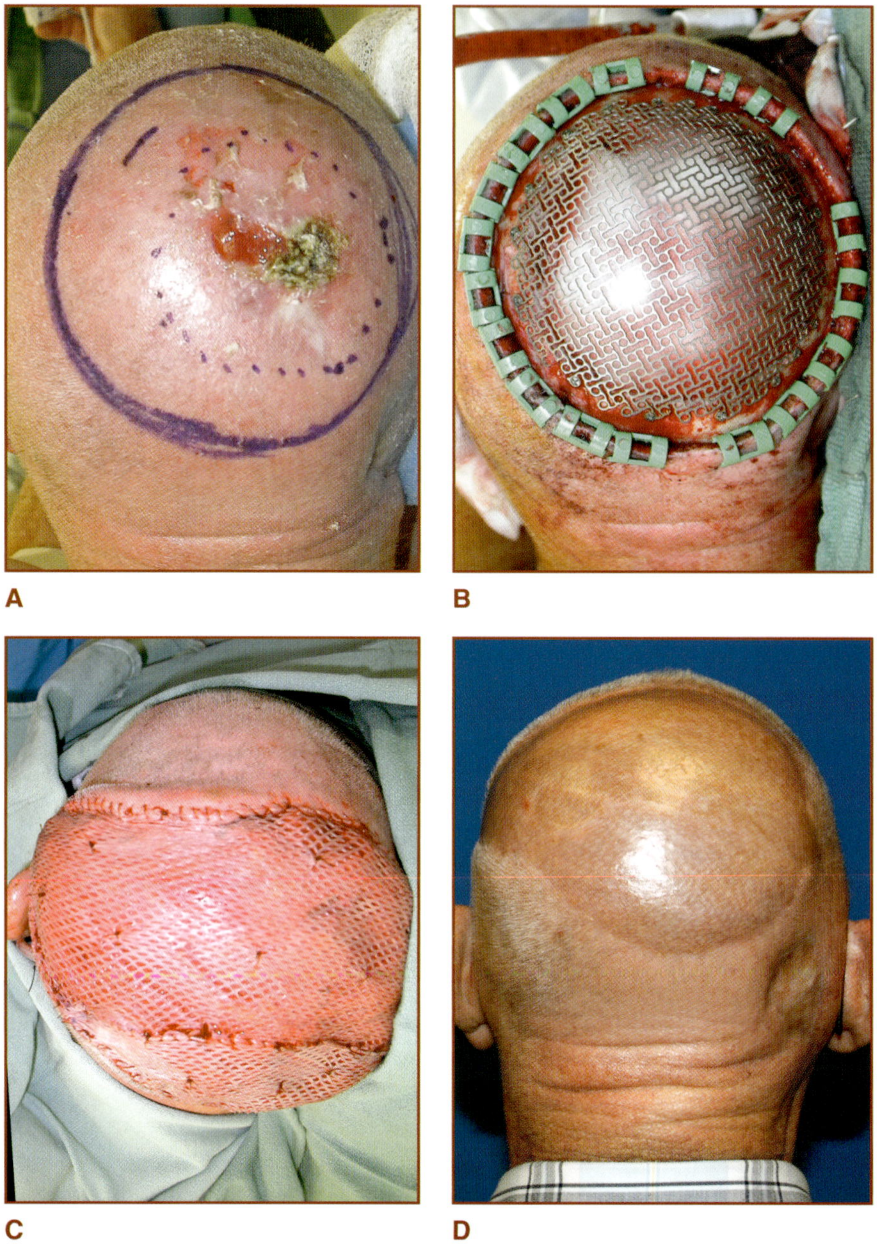

Figure 37–9. **A.** Osteoradionecrosis of the calvarium and open wound after radiation therapy for malignant melanoma of scalp. **B.** The skin and necrotic bone were debrided, and the calvarium was reconstructed with titanium mesh. **C.** A latissimus dorsi muscle free flap and meshed split-thickness skin graft were used for scalp reconstruction. **D.** Postoperative result.

the calvarium and the covering scalp simultaneously. Alternately, calvarial bone pedicled on the superficial temporal vessels by maintaining connections with the superficial temporal fascia and pericranium have been described for small calvarial defects.[72] Of course, such a flap still would still require healthy, well-vascularized coverage with a tension-free closure.

Hair Replacement After Scalp Reconstruction

Hair transplantation can be used to augment reconstructive techniques by camouflaging areas of alopecia that may not be amenable to excision and direct repair or replacement with local hair-bearing flaps. Micrografts (one- to two-hair follicular unit grafts) and minigrafts (three- to four-hair follicular unit grafts) are most commonly used.[73–76] Because of the low metabolic requirement necessary for survival of these small follicular units, growth in areas of tissue fibrosis and even in split-thickness skin grafts is possible. Reports of 85% survival and hair growth in compromised tissue has been published compared with 95% in healthy unscarred tissue.[77]

In addition, survival of follicular unit grafts transplanted into free flaps, such as a skin grafted muscle free flap, approximates 90% and is similar to that of the native scalp.[78] Hair transplantation techniques are usually used in the secondary setting after the initial reconstruction has healed. The grafts are most often harvested from the occipital scalp below a horizontal line that connects the superior aspect of the ears or from the temporal region 5 cm above the superior auricular rim.[79] Often, this can be performed under local anesthesia; however, tedious and meticulous harvest and placement are necessary in multiple sessions over a 6- to 18-month period to accomplish the desired aesthetic result.[78]

Conclusions

The management of extensive scalp defects often is challenging, especially in the setting of oncologic resection and treatment. Less invasive techniques such as primary closure, healing by secondary intention, and skin grafting often are risky in cases in which radiation therapy is given either before or after tumor excision. The use of tissue expansion often requires lengthy preoperative planning and procedures, resulting in limited use as a primary procedure because oncologic resections often require immediate coverage. Local flaps from adjacent scalp tissue are useful in smaller defects. The advent of microvascular tissue transfer has allowed for more oncologic freedom in carrying out extensive scalp and composite resections but requires expertise and the availability of a microvascular surgeon. Extensive preoperative, intraoperative, and postoperative planning and coordination across multiple surgical and medical specialties are often required in determining the appropriate method of reconstruction for successful tumor eradication as well as scalp restoration.

References

1. Tolhurst DE, Carstens MH, Greco RJ, Hurwitz DJ. The surgical anatomy of the scalp. *Plast Reconstr Surg.* 1991; 87:603–612.
2. Mimoun M, Chaouat M, Picovski D, et al. The scalp is an advantageous donor site for thin-skin grafts: a report on 945 harvested samples. *Plast Reconstr Surg.* 2006;118: 369–373.
3. Mitz V, Peyronie M. The superficial musculo-aponeurotic system (SMAS) in the parotid and cheek area. *Plast Reconstr Surg.* 1976;58:80–88.
4. Jost G, Levet Y. Parotid fascia and face lifting: a critical evaluation of the SMAS concept. *Plast Reconstr Surg.* 1984;74:42–51.
5. Minor LB, Panje WR. Malignant neoplasms of the scalp. Etiology, resection, and reconstruction. *Otolaryngol Clin North Am.* 1993;26:279–293.
6. Millard DR. The crane principle for the transport of subcutaneous tissue. *Plast Reconstr Surg.* 1969;43:451–462.
7. Seyhan A, Yoleri L, Barutcu A. Immediate hair transplantation into a newly closed wound to conceal the final scar on the hair-bearing skin. *Plast Reconstr Surg.* 2000; 105:1866–1870; discussion 1871.
8. Snow SN, Stiff MA, Bullen R, et al. Second-intention healing of exposed facial-scalp bone after Mohs surgery for skin cancer: review of ninety-one cases. *J Am Acad Dermatol.* 1994;31:450–454.
9. Becker GD, Adams LA, Levin BC. Secondary intention healing of exposed scalp and forehead bone after Mohs surgery. *Otolaryngol Head Neck Surg.* 1999;121:751–754.
10. Terkonda RP, Sykes JM. Concepts in scalp and forehead reconstruction. *Otolaryngol Clin North Am.* 1997;30:519–539.
11. Jackson IT. (Ed.). *Local Flaps in Head and Neck Reconstruction.* St. Louis, MO: Mosby; 1985.
12. Raposio E, Santi P, Nordstrom RE. Effects of galeotomies on scalp flaps. *Ann Plast Surg.* 1998;41:17–21.
13. Chandawarkar RY, Cervino AL, Pennington GA. Intraoperative acute tissue expansion revisited: a valuable tool for challenging skin defects. *Dermatol Surg.* 2003;29: 834–838.

14. Hoffmann JF. Tissue expansion in the head and neck. *Facial Plast Surg Clin North Am.* 2005;13:315–324.
15. Sasaki GH. Intraoperative sustained limited expansion (ISLE) as an immediate reconstructive technique. *Clin Plast Surg.* 1987;14:563–573.
16. Siegert R, Weerda H, Hoffmann S, et al. Clinical and experimental evaluation of intermittent intraoperative short-term expansion. *Plast Reconstr Surg.* 1993;92: 248–254.
17. Sheridan RL, Choucair RJ, Donelan MB. Management of massive calvarial exposure in young children. *J Burn Care Rehabil.* 1998;19:29–32.
18. Molnar JA, DeFranzo AJ, Marks MW. Single-stage approach to skin grafting the exposed skull. *Plast Reconstr Surg.* 2000;105:174–177.
19. Gurlek A, Alaybeyoglu N, Demir CY, et al. Aesthetic reconstruction of large scalp defects by sequential tissue expansion without interval. *Aesthetic Plast Surg.* 2004;28: 245–250.
20. Manders EK, Graham WP 3rd, Schenden MJ, et al. Skin expansion to eliminate large scalp defects. *Ann Plast Surg.* 1984;12:305–312.
21. van Rappard JH, Molenaar J, van Doorn K, et al. Surface-area increase in tissue expansion. *Plast Reconstr Surg.* 1988;82:833–839.
22. Bilkay U, Kerem H, Ozek C, et al. Alopecia treatment with scalp expansion: some surgical fine points and a simple modification to improve the results. *J Craniofac Surg.* 2004;15:758–765.
23. Leedy JE, Janis JE, Rohrich RJ. Reconstruction of acquired scalp defects: an algorithmic approach. *Plast Reconstr Surg.* 2005;116:54e–72e.
24. Saxby PJ. Survival of island flaps after tissue expansion: a pig model. *Plast Reconstr Surg.* 1988;81:30–34.
25. Antonyshyn O, Gruss JS, Zuker R, et al. Tissue expansion in head and neck reconstruction. *Plast Reconstr Surg.* 1988;82:58–68.
26. Antonyshyn O, Gruss JS, Mackinnon SE, et al. Complications of soft tissue expansion. *Br J Plast Surg.* 1988;41: 239–250.
27. El-Saadi MM, Nasr MA. The effect of tissue expansion on skull bones in the paediatric age group from 2 to 7 years. *J Plast Reconstr Aesthet Surg.* 2008;61:413–418.
28. Lesavoy MA, Dubrow TJ, Schwartz RJ, et al. Management of large scalp defects with local pedicle flaps. *Plast Reconstr Surg.* 1993;91:783–790.
29. Ahuja RB. Geometric considerations in the design of rotation flaps in the scalp and forehead region. *Plast Reconstr Surg.* 1988;81:900–906.
30. Orticochea M. Four flap scalp reconstruction technique. *Br J Plast Surg.* 1967;20:159–171.
31. Orticochea M. New three-flap reconstruction technique. *Br J Plast Surg.* 1971;24:184–188.
32. Arnold PG, Rangarathnam CS. Multiple-flap scalp reconstruction: orticochea revisited. *Plast Reconstr Surg.* 1982;69:605–613.
33. Juri C, Juri J, Colnago A. Monopedicled transposition flap for the treatment of traumatic scalp alopecias. *Ann Plast Surg.* 1980;4:349–356.
34. Juri J, Juri C. Aesthetic aspects of reconstructive scalp surgery. *Clin Plast Surg.* 1981;8:243–254.
35. Juri J, Juri C, Arufe HN. Use of rotation scalp flaps for treatment of occipital baldness. *Plast Reconstr Surg.* 1978; 61:23–26.
36. Juri J, Juri C, Colnago A. Reconstruction of scalp hemi-circumference. *Ann Plast Surg.* 1980;4:304–309.
37. Mehrara BJ, Disa JJ, Pusic A. Scalp reconstruction. *J Surg Oncol.* 2006;94:504–508.
38. Newman MI, Hanasono MM, Disa JJ, et al. Scalp reconstruction: a 15-year experience. *Ann Plast Surg.* 2004;52: 501–506; discussion 506.
39. Baker SR, Johnson TM, Nelson BR. Technical aspects of prolonged scalp expansion. *Arch Otolaryngol Head Neck Surg.* 1994;120:431–436.
40. Byrd HS. The use of subcutaneous axial fascial flaps in reconstruction of the head. *Ann Plast Surg.* 1980;4:191–198.
41. Oishi SN, Luce EA. The difficult scalp and skull wound. *Clin Plast Surg.* 1995;22:51–59.
42. Nair S, Giannakopoulos G, Granick M, et al. Surgical management of radiated scalp in patients with recurrent glioma. *Neurosurgery.* 1994;34:103–106; discussion 106–107.
43. Wells MD. Scalp Reconstruction. In: Mathes SJ, ed. *Plastic Surgery.* Vol. 3. Philadelphia, PA: Elsevier, Inc; 2006: 613–632.
44. Yang D, Morris SF. Trapezius muscle: anatomic basis for flap design. *Ann Plast Surg.* 1998;41:52–57.
45. Lynch JR, Hansen JE, Chaffoo R, et al. The lower trapezius musculocutaneous flap revisited: versatile coverage for complicated wounds to the posterior cervical and occipital regions based on the deep branch of the transverse cervical artery. *Plast Reconstr Surg.* 2002;109:444–450.
46. Mathes SJ, Stevenson TR. Reconstruction of posterior neck and skull with vertical trapezius musculocutaneous flap. *Am J Surg.* 1988;156:248–251.
47. Ozbek MR, Kutlu N. Vertical trapezius myocutaneous flap for covering wide scalp defects. *Handchir Mikrochir Plast Chir.* 1990;22:326–329.
48. Lutz BS, Wei FC, Chen HC, et al. Reconstruction of scalp defects with free flaps in 30 cases. *Br J Plast Surg.* 1998; 51:186–190.
49. Beasley NJ, Gilbert RW, Gullane PJ, et al. Scalp and forehead reconstruction using free revascularized tissue transfer. *Arch Facial Plast Surg.* 2004;6:16–20.
50. Wang HT, Erdmann D, Olbrich KC, et al. Free flap reconstruction of the scalp and calvaria of major neurosurgical resections in cancer patients: lessons learned closing large, difficult wounds of the dura and skull. *Plast Reconstr Surg.* 2007;119:865–872.
51. McCombe D, Donato R, Hofer SO, et al. Free flaps in the treatment of locally advanced malignancy of the scalp and forehead. *Ann Plast Surg.* 2002;48:600–606.

52. Hussussian CJ, Reece GP. Microsurgical scalp reconstruction in the patient with cancer. *Plast Reconstr Surg.* 2002;109:1828–1834.
53. Furnas H, Lineaweaver WC, Alpert BS, et al. Scalp reconstruction by microvascular free tissue transfer. *Ann Plast Surg.* 1990;24:431–444.
54. McLean DH, Buncke HJ Jr. Autotransplant of omentum to a large scalp defect, with microsurgical revascularization. *Plast Reconstr Surg.* 1972;49:268–274.
55. Losken A, Carlson GW, Culbertson JH, et al. Omental free flap reconstruction in complex head and neck deformities. *Head Neck.* 2002;24:326–331.
56. Lipa JE, Butler CE. Enhancing the outcome of free latissimus dorsi muscle flap reconstruction of scalp defects. *Head Neck.* 2004;26:46–53.
57. Gordon L, Buncke HJ, Alpert BS. Free latissimus dorsi muscle flap with split-thickness skin graft cover: a report of 16 cases. *Plast Reconstr Surg.* 1982;70:173–178.
58. Borah GL, Hidalgo DA, Wey PD. Reconstruction of extensive scalp defects with rectus free flaps. *Ann Plast Surg.* 1995;34:281–285; discussion 285–287.
59. Guerrissi JO. Reconstruction of large defects in the scalp with fasciocutaneous flaps. *Scand J Plast Reconstr Surg Hand Surg.* 1999;33:217–224.
60. Lutz BS, Chang SC, Chuang SS, et al. [Supra-fascial elevated free forearm flap—indications, surgical technique and follow-up examination of the donor site defect]. *Handchir Mikrochir Plast Chir.* 1999;31:10–14.
61. Chicarilli ZN, Ariyan S, Cuono CB. Single-stage repair of complex scalp and cranial defects with the free radial forearm flap. *Plast Reconstr Surg.* 1986;77:577–585.
62. Chiu DT, Sherman JE, Edgerton BW. Coverage of the calvarium with a free parascapular flap. *Ann Plast Surg.* 1984;12:60–66.
63. Batchelor AG, Sully LA. Multiple territory free tissue transfer for reconstruction of a large scalp defect. *Br J Plast Surg.* 1984;37:76–79.
64. Heller F, Hsu CM, Chuang CC, et al. Anterolateral thigh fasciocutaneous flap for simultaneous reconstruction of refractory scalp and dural defects. Report of two cases. *J Neurosurg.* 2004;100:1094–1097.
65. Lutz BS, Wei FC. Microsurgical workhorse flaps in head and neck reconstruction. *Clin Plast Surg.* 2005;32:421–430, vii.
66. Ozkan O, Coskunfirat OK, Ozgentas HE, et al. Rationale for reconstruction of large scalp defects using the anterolateral thigh flap: structural and aesthetic outcomes. *J Reconstr Microsurg.* 2005;21:539–545.
67. Yu P. Characteristics of the anterolateral thigh flap in a Western population and its application in head and neck reconstruction. *Head Neck.* 2004;26:759–769.
68. Kimata Y, Uchiyama K., Ebihara S, et al. Anatomic variations and technical problems of the anterolateral thigh flap: a report of 74 cases. *Plast Reconstr Surg.* 1998;102:1517–1523.
69. Koshima I, Fukuda H, Utunomiya R, et al. The anterolateral thigh flap; variations in its vascular pedicle. *Br J Plast Surg.* 1989;42:260–262.
70. Pinar YA, Govsa F. Anatomy of the superficial temporal artery and its branches: its importance for surgery. *Surg Radiol Anat.* 2006;28:248–253.
71. Blake GB, MacFarlane MR, Hinton JW. Titanium in reconstructive surgery of the skull and face. *Br J Plast Surg.* 1990;43:528–535.
72. McCarthy JG, Zide BM. The spectrum of calvarial bone grafting: introduction of the vascularized calvarial bone flap. *Plast Reconstr Surg.* 1984;74:10–18.
73. Lucas MW. Recent advances in hair transplantation. *Skin Pharmacol.* 1994;7:105–108.
74. Vogel JE. Correction of the cornrow hair transplant and other common problems in surgical hair restoration. *Plast Reconstr Surg.* 2000;105:1528–1536; discussion 1537–1541.
75. Barrera A. The use of micrografts and minigrafts for the correction of the postrhytidectomy lost sideburn. *Plast Reconstr Surg.* 1998;102:2237–2240.
76. Barrera A. Face lift and hair transplantation as a single procedure. *Plast Reconstr Surg.* 1999;104:1831–1838.
77. Barrera A. The use of micrografts and minigrafts in the aesthetic reconstruction of the face and scalp. *Plast Reconstr Surg.* 2003;112:883–890.
78. Blackwell KE, Rawnsley JD. Aesthetic considerations in scalp reconstruction. *Facial Plast Surg.* 2008;24:11–21.
79. Lee S, Rafii AA, Sykes J. Advances in scalp reconstruction. *Curr Opin Otolaryngol Head Neck Surg.* 2006;14:249–253.

38

RECONSTRUCTION OF THE CHEEK

ANUJA K. ANTONY
BABAK J. MEHRARA

Introduction

The cheek constitutes a significant portion of the face. The large surface area of the cheek renders it susceptible to sun damage and resultant cancers, which require extirpation and reconstruction. Similarly, traumatic injuries to the cheek are common given its relative prominence. The inherent mobility of the cheek often allows for a simple and straightforward approach for closure after tumor removal, or repair, although more elegant methods of reconstruction may be needed when more substantial defects arise. This chapter outlines the principles of cheek reconstruction, from aesthetic and anatomic considerations to more specific reconstructive options. In particular, meticulous planning is required to restore the natural contour of the cheek, with attention paid to the hair-bearing pattern and skin's color, texture, and tension lines. Ideally, reconstruction is planned with respect to these factors.

Anatomy

The cheek is less amenable to aesthetic unit analysis than other facial regions as shadow lines are less prominent. However, the cheek may be defined as extending from the superior border at the infraorbital crease and zygomatic arch to the inferior border of the mandible, and medially from the nasofacial sulcus and nasolabial border, to the preauricular crease laterally. Jackson[1] has divided the cheek into five reconstructive zones based on anatomic characteristics and reconstructive techniques (lateral, lower, malar, superomedial, and alar base-nasolabial). Likewise, Roth et al[2] has divided the cheek into three overlapping zones, suborbital, preauricular, and buccomandibular, based on reconstructive principles. Such classification schemes can be useful for surgical planning, but application of subunit principles used for other areas of the face (eg, discarding entire units if more than 50% is missing, as in nasal reconstruction) is less suitable. In general, incision planning will consider anatomic boundaries, which can serve as a repository for incisional scars, and lines of tension paramount for scar camouflage.

The motor innervation of the superficial muscles of the face is provided by the facial nerve. The motor nerve deep to the parotid is protected by the parotid's masseteric fascia and superficial lobe. After exiting the parotid gland, the facial nerve divides into five major branches (temporal, zygomatic, buccal, marginal mandibular, cervical) that travel more superficially under the superficial musculoaponeurotic system (SMAS) fascia and the cutaneous layers of the skin. The trigeminal nerve innervates the masseter and temporalis muscles. Sensory innervation to the cheek is provided by the maxillary and mandibular divisions of the trigeminal nerve, as well as minor contributions from the cervical plexus via the anterior cutaneous nerve of the neck and the great auricular nerve. Deeper excisions of the cheek extending into the parotid gland may warrant special consideration with intraoperative nerve stimulation. Sequelae of facial nerve injury in more superficial zones of susceptibility include brow ptosis from injury to the temporal branch as it crosses the zygoma, and inability to depress the lower lip due to injury of the marginal mandibular as it crosses the mandible. Overlapping innervation and the deeper lie of the zygomatic and buccal branches usually mitigates some of the negative consequences resulting from injury secondary to extirpation near these branches.

The arterial supply of the cheek is afforded by a well-arborized blood supply arising from branches of the external carotid, including the facial artery, the superficial temporal artery, and the transverse facial artery. Such abundant blood supply minimizes risk of devascularization to the skin in cases of transection of any one vessel. Venous drainage follows the arterial supply. Lymphatic drainage is provided along facial vessels to the submandibular nodes and the lymphatic channels within the parotid nodes. The central region of the cheek also accommodates the parotid duct as it emerges from the parotid gland to exit intraorally. Any suspected injury to the parotid duct should be investigated to prevent potential for a chronically draining sinus.

Defect Analysis

For any given defect, several reconstructive options may be tenable. Analysis of the defect or anticipated defect is vital to the reconstructive process. Defects may be simple, including only superficial structures such as skin and fat, or may be more complex, involving deeper structures such as facial musculature, nervous components, mucosa, and bone. Such complex defects may arise from more invasive superficial cancers, advanced intraoral cancers, or trauma. A like-for-like approach to replace missing structures with similar donor tissue may be utilized when feasible. Thus, as with other areas of the face, reconstruction for all layers should be planned to reconstruct appropriate lining, support, and coverage. Complex reconstructions may require a staged approach to achieve the best possible aesthetic contour. Facial nerve resection should be anticipated if possible, and tagging of nerve ends at the time of resection can facilitate later identification and repair. Nerve grafts from appropriate donor sites may be required from local (ansa cervicalis, great auricular nerve), or distant (sural nerve) locations. For defects acquired from trauma, coexisting injuries should be ruled out.

Optimal reconstruction should be based on the defect and its relationship to the surrounding structures, hair-bearing features, skin tension lines, natural wrinkles, laxity, and previous scars. Surgical incision planning ideally utilizes skin tension lines and the natural borders of the cheek to conceal scars. Care is taken to avoid distortion to hair-bearing regions (beard, sideburns) and rotating hair-bearing skin into non-hair-bearing regions. Similarly, contour irregularities and color mismatch often can be avoided with careful planning. Cheek reconstruction requires awareness of the surrounding anatomic structures such as the lower eyelid, upper lip, and oral commissure. Distortion of these structures should be avoided if possible because disfigurement may result; in particular, tension in the eyelid region can result in an immediate or delayed ectropion. Longaker and colleagues[3] indicated that incisions along the nasolabial fold or by blepharoplasty should replace vertical incisions placed medial to a line drawn from the lateral canthus, because such incisions provide inferior results and remain obvious on frontal view.

Other considerations include previous radiation, level of contamination, and definitive pathological results. A history of radiation therapy may prohibit local flap reconstruction. Contaminated wounds may require serial debridement and dressing care until an appropriate reduction in bacterial content is achieved. In the same way, confirmed final pathology with negative margins should be realized if technically possible before definitive reconstruction is carried out. However, in the case of extensive resection with exposure of vital structures, frozen sections may be beneficial in proceeding with the reconstruction.

Reconstructive Options

Closure by Secondary Intention

Secondary intention healing may be useful for small superficial defects sometimes seen after Mohs micrographic resection. These defects usually are in the epidermis or superficial dermis without exposure of subcutaneous fat. Selected, slightly deeper defects along the borders of the cheek or in concave regions (infraorbital, preauricular) also may fare reasonably well with this method of healing. This method of obtaining closure may be the simplest option but has limited applicability for larger, more conspicuous defects. Closure by secondary intention may result in unstable coverage with contour irregularities and distortion of adjacent structures, yielding a suboptimal aesthetic and functional outcome. Furthermore, larger defects may require a protracted period of time to achieve closure, with associated time-consuming wound management and dressings.

Primary Closure

For small defects of the cheek, primary closure is often the reconstructive method of choice. With this method of closure, typically an elliptical excision is planned with the resultant scar kept along lines of minimal tension or natural cheek borders (eg, nasolabial fold). An excellent result can be obtained if a minimal tension or tension-free closure without excessive distortion of surrounding structures can be achieved. In elderly patients with increased skin laxity, significant defects can be closed with tissue undermining. Primary closure offers the benefits of relative ease of closure, rapid healing time, reduced donor tissue deformity, and avoidance of interpolating tissue from distant sites. Disadvantages include possible creation of a long, linear scar and dog-ears, which may require further lengthening of the scar for excision.

Skin Grafts

In some instances, a full-thickness skin graft can be a reasonable option for obtaining wound closure. In particular, when presented with a high-risk patient with multiple comorbidities or defects awaiting final pathologic results, a skin graft may be utilized for temporary (eg, for tumor surveillance, prior to definitive reconstruction) or permanent closure. Similarly, areas of the cheek that are not noticeable at conversational distance (ie, preauricular area) are well treated with full-thickness skin grafts. The use of skin grafts in other areas, however, may result in discrepancies in skin color or texture and secondary graft contracture. Graft contracture is particularly a problem with split-thickness or very thin full-thickness grafts. In addition, skin grafts are typically associated with shiny, patchlike areas and poor contour match. However, careful attention to harvest site depth and location may facilitate improved results. Similarly, harvesting grafts from the preauricular/postauricular, neck and upper back regions may enhance color and texture match to the native excised skin.

Advancement Flaps

Advancement flaps are random pattern flaps based off blood supply from the subcutaneous plane and typically carried out as a V-Y advancement or with excision of Burrow's triangles (Fig 38–1). A Burrow's advancement flap with a component of rotation can be helpful for preauricular defects, providing a vertical incision line in or parallel to the preauricular sulcus. Similarly, defects arising from the alar base or medial cheek may be reconstructed using these local flaps, as they reduce potential distortion from a primary closure. Near the eyelid margin or nasal base, anchoring of the flap to periosteum (maxillary, zygomatic) may prevent subsequent ectropion or nostril flare. Typically, defects are best excised as a rectangle or square to prevent trapdoor deformity and a flap base-to-length width of 1 to 1 can be considered safe to avoid tip necrosis. Furthermore, flap length is often estimated such that minimal tension on the closure results.

An advancement flap termed the *cervicofacial hike* described by Roth et al,[2] based on the SMAS blood supply similar to the deep plane rhytidectomy, advances the cheek unit superiorly while incorporating blepharoplasty incisions to remove

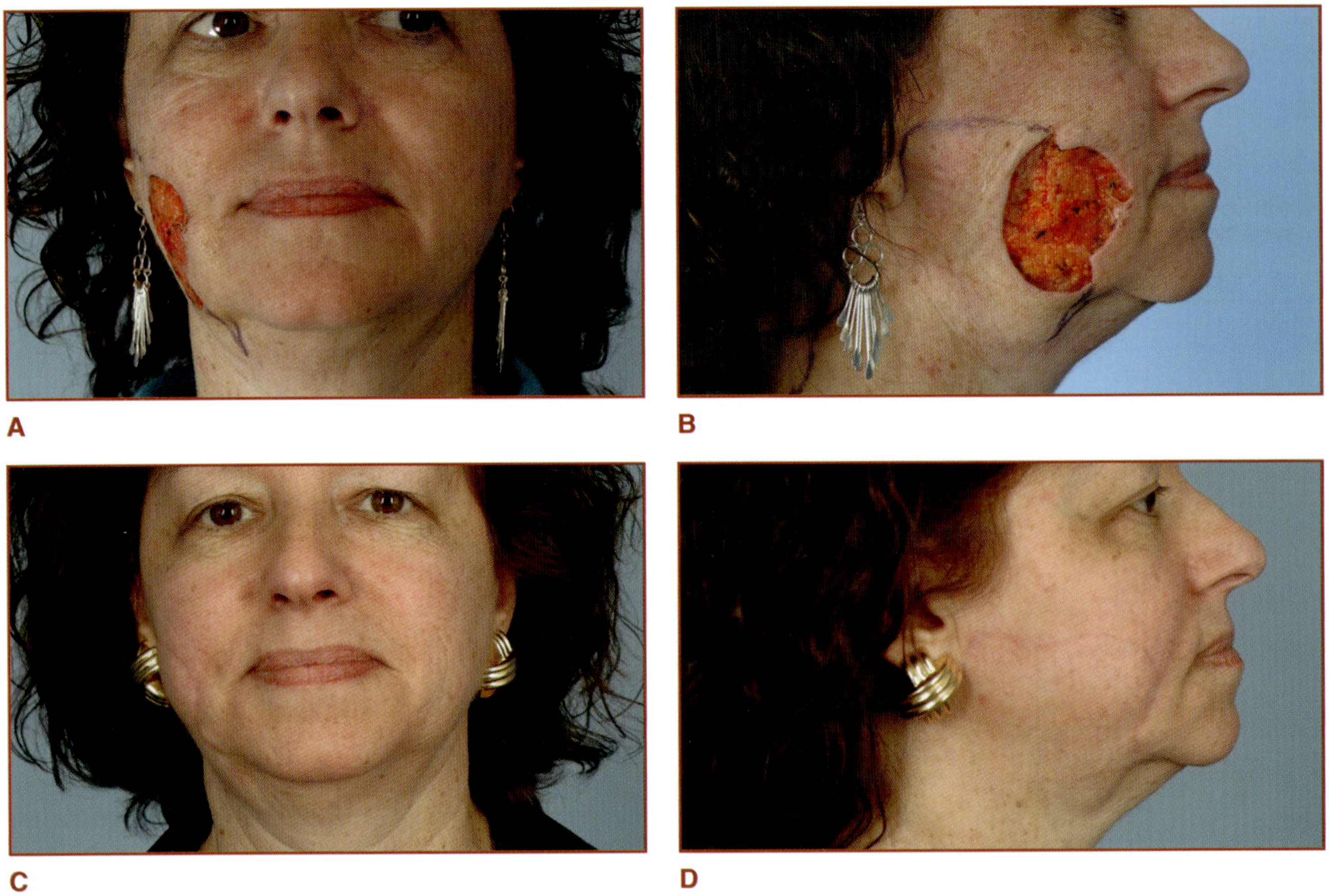

Figure 38–1. Advancement flap closure of medium sized cheek defect. **A** and **B.** Preoperative views after excision with final negative margins for malignant melanoma in situ. **C** and **D.** Postoperative result at 8 months.

residual dog-ears in a cosmetically acceptable fashion. The vertically advanced flap must be slightly overcorrected by anchoring the flap to the periosteum just above the recipient defect, thereby removing all tension from the skin and preventing ectropion.[3] Alternatively, the blepharoplasty incisions may facilitate tension-free closure by transposing redundant upper eyelid skin to the lower lid tissue defect. A vertical spreading technique in the region of the facial nerve is performed to prevent injury from sharp dissection, while still allowing for cheek advancement.

Transposition Flaps

Transposition flaps provide a method of borrowing skin from a reservoir of excess tissue to repair a defect in an area of relative tissue deficiency. The residual skin laxity in the initial donor site allows for a primary closure after flap transfer. The more common transposition flaps, banner flaps, bilobed flaps, and rhomboid flaps, are useful for medium to large cheek defects. Placement of donor scars along relaxed skin tension lines or aesthetic unit boundaries can yield good results, as they accomplish redistribution and redirection of tension. In addition, careful selection of patients can reduce potential pitfalls (pin cushioning, hair distortion, complex scars).

Banner Flaps

Banner flaps are a popular version of the transposition flap. Here, a finger-shaped random pattern flap from adjacent lax skin is transferred such that the

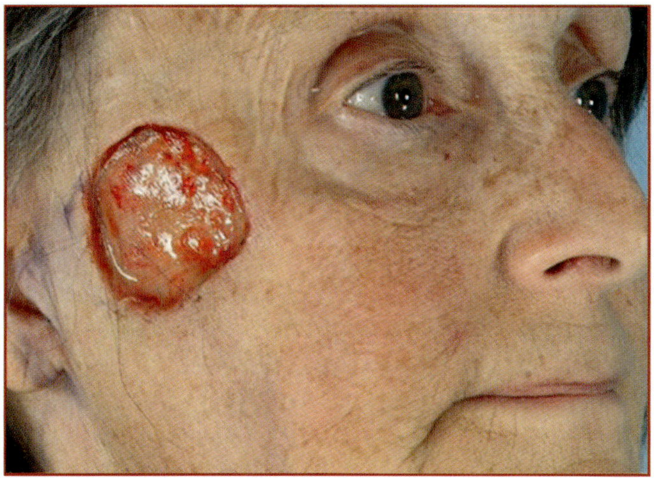

A

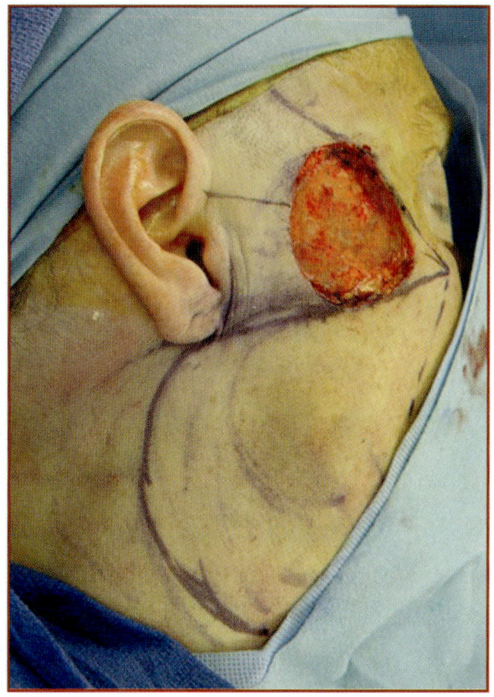

B

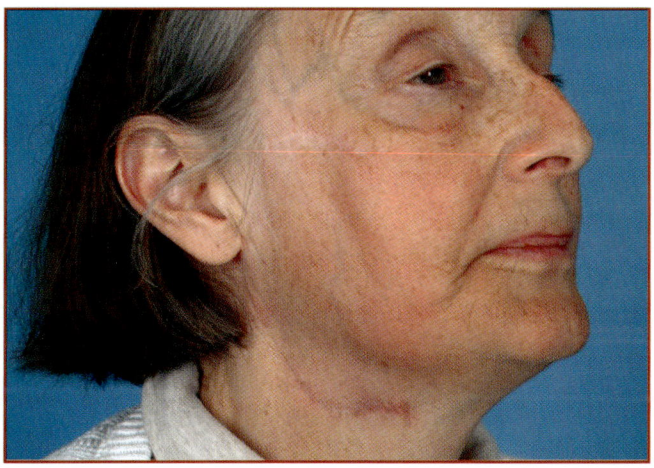

C

Figure 38–2. Rotation flap closure of lateral cheek defect. **A** and **B.** Preoperative views after excision with negative margins. **C.** Postoperative result at 18 months.

resulting secondary scar is placed in a skin fold or crease (Fig 38–2). The donor defect ideally is placed into the junction of two neighboring aesthetic units. Wide undermining helps to reduce tension on the closure. Smaller banner flaps can lead to pincushioning, which is troublesome to treat. Additionally, dynamic movements of the face may draw attention to resultant scars.

Bilobed Flaps

Bilobed flaps are a double-lobed modification of the banner transposition flap that use a secondary flap to close the defect created by the primary flap. The use of the second flap utilizes the laxity of a more distant site from the original defect. In general, bilobed flaps are not often used in cheek reconstruction due to extensive scarring and potential pin-cushioning of the flap that may occur. Larger single-lobed flaps (ie, banner flaps) can be designed to mitigate these issues.

Rhomboid Flaps

Rhomboid flaps may be useful for defects of the lateral, lower cheek, and temporal areas, and can be used in the infraorbital region to minimize ectropion. Rhomboid flaps are a modification of the banner flap and can be difficult to design but are thought to have a decreased tendency for trapdoor scarring or pin-cushioning. Furthermore, rhomboid flap design requires excision of a greater amount of "normal" surrounding skin to avoid dog-ears, therefore resulting in longer incision. Flap geometrics typically dictate designing a rhombus with 60- and 120-degree angles. The donor flap bisects the 120-degree angle such that the donor incision is enclosed within an area of relaxed skin tension lines (normal facial rhytids) and maximal distensibility. Fashioning the flap in this way facilitates transfer of redundant skin to the defect and primary closure of the donor site and requires wide undermining.

Rotational Flaps

For moderate to large defects of the cheek, rotational flaps are the cornerstone of soft tissue repair. By taking advantage of the laxity encountered in the neck and preauricular regions, rotation flaps provide a useful means of importing soft tissue for full-thickness skin and subcutaneous tissue defects, particularly those that are more extensive. These flaps usually are modifications of the Mustarde (cheek rotation flap used to reconstruct the eyelid), cervicofacial, or Juri flaps. However, drawbacks to these flaps arise from random, unpredictable perfusion with skin loss at the distal flap tip, dog-ears along the axis of rotation, and gravitational or cicatricial forces acting on the lower eyelid causing ectropion.[3] Additionally, when using these flaps to cover excisions of greater depth, contour abnormalities may result.

Cervicofacial Flaps

Perhaps one of the most popular cheek rotation flaps is the Juri type cervicofacial rotation advancement flap, as described by Juri and Juri in 1979.[4] These inferiomedially based flaps allow for transfer of large amounts of soft tissue from the loose preauricular and neck regions to upper medial region defects of the cheek (Fig 38–3). Incisions for the flap begin at the superior margin of the defect and extends along the outer canthus and up toward the zygomatic arch. The incision proceeds along the preauricular crease, below the ear and into the retroauricular hairline to the mid-posterior line of the neck. Advancement and rotation of the flap, as well as primary closure of the donor site, is achieved via wide subcutaneous undermining of the skin flap. Anchoring of the flap to the zygoma and lateral orbital wall with permanent suture is recommended to reduce tension on the lid margin that otherwise would lead to ectropion. Concurrent lower-lid tightening procedures (canthoplasty, canthopexy) may be considered for disproportionate lid laxity, but usually are not necessary if the flap is anchored above the lateral canthus. Tailoring of redundant skin at the nasolabial fold is done carefully to prevent narrowing of the flap base. A full-thickness skin graft, usually excised from the dog-ear of the flap, may be required for donor defect closure in the preauricular area, as this area provides maximal camouflage. Potential drawbacks of the cervicofacial flap, as with other flaps of this type, include distal skin flap necrosis (particularly troublesome in smokers); shifts in the normal hair-bearing pattern; and lid-related issues, including ectropion and prolonged edema. In addition, underlying hematoma should be watched for closely and may require drainage to avert skin necrosis. Rarely, facial nerve sequelae may result.

Alternatively, an inferolaterally based cervicofacial flap may be used for cheek defects. The inferolaterally based rotation flaps transfer lax skin from the jowls and nasolabial fold to reconstruct upper medial defects. The incision can be extended along the mandible and backcut to assist with closure or along a contralateral neck crease to improve flap reach. Incisions that cross the mandible may require Z-plasty to prevent scar contractures. The inferolaterally-based flap has a lesser tendency to develop distal end necrosis than its inferomedially based counterpart; however, the centrally placed facial scar is a disadvantage. Similar to the Juri flap, anchoring of the flap to underlying bone/periosteum renders the flap less susceptible to gravity-induced tension on the lid margin over time and subsequent ectropion. Additionally, resections adjacent to the lid margin may incur setbacks with lid edema, pin cushioning, and nasolabial fold asymmetry. Composite elevation of the skin flap has been described to improve flap circulation and reliability.[3,5] Flap elevation proceeds deep to the SMAS with vertical spreading to reduce injury to the facial nerve branches. This adaptation allows for a larger

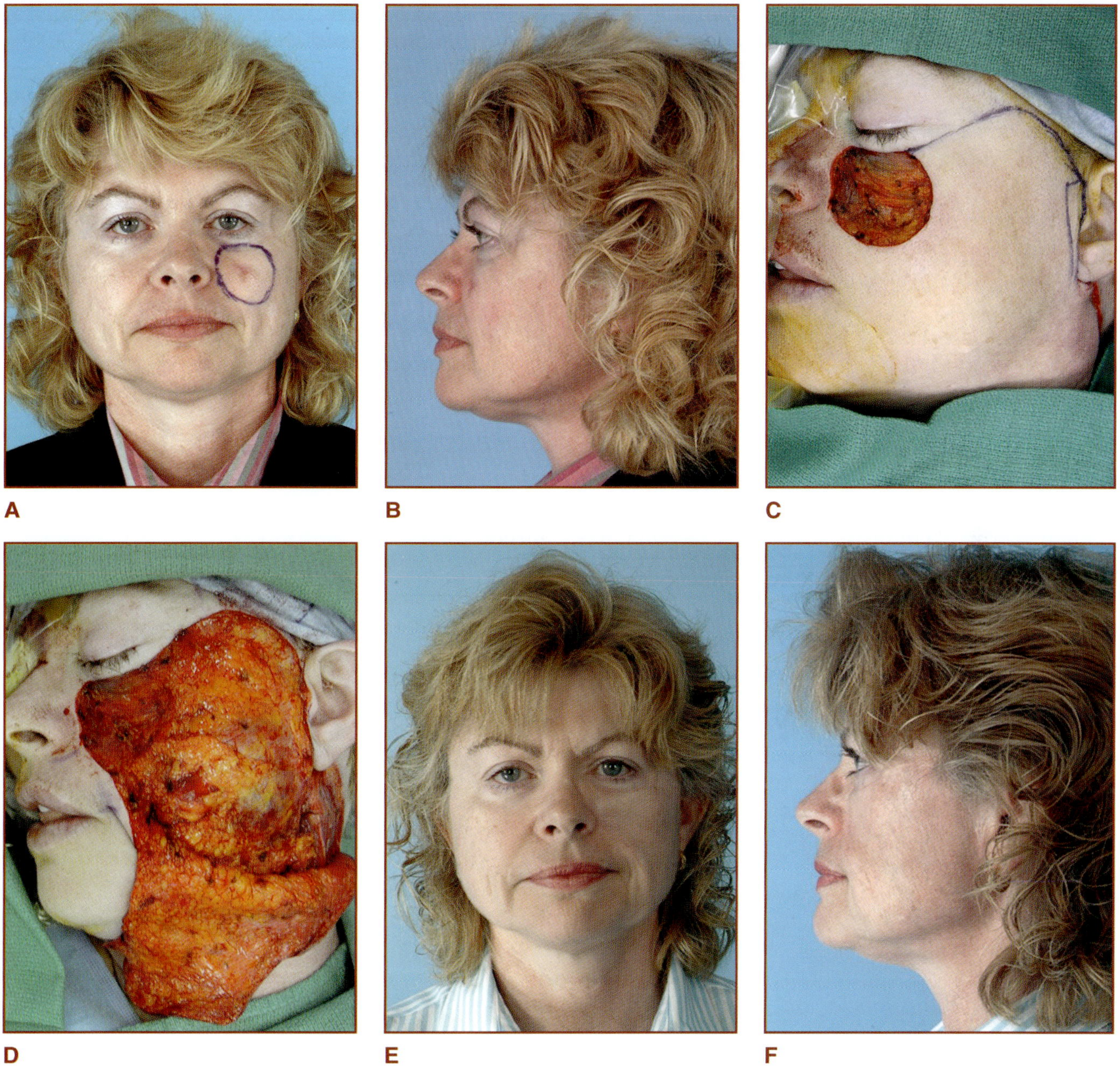

Figure 38–3. Cervicofacial flap closure of medial cheek defect. **A** and **B.** Preoperative markings of a squamous cell cancer of the medial cheek. **C** and **D.** Intraoperative resection and flap elevation. **E** and **F.** Postoperative result at 8 months.

flap design in smokers and patients with reduced skin quality. Additionally, these thicker flaps may mask potential contour deformities from deeper resections but may require secondary thinning if used for more superficial defects.

Cervicopectoral Flaps

For lower lateral cheek defects, a cervicopectoral flap may be employed to mobilize redundant tissue in the neck and chest regions for reconstruction.[6] In general, a line drawn from the tragus to the lateral commissure defines the upper border of defects suitable for coverage with the cervicopectoral flap. Defects chosen for reconstruction that extend above this line are at increased risk of developing skin necrosis. The flap design incorporates the posterior margin of the defect and continuation along the ear lobe, the retroauricular hairline and into the neck, approximately 2 to 3 cm posterior to the anterior border of the trapezius and along the deltopectoral groove. The flap can be enlarged by carrying the incision along the pectoralis major border and across the chest. Blood supply to the cervicopectoral flap is mainly from the internal mammary perforators with secondary contribution from the thoracoacromial perforators. This flap begins in the subcutaneous plane in the cheek and lower mandible and deep to the platysma at 3 to 4 cm below the mandibular border. To improve reach, the platysma may be safely transected at this level and the flap can be advanced and rotated to close the defect. V-to-Y closure is accomplished in the region lateral to the pectoralis muscle. Back-cutting of the skin flap or skin grafting of the donor site may be utilized as necessary to achieve closure.

Musculocutaneus Flaps

Pectoralis Major Flaps

The pectoralis major flap may be utilized as a muscle or musculocutaneus flap for lower lateral cheek defects on occasion. The pectoralis muscle originates from the sternum, clavicle, and anterior border of the first through sixth ribs. The muscle fibers travel transversely and laterally to insert on the humerus. The blood supply to the pectoralis flap is derived from the thoracoacromial vessels, which exit from below the clavicle. These vessels can be located easily with a Doppler probe along a line envisioned from the xiphoid to the acromion. The pectoralis flap is hardy, but the distal skin paddle may become ischemic, particularly in patients with lax skin.

The pectoralis flap has a tendency to be bulky and is better suited to composite defects involving skin, subcutaneous tissue, muscle, and/or parotid gland structures. It also has been described for intraoral and extraoral coverage as a double-paddle pectoralis flap for through-and-through defects, though it may be cosmetically disfiguring due to bulk.[7] Skin paddle design for the musculocutaneus version is most reliable when vertically oriented and encompassing periareolar perforators. The recommended width of the elliptical skin paddle is 6 to 8 cm for tension-free closure. Restricting the superior extent of the paddle to the level of the second intercostal internal mammary perforators allows for future use of the deltopectoral flap.

Trapezius Flap

The trapezius flap also has been described for lower lateral cheek defects and as a folded flap for through-and-through defects.[8] The trapezius extends from the occipital bone and lower thoracic vertebrae to the scapula. It is innervated by the third and fourth cervical nerves and the spinal accessory nerve. The pedicle for the trapezius flap is the transverse cervical artery and vein, with a variable contribution to the distal portions of the muscle arising from the dorsal scapular artery and vein. Care must be taken to preserve vessel anatomy during dissection to reduce risk of ischemia from inadvertent division. The reach of the trapezius flap is often restricted and generally limits its usefulness in most cheek reconstructions save for those that involve inferior and lateral defects.

Tissue Expansion

When timing of the reconstruction is more flexible, tissue expansion presents as a reasonable method of recruiting tissue. In addition, defects treated with skin grafts or myocutaneous flaps with a skin paddle may result in poor color match, poor scar, or shifts in hair pattern. Tissue expansion assists with secondary revision by expanding adjoining tissue with like color, texture, and hair-bearing features without additional donor defects.

Although tissue expansion offers these theoretical advantages, actual practice may be confounded by a high rate of complications.[9] Despite these difficulties, a successful reconstruction can be achieved with salvage of the expanded tissue. Exercising judgment with regards to the optimal patient candidate as well as ideal expander selection and placement is important for achieving successful tissue expansion.[10]

Several rules of thumb, as outlined by Wiselander[10] in his experience of over 100 patients, can be applied to this regard: expander dimensions should be as large as or larger than the defect; use of small, distant access incisions; avoidance of straight incisions adjacent to the lesion; and distant placement of fill valves (less than 7 cm) lateral or inferior to the pocket. Expanders are filled to tissue tolerance to decrease the risk of seroma and hematoma formation. Typically, postoperative expansion is delayed 10 to14 days, and expanders are overfilled 30% to 50% by completion of the expansion process. At the time of flap transposition, capsulotomy, without capsulectomy, is preferred.

Microsurgical Reconstruction

Free tissue transfer usually is needed for complex defects inadequately served by local tissue options (such as in patients who have undergone radiation therapy). Particularly for complex facial defects involving multiple layers, larger defects with major skin resection, or congenital or acquired contour abnormalities, microsurgical tissue transfer can furnish abundant tissue for reconstruction.

Although numerous microsurgical flaps have been described for cheek reconstruction, for practical purposes, the following flaps are most beneficial: the anterolateral thigh, radial forearm, parascapular, rectus abdominus, and free fibula flaps. The ultimate choice of free flap depends on the individual defect, including external skin requirements (size, location, thickness of skin defect), composite tissue needs (bone, lining), and pedicle length required for recipient vessel anastomosis.

Anterolateral Thigh Flap (ALT)

The anterolateral thigh flap can provide an abundant source of pliable, thin tissue, depending on the patient's body habitus. This fasciocutaneous flap is based on perforating vessels that arise from the descending branch of the lateral circumflex femoral artery and vein. The flap also can be harvested with a portion of the vastus lateralis for additional bulk in composite reconstruction (Fig 38–4). Perforator number and orientation in a patient with a thin body habitus may allow for a double-paddle flap reconstruction for through-and-through defects. Perforator variability is more commonly encountered than in the radial forearm flap; however, donor site scarring is in general more acceptable. In addition, flap harvest can easily be performed simultaneously with tumor resection. The distant location of the flap, however, affords less agreeable color and hair pattern match compared with local flap options.

Radial Forearm Flap

The radial forearm flap is a robust flap that provides a reasonable amount of thin, pliable skin and a lengthy and reliable pedicle. This fasciocutaneous flap can be harvested with the two venous systems, a sensory nerve, and/or a portion of bone if required. The dual venous output of the flap is supplied by the cephalic vein and vena comitans of the radial artery; the skin paddle design is adjusted to capture the cephalic vein. The lateral antebrachial cutaneous nerve can be included in the dissection to make the flap sensate. The flap has been used with multiple skin islands for through-and-through defects or complex reconstructions and can be folded over and partially de-epithelized for increased bulk. A small portion of the radial bone may be harvested with the flap. Concern over subsequent radius fracture has limited bone resection with the flap, although prophylactic plating to reduce this risk and restore biomechanical stability postharvest has been described.[11] Similar to the anterolateral thigh flap, downsides to the radial forearm flap include poor color, texture, and hair-pattern match. Furthermore, the donor site disfigurement may be unacceptable in some patients, particularly for female patients.

Parascapular Flap

The parascapular fasciocutaneous flap provides more bulk than the radial forearm flap and can be useful

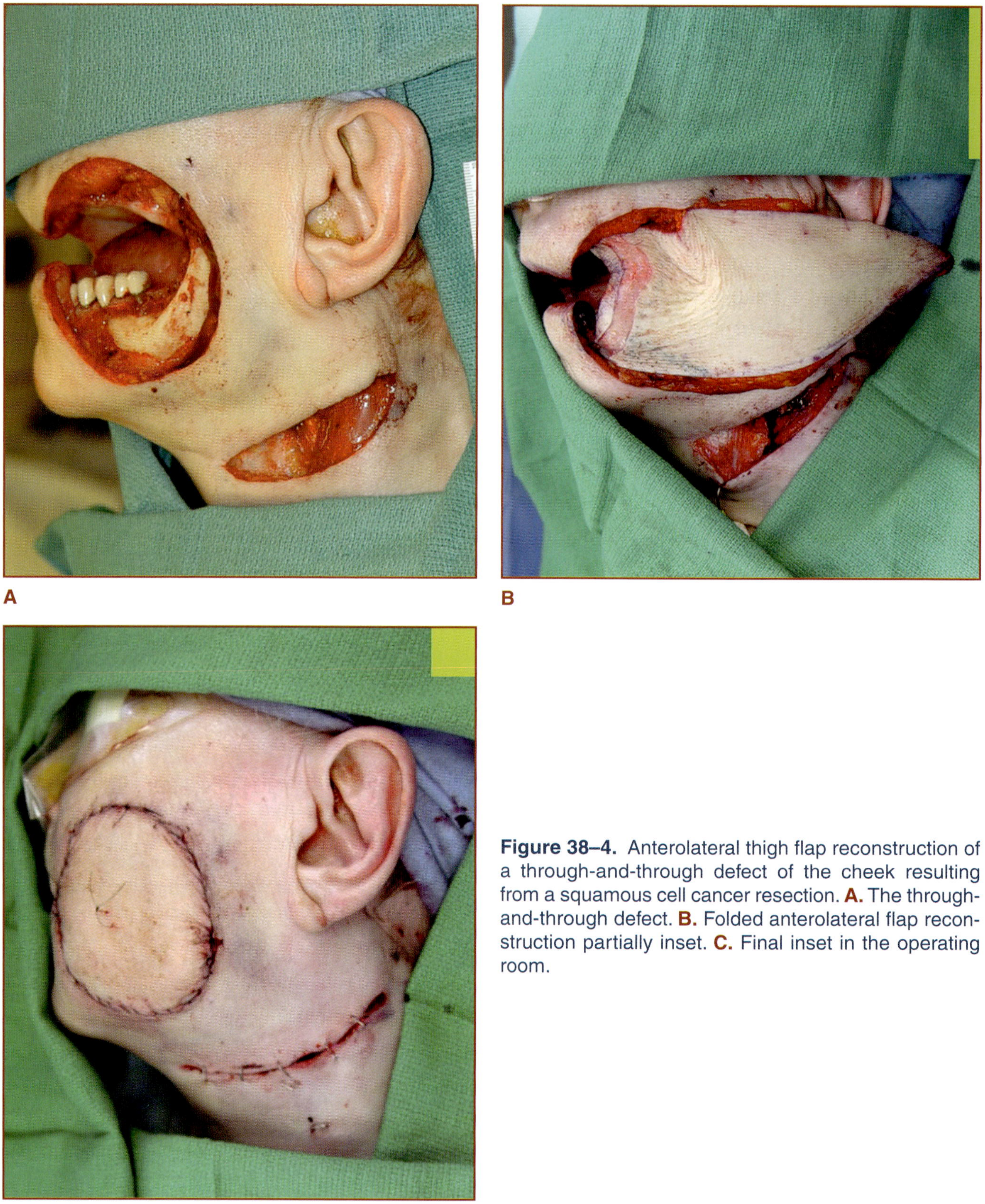

A

B

C

Figure 38–4. Anterolateral thigh flap reconstruction of a through-and-through defect of the cheek resulting from a squamous cell cancer resection. **A.** The through-and-through defect. **B.** Folded anterolateral flap reconstruction partially inset. **C.** Final inset in the operating room.

for composite resections. For larger defects, the latissimus dorsi muscle and a portion of the scapular bone can be harvested as well. This flap has the benefit of improved color match and minimal donor deficits compared with other microvascular options. However, the pedicle is relatively short and semilateral positioning is required for flap harvest making concurrent harvest and tumor ablation challenging.

Rectus Abdominis Flap

The rectus abdominis flap or deep inferior epigastric flaps are useful for complex defects of the cheek and is based on the deep inferior epigastric vessels. The long pedicle length and reliable skin paddle make this flap a workhorse for head and neck reconstruction. However, the flap may be bulky, particularly in overweight patients. In addition, the color match to the facial skin is not optimal. The perforator flap modification may reduce risk of hernia and donor site morbidity.[12]

Fibula Osteocutaneous Flap

The fibula flap affords vascularized skin, soft tissue, muscle, and bone for composite reconstructions. The peroneal vessels supply septocutaneous perforating vessels to support a skin island. Portions of the soleus and flexor hallucis longus muscle can be simultaneously harvested. Typically, segmental composite defects involving the mandible and overlying cheek skin are most appropriate for this type of flap. The distant donor site location facilitates a two-team approach with simultaneous tumor resection and flap harvest.

Other Considerations in Cheek Reconstruction

As smoking impairs the microcirculation and retards the healing response of the body, smokers should be advised to discontinue tobacco or nicotine-containing products 4 to 6 weeks prior to surgery. However, even this length of abstinence likely does not normalize skin perfusion in smokers. In fact, the damage that occurs to the skin circulation from long-term smoking may be irreversible even after prolonged periods of time. Anticoagulant medications should be stopped 1 to 2 weeks prior to surgery, if possible.

Complications and Side Effects

Scarring is not uncommon after any surgical intervention. Awareness of existing facial wrinkles and skin's natural tension lines can assist with scar camouflage. Scars that transverse natural skin lines or become wide and thickened can be reoriented and revised as needed after maximal scar reorganization has taken place (6 to 12 months). Scar also may result from necrosis due to excess tension, poor circulation due to smoking, or poor flap planning. Careful planning should be carried out to reduce tension on wound closure, identify ideal scar placement, and utilize optimal postoperative scar management (removing sutures in a timely fashion, postoperative taping). Silicone dressing application can be useful for hypertrophic scarring. Topical ointments generally are not recommended.

Similarly, excess tension may result in distortion of facial features. Careful planning, undermining of surrounding skin and adequate anchoring of susceptible structures (canthopexy, canthoplasty) can minimize this risk. Skin grafting as needed to assist with donor site closure (eg, cheek-ear junction of cervicofacial flap) also may prevent unnecessary tension and subsequent anatomic distortion.

Additionally, the inherent vascularity of the face lends itself to bleeding-related complications after cheek reconstruction. Meticulous technique to achieve hemostasis should be performed. Adequate blood pressure management with a controlled wake-up from anesthesia may prevent postoperative hematoma formation. Advising the patient to sleep with the head elevated and to avoid activities that may increase intracranial and/or facial pressure (eg, straining, bending over) is beneficial. Surgical drains are routinely employed, but should not be used to compensate for diligent adherence to routine postoperative management.

Finally, facial nerve injury may result during reconstruction. This outcome is fortunately rare with careful technique but, if noted early in the postoperative period, may require re-exploration and repair of the injured nerves.

Conclusions

Cheek reconstruction can be successfully carried out with adequate planning. Numerous options for reconstruction exist; however, tailoring of local or distant options for individual defects will depend on patient characteristics, composite tissue needs of the defect, and donor tissue location and availability for optimal results.

References

1. Jackson I. Cheek reconstruction. In: *Local Flaps for Head and Neck Reconstruction*. St. Louis, MO: Quality Medical Publishing; 2002:327–412.
2. Roth DA, Longaker MT, Zide BM. Cheek surface reconstruction: best choices according to zones. *Oper Tech Plast Reconstruct Surg*. 1998;5:26–36.
3. Longaker MT, Glat P, Zide BM. Deep-plane cervicofacial "hike": anatomic basis with dog-ear blepharoplasty. *Plast Reconstr Surg*. 1997;99:16–21.
4. Juri J, Juri C. Advancement and rotation of a large cervicofacial flap for cheek repairs. *Plast Reconstr Surg*. 1979; 64:692–696.
5. Kroll S, Reece GP, Robb G, Black J. Deep-plane cervicofacial rotation-advancement flap for reconstruction of large cheek defects. *Plast Reconstr Surg*. 1994;94:88–93.
6. Shestak KC, Roth AG, Jones NF, Myers EN. The cervicopectoral rotation flap: a valuable technique for facial reconstruction. *Br J Plast Surg*. 1993;46:375–377.
7. Ord RA, Avery BS. Side-by-side double paddle pectoralis major flap for cheek defects. *Br J Oral Maxillofac Surg*. 1989;27(3):177–185.
8. Guillamondegui OM, Campbell BH. The folded trapezius flap for through-and-through cheek defects. *Otolaryngol Head Neck Surg*. 1987;97(1):24–27.
9. Antonyshyn O, Gurss JS, Zuker R, Mackinnon SE. Tissue expansion in head and neck reconstruction. *Plast Reconstr Surg*. 1988;82:58–68.
10. Wieslander J. Tissue expansion in the head and neck. *Scand J Plast Reconstr Hand Surg*. 1991;25:47–56.
11. Karamanoukian R, Gupta R, Evans GR. A novel technique for the prophylactic plating of the osteocutaneous radial forearm flap donor site. *Ann Plast Surg*. 2006;56: 200–204.
12. Max LX, Selber JC Serletti JM. Abdominal wall following free TRAM or DIEP reconstruction: a meta-analysis and critical review. *Plast Recon Surg*. 2009;124(3):752–764.

39

PROSTHETIC REHABILITATION

THERESA M. HOFSTEDE
PATRICIA C. MONTGOMERY
RHONDA F. JACOB
PEGGY J. WESLEY
JACK W. MARTIN
MARK S. CHAMBERS

Introduction

Facial defects resulting from ablation of malignant cutaneous lesions can be disfiguring and compromise a patient's quality of life. Most patients desire surgical reconstruction or prosthetic rehabilitation to restore their appearance and confidence. Although surgical reconstruction with healthy native tissue is preferred, it may not always be feasible owing to limited adjacent tissue, radiation-associated tissue damage, comorbid conditions of the patient, or need to routinely examine the postsurgical defect. The prosthetic rehabilitation of facial defects can provide an aesthetic alternative to surgical reconstruction. The maxillofacial prosthodontist and the anaplastologist have been trained specifically to fabricate such prostheses.

Conventional facial prostheses include the nasal, orbital, and auricular prostheses, all of which are designed for patients who have undergone ablative resections. These removable facial prostheses are custom-made for patients to replicate their presurgical anatomic contours, skin tones, and skin texture; hence, the aesthetics and facial profile can be excellent. If postsurgical healing is optimal and the tissue is healthy with good proximal and internal defect contour, a facial prosthesis can be fabricated within a reasonable time frame to replace the lost structure. However, prosthetic rehabilitation can be delayed if the tissues are inflamed, have poor wound healing, have bulky or convex contour, or are very mobile or compressible. Additional surgery may be required to modify the contour of the recipient tissue surface to better accept the prosthesis. Postoperative radiation and/or chemotherapy also can extend healing time and delay prosthetic fabrication. Mobile underlying tissue can create a problem for prosthetic retention, resulting in detachment with excessive skin movement. Medical-grade adhesive tapes or glues used for retention can irritate the underlying tissue. The elastomeric silicone rubber material, from which most prostheses are made, will discolor over time, as well as tear at the edges due to everyday use and cleaning. A facial prosthesis requires diligent hygiene and daily maintenance. Typically, a facial prosthesis is remade or revised on a yearly basis.

Preoperative Evaluation

The maxillofacial prosthodontist and anaplastologist should be active members of the head and neck multidisciplinary team. Evaluation of the patient prior to the ablative surgical procedure allows for a two-way discussion of available facial rehabilitation options and for the future fabrication of a facial prosthesis. This appointment establishes an interpersonal relationship between the patient and their providers. The expectations and desires of the patient can be determined and discussed. Explanation of the benefits and limitations of prosthetic rehabilitation and surgical reconstruction must be discussed prior to surgery. The expected surgical defect, the possibilities for surgical reconstruction, and the patient's desire regarding prosthetic rehabilitation must be considered during the treatment-planning stage. The patient is advised of the time required and steps involved in the fabrication, as well as the maintenance and the longevity of the prosthesis. The materials used in the fabrication and their limitations also must be discussed. The removable nature of the prosthesis should be stressed because many patients believe these prostheses are permanent and fixed to the underlying tissue surface. Sample prostheses are shown to the patient so that he or she may have a good appreciation of the texture and contour of the completed prosthesis. Every prosthesis is custom-made for each patient. As such, presurgical documentation should include a facial and oral examination that will impact the final prosthetic treatment.

Presurgical facial photographs are beneficial to document the progression of treatment. Also, presurgical contours and skin tones can be documented in photographs. Presurgical impressions and their resultant models can be beneficial if there is minimal tissue distortion by the tumor. These stone models will record the tissue contours and can be used as a reference for prosthesis fabrication postsurgically. If there is excessive distortion or a tissue defect from the tumor, an impression or cast of the structure may have little value.

Postsurgical Evaluation

Postsurgical examination is necessary to evaluate the healing and anatomic features of the surgical site. The presence of a split-thickness skin graft, pedicled or microvascular free flap, exposed bone, or granulation tissues can be evaluated. Gentle palpation of the surgical site can identify areas of tenderness, edema, friable, and bleeding tissue as well as tissue tone and mobility. The mobility of tissues adjacent to the defect can be evaluated by having the patient move the muscles of facial expression. The tissues overlying these muscles are routinely engaged for retention of the prosthesis, and excessive movement may pose difficulties with prosthesis retention in the future. If the anatomic structures of the surgical site are not appropriate for prosthesis fabrication, additional preprosthetic surgery may be required.

The need for postoperative chemotherapy or radiation therapy will delay the start of facial prosthetic rehabilitation due to treatment related morbidities, specifically, edema, discomfort, dermatitis, fibrosis, and flap atrophy. The start of definitive prosthetic treatment must be delayed until the supporting tissues have completely stabilized. Initial planning for the prosthetic rehabilitation and current limitations of the tissues and the need for additional surgery can be discussed with the patient at the postsurgical appointment.

Surgical Enhancements to Improve Prosthetic Treatment

The success or failure of a facial prosthesis is directly related to the foundation of supporting tissues to which it attaches. The following surgical enhancements can help to improve this success.[1] First, the bony margins should be smoothed and rounded at the conclusion of the ablative surgical procedure because they may irritate the overlying tissue and may cause discomfort with placement and removal of the prosthesis. Any sharp bony areas may be particularly problematic in irradiated tissues. Ideally, all sharp bony prominences should be removed prior to prosthesis fabrication (Fig 39–1).

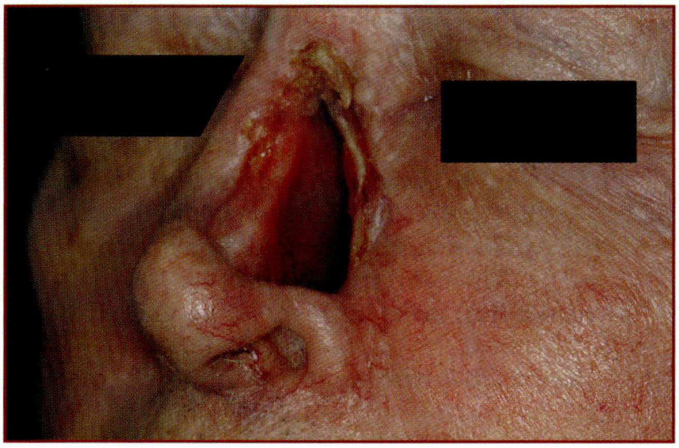

Figure 39–1. A postsurgical view following a partial rhinectomy revealing exposed bone along the margins of the defect. Surgical removal of the exposed bone is required prior to facial prosthesis fabrication. Elevation of the muscles around the perimeter of the defect and placement of a split-thickness skin graft would provide a durable and immobile surface ideal for prosthetic placement.

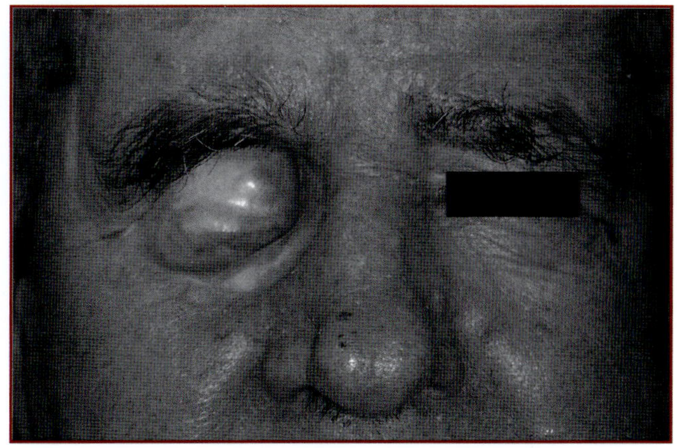

Figure 39–2. A well-healed split-thickness skin graft lines this bony orbital defect. This concave site with its resilient and immobile skin graft provides an ideal surface for prosthesis placement.

Second, any exposed bone or periosteum that is not covered with tissue should be grafted with a split-thickness skin graft. A skin graft that is firmly attached to the underlying bone will provide a thin immobile site for prosthesis placement. A healed skin graft will withstand the various forces of a facial prosthesis better than respiratory mucosa or granulation tissue will. Similarly, the durability of a skin graft will allow for manual cleaning of the defect, without tissue breakdown. The skin graft will also reduce mucous secretions and thus moisture contamination. Excessive secretions can significantly decrease prosthetic retention, particularly if adhesives or tapes are utilized (Fig 39–2).

Third, tissue tags that are not supported by bone or cartilage should be removed. These loose tags are difficult to capture in their passive position within an impression and may not have consistent contours over time, resulting in an ill-fitting prosthesis. Tissue tags may be in an unnatural position, and require overcontouring of the prosthesis to conceal them (Fig 39–3).

Fourth, in cases in which free tissue transfer flaps or pedicled flaps are used for surgical reconstruction, the bulkiness of the flap should be minimized. These flaps are ideal for covering sinus cavities and protecting vital underlying structures. However, to provide a well-contoured facial prosthesis, a slightly concave defect is ideal, particularly in orbital and midfacial reconstructions. Surgical debulking of the flap tissues may be necessary as a secondary procedure to facilitate effective prosthetic treatment (Fig 39–4).

Fifth, tissue transfers with an osseous component require careful treatment planning prior to the surgery. Inappropriate placement of an osseocutaneous flap can preclude placement of a facial prosthesis. Presurgical stereolithographic models can be utilized to preplan the surgical reconstruction and to fabricate surgical guides.[2] Close communication between the reconstructive surgeon, head and neck oncologic surgeon, maxillofacial prosthodontist, and anaplastologist is essential for an optimal outcome.

Biomaterials

Through the ages, numerous materials have been used for the fabrication of facial prostheses. In ancient Egypt, auricular, nasal, and orbital prostheses have been found in excavated tombs. Gold and silver facial

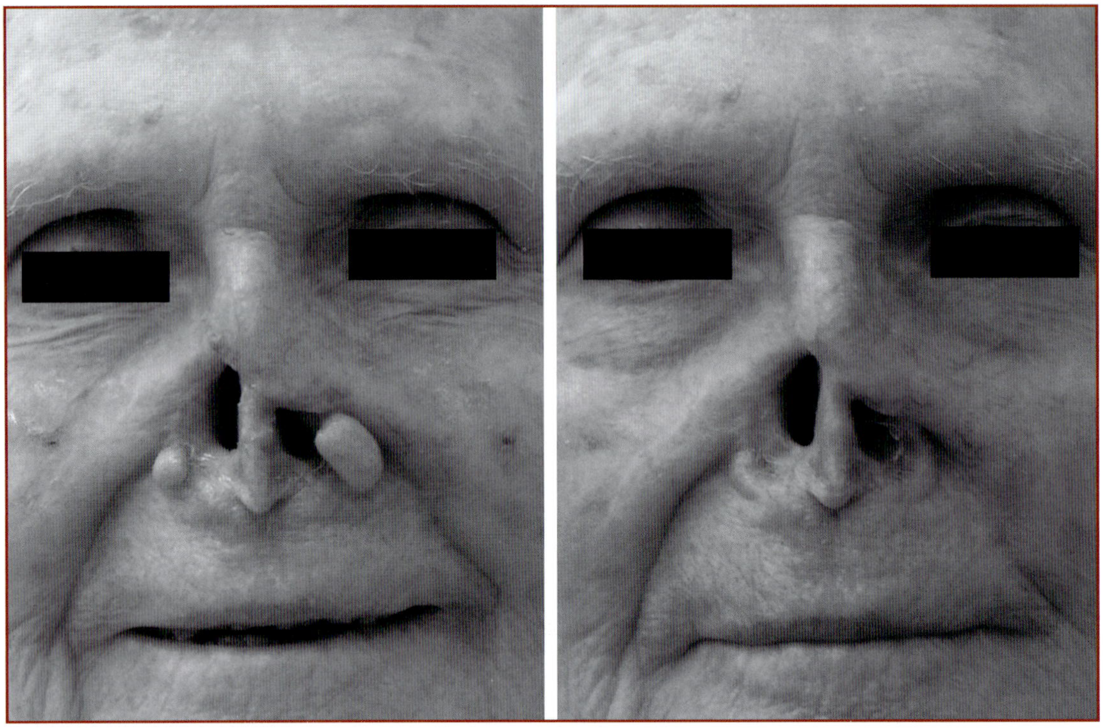

Figure 39–3. Residual nasal alar tags following a partial rhinectomy are unsupported and provide little support or retention for the prosthesis (*left*). Removal of the alar tissue tags provides a better tissue surface for nasal prosthesis fabrication (*right*).

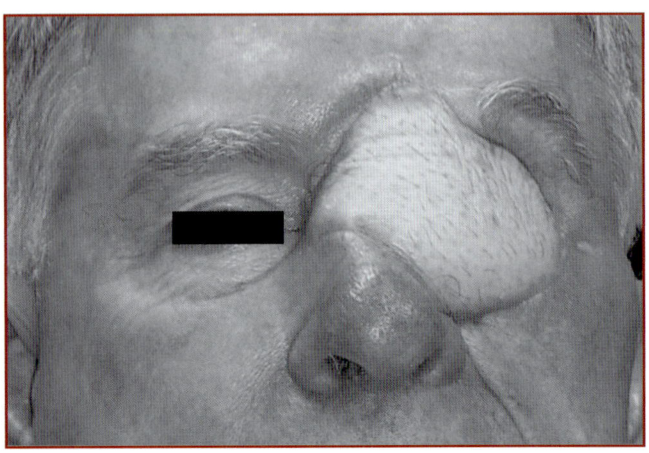

Figure 39–4. An orbital defect that has been reconstructed with a microvascular free tissue transfer flap. The bulkiness of this flap creates an excessively convex tissue contour that precludes placement of a facial prosthesis. Debulking of the flap is necessary prior to facial prosthetic rehabilitation.

masks were used during the Greek and Roman period.[3] During the modern ages, various materials such as porcelain, paper mache, wood, silver, and gold were used in the fabrication of facial prostheses. With developments in polymer chemistry, the 1900s saw a significant improvement in maxillofacial prosthetic materials. Initially, vulcanite rubber was used but was replaced by latex, acrylic resins, and polyvinylchloride materials.[4]

Since the 1960s, elastomeric polymers, such as silicone rubber, have been the most commonly used biomaterial in facial prosthesis fabrication.[4] Silicone rubber provides reasonable durability, ease of manipulation, and flexibility that is similar to that of skin. This biomaterial can be colored both intrinsically and extrinsically and can produce excellent color and surface texture, thus creating a lifelike prosthesis. Its flexibility in thin dimensions allows it to move with the tissues during normal use without detaching.

Limitations of this prosthetic material include the following: poor edge strength, limited longevity of the prosthesis, discoloration over time, and ability to support fungal growth. The average life span of a facial prosthesis has been found to be 10 months.[5] Prostheses fabricated with silicone rubber frequently are lined internally with a polyurethane sheet.[6] This liner improves tear resistance, provides an impervious layer that reduces fungal growth, allows thinner margins, and provides a smooth surface to accept adhesives or tape.

Acrylic resins are also routinely utilized in facial prosthesis fabrication. This material is made of a heat-polymerized methyl methacrylate that is identical to denture acrylic resins. Acrylic resins provide a hard, rigid, and durable prosthesis that maintains its shape and coloration over time. This material can be used for the entire facial prosthesis; however, its rigidity limits its use to areas with little or no facial movement. The material frequently is used for fabrication of a substructure that will assist in the retention of silicone rubber facial prosthesis (Fig 39–5). It also typically is used to fabricate prosthetic eye globes (ocular prostheses), which are a component of the orbital prosthesis.

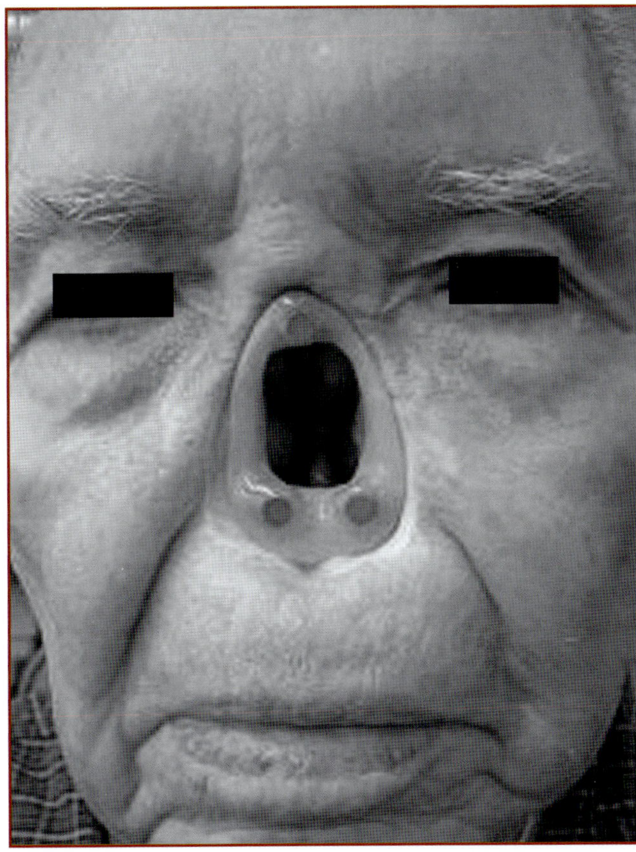

Figure 39–5. A removable acrylic resin substructure conforms to the internal aspect of the nasal defect and is retained and supported by these tissues. Three embedded magnets attach to counter magnets on the undersurface of the nasal prosthesis. This acrylic substructure provides improved stability and retention to the overlying nasal prosthesis. The magnets aid with orientation of the nasal prosthetic.

Ideal Properties of Facial Prosthetic Material

Facial prosthetic materials fall short of truly replicating the qualities of human tissues. The characteristics of an ideal facial prosthetic material are summarized in Table 39–1.[4]

Methods of Fixation

Predictable prosthesis retention is an important factor for patient confidence and acceptance. Retention of a facial prosthesis can be accomplished in various ways, including medical-grade adhesives, double-sided tapes, acrylic substructure with magnets embedded in the acrylic, anatomic undercuts, and craniofacial endosteal implants.[7] The method of retention often is dictated by the underlying tissue quality, its mobility, and the contours. Ideally, the tissue should be nonfriable and have little movement.

Double-sided adhesive tape is commonly used to retain facial prostheses.[5] This tape provides good retention and has ease in application and removal. Tape has the advantage of working in moist conditions and does not leave a residue on the skin. It can, however, irritate the underlying skin with frequent removal. A polyurethane liner on the tissue side of the prosthesis is required as this will limit prosthesis damage during removal of the tape.[6] The limited

Table 39–1. Characteristics of an Ideal Facial Prosthetic Material

Does not irritate the underlying or supporting tissues
Soft and pliable, allowing it to harmonize with facial movement yet maintain its form (regarding the replacement of structures covered by skin)
Sufficiently lightweight—it will not detach during normal wear
Intrinsic skin colors that allow extrinsic coloration
Hygienic, nonporous, and able to withstand daily cleansing with approved solutions
Resistant to deterioration with normal wear, with good tear resistance and durability
Limited thermal conductivity
Easy to manipulate without expensive or complicated processing equipment
Surface accepts adhesives for retention and colorants for characterization
Reasonably inexpensive and readily available

flexibility of tape limits its use to defects where the underlying tissue has little movement.[8]

Medical-grade water-based adhesives also are commonly used for prosthesis retention. These adhesives are applied to both the tissue surface of the prosthesis and the skin prior to placement. Medical grade adhesive is gentler to the tissues than tape and can be removed easily with warm soapy water. The length of retention varies with tissue movement, perspiration, and moisture, environmental conditions, and proper placement. Medical-grade adhesive can retain a prosthesis for up to 10 hours.[1]

Dependence on adhesives can be reduced by utilizing tissue undercuts or creating substructures that retain the prosthesis with magnets.[9,10] These substructures typically are fabricated with acrylic resins and can be mechanically retained in the surgical defect. Small samarium cobalt magnets are embedded into the acrylic resin and the corresponding silicone prosthesis (see Fig 39–5). This combination aids in retention as well as proper orientation of the prosthesis during placement. Surgical defects must be individually assessed for adequate tissue surface and space before a substructure can be utilized (Fig 39–6).

Osseointegrated titanium implants have provided long-term success in intraoral dental prosthetic reconstructions.[11,12] Similarly, craniofacial implants have been utilized to restore facial defects with great success.[13–18] Osseointegration involves a direct bond between the titanium oxide on the surface of the implant and the surrounding bone. Typically, craniofacial implants are fabricated of commercially pure titanium, cylindrical in shape, and threaded along the long axis. The dimensions of craniofacial implants are approximately 3 to 5 mm in length, with a diameter of 3 to 4 mm. The transmucosal section (abutment) of the implant allows attachment of the facial prosthesis.

Accurate positioning of implants into the underlying bone is vital to the overall success of the prosthetic rehabilitation. Poorly located implants may not be usable because they result in an overcontoured and/or malpositioned prosthesis. The implants also must be placed in a location to allow access for patient cleaning of the defect and transmucosal tissues around the implant. Implants can be placed immediately after the surgical ablation or as a delayed procedure following healing. If postoperative radiation is planned, it is advisable to place the implants prior to radiation, because there are greater failure rates for implants placed in irradiated bone.[19]

If delayed implant placement is planned, surgical guides can be made prior to the procedure by the maxillofacial prosthodontist or anaplastologist. These guides can greatly improve implant positioning and thus prosthetic success.[20] These surgical guides can be fabricated of acrylic resin from an impression of the surrounding skin. They must be made to rest accurately in a reproducible position on the skin. Implant locations are indicated by strategically placed perforations in the surgical guide. During the procedure, the surgical guide is placed on the skin and the position of the implants is marked on the skin and transferred to the bone with an ink-soaked needle. Once the flap is raised, the implant position can be confirmed by repositioning the needle into the flap until it touches the bone, then re-marking the bone.[20] Stereolithographic models made from computed tomography (CT) scans also can be used

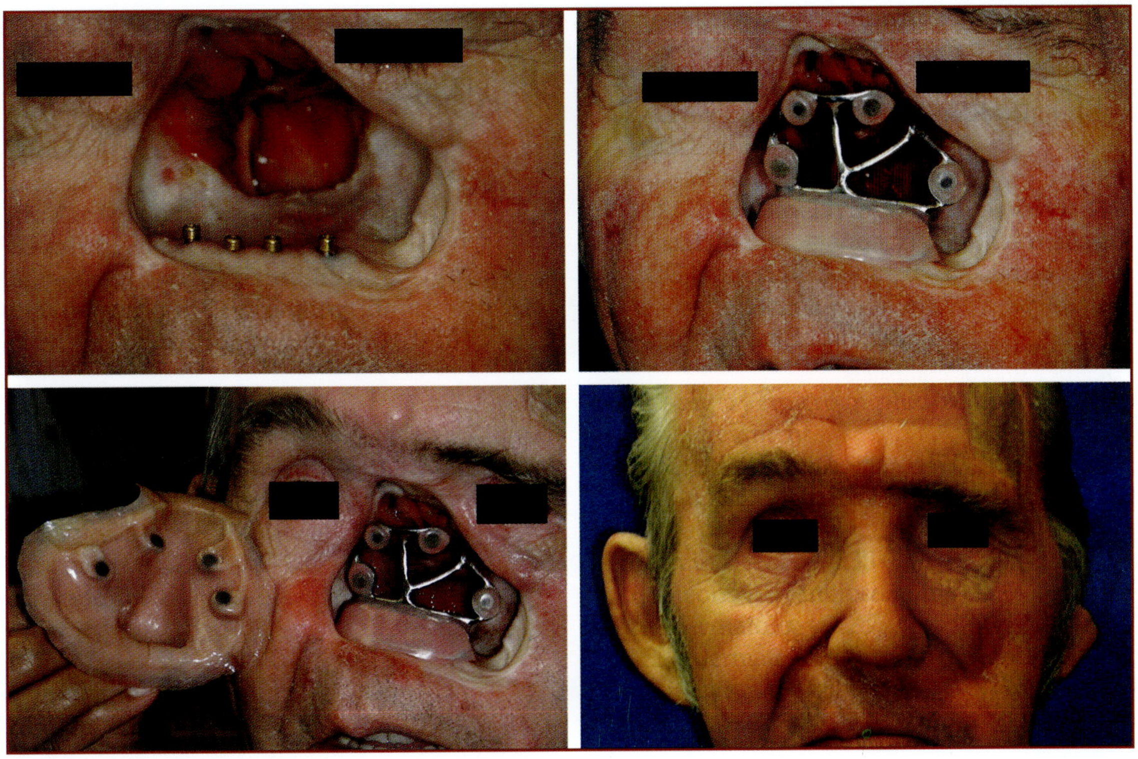

Figure 39–6. A healed midfacial defect following surgical ablation of cutaneous squamous cell carcinoma (*upper left*). The removal of the bony structures inside the nasal cavity and placement of a split-thickness skin graft provides adequate space for a substructure. Implants are placed vertically into the maxillary alveolar bone of this edentulous patient to support the substructure. A removable acrylic and metal substructure connects to the implants (*upper right*). The substructure contains four magnets that correspond to counter magnets in the facial prosthesis (*lower left*). This prosthesis is retained by the magnets and the implant-retained substructure. Final prosthesis in position (*lower right*).

to fabricate surgical guides. The models are useful to evaluate the bone contours and thickness. Surgical guides made from these models rest directly on the bone intraoperatively.

Craniofacial implants should be placed in sterile conditions under local or general anesthesia. A full-thickness flap is raised at the surgical site and the implant locations are selected. A surgical guide or template is invaluable at this stage to ensure correct positioning of the implants. Osteotomies are prepared to a specific length and diameter using a rotary drill with copious saline irrigation. The implant is positioned manually with a torque wrench until all the exposed threads are covered with bone. A cover screw is placed onto the top of the implant to prevent tissue from growing into the internal attachment. The reflected soft tissues are closed primarily and the implants are left to heal, unloaded, for 3 to 6 months. A second surgery is required to uncover the implants and attach the transmucosal or transcutaneous abutments.

This osseointegrated implant connects to a restorative abutment, which provides the retentive element (clip, magnet, or bar) that attaches to the prosthesis. This technology helps to overcome some of the challenges associated with facial prostheses. The benefits of implant-retained prostheses are depicted in Table 39–2.[21,22]

Table 39–2. Benefits of an Implant-Retained Prosthesis

Improved prosthesis retention and stability
Reduction of skin reactions to tapes and adhesives
Precise and reproducible prosthesis placement
Improved patient comfort and confidence
Improved aesthetics from thin prosthetic margins
Reduced maintenance—no need for placement and removal of tapes and/or adhesives
Improved prosthetic longevity due to less required manipulation and cleaning, with subsequent damage

Types of Prostheses

Nasal Prosthesis

Patients who undergo a partial or total rhinectomy as a result of cutaneous malignancies may benefit from prosthetic reconstruction. Partial or total nasal prostheses are commonly used to replace ablated nasal tissues. They frequently are retained with medical-grade adhesives or tapes. The mobility of the skin surrounding the defect can significantly impact the retention of the nasal prosthesis. If there is a concave, skin graft-lined opening into the nasal cavity, an acrylic substructure with magnets may be fabricated to rest in the defect and retain the silicone prosthesis with magnets (see Fig 39–5). Endosteal implants can be used, in limited situations, to retain nasal prostheses. Much of the bone surrounding the nasal defect has a complex architecture and typically is too thin to support the craniofacial implants.[13] Implants can be placed diagonally into the anterior nasal spine such that they engage the maxillary basal bone, but placement can be limited by the presence of teeth. Implants that exit through the mobile skin tissue of the upper lip often have chronic irritation. The implants should be placed in the anterior part of the nasal floor and be spaced 8 to 10 mm apart and exit through immobile tissue. Chronic dermatitis of the skin surrounding the implants is a common complication that may lead to implant failure.[23] Implants placed in the glabella region have high failure rates.[24]

Surgical enhancements can optimize prosthetic reconstruction of the nasal region. All unsupported tissue tags including alar tags should be removed (see Fig 39–3).

Second, the nasal bone should be left in place because it will help to provide a vertical support for a prosthesis. It will also help to retain eyeglasses. Third, the cartilaginous part of the nasal septum should be reduced to provide a concave defect. This may allow space for a substructure that can help retain the prosthesis. This also will reduce the mucous discharge that may contaminate the prosthesis and its adhesive bond.

Fourth, skin grafting of exposed bone provides a good surface for adhesion of the prosthesis because it has no hair growth or glandular secretions. A skin graft around the periphery of the defect reduces the movement of the muscles. Fifth, maintaining the anterior nasal spine and lip attachments can prevent migration of the lip superiorly (Fig 39–7).[25]

Auricular Prosthesis

Patients with a subtotal or total auriculectomy may benefit from prosthetic rehabilitation. The total auriculectomy site offers advantages over the partially resected site because it allows freedom with the location, size, and shape of the prosthesis. The recipient site should be concave or flat to provide natural aesthetics and contours. Bulky reconstruction flaps must be thinned prior to prosthetic treatment. Ideally, the tissues of the recipient site should be devoid of hair to provide an adequate surface for adhesive or tape attachment. A split-thickness skin graft over bone provides such a surface.

The tissue remnants following a partial resection may be distorted, malpositioned, and unsupported, which compromises aesthetics, bilateral symmetry, and final prosthetic results. Malpositioned tissue remnants can compromise aesthetics and bilateral symmetry. The tragus is the ideal tissue to be spared during an auriculectomy. The tragus is not easily distorted following surgery due to its rigid supporting cartilage. It aids the patient in orienting the prosthesis into position and provides an area to con-

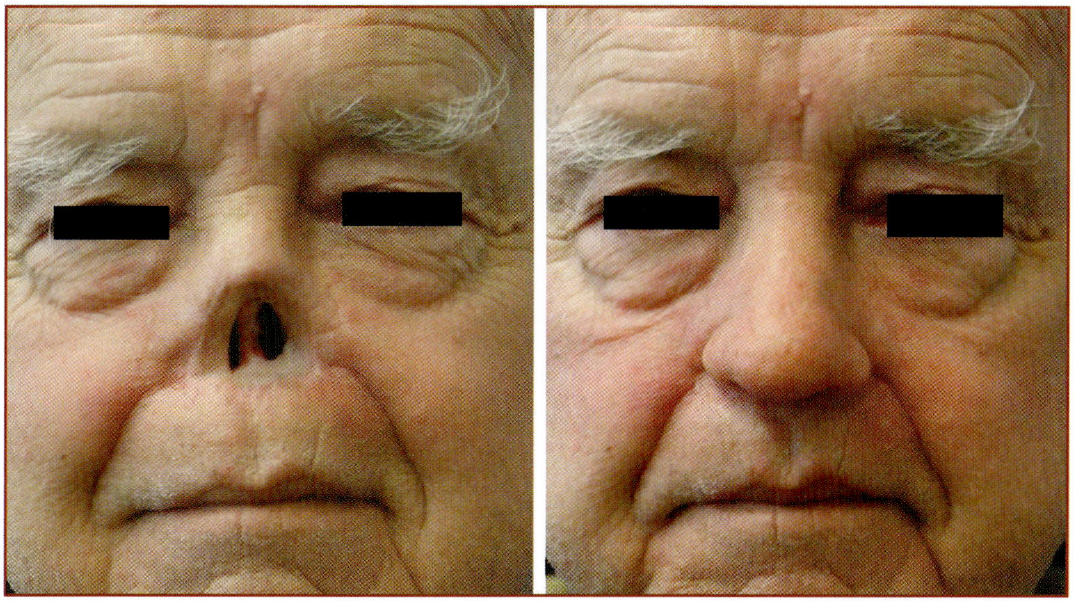

Figure 39–7. Well-healed nasal defect with a split-thickness skin graft in position (*left*). The nasal bone remains in position, which will help support eye glasses and a nasal prosthesis. Nasal prosthesis in position (*right*).

ceal the anterior margin of the auricular prosthesis. The superior aspect of the auricle has cartilaginous support but often becomes displaced and distorted following surgery. If the root of the helix adjacent to the tragus is maintained, the helix will provide a vertical support for the prosthesis and eyeglasses (Fig 39–8).

Tissues of the ear that lack cartilaginous support, such as the inferior half of the pinna and lobe, have little benefit for prosthesis retention or orientation. These tissues are not stable, are difficult to capture in the impression, and do not provide a reliable surface for prosthesis placement and retention (Fig 39–9).

Craniofacial implants placed (in nonirradiated bone) in the auricular region are very successful, with success rates exceeding 95%.[26,27] Two implants typically are adequate to retain an auricular prosthesis. The implants must be positioned such that the implants and their retentive abutments will be under the antihelix part of the prosthetic ear. This position is the thickest part that allows adequate space to conceal the implant abutments and its prosthetic attachments. The implants should be placed 15 to 18 mm from the external auditory meatus. For

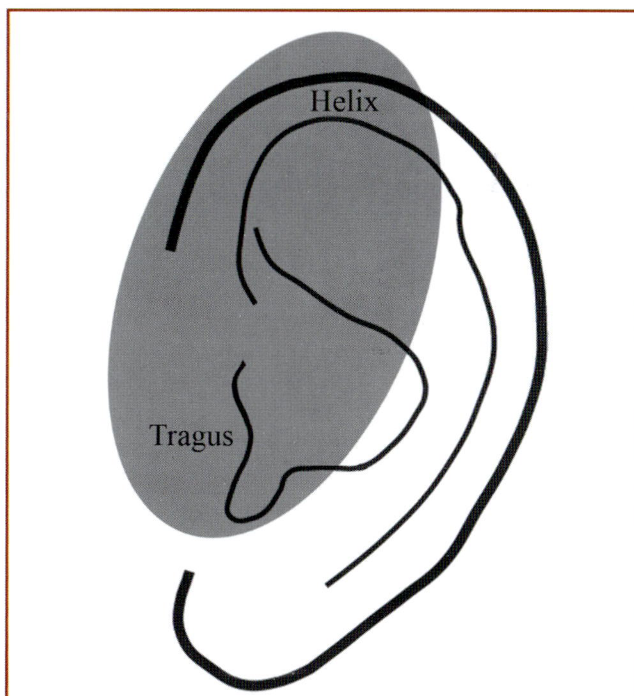

Figure 39–8. Diagram with the shaded area denoting the ideal postsurgical auricular remnant with the tragus and root of the helix remaining.

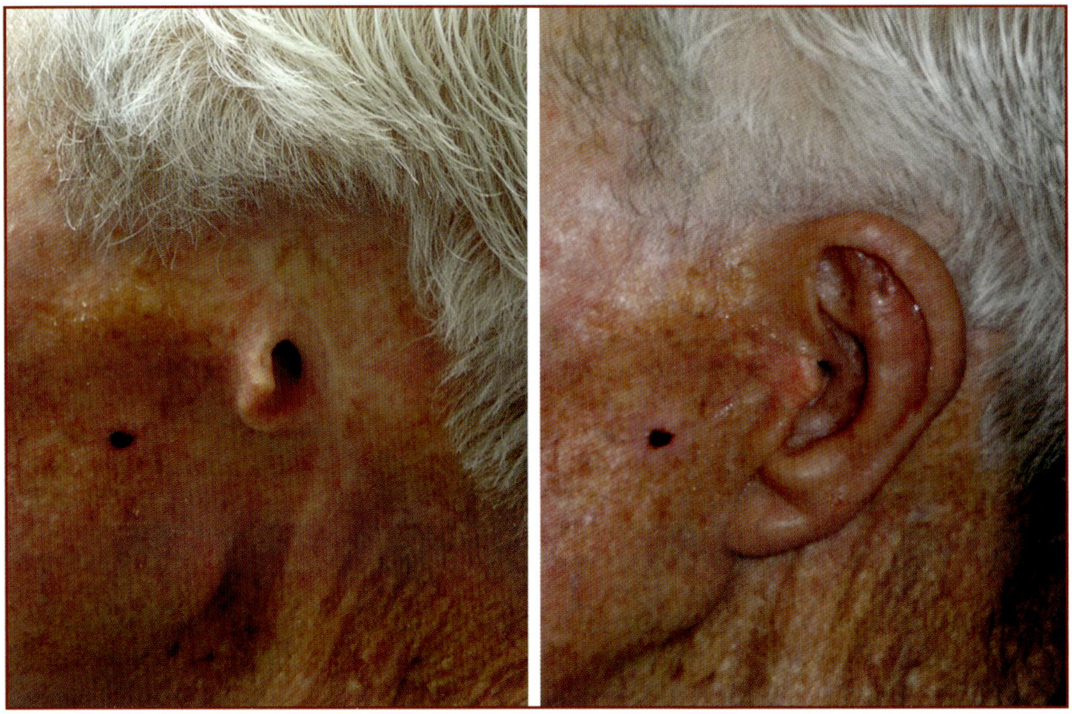

Figure 39–9. Auricular defect with ideal tissue characteristics for prosthesis attachment (*left*). Final prosthesis in position (*right*). The remaining tragus helps to conceal the anterior border of the prosthesis as well as aid in positioning.

the right ear, the implants should be positioned in the 9 o'clock and 11 o'clock positions. Implants for the left ear should be in the 3 o'clock and 1 o'clock positions.[28]

Orbital Prosthesis

Prosthetic rehabilitation following an orbital exenteration remains one of the most artistically challenging. Optimal aesthetic results require an ideal recipient site for the orbital prosthesis. The head and neck oncologic surgeon and reconstructive surgeon can improve the prosthetic outcome with a well-planned surgical technique. If possible, the eyelids should be resected and eyebrows maintained. The periorbital bony rim can greatly improve the support of the prosthesis. If these orbital bones are resected during the ablative surgery, all sharp margins should be smoothed and rounded to minimize tissue irritation. If the inferior bony margin of the orbit is resected, the prosthesis will have poor support and may droop. Therefore, reconstruction of the inferior margin is preferred. Large bulky flaps used to reconstruct the internal aspect of the orbital cavity will preclude prosthetic reconstruction (see Fig 39–4). Debulking of the flap will be necessary prior to prosthesis fabrication. The ideal site for an orbital prosthesis is the concave bony orbit that has been lined by a split-thickness skin graft following exenteration.

This postsurgical anatomy provides a solid supporting foundation with cleansible, nonmobile tissues. It also provides depth that is required for appropriate lifelike contours (see Fig 39–2). If the resection extends beyond the internal tissue of the orbit, to the more mobile periorbital skin tissue, retention can be even more challenging. An internal substructure fabricated with acrylic resin or silicone can engage undercuts in the orbital cavity. This substructure has embedded magnets that connect to the counter magnets in the prosthesis. Craniofacial osseo-integrated implants also can be utilized to aid in the retention of prostheses. The malar body, supraorbital rim, and lateral rim are the favored sites for implant placement. These implants should be placed such that they can be concealed by the prosthesis. Ideally, the implants should be placed prior to any postoperative radiation therapy to minimize the risk of osteoradionecrosis (Fig 39–10).

Technique for Fabrication of a Facial Prosthesis

Fabricating a facial prosthesis involves a variety of materials and techniques that are unique to the knowledge and experience of an anaplastologist and a maxillofacial prosthodontist. No one definitive technique is used because patient needs vary depending on the defect and the desired final outcome. A thorough assessment of the defect and preprosthetic planning are necessary prior to initiating facial prosthetic rehabilitation.

The process of fabricating a facial prosthesis begins by obtaining an accurate impression or moulage of the defect and surrounding tissue. For a facial impression, the patient should be in an upright sitting position to record the tissue in its most natural position. The two most commonly used impression materials are irreversible hydrocolloid and vinyl polysiloxane. Both of these materials provide accurate reproduction of the facial contours with excellent detail. A resultant model or master cast is obtained from pouring a high-quality stone onto the tissue surface of the impression. The missing

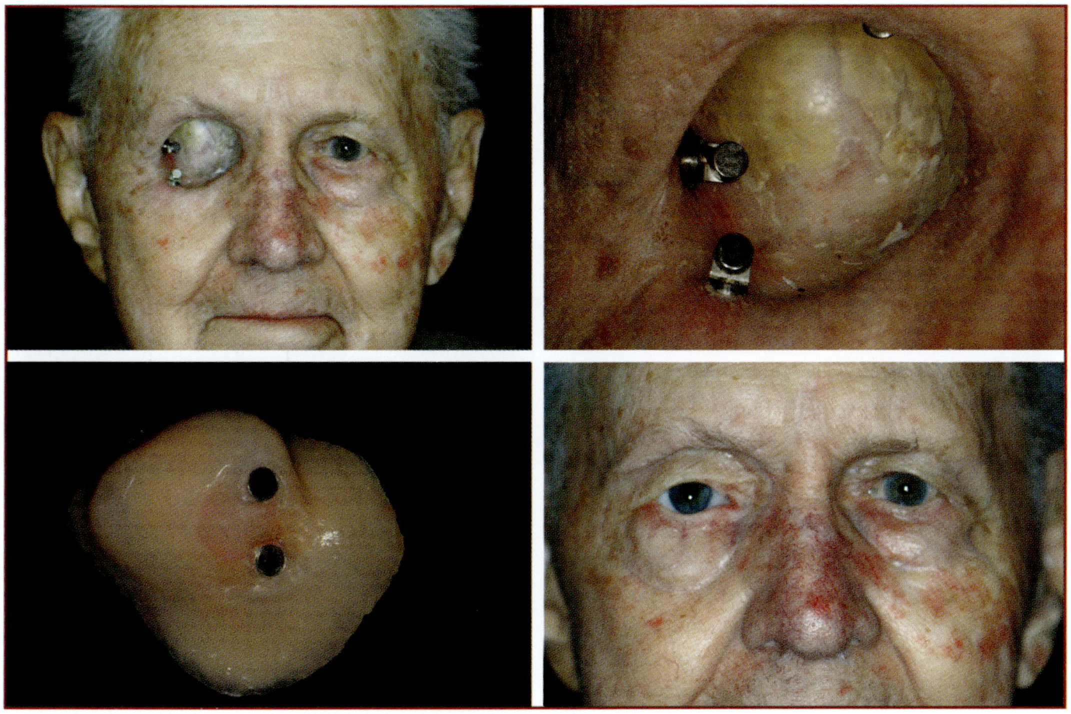

Figure 39–10. Orbital defect following exenteration. Notice implants in position on the lateral rim and supraorbital rim (*upper left*). The implant in the supraorbital rim was not used due to the excessive tissue bulk and movement of the periorbital tissue around the fixture. The lateral implants have magnets attached (*upper right*). The tissue surface of the facial prosthesis has the corresponding magnets embedded in the silicone (*lower left*). These magnets help support and positioning of the facial prosthesis. Final orbital prosthesis in position (*lower right*).

anatomy is then sculpted on the resultant master cast with wax or clay. Sculpting wax is generally preferred for sculpting a nose or an ear, whereas a nonhardening clay modeling compound is preferred for sculpting an eye owing to the intricacies of orbital anatomy. To keep the sculpting from sticking to the cast, a layer of foil is burnished to the back of the sculpting. The fit and accuracy of the sculpting is checked multiple times on the patient. The patient is asked to make facial movements while the sculpted wax or clay is in position. This helps to identify areas that are not in intimate contact with the underlying tissue. The master cast is adjusted to reflect what was seen on the patient. The wax sculpting is adjusted and then positioned on the patient repeatedly until a good fit is achieved.

Once the wax or clay sculpting is complete, it is processed into silicone. The completed sculpting is sealed onto a master cast and encased in stone. The mold is separated, wax is removed, and then the mold is packed with silicone. This silicone is intrinsically colored with pigments and opaque powders to match the patient's skin tones. Once the silicone is set, the facial prosthesis is removed from the stone assembly, trimmed, cleaned, and refit onto the patient's defect. It is then extrinsically colored with the patient present. In most cases, a nose or ear prosthesis is designed and fabricated within 1 week, whereas an orbital prosthesis usually takes 2 weeks or more to fabricate.

Summary

Prosthetic rehabilitation of postsurgical defects of the head and neck remains an excellent alternative to surgical reconstruction. The most common prostheses include the nasal, auricular, and orbital prosthesis; however, modifications of each prosthesis are made depending on the clinical situation. Although facial prostheses have limitations, they provide a good alternative for patients who cannot have surgical reconstruction or who are awaiting surgical reconstruction. The use of endosteal implants or acrylic substructures can greatly enhance the retention and stability of these prostheses. Coordination of the treatment by the head and neck oncologic surgeon, reconstructive surgeon, maxillofacial prosthodontist, and anaplastologist is essential. Careful presurgical planning, tissue management, and attention to detail during every phase of the treatment can result in superior results. This dedication to teamwork and attention to detail can greatly improve a patient's quality of life and sense of well-being.

References

1. Lemon JC, Chambers MS, Martin JW. Prosthetic rehabilitation of patients with advanced nonmelanoma skin cancer. *Clin Plast Surg.* 1997;24(4):797–815.
2. Al-Sukhun J, Helenius M, Lindqvist C, Ashammakhi N, Tornwall J, Penttila H. Stereolithography and the use of pre-adapted or fabricated plates for accurate repair of maxillofacial defects. *Br J Oral Maxillofac Surg.* Nov 28, 2006. e-pub ahead of print.
3. Conroy BF. The history of facial prostheses. *Clin Plast Surg.* 1983;10(4):689–707.
4. Heller HL, McKinstry RE. Facial Materials. *Fundamentals of Facial Prosthetics.* St. Petersburg, FL: ABI Professional Publications; 1995:84–85.
5. Chen MS, Udagama A, Drane JB. Evaluation of facial prostheses for head and neck cancer patients. *J Prosthet Dent.* 1981;46(5):538–544.
6. Udagama A. Urethane-lined silicone facial prostheses. *J Prosthet Dent.* 1987;58(3):351–354.
7. Lemon JC, Chambers MS. *Conventional methods of retention of facial prostheses.* First International Congress on Maxillofacial Prothesis; 1994.
8. Beumer J 3rd, Curtis TA, Marunick MT. *Maxillofacial Rehabilitation: Prosthodontic and Surgical Considerations.* St. Louis, MO: Ishiyaku EuroAmerica, Inc; 1996:396.
9. Lemon JC, Martin JW, Chambers MS, Wesley PJ. Technique for magnet replacement in silicone facial prostheses. *J Prosthet Dent.* 1995;73(2):166–168.
10. Mekayarajjananonth T, Huband ML, Guerra LR. Clear acrylic resin device for orientation and placement of a small facial prosthesis. *J Prosthet Dent.* 2000;83(6):656–659.
11. Adell R, Eriksson B, Lekholm U, Branemark PI, Jemt T. Long-term follow-up study of osseointegrated implants in the treatment of totally edentulous jaws. *Int J Oral Maxillofac Implants.* 1990;5(4):347–359.
12. Adell R, Lekholm U, Rockler B, Branemark PI. A 15-year study of osseointegrated implants in the treatment of the edentulous jaw. *Int J Oral Surg.* 1981;10(6):387–416.
13. Miles BA, Sinn DP, Gion GG. Experience with cranial implant-based prosthetic reconstruction. *J Craniofac Surg.* 2006;17(5):889–897.

14. Tjellstrom A. Osseointegrated implants for replacement of absent or defective ears. *Clin Plast Surg.* 1990;17(2): 355–366.
15. Tolman DE, Taylor PF. Bone-anchored craniofacial prosthesis study: irradiated patients. *Int J Oral Maxillofac Implants.* 1996;11(5):612–619.
16. Wolfaardt JF, Wilkes GH, Parel SM, Tjellstrom A. Craniofacial osseointegration: the Canadian experience. *Int J Oral Maxillofac Implants.* 1993;8(2):197–204.
17. Parel SM, Tjellstrom A. The United States and Swedish experience with osseointegration and facial prostheses. *Int J Oral Maxillofac Implants.* 1991;6(1):75–79.
18. Tolman DE, Taylor PF. Bone-anchored craniofacial prosthesis study. *Int J Oral Maxillofac Implants.* 1996;11(2): 159–168.
19. Ihde S, Kopp S, Gundlach K, Konstantinovic VS. Effects of radiation therapy on craniofacial and dental implants: a review of the literature. *Oral Surg Oral Med Oral Pathol Oral Radiol Endod.* 2009;107(1):56–65.
20. Reisberg DJ, Habakuk SW. Use of a surgical positioner for bone-anchored facial prostheses. *Int J Oral Maxillofac Implants.* 1997;12(3):376–379.
21. Beumer J 3rd, Curtis TA, Marunick MT. *Maxillofacial Rehabilitation: Prosthodontic and Surgical Considerations.* St Louis, MO: Ishiyaku Euro-America, Inc; 1996:436.
22. Jacobsson M, Tjellstrom A, Fine L, Jansson K. An evaluation of auricular prosthesis using osseointegrated implants. *Clin Otolaryngol Allied Sci.* 1992;17(6):482–486.
23. Scolozzi P, Jaques B. Treatment of midfacial defects using prostheses supported by ITI dental implants. *Plast Reconstr Surg.* 2004;114(6):1395–1404.
24. Nishimura RD, Roumanas E, Moy PK, Sugai T. Nasal defects and osseointegrated implants: UCLA experience. *J Prosthet Dent.* 1996;76(6):597–602.
25. Marunick MT, Harrison R, Beumer J III. Prosthodontic rehabilitation of midfacial defects. *J Prosthet Dent.* 1985; 54(4):553–560.
26. Wright RF, Zemnick C, Wazen JJ, Asher E. Osseointegrated implants and auricular defects: a case series study. *J Prosthodont.* 2008;17(6):468–475.
27. Visser A, Raghoebar GM, van Oort RP, Vissink A. Fate of implant-retained craniofacial prostheses: life span and aftercare. *Int J Oral Maxillofac Implants.* 2008;23(1):89–98.
28. Beumer J, Curtis TA, Marunick MT. *Maxillofacial Rehabilitation: Prosthodontic and Surgical Considerations.* St Louis, MO: Ishiyaku EuroAmerica, Inc; 1996:438.

INDEX

A

ABCDE (*a*symmetry, *b*order irregularity, *c*olor variegation, *d*iameter greater than 6 mm, and *e*volving [increasing] size or color)
  biopsy criteria, 333
  early detection, 24
  melanoma, 16, 17
  pediatric melanoma, 43
  and SSE (self-screening examination), 42
About Face USA, 37
Abraxane, 39
Abrikossoff tumor histopathology, 91
acitretin, 446
ACS (American Cancer Society), 36
  Look Good . . . Feel Better program, 35, 36
  on screening, 42
actinic keratoses (AK)
  acantholytic actinic keratosis, 81
  actinic chelitis, 81
  diclofenac, 446
  5-ALA, 120–121, 447
  5-fluorouracil, topical, 444
  HAK (hyperplastic actinic keratosis), 81
  histopathology, 79–81
    atypical keratinocytes, 79–80
    dermal solar elastosis, 80
    variants, 81
  imiquimod, 445
  lychenoid actinic keratosis, 81
  and NMSC (nonmelanoma skin cancer), 122
  overview, 441–442
  PDT (photodynamic therapy), 207, 208
  pigmented actinic keratosis, 81
  radiotherapy, 449–450
  and SCC (squamous cell carcinoma), 12–13, 48, 49, 51, 79, 80, 122
    excision margins, 443
  treatment, 442
    chemical peel, 447–448
    cryosurgery, 448–449
    laser resurfacing, 447–448
    and MAL (methyl aminolevulinic acid), 447
    medical adjunctive, 444–447
    photodynamic therapy, 447
    procedure-based adjunctive, 447–450
  and xeroderma pigmentosum (XP), 120–121
adenexal neoplasms (malignant) histopathology, 91–93
adjuvant regional radiotherapy
  MCC (Merkel cell carcinoma)
    clinically positive lymph node management, 241
adnexal tumors
  benign, 224–226
  classification, 224
  clinical evaluation, 224
  cylindroma, 226
  ductopapillary apocrine carcinoma, 229
  of hair follicle origin, 224–225
  hidradenocarcinoma, 226–227
  hidradenoma, 225
  malignant, 226–229
    cylindroma, 227
  microcystic adnexal carcinoma (MAC), 92, 228–229, 435
  ocular adnexal carcinomas, 180
  ocular adnexal cutaneous lesions, 173
  outcomes, 230
  overview, 223, 230–231
  pilar tumor, 224–225
  pilomatricoma, 225, 226
  proliferating trichilemmal cyst, 224–225
  sebaceous adenoma, 225
  sebaceous carcinoma, 226
  sebaceous gland origin, 225
  surgery/ocular adnexal tissue protection, 176

adnexal tumors *(continued)*
of sweat gland origin, 225, 226–229, 227
syringoid eccrine carcinoma, 227
syringoma, 225
treatment, 229–230
AIDS
immunosuppression, 298
AIDS immunosuppression, 298
AJCC (American Joint Committee on Cancer). *See* staging *main entry*
Melanoma Task Force
stage III morbidity, 346, 347
tumor miotic rate replacing Clark's level (T1b) disease, 23
albinism, 12, 13, 103
oculocutaneous, 13, 46, 48
oculocutaneous types 1 and 2, 121
overview, 121
and SCC (squamous cell carcinoma), 121
ameloblastoma, 121
American Academy of Dermatology (AAD), 57
cancer screening program, 42
Mohs surgery indications, 434
on UV exposure, 272
anatomy
auricular reconstruction, 531–533 (*See also* auricular reconstruction *main entry*)
blood supply, 533–534
sensory nerve supply, 534–535
basale/stratum germinativum, 1
basement membrane zone, 3
canaliculi, 173
cheeks, 575–576
conjunctiva, 174
conjunctiva ocular melanoma, 409
dermis, 3
epidermis, 1–3
extraocular muscles, 173–174
eyelids, 173
head and neck anatomic zones, 5
lips, 487–488
periauricular lesions, 157
periorbital, 173–174
periorbital sensory nerves, 174
scalp reconstruction
blood supply, 557–559
innvervation, 559–560
layers, 557, 558
skin appendages
embryology, 223
histology, 223–224
stratum corneum, 2
stratum germinativum/basale, 1
stratum granulosum, 2
stratum spinosum, 1
angiosarcoma, head and neck
treatment
radiotherapy, 263
targeted molecular therapy, 264–265
angiosome concept (skin blood supply), 4
antiangiogenic agents, 382
antibiotics, 446, 479, 500, 507
anticoagulants, 585
anti-CTLA-4 (cytotoxic T lymphocyte-associated antigen), 395
antiemetics, 390
apoptosis impairment, 7, 13, 63
APOS (American Psychosocial Oncology Society), 36
arsenic compounds, 13, 48
AS (angiosarcoma), 260
biopsy, 259–260
blood tests, 260
clinical characteristics/presentation, 258–259
cutaneous, 437
demographics, 258
diagnostic tests, 259–260
differential diagnosis, 260
histopathology, 260–261
imaging studies, 260
immunohistochemistry, 261
overview, 257, 266
pathogenesis, 258
patient evaluation
biopsy, 259–260
diagnostic tests, 259–260
history, 259
physical examination, 259
risk factors, 258
staging
AJCC (American Joint Committee on Cancer), 260, 261
treatment
advanced or disseminated disease, 264
chemotherapy, 264
localized disease management, 261–263
Mohs micrographic surgery, 263
outcomes, 261–262
radiation with surgery, 262–263
surgery extent, 263
surgery with radiation, 262–263
targeted molecular therapy, 264–265
asphalt, 48
atypical fibroxanthoma (AFX), 87, 88, 436
auricular lesions

overview, 166
surgical techniques, 161–162 (*See also* surgery *main entry*)
auricular reconstruction. *See also* head and neck reconstructive surgery *main entry*
anatomy, 531–533
blood supply, 533–534
sensory nerve supply, 534–535
auricular defect extent preop studies, 536
blood supply assessment, 536
cartilage harvest site assessment, 536
clinical assessment/preoperative workup, 535–537
defect types, 535
frame reconstruction
alloplastic materials for, 546–547
suture materials in, 547–548
goal setting, 535
larger defect reconstruction with adequate local skin, 548–550
larger defect reconstruction without adequate local skin
tissue expansion, 550
vascularized tissue, 550–551
medical history, patient, 535–536
multidisciplinary management, 535
overview, 553
prosthetics, 551–553
prosthetics team assessment, 536
techniques
Antia-Buch flap (helical rim defects), 544, 545–546
Dieffenbach flap (pinna middle third defects), 546
lobule-only small defect reconstruction, 540, 542, 543
posterior auricular flaps, 544, 545
skin and cartilage small defect reconstruction, 540, 541
skin grafts, 542, 544
skin-only small defect reconstruction, 539–540
vascularized island flap, 546, 547
template fabrication, 536–537
timing of reconstruction, 539
auricular skin cancer. *See also* periauricular lesions
spread mechanisms, 160–161
treatment surgical margins, 161

B

bacitracin, 507
Barrett esophagus, 206
basal cell nevus syndrome/Gorlin syndrome/Gorlin-Goltz syndrome, 12, 13, 48–49, 51, 103, 210, 446
overview, 121
radiation therapy, 48–49 (*See also* ionizing radiation *main entry*)
radiotherapy, 449
and UV radiation, 48–49
basement membrane zone anatomy, 3
Bazex syndrome, 49
BCC (basal cell carcinoma), 85. *See also* NMSC (nonmelanoma skin cancer)
adenoid, 85
aggressive, 124
surgical margins, 133
AJCC histologic grades, 23
AJCC prognostic groups, 23
AJCC staging, 22, 23, 132 (*See also* staging *main entry*)
auricular tumor locations, 157–158
basal cell nevus syndrome/Gorlin syndrome/Gorlin-Goltz syndrome, 48–49, 121
Bazex syndrome, 49
clinical evaluation, 15–16 (*See also* BCC (basal cell carcinoma) *under* clinical evaluation for details)
cumulative chronic sun exposure, 11
and *Drosophila* patched gene (PTCH) mutations, 83
electrodessication and curettage, 161–162, 444
environmental risk factors, 13
epidemiology, 102–103
facial H-zone, central, 125
geographical correlation, 12
and glucocorticoids, 49
hamartomatous, 85
histologic variants, 83–85
histopathology, 82–85
subtypes, 123
HPV (human papillomavirus) oncogenic strains, 49
infiltrative/morpheaform, 15, 16, 84–85, 434–435, 444
interferon alpha-2b, 445
ionizing radiation, 12, 122
metatypical, 84
micronodular, 84, 85, 124, 434–435, 444
NCCN metatypical form categorization, 15
nevi sebaceous, 48
nodular, 85, 123, 209–210
nodulocystic, 83
organ transplant patients, 49
outcomes, 41, 42
overview, 82–83, 443
PDT (photodynamic therapy), 209–210, 444
periauricular lesions histology, 155–156

BCC (basal cell carcinoma) *(continued)*
periorbital lesions, 173
medial canthus surgical management, 177–178
orbital invasion management, 178–179
surgical margins, 176
PET/with or without CT scanning, 20
prognosis, 112–113
radiotherapy
adjuvant radiotherapy, 194
management, 200–203
overview, 191–192, 449–450
radiotherapy alone, 192–194
treatment modality selection, 192–194
Rombo syndrome, 49
SBCC (superfical basal cell carcinoma)
5-ALA, 447
overview, 209
treatment, 210
skull base/subcranial soft tissue extension prognosis, 189
squamous differentiation, 85
with squamous features, 84
staging
AJCC, 22, 23
overview, 21
superficial, 209–210
superficial pattern, 15, 83–84, 85, 123
surgery
and perineural invasion, 146
peripheral margins, 145
surveillance
environmental contaminant concerns, 48
and genetics, 48–49
immunosuppression, 49
ionizing radiation, 48
occupational concerns, 48
phenotype, 46
UV radiation, 48
targeted therapy: hedgehog pathway, 218–219
treatment, 443–444
basosquamous/metatypical, 434–435, 444
cryosurgery, 448
curettage, 21–22
electrodesiccation, 21
follow-up, 23
high-risk, 22–23, 434–435
low-risk lesions (NCCN guidelines), 21–22
Mohs micrographic surgery, 22, 428, 432, 433, 434, 444
radiation, 23
resection, 22
tumorigenesis risk factors, 13
UVB, 46
UV signature mutations, 58
and xeroderma pigmentosum (XP), 120–121
BCG (Bacillus Calmette-Guérin), 387, 388, 421
injection, 23
BDI-II (Beck Depression Inventory-II), self-report screening measure, 35
bevacizumab, 265, 382, 399
biopsy. *See also* sentinel lymph node biopsy (SLNB) *main entry*
AS (angiosarcoma)
patient evaluation, 259–260
clinical evaluation
melanoma, 18
NMSC (nonmelanoma skin cancer), 127
partial thickness, 18
punch, 18, 334
small BCC/SCC, 18
MCC (Merkel cell carcinoma), 236
MM (malignant melanoma) local management
ABCDE (*a*symmetry, *b*order irregularity, *c*olor variegation, *d*iameter greater than 6 mm, and *e* evolving [increasing] size or color) criteria, 333
by narrow margin excision, 333–334, 335
punch/incisional full thickness, 334, 335
shave, 334
SLNB (sentinel lymph node biopsy), 335
NMSC (nonmelanoma skin cancer), 21
aggressive, 127
techniques
NMSC (nonmelanoma skin cancer), 127
bleomycin, 442, 443
overview, 446
blepharoptosis, 174
Bovenoid papulosis, 49
Bowen disease, 13, 14, 81. *See also* SCC (squamous cell carcinoma)
BSI 18 (Brief Symptom Inventory) psychological stress measure, 34

C

C255, 218
CancerCare, 36
Cancer Care for the Whole Patient: Meeting Psychosocial Health Needs (Institute of Medicine), 30, 33, 34, 35
Cancer Information Service, NCI (National Cancer Institute), 36
CancerVax, 389
Canvaxin melanoma cell vaccine, 300–301

carboplatin, 241, 243, 391, 393
carboplatin, paclitaxel, sorafenib, 393
carboplatin and paclitaxel, 393
carcinogenesis. *See* UV carcinogenesis
cardiac fibroma, 121
carmustine, 392, 393
CDK4 (cyclin-dependent kinase 4), 12, 13, 46
CDKN2A/p16 tumor suppressor gene heritable germline mutations, 12, 13, 50
celecoxib, 217–218
cellular growth factor increase, 13
cetuximab, 217–218, 218
Changing Faces, UK support organization, 35, 37
c-Ha-ras mutation, 13
cheek reconstruction. *See also* head and neck reconstructive surgery *main entry*
  anatomy, 575–576
  anticoagulant medications, 585
  bleeding-related complications, 585
  defect analysis, 576
  and facial feature distortion, 585
  facial nerve injury, 585–586
  overview, 575
  reconstructive options
    advancement flaps, 577–578
    anterolateral thigh flap (ALT), 583, 584
    banner flaps, 578–579
    biloped flaps, 579
    cervicofacial flaps, 580–581
    cervicopectoral flaps, 581–582
    closure, 577
    fibula osteocutaneous flap, 585
    flaps, 577–583, 583–585
    microsurgery, 583–585
    musculocutaneus flaps, 582–583
    parascapular flap, 583, 585
    pectoralis major flaps, 582
    primary closure, 577
    radical forearm flap (ALT), 583
    rectus abdominis flap, 585
    rhomboid flaps, 579–580
    rotational flaps, 580–582
    secondary intention closure, 577
    skin grafts, 577
    tissue expansion, 582–583
    transposition flaps, 578–580
  scarring, 585
  with smokers, 585
chemotherapy, 178
  angiosarcoma, head and neck, 264
  chemoradiation
    skull base/subcranial soft tissue extension, 188
  melanoma drug resistance/apoptosis resistance, 286
  NMSC (nonmelanoma skin cancer)
    aggressive, 136
  platinum-based, 444
  with radiotherapy, 136
cisplatin, 136, 241, 243, 264, 294, 391, 392–393, 394
cisplatin, vinblastine, dacarbazine/interferon-2, interferon-alpha, 394
c-KIT receptor tyrosine kinases, 398–399
Clark levels
  melanoma, 16, 17, 23
  SCC (squamous cell carcinoma), 15
clinical evaluation. *See also* FNA (fine-needle aspiration)
  ABCDE (asymmetry, border irregularity, color variegation, diameter less than 6 mm, evolving in size, shape, color shades, and surface features or symptoms), 8, 18
    and malignancy suspicion, 16
    melanoma, 16
  adnexal tumors, 224
  BCC (basal cell carcinoma)
    histomorphologic growth patterns, 15
    infiltrative/morpheaform, 15, 16
    metatypical/basosquamous, 15
    nodular/noduloulcerative, 15, 123
    path of spread, 16
    regional metastasis, 16
    superficial multicentric, 15
  biopsy techniques
    NMSC (nonmelanoma skin cancer), 127
  bony invasion suspicion, 19
  chest x-ray, 19
  contrasted neck CT, 19
  cortical irregularities, 19
  cranial nerve exam, 18
  CT imaging, 19–20
  dermoscopy, 18
  diplopia, 18
  facial weakness, 18
  gadolinium-contrast MRI, 20
  hearing assessment, 18
  high-resolution CT, 19
  high-resolution ultrasound, 20
  high-resolution ultrasound FNA (fine-needle aspiration), 20
  imaging, 19–20, 23
    NMSC (nonmelanoma skin cancer), 127–131
  intraorbital/intracranial MRI, 20
  LDH (serum lactate dehydrogenase) measurement, 19, 23

clinical evaluation *(continued)*
lesions
biopsy: melanoma, 18
biopsy: punch, 18, 334
biopsy: small BCC/SCC, 18
and questions for patient, 13
suspicious, 18–19
and lesions
qualities, 12
lymphadenopathy check, 18
lymphatic drainage patterns, 18
lymph node CT, 20
melanoma, 16–17
MM (malignant melanoma), 16–17
MRI, 20
MRI imaging, 20
and neural foramina widening, 19
and nevi changes, 8, 46–47
otoscopy, 18
overview, 24–25
parotid gland, 18
parotid masses, 12
patient history
basal cell nevus syndrome/Gorlin syndrome/ Gorlin-Goltz syndrome, 12
CDK4 (cyclin-dependent kinase 4), 12, 46
clinical implications, 12
environmental toxin exposure, 12
family history, 12
geographical correlation, 12
geography correlation, 12
ionizing radiation, 12, 47
MC1R (melanocortin-1 receptor), 12, 46
MM (malignant melanoma), 47
and nevi, 12
NMSC (nonmelanoma skin cancer), 126–127
stasis ulcers/sinus tracts, chronic, 12
trauma, 12
ultraviolet exposure, 11–12 (*See also* UV radiation *main heading*)
xeroderma pigmentosum (XP), 12, 46
perineural invasion MRI, 20
perineural invasion suspicion, 19
PET/with or without CT scanning, 20
physical examination, 17–18
DFSP (dermatofibrosarcoma protuberans), 250–251
MCC (Merkel cell carcinoma), 235–236
PNI (perineural invasion), 6
proptosis, 18
SCC (squamous cell carcinoma)
actinic keratoses (AK), 12–13, 14, 48
Bowen disease, 13, 14
differential, 14
invasive, 14–15
keratoacanthoma, 14
sentinel lymph node biopsy (SLNB), 4–5, 20, 21, 134
staging, 20, 21–24 (*See also* staging *main entry for details*)
NMSC (nonmelanoma skin cancer), 106–112, 131–132 (*See also* staging *main entry; individual disease categories*)
trigeminal nerve sensation, 18
coal tar, 13, 48
Coley, William (1862–1936), 297
colorectal carcinoma, 121
COX-2 inhibition, 217–218
COX (cyclooxygenase) inhibition, 136
cranial convexity tumors. *See under* neurosurgical management *main entry*
creosote, 13
cryosurgery, 448–449. *See under* surgery; surgery *main entry*
CTLA-4 (cytotoxic T lymphocyte-associated antigen), 306–307, 382
anti-CTLA-4 (cytotoxic T lymphocyte-associated antigen), 395
cutaneous melanoma. *See also* immunobiology/ melanoma; immunotherapy of melanoma; melanoma; metastatic melanoma local management; metastatic melanoma regional management; metastatic melanoma treatment; MM (malignant melanoma); mucosal melanomas of the head and neck (MMHN); ocular melanoma
AJCC staging criteria, 23, 24
anatomic stage groupings, 24
excision margins, 176
history of sequelae, 48
lymphoscintigraphy/sentinel node biopsy (SLNB), 4–5
TNM staging criteria, 24
tobacco smoking risk factor, 47
and UVB tumor suppressor gene mutations, 58–59
and xeroderma pigmentosum (XP), 120
CVD (cisplatin, vinblastine, dacarbazine), 392–393
cyclophosphamide, 241, 264
cyclophosphamide (CTX), 309

D

dacarbazide, 308
dacarbazine, 389, 390, 391, 392–393, 394, 399
dacarbazine, cisplatin, carmustine, tamoxifen, 393
Darier disease, 81

dasatinib, 421
dermatology for screening follow-up, 49
dermis anatomy, 3
dermoepidermal junction. *See* basement membrane zone
DFSP (dermatofibrosarcoma protuberans)
  chemotherapy, 253–254
  clinical presentation
    metastatic disease, 249
    primary disease, 248–249
  epidemiology, 247–248
  follow-up, 254
  molecular biology/genetics, 249–250
  overview, 247, 254
  pathology, 249–250
  physical examination, 250–251
  staging, 252
  surgery
    Mohs micrographic, 253, 435–436
    reconstruction, 253
    wide local excision, 252–253
  surveillance, 254
  treatment, 252–254
DHA (dihydroxyacetone), 50
diclofenac, 442
  overview, 446–447
diet, 48, 136
diplopia, 174
DNA alkylators, 392
DNA impairment, chemically induced, 13
docetaxel, 264, 391, 393, 444
doxorubicin, 241, 264, 444
doxorubicin, pegylated liposomal, 264, 265
Drosophila patched gene (PTCH) mutations, 83
drugs, 390
  Abraxane, 39
  acitretin, 446
  antiangiogenic agents, 382
  antibiotics, 446, 479, 500, 507
  anticoagulants, 585
  antiemetics, 390
  bacitracin, 507
  bevacizumab, 265, 382, 399
  bleomycin, 442, 443, 446
  C255, 218
  capecitabine, 445
  carboplatin, 241, 243, 391, 393
  carboplatin, paclitaxel, sorafenib, 393
  carboplatin and paclitaxel, 393
  carmustine, 392, 393
  celecoxib, 217–218
  cetuximab, 217–218, 218
  cisplatin, 136, 241, 243, 264, 294, 391, 392–393, 393, 394
  cisplatin, vinblastine, dacarbazine/interferon-2, interferon-alpha, 394
  COX-2 inhibition, 217–218
  CVD (cisplatin, vinblastine, dacarbazine), 392–393
  cyclophosphamide, 241, 264
  cyclophosphamide (CTX), 309
  dacarbazide, 308
  dacarbazine, 389, 390, 391, 392–393, 394, 399
  dacarbazine, cisplatin, carmustine, tamoxifen, 393
  dasatinib, 421
  diclofenac, 442
    overview, 446–447
  DNA alkylators, 392
  docetaxel, 264, 391, 393, 444
  doxorubicin, 241, 264, 444
  doxorubicin, pegylated liposomal, 264, 265
  Erbitux, 218
  erlotinib, 217
  etoposide, 241, 243, 264
  5-fluorouracil, 50, 178, 264, 435, 443, 444–445
  5-fluorouracil, topical, 444–445
  5-fluorouracil cream, 442
  5-fluorouracil solution, 442
  fluorouracil, 445
  C-fluorouracil, 178
  fotemustine, 392
  gemcitabine, 243
  Gleevec, 421
  glucocorticoids, 49
  ifosfamide, 264
  imatinib, 265
  imatinib, 421
  imiquimod, 23, 50, 435, 443, 444, 445
  imiquimod cream, 442
  immunodulators, topical, 441
  immunosuppressive, 456
  interferon, 382–383, 390, 410, 435, 444
  interferon-α, 136, 301, 303, 394
  interferon-alpha, recombinant, 383
  interferon alpha-2a, 443, 444
  interferon alpha-2b, 264
  interferon-alpha2b, 393, 421, 442
  interferon alpha (IFA), 23, 388–389
  interleukin-1, 206
  interleukin-2, 393, 421
  interleukin-2 (IL-2), 265, 304, 305–306, 392, 394–395
  interleukin-2 (IL-2), recombinant, 394–395
  interleukin-6, 206
  interleukin-12 (IL-12), 306–307
  interlukin-2, 265

drugs *(continued)*
ipilimumab, 307
irinotecan, 243
isotretinoin, 51
levamisole, 383
lomustine, 392
melphalan, 23
mensa, 264
methotrexate, 446
mitomycin-C, 410, 436
multikinase inhibitors, 49
mupirocin, 507
neomycin, 507
nilotinib, 421
NSAIDs, 446–447
oblimersen sodium, 382
OK-432, 265
Ontak, 308–309
OSI-774, 217
paclitaxel, 39, 264, 393
prednisone, 444
protein kinase inhibitors, 382
rapamycin, 218, 265
retinoic acid, 136
retinoids, 51, 446
SilverMed, 507
sorafenib, 49, 265, 382, 393
steroids, 456
tamoxifen, 390, 393
tamoxifen, cisplatin, dacarbazine, interleukin-2, interferon-alpha2b, 393
Tarceva, 217
taxanes, 243, 264
tazarotene, 446
temozolomide, 308, 390–391, 393
temozolomide and docetaxel, 393
tetracyclines, 446
tipfarnib, 49
topotecan, single-agent, 243
tretinoin, 446
tretinoin, topical, 443
vinblastine, 392–393, 394
vincristine, 241, 444
vinorelbine, 392
DT (Distress Thermometer) screening tool, 34

E

electrochemotherapy, 446
EMPD (extramammary Paget disease), 86. *See also* Paget disease
histopathology, 85, 92
imiquimod, 445
topical immunodulators, 441
environmental exposure
BCC (basal cell carcinoma), 13
MM (malignant melanoma), 13
SCC (squamous cell carcinoma), 13
UVA, 7
UVB, 7–8, 11, 12, 13
epidemiology, 11
BCC (basal cell carcinoma), 102–103
DFSP (dermatofibrosarcoma protuberans), 247–248
MCC (Merkel cell carcinoma), 105–106
NMSC (nonmelanoma skin cancer)
101-102, overview
aggressive form overview, 119–120
overview, 101–102
periauricular lesions, 156
SCC (squamous cell carcinoma), 103–105
overview, 103
risk factors, 103–105
epidemodysplasia verruciformis (EV), 122
epidermis
anatomy, 1–3
basale/stratum germinativum, 1
physiology, 1–3
stratum spinosum, 1
epidermodysplasia verruciformis, 13, 48. *See also* HPV (human papillomavirus)
Erbitux, 218
erlotinib, 217
esophageal cancer, 206
etiology. *See also* genetics
etoposide, 241, 243, 264
examination, physical. *See* clinical evaluation

F

family history
clinical evaluation, 12
genetics, melanoma, 12, 13
and MM (malignant melanoma), 46
fibrosarcoma, 121
Fitzpatrick's classification of sun-reactive skin types, 3
5-ALA (5-aminolevulinic acid) lipohilic photosynthesizer, 206
5-fluorouracil, 50, 178, 264, 435, 443, 444–445
5-fluorouracil, topical, 444–445
5-fluorouracil cream, 442
5-fluorouracil solution, 442

fluorouracil, 445
C-fluorouracil, 178
FNA (fine-needle aspiration)
high-resolution ultrasound, 20
and regional lymph node suspicion, SCC, 21
fotemustine, 392
Frey syndrome, 164

G

gemcitabine, 243
genetics
albinism, 12, 13
oculocutaneous, 13, 46, 48
oculocutaneous +, 46
basal cell nevus syndrome/Gorlin syndrome/Gorlin-Goltz syndrome, 12, 13, 51, 121
BCC (basal cell carcinoma), 13
CDK4 (cyclin-dependent kinase 4), 12, 46
CDKN2A/p16 tumor suppressor gene heritable germline mutations, 12, 13, 50
D294H variant of MC1R, 46
epidermodysplasia verruciformis, 13
familial atypical mole, 271
genodermatoses, 51
high-risk carrier follow-up, 50
HPV (human papillomavirus), 13, 48, 122
MC1R (melanocortin-1 receptor), 12, 46
melanocyte progression/metastasis, 289–290 (*See also* Melanocyte progression/metastasis *main entry*)
melanocytes, 46
melanocyte self-maintenance/proliferation (mutations), 286–288 (*See also* Melanocyte self-maintenance/proliferation (genetic mutations) *main entry for details*)
melanocyte transformation and cell-to-cell communication changes, 290–292 (*See also* Melanocyte transformation and cell-to-cell communication changes *main entry for details*)
melanocytic lesion genetic alterations/proliferation, 281–286 (*See also* Melanocytic lesion genetic alterations/proliferation *main entry for details*)
melanoma family history, 12, 13, 271
MM (malignant melanoma), 13
Muir-Torre syndrome (MTS)/HNPCC (hereditary nonpolyposis colon cancer), 121
p53 tumor suppressor gene in keratinocyte DNA, 7–8, 93, 104, 120
R151C variant of MC1R, 46
R160W variant of MC1R, 46
risk factors, 13
SCC (squamous cell carcinoma), 13
xeroderma pigmentosum (XP), 12, 13, 46, 271
geographical risk factor, 12, 13
Gilda's Club, 36
Gleevec, 421
Gorlin-Goltz syndrome. *See* basal cell nevus syndrome/Gorlin syndrome/Gorlin-Goltz syndrome
Gorlin syndrome. *See* basal cell nevus syndrome/Gorlin syndrome/Gorlin-Goltz syndrome
grading
SCC (squamous cell carcinoma) histologic, 81
granular cell tumor (GCT) histopathology, 91
granulocyte-macrophage colony stimulating factor (GM-CSF), 306, 388

H

HADS (Hospital Anxiety and Depression Scale), 34
head and neck reconstructive surgery. *See also* auricular reconstruction; cheek reconstruction; cheek reconstruction *main entry;* lip reconstruction *main entry;* nasal reconstructive surgery; periorbital reconstruction *main entry;* scalp reconstruction *main entry;* surgery
armamentarium, reconstructive, 458–469
cartilage grafts, 462–463
composite grafts, 463
flaps
axial pattern, 467
free tissue transfer, 467–468
local random: advancement, 464
local random: overview, 463–464
local random: rhombic, 466
local random: rotation, 464–466
regional pedicled, 467
full-thickness skin graft (FTSG), 461, 462
goals, 455–456
honey for wound care, 507
options
for auricle, 460
for cheek, 460
for lip, 459
for nose, 459
for orbital/periorbital area, 460
for scalp, 461
overview, 455, 469

head and neck reconstructive surgery *(continued)*
planning
and actinic damage, 457
and adjuvant therapy, 456
and advanced or recurrent disease, 456
and cardiovascular disease, 456
and cicatrical contracture, 457
and comorbidities, 456
and critical facial features (lip, ala, eyelid), 457
defect analysis, 456–458
delayed reconstruction, 458
and diabetes, 456
and facial aesthetic units, 457
facial wound elements, 458
history of lesions, biopsies, procedures, 456
layer depth of wound, 458
Mohs micrographic excision, 458
patient factors, 456
single-stage *versus* multistage, 456
and smoking, 456
three-dimensional defect consideration, 458
prosthetic rehabilitation, 456, 468–469
secondary intention healing, 458
shampoo wound care, 507
shortening oil for wound care, 507
single-stage resection/reconstruction of composite facial defects, 467–468
split-thickness skin graft (STSG), 461–462
wound care, 507

H

hemangioendotheliomas, 260
hemangiopericytoma, 260
histology
melanocytic nevi precursor lesions, 317–320 (*See also* precursor lesion histology *under* melanoma *main entry*)
melanoma
acral lentiginous melanoma/mucosal melanoma, 326
Breslow levels of thickness, 323
Clark levels of thickness, 323
clear cell sarcoma (soft parts melanoma), 328–329
dermal component, 323
desmoplastic melanoma, 326–327
features, 323–324
lentigo maligna type, 325
and maturation absence, 324
metastatic, 328
nevoid melanoma, 326
nodular melanoma, 326
overview, 323
partial regression, 323
pathology report elements, 324
perineural invasion, 323–324
satellitosis, microscopic, 324
Spitzoid melanoma/atypical Spitzoid lesions, 327–328
subtypes, miscellaneous, 328
superficial spreading melanoma, 325–326
tumor-infiltrating lymphocytes, 324
ulceration, 323
melanoma precursor lesions, 317–320 (*See also* precursor lesion histology *under* melanoma *main entry*)
melanoma precursor lesions by degree, dysplastic nevi, 320–322 (*See also* dysplastic nevi (melanoma precursors by degree) histology *under* melanoma *main entry*)
MM (malignant melanoma)
metastatic, 328
periauricular lesions, 155–156
skin appendages, 223–224
histopathology
Abrikossoff tumor, 91
adnexal tumors, 224
AK (actinic keratosis), 79–81
angiosarcoma, 90
atypical fibroxanthoma (AFX), 87, 88
and malignant fibrous histiocytoma (MFH), 88
BCC (basal cell carcinoma), 82–85
subtypes, 123
benign fibrous histiocytoma (BFH), 86–87
cellular schwannoma, 91
chondrosarcoma, 90
cutaneous lymphoid hyplasia (CLH), 94–95
cutaneous lymphomas, 95–96
dermafibrosarcoma protuberans (DFSP), 87, 88
dermatofibroma, 86–87
desmoplastic SCC, 124
eccrine neoplasms, 92–93
EMPD (extramammary Paget disease), 85, 86, 92
epidermotropism, 92
epithelial proliferations of skin, 7908
fibrohistiocytic proliferations, 86–89
follicular neoplasms, 91–92
granular cell tumor (GCT), 91
Kaposi sarcoma, 89
leiomyosarcoma, 89–90
lymphoid hyperplasia (reactive), 94–95
malignant adenexal neoplasms, 91–93
malignant fibrous histiocytoma MFH)
and atypical fibroxanthoma (AFX), 88

malignant mixed tumor (MMT), 92–93
malignant pilar tumor, 91–92
malignant pilar tumor (MPT), 91–92
MCC (Merkel cell carcinoma), 93–94, 95
mesenchyman neoplasms, 86–91
microcystic adnexal carcinoma (MAC), 92
mucinous carcinoma (MC), 93
neural tumors, 89–91
NMSC (nonmelanoma skin cancer)
aggressive, 123
osteosarcoma, 90
overview, 97
plexiform schwannoma, 90–91
porocarcinoma, 92
primary cutaneous B-cell lymphomas, 95–96
rhabdomyoblastoma, 90
sasosquamous SCC, 124
SCC (squamous cell carcinoma), 81–82, 123
sebaceous adenoma, 93
sebaceous carcinoma, 93
sebaceous epithelioma, 93
sebaceous neoplasms, 93
spindle cell SCC, 124
trichilemmal carcinoma (TC), 91
vascular tumors, 89
history
ear reconstruction 600 BC–1950s, 531
facial prostheses, ancient Egypt, 589
Greek/Roman gold/silver facial prosthetic masks, 590
head and neck reconstructive surgery
3000 BC earliest dated, 455
Edwin Smith Surgical Papyrus (Egypt) facial trauma management, 455
nasal reconstruction, northern India, 6th century BC, 455
Mohs, Frederic (1910–2002), 425–426
Mohs surgery
controversy, 426
frozen section incorporation into technique, 426
micrographic observation of tumor surgical margins concept, 425–426
HIV, 49, 89, 104, 114
SCC (squamous cell carcinoma), 49
HNPCC (hereditary nonpolyposis colon cancer)/Muir-Torre syndrome (MTS), 121
HPPH (2[1-hexyloxyethyl]-2 devinyl pyroheophorbide, or photochlor), 207
HPV (human papillomavirus), 13, 48. *See also* epidermodysplasia verruciformis
SCC (squamous cell carcinoma), 443
and SCC (squamous cell carcinoma), 122
types, 82
and VC (verrucous carcinoma) of scalp, 82
hydrocarbons, polycyclic aromatic, 48
H-zone (midface: upper lip, nose, medial canthus), 7, 8

I

IFN (interferon) injection, 23
ifosfamide, 264
imatinib, 265, 421
imiquimod, 23, 50, 435, 443, 444
imiquimod cream, 442
immunobiology/melanoma, 299. *See also* cutaneous melanoma; Immunotherapy of melanoma; melanoma; metastatic melanoma local management; metastatic melanoma regional management; MM (malignant melanoma); mucosal melanomas of the head and neck (MMHN); ocular melanoma
immunodulators, topical, 441
immunosuppression, 12, 13, 47
AIDS, 298
prevention of cutaneous cancer, 51
and prevention of cutaneous cancer, 50
and SCC (squamous cell carcinoma), 122
immunosurveillance
and AIDS immunosuppression, 298
immunology terms, 298
MHC (major histocompatability complex), 298, 299
PAMPS (pathogen-associated molecular patterns), 297–298
and posttransplant antirejection therapy, 298
TAAs (tumor-associated antigens), 298
T cells, 297–299
TILs (tumor-infiltrating lymphocytes) T cells, 298–299
TLR (toll-like receptor) eerm line-encoded pattern-recognition receptors, 297
Tregs (immunosuppressive regulatory T cells), 298, 299
Immunosurveillance *main entry. See also* Immunotherapy of melanoma
immunotherapy of melanoma. *See also* cutaneous melanoma; Immunobiology/melanoma; Immunosurveillance *main entry;* melanoma; metastatic melanoma local management; metastatic melanoma regional management; mucosal melanomas of the head and neck (MMHN); ocular melanoma
approaches, 299–310
cancer-testis antigens, 302
differentiation antigens, 302
future, 310–311

immunotherapy of melanoma *(continued)*
history of treatment, 297
immune stimulation, 304
immunology terms, 298
immunostimulatory cytokines
granulocyte-macrophage colony stimulating factor (GM-CSF), 306, 388
interferon-α (IFN-α), 304–305
interleukin-2 (IL-2), 305–306
interleukin-12 (IL-12), 306–307
inhibiting the inhibitors
adoptive immunotherapy, 309–310
with chemotherapy, 308
cyclophosphamide (CTX), 309
cytotoxic T lymphocyte-associated antigen 4 (CTLA-4), 307
ipilimumab antibody, 307–308
Ontak, 308–309
overview, 307
Tregs (regulatory T cells), 308–309
tremelimumab antibody, 307, 308
MAGE-1 cancer-testis antigen, 302
melanoma-associated antigens, 302
for metastatic disease, 394–395 (*See also* drugs *main entry; listings for individual agents*)
overexpressed antigens, 302
radiotherapy potential, 310
tumor-induced immunosuppression mechanisms, 308
tumor-specific antigens, 302
Tyrosinase differentiation antigen, 302
vaccination
allogeneic, 300–301
antigen delivery, 302–303
autologous, 301
with cancer-testis antigens, 302
Canvaxin melanoma cell vaccine, 300–301
dendritic-cell antigen delivery, 303
dendritic-cell (DC) delivery, 303, 421
by DNA, 303
with HSPs (heat shock proteins), 303
and immunostimulatory cytokines, 301
Malacine melanoma cell vaccine, 301
with melanoma-associated antigens, 302
with mutated antigens, 302
and overexpressed antigens, 302
overview, 299–300, 303
tumor antigen peptide delivery, 302–303
tumor cell-based melanoma vaccines, 300–301
immunotherapy of melanomas, Coley, William (1862–1936), 297
interferon, 382–383, 390, 410, 435
interferon-α, 136, 301, 303, 394
interferon-α, recombinant, 383
interferon-α-2a, 443, 444
interferon-α2b, 264, 393, 421, 442
interferon α (IFA), 23, 388–389
interleukin-1, 206
interleukin-2, 393
interleukin-2 (IL-2), 265, 304, 305–306, 392, 394–395
interleukin-2 (IL-2), recombinant, 394–395
interleukin-6, 206
interleukin-12 (IL-12), 306–307
interlukin-2, 265
ionizing radiation, 12. *See also* radiation therapy
BCC (basal cell carcinoma), 122
and prevention of cutaneous cancer, 50
and xeroderma pigmentosum (XP), 48
ipilimumab, 307
irinotecan, 243
isotretinoin, 51
ITEM (immunosuppression, treatment, extracapsular spread, and margins) prognostic scoring system, 113–114

K

KA (keratoacanthoma), 82, 83
Kaposi sarcoma, 89, 101, 260, 264
keratinocytes
atypical, AK, 80, 81
atypical, SCC, 81
basal, 79, 80, 81
Borst-Jadassohn pattern, 81
DNA of, 7
physiology, 1, 2, 7
and SCC, 12–13
and UV immune suppression, 65
keratoacanthomas, 14, 121
K-ras mutation, 13
Kripke, Margaret, 57

L

LAF (Lance Armstrong Foundation), 36
Langerhans cells
physiology, 2
and UV immune suppression, 64–65
UV radiation, 61
leiomyosarcoma
histopathology, 89–90
Let's Face It (University of Michigan), 37
levamisole, 383
Levulan Kerastick, 207
lip reconstruction, 459. *See also* head and neck reconstructive surgery

anatomy, 487–488
options
conversion to full-thickness defect , then local flap reconstruction (partial-thickness defects), 489
defects greater than two thirds of lip (full-thickness defects), 501
defects of one third to two thirds of lip (full-thickness defects), 490–497
defects of up to one-third of lip (full-thickness defects), 490
local flap reconstruction (partial-thickness defects), 489
partial-thickness defects, 488–489
skin grafting (partial-thickness defects), 489
overview, 487, 502
postoperative care, 500
reconstructive strategy, 488
surgical complications, 500, 502
llnevi sebaceous
BCC (basal cell carcinoma), 48
lomustine, 392
Look Good . . . Feel Better program (American Cancer Society [ACS]), 35, 36
lung cancer, 206
lUV radiation
UVB
and immune reaction suppression, 60
lymphatic drainage
buccinator/perifacial lymphatics, 5
cervical lymphatic basins, 6
external jugular lymphatics, 5
lymphatic metastases site clinical predictions, 4
nodal drainage patterns, 5–6
overview, 4–5
periauricular lymphatics, 5
lymphatic mapping
metastatic melanoma regional management in node-negative neck, 348–350
lymphatic metastases site clinical predictions, 4
lymphocytic leukemia, chronic, 126
lymphoproliferative lesions, 173

M

Malacine melanoma cell vaccine, 301
MAL (methyl aminolevulinic, 447
management. *See* treatment
mandible ondontogenic keratocysts, 121
Marjolin ulcer +, 12, 13
MC1R (melanocortin-1 receptor), 12, 13, 46
MCC (Merkel cell carcinoma), 173
anatomic distribution, 234
biopsy, 236
clinically positive lymph node management
adjuvant chemotherapy, 241
adjuvant regional radiotherapy, 241
therapeutic dissection, 240–241
clinical presentation, 235
epidemiology, 105–106, 233
etiology, 234–235
FNA (fine-needle aspiration), 236
follow-up, 244
histologic workup, 236–237
histopathology, 93–94, 95
Mohs surgery (micrographic/histographic), 437
overview, 233
pathogenesis, 234–235
patient history, 235
physical examination, 235–236
primary tumor management
surgical margins, 239
wide local excision, 239
prognosis, 114–115
radiographic workup, 237
radiotherapy, 240
regional disease management, 240–243
risk factors, 234–235
sentinel lymph node biopsy (SLNB), N0 neck, 241–243
stage IV disease management, 243
staging, 106
AJCC (American Joint Committee on Cancer), 112, 238–239
MSKCC (Memorial Sloan Kettering Cancer Center), 111–112, 238
surveillance, 244
tumor biology, 233–234
medulloblastoma, 121
melanin reactive oxygen species, 13
melanocyte progression/metastasis
IGFBP7, 289–290
PL3K-AKT (phosphatidylinositol-3-kinase-AKT) pathway, 289
mTOR, 289
PTEN, 289
melanocytes +, 2, 13, 46
melanocyte self-maintenance/proliferation (genetic mutations)
apoptosis resistance, 286–288
Bcl-2 family, 286–287
overview, 286
Apaf-1, 288
overview, 286

melanocyte stem cells
CD20, 293–294
label-retaining cells, 294
side-population cells, 294
melanocyte transformation and cell-to-cell communication changes
cadherins
β-catenin, 290–291
epithelial-mesenchymal transcriptional regulators, 292
notch-1 genes, 292
overview, 290
melanocytic lesion genetic alterations/proliferation
cyclin D1 extracellular signal mediation/sensing, 286
illustrative summary, 282
key regulatory pathway somatic mutation importance, 281–282
melanoma susceptibility genes
CDK4 high-penetrant melanoma-predisposing gene, 285
CDKN2A (cyclin-dependent inhibitor 2A) high-penetrance gene, 284–285
MC1R (melanocortin-1 receptor) low penetrance, 285
MITF (microphthalmia transcription factor), melanocyte development/survival implication, 285–286
RAS-RAF-MEK-ERK pathway/cascade
$BRAF^{V600E}$/basal kinase activity increase, 283, 284, 289
NRAS, first gene found as altered, 282–283
receptor tyrosine kinases
cKIT and individualized therapy, 284
cMET HGF receptor/proto oncogene, 284
melanocytic nevi, 50
melanoma. *See also* cutaneous melanoma; immunobiology/melanoma; immunotherapy of melanoma; MM (malignant melanoma); mucosal melanomas of the head and neck (MMHN)
ABCDE (asymmetry, border irregularity, color variegation, diameter less than 6 mm, evolving in size, shape, color shades, and surface features or symptoms), 16, 17
acral lentiginous, 17
amelanotic, 17
tumor initiation/progression from genetic hits illustrated, 288
auricular tumor locations, 157–158
chest x-ray, 19, 23
cisplatin-resistant, 294
Clark levels, 16, 17, 23
of thickness, 323
clinical evaluation, 16–17
CT, 23
dermoscopy, 18
desmoplastic, 17
drug resistance/apoptosis resistance, 286
dysplastic nevi (melanoma precursors by degree) histology
classification, 320–322
"Dysplastic Nevus: The Eye of the Hurricane" (Arumi-Uria), 320
NIH 1992 consensus conference terminology for, 320–321
and episodic UV exposure risk, 11
genetic factors
familial atypical mole, 271
melanoma syndrome, 271
histology
acral lentiginous melanoma/mucosal melanoma, 326
Breslow levels of thickness, 323
clear cell sarcoma (soft parts melanoma), 328–329
dermal component, 323
desmoplastic melanoma, 326–327
features, 323–324
lentigo maligna type, 325
and maturation absence, 324
metastatic, 328
nevoid melanoma, 326
nodular melanoma, 326
overview, 323
partial regression, 323
pathology report elements, 324
perineural invasion, 323–324
satellitosis, microscopic, 324
Spitzoid melanoma/atypical Spitzoid lesions, 327–328
subtypes, miscellaneous, 328
superficial spreading melanoma, 325–326
tumor-infiltrating lymphocytes, 324
ulceration, 323
and immunobiology, 299 (*See also* Immunotherapy of melanoma *main entry*)
incidence, 269–270
initial evaluation guidelines, 277
LDH (serum lactate dehydrogenase) measurement, 19, 23
lentigo maligna (melanoma in situ), 16, 17, 81, 323, 325, 326, 336, 337–338, 340, 437–438
melanocytic nevi precursor lesions

histology, 317–320 (*See also* precursor lesion histology *in this section*)
and micrometastes, 23
and microscopic nodal metastases, 23
mortality, 270
MRI, 23
NAD (nevus with architectural disorder) (*See* dysplastic nevi (melanoma precursors by degree) histology *in this section*)
nevi, 271
nodular, 16–17
overview, 269, 277
pathogenesis overview, 294
periauricular lesions
rate of metastatic spread, 160
periorbital lesions
medial canthus surgical management, 178
PET, 23
PET-CT, 23
pigment characteristics, 271
precursor (by degree) lesion histology, dysplastic nevi, 320–322 (*See also* dysplastic nevi (melanoma precursors by degree) histology *in this section*)
precursor lesion histology, 317–320
benign melanocytic nevi, 317–319
blue nevus, 319
blue nevus, cellular, 319
combined nevus, 319
compound nevi (benign), 319
congenital nevi, 320
halo nevi, 319
intradermal nevi (benign), 318
junctional nevi (benign), 317–318
so-called nevi of special sites, 319
Spitz nevi, 319–320
prevention, 272
prognosis, 273–276
rate increase, 41
risk factors, 270
staging
AJCC, 24, 273, 274, 374–376
exceptions to AJCC criteria, 23
I and II: localized, 273, 275
III: regional metastatic, 275
from immunohistochemical staining, 23
IV: distant metastatic, 275–276
of newly diagnosed patients, 276
and sunburn number, 12
and sunscreens, 272
thin
early detection, 42
treatment
BCG (Bacillus Calmette-Guérin) injection, 23
and Breslow thickness, 23
chemotherapy, 23
and Clark level, 23
IFN (interferon) injection, 23
imiquimod, 23
local ablation, 23
melphalan, 23
miotic rate, 23
and mitotic rate, 23
radiation, 23
and satellitosis, 23
and ulceration status, 23
and UV exposure, 271
UV signature mutations, 58–59
melphalan, 23
meningioma, 121
mensa, 264
mesenchyman neoplasms
histopathology, 86–91
metastatic melanoma local management. *See also* cutaneous melanoma; immunobiology/melanoma; immunotherapy of melanoma; mucosal melanomas of the head and neck (MMHN)
metastatic melanoma regional management. *See also* cutaneous melanoma; immunobiology/melanoma; immunotherapy of melanoma; MM (malignant melanoma); mucosal melanomas of the head and neck (MMHN)
in node-negative neck
and AJCC staging, 344–346
curative SLNB/lymphatic mapping patient selection, 352–353
ELND (elective [or immediate or prophylactic] lymph node dissection), 346–348, 348
future of, 364
intraoperative assessment, sentinel lymph nodes, 351
lymphatic mapping/SLNB: after wide local excision, 353
lymphatic mapping/SLNB: desmoplastic melanoma, 353–354
lymphatic mapping/SLNB: following wide local excision, 353
lymphatic mapping/SLNB: imaging considerations, 354
lymphatic mapping/SLNB: integration of nuclear medicine, surgery, and pathology, 354–355
lymphatic mapping/SLNB: in-transit metastasis risk, 362

metastatic melanoma regional management; in node-negative neck *(continued)*
lymphatic mapping/SLNB: morbidity, 362
lymphatic mapping/SLNB: preoperative lymphoscintigraphy, 355–358
lymphatic mapping/SLNB after wide local excision, 353
lymphatic mapping/SLNB complications, 362
lymphatic mapping/SLNB intraoperative considerations, 358–361
lymphatic mapping/SLNB (sentinel lymph node biopsy), 348–350, 352–353
lymphatic mapping/SNLB operating room positioning strategies, 361
non-sentinel lymph node involvement following completion lymph node dissection (CLND), 349–350
overview, 343
reverse-transcriptase-polymerase chain reaction (RT-PCR), 351
sentinel lymph node biopsy role, 350
sentinel lymph node pathologic analysis, 350–351
sentinel lymph node potential cure role, 352
submicroscopic disease clinical relevance, 351
TLND (therapeutic [or delayed] lymph node dissection), 346–348, 348
in node-positive neck
AJCC staging, 374–375
biochemotherapy, 382
diagnostic evaluation, 373–374
extent of tumor in lymph nodes, 377–379
imaging, 373–374
location of palpable nodes, 379–380
lymph node tumor burden, 374
and number of involved nodes, 374–375
overview, 373, 383
and primary melanoma location, 376–377
prognosis, 374–376
radical neck dissection (RND), 378, 380
radiotherapy role, 380, 382
satellitosis/in-transit metastases, 375
selective neck dissection (SND), 378–380, 382
targeted molecular therapy, 382
unknown primary melanoma, 376
metastatic melanoma treatment. *See also* cutaneous melanoma; MM (malignant melanoma); mucosal melanomas of the head and neck (MMHN)
adjuvant systemic therapy, 387–389 (*See also* drugs; vaccines; *individual agent listings*)
chemotherapeutic treatment
alkylating agents, 390–391 (*See also* drugs *main entry; listings for individual agents*)
biochemotherapy, 393–394 (*See also* drugs *main entry; listings for individual agents*)
combination, 392–393 (*See also* drugs *main entry; listings for individual agents*)
cytotoxic, 389–390 (*See also* drugs *main entry; listings for individual agents*)
nitrosoureas, 392 (*See also* drugs *main entry; listings for individual agent*)
platinum analogs, 391 (*See also* drugs *main entry; listings for individual agents*)
single-agent, 389–392 (*See also* drugs *main entry; listings for individual agents*)
taxanes, 391 (*See also* drugs *main entry; listings for individuals agents*)
vinca alkaloids, 391–392 (*See also* drugs *main entry; listings for individual agents*)
immunotherapy, 394–395 (*See also* drugs *main entry; listings for individual agents*)
overview, 387, 400
targeted therapy
antiangiogenesis, 399
anti/pro-apoptotic pathways, 399–400
bFGF receptors, 400
c-KIT receptor tyrosine kinases, 398–399
future directions, 400
heat-shock protein 90 (HSP90), 400
PI3K/AKT/mTOR pathway, 397–398
poly (ADP-robose) polymerase (PARP) protein, 400
RAS/RAF/MAPK pathway, 395–397
methotrexate, 446
Metvix, 207
Metvixia, 207
mitomycin-C, 410, 436
MM (malignant melanoma). *See also* cutaneous melanoma; immunobiology/melanoma; melanoma; metastatic melanoma *main entry;* metastatic melanoma regional management *main entry;* metastatic melanoma treatment *main entry;* MM (malignant melanoma) local management *main entry*
AJCC cutaneous groupings, 345
AJCC staging TNM, 24, 344
CDK4 (cyclin-dependent kinase 4), 12, 46
clinical evaluation, 16–17
conjunctive/eyelid preoperative workup, 174–175

contrasted neck CT, 19
environmental risk factors, 13
histology, metastatic, 328
invasive lentigo, 16, 17
MC1R (melanocortin-1 receptor), 12, 46
outcomes, 42
periauricular lesions
incidence of lymph node metastasis, 160
nodal metastasis risk factors, 159
PET/with or without CT scanning, 20
sentinel lymph node biopsy (SLNB), 163–164
prognostic significance, 349
superficial spreading, 16
surveillance
and albinism, oculocutaneous, 46
family history, 46
and genetics, 46
immunosuppression, 47
ionizing radiation, 47
MM history, 47
nevi, 46–47
nevi, congenital (garment), 47
phenotype, 46
tobacco smoking, 47
tumorigenesis risk factors, 13
UVA, 46
MM (malignant melanoma) local management
biopsy
ABCDE (*a*symmetry, *b*order irregularity, *c*olor variegation, *d*iameter greater than 6 mm, and *e* evolving [increasing] size or color) criteria, 333
by narrow margin excision, 333–334, 335
punch/incisional full thickness, 334, 335
shave, 334, 335
SLNB (sentinel lymph node biopsy), 335
local recurrence management
and margin size, 336, 337
overview, 339–340
and tumor depth, 335
overview, 333, 340
primary tumor radiographic assessment, 334–335
radiotherapy
adjuvant radiation, 340
wide local excision
biopsy site (prior) management, 335–336
deeply invasive tumors, 338
lymphatics, 336
margin size, 336–338
margin size: disfigurement compromise dilemmas, 337
margin size: recommendations for tumor thicknesses, 336–338, 337
overview, 335
perineural invasion, 338–339
satellite lesions, 339
site of margin, 337
SLNB (sentinel lymph node biopsy), 336
MM (malignant melanoma) regional management
AJCC (American Joint Committee on Cancer) Melanoma Task Force
stage III morbidity, 346, 347
Mohs, Frederic (1910–2002), 425–426
Mohs surgery (micrographic/histographic). *See also* treatment
atypical fibroxanthoma (AFX), 436
BCC (basal cell carcinoma), 22, 428, 432, 433, 434–435, 444
contraindications, 438
cutaneous AS (angiosarcoma), 437
and dermatology, 428
DFSP (dermatofibrosarcoma protuberans), 253, 435–436
fundamentals, 428
history
controversy, 426
micrographic observation of tumor surgical margins concept, 425–426
Mohs, Frederic (1910–2002), 425–426
indications for
clinical features, 434
histologic considerations, 434–438
overview, 433–434
lentigo maligna (melanoma in situ), 437–438
margin control
Mohs surgery, 428
overview, 426
MCC (Merkel cell carcinoma), 437
microcystic adnexal carcinoma (MAC), 435
NMSC (nonmelanoma skin cancer), 436–437
patient considerations, 438
patient evaluation/selection, 428–430
and reconstruction, 458
SCC (squamous cell carcinoma), 21, 434, 435
SCIS (SCC in situ), 443
sebaceous carcinoma, 436
technique
biopsy site identification, 430
outer margin determination, 430, 431
specimen maneuvers, 430, 432
tissue processing/assessment, 430, 432
treatment alternatives, 438–439
tumor clearance/reconstruction, 432–433

mucosal melanomas of the head and neck (MMHN). *See also* cutaneous melanoma; immunobiology/melanoma; immunotherapy of melanoma; melanoma; metastatic melanoma local management; metastatic melanoma regional management; metastatic melanoma treatment; ocular melanoma
clinical features/evaluation
biopsy, 416
histopathologic, 416
imaging, 416
intracellular melanin, 416
oral cavity benign pigmented lesions, 415
physical examination findings, 414–415
staging: TNM, 416–418
epidemiology, 414
etiology, 413–414
overview, 413, 421–422
and tobacco smoking, 414
treatment
chemotherapy, 421
immunotherapy, 421
neck dissection, 420
orbit management, 420
overview, 418–420
radiation therapy: adjuvant, 421
radiation therapy: overview, 420
radiation therapy: primary, 421
systemic, 421
Muir-Torre syndrome (MTS), 82, 121, 436
Muir-Torre syndrome (MTS)/HNPCC (hereditary nonpolyposis colon cancer), 121
mupirocin, 507
mustard gas, 13

N

nasal reconstructive surgery, 459. *See also* head and neck reconstructive surgery
allografts, 481
composite grafts, 473, 474
external skin replacement, 473–481
flaps
bilobed, 475, 476
cheek advancement, 481
FAMM (facial artery muculomucosal), 482–483
forehead, 475, 478–479
local, 473–475
nasolabial, 479–481, 479–481′
regional, 475, 478–481
septal/vestibular, 482–483
single-lobe transposition/banner, 475
skin for nasal lining, 483–484
nasal lining, 482–484
nasal support, 481
overview, 471, 484
skin grafts, 473
structural grafts, 481–482
total reconstruction, 484
National Comprehensive Cancer Network
SCC (squamous cell carcinoma) surgical margins, 161
NCCN (National Comprehensive Cancer Network)
low-risk BCC skin lesion treatment, 21–22
MCC guidelines, 236
metatypical BCC categorization, 15
"Practice Guidelines in Oncology for Distress Management," 34, 35
on psychological distress of cancer, 29
NCCS (National Coalition for Cancer Survivorship), 37
NCI (National Cancer Institute)
Cancer Information Service, 36
SEER (Surveillance, Epidemiology, and End Results) program, 30, 42
neomycin, 507
nerve involvement
facial nerve, 6, 7
PNI (perineural invasion), 6
trigeminal nerve, 6, 7
neurosurgical management
cranial convexity tumors
en bloc resection, 183–185
layer-by-layer tissue removal, 185
prognosis, 187
reconstruction, 186–187
vascular structure management, 185–186
overview, 183
skull base/subcranial soft tissue extension
craniofacial resection, 189
invasive cutaneous malignancy, 189
overview, 189
perineural invasion, 187–188
prognosis, 188–189
neurotropism, 6–7
nilotinib, 421
NMSC
aggressive
characteristics, 146
NMSC (nonmelanoma skin cancer). *See also* BCC (basal cell carcinoma); SCC (squamous cell carcinoma)
aggressive, 21

adjuvant therapies, 135–136
angled images through oral cavity, 128
biopsy techniques, 127
and chronic lymphocytic leukemia, 126
elective neck dissection, 134
facial H-zone, central, 125–126, 146
features of, 124–126
histopathology, 123
imaging, 127–131
lesion size, 124–125
location, 125–126
metastases, regional, 126
metastasis to parotid, 126
metastatic adenopathy imaging, 127–128
MRI advantages/disadvantages, 128–129
N0 neck treatment, 133–134
N+ neck treatment, 134–135
nodal staging on initial CT neck scan with contrast, 127
overview, 119–120, 136–137
patient history, 126–127
PET imaging use, 129–130
PNI (perineural invasion), 125, 126
PNI (perineural invasion) MRIs exploration, 128–129
on preauricular skin, 126
primary lesion treatment, 132–133
radiotherapy, 135–136
recurrence, 125
sentinel lymph node biopsy (SLNB), 134
subdermal infiltration CT evaluation, 128
surgical margins, 133
on temporal skin, 126
and transplant patients, 126
treatment, 132–136
tumor thickness, 125
and AK (actinic keratosis), 122
biopsy, 21
bony ear canal tumor involvement, 163
epidemiology (*See* epidemiology *main entry*)
etiology, 120–122
features of, 123
5-ALA, 447
histopathology, 79–97 (*See also* histopathology)
and HPV (human papillomavirus), 122
and immunosuppression, 122
Mohs surgery (micrographic/histographic), 436–437
molecular biology, 120
and organ transplantation, postsurgery, 122
outcomes, 41
overview, 101
parotidectomy, 164
patient psychosocial issues, 33
periauricular lesions
immunosuppression, 160
incidence of lymph node metastasis, 160
nodal metastasis risk factors, 159, 160
precursor lesions, 122
prevention, 136
and previous skin malignancy, 122
prognosis, 112–115 (*See also individual cancers*)
radiotherapy, 449–450
rate increase, 41, 42
regional metastases risk factors, 123
retinoids, 446
staging, 20 (*See* staging *main entry*)
surveillance, 48–49
treatment
anatomic/physiologic/cosmetic considerations, 150–153
chemical peel, 447–448
cryosurgery, 448–449
5-ALA, 447
forehead/scalp considerations, 151–152
laser resurfacing, 447–448
and MAL (methyl aminolevulinic acid), 447
medical adjunctive, 444–447
midface considerations, 152–153
nonsurgical overview, 441
nose/upperlip considerations, 152–153
photodynamic therapy, 447
procedure-based adjunctive, 447–450
and xeroderma pigmentosum (XP), 120–121
nonhealing wounds, chronic, 48
NSAIDs, 446–447

O

oblimersen sodium, 382
ocular adnexal carcinomas, 173
ocular adnexal cutaneous lesion overview, 173
ocular melanoma. *See also* cutaneous melanoma; immunobiology/melanoma; immunotherapy of melanoma; mucosal melanomas of the head and neck (MMHN)
and adenocarcinoma, 412
brachytherapy, 410, 411, 412
chemoembolization, 411
chemotherapy, 410, 411 (*See also* drugs *main entry; listings for individual agents*)
and CHRPE (congenital hypertrophy of the retinal pigment epithelium), 412

ocular melanoma *(continued)*
  of conjunctiva
    anatomy, 409
    clinical features, 410
    differential diagnosis, 409
    lid-sparing management, 410
    management, 410
    sentinel lymph node biopsy (SLNB), 410
  cryotherapy, 410
  enucleation, 411
  external beam radiation, 411
  fine needle aspiration, 411
  laser therapy, 411
  melancocytomas, 412
  metastatic eye/orbit lesions, 411–412
  overview, 409, 412
  PAM (primary acquired melanosis)
    overview, 409–410
  teletherapy, 411
  of uvea
    clinical presentation, 410–411
    management, 411
    risk factors, 410
    special considerations, 411
Ontak, 308–309
organ transplant patients, 49
  and cutaneous cancer prevention, 50, 51
OSI-774, 217
osteoradionecrosis (ORN), 194
ovarian desmoid tumors, 121
ovarian fibroma, 121

P

p21 mutation, 13
p53 mutation, 13
p53 tumor suppressor gene, 93, 104, 120
paclitaxel, 39, 264, 393
Paget disease. *See also* EMPD (extramammary Paget disease)
PAMPS (pathogen-associated molecular patterns), 297–298
paraffin, 13
parotidectomy, MM (malignant melanoma), 164–165
Patient-Centered Communication in Cancer Care (National Cancer Institute), 34
PDT (photodynamic therapy), 50
  for actinic keratoses (AK), 207, 208
  auto-oxidation, or photobleaching, 207
  BCC (basal cell carcinoma), 435
  for BCC (basal cell carcinoma), 209–210, 444
  cosmetic results, 210
  dosimetry, 207–208
  5-ALA (5-aminolevulinic acid) lipohilic photosynthesizer, 206, 447
  fluence, 207
  history, 205–206
  HPPH (2[1-hexyloxyethyl]-2 devinyl pyroheophorbide, or photochlor), 207
  irradiance, 207
  Levulan Kerastick, 207
  light sources, 207–208
  MAL (methyl aminolevulinic), 207
  mechanism of action, 206
  Metvix, 207
  Metvixia, 207
  for NMSC (nonmelanoma skin cancer), 207, 208
  overview, 210–211
  photosensitizers, 206–207
  porfimer sodium photosensitizers, 206
  for SCC (squamous cell carcinoma), 209
People Living with Cancer, 37
periauricular lesions. *See* auricular skin cancer
  anatomy, 157
  auricular tumor locations, 157–158
  and burn chondritis, 155
  epidemiology, 156
  histologic types, 156
  histology, 155–156
  and lupus erythematosus, chronic scarring, 155
  nodal metastasis risk factors
    desmoplasticity, 160
    differentiation degree, 160
    immunosuppression, 160
    invasion depth, 159–160
    lesions, 159
    positive margins, 160
    recurrence, 160
    tumor thickness, 159
  overview, 155, 166
  prognosis, 156
  staging, 158–159
  surgical techniques, 161–162 (*See also* surgery *main entry*)
periorbital lesions, 7
  at-risk nodal basins, 175
  BCC (basal cell carcinoma), 173
  intraoperative issues, 176–179
  medial canthal lesions, 173
  overview, 173, 180–181
  preoperative issues, 174–176
  radiation therapy, 179–180
  SCC (squamous cell carcinoma), 173

surgery reconstruction, 180 (*See also* periorbital reconstruction; periorbital reconstruction *main entry*)
surveillance, postoperative, 180
periorbital reconstruction
canalicular repair, 525–526
defect assessment, 505–506
defects not involving eyelid margin
second-intention wound healing, 506–507
eyelid margin involved defects
free mucosa-lined grafting, 523–525
lateral periosteal flap, 518–519
lateral semicircular rotational flap, 518
modified Hughes procedure (tarsoconjunctifal bridge flap), 521–523
overview, 517–518
sharing tarsoconjunctival bridge flap, 521–523
sliding tarsoconjunctival flap, 520–521
upper eyelid defects, 523–525
flap repair, large nonmarginal periocular defects, 514–515
full-thickness skin grafting, 507–509
medial canthal reconstruction, 525
overview, 505
skin flaps
advancement flaps, 511
advancement flaps: cheek, 515, 516
advancement flaps: eyebrow, 515, 516
advancement flaps: eyelid-cheek complex, 516
advancement flaps: forehead, 515, 516
advancement flaps: glabella, 515
advancement flaps: lower eyelid, 515, 516
rotation-advancement flaps, 515
rotation flaps: glabellar, 511–512
sliding cutaneous flaps: modified ellipses, 509–511
sliding cutaneous flaps: simple ellipses, 509
transposition flaps: bilobed, 513–514
transposition flaps: overview, 512–513
pesticides, 48
photoimmunology, human
sunscreen photobiology, 68–69
photoprotection, 50
PHQ-9 (Patient Health Questionnaire-9), depression measure, 35
physical examination. *See* clinical evaluation
physiology
epidermis, 1–3
keratinocytes, 1, 2, 7
Langerhans cells, 2
melanocytes, 2
Merkel cells, 3
PI3K/AKT/mTOR pathway, 397–398
pitch (viscous substance), 13
PNI (perineural invasion), 6–7
NMSC (nonmelanoma skin cancer), aggressive, 125, 126
NMSC (nonmelanoma skin cancer) aggressive, 128–129
SCC (squamous cell carcinoma), 125
porfimer sodium photosensitizers, 206
"Practice Guidelines in Oncology for Distress Management," 35
"Practice Guidelines in Oncology for Distress Management" (NCCN), 34
prednisone, 444
prevention of cutaneous cancer
and actinic keratoses (AK), 50
and adolescents, 50
and cryosurgery, 50
5-fluorouracil, 50
genetic counseling, 50
imiquimod, 50
and immunosuppression, 50, 51
and ionizing radiation, 50
organ transplant patients, 50, 51
photoprotection, 50
SunSmart (educational program), 50
SunWise (young children education), 50
prosthetic rehabilitation
acrylic resin biomaterials, 591
biomaterials, 589–591
craniofacial implant placement, 593
delayed implant placement preprocedure surgical guides, 592–593
double-sided adhesive tape fixation, 591–592
elastomeric polymer biomaterials, 590–591
fixation, 591–592
ideal characteristics of facial prosthetic materials, 591, 592
implant-retained prostheses, 593–594
medical-grade water-based adhesive fixation, 592
nasal prostheses, 594, 595
orbital prostheses, 596–597
osseointegrated implants, 593–594
overview, 587–588, 598
polyeurethane sheet liner biomaterials, 591
polyeurethan sheet liner, 591
preoperative evaluation, 588
silicone rubber biomaterials, 590–591
surgical enhancements to improve prosthetic treatment, 588–589
types, 594–597
protein kinase inhibitors, 382

psychosocial issues
About Face USA, 37
APOS (American Psychosocial Oncology Society), 36
barriers to dealing with, 33
BDI-II (Beck Depression Inventory-II), 35
of body image, 31–32
BSI 18 (Brief Symptom Inventory) psychological stress measure, 34
CancerCare, 36
Cancer Care for the Whole Patient: Meeting Psychosocial Health Needs (Institute of Medicine), 30, 33, 34, 35
Cancer Information Service, NCI (National Cancer Institute), 36
cancer-specific concerns, 29–30
Changing Faces, UK support organization, 35, 37
concerns other than psychiatric conditions, 30
DSM-IV depressive episode criteria, 35
DT (Distress Thermometer) screening tool, 34
of facial disfigurement, 30–31
and family members, 30
of future tumors, 33
Gilda's Club, 36
HADS (Hospital Anxiety and Depression Scale), 34
of head/neck skin cancer patients, 30–33
identification of needs, 34–35
as integral in oncology care, 33
LAF (Lance Armstrong Foundation), 36
Let's Face It (University of Michigan), 37
Look Good . . . Feel Better program (American Cancer Society [ACS]), 35, 36
medical misperceptions about, 33
meeting patient/family needs, 33–34
model for addressing patient needs (IOM), 33–34, 35
NCCN (National Comprehensive Cancer Network) on, 29
NCCS (National Coalition for Cancer Survivorship), 37
NCI (National Cancer Institute) Cancer Information Service, 36
oncologist-mental health provider collegiality, 35
overview, 29, 37–38
Patient-Centered Communication in Cancer Care (National Cancer Institute), 34
People Living with Cancer, 37
PHQ-9 (Patient Health Questionnaire-9), depression measure, 35
"Practice Guidelines in Oncology for Distress Management" (NCCN), 34
and provider-patient communication, 34
recurrence anxiety, 33
SCI (Skin Cancer Index), 33
SEER (Surveillance, Epidemiology, and End Results) National Cancer Institute program, 30
strategies for addressing, 35–37
suicide rate of patients, 30
The Wellness Community, 37

R

radiation. *See* ionizing radiation; UV radiation
radiotherapy. *See also* ionizing radiation
actinic keratoses (AK), 449–450
adjuvant, 165–166
adnexal tumors, 230
AS (angiosarcoma), 263
angiosarcoma, head and neck, 263
basal cell nevus syndrome/Gorlin syndrome/Gorlin-Goltz syndrome, 48–49, 449
BCC (basal cell carcinoma)
adjuvant radiotherapy, 194
management, 200–203
overview, 191–192, 449–450
radiotherapy alone, 192–194
treatment modality selection, 192–194
cervical lymph node metastasis, postoperative, 194
chemoradiation
skull base/subcranial soft tissue extension, 188
with chemotherapy, 136
dose-fractionation schedules, 198
electron beam, 449
field arrangement, 197
head and neck reconstruction surgery planning, 456
high-energy photons, 449
high-energy photon treatment, 197
immunotherapy of melanoma, 310
and immunotherapy of melanoma, 310
IMRT (intensity-modulated radiotherapy), 197
insterstitial brachytherapy, 449
lead masking, 196
lead masking/margins, 196–197
MCC (Merkel cell carcinoma), 240
adjuvant regional, 241
MCC (Merkel cell carcinoma), adjuvant regional
clinically positive lymph node management, 241
melanoma drug resistance/apoptosis resistance, 286
metastatic melanoma regional management
in node-positive neck, 380, 382

metastatic melanoma regional management, node-negative neck
radiotherapy role, 362–363, 380, 382
metastatic melanoma regional management in node-positive neck, 380, 382
MM (malignant melanoma) local management
adjuvant radiation, 340
as primary therapy, 340
NMSC (nonmelanoma skin cancer), 135–136, 165–166, 449–450
aggressive, 135–136, 136, 165–166
NMSC (nonmelanoma skin cancer), aggressive, 135–136
ocular protection, 197
orthovoltage, 449
orthovoltage *versus* electron beam, 195, 197
osteoradionecrosis (ORN), 194
and otorrhea, 162
outcomes following, 200–203
parotid lymph node metastasis, 194, 198–200
and parotid metastases, 136
periorbital lesions, 179–180
primary lesion management, 200–203
primary lesion techniques, 195–198
proton beam, 449
recurrence surveillance/management, 200
regional disease management, 200–203, 241, 380, 382
SCC-related, 82, 105
SCC (squamous cell carcinoma), 21, 113
adjuvant radiotherapy, 194
management, 200–203
overview, 191–192, 449–450
radiotherapy alone, 192–194
treatment modality selection, 192–194
xeroderma pigmentosum, 449
rapamycin, 218, 265
RAS/RAF/MAPK pathway, 395–397
RAS-RAF-MEK-ERK pathway/cascade, 282–283
NRAS, first gene found as altered, 282–283
reconstruction technique
and cartilage, 538
overview, 538
and skin, 538
redox-active metal exposure, 13
retinoic acid, 136
retinoids, 51, 136
reverse-transcriptase-polymerase chain reaction (RT-PCR), 351
risk factors, skin cancer, 8, 12. *See also* patient history *under* clinical evaluation
BCC (basal cell carcinoma), 13
environmental, 13
genetic, 13
host issues, 13
MM (malignant melanoma), 13
molecular, 13
SCC (squamous cell carcinoma), 13
in tumorgenesis, 13
Rombo syndrome, 49

S

SBCC (superfical basal cell carcinoma). *See under* BCC (basal cell carcinoma)
cryosurgery, 448–449
scalp reconstruction. *See also* head and neck reconstructive surgery *main entry*
anatomy, 557–560
blood supply, 557–559
innvervation, 559–560
layers, 557, 558
hair replacement following, 571
overview, 557, 571
process
calvarial reconstruction, 569–570
healing by secondary intention, 560–561
local flaps, 562–564
microvascular free flaps, 566–569
overview, 560
primary closure, 561
regional flaps, 564–566
skin grafting, 561, 562
tissue expansion, 561–562
SCCIS. *See* SCIS (SCC in situ)
SCC (squamous cell carcinoma). *See also* Bowen disease; NMSC (nonmelanoma skin cancer)
acantholytic, 82, 435
actinic keratoses (AK), 13, 14, 48
adenoid, 82
aggressive, 124
surgical margins, 133
AJCC histologic grades, 23
AJCC prognostic groups, 23
AJCC staging, 22, 23, 132 (*See also* staging *main entry*)
and AK (actinic keratosis), 79–81, 80
and albinism, 121
auricular tumor locations, 157–158
Bovenoid papulosis, 49
Bowen disease, 122
Bowenoid papulosis, 122
and cigarette smoking, 48, 104–105
Clark levels, 15

SCC (squamous cell carcinoma) *(continued)*
clinical evaluation, 12–15 (*See also* SCC (squamous cell carcinoma) *under* clinical evaluation *for details*)
contrasted neck CT, 19, 20
cumulative chronic sun exposure, 11
desmoplastic, 124, 435
elective neck dissection, 134
environmental risk factors, 13, 103–104
and eosinophilic cytoplasm, 81
epidemiology, 103–105
epidemodysplasia verruciformis (EV), 122
epidermodysplasia verruciformis, 48
geographical correlation, 12
grading, 107–111 (*See also* grading *main entry*)
histologic, 81
grading, histologic (*See also* grading)
histologic variants, 82
histopathology, 81–82, 123
HIV patients, 49
HPV (human papillomavirus)
oncogenic strains, 49, 443
and HPV (human papillomavirus), 122
HPV (human papillomavirus) and risk, 104
and immunohistochemical studies, 81
immunosuppression risk factor, 104
and immunosuppression therapy, 122
interferon alpha-2b, 445
invasive, 14, 81
ionizing radiation, 12
KA (keratoacanthoma), 14, 82, 83, 435
and keratin pearls, 81
and light microscopy, 81
lymph node spread, 6
Marjolin ulcer, 434
metastatic disease risk factors, 105
Mohs micrographic surgery, 21, 428, 434
and nuclear pleomorphism, 81
O'Brien et al. nodal staging (P and N), 109–111
organ transplant patients, 49
outcomes, 41, 42
overview, 442–443
PDT (photodynamic therapy), 209, 210
periauricular lesions
epidemology, 156
histology, 155–156
incidence of lymph node metastasis, 160
nodal metastasis risk factors, 159, 160
prognosis, 156
and perineural invasion risk, 81
periorbital lesions, 173
medial canthus surgical management, 178, 179
surgical margins, 176
PNI (perineural invasion), 125
and polycyclic aromatic hydrocarbons, 105
probable location, lesions of origin, metastatic SCC, 7
prognosis
and combined modality treatment, 113
and immunosuppression, 113
ITEM (immunosuppression, treatment, extracapsular spread, and margins) scoring system, 113–114
radiotherapy
adjuvant radiotherapy, 194
overview, 191–192, 449–450
radiotherapy alone, 192–194
regional management, 200–203, 241
treatment modality selection, 192–194
recurrence, 125, 166
risk factors, 103–105, 443
sarcomatoid, 82
sasosquamous, 124
SCIS (SCC in situ), 81, 435, 442, 443 (*See also* Bowen disease)
bleomycin, 446
5-ALA, 447
5-fluorouracil, topical, 444–445
imiquimod, 445
and skin adnexa, 435
and solid organ transplant recipients, 443
and sorafenib, 49
spindle cell, 82, 124, 435
surgery
deep margins, 146
N1 disease, 21
N2c disease, 21
N2 disease, 21
peripheral margins, 145
surveillance
environmental contaminant concerns, 48
and genetics, 48
immunosuppression, 49
ionizing radiation, 48
occupational concerns, 48
phenotype, 46
precursor lesions, 48
UV radiation, 48
systemic cytotoxic therapies, 216
targeted therapy: EGFR (anti-epidermal growth factor receptor), 216–217
targeted therapy: mTOR (rapamycin) molecular target, 218
targeted therapy: radiotherapy with EGFR inhibition targeted therapy, 218

targeted therapy: tyrosine kinase inhibitors, 217–218
tipfarnib, 49
treatment
combined modality treatment, 113
cryosurgery, 448
curettage, 21
electrodesiccation, 21
follow-up, 21
local, high-risk lesions, 21
local, low-risk lesions, 21
Mohs micrographic surgery, 21, 428, 434, 435
radiation therapy, 21, 113 (*See also* ionizing radiation *main entry*)
surgical resection, 113
suspicious regional lymph node involvement, 21
tumorigenesis risk factors, 13
UVB, 46
UV signature mutations, 58
VC (verrucous carcinoma), 82, 435
and HPV (human papillomavirus), 82
and xeroderma pigmentosum (XP), 120–121
SCI (Skin Cancer Index), psychosocial measure, 33
SCIS (SCC in situ), 81, 435, 442, 443. *See also* Bowen disease
bleomycin, 446
5-ALA, 447
5-fluorouracil, topical, 444–445
imiquimod, 445
Mohs surgery (micrographic/histographic), 443
SCC (squamous cell carcinoma) excision margins, 443
treatment, 442, 443
cryosurgery, 448–449
screening. *See also* surveillance
ABCDE (asymmetry, border irregularity, color variegation, diameter less than 6 mm, evolving in size, shape, color shades, and surface features or symptoms), 42
ACS (American Cancer Society) on, 42
American Academy of Dermatology
cancer screening program, 42
atypical views, 44–45
baseline photography, 45
best practices, 41, 42
CSLM (confocal scanning laser microscopy), reflectance, 45–46
and dermoscopy/dermatoscopy, 43, 45
digital, 45
difficulty range, 43–45
Internet image sharing, 45
multispectral digital dermoscopy, 45
overview, 41
PCP (primary care physician) training need, 43
by physicians, 43–44
rationale, 41
research needs, 42
and specialized software, 45
SSE (self-screening examination), 42–43
techniques, 42–46
teledermascopy, 45
thoroughness, 43–44
tools, 44–46
USPSTF (U.S. Preventive Services Task Force), Department of Health and Human Services (DHHS), 41–42
whole body photography, 45
sebaceous carcinoma, 93, 226, 436
sebaceous tumors, 121
SEER (Surveillance, Epidemiology, and End Results) National Cancer Institute program, 30
and psychosocial issues, 30
and screening, 42
sentinel lymph node biopsy (SLNB). *See also* biopsy *main entry;* surgery
clinical evaluation, 4–5, 20, 21, 134
conjunctival malignancy, 175
cutaneous melanoma, 4–5
eyelid malignancy, 175
goals/benefits, 348
MCC (Merkel cell carcinoma), 236
metastatic melanoma regional management
in node-negative neck, 348–350
metastatic melanoma regional management, node-negative neck
after wide local excision, 353
complications, 362
desmoplastic melanoma, 353–354
imaging considerations, 354
integration of nuclear medicine, surgery, and pathology, 354–355
in-transit metastasis risk, 362
intraoperative considerations, 358–361
lymphatic mapping/SLNB: after wide local excision, 353
morbidity, 362
operating room positioning strategies, 361
patient selection, 352–353
preoperative lymphoscintigraphy, 355–358
SLNB possible curative role, 352
vital blue dye complications, 362
metastatic melanoma regional management in node-negative neck
goals/benefits, 348
validation, 348–349

sentinel lymph node biopsy (SLNB) *(continued)*
and metastatic melanoma regional management in node-negative neck, 350
MM (malignant melanoma), 163–164
NMSC (nonmelanoma skin cancer), 163–164
aggressive, 134
of ocular conjunctiva, 410
prognostic significance, 349
treatment, 147–148
validation, 348–349
sentinel node biopsy (SLNB)
cutaneous melanoma, 4–5, 25, 349
and lymph nodes, nonmelanoma skin cancer, 106, 147
and potential cure, 352
therapeutic efficacy, 352
Sezary syndrome, 96
SilverMed, 507
skin. *See also* basement membrane zone; dermis; epidermis; lymphatic drainage
anatomy, 1–3
architecture schematic overview, 2
blood supply, 4
cytologic constituents' schematic overview, 2
Fitzpatrick's classification of sun-reactive skin types, 3
nonchronic sun-damaged BRAF mutation, 283
physiology, 1–3
sun-reactive skin types, Fitzpatrick's classification, 3
skull base/subcranial soft tissue extension. *See under* neurosurgical management
small blue cell tumors differential diagnosis, 237
smoking
cigarette, 47, 48, 104–105
solar keratoses. *See* actinic keratoses (AK)
sorafenib, 265, 382, 393
staging, 20
AJCC
DFSP (dermatofibrosarcoma protuberans), 252
MCC (Merkel cell carcinoma), 238–239
periauricular lesions, 158–159
AJCC (American Joint Committee on Cancer)
AS (angiosarcoma), 260, 261
BCC (basal cell carcinoma), 22, 23, 132
carcinoma anatomic stages, 23
carcinoma histologic grades, 23
carcinoma prognostic groups, 23
and clinically negative neck, 344–346
example of 7th staging manual high-risk features, 106
eyelid TNM, 175–176, 193
MCC (Merkel cell carcinoma), 112
melanoma, 273–276
melanoma anatomic stages, 25
melanoma (cutaneous) groupings, 345
melanoma TNM, 24, 344
mucosal melanoma of head and neck TNM, 417–418
SCC (squamous cell carcinoma), 22, 23, 132
nodal staging, 108
T classification, 107–109
T classification, melanoma, 24
T classification, SCC, 107, 108
TNM (tumor, node, metastasis), 106, 131–132
BCC (basal cell carcinoma)
overview, 21
MCC (Merkel cell carcinoma), 106
MSKCC (Memorial Sloan Kettering Cancer Center)
MCC (Merkel cell carcinoma), 111–112, 238
NMSC (nonmelanoma skin cancer), 20
O'Brien et al. (P and N)
SCC (squamous cell carcinoma), nodal staging, 109–111
SCC (squamous cell carcinoma)
AJCC, 22, 23
N1S3 (Australia), 21
overview, 21
TNM classification, 24, 106, 131–132
steroids, 456
sunscreens
and melanoma prevention, 272
photobiology, 68–69
photoimmunology, human, 68–69
UVA/UVB, 69
SunSmart (educational program), 50
SunWise (young children education), 50
surgery. *See also* auricular reconstruction; cheek reconstruction; cheek reconstruction *main entry;* head and neck reconstructive surgery; lip reconstruction *main entry;* nasal reconstructive surgery; neurosurgical management; periorbital reconstruction *main entry;* scalp reconstruction *main entry;* sentinel lymph node biopsy (SLNB); treatment; treatment *main entry*
adnexal tumors, 229–230
AS (angiosarcoma)
localized disease, 261–263
for at-risk cervical lymphatic basins, 148
auricular
surgical margins, 161
auriculectomy, 162, 163, 164, 166
BCC (basal cell carcinoma)
and perineural invasion, 146

peripheral margins, 145
resection, 22
surgical margins, 161
for bony ear canal tumor involvement, 163
cervical lymph node metastasis, 194
cryosurgery, 50, 448–449
and cutrettage/electrodessication, 143, 444
or cutrettage/electrodessication, 161–162
cutaneous auricle malignancy
surgical margins, 161
cutaneous melanoma
excision margins, 176
DFSP (dermatofibrosarcoma protuberans)
Mohs micrographic, 253
reconstruction, 253
wide local excision, 252–253
ELND (elective [or immediate or prophylactic] lymph node dissection), 346–348, 348, 352
excision, standard, 162
intraoperative assessment, sentinel lymph nodes, 351
LTBR (lateral temporal bone resection), 163
lymphadenectomy, 135, 137, 346, 348, 374, 376, 377, 379, 380, 382
cervical, 164
completion, 349–350
MCC (Merkel cell carcinoma)
margins, 239
Mohs micrographic surgery, 239–240
therapeutic lymph node dissection, 240–241
wide local excision, 239
modified radical neck dissection (MRND), 378–380
Mohs micrographic surgery, 21, 22, 143–144, 162, 443
MCC (Merkel cell carcinoma), 239–240
mucosal melanomas of the head and neck (MMHN) neck dissection, 420
NMSC (nonmelanoma skin cancer)
anatomic/physiologic/cosmetic considerations, 150–153
forehead/scalp considerations, 151–152
midface considerations, 152–153
nose/upperlip considerations, 152–153
peripheral margins, 145
resection margins, 145
NMSC (nonmelanoma skin cancer), aggressive
deep margins, 146–147
frozen section margin assessment, 147
overview, 145–146
and perineural invasion, 146
surgical margins, 133
ocular adnexal tissue protection, 176
parotidectomy, 135, 194, 379, 383
elective, 150
facial nerve preservation, 377
MM (malignant melanoma), 164–165
nerve-sparing, 105
NMSC (nonmelanoma skin cancer), 164
radical, 148
superficial, 21, 134, 148, 163, 164
total, 380
parotidectomy/neck dissection, 6, 7
for parotid metastases, 148–150
periauricular surgical margins, 161
periorbital lesions
BCC margins, 176
conjunctiva management, 178
delicate structure protection, 176
excision margins, 176–177
eyelid malposition risk, 179
intraoperative issues, 176–179
lid margin management, 177
orbital invasion management, 178–179
reconstruction, 180
SCC margins, 176
radical neck dissection (RND), 378, 380
reconstruction, surgical defect, 150
SCC (squamous cell carcinoma)
N1 disease, 21
N2c disease, 21
N2 disease, 21
and perineural invasion, 146
peripheral margins, 145
resection, 113
surgical margins, 161
selective neck dissection (SND), 378–380, 382
TLND (therapeutic [or delayed] lymph node dissection), 346–348, 348
TMJ resection, 163
surveillance. *See also* Immunosurveillance *main entry;* screening
actinic keratoses (AK), 48
and albinism
oculocutaneous, 46, 48
retinoblastoma, 46
BCC (basal cell carcinoma)
environmental contaminant concerns, 48
genetics, 48–49
immunosuppression, 49
ionizing radiation, 48
occupational concerns, 48
phenotype, 46
UV radiation, 48
CDK4 (cyclin-dependent kinase 4), 46

surveillance *(continued)*
family history, 12, 13, 46
follow-up, 49
and genetics, 12, 46, 48
immunosuppression, 47, 49
ionizing radiation, 47, 48
MC1R (melanocortin-1 receptor), 46
methods, 49
MM (malignant melanoma)
and albinism, oculocutaneous, 46
family history, 46
and genetics, 46
immunosuppression, 47
ionizing radiation, 47
nevi, 46–47
nevi, congenital (garment), 47
phenotype, 46
tobacco smoking, 47
MM patient history, 47
and multikinase inhibitors, 49
nevi, 46–47
nevi, congenital (garment), 47
nevi sebaceous, 48
NMSC (nonmelanoma skin cancer), 48–49
occupational concerns, 48
overview, 46
phenotype, 48
precursor lesions, 48
SCC (squamous cell carcinoma)
environmental contaminant concerns, 48
immunosuppression, 49
ionizing radiation, 48
occupational concerns, 48
phenotype, 46
precursor lesions, 48
UV radiation, 48
UV radiation, 46, 48
xeroderma pigmentosum (XP), 46

T

tamoxifen, 393
tamoxifen, cisplatin, dacarbazine, interleukin-2, 393
tanning beds, 7, 11, 12, 46, 48, 50
Tarceva, 217
targeted therapy. *See also* treatment; treatment *main entry*
and adjuvant agents, 215
AS (angiosarcoma), 264
C255, 218
celecoxib, 217–218
cetuximab, 217–218, 218
chemotherapy, targeted
EGFR (anti-epidermal growth factor receptor), 216
combination anti-EGFR therapy and other targeted agents, 217–218
COX-2 inhibition, 217–218
and EGFR (anti-epidermal growth factor receptor), 216
Erbitux, 218
erlotinib, 217
hedgehog pathway
BCC (basal cell carcinoma), 218–219
mTOR (rapamycin) molecular target
SCC (squamous cell carcinoma), 218
OSI-774, 217
overview, 215, 219
postoperative adjuvant chemotherapy, 216
postoperative adjuvant radiotherapy guidelines
NCCN (National Comprehensive Cancer Network), 216
radiotherapy with EGFR inhibition, 218
SCC (squamous cell carcinoma), 218
Tarceva, 217
target population, 215
taxanes, 243, 264
tazarotene, 446
T cells
natural killer T (NKT) cells, 67–68
T helper cells, 60
T regulatory cells, 67
temozolomide, 308, 390–391, 393
temozolomide and docetaxel, 393
tetracyclines, 446
thermal burns, 48
tipfarnib, 49
tobacco smoking, 47, 414, 456, 585
topotecan, single-agent, 243
trauma, 12, 13
treatment. *See also* Mohs surgery (micrographic/histographic); surgery; surgery *main entry;* targeted therapy; targeted therapy *main entry*
actinic keratoses (AK), 442
chemical peel, 447–448
cryosurgery, 448–449
laser resurfacing, 447–448
and MAL (methyl aminolevulinic acid), 447
photodynamic therapy, 447
procedure-based adjunctive, 447–450
adnexal tumors, 229–230
angiosarcoma, head and neck
advanced/disseminated disease management, 264

for at-risk cervical lymphatic basins, 148
BCC (basal cell carcinoma), 443–444
  curettage, 21–22
  electrodesiccation, 21
  follow-up, 23
  high-risk forms, 22–23, 434–435
  low-risk lesions (NCCN guidelines), 21–22
  Mohs micrographic surgery, 22, 428, 432, 433, 434
  radiation, 23
  resection, 22
BCC (basal cell carcinoma), invasive
  cryosurgery, 448
cryosurgery, 448–449
DFSP (dermatofibrosarcoma protuberans), 252–254
follow-up
  BCC (basal cell carcinoma), 23
  SCC (squamous cell carcinoma), 21
melanoma
  BCG (Bacillus Calmette-Guérin) injection, 23
  and Breslow thickness, 23
  chemotherapy, 23
  and Clark level, 23
  IFN (interferon) injection, 23
  imiquimod, 23
  local ablation, 23
  melphalan, 23
  miotic rate, 23
  and mitotic rate, 23
  radiation, 23
  and satellitosis, 23
  and ulceration status, 23
metatastic melanoma, 387–401 (*See also* metastatic melanoma treatment *main entry for details*)
nevi removal questions, 49
NMSC (nonmelanoma skin cancer)
  anatomic/physiologic/cosmetic considerations, 150–153
  chemical peel, 447–448
  cryosurgery, 448–449
  5-ALA, 447
  forehead/scalp considerations, 151–152
  laser resurfacing, 447–448
  and MAL (methyl aminolevulinic acid), 447
  midface considerations, 152–153
  nonsurgical overview, 441
  nose/upperlip considerations, 152–153
  photodynamic therapy, 447
observation, 147–148
for parotid metastases, 148–150
PDT (photodynamic therapy), 50
regional disease, 147–150
  SBCC (superfical basal cell carcinoma), 210 (*See also* SBCC (superficial basal cell carcinoma *under* BCC (basal cell carcinoma) *main entry*)
    cryosurgery, 448–449
  SCC (squamous cell carcinoma)
    combined modality treatment, 113
    curettage, 21
    electrodesiccation, 21
    follow-up, 21
    local, high-risk lesions, 21
    local, low-risk lesions, 21
    Mohs excision, 21, 428, 434
    Mohs micrographic surgery, 21, 428, 434
    radiation therapy, 21, 113 (*See also* ionizing radiation *main entry*)
    surgical resection, 113
  SCC (squamous cell carcinoma), invasive, cryosurgery, 448
  SCIS (SCC in situ), 442, 443
    cryosurgery, 448–449
  sentinel lymph node biopsy (SLNB), 147–148
tretinoin, 446
tretinoin, topical, 443

U

ultraviolet. *See* UV radiation
UV carcinogenesis. *See also* UV radiation
  indirect DNA damage, 58–59
  SCUP (Skin Cancer Utrecht-Philadelphia), 58 (*See also* UVB *under* UV radiation *main entry*)
  signature mutations, UVB, 58–59
  sunlight/skin cancer induction
    signature mutations, 58–59
UV immune suppression. *See also* UV carcinogenesis
  cellular targets in the skin
    keratinocytes, 65
    Langerhans cells, 64–65
    mast cells, 65–67
    overview, 63–64
  contact hypersensitivity, 59–60
  delayed type hypersensitivity studies, 59–60
  epidermal UV photoreceptors
    DNA, 60–61
    lipids, 62–63
    trans-UCA (urocanic acid), 62
  overview, 59
  T helper cells, 60
  UV-induced immune regulatory cells
    B cells, 68
    natural killer T (NKT) cells, 67–68
    T regulatory cells, 67

UV radiation. *See also* UV carcinogenesis
chronic, 13
cumulative effects, 11
as etiology, 120
and gender, 48
Langerhans cells, 61
and melanoma, 271
MM (malignant melanoma), 46
photoprotection, 50
sunburn number as melanoma risk, 12
surveillance, 46, 48
tanning beds, 7, 11, 12, 46, 48, 50
UVA, 11, 46
DNA damage, 59, 120
and immune reaction suppression, 60, 66, 68
and sunscreens, 69
UVB, 12, 13, 46
DNA damage, 59, 120
SCUP (Skin Cancer Utrecht-Philadelphia), 58
signature mutations, 58–59
and sunscreens, 69

V

vaccines
BCG (Bacille Calmette-Guérin), 387
BCG (Bacillus Calmette-Guérin), 23, 388, 421
CancerVax, 389
Canvaxin melanoma cell vaccine, 300–301
Malacine melanoma cell vaccine, 301
vasoformative tumors. *See* AS (angiosarcoma)
VC (verrucous carcinoma)
and HPV (human papillomavirus), 82
vinblastine, 392–393, 394
vincristine, 241, 444
vinorelbine, 392
visceral malignancy, 121

W

Web sites
About Face USA, 37
ACS (American Cancer Society), 36
American Academy of Dermatology, 57
APOS (American Psychosocial Oncology Society), 36
CancerCare, 36
Cancer Information Service, NCI (National Cancer Institute), 36
Changing Faces, UK support organization, 37
Gilda's Club, 36
LAF (Lance Armstrong Foundation), 36
Let's Face It (University of Michigan), 37
Look Good . . . Feel Better program (American Cancer Society [ACS]), 36
melanoma risk tool, 46
NCCS (National Coalition for Cancer Survivorship), 37
NCI (National Cancer Institute) Cancer Information Service, 36
People Living with Cancer, 37
The Wellness Community, 37

X

xeroderma pigmentosum (XP), 12, 13, 46, 48, 103, 120–121, 271
and ionizing radiation, 48
isotretinoin, 51
radiotherapy, 449